Text and Atlas of Wound Diagnosis and Treatment

Third Edition

NOTICE

Text and Atlas of Wound Diagnosis and Treatment

Third Edition

Edited by

Rose L. Hamm, PT, DPT, FACCWS

Adjunct Associate Professor of Clinical Physical Therapy
University of Southern California
Los Angeles, California

McGraw Hill

New York Chicago San Francisco Athens London Madrid
Mexico City Milan New Delhi Singapore Sydney Toronto

Text and Atlas of Wound Diagnosis and Treatment, Third Edition

1 2 3 4 5 6 7 8 9 DSS 28 27 26 25 24 23

ISBN 978-1-264-92310-6
MHID 1-264-92310-4

This book was set in Minion Pro by MPS Limited.
The editors were Michael Weitz and Kim J. Davis.
The production supervisor was Catherine Saggese.
Project management was provided by Monika Chaudhari, MPS Limited.

This book is printed on acid-free paper.

Library of Congress Control Number: 2023944348

The third edition of the
Text and Atlas of Wound Diagnosis and Treatment
is dedicated to the amazing AUTHORS
whose passion for taking care of patients with wounds
is evident in their unlimited energy and expertise.
Each one has had a distinctive and profound influence
on my professional career, for which I am eternally grateful.

Contents

Contributors

Joseph N. Carey, MD
Associate Professor of Surgery
Division of Plastic and Reconstructive Surgery
Keck School of Medicine
University of Southern California
Los Angeles, California

Zachary J. Collier, MD, MS
Global Surgery Fellow
Division of Plastic and Reconstructive Surgery
University of Southern California
Los Angeles, California

Alexander DiBartolomeo, MD
Resident Physician
Division of Vascular Surgery and Endovascular Therapy
Department of Surgery
University of Southern California
Los Angeles, California

Sonya Dick, PT, DPT, CWS
Adjunct Assistant Professor
Department of Neuroscience
University of Kentucky College of Medicine
Bowling Green, Kentucky

Aimée D. Garcia, MD, CWS, FACCWS
Associate Professor
Department of Medicine
Geriatrics Section
Baylor College of Medicine
Houston, Texas

Karen A. Gibbs, PT, PhD, DPT, CWS
Professor
Department of Physical Therapy
Texas State University
Round Rock, Texas

Jaimee Haan, PT, MBA, CWS
Executive Director
Rehabilitation, Wound Management and Fitness
Academic Health Center
Indiana University Health
Indianapolis, Indiana

Nicholas D. Hamelin, MD, DMV, MBA, FRCSC
Service de Chirurgie plastique
Département de Chirurgie
Hôpital Pierre Boucher
Longueuil, Québec, Canada

Rose L. Hamm, PT, DPT, FACCWS
Adjunct Associate Professor of Clinical Physical Therapy
University of Southern California
Los Angeles, California

Daryl Lawson, PT, MPT, DSc
Associate Professor
Department of Physical Therapy
Western Michigan University
Kalamazoo, Michigan

Sharon Lucich, PT, CSPHA
Senior Clinician
Department of Clinical Affairs
EHOB, Inc.
Indianapolis, Indiana

Tammy Luttrell, PhD, MSPT, CWS, FCCWS
Burn and Reconstructive Center Sunrise Hospital
Las Vegas, Nevada

Haig Manoukian, BS
Medical Student I
Sidney Kimmel Medical College
Thomas Jefferson University
Philadelphia, Pennsylvania

James McGuire, DPM, PT, CPed, FAPWHc
Director of Leonard Abrams Center for Advanced Wound Healing
Temple University
School of Podiatric Medicine
Philadelphia, Pennsylvania

Christian Ochoa, MD
Associate Professor of Surgery
Associate Program Director
Division of Vascular Surgery
Keck School of Medicine
University of Southern California
Los Angeles, California

Brian H. Odom, PT, PhD, CWS
Assistant Professor
Department of Physical Therapy
University of Central Arkansas
Conway, Arkansas

Marisa Perdomo, PT, DPT, CLT-Foldi, CES
Board Certified Oncology Physical Therapy Specialist
Assistant Professor
Division of Biokinesiology and Physical Therapy
University of Southern California
Los Angeles, California

Vincent L. Rowe, MD
Professor and Chief
Division of Vascular and Endovascular Surgery
David Geffen School of Medicine at UCLA
Los Angeles, California

Lee C. Ruotsi, MD, CWS-P, ABWMS, UHM
Medical Director
Saratoga Hospital Center for Wound Healing and Hyperbaric Medicine
Saratoga Springs, New York

Pamela Scarborough, PT, DPT, MS, CWS, FAAWC
Vice President, Clinical Affairs
RestorixHealth
Metairie, Louisiana

Jayesh B. Shah, MD, MHA, CWSP, FUHM, FACHM, FACP, FACCWS
Assistant Professor, Department of Community Medicine
UT Health
Associate Professor
University of Incarnate Word School of Osteopathic Medicine
President
South Texas Wound Associates, PA
Medical Director
NE Baptist and Mission Trail Baptist Wound Healing Centers
San Antonio, Texas

Cynthia Sung, MD
PGY-1
Plastic Surgery
Indiana University School of Medicine
Indianapolis, Indiana

Dot Weir, RN, CWON, CWS
Clinician
Saratoga Hospital Center for Wound Healing and Hyperbaric Medicine
Saratoga Springs, New York

Deborah M. Wendland, PT, DPT, PhD, CPed
Associate Professor
Department of Physical Therapy
Mercer University
Atlanta, Georgia

Stephanie Woelfel, PT, DPT, CWS
Associate Professor of Clinical Physical Therapy & Surgery
Division of Biokinesiology & Physical Therapy
Department of Surgery
University of Southern California
Los Angeles, California

Alex K. Wong, MD, FACS
Professor
Division of Plastic Surgery
City of Hope National Medical Center
Duarte, California

Foreword

It is with great pleasure that I offer you, the reader, a few comments on the newest edition of this well written, wonderfully illustrated, textbook. In my opinion, this is the only textbook that truly provides insight into anatomy, physiology, diagnosis, and treatment of nonhealing wounds through a true interdisciplinary lens. Over a span of almost 30 years, I have been fortunate to practice with a balanced team of nurses, physical therapists (PTs), physicians, nurse practitioners (NPs), support staff, students, residents, and fellows. Our challenge, however, was to find a book that the entire team could use as a basis for our didactic content. How could a book strike a balance of content and depth, given the wide educational backgrounds of such a diverse team? Look no further, this is your book!

In 2008 at the University of Illinois Chicago, I started the first one-year clinical fellowship in wound care. We now have a full physical therapy wound team, NPs, WOCNs, and students rounding at a subacute unit, inpatient acute care, and outpatient wound clinics. This textbook literally covers our core content and is the didactic basis for our program. The first three chapters, which cover anatomy, wound healing physiology, and the overall work-up of a patient with a wound, must be completed by the fellow in the first month of the program. The tables, illustrations, and level of depth at a biochemical and cellular level, I believe, help new wound management providers develop an appreciation of the scope of knowledge necessary to provide wound care. Too often students come to our service hoping to figure out, "What dressing should I use?" While that question needs to be asked, it should follow a thorough history, physical, lab testing, and generation of a differential diagnosis, no different than for any other field of medicine. The section on wound diagnosis allows the reader to take a deep dive into various wound etiologies. We have our fellows read the respective chapter in this section prior to their clinical rotation, for example, in plastic or vascular surgery. The new chapter on pediatric wounds is a welcome addition to this text.

The section on wound bed preparation allows the reader to gain an understanding of all forms of debridement and how to manage these wounds with the correct dressings post procedure. The field of wound bed preparation has come a long way over the past 20 years, and with new diagnostic tools becoming available will continue to develop into the future.

Finally, the section on adjunctive therapies is informative and comprehensive. I believe this is a section physicians should really master. I have been amazed at how few of my colleagues understand the huge role these techniques play for patients with hard-to-heal wounds. Many years ago, I was introduced to Luther Kloth, PT, PhD from Marquette. After a visit to his lab, my team adopted PT-based modalities and encouraged others to broaden their knowledge in this critically important area. Finally, I am pleased to see a chapter on exercise therapy. So much of our time is focused on treating that we tend to forget about preventing initial wounds and wound recurrence. Helping our patients help themselves should take a bigger role in our wound care centers.

In summary, I am a major fan of this book and I know you will be as well; happy reading, and let's all continue to heal our patients. This book gives us much needed ammunition.

William J. Ennis, DO

Preface

Since the second edition of the *Text and Atlas of Wound Diagnosis and Treatment* was published, I have read two books that had a profound effect on how I view the science of wound healing. *The Beautiful Cure: The Revolution in Immunology and What It Means for Your Health* by Daniel Davis and *The Language of God: A Scientist Presents Evidence for Belief* by Francis Collins—both are captivating reads about the miraculous human body and how it functions. Reading these books increased the awe, both medical and spiritual, I have always felt as I witnessed wound healing in my patients. The understanding of the cellular and acellular components of tissue and how they communicate for both normal and pathological physiology has exploded over the past few years (and I do mean relatively few!). That deeper knowledge has helped the profession (1) to understand how some of the clinical interventions that have been used for decades actually facilitated healing that has been observed clinically (ie, electrical stimulation and ultrasound); and (2) to discover and develop new interventions and diagnostic technologies that are now considered standard care within the wound care community (ie, fluorescence imaging and cellular/acellular matrix products).

These changes are incredibly exciting and at the same time challenging for clinicians as we make decisions on a case-by-case, day-by-day basis for our patients. The options sometimes seem limitless! And as an educator, how can I possibly teach all of this to my students in a two-unit course, much less in a 16-hour module? Thus, my goals for this third edition are (1) to present the new technologies in a concise way that is relative to the basics of wound healing; and (2) to maintain the book's relevance to all of the medical specialties on the wound care team.

When I read Dr. Ennis' statement that the book is required reading for his fellows, I was humbled, grateful, and excited that he felt it was indeed applicable to all disciplines. As I pondered, researched, and sometimes sweated over revisions, the words in his foreword became the yardstick as to whether something should stay, change, be deleted, or be enhanced. Would it improve a fellow's understanding of wound healing and the physiology of specific interventions? His words became the conscience of the revision process!!! I pray that each decision was the correct one.

The two new chapters on Pediatric Wounds and Exercise for the Patient with a Wound are topics that are seldom discussed at length, and certainly not included in a comprehensive wound care textbook. The authors of these chapters were quick to jump on board the project and have done an outstanding job of making them fit the format of the book. I hope that both of them are helpful to you in your practice.

The reception of the first two editions of the *Text and Atlas* has far exceeded any dreams that I had when the first edition was imagined 10 years ago. My life has changed probably more than the book's content, but my passion for caring for patients (friends and family now that I am retired from clinical practice) with wounds has never waived nor diminished. I thank each and every one of you for your support in this journey, for the constructive and positive feedback you have provided, and for sharing the vision of a true medical wound management specialty. Blessings to you all from the depth of my heart and soul.

Rose L. Hamm, PT, DPT, FACCWS

Acknowledgments

First and foremost, my deepest appreciation goes to the incredible authors who agreed to continue their contributions in the update of this edition. Of the original 21 authors of the first edition, 16 have remained actively involved in the third edition, and 9 new experts have added to the chapters. Their expertise in caring for patients with wounds and their dedication to education flows from their words, photographs, graphs, and tables in such a way that will continue to have a ripple effect in patient care. I am especially grateful to Brian Odom, Stephanie Woelfel, and Deborah M. Wendland who dug deep to start their chapters from scratch! And deep appreciation goes to Dr. Ennis who inspired me with his words of support and confidence and confirmed that the third edition was a must-do.

The editorial staff at McGraw Hill have been supportive and encouraging from the very beginning. Michael Weitz never stops dreaming with me and reminding me with the statistics that this textbook continues to have worldwide impact on patient care. Kim Davis has been meticulous in keeping up with the book's details and timeline, always with grace and understanding. Melinda Avelar managed the contributor agreements (no small task) and distributes books to the authors after publication, as well as educators who need trial copies. Kudos to Catherine Saggese who orders the paper for the book, manages and pays the compositor, and takes care of a myriad of other details. I have actually received compliments from other authors about the quality of paper, photographs, etc., in the text, and to Catherine and the printers goes the credit. Although Catherine is behind the scenes (meaning I never get an email from her!), she does a lot to keep the production on track. And to each and every sales rep who has taken the textbook to the educational marketplace, you have my sincere thanks.

The covers of all three editions have been designed to reflect an emphasis that I tried to make in the content. The first edition focused on the cellular components that affect tissue healing; the second edition emphasized the importance of an interdisciplinary team to care for patients; and this third edition aims to illustrate the emergence of technology in diagnosis and prognosis of wounds. Anthony Landi has been of tremendous help in making my subtle messages come alive. Thank you, Anthony!!!

Monika Chaudhari and the team at MPS Limited were awesome in catching every inconsistency, grammar and spelling mistake, and reference error. They have, pun intended, saved my skin in more places than I would like to admit!!! They were also sensitive to my suggestions for figure and table placement in order to make the book as reader-friendly as possible. The MPS team was also responsible for pursuing permissions when necessary, and my gratitude goes to Prabhat Singh, Ankita Mapwal, Sumit Pandey, Rahul Raj, and Julissa Ramos for keeping us out of trouble!

As I was writing all three editions, there were two past professors from graduate school who were constantly sitting on my shoulder and acting as my conscience as I put the words, sentences, paragraphs, and pages together, and I wish to reiterate my gratitude to them. Dr. Carolee Winstein was my first professor in graduate school, a most daunting experience I must say. She was the consummate professor who taught me, not just the material of the class, but HOW to be a good student, and specifically how to critically read journal articles for their credibility and applicability. Dr. Michael Schneir, a professor in the Herman Ostrow School of Dentistry at USC, taught me scientific writing, first in a class and then in one-on-one sessions as I prepared my first teaching document for publication. I read and reread every revision through his eyes, with his enormous textbook at my side. To both of these magnificent educators, I say thank you for all that you taught me and for being everlasting mentors.

My gratitude is never-ending to my family and friends who were also quick to ask, "How is the book coming along?" Their support and encouragement boosted me when I thought my enthusiasm was waning and kept me going to the bittersweet end of the project.

Any successful venture takes a team working together, each member with its own special skills and talents, and the **team** that created this third edition of the *Text and Atlas of Wound Diagnosis and Management* has been stellar. May each and every reader feel the passion and expertise that is reflected in these pages, and use it to help their patients reach their full healing and functional potential. This has been a labor of love from all of the team members, and my love and gratitude to them is eternal.

Rose L. Hamm, PT, DPT, FACCWS

PART ONE
Integumentary Basics

CHAPTER ONE

Anatomy and Physiology of the Integumentary System

Rose L. Hamm, PT, DPT, FACCWS

CHAPTER OBJECTIVES

At the end of this chapter, the learner will be able to:

1. **Identify each layer of the skin and its components and discuss their functions.**
2. **Relate the function of each cell type to the overall function of the integumentary system.**
3. **Recognize the role of noncellular components of skin in maintaining an integumentary system capable of healing.**
4. **Diagnose tissue injury based on the depth of skin loss.**

SKIN

Skin is an important part of one's personality and character; a lot can be learned by observing an individual's skin and its abnormalities. Wrinkles are an indication of one's mood, age, social habits, or overexposure to the sun. The skin color reflects one's ethnicity as a result of the melanin content; the skin texture can reflect one's life occupation that involves repeated mechanical forces or weather exposure. Skin reflects one's emotions as it moves fluidly with the underlying muscles and connective tissue. Skin abnormalities can be a response to a disease process, injury, allergy, or medication. But what does the skin have to do with wound healing? In order to be considered closed, a wound has to have full re-epithelialization, defined as new skin growth, and no drainage or weeping from the healed tissue. An appreciation for the anatomy and physiology of the integumentary system and the skin's role in healing is needed to understand wound closure, complete with optimal aesthetics and function.

ANATOMY OF THE SKIN

The skin is a complex, dynamic, multilayered organ that covers the body, making it an individual's largest single organ. It comprises 15–20% of the total body weight; if laid out flat, the skin would cover a surface of 1.5–2 m^2.[1] Embedded in the layers, which are made primarily of collagen matrices, are a plethora of cells, blood vessels, nerve endings, and adnexal structures (hair follicles, arrector pili, sebaceous glands, sweat glands, and nails), each performing a specific task that as a whole enables the skin to protect and preserve the rest of the body (**TABLE 1-1**). Both the cellular and noncellular components of the epidermis and dermis are described in **TABLES 1-2** and **1-3**.

The layers of the skin are organized into the outermost *epidermis* and the underlying *dermis*. Beneath the dermis is a structure called the *hypodermis* or subcutaneous layer, and although it is not a true part of the skin, it is frequently referred to as a third layer of the skin (**FIGURE 1-1**). The junction of the epidermis and dermis is reticular, with an individualized pattern that forms dermatoglyphs, or the fingerprints and footprints, of the hands and feet.[1] The reticular structure helps the skin to withstand the repeated friction and shear forces that occur with activities of daily living; however, as the skin ages the ridges flatten out and the skin is more susceptible to frictional tears and blistering. Between the epidermis and dermis is a laminar adhesive layer termed the *basement membrane* that binds the two layers of skin.

Epidermis

The layers of the epidermis are, from innermost to the surface, *stratum basale, stratum spinosum, stratum granulosum, stratum lucidum,* and *stratum corneum*; in totality the layers are 50–150 μm in thin skin, 400–1400 μm in thick skin[1,2] (**FIGURE 1-2**). The primary cells composing the epidermal layers are keratinocytes, with melanocytes, Langerhans cells, and Merkel cells embedded in layers. Although they are mitotically active in the stratum basale, through a process termed *stratification*, keratinocytes migrate outward to the avascular stratum spinosum and begin to flatten out and become less active. When they reach the outer stratum corneum, the keratinocytes are termed *corneocytes*, the dead flat cells that form the outer protective layer of the skin.

The keratinocytes are composed of keratin protein filaments that are present in greater concentrations as the cells migrate toward the stratum corneum. In the stratum basale, the keratinocytes are bound to the basal lamina by *hemidesmosomes*; and in all the epidermal layers, they are bound to each other by *desmosomes*. These cell-to-cell adherent discs are composed of transmembrane glycoproteins, termed *cadherins*, and include four desmoglein proteins (**FIGURE 1-3**).[3,4]

As the keratinocytes move into the stratum spinosum, they become active in keratin or protein synthesis. The keratin forms intermediate filaments that bundle together to form

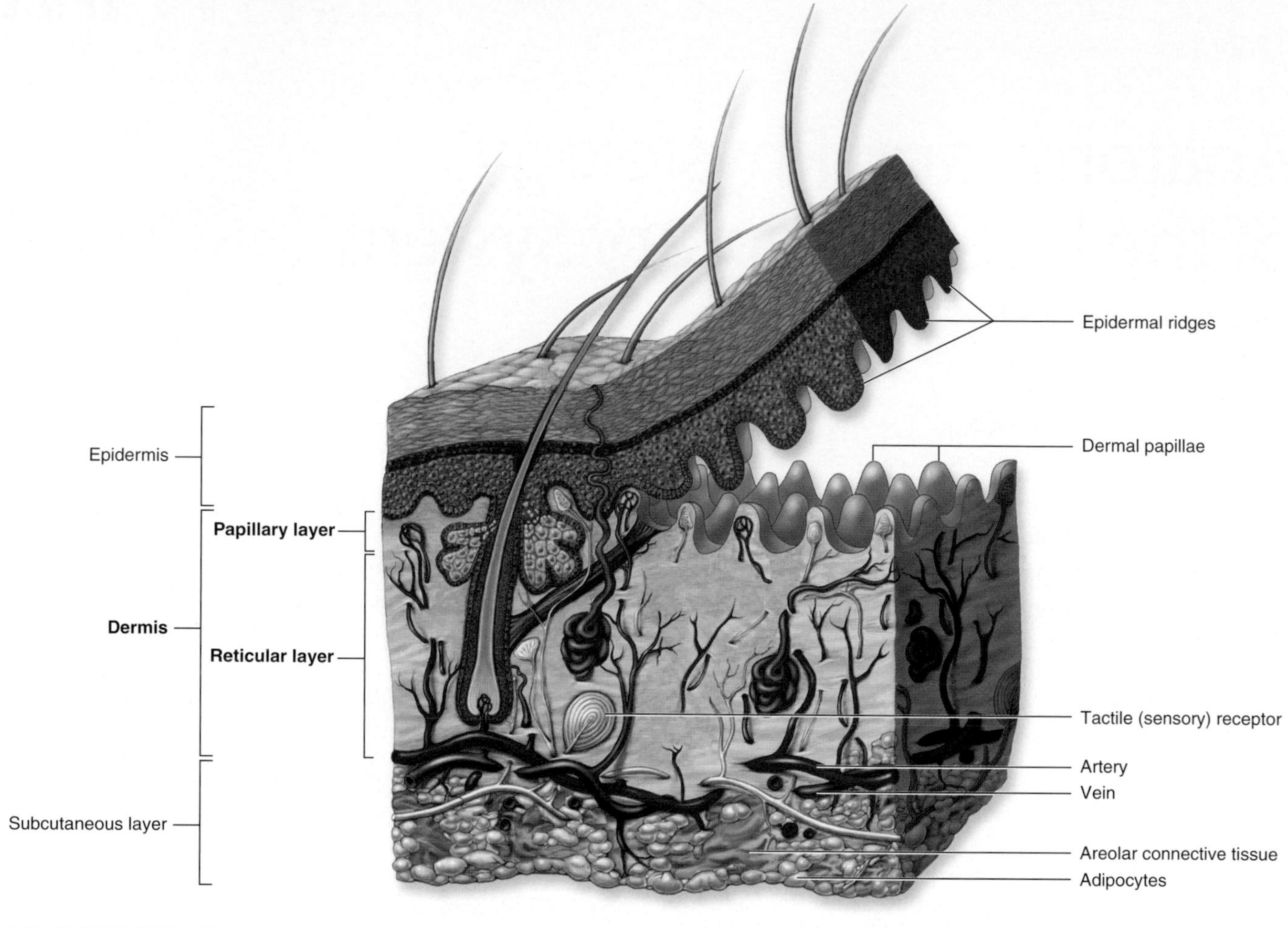

FIGURE 1-1 Anatomy of the skin. (Reproduced with permission from Mescher AL, ed. *Junqueira's Basic Histology: Text and Atlas.* 16th ed. New York, NY: McGraw Hill; 2021.)

TABLE 1-1 Adnexal Structures of the Skin

Adnexal Structures	Description	Location	Function
Hair follicle	Tube-like structure that surrounds the hair shaft with the following layers: Papilla at the base, made of connective tissue Hair matrix around the papilla External and internal root sheath Bulge containing stem cells	Originates in dermis, extends through the epidermis to the outer surface of skin; does not exist on the soles of the feet and palms of the hands	Hair contributes to one's appearance and protects the top of the head from UV sun rays
Arrector pili	Bundle of muscle fibers	Attached to the hair follicle in mid-dermis	Controls the response of the hair follicle to changes in temperature or emotions (goose bumps)
Sebaceous gland	Multilobed glands with multiple glands connecting to one duct	Attached to and opens into the hair follicle; also exists in skin where there is no hair	Produces sebum, an oily substance which lubricates the skin and hair
Sweat glands	Eccrine—composed of water and small amounts of minerals, metabolites, and unmetabolized drugs Apocrine—oily, odorless substance with primarily proteins, lipids, and steroids	Present at birth, cover entire body surface Dormant until puberty; present in hairy parts of axilla, mammary, perineal, and genital regions	Temperature regulation Detoxification of harmful molecules Control water output Direct secretion of Na^+ and Cl^- during exercise Secrete up to 30% of the bodily waste
Nails	Keratin	Distal digits	

Data from Garza L. Developmental biology of the skin. In: Kang S, Amagai M, Bruckner AL, et al, eds. *Fitzpatrick's Dermatology*, 9th ed. New York, NY: McGraw Hill; 2019. Available at: https://accessmedicine.mhmedical.com/content.aspx?bookid=2570&sectionid=210415357. Accessed September 21, 2022; Chen Y, Kuan W, Liu C. Comparative study of the composition of sweat from eccrine and apocrine sweat glands during exercise and in heat. *Int J Environ Res Public Health*. 2020;17(10):3377.

TABLE 1-2 Cellular Components of the Skin

Cell Name	Description	Location	Function
EPIDERMIS			
Keratinocytes—dead	Flat, elongated, nonnuclear	Stratum corneum of epidermis	Provide mechanical strength[2]
Squames	Horny, cornified cells	Surface of stratum corneum	Sloughing layer of epidermis
Keratinocytes—living	Polyhedral, slightly flattened	Stratum spinosum of epidermis	Synthesize keratin filaments; phagocytose the tips of melanocytes to release melanin; hold and transport water and urea; participate in innate and adaptive immunity through antimicrobial peptide secretion
Keratinocytes—living	Flattened polygonal	Stratum granulosum	Keratinization at terminal differentiation of the epithelial cells
Eosinophilic keratinocytes	Flat, no nuclei or organelles; densely packed keratin filaments embedded in a dense matrix	Stratum lucidum (only in soles of the feet and palms of the hands)	Provide dense, thick layer of skin that resists friction
Melanocytes	Round cell bodies with long, irregular dendritic extensions	Between the stratum basal and stratum spinosum; in hair follicles[1]	Produce melanin, the pigment that gives color to the skin
Langerhans cells (dendritic cells)	Round cell bodies with long dendritic extensions into intercellular spaces	Stratum spinosum with cytoplasmic processes extending between the keratinocytes of all the epidermal layers	Bind, process, and present antigens to the T-lymphocytes
Lymphocytes	Dendritic	Epidermis	Recognize epitopes; produce cytokines
Merkel cells	Dendritic; have contact with unmyelinated sensory fibers in basal lamina	Stratum basale of highly sensitive areas; base of hair follicles	Mechanoreceptors for touch
Basal cells	Cuboid or columnar, contain keratin in progressively increasing amounts as the cells migrate toward the stratum corneum	Stratum basale	Continuous production of epidermal cells
DERMIS			
Stem cells		Stratum basale, bulge of the hair follicle	Production of keratinocytes
Fibroblasts	Elongated, irregular shape with large, ovoid nucleus	In the connective tissue of the papillary layer of dermis	Synthesize collagen, elastin, GAGs, proteoglycans, and glycoproteins
Mast cells	Large, oval, or round; filled with basophilic secretory granules	Near the capillaries in the dermis	Produce histamine and heparin
Macrophages	Large cells with off-center, large nuclei	In the connective tissue of the papillary layer of dermis; become Langerhans cells in the epidermis	Phagocytosis, produce enzymes and cytokines that facilitate wound healing; immune processes
Leukocytes	Spherical white blood cells	Papillary layer of dermis	Phagocytose foreign material and dead cells
Free nerve cell endings	Unencapsulated receptors	Papillary layer of dermis into lower epidermal layers	Detect temperature changes, pain, itching, light touch
Tactile discs	Unencapsulated receptors	Papillary layer of dermis	Receptors for light touch
Root hair plexus	Web of sensory fibers	Reticular layer of dermis	Detect movement of the hairs
Meissner corpuscles (tactile corpuscles)	Elliptical encapsulated nerve endings	Reticular layer of dermis	Detect texture and slow vibrations[25]
Pacinian corpuscles (lamellated)	Large oval nerve endings with outer capsule and concentric lamellae of flat Schwann-type cells and collagen around an unmyelinated axon	Reticular layer of the dermis, hypodermis	Detect coarse touch, deep pressure, fast vibration[25]
Ruffini corpuscles	Enlarged dendritic endings with elongated capsules	Reticular layer of the dermis	Detect sustained pressure[25]
Adipocytes	Globular cells containing fat molecules	Hypodermis	Produce and store lipids that can be used for energy, provide insulation, produce cytokines for cell-to-cell communication (restin, leptin, adiponectin)

Data from Mescher AL. *Junqueira's Basic Histology: Text & Atlas.* 15th ed. New York, NY: McGraw Hill; 2018.

TABLE 1-3 Noncellular Components of the Skin

Structure Name	Description	Location	Function
EPIDERMIS			
Basement membrane	Composite structure of basal lamina and reticular lamina	Between the stratum basale and the papillary layer of the dermis	Binds the dermis and epidermis; allows diffusion of nutrients from the dermis to the epidermis
Basal lamina	Felt-like sheet of extracellular matrix composed of laminin, Type IV collagen, and entactin	In the basement membrane	Attach to reticular fibers in the connective tissue to bind the layers of skin
Reticular lamina	Fibers composed of Type III collagen	Below the basal lamina in the basement membrane	Attach to the basal lamina with reticular fibers
Vitamin D_3	Also known as cholecalciferol; technically a hormone and not a vitamin	Keratinocytes	Metabolizes calcium, bone formation; up-regulates antimicrobial peptide synthesis for immune system
Desmosomes	A disc-shaped structure on the surface of one cell that connects with an identical structure on an adjacent cell	Between epithelial cells	Provide a strong bond between the cells
Hemidesmosomes	Half of a desmosome structure; contain integrins	Between the cells of the stratum basale and the basement membrane	Bind the basal cells to the basement membrane
Corneodesmosomes	Specialized protein structures modified from desmosomes	Between the keratinocytes, or corneocytes, in the stratum corneum	Bind the cells in the outer layer of skin, are degraded as the cells migrate to the epithelial surface so that outer keratinocytes are sloughed
Integrins	Transmembrane proteins	In the hemidesmosomes	Receptor sites for macromolecules of laminin and for Type IV collagen
Keratins	Filament proteins	In all epithelial cells and hard structures (eg, nails)	Strengthen epidermis, protect against abrasion, prevent water loss
Tonofibrils	Bundles of keratin filaments	Converge and terminate at desmosomes located in areas subject to continuous mechanical forces, eg, soles of the feet	Protect the skin from effects of continuous friction and pressure
Keratohyalin granules	Contain dense masses of filaggrin	In the cytoplasm of the stratum granulosum cells	Link with the keratins of tonofibrils to facilitate keratinization
Filaggrin	Protein monomers that bind to keratin fibers in the stratum corneum	In the keratohyalin granules of stratum granulosum cells	Help regulate epidermal homeostasis; assist in water retention in the skin
Lamellar granules	Small ovoid structures containing lamellae of lipids	In the stratum granulosum cells	Form lipid envelopes around the cells to prevent water loss from the skin
Melanin	A brownish-black pigment produced by the melanocytes	In the stratum basale cells and hair follicles	Provides color to the skin, protects from UV exposure
Carotene	Unsaturated hydrocarbon absorbed from the diet and stored in the fat	In the stratum basale cells	Stores vitamin A, provides pigment
Melanosomes	Mature elliptical-shaped protein vesicles	In the melanocytes of the stratum basale and stratum spinosa	Store melanin
DERMIS			
Connective tissue	Extracellular matrix composed of protein fibers and ground substance	Dermal layer and hypodermis	Gives form to all organs, connects and binds tissues and cells, allows diffusion of nutrients and waste products
Anchoring fibrils	Filaments of Type VII collagen	Between the basal lamina and the papillary dermis	Bind the dermis to the epidermis
Elastic fibers	Thin collagen fibers that form networks with other collagen bundles	Dermis	Provide elasticity and flexibility to the skin
Ectosomes	Extracellular vesicles (100–500 nm) generated by the plasma membrane, originate outside the cell	Extracellular matrix	Composed of the proteins, mRNA, and miRNA that are typical of the cell of origin; release molecules that activate cell-surface molecules such as receptors and enzymes, thus contribute to intercellular communication and signaling
Exosomes	Extracellular vesicles (50–150 nm) that originate from exocytosis of multivesicular bodies (MVBs) and then interact with other intracellular vesicles and organelles	Extracellular matrix	Contain constituents of cells such as DNS, RNA, lipids, metabolites, and certain proteins; contribute to intercellular communication and signaling

Data from Mescher AL. *Junqueira's Basic Histology: Text & Atlas*. 16th ed. New York, NY: McGraw Hill; 2021.

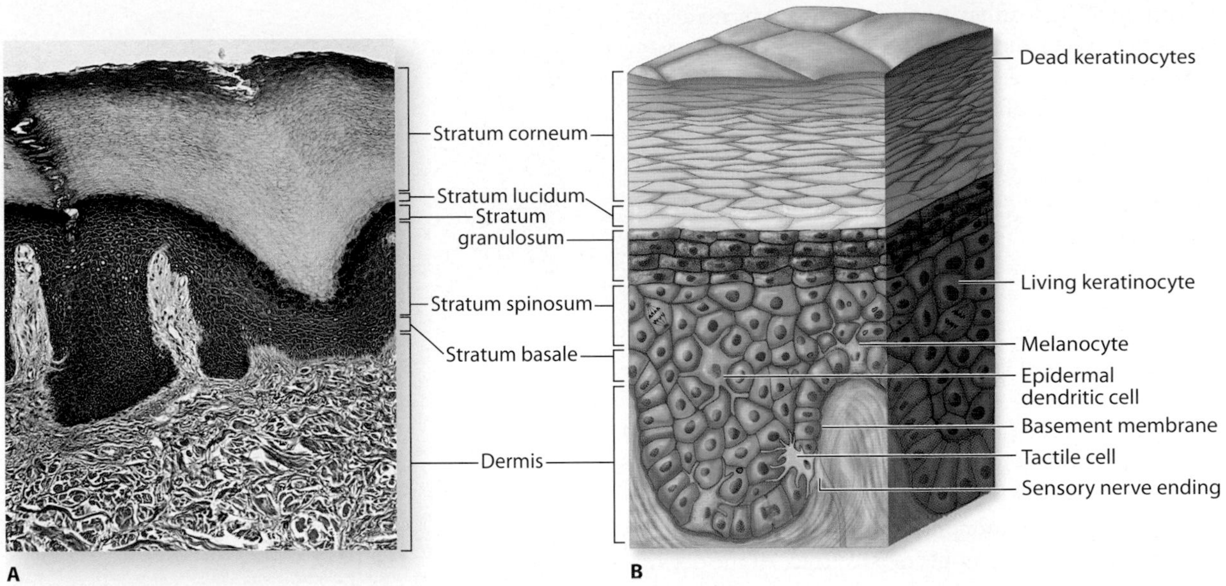

FIGURE 1-2 Layers of the epidermis.

Stratum basale—composed of a single layer of cuboid cells, attached to the underlying dermis by the basement membrane. The stratum basale is constantly producing epidermal cells (keratinocytes) from stem cells located in both the basal layer and the bulge of the hair follicles in the dermis.
Stratum spinosum—composed of slightly flattened cells that are responsible for protein synthesis, primarily keratin that forms bundles called *tonofibrils*. This is the thickest layer of the epidermis.
Stratum granulosum—composed of 3–5 layers of flattened cells that are undergoing terminal differentiation as they approach the outermost layer of skin. The intercellular spaces are filled with a lipid-rich material that forms a sheet or envelope around the cells, thereby making skin a barrier to both water loss and extrinsic foreign material.
Stratum lucidum—composed of flattened eosinophilic cells, creating a clear or translucent layer located only in the soles of the feet and palms of the hands. Cells contain densely packed keratin and are connected by desmosomes. Provides thickness and strength to withstand friction to the soles and palms.
Stratum corneum—composed of 15–20 layers of dead keratinized cells that are continuously being shed in a process called *desquamation*.

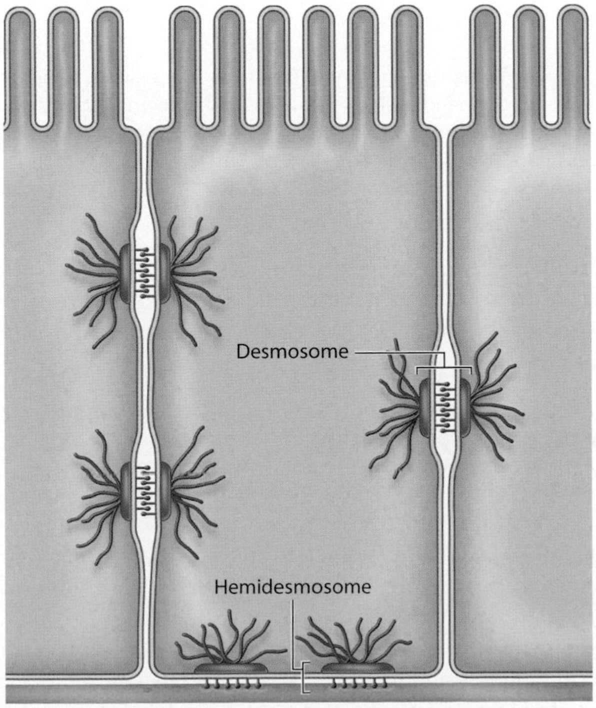

FIGURE 1-3 Cell adherence with desmosomes and hemidesmosomes. *Desmosomes* are adherent glycoprotein discs that bind keratinocytes to each other. *Hemidesmosomes* are adherent glycoprotein half-discs that bind keratinocytes to the basement membrane between the stratum basale and the dermis.

tonofibrils that converge on the hemidesmosomes and desmosomes to give the skin strength to withstand friction or shear force. They also have a role in maintaining the structure and mechanical properties of the keratinocyte.[5] As the keratinocytes migrate into the stratum granulosum, *filaggrin* (derived from "filament-aggregating protein") binds to the tonofibrils, thereby forming an insoluble keratin matrix that "acts as a protein scaffold for the attachment of cornified-envelope proteins and lipids that together form the stratum corneum."[6] Also in the stratum granulosum, *lamellar granules* containing many lamellae of lipids undergo exocytosis and release a lipid-rich material into the intercellular spaces and thereby form envelopes around the protein-filled cells that are undergoing keratinization.[1] This combination of tightly adhered filaments and lipid-rich envelopes contributes to the skin's ability to serve as both a barrier to loss of water from the body and protection from extrinsic foreign material.

The stratum lucidum is present primarily in the thick, hairless skin of the palms and soles (termed *glabrous skin*) and consists of dead, clear keratinocytes, thus the term "clear layer." The stratum lucidum is between the stratum granulosum and the stratum corneum and provides the palms and soles more protection from friction and serves as a greater moisture barrier.

When the keratinocytes enter the stratum corneum, they are flat, stacked, and embedded in lipid layers to form the main protective shield of the skin. The keratinocytes are held together with modified adhesive desmosomes, termed *corneodesmosomes*.[7] When the keratinocytes migrate to the surface they are termed corneocytes. The corneodesmosomes are degraded in a process carefully controlled by a number of proteases and their inhibitors, and as a result the corneocytes desquamate, or slough off.[8,9] Over a period of 28 days, the entire process of migration and desquamation is completed and the epidermis is renewed.

Dermis

The dermis (composed of collagen fibers, extracellular matrix [ECM], cells, and adnexal structures) binds the epidermis to the hypodermis or subcutaneous tissue. The ECM of the dermis is composed of collagen (mostly Type I), elastic fibers, and ground substances such as glycosaminoglycans (GAGs) and proteoglycans.[10] These components give the skin its elasticity and its tensile strength.[11] The uppermost surface of the dermis is reticular and interdigitates with the ridges of the epidermis; the structures are termed *epidermal pegs* and *dermal papillae* (**FIGURE 1-4**).

Between the dermis and epidermis is the basement membrane, consisting of the basal lamina and the reticular lamina. Structurally, the basement membrane protein is composed primarily of Type IV collagen, perlecan, and laminin 332 (specific ECM proteins).[12] Besides holding the two layers together, the basement membrane controls cell traffic and diffusion of bioactive materials in both directions through its pores, and thus allows the nutrients from the dermal vasculature to pass through to the avascular epidermis.[11,13] The basement membrane also binds a variety of cytokines and growth factors, controls their release, and thus plays an important role in tissue repair.[11]

The acellular dermal components (**TABLE 1-3**) include the ECM, anchor fibrils of Type VII collagen linking the dermal papillae and the basal lamina, and the elastic fibers that are intertwined with the other collagen fibers to give flexibility and elasticity to the skin. Exosomes and ectosomes are two extracellular vesicles located within the ECM and play key roles in intercellular communication.[14,15] Hyaluronan (previously known as hyaluronic acid and renamed because it is not an acid) is an anionic nonsulfated GAG located in the ECM which contributes to cellular proliferation and migration; it is thus an integral part of wound healing.[16,17]

The cellular components of the dermis are listed in **TABLE 1-2** and their role in dermal physiology is discussed in the section "Functions of the Skin." The papillary layer contains the fibroblasts, mast cells, and macrophages, as well as some extravasated leukocytes.[1] The reticular layer is composed of dense, mainly Type I, collagen and contains the vasculature, nerve endings, glands, hair follicles, and more elastic fibers.

The hypodermis, or subcutaneous layer, is the tissue that binds the skin to the underlying structures. It is composed of loose connective tissue, vascular supply, and adipose cells that vary in number at different body areas and also among individuals. The hypodermis provides protection and insulation to the body, and it allows the skin to move freely over the underlying structures, thereby facilitating fluid muscle and joint movement.

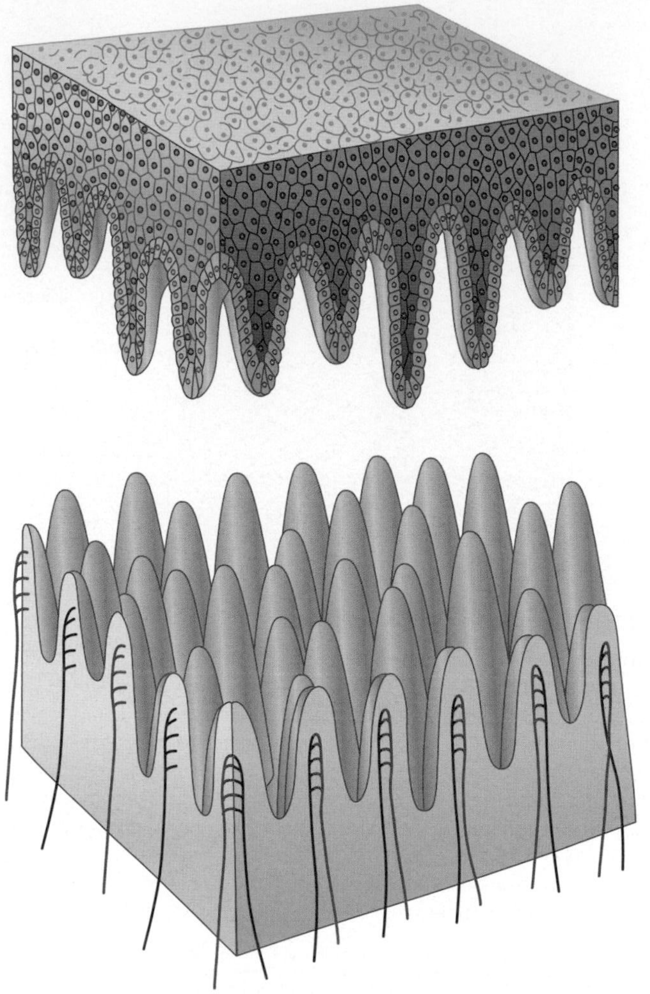

FIGURE 1-4 Dermal/epidermal junction. The epidermal/dermal junction is composed of dermal papillae and epidermal pegs that interdigitate to create a bond that will withstand friction and shear forces on the skin. The junction flattens with age, making geriatric skin more susceptible to skin tears.

SKIN MATURATION

Dermal evolution over the human life span can be represented by the six stages described in **TABLE 1-4**. The development of neonatal skin and its healing projectory is exquisitely covered in Chapter 8, Pediatric Wounds. Adult skin changes usually begin at about 50 years of age and are characterized by wrinkles, sunspots or hyperpigmentation, hypopigmentation in darker skin, uneven skin color, sagging skin, less elasticity, and rhytides (defined as the fine lines and minor creases that precede wrinkles).[18,19] The cutaneous changes are influenced by both intrinsic and extrinsic factors and vary among individuals based on lifestyle as

TABLE 1-4 Stages of Skin Development and Maturation across the Life Span

Developmental Age	Developmental Phase	Skin Description
5–8 weeks gestational age	Cellular dermis	Dermal cells are an open network; ECM is mostly hyaluronic acid that holds water; thin collagen fibrils of Type I and III are first to appear
9–12 weeks gestational age	Transition dermis	Development of blood vessels and nerves demarcate dermis from subcutaneous tissue; collagen fibrils increase and form bundles; ECM organizes to differentiate papillary and reticular dermis
13 weeks gestational age and later	Fibrous dermis	Rete pegs form to further differentiate papillary and reticular dermis; fibroblasts begin to appear; collagen fiber density increases with a greater ratio of Type III collagen
Child	Immature dermis	Dermis is immature and thin; average thickness of reticular dermis is 1.6 mm and increases with age; fibroblast density decreases; progenitor cells in the hair follicle bulge decrease and thus affect healing process
Adult < 50 years age	Mature dermis	Reticular dermal thickness increases to about 3.2 mm; dermal ECM thickens to form 70–80% of the skin weight; water content interacts with GAGs to give skin more stiffness
Adult > 50 years age	Degraded dermis	Skin begins to degenerate; ECM becomes thinner; epidermal-dermal rete pegs flatten; thickness of collagen bundles decreases and space between bundles increases; cellular contacts decrease; number of senescent cells increases; possible deregulation of the MMP/TIMP balance occurs; elastin network atrophies so skin has less elasticity

Data from Haydont V, Bernard BA, Fortunel NO. Age-related evolutions of the dermis: clinical signs, fibroblast and extracellular matrix dynamics. *Mech Ageing Dev*. 2019;177:150-156.

well as underlying structural and functional differences due to ethnic origin.[19] The intrinsic changes, which are a result of oxidative stress and molecular damage, include rhytides, fat atrophy with soft tissue redistribution and sagging, and areas of pigmentation heterogeneities (either hyper- or hypopigmentation)[19] (**FIGURE 1-5**). In addition, the aging skin will have decreased thickness, decreased number of most cell types, and decreased microcirculation, all of which can affect wound healing.[20]

The extrinsic factors that influence skin aging relate to environmental exposure, health, and lifestyle, with cumulative sun exposure being the most important factor. Other extrinsic factors include tobacco use, excessive alcohol use, poor nutrition, and exercise.[19] Skin changes as a result of these extrinsic factors include deep wrinkling, telangiectasia dark spots, and loss of elasticity (**FIGURE 1-6**). Darker skin with more melanin has been shown to be less susceptible to sun-induced skin damage, changes due to aging tend to be less severe, and changes tend to occur 10–20 years later than in age-matched fair skin.[21] The increased amount of melanin in darker skin does, however, make it more vulnerable to dyspigmentation.[19]

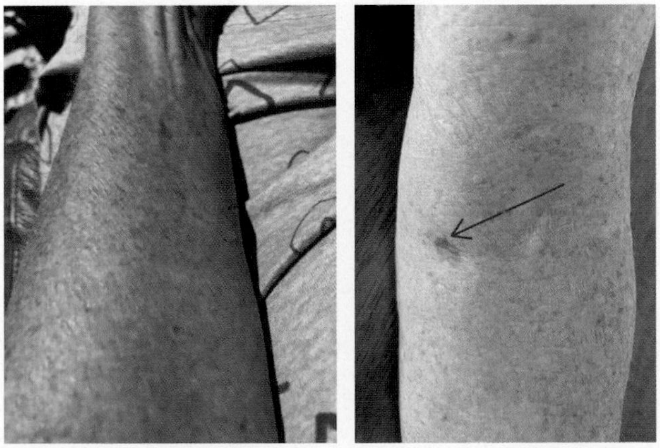

FIGURE 1-5 Signs of aging skin seen on areas of the body that are not usually exposed to the sun include rhytides or fine wrinkles and areas of hyperpigmentation. These subtle changes occur about 10 years later in skin of color, and may appear as hypopigmentation in darker skin.

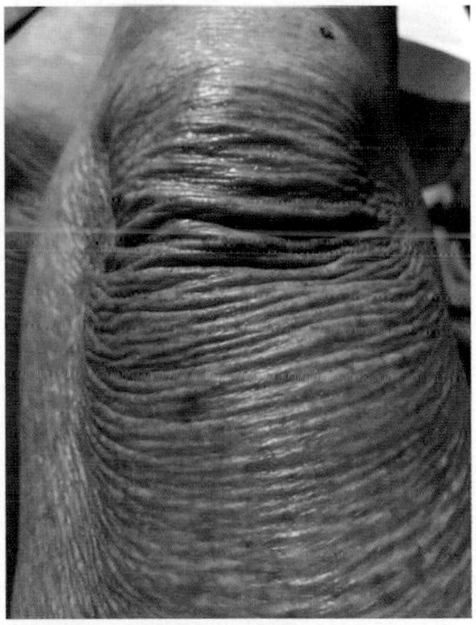

FIGURE 1-6 Deep wrinkles, sun spots or hyperpigmentation, and sagging skin as a result of cumulative sun exposure on the knee and lower thigh.

SKIN PHYSIOLOGY

Vascular Supply

The dermis contains two microvascular blood vessel plexuses, as well as lymphatic vessels, that are parallel to the skin surface (see **FIGURE 1-1**). The larger arterioles and venules are in the deep reticular layer, and the smaller vessels extend into the papillary layer and terminate in capillary loops.[22,23] Blood flow through the capillary loops is controlled by highly innervated arterioles,[24] and their close proximity to the basement membrane allows the blood supply to feed the deep keratinocytes of the epidermis. Between the larger deep plexus and the capillary loops are numerous *arteriovenous anastomoses* (AVAs) or shunts that play a major role in maintaining constant body temperature during hot and cold weather conditions. Lymphatic terminal vessels, little sacs interspersed with the capillary loops, are controlled by a filament anchored to the connective tissue. As the filament moves, it opens a flap to the lymphatic vessels, thereby facilitating transport of excess interstitial fluid, protein molecules, and fat molecules out of the dermis. (Refer to Chapter 5, Lymphedema.)

Nerve Supply

Because of its large and superficial surface area, the skin contains the sensory receptors necessary for the body to process the external environment (**FIGURE 1-7**). The nerve endings

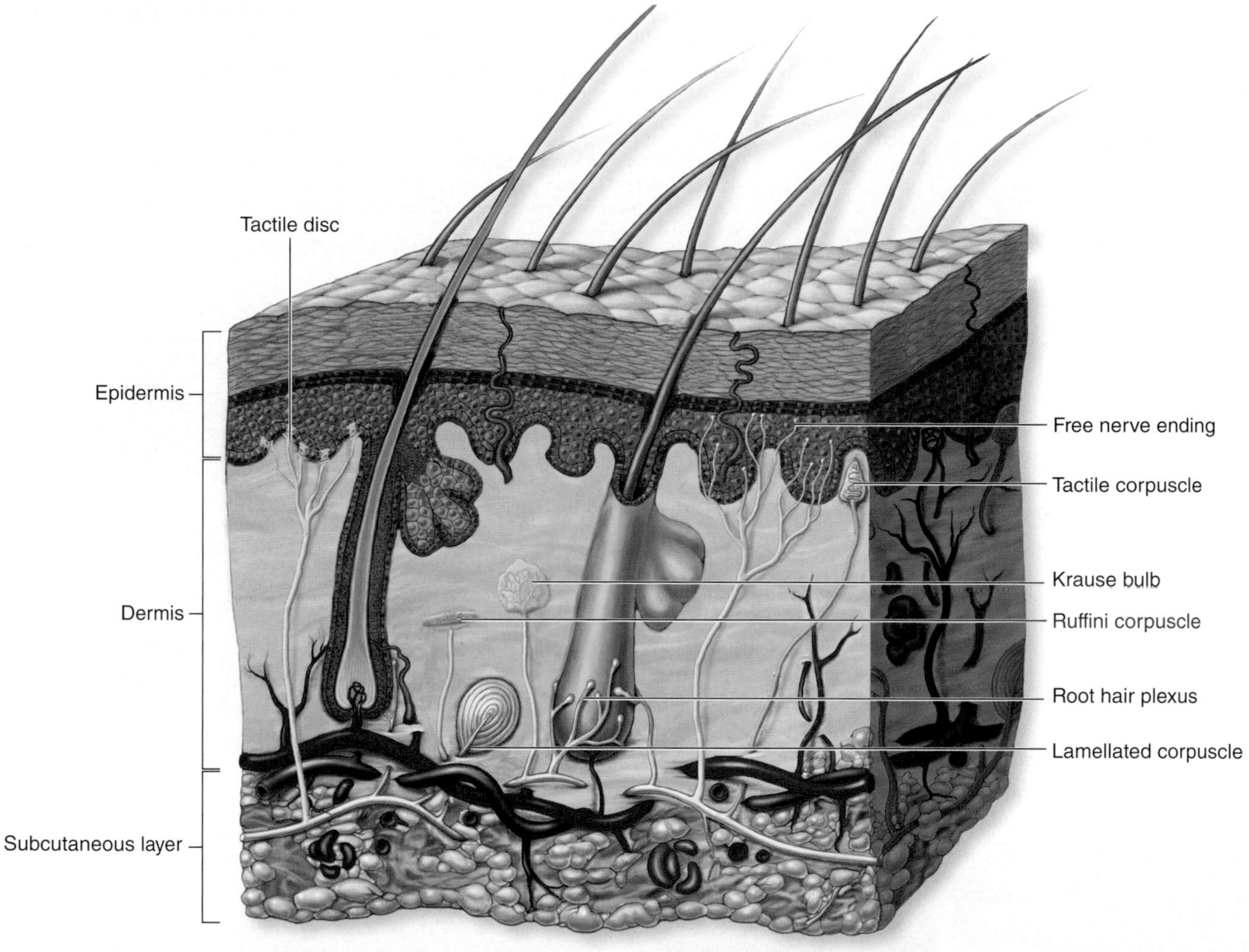

FIGURE 1-7 Sensory nerves within the dermal reticular layer. (Reproduced with permission from Mescher AL. Skin. In: Mescher AL. eds. *Junqueira's Basic Histology: Text and Atlas.* 16th ed. New York, NY: McGraw-Hill; 2021.)

Free nerve endings—unencapsulated nerve endings resembling the roots of a tree that are in the stratum basale of the epidermis; function as thermoreceptors, nociceptors, or cutaneous mechanoreceptors. The nerves lose the Schwann cell covering when they cross the dermal/epidermal junction into the stratum basale.
Tactile or Merkel disc—unencapsulated nerve ending close to the dermal/epidermal junction that is a receptor for light touch.
Meissner corpuscle—encapsulated unmyelinated nerve ending in the dermal papillae that responds to texture and slow vibrations. The corpuscle is a single nerve fiber surrounded by lamella of flattened connective tissue cells, giving it a bulbous appearance. Meissner corpuscles are located most densely in glabrous skin.
Pacinian corpuscle—oval-shaped mechanoreceptor that consists of a single unmyelinated nerve fiber in a fluid-filled cavity surrounded by lamella of thin, flat, modified Schwann cells and wrapped in a layer of connective tissue, giving it the appearance of an onion. Pacinian corpuscles detect deep pressure and high-frequency, fast vibration.
Krause bulb—encapsulated nerve fiber located in the middle dermal layer; both a mechanoreceptor and a thermoreceptor, detecting light pressure, soft low vibrations, and cold.
Ruffini corpuscle—encapsulated elongated dendritic nerve ending located in the deep dermis and hypodermis; both a mechanoreceptor and thermoreceptor, detecting sustained pressure, stretching, and heat.
Root hair plexus—a network of sensory fibers around the root of the hair follicles in the deep dermis; detects and transmits any hair movement.

are either unencapsulated (have no glial or collagenous covering) or encapsulated (have a covering of glia and connective tissue capsules).[1,25] When the nerves cross the dermal/epidermal junction, they lose the Schwann cell covering and exist in the epidermal pegs as free nerve endings. Also in the granulosum basale are unencapsulated mechanoreceptors termed *tactile* or *Merkel cells* that contribute to the encoding of information about the texture and shape of an object.[26] Recent studies have shown that there are synaptic-like contacts between the keratinocytes and the free nerve endings in the epidermis, indicating that the keratinocytes have a key role in the transduction of nociceptive information and cutaneous perception of pain, temperature, and itch.[26–28] This knowledge provides more insight into the sensory loss that occurs with dermal tissue injury.

Skin Nutrition

Much has been written, and even more spent, on nutrients, supplements, and topicals to maintain skin nutrition and ergo youth. While there are no double-blind, placebo-controlled studies to support what is called the "inside-out" approach to maintaining skin integrity, there are certain vitamins and antioxidants that are known to play a role in skin health, in large part by their antioxidant effects.[29] These substances and their functions are listed in **TABLE 1-5**. In addition, the following micronutrients are essential to skin health: selenium, zinc, copper, silicon, and polyphenols.[30] These micronutrients cannot be synthesized in humans and thus need to be obtained from one's diet, or from supplements when deficient.

Skin Renewal

The skin is continuously renewing itself through synthesis of new keratinocytes in the stratum basale and sloughing of the corneocytes from the stratum corneum, a process that takes approximately 28 days.[10,31] Fully differentiated cuboidal keratinocytes in the basal layer migrate through the spinous and granular layers toward the surface, and in the process accumulate keratin and lipids. The cells then undergo terminal differentiation to form the stratum corneum.[10] The functions of keratinocytes are listed in **TABLE 1-1**, and their role in wound healing is discussed in Chapter 2, Healing Response in Acute and Chronic Wounds.

TABLE 1-5 Nutrients Important to Maintenance of Skin Health

Nutrient	Function	Source
Vitamin D	Maintains the bony structure Maintains calcium homeostasis May help modulate the skin's immune response May promote healing of DFUs by up-regulating cathelicidin in keratinocytes	Synthesis in skin as a result of exposure to sunlight Enriched milk, orange juice, cereal Fatty fish (salmon, mackerel), cod liver oil Eggs and cheese
Vitamin C (ascorbic acid)	Eliminates free radicals (antioxidant) Promotes collagen synthesis Promotes wound healing May promote fibroblast proliferation May inhibit melanogenesis	Vegetables Citrus fruits
Vitamin E	Lipid-soluble, membrane-bound antioxidant May protect against UVB effects	Vegetables, oils, seeds, corn, soy, whole wheat flour, margarine, nuts, some meat and dairy products
Vitamin A (derived carotenoids)	Antioxidants Promotes collagen deposition Protects against UV radiation	Yellow and orange vegetables Salmon Leafy green vegetables
Vitamin F (essential fatty acids)	Formation of cell walls May protect against UV radiation May mitigate inflammation	Oils from flaxseed, canola, hemp seed, chia seed, walnuts, sesame seeds, avocados, salmon, albacore tuna, olive oil
Coenzyme Q10	Endogenous antioxidant	Synthesized by the body, present in all cells Fatty fish, liver, whole grains
Plant-derived antioxidants	Prevent lipid peroxidation	Soy, curcumin, silymarin, ginkgo, green tea, pomegranate
Collagen peptides	Decreases MMPs Promote fibroblast growth Stimulate hyaluronic acid production	Fish

Adapted from Draelos ZD. Nutrition and enhancing youthful-appearing skin. *Clin Dermatol*. 2010;28:400-408; Michalak M, Pierzak M, Krecisz B, Suliga E. Bioactive compounds for skin health: a review. *Nutrients*. 2021;13(1):203; Muzumdar S, Ferenczi K. Nutrition and youthful skin. *Clin Dermatol*. 2021;39(5):796-808.

FUNCTIONS OF THE SKIN

Protection from Environment

The dense, adhered structure of the skin provides protection from the environment by preventing the penetration of some microbes and other foreign bodies, by absorbing shock as a result of the cushioning hypodermis, by serving as a barrier to excessive water absorption or loss, and by containing specialized structures and cells with other protective functions (eg, lymphocytes and antigen-presenting cells that respond to invading microorganisms and thereby mount an immune response).[1] Most of the physical protection comes from the epidermis which is relatively impermeable due to the physiochemical properties and architectural arrangement of the keratinocytes.[32] The keratin, which provides much of the defensive nature of the epidermis due to its strength and stability, is composed of (1) chains of keratin molecules arranged in filaments which are in turn bundled into fibrils and (2) a matrix between the filaments which contains globular keratin protein. The intercellular spaces of the epidermis are filled with lipid-rich fluid which gives the skin its "waterproof" effect. When the skin is damaged by disease or lost as a result of injury, its functions are compromised and can have detrimental, even fatal, effects on the body.

Sensation

Sensation is both informative and protective. Stimuli received in the skin and transmitted to the brain can initiate a motor response that moves the person away from noxious stimuli. Embedded in the dermis are numerous nerve endings, illustrated and summarized in **FIGURE 1-7**. The most prevalent diagnosis resulting in the loss of tactile, pressure, and pain sensation in the skin is diabetic polyneuropathy, a major contributing factor to the formation of diabetic foot wounds. The lack of sensation allows trauma, even repeated trauma, to occur unnoticed and thereby results in wounds that are difficult to heal. This is just one example of how the failure of the skin sensory function may be a primary cause of wounds.

Prevention of Fluid Loss

The dense, extensively cross-linked lipid and protein matrix in the stratum corneum serves as a barrier to fluid loss, thereby helping to maintain homeostasis. This protection is enhanced in the palms and soles by the presence of the stratum lucidum. In addition, "natural moisturizing factors" (including free amino acids, lactic acid, urea, and salts) attract and hold water in the stratum corneum which is normally approximately 30% water.[33] This property of maintaining the water content is termed *hygroscopy*. The amino acids are a result of filaggrin degradation by proteolytic enzymes.[33] Injury to the skin or atmospheric conditions that result in loss of water can cause dry skin, irritant dermatitis, or cracking which results in fissures that allow noxious stimuli to enter the skin layers and may in turn lead to cellulitis. Water loss from the skin surface occurs by the following three physiologic mechanisms: (1) diffusion, also known as transepidermal water loss, which occurs at different rates depending upon the age (greater in premature infants than mature infants and adults), body region (greater in abdomen and lower back than in extremities), and disease conditions (psoriasis or erythroderma); (2) sweat gland excretion (increases with strenuous exercise, raised temperature, or emotional stress); and (3) desorption, or evaporation of water that has been absorbed by the stratum corneum.[32] Moisturizers used to rehydrate and repair the skin may use some of the same compounds that are in normal skin (eg, hyaluronan).

Immunity

In addition to the physical barrier to environmental microbes, the skin has three properties that contribute to its role in the body's immune system: (1) Langerhans cells, (2) antimicrobial peptides and lipids, and (3) an acidic pH.

Langerhans cells are dendritic cells primarily in the stratum spinosum that are alerted by any foreign microbes which enter the epidermis. Subsequently these cells bind, process, and present the antigens to the T-lymphocytes which are also in the epidermis, thereby initiating an immune response.[1] *Antimicrobial peptides* are innate protein fragments that prick the microbe cell membrane and destroy its integrity, rendering it inactive. Some antimicrobial peptides are present in both healthy and infected tissue (eg, human β-defensin or HBD 1 and RNase 7), whereas others are present only in the event of epidermal penetration by the microbes (eg, psoriasin S100A7, HBD 2, and HBD 3). Lysozyme, dermcidin, and LL-37 are antimicrobial peptides found in the hair follicles and eccrine glands.[2] These same peptides signal and recruit the immune cells (T-lymphocytes, macrophages, neutrophils, and other dendritic cells) needed to phagocytose the attacked microbes or present antigens to the host immune system. See Chapter 2 for a more detailed discussion of peptides and their role in wound healing.

The skin has a slightly *acidic pH* (4.2–6) that serves as a barrier to exogenous bacteria. The "acid mantle" of the stratum corneum is a combined result of free fatty acids, oils produced by the sebaceous glands (sebum), secretions from the eccrine sweat glands, and proton pumps (by pumping H^+ ions out of cells onto the skin).[34] This acidic layer is a hostile environment for the bacteria, inhibits their replication, and thus serves as a natural immune mechanism.[35]

Thermoregulation

Thermoregulation as a response to changes in the environmental temperature is maintained by the dermal vasculature and by the sweat glands. When a person is inactive, normal skin blood flow is 30–40 mL/min/100 g of skin. During cold stress when the core body temperature drops, the hypothalamus sends impulses to the skin causing the arterioles and the arteriovenous anastomoses (AVAs) to constrict, thereby reducing the flow of blood to the skin and preserving inner body heat.[32] In extreme conditions, the flow can be reduced almost to zero, at which point the AVAs will dilate to maintain tissue temperature and viability. (Examples are when the skin turns erythematous upon application of a cold pack or when the nose turns red in extremely cold weather.) On the contrary, during times of heat stress, the hypothalamus sends signals to the same vessels causing them to dilate and allow more blood to circulate near the skin surface thereby dissipating the heat. The catalyst for the vasoconstriction or vasodilation is a dual sympathetic neural control. Glabrous (nonhairy) skin arterioles have sympathetic, norepinephrine innervation; nonglabrous (hairy) skin has both noradrenergic and cholinergic innervations. Nonglabrous skin vasculature also responds to the effects of local temperature changes (eg, with application of hot or cold packs).[24]

During periods of heat stress due to exercise or when the environmental temperature is higher than the blood temperature, thermoregulation is enhanced by the evaporation of fluid from the eccrine sweat glands. Initially the fluid produced is isotonic, but as it progresses toward the outer layer of the skin it becomes hypotonic by the reabsorption of the Na^+ ions.[33]

Protection from Ultraviolet Rays

The presence of melanin in the skin provides color variation among individuals and protects the underlying tissue from the effects of ultraviolet rays. This is accomplished through the activity of the epidermal-melanin unit, composed of the melanocytes that *produce* melanin and keratinocytes that *store* melanin.[1] Melanocytes produce melanosomes, which are highly organized organelles in which melanin synthesis takes place. Melanin is synthesized through a multistep process in which tyrosinase converts tyrosine into dihydroxyphenylalanine (DOPA) that is further transformed into melanin.[36] The melanin then migrates into the dendrites of the melanocytes. The dendritic ends of the keratinocytes phagocytose the melanocyte tips, allowing the melanin to enter into the keratinocyte where it is stored in quantities sufficient to absorb and reflect UV rays, thereby protecting the cellular DNA from the harmful effects of UV radiation. The number of melanocytes is consistent among all skin types; however, the number, size, and manner in which the melanosomes are distributed in the keratinocytes varies.[36] Each melanocyte communicates with 30–40 keratinocytes. As the keratinocytes migrate toward the surface of the epidermis, the melanosomes start to degrade, causing the melanin pigmentation of the skin.[37] Increases in both melanin production and accumulation result from increased exposure to sunlight, and is evidenced by the darker color of ethnic groups who originated in geographical areas near the equator.[1,38] It is important to note that the differences in skin color can affect the way wounds present differently, eg, in pressure injuries, which will be discussed in more detail in Chapter 3.

Several classifications of skin color have been developed, beginning with the *Fitzpatrick classification* of skin phototyping which was first introduced in 1975 (**TABLE 1-6**). This system, based on an individual's ethnicity and tendency to sunburn and tan in the non-Hispanic white population, was initially intended to be used to calculate the initial dose of phototherapy for psoriasis.[39,40] The Fitzpatrick classification, although still used to classify natural pigmentation of the skin and the effects after UV exposure, does have inaccuracies and limitations. It does not accurately reflect the occurrence of skin cancer or the likelihood of sunburning.[41] Although it is still used for research, the Fitzpatrick classification has since been modified and other systems have been developed. The *Obagi system*, which is also based on skin color and used primarily for determining treatment or predicting outcomes of dermatologic interventions, has the following three classifications:

- Original: skin on individuals not racially or ethnically mixed, eg, original light white, original dark black, and original yellow-toned Asian
- Deviated: skin on individuals racially or ethnically mixed
- Complex: skin on individuals racially or ethnically mixed with variable skin tones[42]

The Genetico-Racial Skin Classification is based on an individual's racial origin and consists of five "north to south" categories, going from coldest to warmest climates vertically across Europe and Africa and three categories in Asia. In Europe and Africa, the roots are Nordic, European, Mediterranean, Indo-Pakistani, and African, and in Asia, northern, central, and southern. The classification considers both skin color and facial features and is intended to be used for prediction of skin treatment outcomes.[43,44]

Regardless of the classification system, changes in skin vary with the skin color and must be recognized when diagnosing skin disorders such as sunburn, pressure injuries, and malignancies.[40,41]

TABLE 1-6 Fitzpatrick Classification of Skin Types

Skin Type	Typical Features	Tanning Ability
I	Pale white skin, blue/green eyes, blond/red hair	Always burns, does not tan
II	Fair skin, blue eyes	Burns easily, tans poorly
III	Darker white skin	Tans after initial burn
IV	Light brown skin	Burns minimally, tans easily
V	Brown skin	Rarely burns, tans darkly easily
VI	Dark brown or black skin	Never burns, always tans darkly

Note: Fitzpatrick classification of skin types is based upon the risk of burning with exposure to UVA and was initially used to determine the amount of UVA to use in treating skin disorders. It has also been used to predict risk of skin cancer; however, it does not take into account other factors that contribute to skin cancer, eg, genetics and sun exposure.

Synthesis and Storage of Vitamin D

Vitamin D is necessary for calcium metabolism and bone formation; vitamins D_2 and D_3 are both prohormone secosteroids (vitamin D_2 is ergocalciferol; vitamin D_3 is cholecalciferol). The skin is the primary source of vitamin D_3 synthesis in the stratum basale and stratum spinosum.[45] Keratinocytes express vitamin D hydroxylase enzymes that convert provitamin D_3 (7-dehydrocholesterol) to vitamin D_3. This process is stimulated by exposure to sunlight, occurs rapidly, and peaks within hours of exposure. Vitamin D_3 is bound to a vitamin D–binding protein that carries it from the epidermis through the bloodstream and to the liver and kidneys where it is hydroxylated into an active form for calcium metabolism. The process of vitamin D synthesis is less effective as the skin ages, which can lead to an increased risk of osteoporosis.[32]

Vitamin D also contributes to the role of epidermis in immunity by upregulating the expression of antimicrobial peptides, and when the vitamin is deficient in the epidermis, there is a concordant increased risk of infection.[46,47]

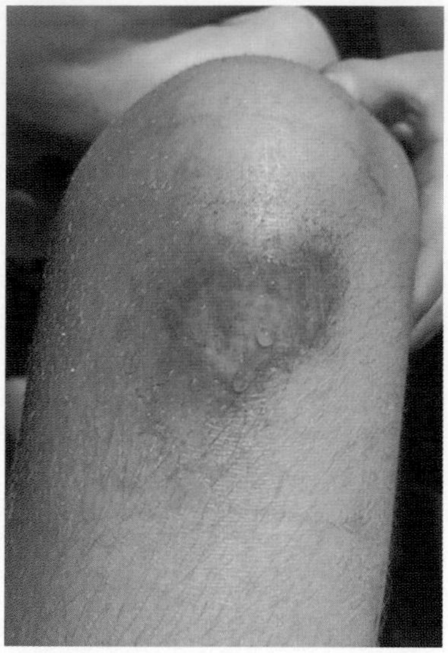

FIGURE 1-8 Erosion. The loss of the superficial epidermis only, with no involvement of the dermis.

Aesthetics and Communication

Skin color, texture, and hyper/hypopigmentation are major components of an individual's appearance and contribute to sexual attraction. Apocrine sweat glands, located primarily in the axillary and perineal regions, are dependent upon sex hormones for development and their secretions contain sex pheromones that can influence social behavior.

DEFINITIONS OF SKIN LOSS

Regardless of its etiology, every wound can be classified by the depth of tissue injury or loss as defined by the following terms.

Erosion is the loss of the superficial epidermis only, with no involvement of the dermis (**FIGURE 1-8**). These wounds will probably not bleed, although there may be increased redness of the skin due to the proximity of dermal vasculature and capillary loops in the dermal papillae. Examples of erosion are superficial burns (previously termed *first degree*) and abrasions. Repair is accomplished by a local inflammatory response and epidermal replacement by migrating keratinocytes.

Partial thickness wounding is the loss of the epidermis and part of the dermis (**FIGURE 1-9**). These wounds will bleed due to interference with the microvascular structure in dermal tissue. Examples of partial thickness skin loss are Stage II pressure ulcers, superficial and deep partial thickness burns (previously termed *second degree*), superficial skin tears, and deep abrasions. Repair is accomplished by re-epithelialization as a result of epithelial cell migration from the wound edges, hair follicles, and sebaceous glands.

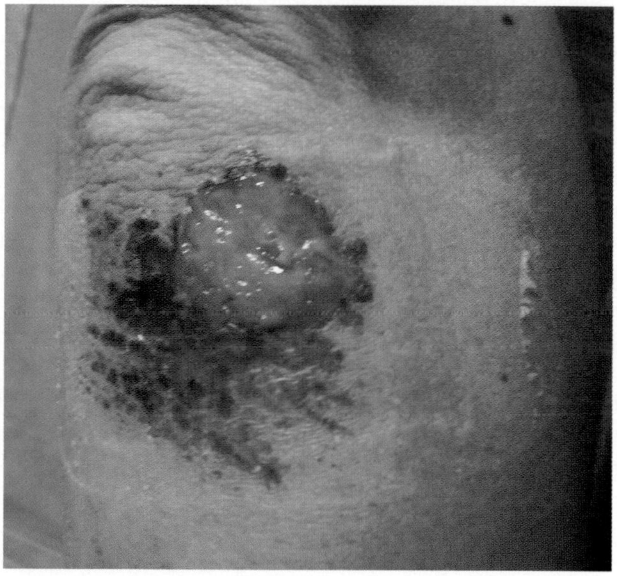

FIGURE 1-9 Partial-thickness skin loss. The loss of the epidermis and part of the dermis.

Full thickness wounding is the loss of the epidermis and dermis, extending into the subcutaneous tissue and in some cases involving bone, tendon, or muscle (**FIGURES 1-10** and **1-11**). Examples are full thickness burns (previously termed *third degree*), Stage III and IV pressure ulcers, surgical incisions, traumatic wounds that are full thickness, and wounds that require debridement of necrotic tissue into the subcutaneous tissue. Repair occurs through the secondary intention healing process, discussed at length in the next chapter.

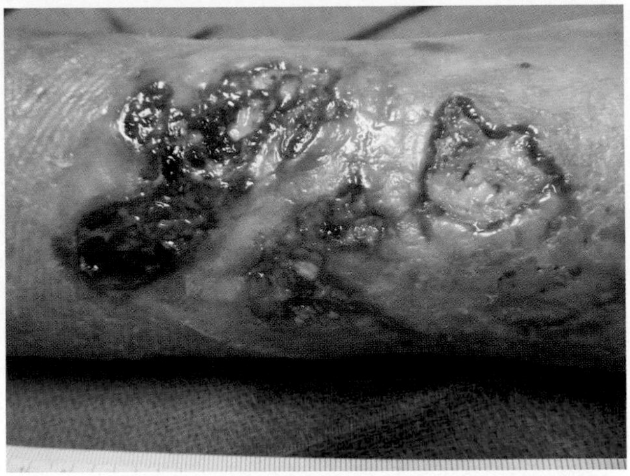

FIGURE 1-10 Full-thickness skin loss. The loss of the epidermis and dermis, extending into the subcutaneous tissue or hypodermis.

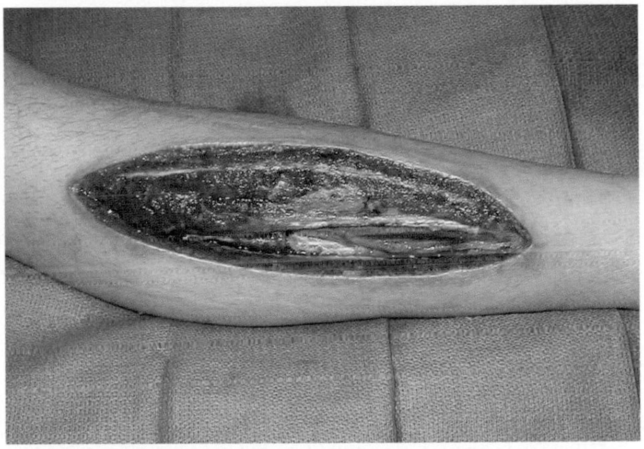

FIGURE 1-11 Full-thickness skin loss with involvement of muscle, bone, and tendon.

SUMMARY

The skin is a complex, multilayered organ that functions both independently to provide the body with its protective functions and interactively with other structures and organs to ensure total health. The cellular and acellular skin components exist at all times to maintain homeostasis; however, injury or disease processes can stimulate the cells to be present in greater numbers, to be more active, and to have greater influence on other processes in order to accomplish tissue repair and regeneration. The adaptive processes that lead to wound healing after tissue injury are the focus of Chapter 2.

STUDY QUESTIONS

1. The primary characteristic of the skin that enables it to withstand friction and shear forces is
   a. The number of layers in the epidermis.
   b. The amount of water and lipids in the interstitial spaces.
   c. The reticular formation of the dermal/epidermal junction.
   d. The nerve supply that alerts the body to abnormal mechanical forces.
2. Fibroblasts, mast cells, and macrophages, all necessary for skin renewal and regeneration, are located primarily in which layer of the skin?
   a. Stratum basale of the epidermis
   b. Papillary layer of the dermis
   c. Reticular layer of the dermis
   d. Throughout all the layers of the dermis and epidermis
3. The epidermal layer that is located in the palms and soles, giving them additional strength and thickness, is the
   a. Stratum basale.
   b. Stratum granulosum.
   c. Stratum corneum.
   d. Stratum lucidum.
4. The epidermis prevents loss of fluid because of its dense matrix of
   a. Lipids and proteins.
   b. Corneocytes.
   c. Dermosomes.
   d. Vitamin complexes.
5. Langerhans cells contribute to innate immunity by
   a. Pricking the bacteria cell wall and causing cytoplasmic leaks.
   b. Presenting antigens to the T-leukocytes.
   c. Phagocytosis of dead tissue that feeds bacteria.
   d. Creating an acidic environment on the skin surface.
6. Which cells are responsible for storing melanin in the form of melanosomes?
   a. Corneocytes
   b. Keratinocytes
   c. Melanocytes
   d. Monocytes
7. The structures that bind the keratinocytes and are subsequently degraded to allow desquamation of the stratum corneum are termed
   a. Desmosomes.
   b. Hemidesmosomes.
   c. Corneodesmosomes.
   d. Melanosomes.
8. The extracellular vesicle that plays a key role in communication and signaling between cells is termed
   a. Exosome.
   b. Hyaluronan.
   c. Organelle.
   d. Perlecan.

Answers: 1-c; 2-b; 3-d; 4-a; 5-b; 6-b; 7-c; 8-a

REFERENCES

1. Mescher AL. *Junqueira's Basic Histology Text & Atlas*. 16th ed. New York, NY: McGraw Hill; 2021.
2. Brogden NK, Mehalick L, Fischer CL, Wertx PW, Brogden KA. The emerging role of peptides and lipids as antimicrobial epidermal barriers and modulators of local inflammation. *Skin Pharmacol Physiol*. 2012;25(4):167-181.
3. Brennan D, Peltonen S, Dowling A, et al. A role for caveolin-1 in desmoglein binding and desmosome dynamics. *Oncogene*. 2012;31(13):1636-1648.
4. Bruckner-Tuderman L, Payne AS. Epidermal and dermal adhesion. In: Kang S, Amagai M, Bruckner AL, et al, eds. *Fitzpatrick's Dermatology*. 9th ed. New York, NY: McGraw Hill; 2019. Available at: https://accessmedicine.mhmedical.com/content.aspx?bookid=2570&sectionid=210416355. Accessed June 23, 2023.
5. Yoon KH, Yoon M, Moir RD, Khuon S, Flitney FW, Goldman RD. Insights into the dynamic properties of keratin intermediate filaments in living epithelial cells. *J Cell Biol*. 2001;153(3):503-516.
6. Sandilands A, Sutherland C, Irvine AD, McLean WHI. Filaggrin in the frontline: role in skin barrier function and disease. *J Cell Sci*. 2009;122(9):1285-1294.
7. Ishida-Yamamota A, Igawa S, Kishibe M. Order and disorder in corneocyte adhesion. *J Dermatol*. 2011;38(7):645-654.
8. Ishida-Yamamoto A, Igawa S. The biology and regulation of corneodesmosomes. *Cell Tissue Res*. 2015;360(3):477-482.
9. Danzberger J, Donovan M, Rankl C, et al. Glycan distribution and density in native skin's stratum corneum. *Skin Res Technol*. 2018;24(3):450-458.
10. Abdo JM, Sopko NA, Milner SM. The applied anatomy of human skin: a model for regeneration. *Wound Med*. 2020. Available at: https://doi.org/10.1016/j.wndm.2020.100179. Accessed June 23, 2023.
11. Breitkreutz D, Koxholt I, Thiemann K, Nischt R. Skin basement membrane: the foundation of epidermal integrity—BM functions and diverse roles of bridging molecules nidogen and perlecan. *Biomed Res Int*. 2013;2013:179784.
12. Sercu S, Zhang M, Oyama N, et al. Interaction of extracellular matrix protein 1 with extracellular matrix components: ECM1 is a basement membrane protein of the skin. *J Invest Dermatol*. 2008;128(6):1397-1408.
13. Oakford ME, Dixon SV, August S, et al. Migration of immunocytes across the basement membrane in skin: the role of basement membrane pores. *J Invest Dermatol*. 2011;131:1950-1953.
14. Kalluri R, LeBleu VS. The biology, function, and biomedical applications of exosomes. *Science*. 2020;367(6478):eaau6977.
15. Medlolesi J. Exosomes and ectosomes intercellular communication. *Curr Biol*. 2018;28:R435-R444.
16. Laurent TC, Laurent UBG, Fraser JRE. The structure and function of hyaluronan: an overview. *Immunol Cell Biol*. 1996;74(2):A1-A7.
17. Gao F, Yang CS, Mo W, Liu YW, He YQ. Hyaluronan oligosaccharides are potential stimulators to angiogenesis via RHAMM mediated signal pathway in wound healing. *Clin Invest Med*. 2008;31(3):E106-E116.
18. Haydont V, Bernard BA, Fortunel NO. Age-related evolutions of the dermis: clinical signs, fibroblast and extracellular matrix dynamics. *Mech Aging Dev*. 2019;177:150-156.
19. Vashi NA, de Castro Maymone MB, Kundu RV. Aging differences in ethnic skin. *J Clin Aesthet Dermatol*. 2016;9(1):31-38.
20. Bentov I, Reed MJ. Anesthesia, microcirculation, and wound repair in aging. *Anesthesiology*. 2014;120(3):760-772.
21. Kaidbey KH, Agin PP, Sayre RM, Kligman AM. Photoprotection by melanin: a comparison of black and Caucasian skin. *J Am Acad Dermatol*. 1979;1(3):249-260.
22. Cracowski J, Roustit M. Human skin microcirculation. *Compr Physiol*. 2020;10(3):1105-1154.
23. Braverman IM. The cutaneous microcirculation. *J Investig Dermatol Symp Proc*. 2000;5(1):3-9.
24. Petzelbauer P, Loewe R, Pober JS. Cutaneous vasculature. In: Kang S, Amagai M, Bruckner AL, et al, eds. *Fitzpatrick's Dermatology*. 9th ed. New York, NY: McGraw Hill; 2019. Available at: https://accessmedicine.mhmedical.com/content.aspx?bookid=2570&sectionid=210415779. Accessed June 23, 2023.
25. Somatosensory neurotransmission: touch, pain, & temperature. In: Barrett KE, Barman SM, Boitano S, Reckelhoff JF, eds. *Ganong's Medical Physiology Examination & Board Review*. New York, NY: McGraw Hill; 2017. Available at: https://accessmedicine.mhmedical.com/content.aspx?bookid=2139&sectionid=160312109. Accessed June 23, 2023.
26. Talagas M, Lebonvallet N, Berthod F, Misery L. Cutaneous nociception: role of keratinocytes. *Exp Dermatol*. 2019;28:1466-1469.
27. Talagas M, Lebonvallet N, Leschiera R, et al. Intra-epidermal nerve endings progress within keratinocyte cytoplasmic tunnels in normal human skin. *Exp Dermatol*. 2020;29(4):387-392.
28. Talagas M, Lebonvallet N, Leschiera R, et al. Keratinocytes communicate with sensory neurons via synaptic-like contacts. *Ann Neurol*. 2020;88(6):1205-1219.
29. Draelos ZD. Nutrition and enhancing youthful-appearing skin. *Clin Dermatol*. 2010;28:400-408.
30. Michalak M, Pierzak M, Kręcisz B, Suliga E. Bioactive compounds for skin health: a review. *Nutrients*. 2021;13(1):203.
31. Gonzales KAU, Fuchs E. Skin and its regenerative powers: an alliance between stem cells and their niche. *Dev Cell*. 2017;43(4):387-401.
32. McKnight G, Shah H, Hargest R. Physiology of the skin. *Surgery*. 2021;40(1):8-12.
33. Cramer M, Gagnon D, Laitano O, Crandall CG. Human temperature regulation under heat stress in health, disease, and injury. *Physiol Rev*. 2022;102(4):1907-1989.
34. Schmid-Wendtner MH, Korting HC. The pH of the skin surface and its impact on the barrier function. *Skin Pharmacol Physiol*. 2006;19:296-302.
35. Mojumdar EH, Sparr E. The effects of pH and salt on the molecular structure and dynamics of the skin. *Colloids Surf B Biointerfaces*. 2021;198:111476.
36. Costin GE, Hearing VJ. Human skin pigmentation: melanocytes modulate skin color in response to stress. *FASEB J*. 2007;21(4):976-994.
37. Lin JY, Fisher DE. Melanocyte biology and skin pigmentation. *Nature*. 2007;445(7130):843-850.
38. Thone HY, Jee SH, Sun CC, Boissy RE. The patterns of melanosome distribution in keratinocytes of human skin as one determining factor of skin colour. *Br J Derm*. 2003;149(3):498-505.
39. Gupta V, Sharma VK. Skin typing: Fitzpatrick grading and others. *Clin Dermatol*. 2019;37(5):430-436.
40. Zaidi Z. Skin of color: characteristics and disease. *J Pakistan Med Assoc*. 2017;67(2):292-298.
41. Goon P, Banfield C, Bello O, Levell NJ. Skin cancers in skin types IV-VI: does the Fitzpatrick scale give a false sense of security? *Skin Health Dis*. 2021;1(3):e40.

42. Rullan P, Karam AM. Chemical peels for darker skin types. *Facial Plast Surg Clin North Am.* 2010;18(1):111-131.
43. Fanous N, Yoskovitch A. New classification scheme for laser resurfacing and chemical peels: modifications for the different ethnic groups. *Facial Plast Surg Clin N Am.* 2002;10:405–413.
44. Fanous N, Cote V, Fanous A. The new Genetico-Racial Skin Classification: how to maximize the safety of any peel or laser treatment on any Asian, Caucasian, or black patient. *Can J Plast Surg.* 2011;19(1):9-16.
45. Saponaro F, Saba A, Zucchi R. An update on vitamin D metabolism. *Int J Mol Sci.* 2020;21(18):6573.
46. Segaert S, Simonart T. The epidermal vitamin D system and innate immunity: some more light shed on this unique photoendocrine system? *Dermatology.* 2008;217:7-11.
47. Bartley J. Vitamin D: emerging roles in infection and immunity. *Expert Rev Anti Infect Ther.* 2010;8(12):1359-1369.

Healing Response in Acute and Chronic Wounds

Tammy Luttrell, PhD, MSPT, CWS, FCCWS
Illustrations by Shelby Luttrell

CHAPTER OBJECTIVES

At the end of this chapter, the learner will be able to:

1. **Describe the sequence of normal acute wound healing.**
2. **Identify the cells that direct activity in the healing cascade.**
3. **Describe the chemical messengers necessary for timely wound healing (including the cells of origin, target cells, and actions).**
4. **Classify the primary enzymes produced during healing (including the cells of origin and actions).**
5. **Describe the innate and adaptive immune responses that occur during wound healing.**
6. **Describe the functions of platelets, monocytes, and fibroblasts and how they change during the course of wound healing.**
7. **Explain the differences between acute and chronic wound healing.**

INTRODUCTION

Perhaps the hamartia, or the flaw, in the study of wound healing is the tendency to oversimplify the elegant system that ensures healing, both anatomically and functionally. The multitude of processes involved in wound closure and the commensurate return of function are equally marvelous.

The illustrations in this chapter introduce the interplay of cellular and molecular signaling in conjunction with vascular events that occur during the healing process. The figures demonstrate how cells involved in the repair process are directed, based upon global and local stimuli that may be cytokine, chemokine, pH, or galvanically driven.[1,2] If invaders or pathogens (eg, bacteria, fungi, viruses, or debris) are present, innate immune cells migrate and proliferate to the site of injury.[3] These cells include macrophages, neutrophils, natural killer (NK) cells, and gamma delta T cells. If the invader is a repeat offender that the host has successfully fended off previously, adaptive immune responses (B-cell clonal expansion) are triggered.[3–5] Simultaneously, debris (necrotic and/or injured cells) is removed and a new wound bed excavated via proteases and extracellular matrix (ECM) degradation. This serves two purposes: (1) the clearance of cell and invader refuse and (2) the provision of pathways for cellular migration and proliferation, which constitute repair.[2]

CELLULAR SIGNALING

The signaling in wound healing, renewal, and regeneration is a product of many factors, including the concentration and timing of chemical signal delivery, target cell receptor availability, active form after cleavage, degradation rate, messenger half-life, pH and presence of enzymes (eg, proteases) in the wound milieu, hydrophobicity, and hydrophilicity. Scaffold-binding (via heparin activation or other mechanisms), fiber type (whether fibrin or collagen), cell shape, adhesion interfaces (via integrins), and storage of growth factors all contribute to the timing and intensity of cell signaling during wound healing. These factors work together to drive growth factor, cytokine, and chemokine bioavailability, thus resulting in wound healing.

Vascular changes occur as a result of endothelial cell activation, migration, and capillary expansion in response to tissue hypoxia and increased lactic acid concentration.[6–8] Phenotypical changes in prominent cells (platelets, macrophages, and fibroblasts) are important in directing healing through the influence and production of many of the chemical messengers. The macrophages have a pronounced cellular functional metamorphosis and are the central orchestrators of the healing process. Cellular roles pertinent to wound healing are described in **TABLE 2-1** along with the cellular communication and signaling that occur to effect progression through the healing process.

The pivotal cells and phases of healing are described in **TABLE 2-2**, which provides a cross-reference of healing phases with key cells and signals, as well as a chronological timeline, thus providing the reader an appreciation of the overlapping and essential functions directed in sequence as opposed to an isolated view of cell function. Although exceedingly complex, the elegance of the healing response lies both in the ability of multiple systems to evoke healing and in the use of paracrine, autocrine, and juxtacrine mediators to effect expedient resolution of tissue injury.

Recent studies show that many of the cell mediators are not expressed individually by a cell, but are collectively "packaged" in small, 50 nm to 150 nm, membrane-bound, extracellular vesicles called exosomes.[53] The power of the extracellular

TABLE 2-1 Important Cells in Wound Healing

Endothelial Cells Description		**Cell Graphic**
PRIMARY ACTION	EFFECT	MECHANISM/SIGNAL
Reestablishment of ECM	Fibroblast proliferation	Acidic fibroblast growth factor (aFGF)
Facilitate in angiogenesis	Facilitation of the reestablishment of the vascular base including the reabsorption of excess capillaries VEGF is a potent stimulator of angiogenesis	Basic fibroblast growth factor (bFGF) VEGF—upregulated in the presence of nitric oxide
Angiogenesis	Angiogenesis is further facilitated by the secretion of PDGF and the upregulation of target cell receptors for PDGF (PDGFRs). Cells primed with PDGFRs include circulating progenitor cells, both endothelial and pericyte cells[9]	Platelet-derived growth factor (PDGF). (This is a family of growth factors, with five members.)[10]
Epithelial Cells Description		**Cell Graphic**
PRIMARY ACTION	EFFECT	MECHANISM/SIGNAL
Attracts platelets	Chemo attraction to injury site	PDGF
Increases vascular permeability	In response to injury, increased vascular permeability allows movement of other key cells (neutrophils, macrophage) into the interstitial space	VEGF
Increase other cells' motility and proliferation	Pleiotropic cell motility and proliferation. Regeneration of the epidermis and other mesenchymal cells	TGF-α
Stimulates angiogenesis	Facilitation of the reestablishment of the vascular base including the reabsorption of excess capillaries	Basic fibroblast growth factor (bFGF) VEGF TNF-α
Formation of granulation tissue during proliferation	Increased granulation tissue in wound bed/base	Insulin-like growth factor (ILGF)
Final re-epithelialization	Reestablishes epithelial barrier	ILGF
Fibroblasts Description		**Cell Graphic**
PRIMARY ACTION	EFFECT	MECHANISM/SIGNAL
Proinflammatory	Stimulate neutrophil development	IL-1—amplifies inflammatory response by increasing synthesis of itself (IL-1) and IL-6
Site-specific migration	Respond to aFGF and bFGF	
Both a constructor and a component of granulation tissue	Elastin production GAGs Adhesive glycoproteins produced on the cell surface anchor the fibroblasts to other cells and proteins in the extracellular matrix	Connective tissue growth factor (CTGF)[11,12]
Change phenotype	During late stage proliferation, fibroblasts morph into myofibroblasts to help bridge the "gap" between the wound edges[13–15]	Differentiation initiated by TGF-β[13]
Collagen production	Direct collagen matrix	Production of fibrin, fibronectin
Recruitment of other key cells	Endothelial cells Keratinocytes[16]	Activated macrophage induce in vitro keratinocyte growth factor (KGF)
Epithelialization	Directs epithelialization and enables cellular migration	KGF2
Differentiate into Myofibroblasts	Epidermal cell motility and proliferation to reestablish intact skin	KGF
Scar contraction	The myofibroblasts pull the newly formed regranulated/scar base together	Actin (REF)
Granular tissue formation and remodeling	Remodeling of the ECM Inhibits and shuts down the tissue MMPs	ILGF-1 TGF-β

(*Continued*)

TABLE 2-1 Important Cells in Wound Healing (*Continued*)

Keratinocytes Description: ▪ Basal cells = Basal Keratinocytes		**Cell Graphic**
PRIMARY ACTION	EFFECT	MECHANISM/SIGNAL
Entry to site a few hours after injury	Migrate over wound bed at the interface between the wound dermis and the fibrin clot	Facilitated by production of specific proteases (eg, collagenase by epidermal cells, which degrades the ECM)[17–19]
↑ Keratinocyte recruitment	Stimulate keratinocytes and induce keratinocyte site-specific proliferation	IL-6
Vitamin D_3 synthesis	Key to antimicrobial peptide production	Only cell in the body, which can complete both hydroxylation steps to activate Vitamin D_3
De novo hair follicle formation	Can contribute to hair follicle formation	Site of epidermal stem cells' continued proliferation of keratinocytes
Recruit macrophage	Migration to and cross talk with macrophage	Cytokines, chemokines, interleukins, growth factors[20,21]
Migration and proliferation	Cross talk with macrophage	Activation of epithelial growth factor receptor (EGFR) expressed on keratinocytes Macrophage-produced EGF
Neo-angiogenesis	Provide nutrients and oxygen for new tissue synthesis	Production of VEGF (↑ VEGF indirectly promoted by macrophage secretion of TNF-α and TGF-β)[22]
Macrophage Description: ▪ Mononuclear phagocytes ▪ Mature continuously from monocytes[5,23]		**Cell Graphic**
PRIMARY ACTION	EFFECT	MECHANISM/SIGNAL
Early surveillance	Bacterial replication activates Binding of bacterial components via membrane proteins, for example, toll-like receptor 4 (TLR4), and causes the release of proinflammatory cytokines[24]	Release of IL-1β, IL-6, TNF-α17
Phagocytosis	Binding of bacterial components Binding of immunoglobulins[24]	Presence of pathogens, apoptotic cells (including neutrophils)[4]
Wound debridement	Clearing of damaged vessels, necrotic cells, and ECM Proinflammatory	Granulocyte-macrophage colony-stimulating factor (GM-CSF) Granulate colony-stimulating factor (G-CSF) Enzymes produced by the macrophage include collagenase and elastase
Recruitment of other cells	Essential for entry of angioblasts, keratinocytes, endothelial cells, and fibroblasts	Cytokines, chemokines, fibronectin, IL-1, IFN-γ, TNF-α, and growth factors including PDGR, TGF-β, EGF, and IGF-16
Inflammation	Wound-associated macrophage central role in the control of inflammation. Upregulation of MMP transcription and nitric oxide (NO) synthesis. TNF-α induces MMP transcription and stimulates the production of NO. Promotes wound closure in normal conditions but are also associated with fibrosis and scar formation[5]	IL-1β IL-6 TNF-α17
Plastic cells	Switch from one functional subpopulation to another depending on the stimulus received[25]	Bacteria, quorum sensing, wound milieu[25]
Coordination of neo-angiogenesis	New vessel formation in the wound bed and surrounding periphery	Stimulates VEGF production by keratinocytes[22]
Stimulate matrix production and regulation	Initially collagen type III is deposited in the wound; however, macrophages are key in each step as listed below. 1. Enzymatically—collagenase and elastase are produced to degrade the ECM 2. Cytokines TNF-α, IL-1, and IFN-γ are produced, all of which are proinflammatory 3. Growth factor production TGF-β, EGF, and PDGF 4. Prostaglandin production PGE2	Growth factor TGF-β1 and TGF-β2 are associated with inflammation and TGF-β3 is associated with scar-free wound healing[26]
Remodeling	Re-epithelialization from the very first day! Wound-activated macrophage (WAM) promotes key cell (keratinocyte and endothelial and epithelial cells) migration via the release of proteases to selectively degrade the ECM[27]	Collagenase secretion Lytic enzyme secretion TGF-β

(*Continued*)

TABLE 2-1 Important Cells in Wound Healing (*Continued*)

Platelets Description:

- Anucleate cellular fragments
- Synthesis controlled by IL-6, IL-3, IL-11, and thrombopoietin
- Circulate in the INACTIVE form
- Once stimulated platelets undergo major shape changes and develop cell surface receptors for clotting factors. This allows binding to themselves (platelet–platelet) and with the subendothelium

Cell Graphic

PRIMARY ACTION	EFFECT	MECHANISM/SIGNAL
Immediate entry into site	Release prothrombin and thrombin to bind-free floating fibrin (from the liver that is found in circulating plasma)	Change in platelet cell shape Change in cell receptors—Receptors displayed on the platelet surface for fibrin and clotting factors, specifically the von Willebrand adhesion factor (Factor VIII)
Entry to site a few hours after injury	Migrate over wound bed at the interface between the wound dermis and the fibrin clot	Facilitated by production of specific proteases (eg, collagenase by epidermal cells, which degrades the ECM)[17–19]
Increases chemotaxis of neutrophils, macrophages, and fibroblasts	Recruitment of macrophage to site of injury to clear and contain invader	Platelet-derived growth factor (PDGF) Tissue growth factors (TGF-β1 and TGF-β2 from platelets)
Delays new vessel formation until clot stable and debris cleared	Inhibits angiogenesis	Endostatin[28]
Proliferation	Extracellular matrix (ECM) synthesis and remodeling	Tissue growth factors (TGF-β1 and TGF-β2 from platelets)
Increased epidermal cell motility	Important in neo-angiogenesis and proliferation phase for reestablishment of epidermal barrier	TGF-β1 and TGF-β2 (from platelets)
Significant source of growth factors	Platelet-derived growth factor (PDGF) TGF-β1 and TGF-β2 Keratinocyte growth factor (KGF) Epidermal growth factor (EGF) Insulin-like growth factor (IGF)	

Polymorphic Neutrophilic Leukocytes (PMNs) Description:

- Neutrophils—classically underappreciated professional phagocytes[4]

Cell Graphic

PRIMARY ACTION	EFFECT	MECHANISM/SIGNAL
Short life span	Survive <24 hours[4,29]	Migrate from capillaries to interstitial space in response to chemokines[30]
Site-specific migration	Respond to infection ↑ in adhesiveness ↑ in cell motility ↑ in chemotactic response	↑ Vascular permeability Local prostaglandin release Presence of chemotactic substances (complement IL-1, TNF-α, TGF-β, platelets)[29,31–34]
First inflammatory cells recruited to the clot	Emigrate to the new wound and soon after enter apoptosis	Cytokine release[35,36]
Phagocytosis	Free radical production Scavenging of necrotic debris, bacteria, and foreign bodies	Release of oxygen radicals including H_2O_2, O_2^-, OH^- Superoxidase, NADH[30,37–43] Nitric oxide
Entrapment	Trap invading bacteria for phagocytosis by macrophage. DNA NETs contain decondensed chromatin, bound histones, azurophilic granule proteins, and cytosolic proteins[44,45]	DNA neutrophil extracellular traps (NETs)[45]
Lysis of invaders	Major source of proteases	Release proteases
Recruitment of other key phagocytic cells Resolution of inflammation	Particularly recruit and intensely stimulate macrophage.[46] In fact, the final stage of neutrophil differentiation is the induction of apoptosis, which causes the recognition by phagocytes/macrophages. This assists with clearing invaders and promotes inflammation, endothelial activation,[47] and eventually the resolution of inflammation[48–50]	Apoptosis (programmed cell death) of neutrophils[49–51] TNF-α (cachectin)

The primary cells that drive the wound healing cascade of cellular and acellular processes, their effects, and their mechanisms of action or of signaling other cells to act are summarized.

TABLE 2-2 Phases of Wound Healing

Clinical Presentation	Normal	Predominant Cell/Tissue Type
Hemostasis (<1 hour) 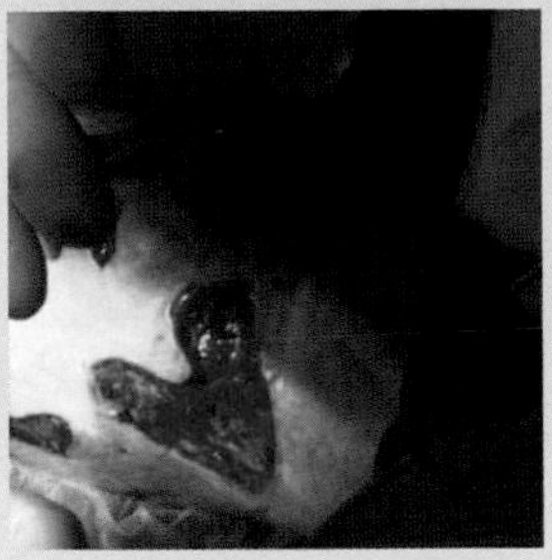	Cellular Activity Clot formation ▪ Stop bleeding ▪ Contain invader ▪ Begin attracting phagocytes	Predominant Tissue Type/Cell Platelet 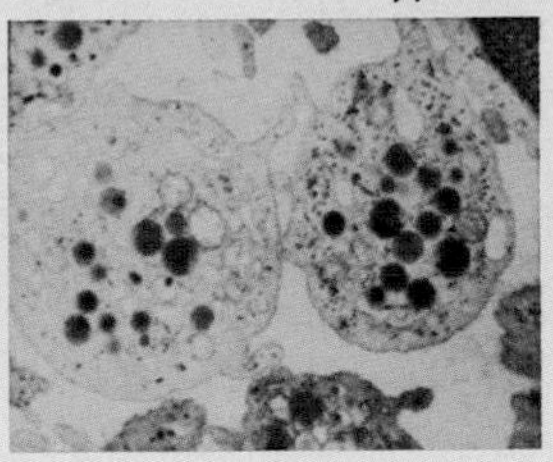
Vascular events	▪ Transient arteriole constriction ▪ Fibrin from liver transported ▪ Vascular permeability increases after bleeding is controlled to allow passage of other key cells including neutrophils and macrophage into the interstitial space	
Cellular events	▪ Neutrophil influx ▪ Platelet aggregation in collagen ▪ Release of platelet α-granules and dense bodies	
Cell signaling	▪ Clotting cascade: von Willebrand adhesion factor (glycoprotein)—binds factor VIII, which initiates the clotting cascade via prothrombin and thrombin conversion ▪ TGF-β1 and TGF-β2 are released from platelets and stimulate the chemotaxis of fibroblast and macrophage ▪ Increased release of IL-1 from antigen-presenting cells (APCs) that are key to identifying the invader (REF). The increased release of IL-1 from APCs (dendritic cells, macrophage) and monocytes stimulates those same cells (autocrine) to produce IL-8. The chemical messenger, IL-8, attracts neutrophils and increases the "sticky" or adhesion factors along the endothelium to assist in this process	
Clinical signs	▪ Clot formation ▪ Hemostasis achieved ▪ Fibrous scab formation ▪ Peri-injury including inflammation and edema	
Inflammation (1 hour–4 days) 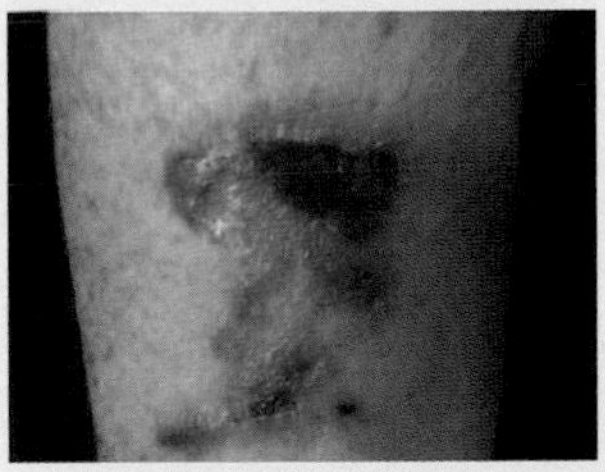	Reactive Chemotaxis/Scavenge ▪ Damage control ▪ Recruit immune system ▪ ↑ Circulation to injury site ▪ Initiate healing sequence	Predominant tissue type/cell macrophage (WAM) 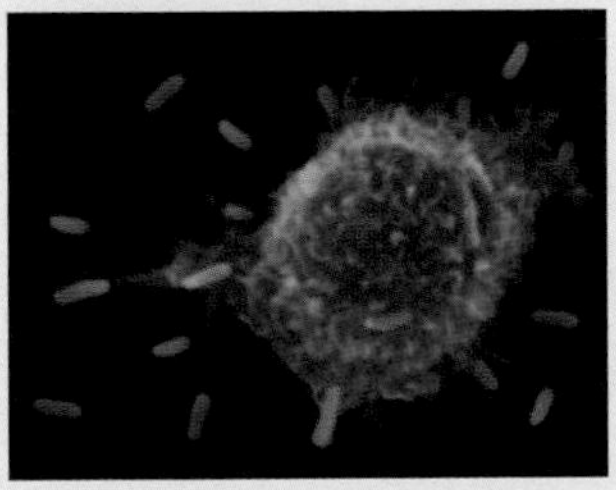
Vascular events	▪ Vasodilation ▪ ↑ Permeability ▪ Stasis	
Cellular events	▪ Migration and accumulation of leukocytes, PMNs, and macrophage ▪ ↑↑ Tissue permeability ▪ ↑ Neutrophils ▪ ↑ Macrophage	

(*Continued*)

TABLE 2-2 Phases of Wound Healing (*Continued*)

Clinical Presentation	Normal	Predominant Cell/Tissue Type
Cell signaling	▪ Platelet α-granules released, which contain PDGF, TGF-β, IGF-1, fibronectin, fibrinogen, thrombospondin, and vWF ▪ Platelet dense bodies (vasoactive amines, serotonin) release ▪ IL-1 (produced by macrophage) ▪ Activates B cells (adaptive immune system/memory cells) • ↑ Clonal expansion of appropriate B cells • ↑ Transmigration from the blood to the tissues • ↑ Expression of adhesion molecules in endothelium, which helps neutrophils "stick" to the endothelium near the site of injury • ↑ Body temperature via the hypothalamus "endogenous pyrogen" ▪ IFN-γ production elevated (produced by Th1/innate immune system neutrophils) • ↑ Creates "angry" macrophages, which ↑ phagocytosis • ↑ Antigen identification/presentation by APCs • ↑ Macrophage phagocytosis • ↑ INHIBITS fibroblast and ECM production	Predominant tissue type/cell macrophage (WAM)
Clinical signs	▪ Rubor (redness) ▪ Tumor (swelling) ▪ Calor (heat) locally AND ↑ core temperature ▪ Dolor (pain)	
Proliferation (4–12 days) **Extracellular matrix** 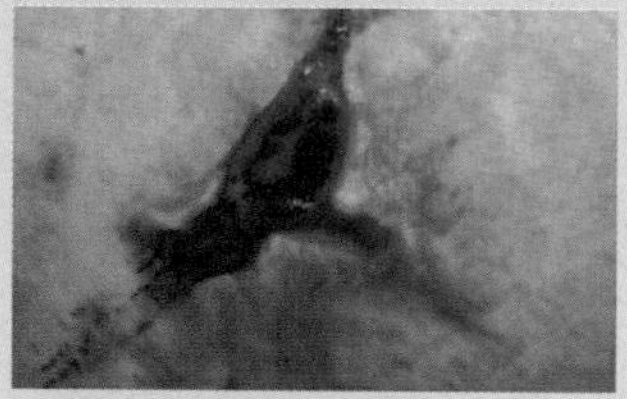	Repair 80% completed laminin ▪ Anatomical cover ▪ ECM ▪ Endothelium ▪ New epithelial barrier in place ▪ Key protein in basal lamina (one of the layers of the basement membrane) ▪ Family of glycoproteins integral part of structural scaffolding ▪ Form independent networks via type IV collagen, entactin, fibronectin, and perlecan ▪ Bind to cell membranes, contribute to cell attachment and differentiation ▪ Specific peptide sequence promotes adhesion of endothelial cells[52]	▪ Extracellular matrix ▪ Fibroblast to myofibroblast ▪ Epithelial cells ▪ Anti-inflammatory macrophage (M2)
Vascular events	▪ Proliferation of new small blood vessels ▪ Proliferation of new ECM and epidermal cells	
Cellular events	▪ Increased mitotic activity (cellular division) of basal epithelial layer ▪ Fibroblast and vascular endothelial proliferation ▪ Proteoglycan, collagen, and ultimately ECM (fibronectin and laminin) synthesis	
Cell signaling	▪ VEGF—vasoendothelial growth factor-angiogenesis (acts through VEGFR-2 primarily) ▪ Proliferation and motility of endothelial cells ▪ aFGF/bFGF—acidic and basic fibroblast growth factor facilitates both fibroblast proliferation and wound vascularization and angiogenesis ▪ Endothelial precursor/progenitor cells ▪ TGF-β1 and TGF-β2 (from platelets)—important for extracellular matrix (ECM) synthesis and remodeling. Also, important in neo-angiogenesis and increased epidermal cell motility to reestablish the epidermal barrier IL-10 (produced by macrophage and keratinocytes) • ↓↓ Synthesis of IL-6 (proinflammatory cytokine) • ↓ Neutrophil/leukocyte migration • ↓ Macrophage cytokine production • Downregulation of neutrophils (Th1 innate immune system cells) • Downregulation of MHC II on APCs—because the invader has presumably been "cleared" and there is no need to continue to stimulate the innate and adaptive immune system cells ▪ TNF-α (from neutrophils)	

(*Continued*)

TABLE 2-2 Phases of Wound Healing (*Continued*)

Clinical Presentation	Normal	Predominant Cell/Tissue Type
Clinical signs	▪ Formation of granulation tissue ▪ Silvery clear covering of wound (new epithelium)	▪ Fibroblast—myofibroblast ▪ Anti-inflammatory macrophage
Maturation and remodeling 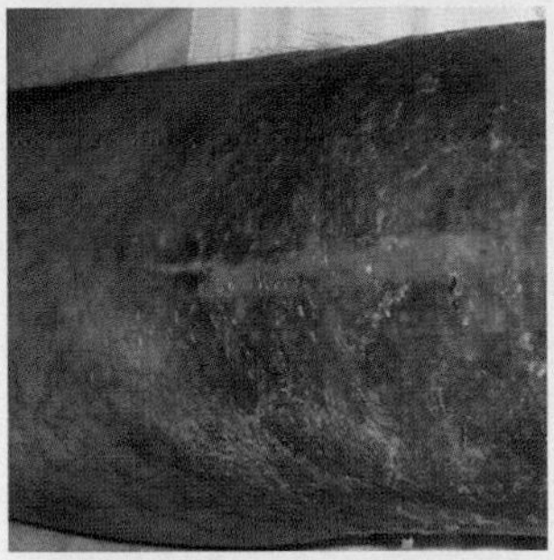	Contraction Fibroblasts differentiate to myofibroblast Migration of melanocytes functional/scar remodel ▪ Function ▪ Thermoregulatory ▪ Range of motion ▪ No reoccurrence of wound	
Vascular events	▪ Removal/Reabsorption of extraneous capillaries	
Cellular events	▪ Macrophages secrete collagenase and lytic enzymes ▪ Fibroblasts secrete TIMPs which inhibit MMPs, the enzymes that degrade the ECM ▪ ↑ Tensile strength/fibrosis occurs ▪ Collagen type III replaced by collagen type I, which increases wound strength	
Cell signaling	▪ Tissue inhibitors of metalloproteinases (TIMPs) counteract MMPs so remodeling proceeds in concert ▪ TGF-β1 and TGF-β2 (produced by the platelets) • ↑ Fibroblast synthesis • ECM synthesis and remodeling	
Clinical signs	Blanching	

The phases of wound healing include hemostasis, inflammation, proliferation, and maturation and remodeling. Each phase is shown with the primary cells that are pertinent in communication, signaling, and/or tissue production. Vascular events, cellular events, cell signaling, and clinical symptoms that occur in each phase are described.

signaling of exosomes is evidenced by the robust autocrine and paracrine signaling observed. The function of exosomes is twofold. First, the vesicle structure protects the small-molecule RNA, cytokines, chemokines, and peptides. Second, it delivers a robust heterogenic signal resulting in the choreographed effect which can be either proinflammatory or proliferative, and delivered with multiple signaling vehicles (peptide, cytokine, chemokine, or si-RNA). The signals within the vesicle can upregulate or downregulate expression of adjacent or distant cell phenotypes. The cell phenotype drives the type(s) of exosome(s) expressed (**FIGURE 2-1**). This is a seminal discovery that will continue to drive and improve the understanding of wound healing and treatment.

In the laboratory, mesenchymal cell (MSC) exosomes have been isolated and demonstrated to be proliferative, anti-inflammatory, and reparative. With the successful reliable replication of this laboratory research and the elucidation of MSC-exosome effects, it has become apparent that MSC exosomes can positively affect healing at all stages. For human clinical trials, MSC exosomes represent a possible therapeutic opportunity for the facilitation of successful wound healing.[54] Thus far human trials have shown more robust wound healing with less scarring.

Intracellular signaling is a function of organelles contained within the cell membrane. The organelles communicate with one another through vesicular trafficking pathways and membrane contact sites, exchanging metabolites, lipids, and proteins. The signaling that occurs between organelles drive organelle division which drives cellular biogenesis and growth.[55,56]

Cells exhibit various levels of activity in response to many factors. **FIGURE 2-2** illustrates four recognized levels of cellular activity and the associated effect on local tissue environment. Cells that exist in a *senescent state* (defined as resistant to apoptosis or programmed cell death) disrupt normal tissue differentiation, drain the metabolism, and secrete cell products that negatively impact the wound environment. Cells in a *baseline state* have normal mitotic and metabolic activity, actively survey and monitor adjacent tissues, and do not impact surrounding tissues negatively. An *upregulated state* has a higher level of metabolic activity and purposefully responds in concert with other cells in reaction to injury, presence of pathogens, or both. A cell that is *out of control* exhibits an overproduction of cellular byproducts, is not coordinated with any other cells, and does not respond to feedback inhibition. The cartoons representing each level of cell activity

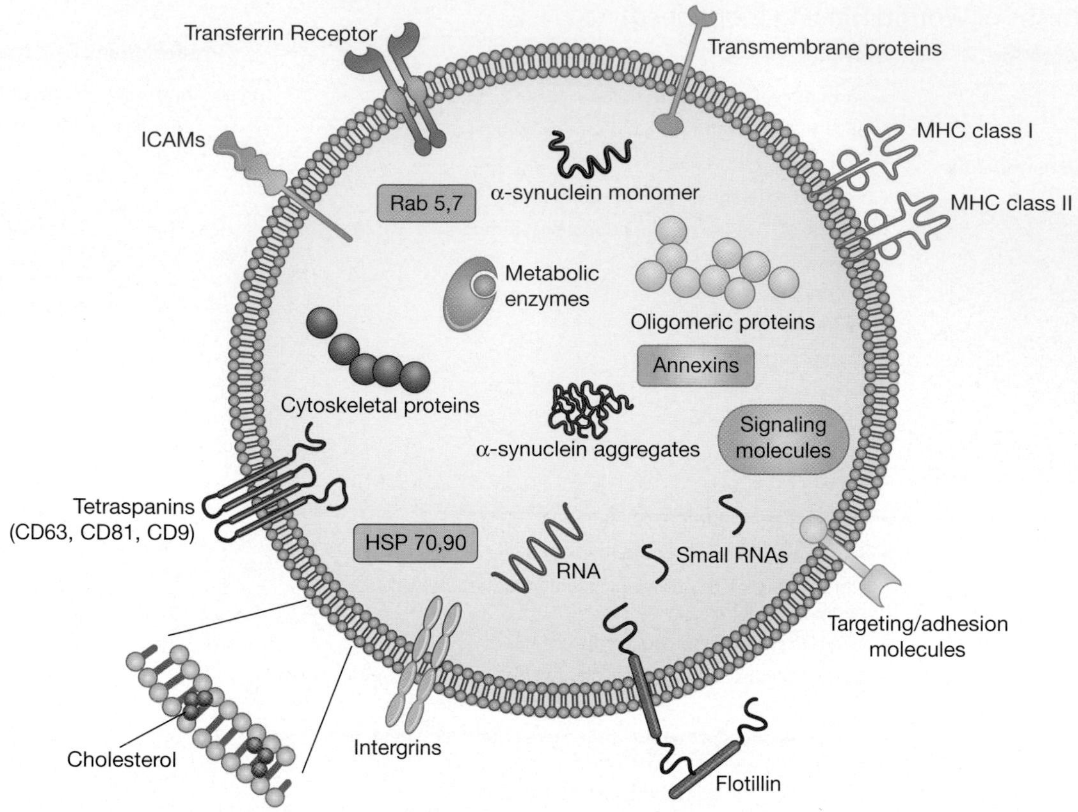

FIGURE 2-1 Representation of an exosome and the contents. Exosomes contain peptides, small-molecule RNA, and signaling proteins including cytokines, chemokines, and growth hormones. On the outer membrane of the exosomes are transmembrane proteins that are often indicative of the cells from which the exosomes originate.

are overlaid in some of the diagrams to illustrate the cellular state in normal and disrupted wound healing. *Both the correct cells and the appropriate level of cellular activity are required to ensure wound healing.*

FIGURE 2-3 illustrates the sequence of cell migration, proliferation, and signaling in the context of cell communication and vascular events, all working in unison to culminate in tissue healing.

HEALING RESPONSE

Healing occurs by one of the following four mechanisms: (1) continuous cell cycling, (2) cell proliferation, (3) regeneration, or (4) fibroproliferative response. Normal intact skin is representative of *continuous cell cycling* whereby labile cells are constantly undergoing a balance of proliferation and programmed apoptosis throughout life, thereby resulting in a steady state. The basal keratinocytes continuously undergo mitosis (cell division), followed by migration to the skin surface and subsequent desquamation or sloughing. *Cell proliferation* occurs when the damaged or lost tissue is replaced by the expansion of remaining healthy cells that undergo mitosis. The structure is not completely duplicated; however, function is approximated.

Regeneration occurs with the loss of a structure. The acute injury that undergoes regeneration stimulates complete duplication in both structure and function of the lost tissue. The liver, hematopoietic tissue, gastrointestinal tract epithelium, and epidermis are examples of tissue that are capable of regeneration. *Fibroproliferative healing* typically occurs in dermal wound healing. The lost tissue is not replaced, but rather a "patch" is constructed that restores the skin covering, integrity, and function. Inflamed tissue that fails to progress to healing results in tissue fibrosis. Divisions of wound healing are graphically depicted in **FIGURE 2-4**.

Categories of Healing Responses

Wound healing is classified either by category or by depth. Four categories describe wound healing—categories 1 to 3 describe healing of full-thickness wounds, category 4 refers to partial-thickness skin wounds.[57,58]

Category 1 *Primary Intention* healing occurs when a clean surgical incision is created and the resulting wound is free from contamination of bacteria, fungi, or foreign bodies. There is minimal tissue loss and the edges are safely approximated and secured with sutures, staples, or surgical glue. The clotting cascade at the wound surface is largely not initiated and the resulting fibrous scab is absent because of the minimal mortality of cells central to wound healing. The cell signaling cascades which are usually launched in an acute penetrating injury are not activated. The incisional wound resolves in an

Figure Key	Numeric Code	Cell Activity Level	Key Events or Conditions

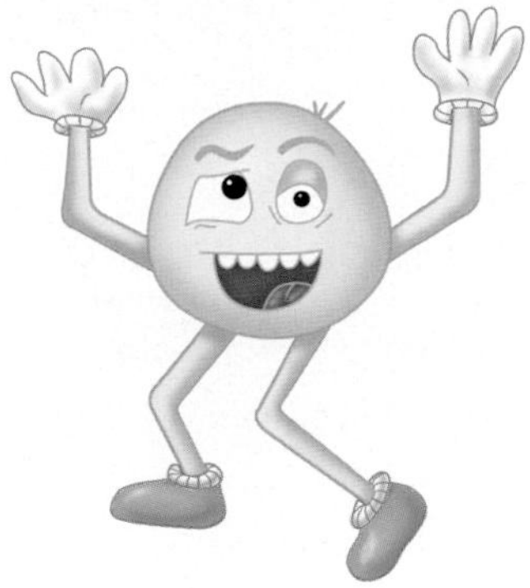	2	Running out of control	State:
			• No feedback inhibition
			• Not coordinated with any other cells in wound milieu
			
			Result:
			• Overproduction of cell byproducts
			• Delayed execution of sequential steps for wound healing
			• Increase in cell necrosis
			  ◦ Necrosis creates increased cell debris and and burden which must be removed by macrophage and neutrophils. This is compared to apoptosis, or programmed cell death, which does not increase cellular debris.
			  ◦ Excess cell debris provides an additional food source for bacterial invaders.

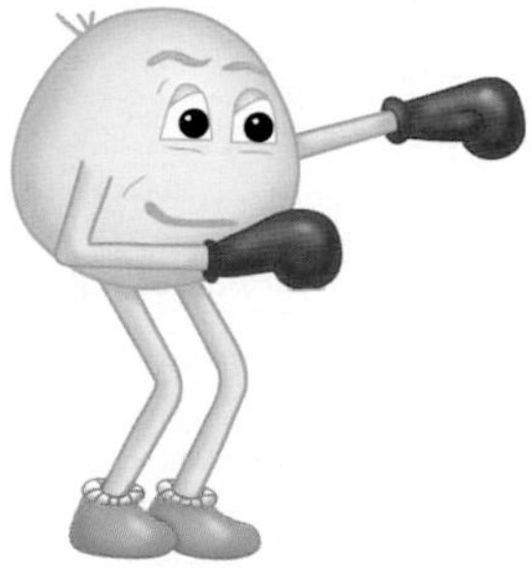	1	Upregulated	State: • Appropriate elevated response in concert with other cells • In response to injury or invader (bacterium, fungi, virus, microbe) Result: • Elevated cellular products • Facilitates sequential steps for wound healing • Decrease in cellular debris
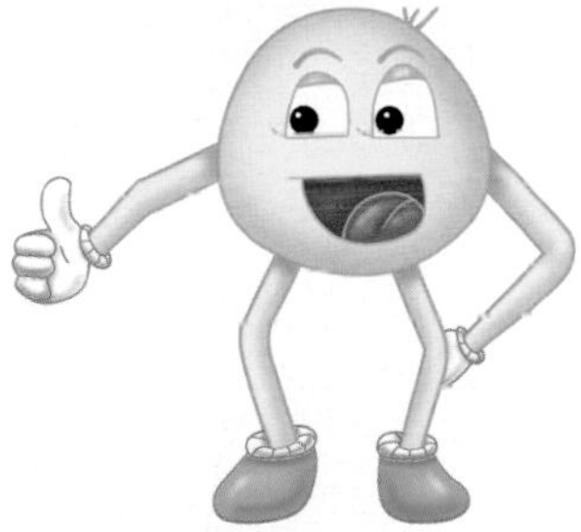		Baseline	State: • Surveilance state. Geographically localised and poised to respond to intruders or injury Result: • Actively monitoring milieu and adjacent cell states • Normal mitosis occurring
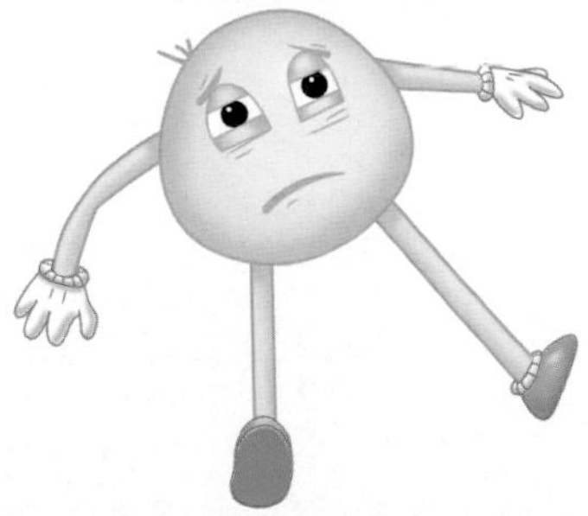	−1	Senescent	State: • Depressed, unresponsive • Not able to be stimulated into appropriate action • Associated with aging or chronic wound environment Result: • Altered cell receptor display and secretion of cell products/ gene expression • Metabolic drain-senescent cells consume energy yet do not contribute to local cell health • Resistant to apoptosis

FIGURE 2-2 Levels of cellular activity. This figure provides an explanation of various cell activity levels and the observed cellular events associated with that level of cellular activity. The cartoons illuminate the cell state and are used throughout the chapter to illustrate whether the level of activity is appropriate or inappropriate, as well as the ramifications.

orderly, sequenced manner over the course of approximately 2 weeks (**FIGURE 2-5**).[59]

Category 2 *Delayed Primary Intention* healing occurs when wound edges are not approximated because of concern for the presence of pathogens or debris, an existing abscess, or loss of extensive tissue (**FIGURE 2-6**). There is an initial release of multiple proinflammatory cytokines, chemokines, and growth factors. Any foreign debris is walled off by macrophages that may metamorphose into epithelioid cells, which in turn become encircled by layers of mononuclear leukocytes, thus forming a granuloma with the foreign body or pathogen at the

FIGURE 2-3 Cell migration, proliferation, and signaling in the wound healing process

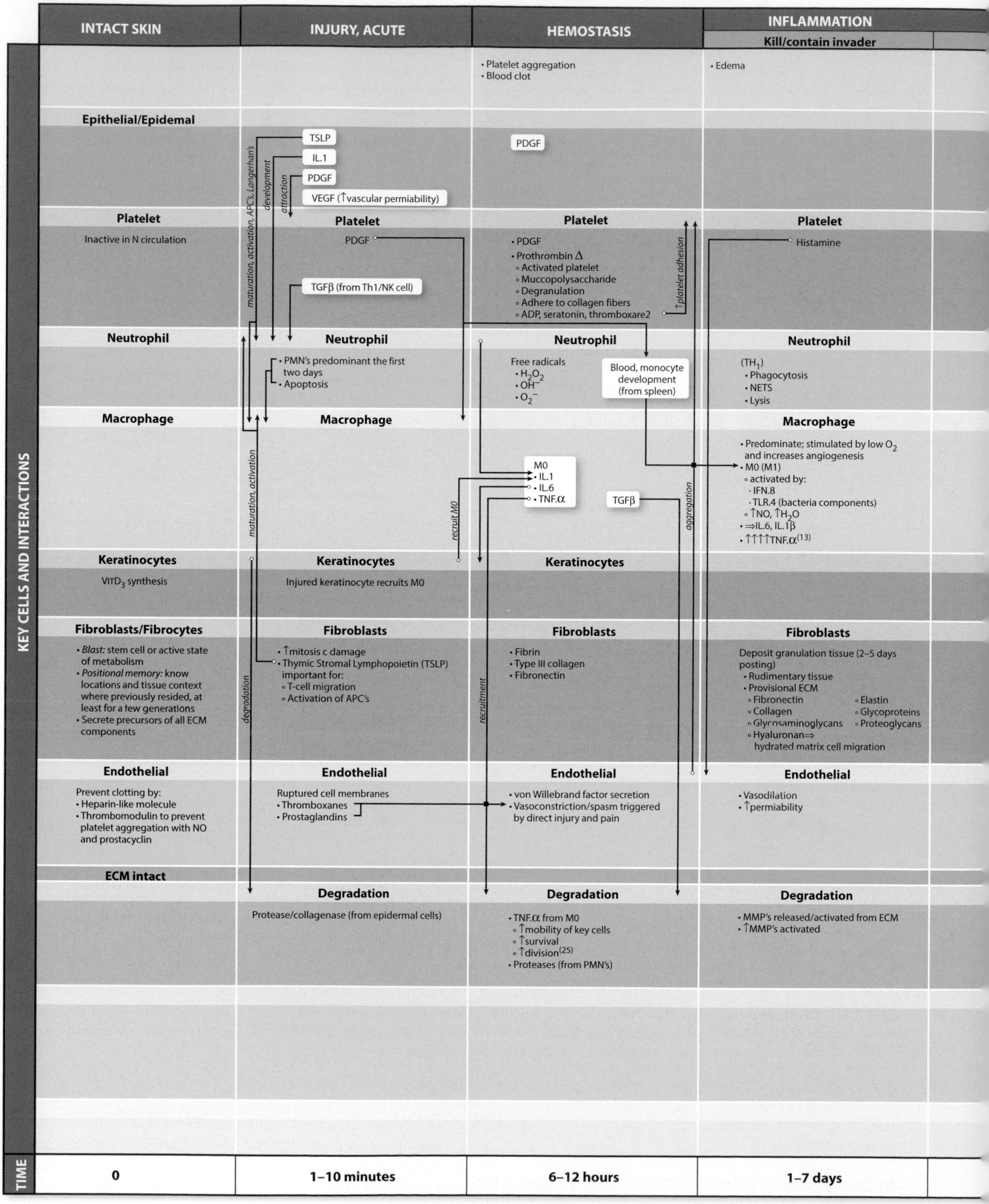

The healing map is a summary of both the acellular and cellular components of wound healing. This illustration is parsed by phases of healing along the horizontal axis, while the primary cells of importance are along the vertical axis.

FIGURE 2-3 *(Continued)*

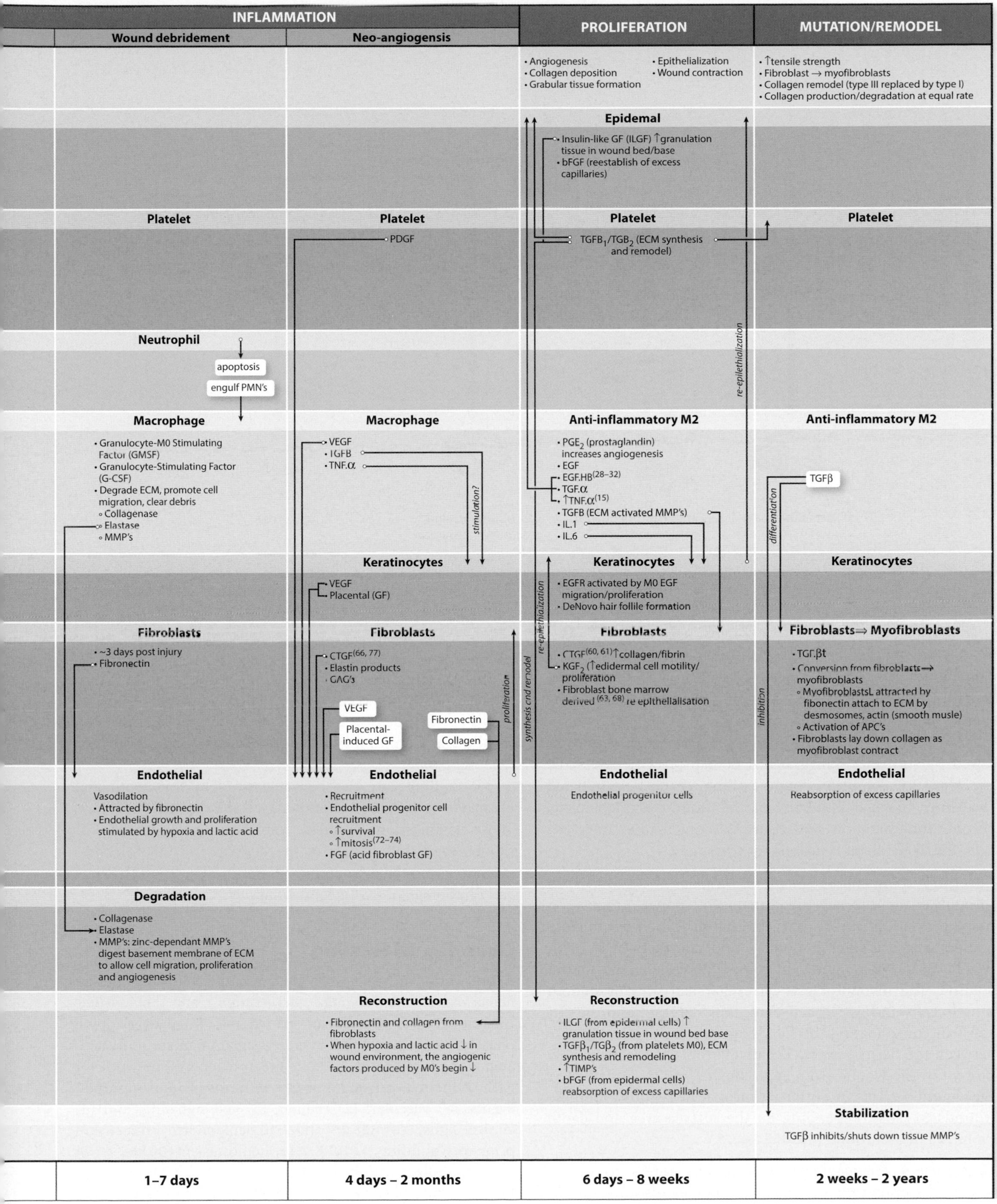

The cytokines, chemokines, and growth factors important at each phase are depicted along with the directional impact exerted on healing by each of these components. The direction is indicated by color-keyed arrows.

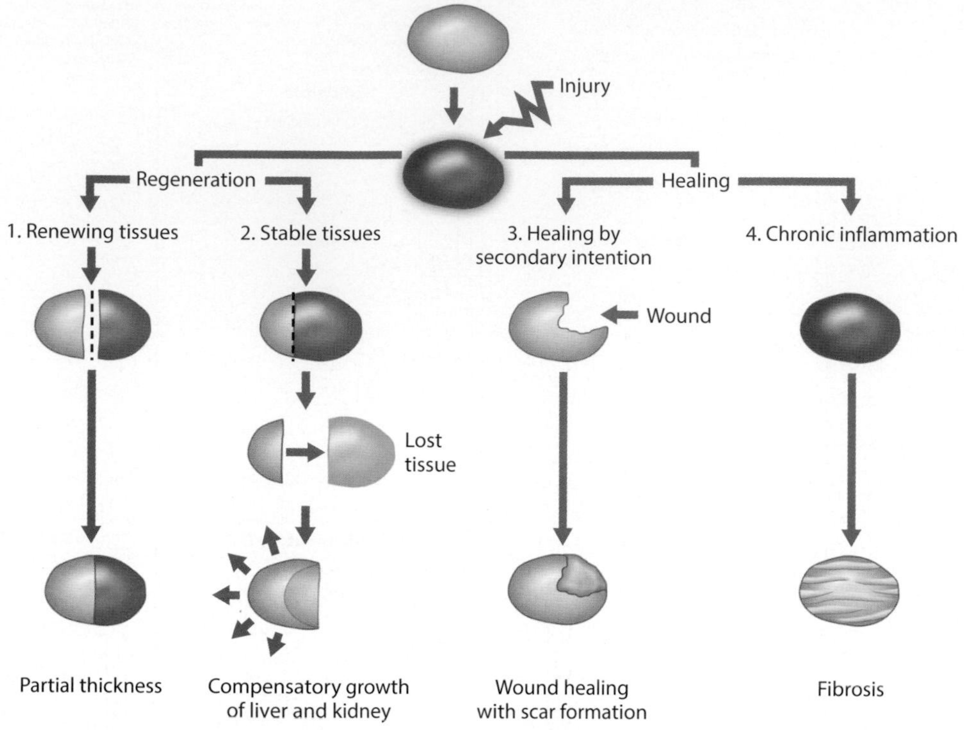

FIGURE 2-4 Divisions of wound healing. The body responds to tissue injury in mechanisms that result in tissue regeneration, thus restoring both structure and function of that specific tissue. The four pathways of response are regeneration, compensatory growth, renewal, and fibrosis. When regeneration of epithelium or the underlying tissue fails to occur in a timely fashion, a state of chronic inflammation usually results.

center and walled off from the host tissue. In these wounds the inflammatory response is more intense and is accompanied by increased granular tissue formation.[59]

Surgical removal of the granuloma, abscess, or debris followed by suturing, skin grafting, or flap placement may be necessary for complete wound healing. If the host-initiated cleansing, (termed *autolysis)* of the wound is incomplete, chronic inflammation can ensue. Without further intervention, the likely result is prominent scarring.

Category 3 *Secondary Intention healing* is accomplished through an appropriate inflammatory response, granulation tissue formation, and re-epithelialization. When left to close without surgical intervention, wound contraction by myofibroblasts plays a significant role in decreasing the wound volume. The myofibroblasts have characteristics of smooth muscle cells and, when activated, they contract and thereby assist in consolidating the ECM and decreasing the distance between the dermal edges. The myofibroblasts are maximally present in the wound from approximately 10 to 21 days after the wound occurs.[14] Additional time may be required for these wounds to close, depending on the surface area and depth (volume) of the wound (**FIGURE 2-7**).[59]

Category 4 *Partial-thickness wounding* refers to partial loss of the epidermis or loss of the epidermis and superficial dermis (the basement membrane is intact, and the hypodermis is not exposed), and healing is accomplished by epithelial cell mitosis and migration. Wound contracture is not an expected or common occurrence during the healing of partial-thickness wounds, as the subdermal layers are not involved and minimal to no granulation tissue is formed (**FIGURE 2-8**).[59]

Wounding can also be categorized by the depth and involvement of tissue lost or damaged as a result of the injury. These classifications progress from the most superficial erosion, to partial thickness of the dermis, and full thickness extending into the hypodermis. (Refer to Chapter 1, Anatomy and Physiology of the Integumentary System.)

Overview of Healing

Acute wound healing is divided into the following phases: *hemostasis*, *inflammation*, *proliferation*, and *remodeling*. Inflammation is further subdivided into three overlapping phases: kill/contain the invader, inflammation, and neoangiogenesis. **FIGURES 2-9** to **2-14B** provide a framework for each of the major healing phases in terms of four important events: (1) vascular, (2) cellular, (3) cell signaling, and (4) clinical signs. **FIGURES 2-9** and **2-10** depict normal intact skin prior to wounding; **FIGURE 2-11**, hemostasis; **FIGURES 2-12A** to **2-14B**, inflammation; and **FIGURES 2-15A** to **2-17**, proliferation. The interplay between each of the four phases is both complex and transitional such that within any wound, signs of more than one phase may be present. Vascular, cellular, and

FIGURE 2-5 Healing by primary intention

Incision causes only focal disruption
- Epithelial basement membrane continuity largely maintained
- Death of a relatively few epithelial and connective tissue cells

Epithelial regeneration predominates over fibrosis

Small scar is formed
- Minimal wound contraction occurs

Filling of narrow incisional space
- First fibrin- and clotted blood
- Followed by rapid invasion of granulation tissue
- Covered by new epithelium

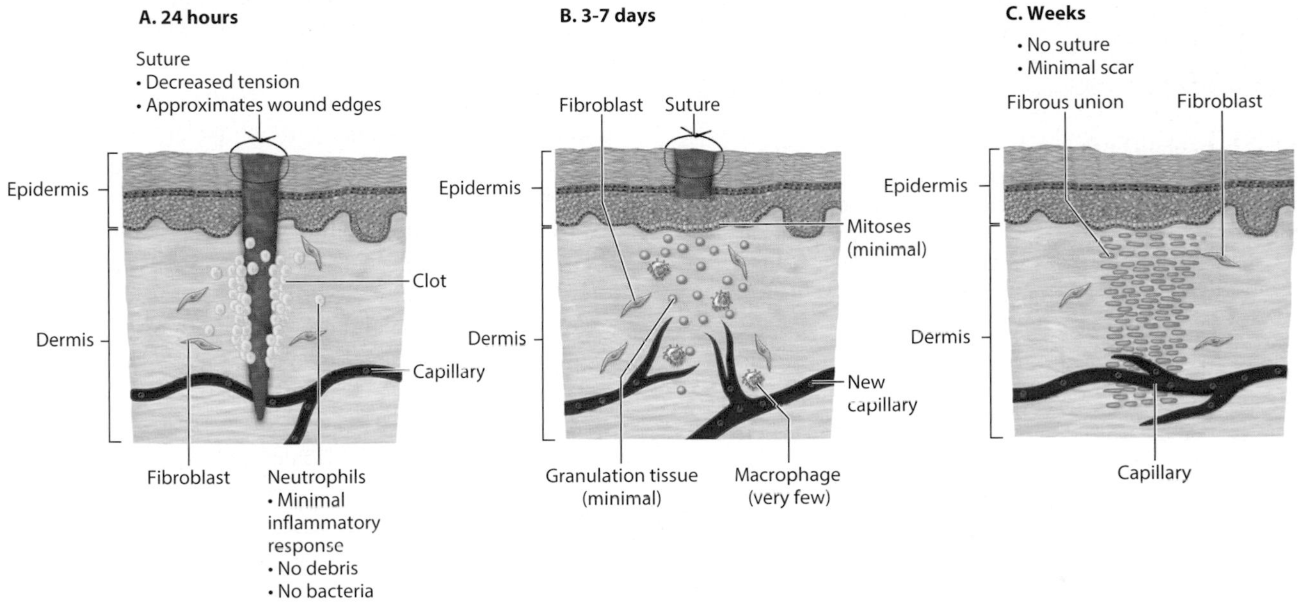

A–C. The series of three images illustrate the tissue response to an incision. Focal disruption and tissue stabilization by suture result primarily in epithelial regeneration.

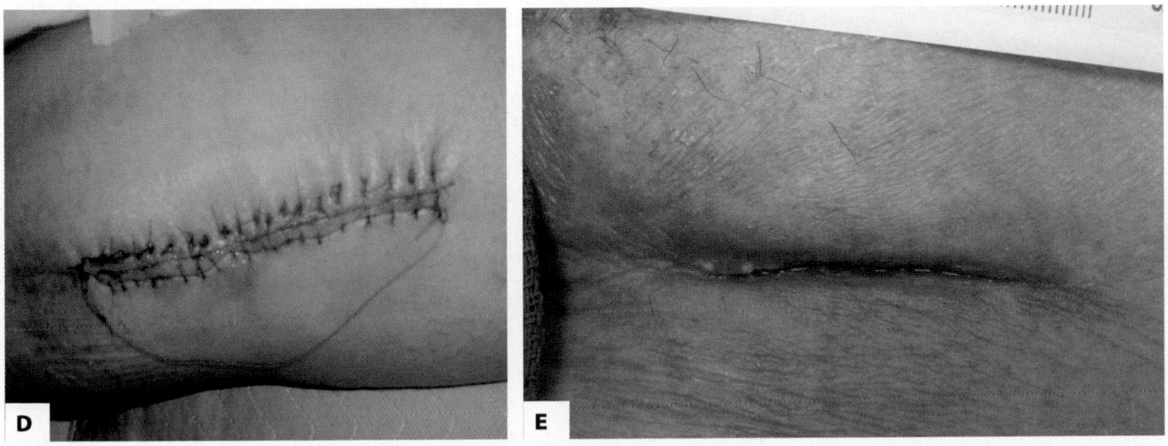

D. Sutures are used to close a surgical incision by primary intention. Healing is achieved when the new epithelium bridges the gap between the two edges, and minimal scar is formed. **E.** The left aspect of this groin incision illustrates closure by primary intention where the epithelium has bridged the incision. In the remaining part, the incision has separated in part because of the amount of moisture that has dissolved the superficial sutures without full skin growth. The incision is termed *separated* if the gap is less than 1 cm; *dehiscence*, if more than 1 cm.

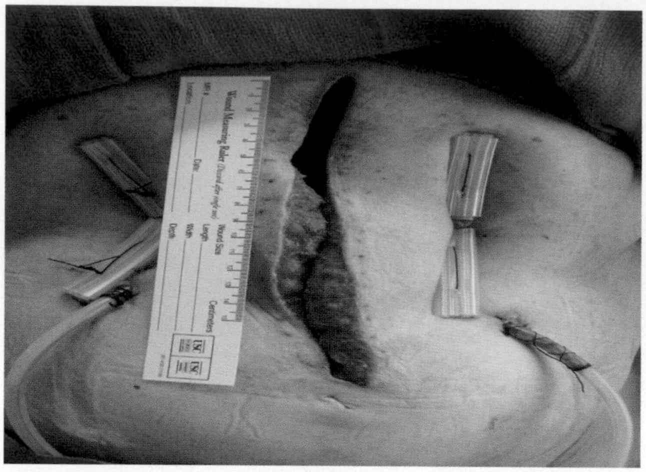

FIGURE 2-6 Healing by delayed primary intention. Large wounds can be partially closed with retaining sutures, or in the case of this abdominal wound, with tension sutures. This technique is used if approximating the edges puts too much strain on the periwound skin and subcutaneous tissue or if there is concern for infection and drainage that needs to be removed in order to prevent abscess formation.

tissues changes that occur during the four phases include the following:

1. Vascular: hemostasis, transient vasoconstriction, retrograde degradation of damaged vessels, and the transition to endothelial cell differentiation, migration, and proliferation—also termed *neo-angiogenesis.*
2. Cellular: the directed migration and accumulation of cells known to be necessary for wound healing (eg, neutrophils and macrophages) to the site of injury.[5] Some cells (platelets, macrophages, and fibroblasts) morph in both phenotype and function, depending on the phase of healing and the surrounding stimuli, whether cytokine, chemokine, or ECM activation.[5]
3. Cell signaling: orchestration of healing by the actions of cytokines, chemokines, growth factors, and receptor accessibility on target cells. It is accomplished through the binding of chemical messengers to cell receptors present on the target cell surface. The binding of the chemical messenger (eg, cytokine, chemokine, growth factor, or interleukin) activates or depresses target cell DNA transcription and protein translation of important activities that are performed by the target cell. These

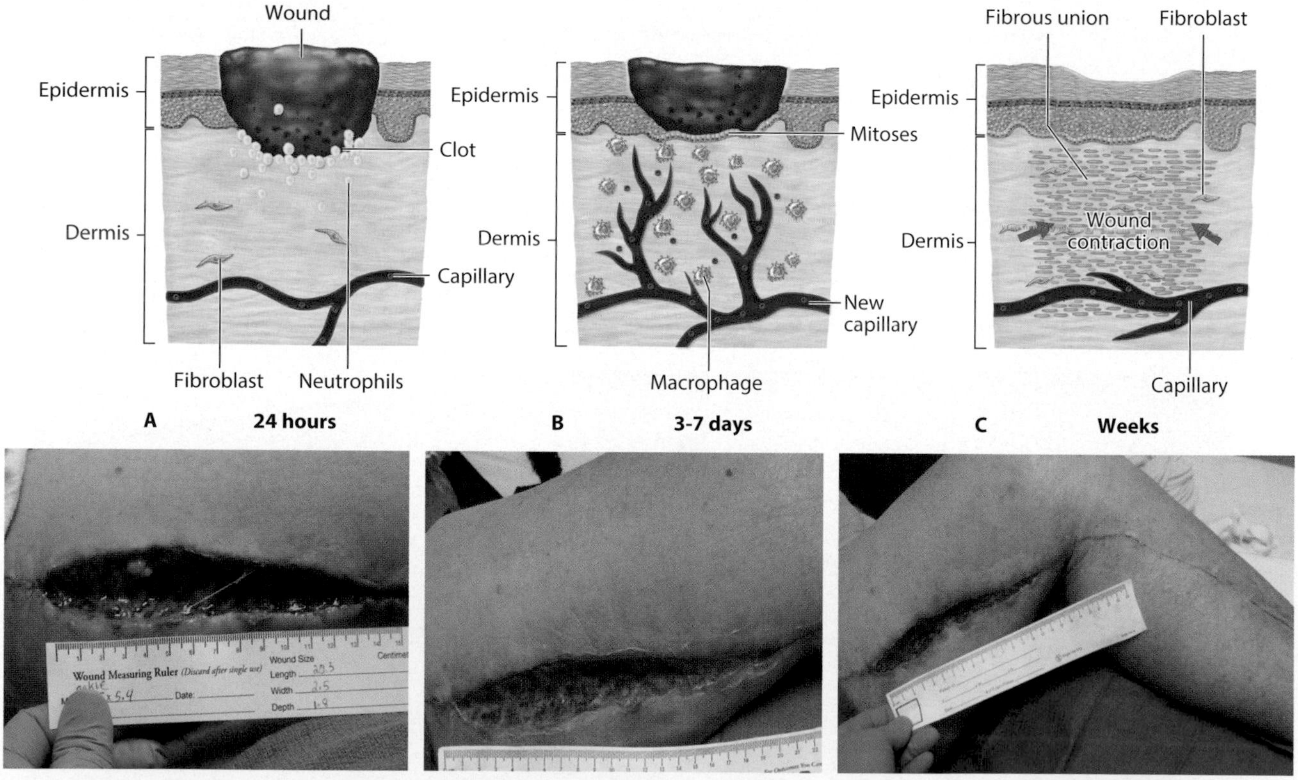

FIGURE 2-7 Healing by secondary intention. When there is extensive tissue loss or contamination, the repair process increases in complexity as illustrated by a robust inflammatory response and an abundance of granulation tissue. **A–C.** The series of three illustrations highlights these attributes along with wound contraction through the action of myofibroblasts. **A.** Dehisced surgical incision on the medial thigh, approximately 24 hours after the site was irrigated and drained surgically. The wound is in the inflammatory phase of healing. **B.** The same wound 2 weeks later is in the proliferative phase with granulation visible throughout the wound bed. **C.** Two weeks later the wound is significantly smaller, and the incision along the lower leg is observed to be closed and remodeling. The wound completed closure by secondary intention without further surgical intervention.

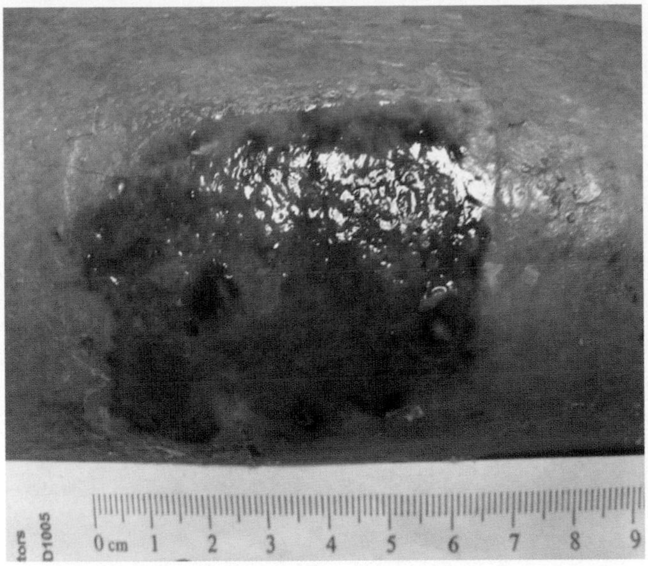

FIGURE 2-8 Healing of a partial-thickness wound. Re-epithelialization can be seen at the wound edges, as well as on the small "epithelial island" at the lower edge. The island indicates that the epithelial cells in that region are migrating from the hair follicle rather than the edge and is commonly seen in partial-thickness wounds.

activities include (a) the production of additional chemical messengers, (b) a change in cell phenotype and function, or (c) binding to adjacent ECM sites. Cell signaling occurs between cells (cell to cell) and between the cell and wound matrix (cell to matrix).[60] The communication that occurs between cells and ECM is bidirectional or reciprocal, meaning that the signal goes both ways to regulate tissue responses to healing, and is termed dynamic reciprocity (DR). The principles of DR occur across all the wound healing phases.[61,62]

4. Clinical signs and symptoms: changes observed in the local periwound environment (pain, redness, and edema) or systemic symptoms detected in the patient (fever, chills, increased heart rate, or pain).

Cytokines are small proteins or glycoproteins that are secreted by numerous cells and alter the function of the target cell. The target cell for the cytokine/interleukin may be itself (autocrine) or a neighboring cell (juxtacrine). Cytokines can be either proinflammatory or anti-inflammatory.

Interleukins are a group of cytokines that were first observed being expressed by white blood cells (leukocytes).[1] The term *interleukin* derives from *inter* as a means of communication, and *leukin,* deriving from the fact that leukocytes produce many of these proteins and are the target of their action. The name is something of a relic as it has been determined that interleukins are in fact produced by a wide variety of body cells. The function of the immune system depends in a large part on interleukins, the majority of which are

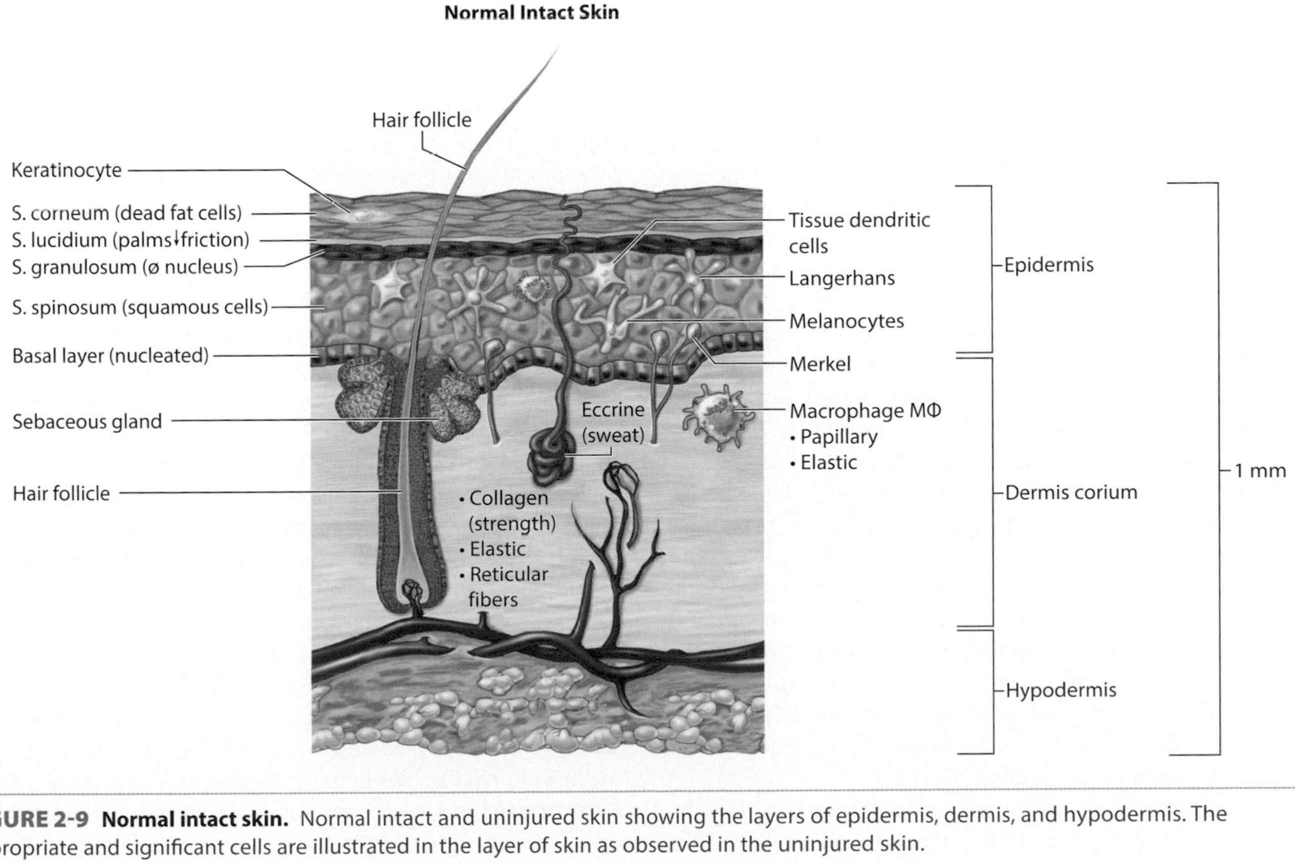

FIGURE 2-9 Normal intact skin. Normal intact and uninjured skin showing the layers of epidermis, dermis, and hypodermis. The appropriate and significant cells are illustrated in the layer of skin as observed in the uninjured skin.

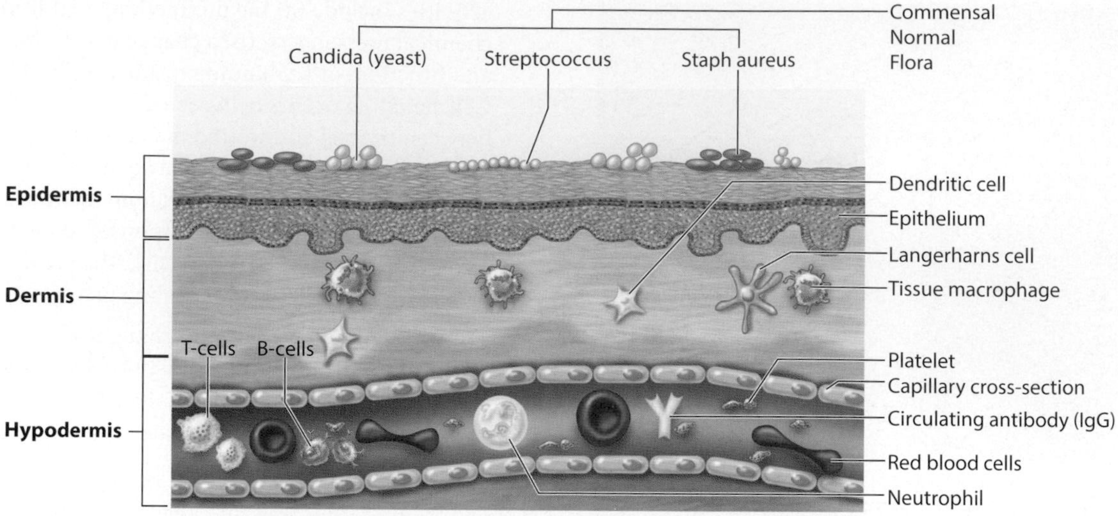

Key

Cell	Macrophage	NK	Platelets	RBC	PMN
State	Baseline	Baseline	Baseline	Baseline	Baseline

FIGURE 2-10 Baseline state of the skin prior to injury. The cells of the skin involved in the immune system are constantly on the attack against invaders that may cause infection, and when injury occurs they are mobilized to be even more active.

synthesized by helper CD4+ T-lymphocytes, as well as monocytes, macrophages, and endothelial cells.[3]

TABLE 2-3 lists the cytokines important to wound healing. The proinflammatory cytokines necessary for wound healing are TNF-α, IL-1, IL-2, IL-6, IL-8, and IFN-γ. In general, IL-4 and IL-10 are considered anti-inflammatory. Receptor expression on target cells can be either up- or downregulated. Each of the signals and the complex interplay serves to enhance, depress, or change entirely the cell function while ensuring that the process culminates in functional wound healing.

Growth factors are soluble polypeptides, produced in both normal and wounded tissues, which stimulate cell migration, proliferation, and alterations in cellular function. They are extremely potent and can exert significant effects in nanomolar concentrations. Growth factors bind to specific cell receptors and have one of two different effects: (1) the stimulation of DNA transcription or (2) the regulation of cell entry in the cell cycle (mitosis). Growth factors that are important in wound healing are listed in **TABLE 2-4**.

Cell-to-wound matrix communication occurs extensively during debridement and angiogenesis. Matricellular proteins (defined as dynamically expressed nonstructural proteins in the ECM that are rapidly turned over and have regulatory roles) destabilize the cell–matrix bonds and interactions, in essence creating a more fluid environment for cell migration.[63] Proteinases, both plasminogen activators and matrix metalloproteinases (MMPs), act to dissolve the wound matrix both immediately after injury and during the proliferative and remodeling phases. This is necessary during angiogenesis for the directed migration of endothelial cells.

The intricacies of cellular communication involve the components of the ECM, including fibrous structural proteins, water-hydrated gels, and adhesive glycoproteins (**FIGURE 2-18**). The fibrous structural proteins include the collagens and elastins, which give tensile strength and recoil to the tissue. Water-hydrated gels that permit resilience and lubrication are categorized as proteoglycans and hyaluronans. Adhesive glycoproteins connect the matrix elements to one another and to cells.

Collagen, one of the two fibrous structural proteins, is composed of three separate polypeptide chains braided into a rope like a triple helix (**FIGURE 2-19**). There are approximately 50 types of identified collagen. Some collagen types (eg, I, II, III, V) form fibrils by virtue of lateral cross-linking of the triple helix and are a major portion of connective tissue in healing wounds and particularly in scars. The cross-linking is a result of a covalent bond catalyzed by the enzyme lysyl oxidase, a process that is dependent on vitamin C. Types of collagen important to wound healing include the following: Type I, skin and bone; Type IV, basement membrane; and Type VIII, dermal–epidermal junction.

Elastin (present mainly in the skin, large vessels, ligaments, and uterus) consists of a central core of elastin surrounded by a mesh-like network of fibrillin glycoprotein. Fibroblasts secrete fibrillin into the ECM where it becomes assimilated into insoluble microfibrils and provides a platform for elastin deposition (**FIGURE 2-20**).

Proteoglycans form extremely hydrated compressible gels that provide both resilience and lubrication (eg, in the skin, cartilage, and joints). Proteoglycans consist of glycosaminoglycans (GAGs) and hyaluronan. GAGs are long polysaccharide chains like heparin sulfate and dermatan sulfate. Hyaluronan binds water and forms a very viscous, gelatin-like matrix. Proteoglycans function to provide compressibility,

FIGURE 2-11 Hemostasis

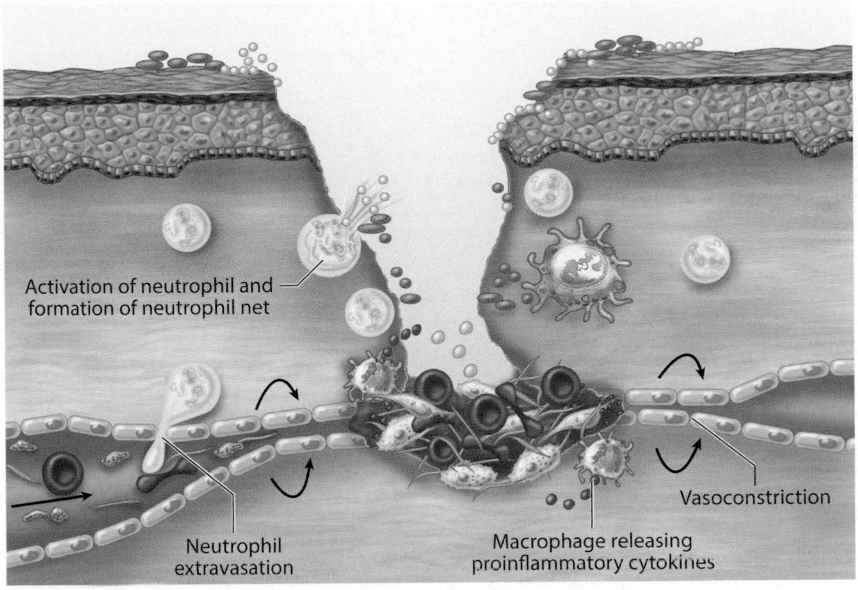

Key A

Cell	Macrophage	NK	Platelets	RBC	PMN
State	Upregulated M1	Upregulated	Upregulated	Upregulated	Upregulated

A. Hemostasis is the first phase of wound healing and is characterized by vasoconstriction of the injured vessel followed by vasodilation of the adjoining vasculature. Platelets aggregate and, along with fibrin, form a stable clot. At the wound site, platelets release molecules to stimulate platelet aggregation and growth of tissues important to healing. In the dermis and epidermis, PMNs and macrophages aggregate to kill and contain pathogenic invaders. The brown cells represent the pathogens.

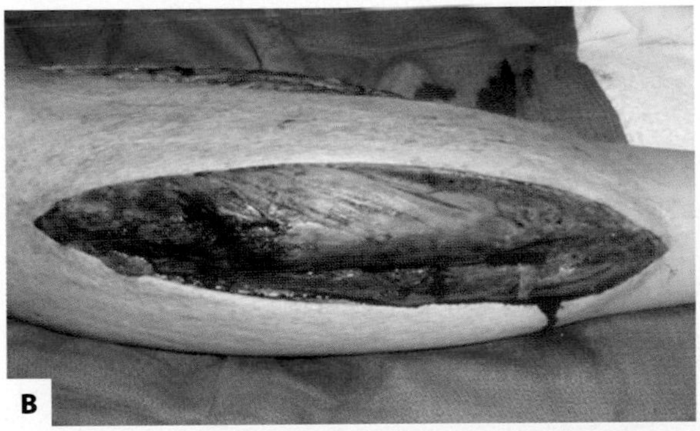

B. The fasciotomy wound has not yet achieved hemostasis, as evidenced by the bleeding occurring at the inferior undermining of the wound.

serve as a reservoir for growth factors that are secreted into the ECM, and are an important component of cell membranes. Thus they have roles in proliferation, migration, and adhesion (**FIGURE 2-21**).

The adherent components of the ECM are the adhesive glycoproteins (fibronectin and laminin) and adhesion receptors (immunoglobulin, selectin, cadherins, and integrins). Laminin and fibronectin together adjoin to collagen and connect to the plasma membrane of cells primary to tissue healing, and thereby reestablish both strength and function to the new replacement tissue. **FIGURE 2-22** depicts the adhesion receptors, which are paramount to ECM function and structure.

PHASES OF ACUTE WOUND HEALING

Wound healing initially appears very simple.[64–66] The human body is designed to heal, repair, and in some cases regenerate lost tissue through a well-orchestrated sequence of events. When it proceeds as planned, healing is complex but rapid and

FIGURE 2-12A Inflammatory phase: contain and kill the invader

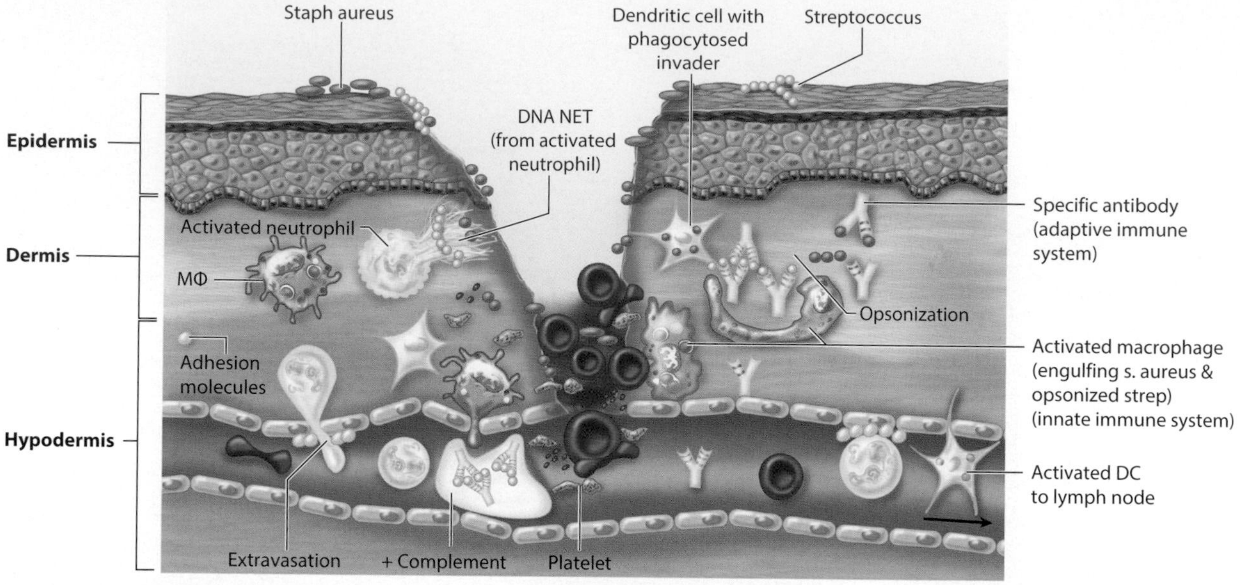

(1a) Clear invader (innate)
- Antimicrobial peptides & proteins
- Phagocytosis (macrophage / NK cells)
- Complement cascade
- Activation γ; α T-cells
- Neutrophil activator—DNA NET / Trap

(1b) Clear invader (adaptive)
- Dendritic cells
  - Pick up antigen (bacterium)
  - Traffic to lymph node to present Ag
  - Activate memory B cells—clonal expansion
- Antibodies released from B cells
  - (prior exposure to known invader)

(2a) Inflammation response iniated
- Platelets release aracadonic acid
- Clot formation fibroblast
- Wound debridement

Key

Cell	Macrophage	NK	Platelets	RBC	PMN	Fibroblast
State	Upregulated M1	Upregulated	Baseline	Baseline	Upregulated	Upregulated

A

Inflammation is the second phase and has three subphases: killing and containing the invader, wound debridement, and neo-angiogenesis. During the process of killing and containing the invader both the innate and the adaptive immune systems are triggered and an inflammatory response initiated.

FIGURE 2-12B Inflammation: killing the pathogens

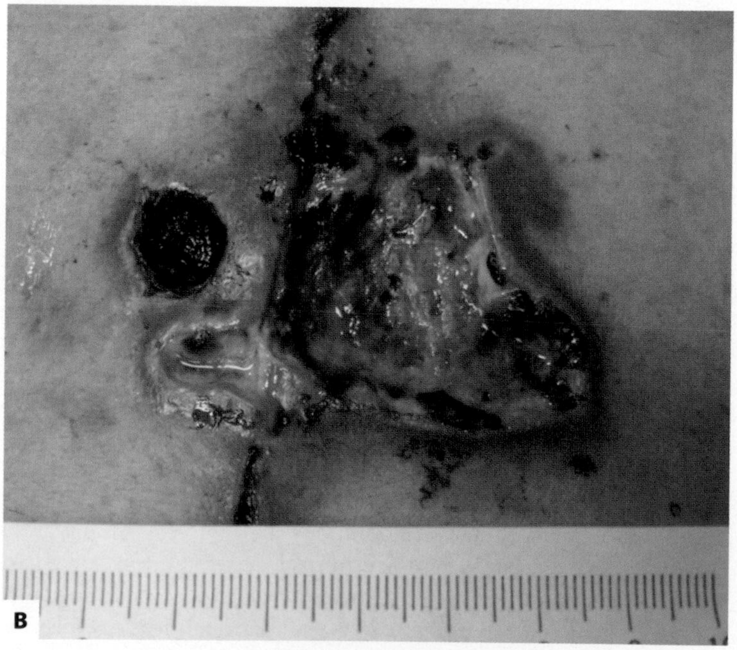

B

Wound in the inflammatory phase when high levels of phagocytic cells are present to break down the necrotic tissue and attack the pathogens. Slough, a byproduct of the autolytic process, is visible at the edges and in the right side of the wound.

FIGURE 2-13 Inflammatory phase: wound debridement

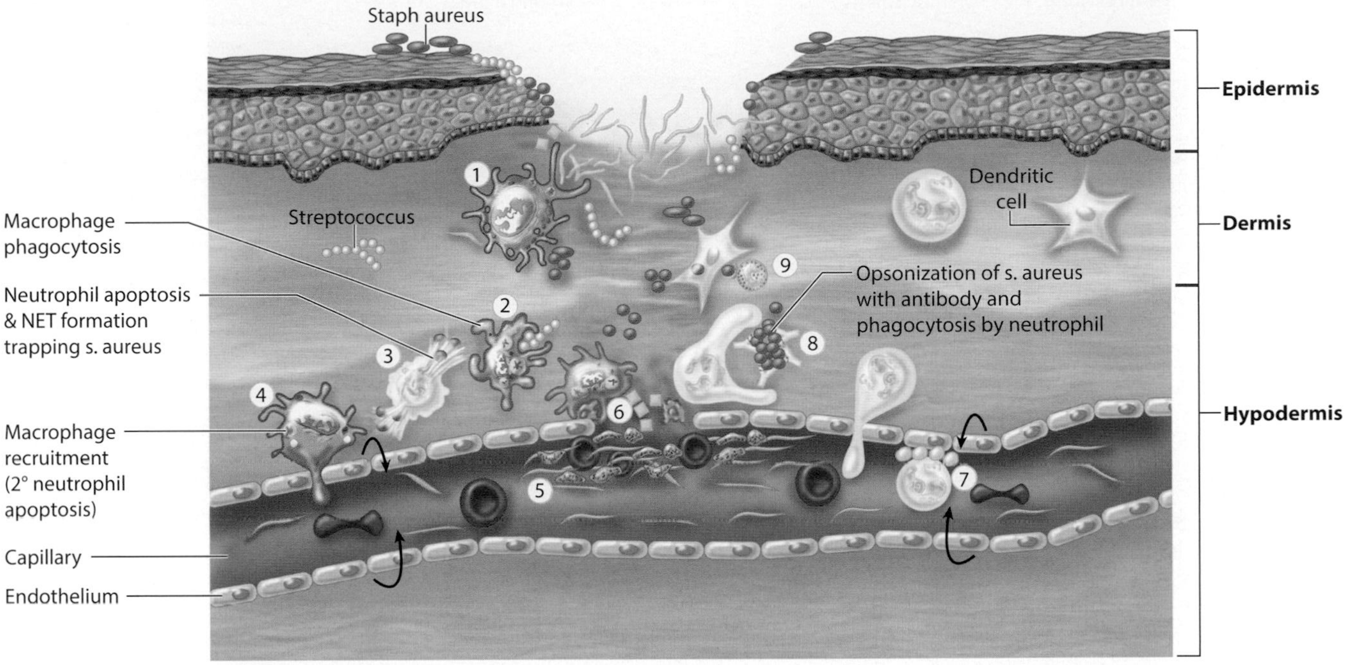

Key

Cell	Macrophage	NK	Platelets	RBC	PMN	Fibroblast	Endothelial
State	Upregulated M1	Upregulated	Baseline	Baseline	Upregulated	Upregulated	Upregulate

A

A. During the wound debridement phase of inflammation, macrophages are activated and begin phagocytosis of cellular debris while releasing enzymes to liquefy the ECM.

1. Activated macrophage phagocytosis of cellular debris and release of enzymes.
2. Macrophage phagocytosis of *Streptococcus*.
3. Apoptosis of neutrophils, formation of neutrophil NETs, trapping *Staphylococcus aureus* in preparation for phagocytosis by macrophages.
4. Macrophage recruitment, secondary to neutrophil apoptosis.
5. Platelet aggregation and entrapment in fibrin.
6. Macrophage phagocytosis of cellular debris and release of cytokines.
7. Adhesion of neutrophils to endothelium in preparation for exocytosis.
8. Opsonization of *Staphylococcus aureus* with antibody and phagocytosis by neutrophils.

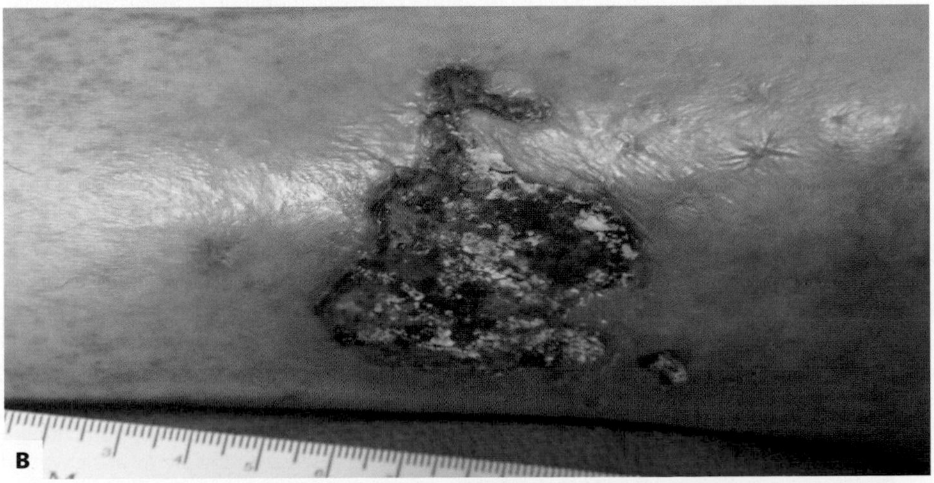

B

B. The necrotic tissue, termed *eschar*, on the wound surface will be attacked from the lower side by the macrophages and other phagocytic cells.

FIGURE 2-14A Inflammatory phase: neo-angiogenesis

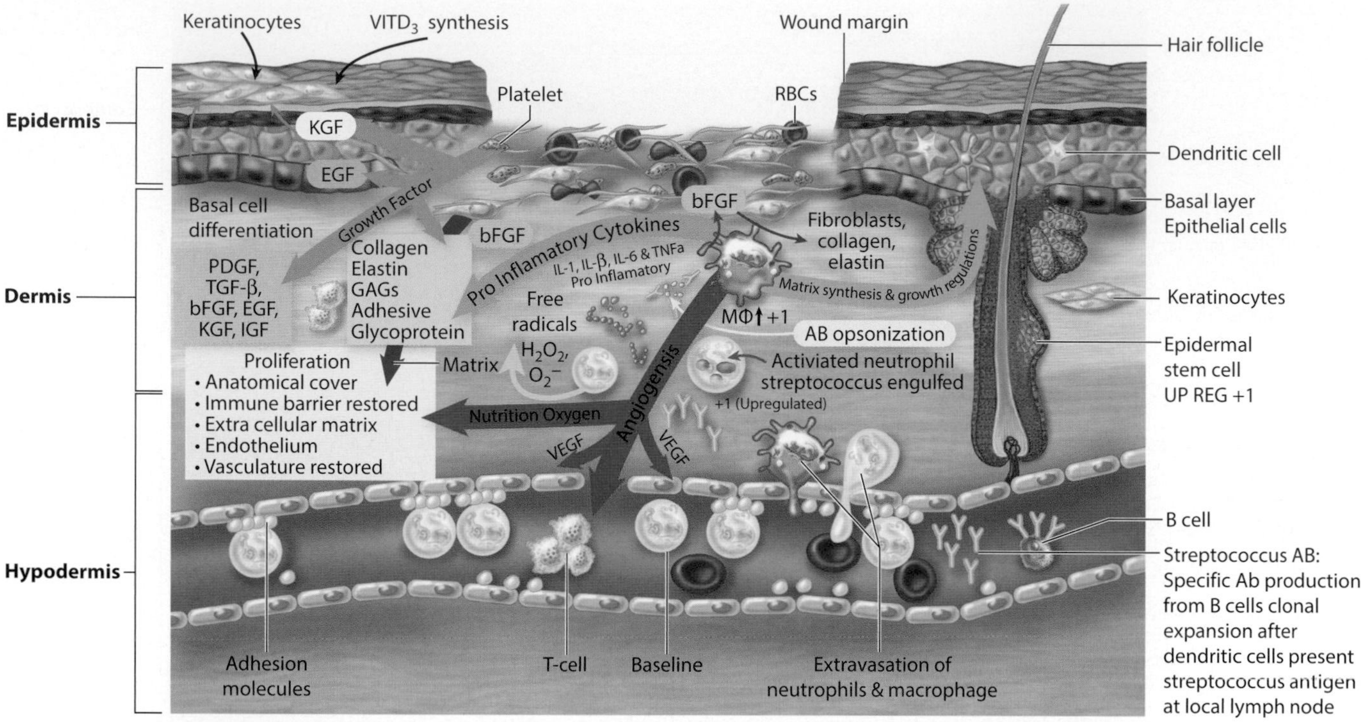

Key

Cell	Macrophage	NK	Platelets	RBC	PMN	Fibroblast	Endothelial	Epithelial
State	Upregulated M1	Upregulated	Baseline	Baseline	Baseline	Upregulated	Upregulated	Upregulated

A

In preparation for proliferation, angiogenesis begins to (1) support new tissue formation and (2) facilitate the removal of debris and waste products as a result of the destruction of cells and tissue.

1. Growth factors are released from the platelets, including PDGF, TGF-β, bFGF, EGF, KGF, and IGF.
2. ECM matrix formation begins accelerating with the formation and release of collagen, elastin, GAGs, and adhesive glycoproteins.
3. Proinflammatory cytokines from the macrophages and other sources (including IL-1, IL-1β, IL 6, and TNF-α) are being downregulated and have a diminishing effect.
4. Neutrophils release free radicals (including H_2O_2, O_2^-, and OH^-), which are destructive to bacteria in the wound milieu.
5. Clonal expansion of specific B cells begins after the dendritic cells present *Streptococcus* antigen in local lymph nodes.
6. Antibodies released by B cells opsonize specific target cells and provide a further signal for neutrophil engulfment.
7. Macrophages release VEGF to stimulate endothelium progenitor cell recruitment and differentiation as well as endothelial mitosis.
8. The foundation of proliferation is accomplished, including the following actions: covering of the anatomical structures, restoration of immune barrier, construction of ECM, fabrication of endothelium, and restoration of circulation with vascular reconstruction.

FIGURE 2-14B Neo-genesis.

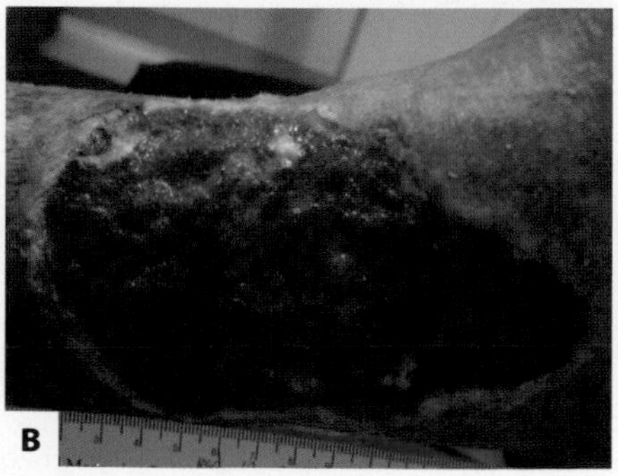

B

Healthy extracellular matrix supports the growth of new capillaries as seen in this lateral ankle wound. The capillaries give the surface of the wound a bumpy, granular appearance, thus the nomenclature "granulation."

FIGURE 2-15A Proliferation

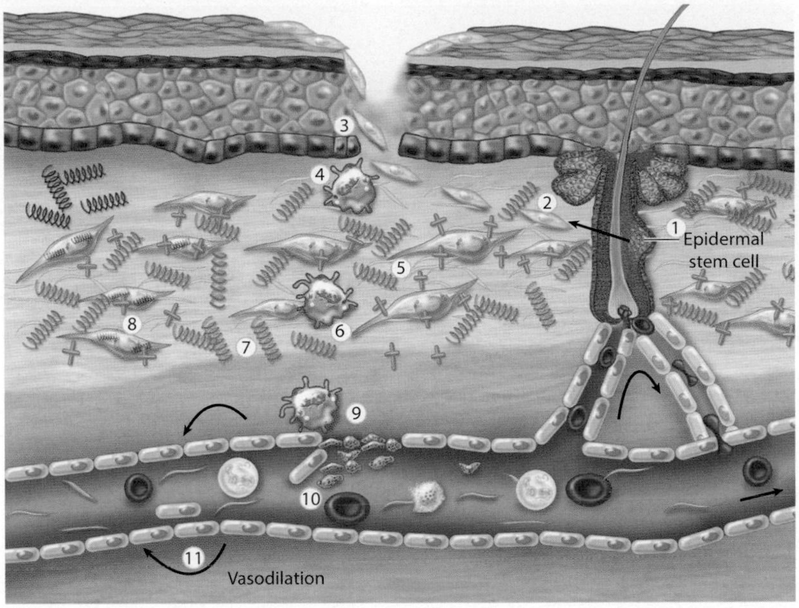

Key A

Cell	Macrophage	NK	Platelets	RBC	PMN	Fibroblast	Endothelial	Epithelial
State	Upregulated M2 Anti-Inflammatory	Baseline	Upregulated	Baseline	Baseline	Upregulated-change to Myofibroblast	Upregulated	Upregulated

Proliferation is a complicated and intricate process composed of the following:

1. Epidermal stem cell activation.
2. Keratinocyte migration from epidermal stem cells.
3. Increased mitosis of basal epithelial cells.
4. Macrophage scavenging cellular debris, and collagen for remodeling while simultaneously releasing enzymes.
5. Laminin attaches to collagen and fibroblast cells via adhesins.
6. Macrophage continues to phagocytose fibrocytes and collagen to facilitate migration.
7. Elastin (pink) and collagen (silver) are important components in the restoration of function.
8. Fibroblast differentiates into myofibroblast evidenced by the presence of α contractile fibers.
9. Macrophage phagocytosis of the old clot (old fibrin, platelets, and RBCs).
10. Endothelial progenitor cells are attracted by VEGF and other factors.
11. Vasodilation facilitates the process of tissue construction.

FIGURE 2-15B Proliferation

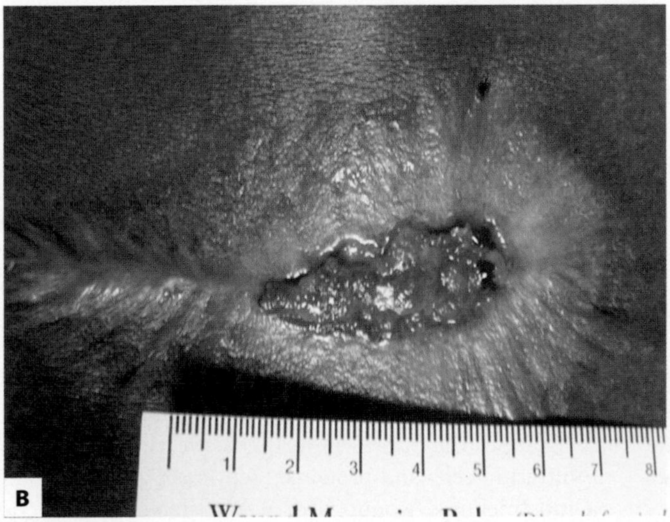

In addition to the visible bright-red granulation tissue in the wound, the results of myofibroblasts can be seen around the edges where the wound bed has contracted and re-epithelialized. The top edge is rolled with senescent cells at the edge of the wound bed, a condition termed *epibole*.

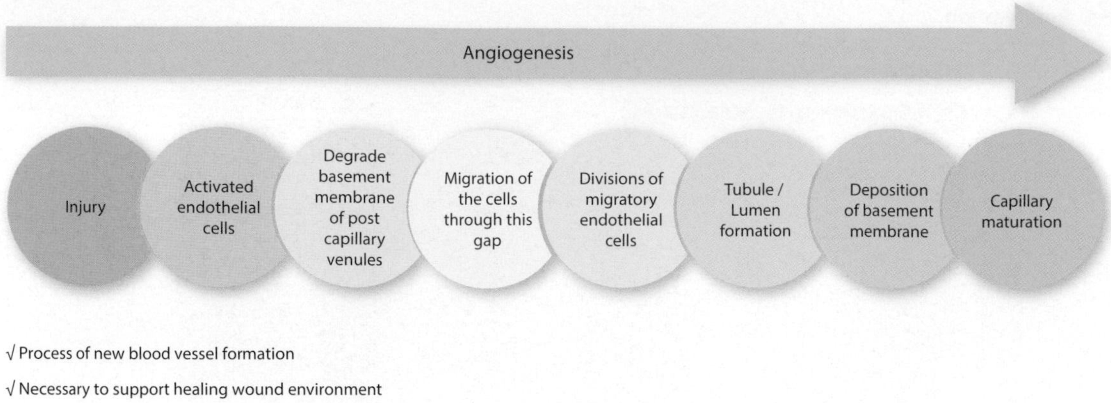

FIGURE 2-16 Angiogenesis. Angiogenesis is the process of new blood vessel formation. The flowchart demonstrates that angiogenesis begins immediately after injury and proceeds through a very orderly sequence, stimulating the extravasation and migration of cells through gaps in the endothelium and progressing through the formation of endothelial cells. The formation of tubules and lumen provides the basis for basement membrane deposition and capillary maturation. Angiogenesis ensures nutrition availability and removal of waste products throughout the healing process.

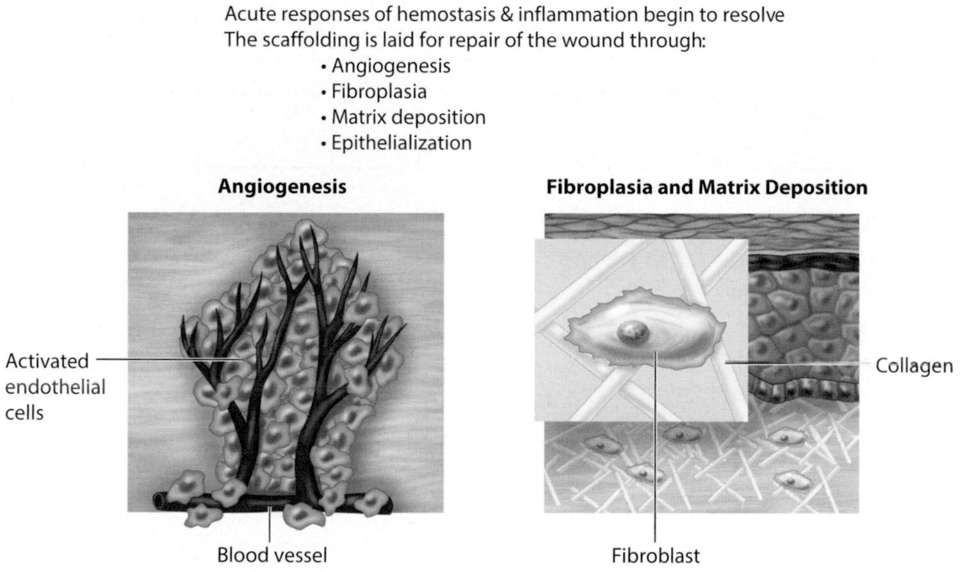

FIGURE 2-17 Proliferation. Proliferation is composed of four broad processes: angiogenesis, fibroplasia, matrix deposition, and epithelialization.

efficient. The four phases of wound healing are delineated by the pertinent vascular, cell-signaling, cellular activity, and clinical responses as previously defined (**FIGURES 2-11** to **2-15B**).

1. Hemostasis—Clot Formation

Small blood vessels initially respond to acute injury with vasoconstriction which stems further blood loss and tissue injury (**FIGURE 2-23**). Activated platelets adhere to the endothelium and eject adenosine diphosphate (ADP) which promotes the clumping of thrombocytes and further ensures clot formation. The clot, composed of various cell types (red blood cells, white blood cells, and platelets), is stabilized by fibers of fibrin.[67] (See **FIGURES 2-24** and **2-25**.)

Alpha granules containing platelet-derived growth factor (PDGF), platelet factor IV, and transforming growth factor β (TGF-β) are released from the platelets. Dense bodies contained within the thrombocytes release vasoactive amines, including histamine and serotonin. PDGF is chemotactic for fibroblasts, and in coordination with TGF-β modulates mitosis of fibroblasts,[68] thereby increasing the number of fibroblasts in close proximity to the wound. Fibrinogen is cleaved into fibrin which undergirds the structural support for the completion of the coagulation process and provides an active lattice for the important cellular components during the inflammatory phase. The fibrin will further serve as a scaffold for other infiltrating cells and proteins. (See **TABLE 2-5**.[3,10,69]) Clinically, a full-thickness wound bed with a stable clot functions to

TABLE 2-3 Principal Sources and Primary Activities of Interleukins and Cytokines

	Principal Source	Primary Activity	Comments
INTERLEUKINS			
IL-1α and IL-1β	Epithelial cells, fibroblasts, platelets, macrophages, and other antigen-presenting cells (APCs)	Costimulation of APCs and T cells, inflammation and host fever, hematopoiesis	Acute phase response
IL-2	Activated Th1 cells and NK cells	Proliferation of B cells and activated T cells, NK cell function Regulate WBCs	
IL-4	Th2 and mast cells, basophils	B-cell proliferation, eosinophil and mast cell growth and function, IgE and MHC class II expression on B cells, inhibition of monokine production Th0 differentiated to Th2 cells, Th2 cells produce ↑ IL-4 Promotes macrophage 0 to differentiate to M2 macrophage; M2 macrophages are considered repair macrophages and coupled with the secretion of IL-10, TGF-β resulting in decreased inflammation and diminution of pathological inflammation	
IL-6	Activated Th2 cells, APCs, adipocytes, macrophages, hepatocytes, PMNs, and fibroblasts	Acute phase response, B-cell proliferation, thrombopoiesis. IL-6 works synergistically with IL-1β and TNF on T cells ↑ Production of neutrophils in bone marrow	Both pro- and anti-inflammatory Also considered a myokine—produced in response to repetitive muscle contraction
IL-8	Macrophages, epithelial, endothelial, fibroblasts, and other somatic cells	Chemoattractant for neutrophils and T cells Induces phagocytosis. IL-8 can be secreted by any cell with toll-like receptors that are involved in the innate immune response. Usually, it is the macrophage that "see" the invader first Promotes angiogenesis	Capable of crossing blood–brain barrier
IL-10	Activated Th2 cells, CD8+, T and B cells, macrophages, monocytes, and mast cells	Inhibits cytokine production, promotes B-cell proliferation, survival and antibody production, suppresses cellular immunity and mast cell growth Downregulation of MHC class II receptor expression	Anti-inflammatory Also known as human cytokine inhibitory factor Inhibition of TNF-α, IL-1, and IL-6 production and inhibition of PMN activation
IL-12	B cells, T cells, macrophages, dendritic cells	Proliferation of NK cells ↑ Cytotoxic activity of NK cells Th0 to Th1 IFN-γ production, promotes cell-mediated immune functions Antiangiogenesis via ↑ production of IFN-γ	Two different protein chains, which form three distinct dimers: AA, AB, BB
IL-13	Th2 cells, B cells, macrophages	Stimulates growth and proliferation of B cells, inhibits production of macrophage inflammatory cytokines Induces MMPs Induces IgE secretion from activated B cells	
IL-18	Macrophages	Increases NK cell activity, induces production of IFN-γ Induces cell-mediated immunity Stimulates NK cells and T cells to release IFN-γ	Proinflammatory Also known as IFN-γ-inducing factor
INTERFERONS			
IFN-α, IFN-β, IFN-γ	Macrophages, neutrophils	Antiviral effects, induction of MHC class I on all somatic cells, activation of NK cells, and macrophages	
IFN-γ	Activated Th1 and NK cells, cytotoxic T cells	Induces expression of MHC class I on all somatic cells, induces MHC class II on APCs and somatic cells, activates macrophages, neutrophils, NK cells, promotes cell-mediated immunity, antiviral effects Activates inducible NO synthesis ↑ Production of IgG2g, IgG3 from activated plasma B cells ↑ MHC I and ↑ MHC II expression by APCs Promotes adhesion binding for leukocyte migration Retards collagen synthesis and cross-linking; stimulates collagenase activity	Also called macrophage activating factor Critical for both innate and adaptive immunity Antiviral IFN-γ binds to glycosaminoglycan heparin sulfate at the cell surface, binding in general inhibits biological activity

(Continued)

TABLE 2-3 Principal Sources and Primary Activities of Interleukins and Cytokines (*Continued*)

	Principal Source	Primary Activity	Comments
ADIPOCYTOKINES			
C-reactive protein	Hepatocytes, adipocytes Synthesized by the liver in response to factors released by macrophage and adipocytes (eg, IL-6)	CRP is a ligand-binding protein (calcium dependent), which facilitates the interaction between complement and both foreign and damaged host cells Enhances phagocytosis by macrophage Modulates endothelial cell functions by inducing the expression of adhesion/"sticky" molecules (ICAM-1, VCAM-1) Attenuates nitric oxide production by downregulating NOS expression CRP's level of expression is regulated by IL-6	First pattern recognition receptor (PRR) to be identified. Acute phase protein. Physiological role is to bind phosphocholine expressed on the surface of dead or dying cells and some types of bacteria in order to activate the complement system via C1Q complex; therefore, phagocytosis is enhanced. Opsonic-mediated phagocytosis helps amplify the early innate immune response
Prostaglandin	Leukocytes and macrophage	Either constriction or dilation of vascular smooth muscle Acts on platelets, endothelium, and mast cells Causes aggregation or disaggregation of platelets Regulates inflammatory mediation Controls cell growth Acts on thermoregulatory center of hypothalamus to produce fever Enzymatic pathway to convert the intermediate arachidonic acid to prostaglandin is found in active WBCs and macrophage	Prostaglandins are potent but have a short half-life before being activated or excreted. Therefore, send only autocrine (acting on the same cell from which it is synthesized) or paracrine (local adjacent cells)

TABLE 2-4 Cell Source and Function of Growth Factors Involved in Wound Healing

Growth Factors	Source	Functions
Platelet-derived growth factor (PDGF)	Platelets, macrophages, endothelial cells, keratinocytes	Chemotactic for PMNs, macrophages, fibroblasts, activates PMNs, macrophages, and fibroblasts; mitogenic for fibroblasts, endothelial cells; stimulates production of MMPs, fibronectin, and HA; stimulates angiogenesis and wound contraction; remodeling
Transforming growth factor-β (including isoforms β1, β2, and β3) (TGF-β)	Platelets, T-lymphocytes, macrophages, endothelial cells, keratinocytes, fibroblasts	Chemotactic for PMNs, macrophages, lymphocytes, and fibroblasts; stimulates TIMP synthesis, keratinocyte migration, angiogenesis, and fibroplasia; inhibits production of MMPs and keratinocyte proliferation; induces TGF-β production
Epidermal growth factor (EGF)	Platelets, macrophages	Mitogenic for keratinocytes and fibroblasts; stimulates keratinocyte migration
Transforming growth factor-α (TGF-α)	Macrophages, T-lymphocytes, keratinocytes	Similar to EGF
Fibroblast growth factor-1 and -2 family (FGF)	Macrophages, mast cells, T-lymphocytes, endothelial cells, fibroblasts	Chemotactic for fibroblasts; mitogenic for fibroblasts and keratinocytes; stimulates keratinocyte migration, angiogenesis, wound contraction, and matrix deposition
Keratinocyte growth factor (also called FGF-7) (KGF)	Fibroblasts	Stimulates keratinocyte migration, proliferation, and differentiation
Insulin-like growth factor (IGF-I)	Macrophages, fibroblasts	Stimulates synthesis of sulfated proteoglycans, collagen, keratinocyte migration, and fibroblast proliferation; endocrine effects similar to those of growth hormone
Vascular endothelial cell growth factor (VEGF)	Keratinocytes	Increases vasopermeability; mitogenic for endothelial cells

mitigate blood loss. Clear proteinaceous exudate may or may not be present.

2. Inflammation

Inflammation presents clinically as rubor (redness), tumor (swelling), calor (heat), and dolor (pain). The orchestrated arrival and departure of important cell mediators are depicted in **FIGURE 2-26**. Key changes that permit the initiation of inflammation and result in the clinical findings associated with inflammation are summarized in **TABLE 2-6**. The processes involved in both innate and adaptive immunity are activated and prevalent.

Kill and Contain Invader Cells involved in immunity arrive, depart, upregulate, or downregulate during the phases of healing. Within the first 6–8 hours after injury, polymorphonucle-

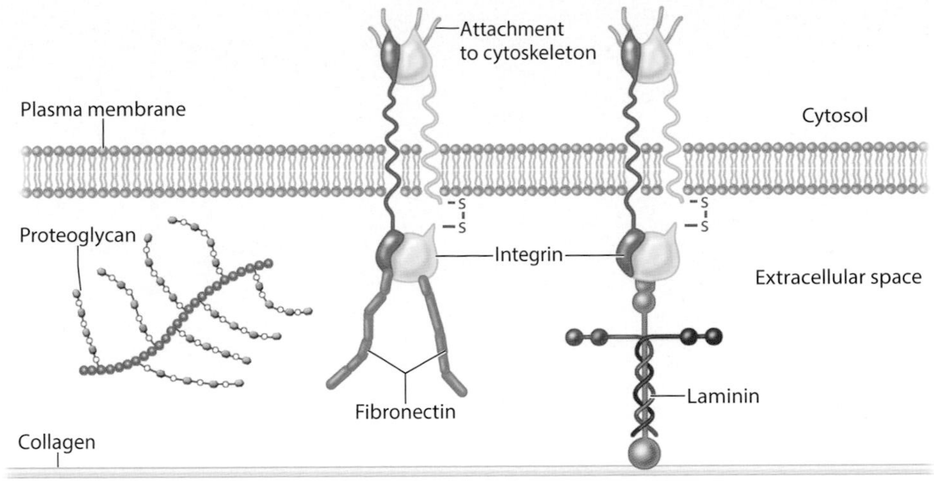

FIGURE 2-18 Extracellular matrix. The extracellular matrix (ECM) is complex and intimately involved in healing by regulating growth factor activation, cell signaling, and cell-to-matrix signaling. This figure illustrates the intricate positioning and connections of the glycoproteins, integrins, and proteoglycans that compose the ECM. It serves as the scaffolding upon which the body builds replacement tissue.

ar leukocytes (PMNs) or *neutrophils* flood the wound. TGF-β (released from platelets) facilitates PMN migration and extrusion from surrounding intact blood vessels to the interstitial wound space. PMNs are phagocytic cells, functioning to cleanse the wound of debris, including both necrotic cells and pathogens (**TABLE 2-7**). The highest number of PMNs within the wound is observed between 24 and 48 hours after injury. By 72 hours, PMN numbers are significantly reduced, just as macrophages are infiltrating (**FIGURE 2-27**).[46,58,70] Factors that promote neutrophil adherence and migration are a combination of cellular activity, chemokines, cytokines, and proteases (**FIGURE 2-27**).

Mast cells are activated by antibodies and move rapidly from vascular circulation to the site of injury. Upon activation, mast cells become "sticky" and adhere to the endothelial surface (**FIGURE 2-28**). Mast cells can influence the local environment by degranulation or through the products that they synthesize. Histamine, a product of degranulation, increases

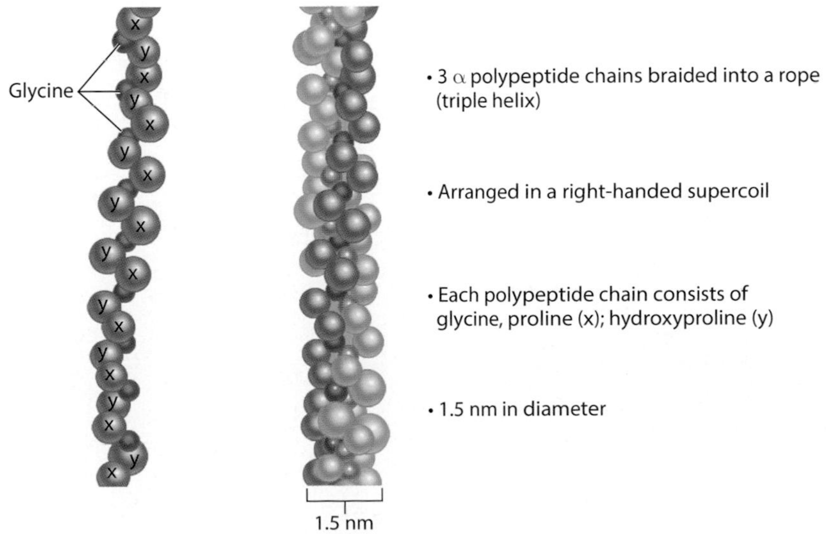

FIGURE 2-19 Collagen triple helix. Collagen triple helix is schematically detailed illustrating the right-handed supercoil. In mature collagen, three polypeptide chains are braided into a triple helix rope. Glycine, proline (x), and hydroxyproline (y) are arranged in a right-handed supercoil that is approximately 1.5 nm in diameter. The three α-chains may be constructed of the same type of collagen (collagen II) or different (collagen I). Some collagen types (eg, collagen I, II, III, V) form fibrils by virtue of lateral cross-linking of the triple helix. Cross-linking is a result of covalent bonds catalyzed by the enzyme lysyl-oxidase, a process that is dependent upon vitamin C. About 50 types of collagen have been identified. Fibrillar collagens are a major component of connective tissue in healing wounds, particularly scars.

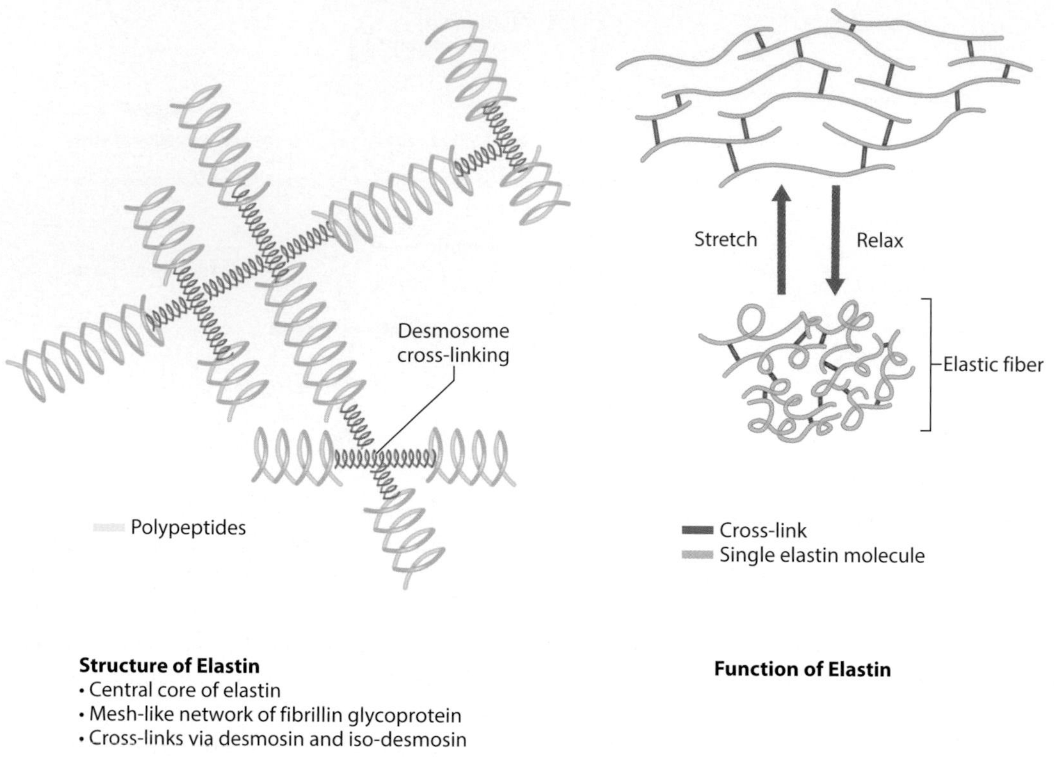

FIGURE 2-20 Elastin structure and function. Upon the release of mechanical stress, changes in the structure of elastin components occur with stretch and recoil. Morphologically, elastin consists of a central core of elastin surrounded by a mesh-like network of fibrillin glycoprotein.

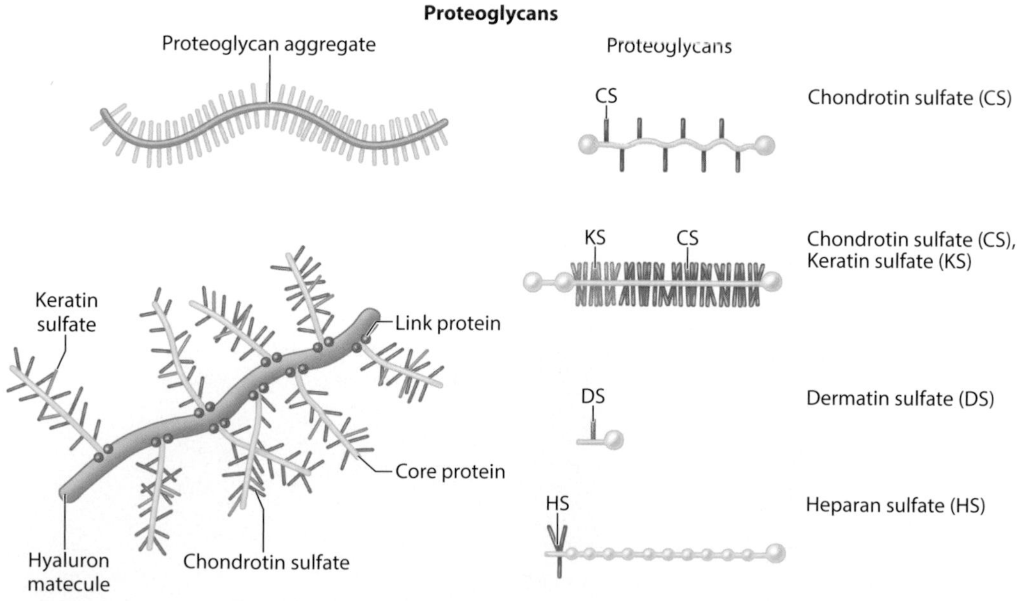

FIGURE 2-21 Proteoglycan structure. Proteoglycans are aggregated in a pinnate, feather-like arrangement. The heterogenic proteoglycans are represented and further subdivided by common types. Proteoglycans form highly hydrated and compressible gels conferring resilience and lubrication (cartilage and joints). They consist of glycosaminoglycans (GAGs), which are long polysaccharide chains designated by their components (eg, heparin or dermatan sulfates). The hyaluronan components bind water and form a viscous gelatin-like matrix. Functionally, the proteoglycans provide tissue compressibility, serve as a reservoir for growth factors (ECM), and are an integral portion in the cell membranes. As part of cellular membranes, these proteins have important roles in proliferation, migration, and adhesion.

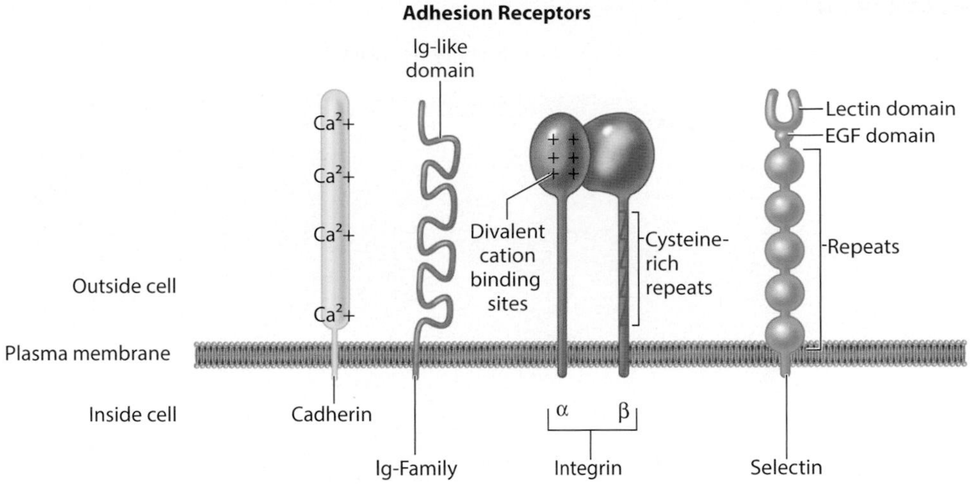

FIGURE 2-22 Adhesion receptors. Adhesive glycoproteins and receptors, fibronectin and laminin, are central ECM components. Their attachment via integrins to cellular matrix cytoskeleton is depicted.

the permeability of endothelial cells, thus facilitating extravasation of PMNs and macrophages. The three major product categories synthesized by mast cells are prostaglandins, thromboxanes, and leukotrienes.[3]

Neutrophils play an important role in the early phagocytosis of pathogens and in the recruitment of macrophages by programmed apoptosis. Neutrophils are also capable of expelling a neutrophil extracellular trap (NET) that is composed of DNA and loosely aggregated chromatin. The NET works somewhat like flypaper, trapping would-be invaders and allowing increased clearance by recruited macrophages or neighboring neutrophils.[45]

Wound Debridement Autolytic wound debridement begins immediately after injury and includes the use of cells and enzymatic proteins to break down necrotic tissue. Cells typically involved in debridement include neutrophils, macrophages, and mast cells.[36,71] Enzymatically active proteins, including proteinases and collagenases, degrade the damaged tissue and ECM, thus providing a migratory path to the site of injury for the key cells needed to complete the healing process.[17,19]

PDGF, released by platelets, is chemotactic for monocytes, causing the monocytes to leave adjacent blood vessels and transform into wound-activated macrophages (WAMs)

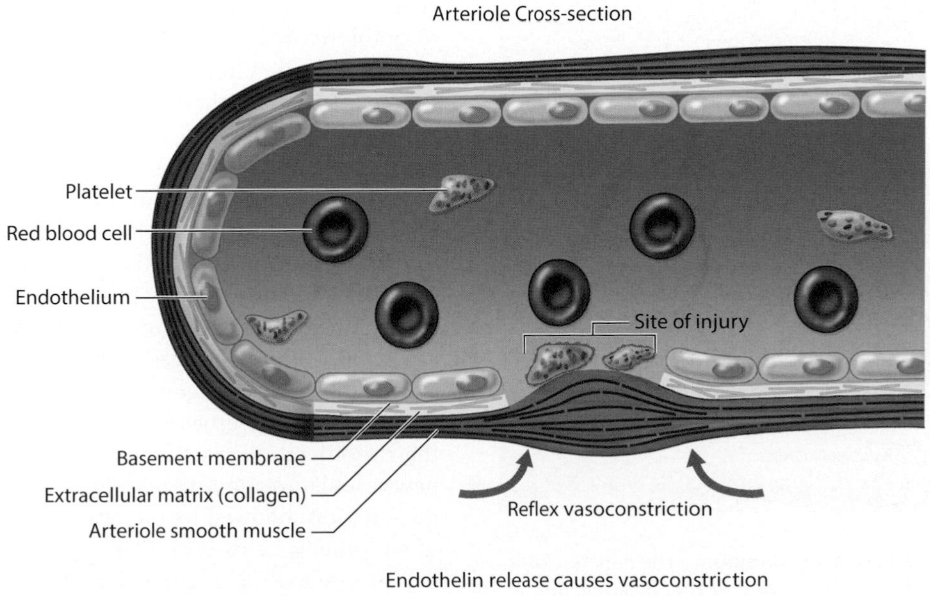

FIGURE 2-23 Vasoconstriction. Cross-section of an arteriole during vasoconstriction. The initial response to injury is reflex vasoconstriction, and the exposed vascular endothelium stimulates platelet adhesion.

FIGURE 2-24 Primary hemostasis

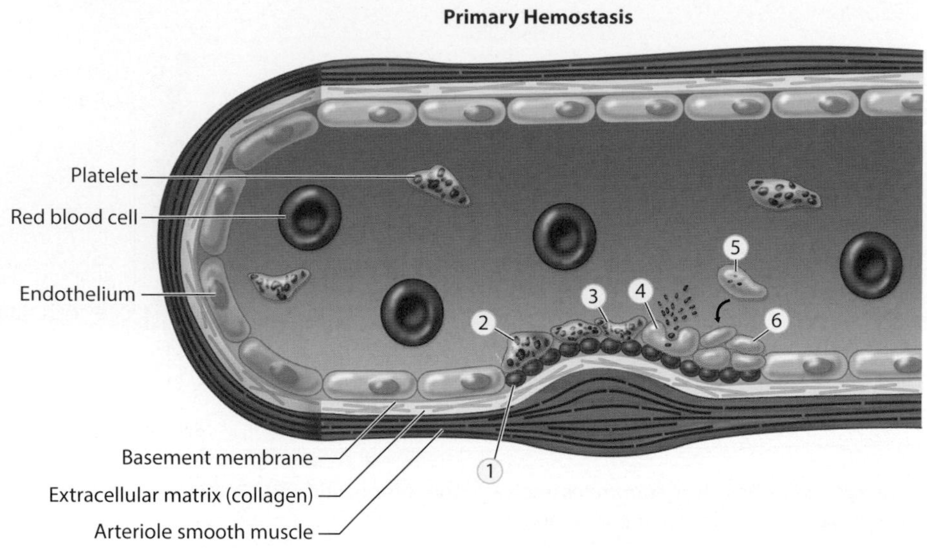

During primary hemostasis:

1. Adhesion molecules are expressed and bind platelets.
2. Platelets adhere to the exposed basement membrane.
3. Granular release (ADP) occurs.
4. Further recruitment of platelets occurs.
5. Complete aggregation with fibrin forms a hemostatic plug.

when they reach the interstitial tissue. WAMs continue the process of debris removal, and more importantly, begin the signaling that will orchestrate the remaining transitions and events central to healing (**FIGURE 2-29**).[27,68] Macrophage numbers remain high for approximately 3–4 days, releasing various tissue growth factors, cytokines, interleukin-1 (IL-1), tumor necrosis factor (TNF), and PDGF.[46] In addition to the phagocytic function, the macrophages provide a unifying script for the multiplication of endothelial cells and the sprouting of new blood vessels, both of paramount importance for continued cell migration and proliferation.[3,5,72–74]

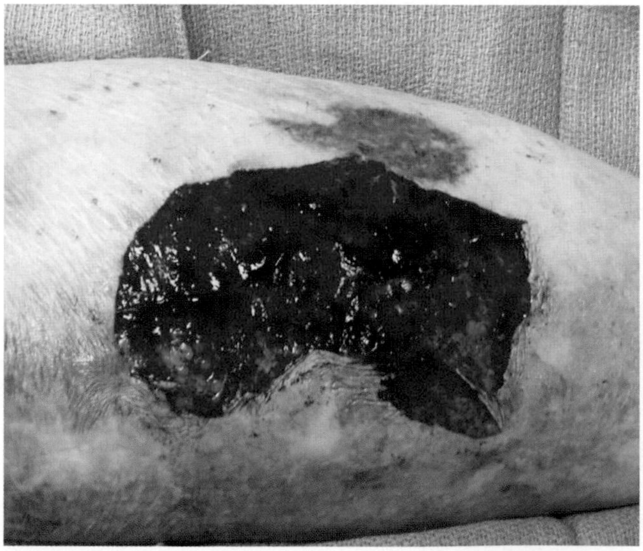

FIGURE 2-25 Stable fibrin clot, or coagulum. The dark red fibrin clots on the surface of this skin tear prevent further bleeding and tissue damage.

The controlled liquefaction of the ECM continues during the debridement process until the damaged cells are removed and the cells needed for repair are in place. The rate of autolytic debridement will decline as debris is cleared, new cells proliferate, and healing ensues. The proinflammatory cytokines and their effects are presented in **FIGURES 2-3** and **2-4**.

Angiogenesis (Early) Just as the re-epithelialization process begins a few hours after wounding, so too does neo-angiogenesis.[75] Keratinocytes from the wound edges migrate beneath the fibrin clot and over the wound. Activated fibroblasts migrate to the site of injury in response to TGF-β1,[11,68,76] and, in combination with macrophages, synthesize granulation tissue.[16,75] Both macrophages and fibroblasts produce vascular endothelial growth factor (VEGF), and fibroblasts produce connective tissue growth factor (CTGF),[77] which results in their proliferation via an autocrine loop.[12] The formation of new vasculature requires both ECM and basement membrane degradation followed by migration, mitosis, and maturation of endothelial cells. Both FGF and VEGF are thought to be key in modulating angiogenesis.[10,28,78–81] The new vessel formation will both (1) supply the oxygen and nutrients required

TABLE 2-5 Platelet Binding and Activation

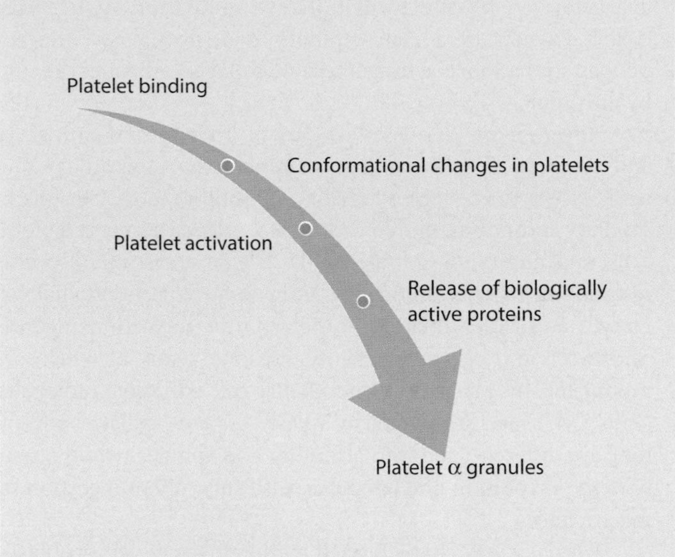

Platelet α-granules secrete:
Platelet-derived growth factor
Transforming growth factor
Insulin-like growth fa ctor
Fibronectin
Fibrinogen
Thrombospondin
von Willebrand factor

The dense bodies contain vasoactive amines like serotonin, which lead to increased vascular permeability and vasodilatation.

The sequence of activities initiated by platelets is described chronologically, as well as the actions driven by the release of substances from platelet alpha granules. The dense bodies contain vasoactive amines (eg, serotonin), which lead to increased vascular permeability and vasodilatation. The platelet binding and activation form a stable blood clot or plug, also termed **coagulum**.[3,19,20]

Phase	Injury	Hemostasis	Inflammation -Early	Inflammation -Late	Degradation	Proliferative granulation, epithelialization contraction	Remodeling	Differentiation -Healed wound
Time after injury	Immed.	5–10 min	12–24 hours	24 hours	2–4 days	3–4 days, Lasts 15–16 days	~21 days	24–42 days
Cell								
Dendritic cell	Sentinel							
γδ T cell	Sentinel							
NK cell								
CD4+ Reg		Entering...				Leaving...		
B cells		Entering...	Antibodies produced - long distance "bombers"		Leaving...			
CD8 + T cells	Immed after..				Leaving...			
Macrophage		Migration	Increasing numbers				Remodeling clean up	
Neutrophil	Sentinel	Increasing in numbers				Leaving...		
Keratinocyte								
Fibroblast								

FIGURE 2-26 Arrival and departure of migratory cells during wound healing. The overall orchestrated arrival and departure of important cells (vertical axis) is correlated with the phases of wound healing (horizontal axis).

TABLE 2-6 Inflammation Overview

- Increased permeability is due to
  - formation of endothelial gaps in venules
  - direct endothelial injury
  - delayed and/or prolonged leakage
  - leucocyte-mediated endothelial injury
  - increased transcytosis and leakage from new vessels
- The combination of intense vasodilation and increased vascular permeability leads to clinical findings of inflammation
  - *rubor* (redness), *tumor* (swelling), *calor* (heat), and (pain)

and (2) remove the waste products of autolysis. **FIGURE 2-30** provides a broad overview of the key events involved in angiogenesis and **FIGURE 2-31** illustrates a well-vascularized granulating wound bed.

3. Proliferation

The proliferation phase of healing consists of four subphases: *angiogenesis*, *fibroplasia*, *matrix deposition*, and *re-epithelialization*.[66,75] **FIGURE 2-17** illustrates a broad overview of the events occurring during the proliferation phase, which is characterized by the formation of granulation tissue. This tissue consists of a rich capillary bed, fibroblasts, macrophages, and a loose arrangement of collagen, fibronectin, and hyaluronan.

Angiogenesis, discussed as part of both the inflammatory and proliferative phases, begins immediately after injury and is necessary to ensure endothelial cell migration that results in capillary sprouting. Injured endothelial cells, adhering red blood cells, and numerous soluble factors trigger a cascade of events resulting in matrix remodeling and concurrent endothelial cell growth and differentiation. Capillary tube formation involves cell-to-cell and cell-to-matrix interactions, many of which are modulated by progenitor endothelial cell adhesion molecules (PECAM-1) and stimulated by VEGF. As new capillaries sprout, they are differentiated into arterioles and venules, while others undergo involution and apoptosis with subsequent ingestion by macrophages.

Fibroplasia is characterized by the presence of fibroblasts, specialized cells that differentiate from resting MSCs located in connective tissue (**FIGURE 2-32**). By approximately the fifth day, fibroblasts migrate into the wound and synthesize new

TABLE 2-7 Polymorphonuclear Cells in Wound Healing

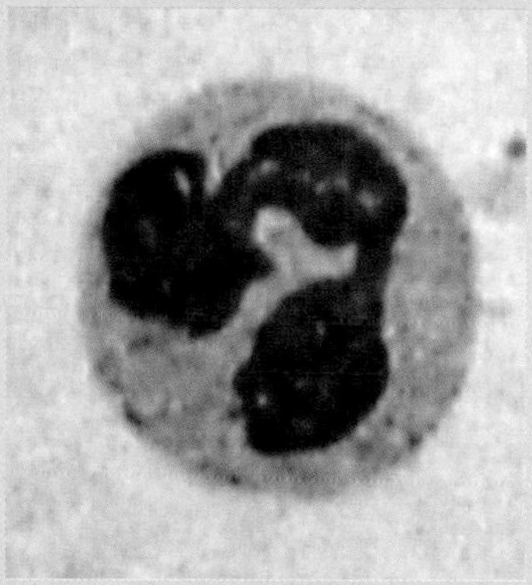

- PMNs are not essential to wound healing
  - Phagocytic role and antimicrobial defense may be taken over by macrophages
  - Sterile incisions will heal normally without the presence of PMNs
- First infiltrating cells to enter the wound site, peaking at 24–48 hours
- Neutrophil migration is stimulated by
  - Increased vascular permeability
  - Local prostaglandin release
- PMNs
  - Major source of cytokines during early inflammation, especially TNF-α
  - Also release proteases such as collagenases
- Following functional activation neutrophils scavenge:
  - Necrotic debris
  - Foreign material
  - Bacteria
- If wound contamination persists or secondary infection occurs, then continuous activation of the complement system and other pathways provides a steady supply of chemotactic factors
  - Result is sustained influx of PMNs into the wound
  - Once wound contamination is resolved, PMN migration halts
- PMNs do not survive longer than 24 hours
- Stimulated neutrophils generate free oxygen radicals
  - Electrons donated by the reduced form of nicotinamide adenine dinucleotide phosphate
  - Electrons are transported across the membrane into lysosomes where superoxide anion (O^{2-}) and hydroxyl (OH^-) are formed
  - Superoxide anion (O^{2-}) and hydroxyl (OH^-) are formed
  - Superoxide anion (O^{2-}) and hydroxyl (OH^-) are very potent free radicals
  - Bactericidal
  - Toxic to neutrophils
  - Toxic to surrounding viable tissues

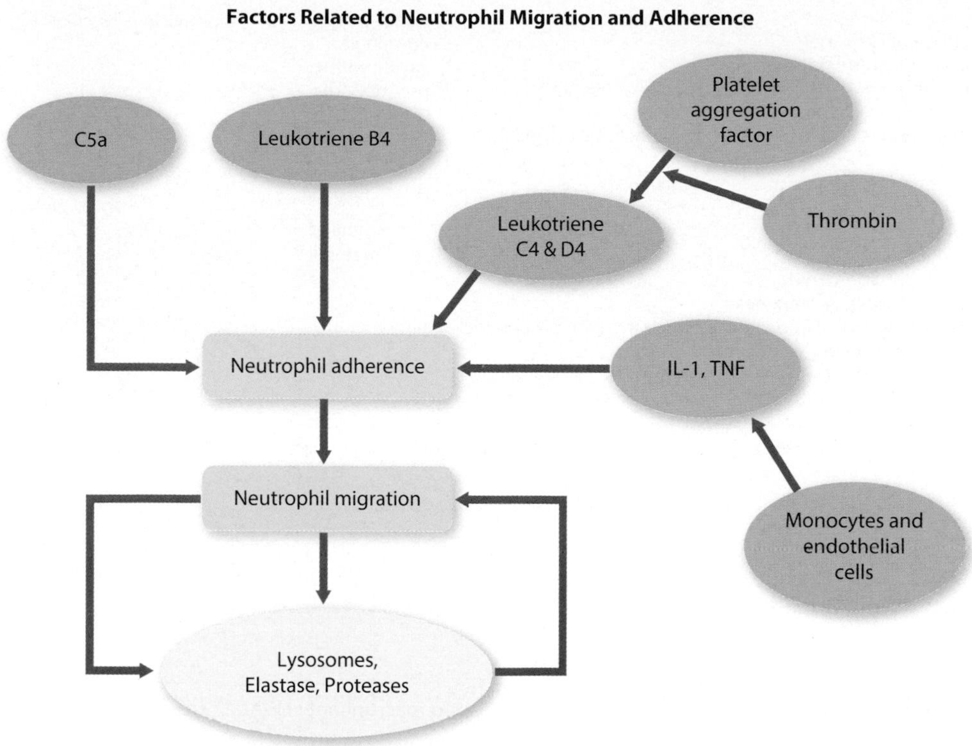

FIGURE 2-27 Factors related to neutrophil migration and adherence. The combination of factors imperative for neutrophil extravasation, migration, and adherence at the site of injury and beyond are depicted.

collagen, either type I or III. (Early in normal wound healing, type III collagen predominates and is later replaced by type I collagen.) The process of collagen formation begins within the fibroblast cell's rough endoplasmic reticulum, where tropocollagen (the precursor to all collagen types) has its proline and lysine hydroxylated. Establishing disulfide bonds allows three tropocollagen strands to form a triple left-handed helix, termed *procollagen*. The procollagen is then secreted

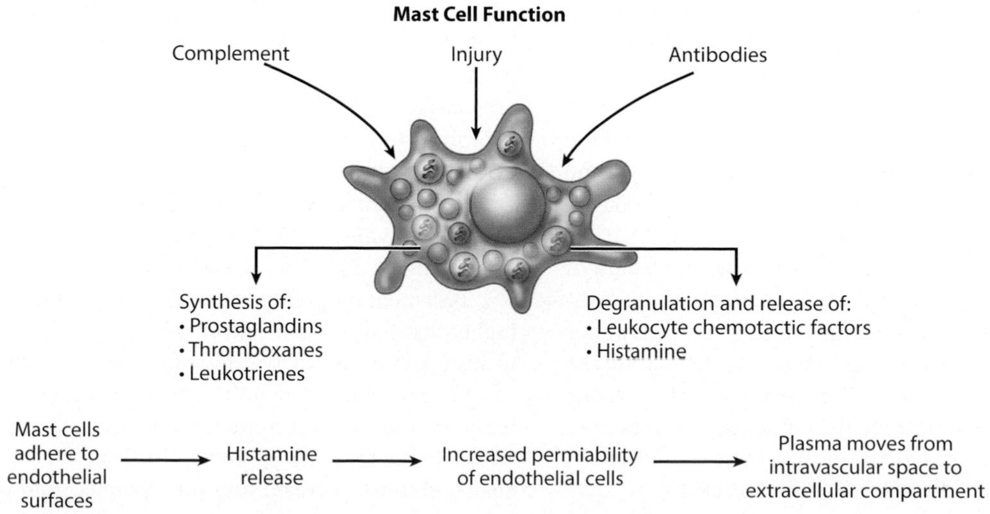

FIGURE 2-28 Mast cell structure and function. Mast cells are early responders along with PMNs and, once activated, mast cells may either (1) synthesize prostaglandins, leukotrienes, and thromboxanes, or (2) degranulate releasing histamine and chemotactic factors for leukocytes. The resulting actions increase permeability of the endothelial cells and provide a means for cells and plasma to move from the intravascular space to the extracellular compartment.

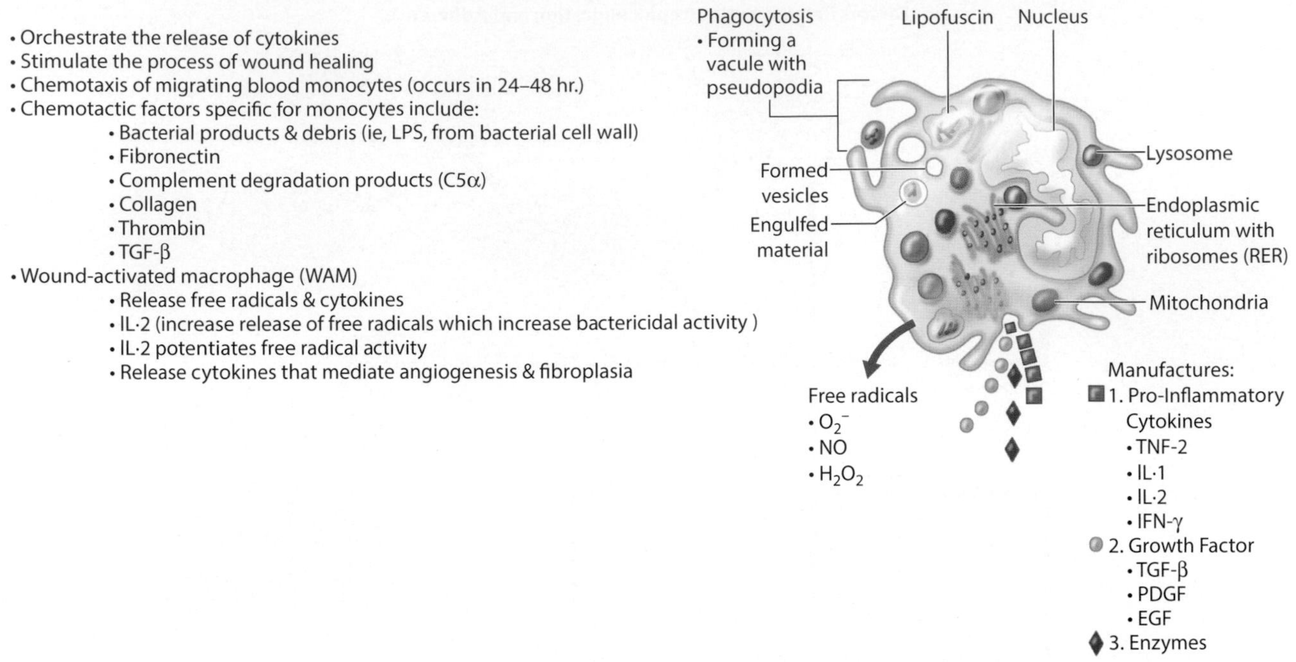

FIGURE 2-29 Wound-activated macrophage functions. Wound-activated macrophages (WAMs) are derived from monocytes that may be activated by integrin expression, a process that promotes adhesion-mediated gene induction in monocytes. The monocytes then transform into WAMs. The changes include pseudopodia, increased number of phagosomes and lysosomes, and appearance of phagolysosomes. Phagocytosis is the primary function, resulting in increased numbers of appropriate cell organelles suited for increased phagocytic activity as well as the manufacture and release of proinflammatory cytokines.

into the extracellular space, passing through the cell wall where peptidases cleave the terminal peptide chains, creating true collagen fibrils (**FIGURE 2-33**).[15,16,72,82,83]

The wound is permeated with GAGs and fibronectin produced by the fibroblasts. The GAGs include heparin sulfate, hyaluronan, chondroitin sulfate, and keratin sulfate. Proteoglycans are GAGs covalently bonded to a protein center. All of these constitute and contribute to *matrix deposition*. The ECM provides both the lattice infrastructure and key binding sites for cells and chemical messengers alike (**FIGURE 2-34**).[14,16,19,84–86] Although labile and stable cells are capable of regeneration, injury to these tissues results in restitution of the normal structure only if the ECM is not damaged. Disruption of the ECM leads to collagen deposition and scar formation.

Re-epithelialization of the wound begins within hours of injury. The wound is rapidly sealed by clot formation and subsequently by the migration of epithelial (epidermal) cells under the clot and across the defect. Keratinocytes located within the basal layer of the remaining and undamaged epidermis migrate to resurface the wound. Keratinocytes undergo a sequence of changes to complete re-epithelialization, which is depicted in **FIGURES 2-35** and **2-36** and summarized in **TABLE 2-8**.

Epidermal cells express integrin receptors, thus allowing them to interact and anchor to ECM proteins. The migrating epidermal cells dissect the wound, separating desiccated eschar from living or viable tissue. The migratory path is determined by both the degradation of injured tissue and the integrins expressed on the epidermal cell surfaces. Epidermal cells also secrete collagenases and metalloprotease-1 (MMP-1) to degrade the ECM ahead of their migratory path, and normal healing/balance studies have demonstrated that the edge-leading epidermal cells can also phagocytize debris. Cells behind the leading cells are stimulated to proliferate, thus resulting in epithelial cells moving in a tumbling motion across the wound surface until contact is established with the opposite edge. If the basement membrane is not intact, it must be repaired prior to epithelial cell migration. Local release of epidermal growth factor (EGF), tissue growth factor alpha (TGF-α), and keratinocyte growth factor (KGF), along with the increased expression of their receptors, may also stimulate this process. **TABLE 2-9** summarizes in detail the growth factors secreted and the cells responsible for their production, as well as the cells influenced by those growth factors.

Basement membrane proteins, such as laminin, appear in a highly ordered sequence proliferating from the wound margin inward. Laminins are a family of glycoproteins that provide an integral part of the structural scaffolding of the basement membrane in almost every animal tissue. Each laminin is a heterotrimer (large protein) assembled from alpha, beta, and gamma chain subunits, secreted and incorporated into cell-associated extracellular matrices. The laminins are unique, in that they can self-assemble, bind to other matrix macromolecules, and have shared cell interactions mediated by integrins and other receptors. Through the interactions with other cells, laminins contribute to cell differentiation, cell shape and movement, and maintenance of tissue phenotypes, as well as promote tissue

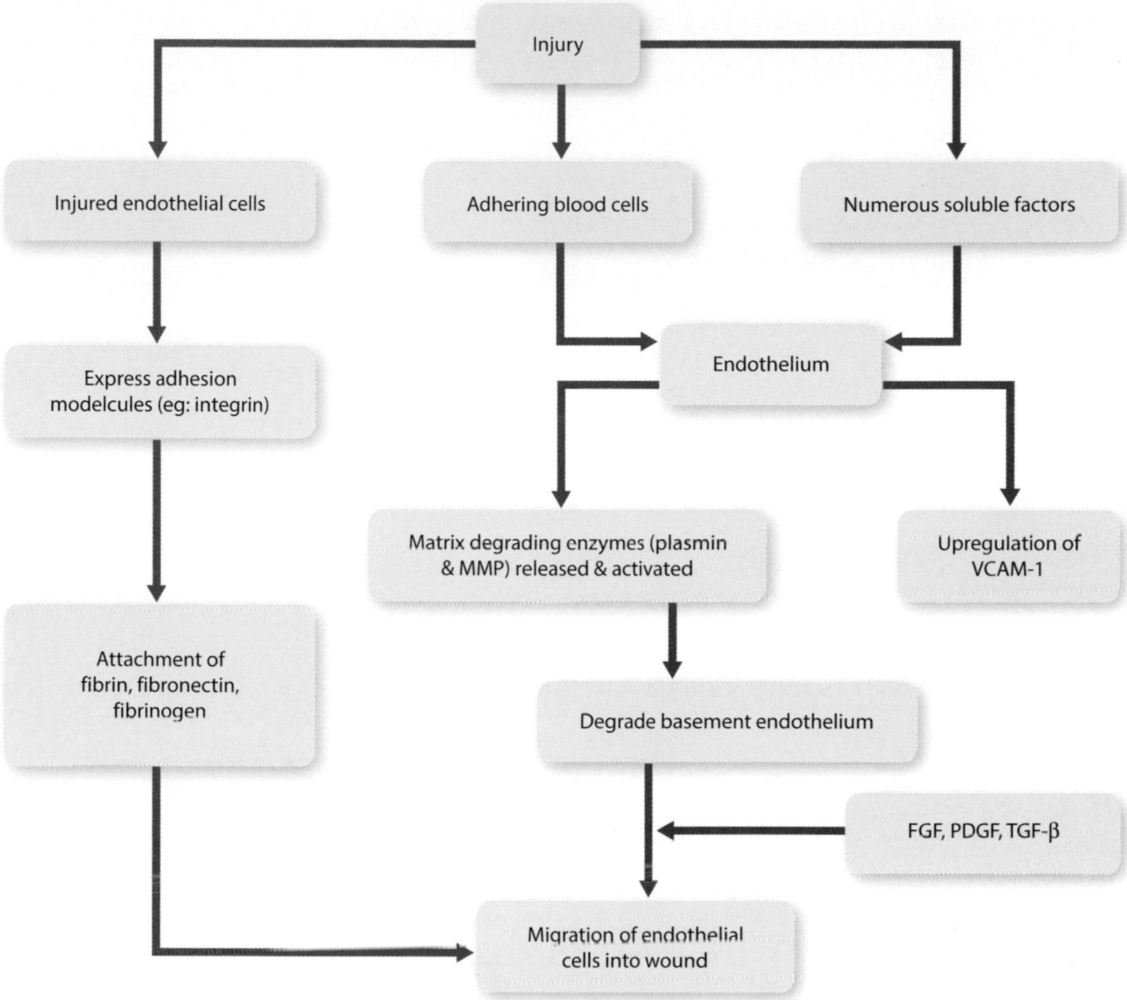

FIGURE 2-30 Angiogenesis overview. Two parallel signaling pathways, one mediated through the injured endothelial cells and the other via the endothelium itself, are necessary for angiogenesis to occur.

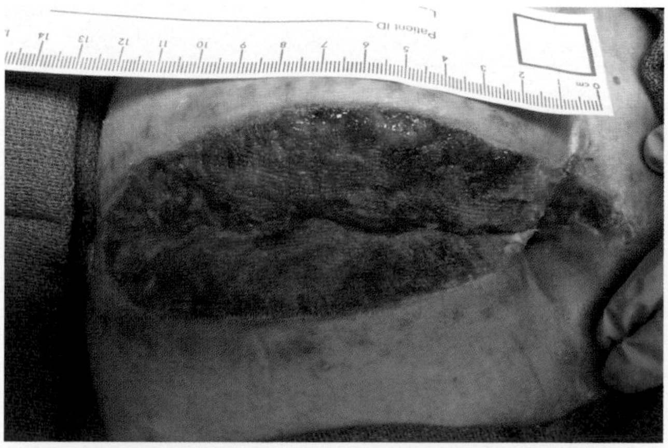

FIGURE 2-31 Granulating wound bed. When the signaling pathways occur in a timely sequence, healthy, beefy red granulation forms in the wound bed, supporting the migration of epithelial cells at the edges.

survival. After the wound is completely re-epithelialized, the cells again become columnar, stratified, and firmly attached to the newly constructed basement membrane and underlying dermis.[17,87] Although the wound may be fully re-epithelialized and closed, it is not referred to as *healed* until the next, final stage of wound healing is completed.

4. Maturation and Remodeling

Restored Function The final stage of the wound healing process consists of *dermal regeneration, wound contraction,* and *programmed involution of the granulation tissue.* Wound contraction occurs in a centripetal fashion, involving the full thickness of the wound and periwound tissue (**FIGURE 2-37**). The primary goal of wound contraction is to aid in the reduction of wound size and reduce the amount of disorganized scar tissue.[88] Wound contraction occurs through complex interactions between the ECM and fibroblasts; aborted cell

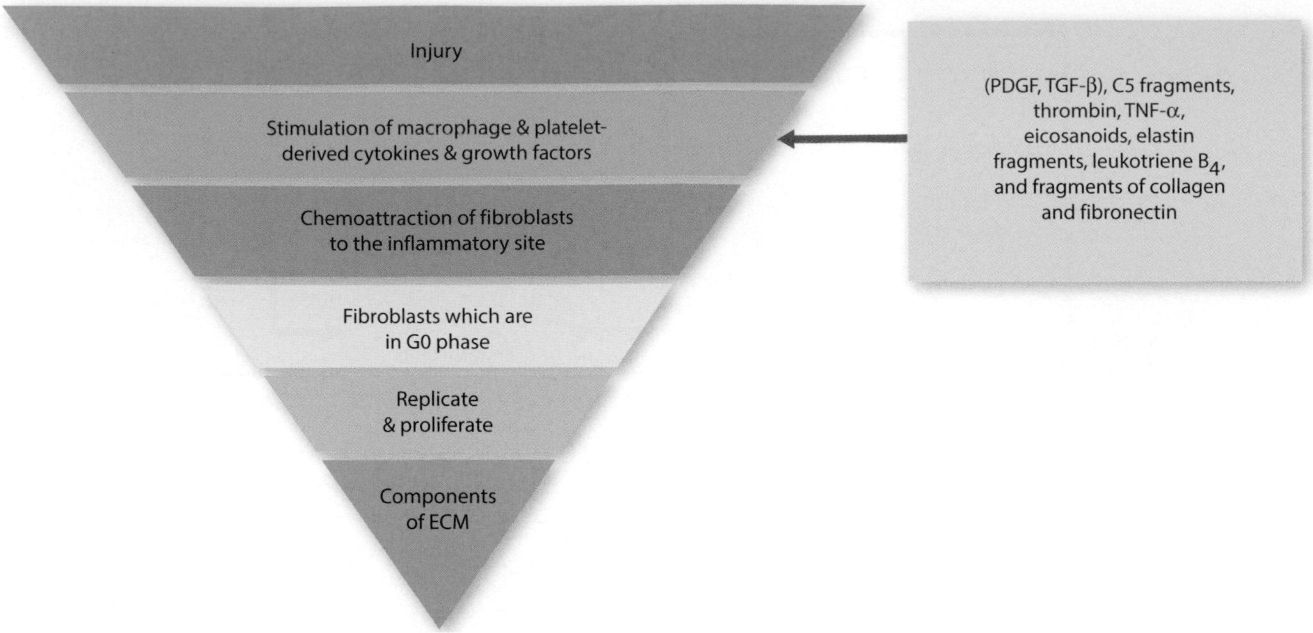

FIGURE 2-32 Fibroplasia overview. The pyramid of activities specific to fibroplasia culminate in the manufacturing of the ECM.

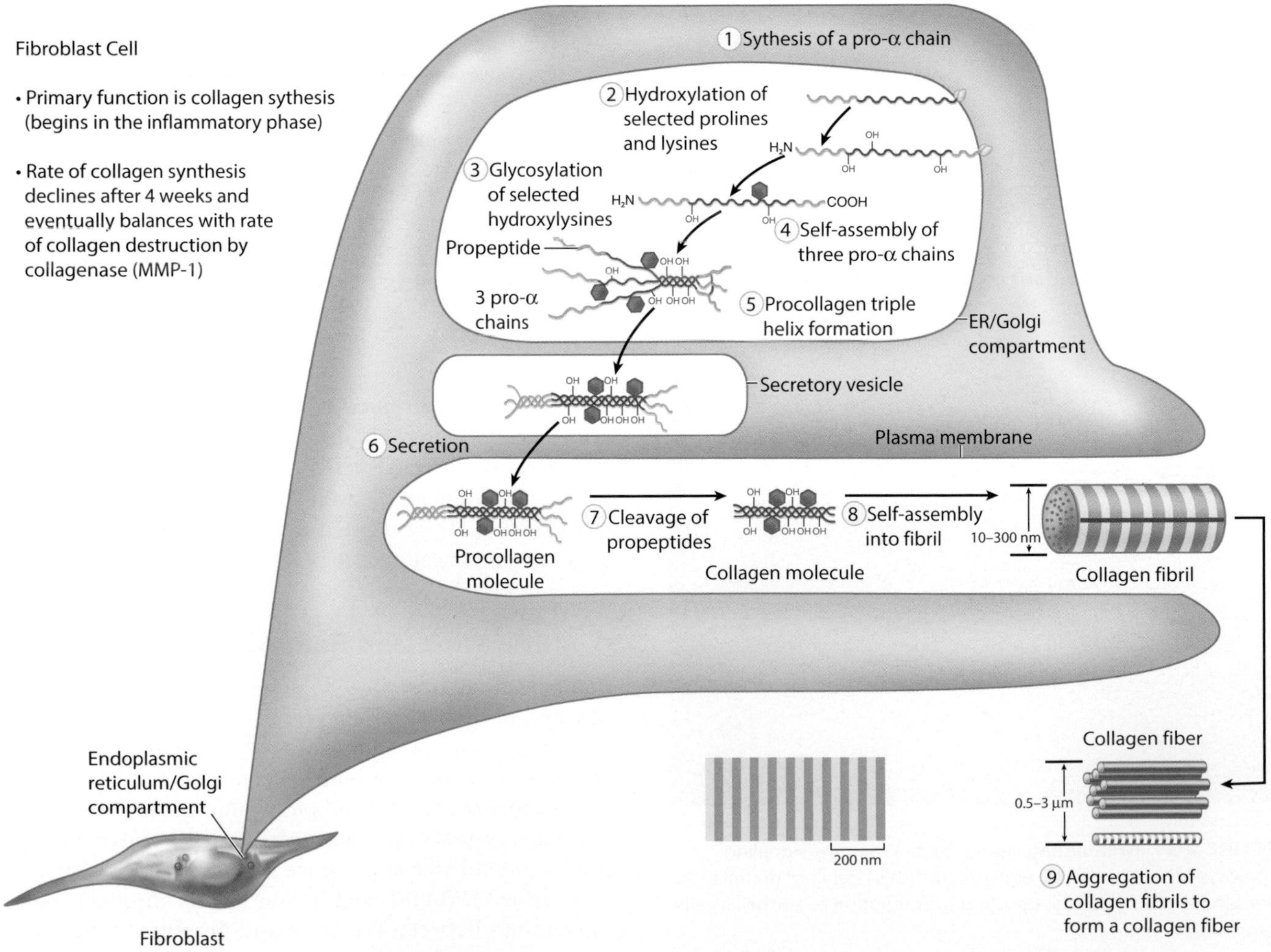

FIGURE 2-33 Collagen synthesis. Collagen synthesis occurs primarily in the fibroblast. This figure illuminates both the intracellular and extracellular steps required to produce collagen fibers, which are an integral part of the ECM.

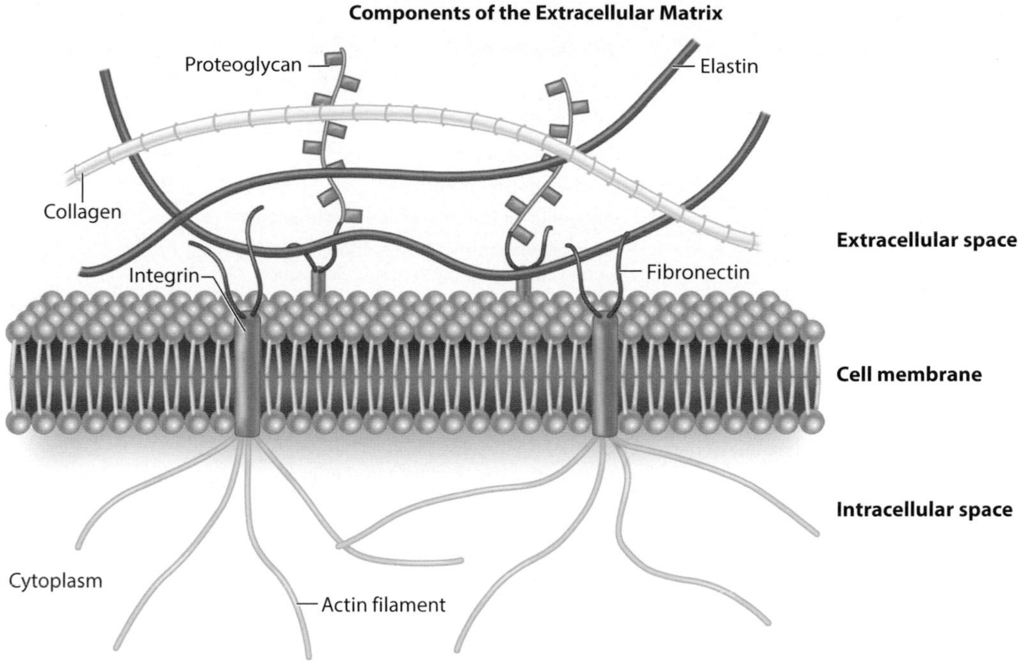

FIGURE 2-34 Components of extracellular matrix. The two primary components of ECM are proteoglycans interlaced with collagen and elastin. The tissue cells are attached to fibronectin through integrins. These integrins are components of the cellular membrane and are attached to actin filaments in the cell cytoplasm.

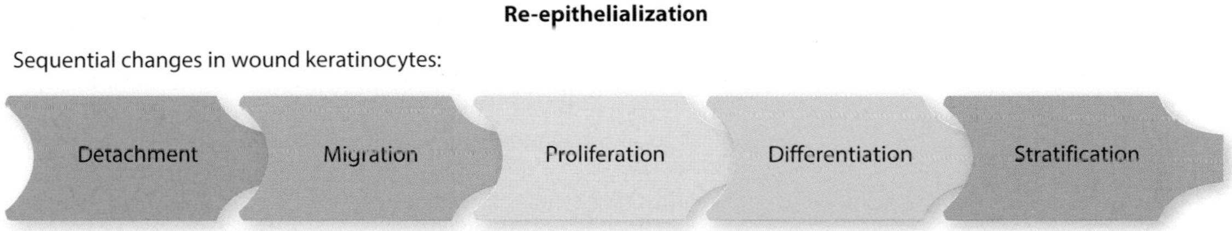

FIGURE 2-35 Re-epithelialization. Re-epithelialization occurs sequentially and is actively displayed in keratinocytes. The keratinocytes detach from the edges, migrate toward the wound center, proliferate, differentiate, and finally stratify to form new epithelium.

TABLE 2-8 Re-epithelialization Highlights

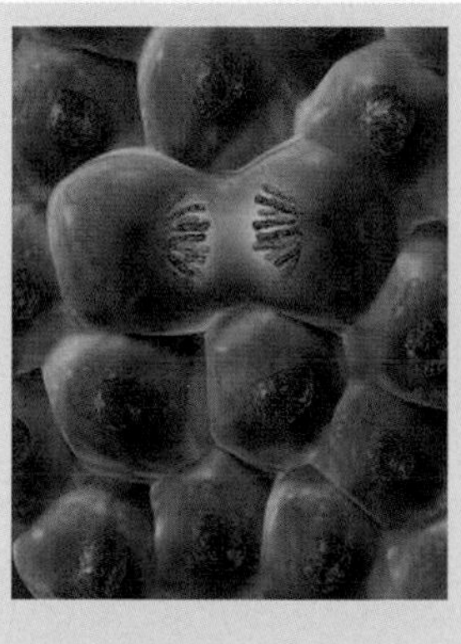	▪ Epidermal cells express integrin receptors that allow them to interact with ECM proteins (fibronectin and others) ▪ Migrating cells dissect the wound by separating the desiccated eschar from viable tissue ▪ Path of dissection is determined by the integrins that the epidermal cells express on their cell membranes ▪ Degradation of the ECM, required if epidermal cells are to migrate between the collagenous dermis and fibrin eschar, is driven by epidermal cell production of collagenase (MMP-I) and plasminogen activator, which activates collagenase and plasmin ▪ Migrating cells are also phagocytic and remove debris in their path ▪ Cells behind the leading edge of migrating cells begin to proliferate. The epithelial cells move in a leapfrog and tumbling fashion until the edges establish contact ▪ If the basement membrane zone is not intact, it will be repaired first ▪ Absence of neighboring cells at the wound margin may be a signal for the migration and proliferation of epidermal cells ▪ Local release of EGF, TGF-α, and KGF and increased expression of their receptors may also stimulate these processes ▪ Basement membrane proteins, such as laminin, reappear in a highly ordered sequence from the margin of the wound inward ▪ After the wound is completely re-epithelialized, the cells become columnar and stratified again while firmly attaching to the reestablished basement membrane and underlying dermis

TABLE 2-9 Growth Factors

Growth Factor	Principal Source	Primary Activity	Comments
Epidermal growth factor (EGF)	Submaxillary gland, Brunner gland, platelets, and macrophage	Promotes proliferation of fibroblast, keratinocyte, and epithelial cells in wound healing	
Fibroblast growth factor (FGF)	Wide range of cells including fibroblast, macrophage, mast cells, and endothelial cells Protein is associated with the ECM	Fibroblast proliferation Chemotactic for fibroblasts Mitogenic for fibroblasts and keratinocytes Stimulates keratinocyte migration, angiogenesis, wound contraction, and matrix deposition	At least 18 family members. Uses five distinct receptors
Insulin growth factor (IGF-1)	Macrophages and fibroblasts	Stimulates synthesis of sulfated proteoglycans, collagen, keratinocyte migration, and fibroblast proliferation Endocrine effects are similar to those of growth hormone Promotes cell proliferation. Related to IGF-2 and proinsulin, also called somatomedin C	
Keratinocyte growth factor (KGF)	Fibroblasts	Stimulates keratinocyte migration, proliferation, and differentiation	
Platelet-derived growth factor (PDGF)	Platelets, endothelial cells, macrophages, keratinocytes, placenta	Promotes proliferation of connective tissue and smooth muscle cells Chemotactic for monocytes, PMNs, and fibroblasts Activates PMNs, macrophages, and fibroblasts Neo-angiogenesis—mitogenic for fibroblasts and endothelial cells Wound remodeling—stimulates production of MMPs, fibronectin, and HA	X-ray crystal structure is very similar to that of VEGF[13,67] Two different protein chains, which form three distinct dimers: AA, AB, BB SMALL-molecule PDGF is active during the initial stages of hemostasis, while LARGE-molecule PDGF is activated during the later stages of proliferation and remodeling
Transforming growth factor β (TGF-β)	Activated Th1 cells (T-helper), natural killer (NK) cells, platelets, macrophages, keratinocytes, and fibroblasts	Anti-inflammatory (suppresses cytokine production and MHC class II expression), promotes wound healing Chemotactic for PMNs, macrophages, lymphocytes, and fibroblasts Inhibits macrophage and lymphocyte proliferation[7] Stimulates TIMP synthesis, keratinocyte migration, angiogenesis, and fibroplasia Inhibits production of MMPs and keratinocyte proliferation Induces TGF-β production	Over 100 different family members Promotes differentiation of fibroblast into myofibroblast[10]
Transforming growth factor α (TGF-α)	Occurs in transformed cells Macrophages, T-lymphocytes, keratin	Important for normal wound healing	Related to EGF
Vascular endothelial cell growth factor (VEGF)	Keratinocytes	Increases vasopermeability, mitogenic for endothelial cells	

locomotion, phenotypic change from fibroblast to myofibroblast, and the expression of TGF-β1 and MMP-3 are all important for the process. Aborted cell locomotion results in the bunching and contraction of collagen fibers. Fibroblasts undergo cellular changes and become myofibroblasts that express α-smooth muscle actin (αSMA). TGF-β1 promotes wound contraction by increasing the expression of β1 integrin. Stromelysin, or MMP-3, through the utilization of integrin β1, allows for the modification of attachment sites between fibroblasts and collagen fibers by degrading the ECM components.

During remodeling, the number of fibroblasts and myofibroblasts decreases, the dense capillary network regresses, and wound tensile strength gradually increases. The early epidermal–dermal interface is fragile because it lacks the interlocking rete pegs, making the newly healed wound at risk for avulsion with minor trauma. Apoptosis of myofibroblasts, endothelial cells, and macrophages results in tissue composed primarily of ECM proteins, particularly collagen type III. Metalloproteinases produced by the epidermal cells, endothelial cells, fibroblasts, and macrophages that remain in the scar continue the process of remodeling, replacing collagen type III with collagen type I.[62,66,69,89] The resulting tissue "patch" has approximately 80% of the tensile strength of the original tissue but will have completely reestablished function.[90–93]

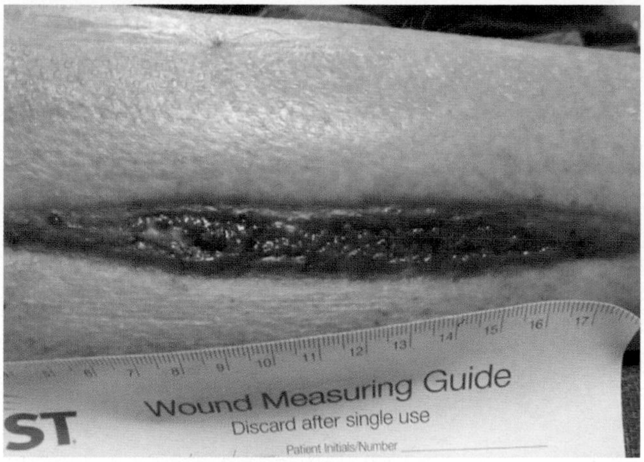

FIGURE 2-36 Re-epithelialization of a wound. Re-epithelialization is visible at the wound edges, especially on both ends where the basement membrane and the new epithelial cells are migrating toward the center. Some of the edges have hypergranulation and may need to be treated with pressure or calcium nitrate in order to decrease the granulation cells so that the epithelial cells can move toward full closure.

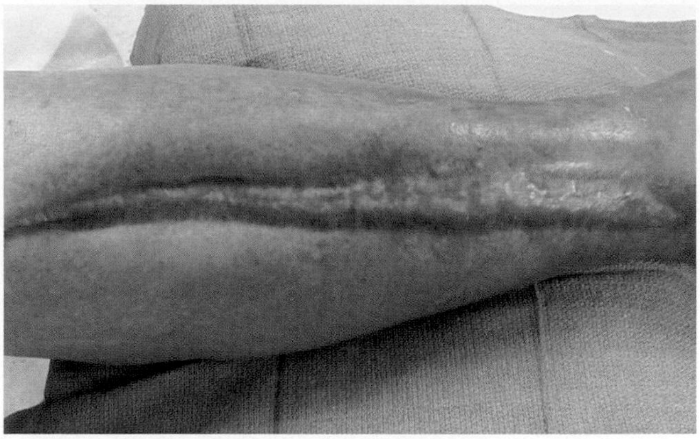

FIGURE 2-37 Maturation and remodeling. A fasciotomy wound on the lower extremity is in the remodeling phase of healing. Although the wound is fully epithelialized, it is not considered healed until the granulation tissue scar recedes, the type III collagen matrix is replaced with type I, and optimal function to the tissue is restored with tensile strength sufficient to prevent epithelial cracking and tearing.

CLEARING AND CONTAINING THE INVADER (IE, PREVENTING INFECTION)

Most pathogenic microorganisms have evolved mechanisms to overcome *innate* immune responses and thus continue to grow. An *adaptive* immune response is required to eliminate the pathogenic invader and prevent subsequent reinfection. Both the innate and adaptive immune responses are active in each phase of wound healing.

Immediately During Clot Formation

In addition to preventing blood and tissue loss, the clot formation recruits the innate immune system to clear debris and pathogens. Platelets are critical in the following three areas: (1) initiation of the clotting cascade, (2) formation of a platelet plug (the outer surface of activated platelets becomes sticky with a mucopolysaccharide coating), and (3) release of cytokines and alpha granules. The fibrin provides an infrastructure for the clot and mechanical entrapment of debris and invaders. TGF-β1 and TGF-β2 are released by the platelets and attract macrophages to the site of injury. Macrophages in turn express IL-1 which stimulates antigen-presenting cells (APCs) to produce IL-8. Subsequently, IL 8 both signals and directs neutrophil migration and margination while simultaneously upregulating "sticky factors" and vascular permeability to expedite the process. The recruitment of both macrophage and neutrophils (PMNs) immediately to the site of injury begins the process of invader identification and clearing.[3]

Innate Immunity

The innate immune response occurs with the migration and extravasation of PMNs from the neighboring vasculature. The extravasation, migration, and proliferation are facilitated by TGF-β1, a growth factor released by the platelets and macrophages that have migrated to the wounded tissue. Neutrophils are the first inflammatory, innate immune system cells to infiltrate a wound; they do so in large numbers in response to the numerous inflammatory cytokines produced by endothelial cells, activated platelets, and degradation products from invading pathogens.[71] Neutrophils undergo programmed cell death (apoptosis) shortly after infiltration, thus releasing additional cytokines that recruit macrophages to the wound site.[46]

Neutrophils, or PMNs, exhibit several important defense mechanisms including (1) NETs, (2) the release of azurophilic pore-forming granules, and (3) phagocytosis and programmed apoptosis.[4] NETs are the result of the neutrophils expelling chromatin, a very sticky substance, and thus serve to mechanically entrap the pathogen (**FIGURE 2-38**). Once entrapped, proteases, elastases, pore-forming granules, and other cytotoxic molecules lyse the invader. Both the entrapment and the lysis of the invader serve to increase the visibility of the intruder to the host immune system.[94] Neutrophils are also capable of direct phagocytosis of an invader. The programmed apoptosis of neutrophils releases proinflammatory cytokines, attracts additional macrophages, and upregulates the key activities of macrophages. Th1 (innate immune system) neutrophils produce interferon gamma (IFN-γ), which both upregulates macrophage activity and alters the macrophage phenotype to a WAM, which characteristically produces increased nitric oxide (NO) and H_2O_2. Both NO and H_2O_2 acidify the environment and the lower pH serves to increase phagocytosis and may thereby increase healing rates.[95] In addition, the WAMs display increased major histocompatibility complex class II (MHC class II) for the presentation of antigens specific to an invader to the adaptive immune system.[96,97] Both neutrophils and macrophages are important to the immediate containment of the invader and the activation of the adaptive (memory/B-cell) immune system of the host.

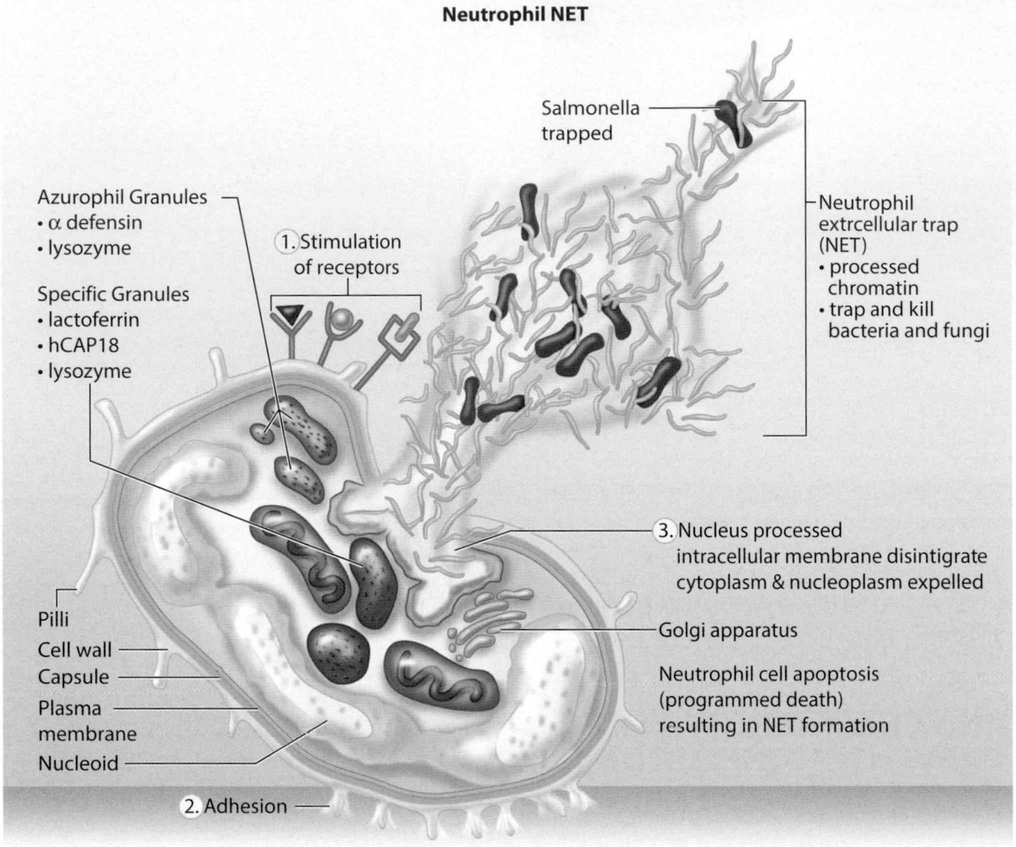

FIGURE 2-38 Neutrophil extracellular traps. Neutrophils expel chromatin, a very sticky substance, which results in the formation of neutrophil extracellular traps (NETs). The NET is expressed in response to the stimulation of receptors, the adhesion of neutrophils, and the disintegration of intracellular membrane and expulsion of cytoplasm and nucleoplasm. The NET mechanism thus serves as a means to trap pathogenic bacteria.

T-lymphocytes are inflammatory immune cells that routinely invade the wound. Although less numerous than macrophages, they bridge the transition from the inflammatory to the proliferative phase and their depletion decreases wound strength and collagen content. T-lymphocytes affect fibroblast function by producing stimulatory cytokines like IL-2, fibroblast activating factor, and inhibitory cytokines (including TGF-β, TNF-α, and IFN-γ). The role of IFN-γ secreted by T-lymphocytes is illustrated in **FIGURE 2-39**. When macrophages are exposed to IFN-γ, their destructive inflammatory capability is amplified and the inflammatory responses are prolonged; thus, the effects of IFN-γ are far-reaching and may be an important mediator of chronic nonhealing wounds.[98]

Adaptive Immunity

Adaptive immunity, or *learned immunity*, is triggered by the first responders, namely macrophages. Macrophages enhance APC's activity, thereby aiding in the presentation of antigens (*anti*body *gen*erator) to the host immune system T cells. Bacterial proteins degraded by host proteases are ingested by macrophages and become antigens, which are then presented by macrophages to T cells via MHC class II receptors on the macrophage surface. Once a T cell binds to the loaded MHC class II receptor, the T cell becomes activated and begins secreting IL-2. IL-2 stimulates T cells to divide and activates the T-cell phenotypic expression of IL-2 receptors, thus resulting in autocrine lymphocyte proliferation and activation (**FIGURE 2-40**).

The dendritic cells, another important APC, migrate to local lymph nodes and present the antigens to resident cells. If the antigen presented is recognized by existing memory B cells, those B cells are activated, and clonal expansion is triggered. In addition, macrophages produce IL-2, a powerful cytokine that drives T cells to become Th2 helper cells, and thereby increases the effectiveness of B cells.[3]

The B cells produce and release antibodies resulting in an increased number of circulating antibodies specific to the pathogen (eg, MRSA, MSSA, VRE). As a result, either neutralization or opsonization can more effectively occur. *Neutralization* occurs with the binding of an antibody to the pathogen, thus blocking access to host cells. *Opsonization* refers to the coating of the pathogen with antibody, thereby increasing the ease of identification and subsequent clearance and phagocytosis.[3] These cellular and acellular events that occur throughout wound healing work to prevent

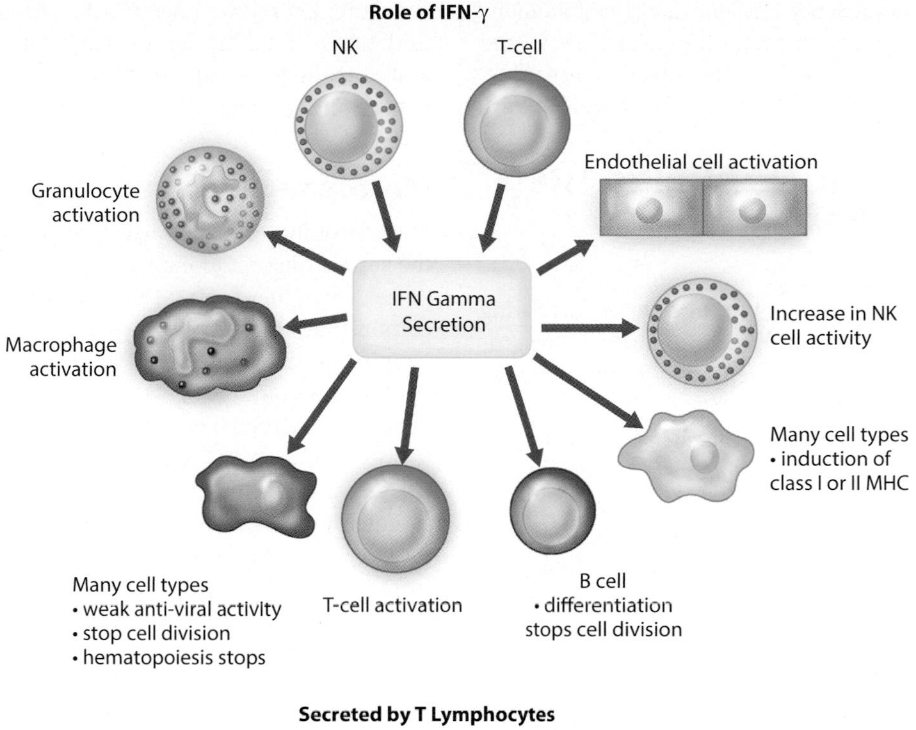

FIGURE 2-39 Role of IFN-γ. IFN-γ is an important cytokine intimately involved in the inflammatory response. IFN-γ stimulates macrophages while simultaneously suppressing collagen synthesis and the release of prostaglandin. At the same time, IFN-γ activates T cells and hence the innate immune response.

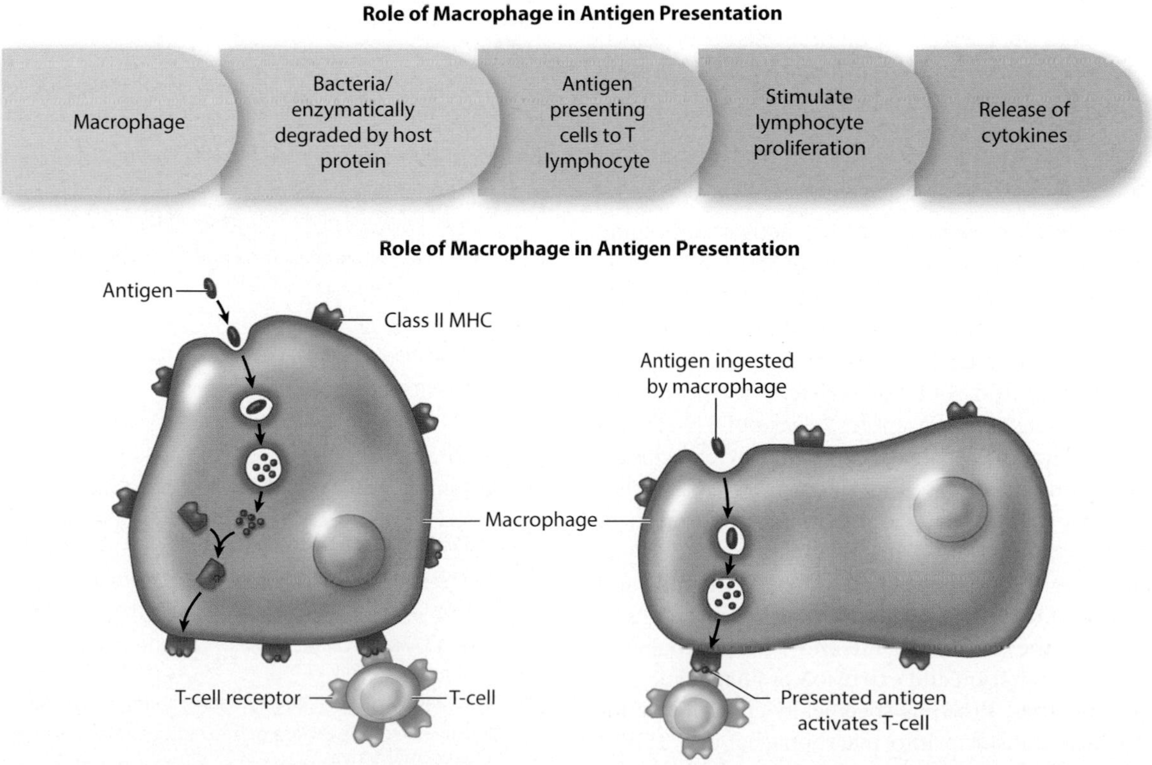

FIGURE 2-40 Role of macrophages in antigen presentation. Macrophages also have a role in presenting antigen. This schematic demonstrates the process by which a macrophage activates the innate immune system. Antigen (bacterial components, PAMPs) uptake by the macrophage is processed and coupled to an MHC class II protein on the cell surface of the macrophage. The antigen–MHC class II complex is recognized by circulating T cells. Once coupled, the T cell is activated and the production of IL-2 results. IL-2 stimulates the expression of T-cell IL-2 receptors and T-cell mitosis.

infection. If the processes are not efficient due to autoimmune deficiencies or too many pathogens for the host to manage, wound healing is impaired and usually stalls in the inflammatory phase, as discussed in Chapter 12, Factors That Impede Wound Healing.

CELL METAMORPHOSIS DURING THE HEALING RESPONSE

Introduction

Typically, a cell has a unique phenotype and set of correlating functions; however, during wound healing, platelets, macrophages, and fibroblasts undergo phenotypic changes with a change in function.

Platelets, although anucleate, provide chemical messengers at the point of initial injury to achieve hemostasis. Alpha granules contained within the platelets release PDGF, platelet factor IV, and TGF-β1, which function during the proliferative phase of healing to accelerate granulation and connective tissue proliferation.[4] *Macrophages*, usually thought of as phagocytes, transition from APCs to phagocytes, to chief-air-traffic-controllers, adapting their cytokine phenotype expression profile to move the healing cascade forward and thus accelerate closure. *Fibroblasts* are vital early during clot construction, granulation tissue formation, and neo-angiogenesis. During the later stages of proliferation and early remodeling, under the influence of TGF-β,[46] fibroblasts change phenotype and become myofibroblasts. The myofibroblasts facilitate centripetal, full-thickness, wound edge approximation, thus decreasing the overall size of the wound. The specific characteristics and effects of these cells are presented in **TABLES 2-1** and **2-9**, which list the growth factors and signaling that occurs throughout wound healing.

Platelets

Platelets at the site of an acute injury are activated, become "sticky," and adhere to the adjacent endothelium while simultaneously ejecting ADP. Together, these two actions promote the initiation of the clotting cascade and the clumping of thrombocytes. The initial goal is clot formation. The further release of alpha granules from the platelets transforms the clot to an "active" state. Alpha granules release PDGF (in two forms: small- and large-molecule PDGF) and platelet factor IV, as well as TGF-β, into the surrounding tissues. PDGF, a chemotactic substance for fibroblasts, draws increased numbers of fibroblasts to the wounded tissue. In coordination with TGF-β, PDGF modulates mitosis of fibroblasts. Both the attraction and increased mitotic activity elevate the number of fibroblasts in direct proximity to the wound.[4] PDGF and TGF-β simultaneously facilitate the migration and extrusion of phagocytic cells from nearby capillaries. PDGF is specifically chemotactic for monocytes (which transform into macrophages) and TGF-β for PMNs. This initiates the cleaning of the wound.

During the proliferative phase when new tissue formation begins, large-molecule PDGF is again key by promoting neo-angiogenesis. In summary, the platelets perform the following functions: (1) serve as a component of the physical clotting structure, (2) release chemical messengers important for the initiation of autolytic debridement by macrophage and PMNs, and (3) continue to function during the proliferative phase by stimulating angiogenesis via PDGF release.[99]

Macrophages

The morphing of macrophages begins when monocytes leave the vessels adjacent to injured tissue and transition into macrophages when they enter the interstitial tissue. Macrophages then demonstrate myriad phenotypes, levels of activation, and differentiation based on the phase of wound healing. Their ability to differentiate into M1, WAM, or M2 repair macrophages highlights the macrophages' complex plasticity and responsiveness to the wound (**TABLE 2-10** and **FIGURE 2-41**). The phenotypic changes are not merely a passive result of the wound milieu or environment; macrophages are actively directed and either delay or advance the healing process. Macrophages transition from an innate immune cell (phagocyte and APC) and then differentiate into a proinflammatory cell, an immune-regulatory cell (during proliferation and re-epithelization), or a phagocytic cell aiding in tissue remodel. See **TABLE 2-11** for a summary of the important proinflammatory and anti-inflammatory cytokines produced by macrophages to direct wound healing in both the inflammatory and resolution phases.[100]

TABLE 2-10 Macrophage Function

Macrophages are the second inflammatory cells to invade a wound and transform into wound-activated macrophages (WAMs).
▪ Second population of inflammatory cells to invade the wound • Chemotaxis of migrating blood monocytes occur in 24–48 hours
▪ One cell that is truly central to wound healing • Orchestrate the release of cytokines • Stimulates many of the subsequent processes of wound healing
▪ Chemotactic factors specific for monocytes include • Bacterial products • Fibronectin • Complement degradation products (C5a) • Collagen • Thrombin • TGF-β
▪ Transformation into wound-activated macrophage (M1) • Activated integrin expression promotes adhesion-mediated gene induction in monocytes • Induces transformation into wound macrophages • Activates lysis of bacterial debris (lipopolysaccharide) • Activates monocytes to release • Free radicals • Cytokines that mediate angiogenesis and fibroplasia • IL-2 increases the release of free radicals and thus enhances bactericidal activity • Activity of the free radicals is potentiated by IL-2
▪ WAMs (M1) phenotypically demonstrate • Increased phagocytic activity • Elevated selective expression of proinflammatory cytokines

FIGURE 2-41 Role of macrophage transition and differentiation in wound healing

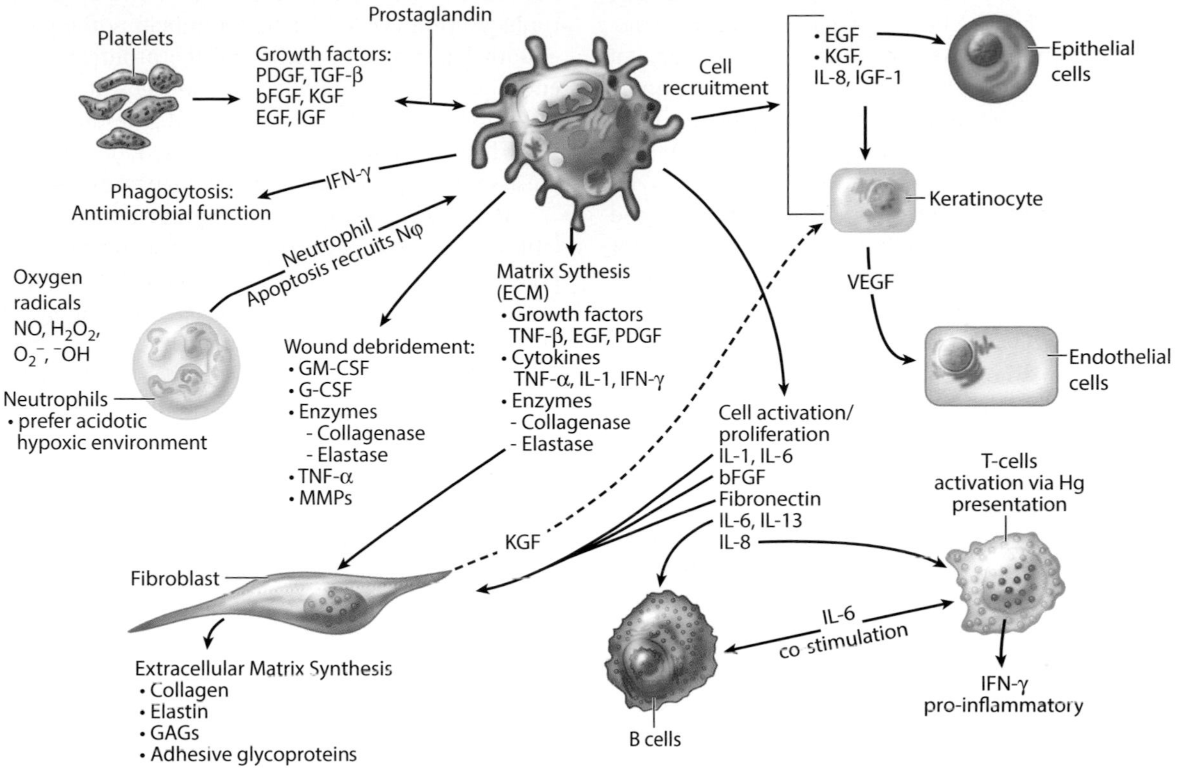

Macrophages are central to wound healing and direct:

1. Production of growth factors
2. Phagocytosis
3. Wound debridement
4. Matrix synthesis
5. Cell activation and proliferation
6. Cell recruitment

TABLE 2-11 Cytokine Activity in Wound Healing

Proinflammatory Cytokines		
CYTOKINE	CELL SOURCE	BIOLOGIC ACTIVITY
TNF-α	Macrophages	PMN margination and cytotoxicity, with or without collagen synthesis; provides metabolic substrate
IL-1	Macrophages Keratinocytes	Fibroblast and keratinocyte chemotaxis, collagen synthesis
IL-2	T-lymphocytes	Increases fibroblast infiltration and metabolism
IL-6	Macrophages PMNs Fibroblasts	Fibroblast proliferation, hepatic acute phase protein synthesis
IL-8	Macrophages Fibroblasts	Macrophage and PMN chemotaxis, keratinocyte maturation
IFN-γ	T-lymphocytes Macrophages	Activates macrophages and PMNs, retards collagen synthesis and cross-linking, stimulates collagenase activity
Anti-inflammatory Cytokines		
CYTOKINE	CELL SOURCE	BIOLOGIC ACTIVITY
IL-4	T-lymphocytes Basophils Mast cells	Inhibition of TNF, IL-1, IL-6 production; fibroblast proliferation, collagen synthesis
IL-10	T-lymphocytes Macrophages Keratinocytes	Inhibition of TNF, IL-1, IL-6 production; inhibition of macrophage and PMN activation

Only a few macrophages are typically located in the dermis and function as surveillance macrophages. Neutrophil apoptosis during the first 24 hours after injury signals macrophages to massively infiltrate the wound. The numbers of macrophages are the greatest and most elevated beginning approximately 2 days after injury. During this phase, macrophages demonstrate increased antigen presentation and phagocytic activity.[46]

The WAMs produce free radicals (NO, H_2O_2, O_2^-) and proinflammatory cytokines, including TNF-α, IL1β, IL-6, or IL-12. These M1 macrophages also overexpress MHC class II molecules which present antigens to T cells and B cells to activate both innate and adaptive immune system responses.[97] The antigen presentation is largely via MHC class II complexes. Antigens presented by MHC class II molecules are derived from extracellular proteins of the pathogen, for example, a bacterium that may be infecting the wound. The loading of the MHC class II complex occurs after phagocytosis by the macrophages. The extracellular proteins are endocytosed and ingested by lysosomes, and signature peptides unique to the specific invader are loaded onto the MHC class II complex and then presented on the macrophage cell surface. Thus, in the early phase of healing the macrophages are both phagocytic and important in stimulating the immune system (**FIGURE 2-42**).

During the inflammatory and proliferative phase when new tissue formation and angiogenesis are occurring, macrophages produce VEGF, thus stimulating the recruitment of endothelial progenitor cells and the proliferation of existing endothelium.[101] In addition, macrophages are also vital to lymphangiogenesis, as $VEGF_c$ and $VEGF_D$ modulate this process. It has been demonstrated that decreased macrophage numbers are associated with decreased lymphangiogenesis.

Remodeling begins with the gradual involution of granulation tissue and simultaneous dermal renewal. During this phase, apoptosis of a significant percentage of macrophages occurs. The remaining macrophages will facilitate the remodeling process by cleaning up the cellular and matrix debris. This ECM debris is largely a result of the cellular apoptosis and the degradation of collagen type III by metalloproteinases produced by epidermal and endothelial cells[75] (**FIGURE 2-41**).

Although the phenotype of undifferentiated macrophages that infiltrate dermal wounds is not fully characterized, the evidence supports the changing role of the macrophage during the phases of healing.[5,102] This suggests that this one cell, the macrophage, has different and diverse roles throughout the phases of skin or wound regeneration.[27,101] **FIGURE 2-41** and **TABLE 2-12** summarize macrophage functions.

In addition, it has now been demonstrated that monocytes not only morph into M1 (inflammatory) or M2 (proliferative)

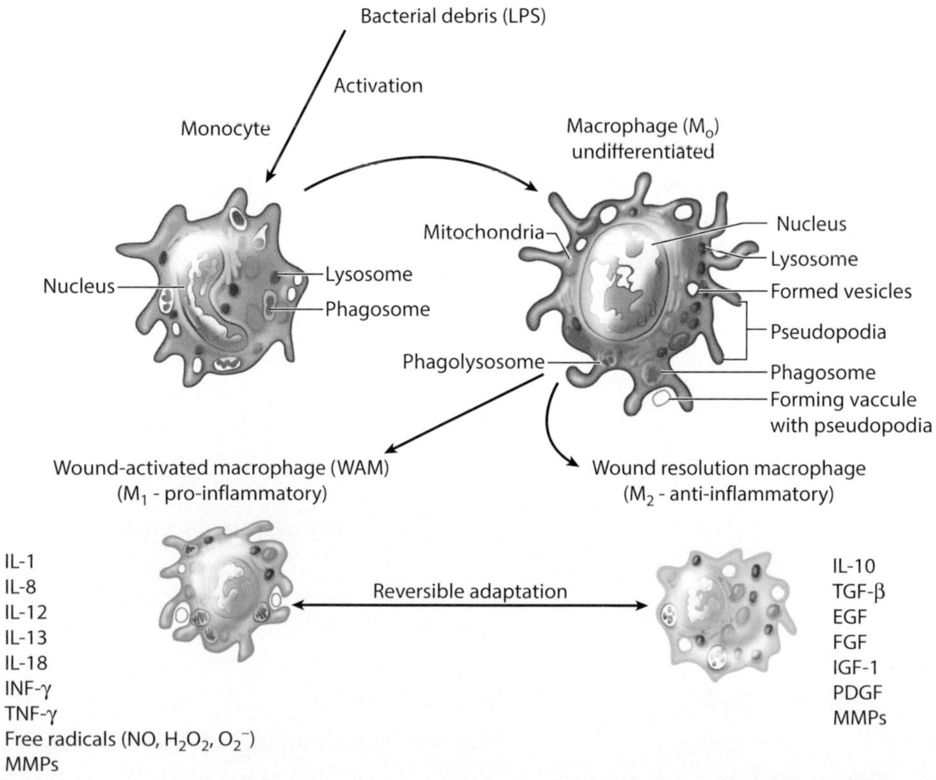

FIGURE 2-42 Phagocytic activity of macrophages. Macrophages originate from the differentiation of monocytes. The undifferentiated macrophage (M_0) can change into either a WAM or an anti-inflammatory macrophage (M_2). There is evidence that phenotypically WAMs can change into M_2 macrophages, and M_2 macrophages can become WAMs. This demonstrates the fluid phenotypic shift that macrophage can undergo in direct response to wound milieu.

TABLE 2-12 Functions of Macrophages in Wound Healing

1. Facilitate apoptosis of polymorphic neutrophilic leukocytes
2. Permit surface recognition of opsonized pathogens and facilitate phagocytosis
3. Produce nitric oxide, which has antimicrobial properties
4. Induce phospholipase; enzymatic degradation of the cell membrane phospholipids ensues, releasing thromboxane A2 and prostaglandin F2α
5. Release leukotriene B4 & C4—potent neutrophil chemoattractant
6. Release proteinases, including matrix metalloproteinases (MMP-1, MMP-2, MMP-3, and MMP-9), which degrade the ECM and are crucial for removing foreign material, promoting cell movement through tissue spaces, and regulating ECM turnover
7. Release growth factors that stimulate fibroblast, endothelial cell, and keratinocyte proliferation

macrophages, they can also differentiate into dendritic cells that present antigens and alter the cell-signaling. When monocytes infiltrate tissues, they differentiate into mo-Macs (monocyte-derived macrophages) or mo-DCs (monocyte-derived dendritic cells) which present antigens to T cells. In persistent chronic inflammation, T-cell stimulation by mo-DCs becomes deleterious. It is known that mo-DCs secrete high amounts of interleukin-23 (IL-23) and stimulate helper-type T cells (T_H17 cells). Blocking monocyte differentiation/phenotype switching is now emerging as a potential therapeutic strategy for inflammatory disorders.[103]

Fibroblasts

Fibroblasts begin to infiltrate the wound during the later inflammation and early proliferation phases and are involved in granular tissue formation, cytokine production to increase keratinocyte proliferation/migration, and differentiation of fibroblasts into myofibroblasts. The primary function of fibroblasts is synthesis of collagen, a process that begins in the inflammation phase and continues throughout the healing process. After the fourth week, the rate of collagen synthesis declines, approaching equilibrium with the demolished collagen as a result of the presence of MMP-1. At this point the wound enters a phase of collagen maturation.

During the maturation phase, fibroblasts undergo a phenotypical change and become activated myofibroblasts, expressing αSMA. During wound contraction, myofibroblasts generate centripetal forces across the wound and throughout the entire depth by contracting the αSMA fibers. The contractile force generated by the myofibroblasts serves to approximate wound edges and continually decrease the wound volume during healing.[104]

Two proposed mechanisms for the phenotypic change from fibroblast to myofibroblast are (1) interstitial flow and (2) TGF-β1. Interstitial flow through shear stress on the cells directly or via strain on fibroblast-to-ECM attachment may further trigger TGF-β1 expression.[105] TGF-β1 expression drives αSMA expression as the fibroblasts differentiate into myofibroblasts and align the matrix fibers.[14–16,106]

CHRONIC WOUNDS

Cutaneous wounds result from a breech in the skin or epithelium and are generally classified as either acute or chronic. Acute wounds are those that resolve without incident in an anticipated time frame, typically 21 days or less, and restore the skin structural and functional integrity.[66] Chronic or hard-to-heal wounds, by contrast, result from an inadequate or disrupted healing process and are defined as those wounds that neither follow a normal trajectory nor restore the skin functional and structural integrity.[107] Chronic wounds can persist for months or years,[108] disrupting patients' lives, interfering with their ability to work, contributing to disfigurement or amputation, and costing the healthcare system billions of dollars each year.[109,110]

Chronic wounds are often cyclical with periods of healing followed by reoccurrence[98] and are known to have multifactorial etiology with impeding factors; **TABLE 2-13** lists the differences in healing that is observed with medications, aging, infection, or diseases. More factors that impede wound healing are discussed in depth in Chapter 12.

Chronic wounds usually stall in a proinflammatory, proteolytic-hostile environment that does not allow cell proliferation, migration, or differentiation. The three primary categories that provide the backdrop for the development of chronic wounds are the presence of foreign bodies, pathogenic invaders (eg, bacteria, virus, fungi, and mycobacterium), or underlying disease processes (eg, diabetes and circulatory disorders).[129] Removal of foreign bodies and sharp debridement can convert the stalled wound to an acute wound and thereby stimulate innate healing processes.[130] Chronic wounds associated with other diseases may or may not be associated with an acute trauma. Lack of acute injury without the expected healing cascade may explain the senescence of important cells. This cell senescence would include macrophages and the associated chemical signaling cascades that normally occur in response to tissue damage. Senescent cells are particularly susceptible and resulting cell-to-cell and cell-to-matrix signaling does not occur, and thus the normal progression of wound healing fails to ensue.[131]

Bacteria infect their host using two seemingly opposite strategies—either the immediate direct kill of the host cell to secure a nutrition source[132–134] or construction of biofilm[135–139] to establish a semipermanent microbial community. Direct kill requires the upregulation of planktonic bacterial genes, which supports "free floating,"[140] while biofilm construction requires expression of genes used to produce or manufacture attachments (integrins, adhesion molecules) to host or ECM structures.[136,141] The bacteria secrete a polysaccharide matrix construct to cover themselves, neighbors, and the progeny of both. This community evades host detection, antibiotic delivery, and innate and adaptive immune responses, thus providing fertile ground for the sharing and swapping of gene cassettes encoded with antibiotic resistance strategies (eg, efflux pump and deactivation).[142–144] In addition, the biofilm prevents the penetration of topical antimicrobials intended to decrease the surface bacteria count. The biofilm community feeds on the increased plasma exudate that is a result of the localized hyperinflammatory state produced by cellular

TABLE 2-13 Differences in Healing When Complicated by Drugs, Aging, Infection, or Disease

			Chronic		
				Disease State	
	Drugs	**Aging**	**Infection**	**Diabetes**	**Vascular**
Hemostasis ▪ Stop bleeding ▪ Contain invader		Clot formation			
Vascular events	Plavix—decreased platelet adhesion and activation. The antiaggregating property of clopidogrel is caused by an inhibition of the binding of ADP to its platelet receptors, and more specifically to the low affinity receptors[111–115]	Arteriosclerosis Atherosclerosis			
Cellular events		Decreased hemoglobin/hemocrit ↓ PDGF receptor expression[75]		↓ PDGF receptor expression[75]	
Cell signaling	Coumadin—interferes with clotting by interfering with the recycling of vitamin K, which interferes with prothrombin function[114]				
Inflammation Kill the invader Clear the debris Create new pathway for cell migration		Reactive chemotaxis			
Vascular events				Disproportionate expression of vascular cell adhesion molecules by endothelial cells. This increases extravasation and inflammatory cell accumulation	
Cellular events	Glucocorticoids are anti-inflammatory. Decrease insulin-like growth factor-1 (IGF-1). Leading to impaired fibroblast function. Cortisol may also lead to increased levels of proinflammatory cytokines and cytokine-induced tissue damage[116]			↑ Infiltration of WAM ↑ ECM (fibrotic) at wound edges[117] Altered sensitivity to VEGF[118]	
Cell signaling		Impaired signaling FGF—FGFR[119,120]	Impaired signaling FGF—FGFR[119,120]	Impaired signaling FGF—FGFR [16,121] Increased and prolonged expression of inflammatory cytokines[122,123]	Impaired signaling FGF—FGFR[72,124]
Proliferation ▪ Anatomical cover ▪ Barrier in place		Regenerative			
Vascular events				Endothelial precursor/progenitor cells ↓↓	
Cellular events	Glucocorticoids inhibit collagen synthesis Vitamin C deficiency inhibits collagen synthesis	ECM synthesis		Decreased EPC recruitment and homing to injured tissues	

(Continued)

TABLE 2-13 Differences in Healing When Complicated by Drugs, Aging, Infection, or Disease (*Continued*)

			Chronic		
				Disease State	
	Drugs	**Aging**	**Infection**	**Diabetes**	**Vascular**
Cell signaling		EGF PDGF FGF TGF IL-1 TNF-α			Epithelial cells lack or have ↓PDGF receptor expression[125]
Maturation		Contracture			
Vascular events					
Cellular events				Poor ECM maturation secondary to elevated ROS from inflammatory cells. Early cell senescence[126]	
Cell signaling				Glycosylation adds to ECM instability and disrupts matrix assembly and interactions between collagen and proteoglycans[127] High glucose levels stimulate MMP production by fibroblasts, macrophage, and endothelial cells[128]	
Remodeling ▪ Function ▪ Thermoregulatory ▪ Range of motion ▪ No reoccurrence of wound		Functional/Scar remodel			

responses largely initiated and sustained by macrophages and neutrophils.[141,142] The very cells designed to identify and eliminate the invaders[145] (macrophage and neutrophils) become the pathogenic invaders' "short-order-cook" by supplying an ongoing stream of nutrition via inappropriate and indiscriminate cell, protein, and plasma destruction.[146]

The chronic wound environment is highly proteolytic, having elevated levels of MMP-2, MMP-8, MMP-9, and elastase.[62,147,148] In this proteolytic environment, protein degradation proceeds in random chaos, failing to initiate the orderly cell migration and proliferation that is necessary for timely healing. Furthermore, the presence of proinflammatory cytokines (eg, TNFα, If-γ, IL-1, IL-6, and IL-8)[149] causes indiscriminant recruitment of neutrophils and macrophages.[5,23,49] The increased concentration of neutrophils[47,149] and macrophages in the context of proinflammatory cytokines also prevents the necessary cellular morphologic changes in key cells required to move the wound environment inflammation to proliferation. .[1,2,150]

In addition to the polysaccharide biofilm encasement and the upregulation of proteases, proinflammatory cytokines, and chemokines along with the excessive accumulation of neutrophils and macrophages, biofilm also induces host cell senescence, thereby protecting the biofilm attachment to the host. Host cell senescence renders the cells unable to undergo cell division, migration, or complete apoptosis. The lack of apoptosis may be the most harmful effect as the controlled, programmed host cell apoptosis initiates anti-inflammatory pathways and cellular cascades that move the healing process from inflammation to proliferation.[21,48–51,87,151,152] The resulting host inflammation is nonfunctional, repetitive, and detrimental to host tissues; however, it serves to nourish the biofilm and the resident bacteria.

Chronic wound etiologies include arterial, diabetic/neuropathic, venous insufficiency, pressure, or nonhealing surgical wounds. However, the variability in the local chronic wound environment is largely due to one of five common factors: diminished perfusion, decreased oxygenation, increased mechanical forces, malnutrition, or systemic disease.[59,153] *It is the presence of these factors and not the age or etiology of the wound that determines its chronicity and make it hard to heal.* Regardless of the etiology, all chronic wounds possess similar cellular and biochemical impairments.[59,154,155]

SUMMARY

Normal wound healing proceeds in an organized fashion progressing from injury through hemostasis to inflammation, proliferation, and remodeling. During the hemostasis phase, coagulation of platelets and the formation of a clot prevent excessive bleeding and form a mechanical trap for pathogens, thus initiating the transition to a proinflammatory environment. The recruitment of neutrophils, leukocytes, and macrophages and the release of growth factors and proinflammatory cytokines are the hallmarks of the transition to inflammation. Completion of the proliferative phase results in the formation of well-vascularized granulation tissue and ECM. Remodeling continues the process of scar contraction by myofibroblast activity, tissue replacement, and controlled collagen replacement. The resulting tissue has physical properties approximating unwounded skin.

Wound healing is integrated and orchestrated with both the innate and adaptive immune systems. Both the innate immune system (eg, neutrophils, macrophages, and leukocytes) and the adaptive immune system (eg, B cells and antibodies) are triggered by early responder cells to protect the host from potentially harmful pathogens. Working together, these cells produce and regulate proteases, growth factors, chemokines, and cytokines to accomplish the regeneration of the skin barrier and to avert infection.

Important events that occur in each healing phase can be described as vascular, cellular, cell signaling, or cell-to-matrix interactions. Initially vasoconstriction occurs during hemostasis. However, during the inflammatory and proliferative phases, angiogenesis and vasodilation predominate in order to supply the nutrients for the repair process and to remove the waste and debris associated with autolytic debridement. Although the cellular and acellular components are largely consistent during the phases of healing, their phenotypes, cellular activities, and numbers vary greatly. Platelets are of primary importance for hemostasis and angiogenesis, macrophages for the inflammatory process, the protein laminin for proper ECM construction and storage of growth factors via ECM attachment, and fibroblasts/myofibroblasts for proliferation and remodeling. The macrophage takes on the most varied phenotypic changes during the healing process, moving from a proinflammatory, WAM in the inflammatory phase to a repair, M2 macrophage, during proliferation and remodeling. Finally, remaining macrophages function as a component of immune surveillance after healing is complete.

Chronic or hard-to-heal wounds occur as a result of either a pathophysiological progression (eg, arterial, venous, or diabetic disease) or an acute injury that fails to heal due to infection, intrinsic processes, or extrinsic inhibiting factors. One or more of the primary pathways traversing the healing process are disrupted. The majority of chronic wounds are characterized by excessive or persistent inflammation, infection, presence of biofilm, and the inability of dermal or epidermal cells to respond to reparative stimuli. Clinical observations include chronic inflammation, edema, increased levels of necrotic tissue, bioburden, a poorly developed ECM, and epithelial overgrowth. These inhibiting factors must be addressed in order for complete healing to occur.

STUDY QUESTIONS

1. A contaminated, full-thickness wound of significant size would most likely undergo which category of healing?
   a. Category 1 (primary healing)
   b. Category 2 (delayed primary healing)
   c. Category 3 (secondary healing)
   d. Category 4 (chronic wound healing)
2. Complete wound healing is the time required for a wound to heal to the point where it
   a. No longer produces pain.
   b. No longer needs a dressing.
   c. Has restored both structural and functional integrity.
   d. Is completely re-epithelialized.
3. Which wound healing phase is characterized by granulation tissue?
   a. Hemostasis
   b. Inflammation
   c. Proliferation/maturation
   d. Remodeling
4. When does inflammation begin?
   a. Immediately after injury
   b. When neo-angiogenesis is evident in the wound bed
   c. When bleeding is fully arrested
   d. When wound contraction is evident
5. When does proliferation begin?
   a. When the epithelial cells begin migration at the wound edges.
   b. When the damaged tissue has largely been replaced and begins to regain strength with the deposition of collagen, primarily type III.
   c. When there is an expansion of blood vessels (angiogenesis) and the initiation of wound contraction to complement closure that is driven by the presence of myofibroblasts.
   d. When capillary buds are first visible in the wound bed.
6. During remodeling, type III collagen is replaced with
   a. Type I collagen.
   b. Type II collagen.
   c. Type IV collagen.
   d. Type V collagen.
7. Which of the following characteristics are typical of most chronic wounds?
   a. Present more than 3 weeks
   b. Presence of necrotic tissue
   c. Presence of pain
   d. Persistent recurrence after re-epithelialization

8. Which cells are the first inflammatory cells to initiate the innate immune process?
   a. Endothelial cells
   b. Macrophages
   c. Neutrophils
   d. Platelets

Answers: 1-c; 2-c; 3-c; 4-a; 5-a; 6-a; 7-b; 8-c

REFERENCES

1. Hart J. Inflammation. 2: Its role in the healing of chronic wounds. *J Wound Care*. 2002;11(7):245-249.
2. Hart J. Inflammation. 1: Its role in the healing of acute wounds. *J Wound Care*. 2002;11(6):205-209.
3. Murphy K, ed. *Janeway's Immunobiology*. 7th ed. New York, NY: Garland Science, Taylor & Francis Group; 2007.
4. Rigby KM, DeLeo FR. Neutrophils in innate host defense against *Staphylococcus aureus* infections. *Semin Immunopathol.* 2012;34(2):237-259.
5. Rodero MP, Khosrotehrani K. Skin wound healing modulation by macrophages. *Int J Clin Exp Pathol.* 2010;3(7):643-653.
6. Bernstein AI, Stout KA, Miller GW. A fluorescent-based assay for live cell, spatially resolved assessment of vesicular monoamine transporter 2-mediated neurotransmitter transport. *J Neurosci Methods*. 2012;209(2):357-366.
7. Hunt AM, Paynter KJ. The role of cells of the stratum intermedium in the development of the guinea pig molar. A study of cell differentiation and migration using tritiated thymidine. *Arch Oral Biol.* 1963;8:65-78.
8. Hunt DP. Measurements of a single galvanic skin response based upon its rate topography. *J Gen Psych.* 1975;93(2nd Half):155-171.
9. Kazlauskas A. The priming/completion paradigm to explain growth factor-dependent cell cycle progression. *Growth Factors.* 2005;23(3):203-210.
10. Figg WD, Folkman J, eds. *Angiogenesis: An Integrative Approach from Science to Medicine.* New York, NY: Springer Science and Business Media; 2008.
11. Grotendorst GR, Okochi H, Hayashi N. A novel transforming growth factor beta response element controls the expression of the connective tissue growth factor gene. *Cell Growth Differ.* 1996;7(4):469-480.
12. Igarashi A, Okochi H, Bradham DM, Grotendorst GR. Regulation of connective tissue growth factor gene expression in human skin fibroblasts and during wound repair. *Mol Biol Cell.* 1993;4(6):637-645.
13. Desmouliere A, Geinoz A, Gabbiani F, Gabbiani G. Transforming growth factor-beta 1 induces alpha-smooth muscle actin expression in granulation tissue myofibroblasts and in quiescent and growing cultured fibroblasts. *J Cell Biol.* 1993;122(1):103-111.
14. Gabbiani G. The myofibroblast in wound healing and fibrocontractive diseases. *J Pathol.* 2003;200(4):500-503.
15. Takehara K. Growth regulation of skin fibroblasts. *J Dermatol Sci.* 2000;24(suppl 1):S70-S77.
16. Werner S, Krieg T, Smola H. Keratinocyte-fibroblast interactions in wound healing. *J Invest Dermatol.* 2007;127(5):998-1008.
17. Pilcher BK, Dumin JA, Sudbeck BD, Krane SM, Welgus HG, Parks WC. The activity of collagenase-1 is required for keratinocyte migration on a type I collagen matrix. *J Cell Biol.* 1997;137(6):1445-1457.
18. Pilcher BK, Gaither-Ganim J, Parks WC, Welgus HG. Cell type-specific inhibition of keratinocyte collagenase-1 expression by basic fibroblast growth factor and keratinocyte growth factor. A common receptor pathway. *J Biol Chem.* 1997;272(29):18147-18154.
19. Sudbeck BD, Pilcher BK, Welgus HG, Parks WC. Induction and repression of collagenase-1 by keratinocytes is controlled by distinct components of different extracellular matrix compartments. *J Biol Chem.* 1997;272(35):22103-22110.
20. McKay IA, Leigh IM. Epidermal cytokines and their roles in cutaneous wound healing. *Br J Dermatol.* 1991;124(6):513-518.
21. Banno T, Gazel A, Blumenberg M. Effects of tumor necrosis factor-alpha (TNF alpha) in epidermal keratinocytes revealed using global transcriptional profiling. *J Biol Chem.* 2004;279(31):32633-32642.
22. Frank S, Hubner G, Breier G, Longaker MT, Greenhalgh DG, Werner S. Regulation of vascular endothelial growth factor expression in cultured keratinocytes. Implications for normal and impaired wound healing. *J Biol Chem.* 1995;270(21):12607-12613.
23. Gordon S, Taylor PR. Monocyte and macrophage heterogeneity. *Nat Rev Immunol.* 2005;5(12):953-964.
24. Martinez FO, Helming L, Gordon S. Alternative activation of macrophages: an immunologic functional perspective. *Annu Rev Immunol.* 2009;27:451-483.
25. Stout RD, Suttles J. Functional plasticity of macrophages: reversible adaptation to changing microenvironments. *J Leukoc Biol.* 2004;76(3): 509-513.
26. Occleston NL, Fairlamb D, Hutchison J, O'Kane S, Ferguson MW. Avotermin for the improvement of scar appearance: a new pharmaceutical in a new therapeutic area. *Expert Opin Investing Drugs.* 2009;18(8):1231-1239.
27. Daley JM, Brancato SK, Thomay AA, Reichner JS, Albina JE. The phenotype of murine wound macrophages. *J Leukoc Biol.* 2010;87(1):59-67.
28. Sanchez-Fidalgo S, Martin-Lacave I, Illanes M, Motilva V.Angiogenesis, cell proliferation and apoptosis in gastric ulcer healing. Effect of a selective cox-2 inhibitor. *Eur J Pharmacol.* 2004;505(1-3):187-194.
29. Rosenbauer F, Tenen DG. Transcription factors in myeloid development: balancing differentiation with transformation. *Nat Rev Immunol.* 2007;7(2):105-117.
30. Kaplan HB, Edelson HS, Friedman R, Weissmann G. The roles of degranulation and superoxide anion generation in neutrophil aggregation. *Biochim Biophys Acta.* 1982;721(1):55-63.
31. Weissman IL, Anderson DJ, Gage F. Stem and progenitor cells: origins, phenotypes, lineage commitments, and transdifferentiations. *Annu Rev Cell Dev Biol.* 2001;17:387-403.
32. Glasser L, Fiederlein RL. Functional differentiation of normal human neutrophils. *Blood.* 1987;69(3):937-944.
33. Zigmond SH. Chemotaxis by polymorphonuclear leukocytes. *J Cell Biol.* 1978;77(2):269-287.
34. Snyderman R, Goetzl EJ. Molecular and cellular mechanisms of leukocyte chemotaxis. *Science.* 1981;213(4510):830-837.
35. Rossi F, Zatti M. Changes in the metabolic pattern of polymorphonuclear leucocytes during phagocytosis. *Br J Exp Pathol.* 1964;45:548-559.
36. Kim SY, Weinstein DA, Starost MF, Mansfield BC, Chou JY. Necrotic foci, elevated chemokines and infiltrating neutrophils in the liver of glycogen storage disease type Ia. *J Hepatol.* 2008;48(3):479-485.
37. Segal AW. How neutrophils kill microbes. *Annu Rev Immunol.* 2005;23:197-223.
38. Segal AW. Structure of the NADPH-oxidase: membrane components. *Immunodeficiency.* 1993;4(1-4):167-179.
39. Segal AW, Abo A. The biochemical basis of the NADPH oxidase of phagocytes. *Trends Biochem Sci.* 1993;18(2):43-47.

40. Babior BM. NADPH oxidase: an update. *Blood*. 1999;93(5): 1464-1476.
41. Clark RA. The human neutrophil respiratory burst oxidase. *J Infect Dis*. 1990;161(6):1140-1147.
42. Smith RJ, Wierenga W, Iden SS. Characteristics of *N*-formyl-methionyl-leucyl-phenylalanine as an inducer of lysosomal enzyme release from human neutrophils. *Inflammation*. 1980;4(1):73-88.
43. Babior BM, Kipnes RS, Curnutte JT. Biological defense mechanisms. The production by leukocytes of superoxide, a potential bactericidal agent. *J Clin Invest*. 1973;52(3):741-744.
44. Papayannopoulos V, Zychlinsky A. NETs: a new strategy for using old weapons. *Trends Immunol*. 2009;30(11):513-521.
45. von Kockritz-Blickwede M, Nizet V. Innate immunity turned inside-out: antimicrobial defense by phagocyte extracellular traps. *J Mol Med (Berl)*. 2009;87(8):775-783.
46. Leibovich SJ, Ross R. The role of the macrophage in wound repair. A study with hydrocortisone and antimacrophage serum. *Am J Pathol*. 1975;78(1):71-100.
47. Haslett C, Savill JS, Meagher L. The neutrophil. *Curr Opin Immunol*. 1989;2(1):10-18.
48. DeLeo FR. Modulation of phagocyte apoptosis by bacterial pathogens. *Apoptosis*. 2004;9(4):399-413.
49. Kennedy AD, DeLeo FR. Neutrophil apoptosis and the resolution of infection. *Immunol Res*. 2009;43(1-3):25-61.
50. Kobayashi SD, Braughton KR, Whitney AR, et al. Bacterial pathogens modulate an apoptosis differentiation program in human neutrophils. *Proc Natl Acad Sci USA*. 2003;100(19):10948-10953.
51. Savill JS, Wyllie AH, Henson JE, Walport MJ, Henson PM, Haslett C. Macrophage phagocytosis of aging neutrophils in inflammation. Programmed cell death in the neutrophil leads to its recognition by macrophages. *J Clin Invest*. 1989;83(3):865-875.
52. Colognato H, Yurchenco PD. Form and function: the laminin family of heterotrimers. *Dev Dyn*. 2000;218(2):213-234.
53. Pegtel DM, Gould SJ. Exosomes. *Annu Rev Biochem*. 2019;88(1):487-514.
54. Vu NB, Nguyen HT, Palumbo R, Pellicano R, Fagoonee S, Pham PV. Stem cell-derived exosomes for wound healing: current status and promising directions. *Minerva Med*. 2021;112(3):384-400.
55. Cohen S, Valm AM, Ippincott-Schwartz J. Interacting organelles. *Curr Opin Cell Biol*. 2018;53:84-91.
56. Jain A, Zoncu R. Organelle transporters and inter-organelle communication as drivers of metabolic regulation and cellular homeostasis. *Mol Metab*. 2022;60(6):101481.
57. Martin JM, Zenilman JM, Lazarus GS. Molecular microbiology: new dimensions for cutaneous biology and wound healing. *J Invest Dermatol*. 2010;130(1):38-48.
58. Hess CT. *Wound Care*. 5th ed. Philadelphia, PA: Lippincott Williams & Wilkins; 2005.
59. Grey JE, Enoch S, Harding KG. Wound assessment. *BMJ*. 2006;332(7536):285-288.
60. Hillyer P, Mordelet E, Flynn G, Male D. Chemokines, chemokine receptors and adhesion molecules on different human endothelia: discriminating the tissue-specific functions that affect leucocyte migration. *Clin Exp Immunol*. 2003;134:431-441.
61. Schultz GS, Davidson JM, Kirsner RS, Bornstein P, Herman IM. Dynamic reciprocity in the wound microenvironment. *Wound Repair Regen*. 2011;19(2):134-138.
62. Brouns JEP, Dankers PYW. Introduction of enzyme-responsivity in biomaterials to achieve dynamic reciprocity in cell-material interactions. *Biomacromolecules*. 2021;22:4-23.
63. Bornstein P. Matricellular proteins: an overview. *J Cell Commun Signal*. 2009;3(3-4):163-165.
64. Annunziata CC, Drake DB, Woods JA, Gear AJ, Rodeheaver GT, Edlich RF. Technical considerations in knot construction. Part I. Continuous percutaneous and dermal suture closure. *J Emerg Med*. 1997;15(3):351-356.
65. Guo S, Dipietro LA. Factors affecting wound healing. *J Dent Res*. 2010;89(3):219-229.
66. Schreml S, Szeimies RM, Prantl L, Landthaler M, Babilas P. Wound healing in the 21st century. *J Am Acad Dermatol*. 2010;63(5): 866-881.
67. Kearney KJ, Ariëns RAS, Macrae FL. The role of fibrin(ogen) in wound healing and infection control. *Semin Thromb Hemost*. 2022;48(2):174-187.
68. Al-Mulla F, Leibovich SJ, Francis IM, Bitar MS. Impaired TGF-beta signaling and a defect in resolution of inflammation contribute to delayed wound healing in a female rat model of type 2 diabetes. *Mol Biosyst*. 2011;7(11):3006-3020.
69. Werner S, Grose R. Regulation of wound healing by growth factors and cytokines. *Phys Rev*. 2003;83(3):835-870.
70. Shaykhiev R, Bals R. Interactions between epithelial cells and leukocytes in immunity and tissue homeostasis. *J Leukoc Biol*. 2007;82(1):1-15.
71. Kim MH, Liu W, Borjesson DL, et al. Dynamics of neutrophil infiltration during cutaneous wound healing and infection using fluorescence imaging. *J Invest Dermatol*. 2008;128(7):1812-1820.
72. Barrientos S, Stojadinovic O, Golinko MS, Brem H, Tomic-Canic M. Growth factors and cytokines in wound healing. *Wound Repair Regen*. 2008;16(5):585-601.
73. Gao Z, Sasaoka T, Fujimori T, et al. Deletion of the PDGFR-beta gene affects key fibroblast functions important for wound healing. *J Biol Chem*. 2005;280(10):9375-9389.
74. Pierce GF, Tarpley JE, Tseng J, et al. Detection of platelet-derived growth factor (PDGF)-AA in actively healing human wounds treated with recombinant PDGF-BB and absence of PDGF in chronic nonhealing wounds. *J Clin Invest*. 1995;96(3):1336-1350.
75. Singer AJ, Clark RA. Cutaneous wound healing. *N Engl J Med*. 1999;341(10):738-746.
76. Postlethwaite AE, Keski-Oja J, Moses HL, Kang AH. Stimulation of the chemotactic migration of human fibroblasts by transforming growth factor beta. *J Exp Med*. 1987;165(1):251-256.
77. Leask A, Abraham DJ. TGF-beta signaling and the fibrotic response. *FASEB J*. 2004;18(7):816-827.
78. Koch AE, Volin MV, Woods JM, et al. Regulation of angiogenesis by C-X-C chemokines interleukin-8 and epithelial neutrophil activating peptide 78 in the rheumatoid joint. *Arthritis Rheumatol*. 2001;44:31-40.
79. Pablos JL, Santiago B, Galindo M, et al. Synoviocyte-derived CXCL12 is displayed on endothelium and induces angiogenesis in rheumatoid arthritis. *J Immunol*. 2003;170:2147-2152.
80. Salcedo R, Ponce ML, Young HA, et al. Human endothelial cells express CCR2 and respond to MCP-1: direct role of MCP-1 in angiogenesis and tumor progression. *Blood*. 2000;96:34-40.
81. Shaykhiev R, Beisswenger C, Kandler K, et al. Human endogenous antibiotic LL-37 stimulates airway epithelial cell proliferation and wound closure. *Am J Physiol Lung Cell Mol Physiol*. 2005;289(5):L842-L848.
82. Braun S, auf dem Keller U, Steiling H, Werner S. Fibroblast growth factors in epithelial repair and cytoprotection. *Philos Trans R Soc Lond B Biol Sci*. 2004;359(1445):753-757.

83. Park HJ, Cho DH, Kim HJ, et al. Collagen synthesis is suppressed in dermal fibroblasts by the human antimicrobial peptide LL-37. *J Invest Dermatol.* 2008;129(4):843-850.
84. Gorin Y, Block K, Hernandez J, et al. Nox4 NAD(P)H oxidase mediates hypertrophy and fibronectin expression in the diabetic kidney. *J Biol Chem.* 2005;280(47):39616-39626.
85. Krivacic KA, Levine AD. Extracellular matrix conditions T cells for adhesion to tissue interstitium. *J Immunol.* 2003;170:5034.
86. Wang X, Waldeck H, Kao WJ. The effects of TGF-alpha, IL-1beta and PDGF on fibroblast adhesion to ECM-derived matrix and KGF gene expression. *Biomaterials.* 2010;31(9):2542-2548.
87. Carretero M, Escamez MJ, Garcia M, et al. In vitro and in vivo wound healing-promoting activities of human cathelicidin LL-37. *J Invest Dermatol.* 2008;128(1):223-236.
88. Yannas IV, Tzeranis DS, So PTC. Regeneration of injured skin and peripheral nerves requires control of wound contraction, not scar formation. *Wound Repair Regen.* 2017;25(2):177-191.
89. Kobayashi SD, Deleo FR. An apoptosis differentiation programme in human polymorphonuclear leucocytes. *Biochem Soc Trans.* 2004;32(Pt 3):474-476.
90. Franz MG, Kuhn MA, Wright TE, Wachtel TL, Robson MC. Use of the wound healing trajectory as an outcome determinant for acute wound healing. *Wound Repair Regen.* 2000;8(6):511-516.
91. Ng GY, Oakes BW, McLean ID, Deacon OW, Lampard D. The long-term biomechanical and viscoelastic performance of repairing anterior cruciate ligament after hemitransection injury in a goat model. *Am J Sports Med.* 1996;24(1):109-117.
92. Noordzij JP, Foresman PA, Rodeheaver GT, Quinn JV, Edlich RF. Tissue adhesive wound repair revisited. *J Emerg Med.* 1994;12(5):645-649.
93. Van Meter BH, Thacker JG, Rodeheaver GT, Edlich RF. Some biomechanical considerations in microsutures. *Ann Plast Surg.* 1994;32(4):401-406.
94. Brinkmann V, Zychlinsky A. Neutrophil extracellular traps: is immunity the second function of chromatin? *J Cell Biol.* 2012; 198(5):773-783.
95. Tarricone A, de la Mata K, Chen S, et al. Relationship between pH shifts and rate of healing in chronic nonhealing venous stasis lower-extremity wounds. *J Foot Ankle Surg.* 2020;59(4):748-752.
96. Bonecchi R, Locati M, Galliera E, et al. Differential recognition and scavenging of native and truncated macrophage-derived chemokine (macrophage-derived chemokine/CC chemokine ligand 22) by the D6 decoy receptor. *J Immunol.* 2004;172(8): 4972-4976.
97. Mantovani A, Sica A, Sozzani S, Allavena P, Vecchi A, Locati M. The chemokine system in diverse forms of macrophage activation and polarization. *Trends Immunol.* 2004;25(12):677-686.
98. Hamidzadeh K, Christensen SM, Dalby E, Chandrasekaran P, Mosser DM. Macrophages and the Recovery from Acute and Chronic Inflammation. *Annu Rev Physiol.* 2017;79:567-592.
99. Etulain J. Platelets in wound healing and regenerative medicine. *Platelets.* 2018;29(6):556-568.
100. Minutti CM, Knipper JA, Allen JE, Zaiss DM. Tissue-specific contribution of macrophages to wound healing. *Semin Cell Dev Biol.* 2017;61:3-11.
101. Lucas T, Abraham D, Aharinejad S. Modulation of tumor associated macrophages in solid tumors. *Front Biosci.* 2008;13:5580-5588.
102. Stout RD, Jiang C, Matta B, Tietzel I, Watkins SK, Suttles J. Macrophages sequentially change their functional phenotype in response to changes in microenvironmental influences. *J Immunol.* 2005;175(1):342-349.
103. Villar J, Cros A, De Juan A, et al. ETV3 and ETV6 enable monocyte differentiation into dendritic cells by repressing macrophage fate commitment. *Nat Immunol.* 2023;24(1):84-95.
104. Feugate JE, Li Q, Wong L, Martins-Green M. The cxc chemokine cCAF stimulates differentiation of fibroblasts into myofibroblasts and accelerates wound closure. *J Cell Biol.* 2002;156(1):161-172.
105. Ng CP, Hinz B, Swartz MA. Interstitial fluid flow induces myofibroblast differentiation and collagen alignment in vitro. *J Cell Sci.* 2005;118(Pt 20):4731-4739.
106. Niu J, Chang Z, Peng B, et al. Keratinocyte growth factor/ fibroblast growth factor-7-regulated cell migration and invasion through activation of NF-kappaB transcription factors. *J Biol Chem.* 2007;282(9):6001-6011.
107. Lazarus GS, Cooper DM, Knighton DR, et al. Definitions and guidelines for assessment of wounds and evaluation of healing. *Arch Dermatol.* 1994;130(4):489-493.
108. Werdin F, Tennenhaus M, Schaller HE, Rennekampff HO. Evidence-based management strategies for treatment of chronic wounds. *Eplasty.* 2009;9:e19.
109. Carrie Sussman BB-J, ed. *Wound Care: A Collaborative Practice Manual for Health Professionals.* 3rd ed. Baltimore, MD: Lippincott Williams & Wilkins; 2007.
110. Sen CK, Gordillo GM, Roy S, et al. Human skin wounds: a major and snowballing threat to public health and the economy. *Wound Repair Regen.* 2009;17(6):763-771.
111. Li N, Wallen NH, Savi P, Herault JP, Herbert JM. Effects of a new platelet glycoprotein IIb/IIIa antagonist, SR121566, on platelet activation, platelet-leukocyte interaction and thrombin generation. *Blood Coagul Fibrinolysis.* 1998;9(6):507-515.
112. Varon D, Jackson DE, Shenkman B, et al. Platelet/endothelial cell adhesion molecule-1 serves as a costimulatory agonist receptor that modulates integrin-dependent adhesion and aggregation of human platelets. *Blood.* 1998;91(2):500-507.
113. Weljie AM, Hwang PM, Vogel HJ. Solution structures of the cytoplasmic tail complex from platelet integrin alphaIIb- beta3-subunits. *Proc Natl Acad Sci U S A.* 2002;99:5878.
114. Gage BF, Fihn SD, White RH. Management and dosing of warfarin therapy. *Am J Med.* 2000;109(6):481-488.
115. Herault JP, Peyrou V, Savi P, Bernat A, Herbert JM. Effect of SR121566A, a potent GP IIb-IIIa antagonist on platelet-mediated thrombin generation in vitro and in vivo. *Thromb Haemost.* 1998;79(2):383-388.
116. Brem H, Tomic-Canic M. Cellular and molecular basis of wound healing in diabetes. *J Clin Invest.* 2007;117(5):1219-1222.
117. Loots MA, Lamme EN, Zeegelaar J, Mekkes JR, Bos JD, Middelkoop E. Differences in cellular infiltrate and extracellular matrix of chronic diabetic and venous ulcers versus acute wounds. *J Invest Dermatol.* 1998;111(5):850-857.
118. Tchaikovski V, Olieslagers S, Bohmer FD, Waltenberger J. Diabetes mellitus activates signal transduction pathways resulting in vascular endothelial growth factor resistance of human monocytes. *Circulation.* 2009;120(2):150-159.
119. Kawano M, Komi-Kuramochi A, Asada M, et al. Comprehensive analysis of FGF and FGFR expression in skin: FGF18 is highly expressed in hair follicles and capable of inducing anagen from telogen stage hair follicles. *J Invest Dermatol.* 2005;124(5):877-885.
120. Komi-Kuramochi A, Kawano M, Oda Y, et al. Expression of fibroblast growth factors and their receptors during full-thickness

skin wound healing in young and aged mice. *J Endocrinol.* 2005;186(2):273-289.
121. Werner S, Breeden M, Hubner G, Greenhalgh DG, Longaker MT. Induction of keratinocyte growth factor expression is reduced and delayed during wound healing in the genetically diabetic mouse. *J Invest Dermatol.* 1994;103(4):469-473.
122. Genco RJ, Grossi SG, Ho A, Nishimura F, Murayama Y. A proposed model linking inflammation to obesity, diabetes, and periodontal infections. *J Periodontol.* 2005;76(11 suppl):2075-2084.
123. Wetzler C, Kampfer H, Stallmeyer B, Pfeilschifter J, Frank S. Large and sustained induction of chemokines during impaired wound healing in the genetically diabetic mouse: prolonged persistence of neutrophils and macrophages during the late phase of repair. *J Invest Dermatol.* 2000;115(2):245-253.
124. Landau Z, David M, Aviezer D, Yayon A. Heparin-like inhibitory activity to fibroblast growth factor-2 in wound fluids of patients with chronic skin ulcers and its modulation during wound healing. *Wound Repair Regen.* 2001;9(4):323-328.
125. Liu ZJ, Velazquez OC. Hyperoxia, endothelial progenitor cell mobilization, and diabetic wound healing. *Antioxid Redox Signal.* 2008;10(11):1869-1882.
126. Ben-Porath I, Weinberg RA. The signals and pathways activating cellular senescence. *Int J Biochem Cell Biol.* 2005;37(5):961-976.
127. Liao H, Zakhaleva J, Chen W. Cells and tissue interactions with glycated collagen and their relevance to delayed diabetic wound healing. *Biomaterials.* 2009;30(9):1689-1696.
128. Dalton SJ, Whiting CV, Bailey JR, Mitchell DC, Tarlton JF. Mechanisms of chronic skin ulceration linsking lactate, transforming growth factor-beta, vascular endothelial growth factor, collagen remodeling, collagen stability, and defective angiogenesis. *J Invest Dermatol.* 2007;127(4):958-968.
129. Kim M, Ashida H, Ogawa M, Yoshikawa Y, Mimuro H, Sasakawa C. Bacterial interactions with the host epithelium. *Cell Host & Microbe.* 2010;8(1):20-35.
130. Sibbald RG, Elliott JA, Persaud-Jaimangal R, et al. Wound bed preparation 2021. *Adv Skin Wound Care.* 2021 Apr 1;34(4):183-195.
131. Regulski MJ. Cellular senescence: what, why, and how. *Wounds.* 2017;29(6):168-174.
132. Aepfelbacher M, Aktories K, Just I. *Bacterial Protein Toxins.* New York, NY: Springer; 2000.
133. Burns DL. *Bacterial Protein Toxins.* Washington, DC: ASM Press; 2003.
134. Alouf JE, Popoff MR. *The Comprehensive Sourcebook of Bacterial Protein Toxins.* 3rd ed. Amsterdam: Academic Press; 2006.
135. An YH, Friedman RJ. *Handbook of Bacterial Adhesion: Principles, Methods, and Applications.* Totowa, NJ: Humana Press; 2000.
136. Costerton JW, Stewart PS, Greenberg EP. Bacterial biofilms: a common cause of persistent infections. *Science.* 1999;284:1318-1322.
137. Dykes GA, Sampathkumar B, Korber DR. Planktonic or biofilm growth affects survival, hydrophobicity and protein expression patterns of a pathogenic *Campylobacter jejuni* strain. *Int J Food Microbiol.* 2003;89(1):1-10.
138. James GA, Swogger E, Wolcott R, et al. Biofilms in chronic wounds. *Wound Repair Regen.* 2008;16(1):37-44.
139. Wolcott RD, Rumbaugh KP, James G, et al. Biofilm maturity studies indicate sharp debridement opens a time-dependent therapeutic window. *J Wound Care.* 2010;19(8):320-328.
140. Pallen MJ, Nelson KE, Preston GM. *Bacterial Pathogenomics.* Washington, DC: ASM Press; 2007.
141. Ammons MC. Anti-biofilm strategies and the need for innovations in wound care. *Recent Pat Antiinfect Drug Discov.* 2010;5(1):10-17.
142. Stewart PS, Costerton JW. Antibiotic resistance of bacteria in biofilms. *Lancet.* 2001;358:135-138.
143. Valencia IC, Kirsner RS, Kerdel FA. Microbiologic evaluation of skin wounds: alarming trend toward antibiotic resistance in an inpatient dermatology service during a 10-year period. *J Am Acad Dermatol.* 2004;50(6):845-849.
144. Park B, Liu GY. Targeting the host-pathogen interface for treatment of *Staphylococcus aureus* infection. *Semin Immunopathol.* 2012;34(2):299-315.
145. Delbridge LM, O'Riordan MX. Innate recognition of intracellular bacteria. *Curr Opin Immunol.* 2007;19(1):10-16.
146. Ratliff CR. Wound exudate: an influential factor in healing. *Adv Nurse Pract.* 2008;16(7):32-35; quiz 36.
147. Gohel MS, Windhaber RA, Tarlton JF, Whyman MR, Poskitt KR. The relationship between cytokine concentrations and wound healing in chronic venous ulceration. *J Vasc Surg.* 2008;48(5):1272-1277.
148. Trengove NJ, Stacey MC, MacAuley S, et al. Analysis of the acute and chronic wound environments: the role of proteases and their inhibitors. *Wound Repair Regen.* 1999;7(6):442-452.
149. Diegelmann RF. Excessive neutrophils characterize chronic pressure ulcers. *Wound Repair Regen.* 2003;11(6):490-495.
150. Worldwide Wound Management, 2009: *Established and Emerging Products, Technologies and Markets in the U.S., Europe, Japan and Rest of World.* 2009. Available at: https://www.prlog.org/10348897-advanced-wound-care-technologies-target-high-costs-according-to-new-medmarket-diligence-report.html. Accessed February 19, 2023.
151. Chamorro CI, Weber G, Gronberg A, Pivarcsi A, Stahle M. The human antimicrobial peptide LL-37 suppresses apoptosis in keratinocytes. *J Invest Dermatol.* 2009;129(4):937-944.
152. Chattree V, Khanna N, Bisht V, Rao DN. Inhibition of apoptosis, activation of NKT cell and upregulation of CD40 and CD40L mediated by *M. leprae* antigen(s) combined with Murabutide and Trat peptide in leprosy patients. *Mol Cell Biochem.* 2008;309(1-2): 87-97.
153. Mustoe T. Understanding chronic wounds: a unifying hypothesis on their pathogenesis and implications for therapy. *Am J Surg.* 2004;187:65S-70S.
154. Fonder MA, Lazarus GS, Cowan DA, Aronson-Cook B, Kohli AR, Mamelak AJ. Treating the chronic wound: a practical approach to the care of nonhealing wounds and wound care dressings. *J Am Acad Dermatol.* 2008;58:185-206.
155. Martin JM, Zenilman JM, Lazarus GS. Molecular microbiology: new dimensions for cutaneous biology and wound healing. *J Invest Dermatol.* 2009;130(1):38-48.

Examination and Evaluation of the Patient with a Wound

Rose L. Hamm, PT, DPT, FACCWS

CHAPTER OBJECTIVES

At the end of this chapter, the learner will be able to:

1. **Perform a subjective evaluation of a patient with a wound.**
2. **Obtain the pertinent medical and surgical history from the patient or medical record.**
3. **Perform an assessment of wound characteristics.**
4. **Determine the tests and measurements needed to establish a diagnosis and care plan.**
5. **Perform a review of systems for a patient with a wound.**
6. **Establish a wound diagnosis (for the four typical wound) etiologies.**
7. **Determine factors that may be inhibiting wound healing.**
8. **Recognize conditions that warrant Immediate medical care and make appropriate referrals.**
9. **Establish goals and outcome measures for a patient with a wound.**

INTRODUCTION

The evaluation of a patient is designed to answer two primary questions: (1) Why does this patient have a wound? and (2) Why is the wound not healing? Answering these questions demands more than a wound assessment, although that is an integral part of the evaluation. It demands an evaluation of the patient, the medical history, and the four systems (integumentary, cardiopulmonary, neuromuscular, and musculoskeletal). Throughout the entire evaluation and treatment process, if the focus is on the patient and not just the wound, there will be a better understanding of *why*. In addition, the time spent obtaining this information will help develop trust and rapport with the patient, and will provide an opportunity to understand the patient goals. Attention to the patient allows the evaluator to recognize emergent or untreated conditions that warrant referral to either the primary care physician or an emergency care facility. Therefore, the focus of this chapter is on "the whole patient and not just the hole in the patient," a phrase first coined by Carrie Sussman, a pioneer in physical therapy treatment of chronic wounds, but a phrase that has been used universally in the era of modern wound management.

SUBJECTIVE HISTORY

Before the wound is uncovered and observed, there are questions that the evaluator can ask the patient (or caregiver) that are helpful in making a diagnosis and understanding why the wound is not progressing. A suggested list of questions is in **TABLE 3-1** and is intended to serve as a guideline for initiating discussion with the patient. As the interview progresses, the evaluator will have additional and more pertinent questions relative to each individual patient. By the time the subjective history is completed, the evaluator will probably have a strong sense of the problems and is on the way to answering the question, *why does this patient have a wound?* Why the wound is not healing often requires "digging deeper." The subjective information also indicates the tests and measurements that are needed to make a definitive diagnosis (eg, laboratory tests, vascular screening, imaging, gait analysis, extremity girth).

If the patient is in an acute care or long-term care facility, a thorough chart review provides information that helps direct the subjective interview, determine the diagnosis, and identify the inhibiting factors. Chapter 12, Factors That Impede Wound Healing, provides a detailed discussion of inhibiting factors and includes a chart of laboratory values that are commonly abnormal for the patient with a wound. If, during the subjective evaluation, any of the signs and symptoms listed in **TABLE 3-2** are observed or reported, the patient is advised to see the primary care physician or go to an emergency care facility. After the subjective evaluation is completed, the wound assessment is initiated.

WOUND ASSESSMENT

In order to perform a complete wound assessment, good lighting and patient positioning for optimal visualization are recommended. Good patient position includes adequate support for the head and neck, covering for both modesty and comfort, and adequate exposure of the wound for both visualization and access (**FIGURES 3-1** and **3-2**).

Although the initial appearance of the wound and periwound skin is observed, the wound assessment is best completed after the wound is cleansed thoroughly with normal saline, sterile water, or an approved cleansing solution. Refer to Chapter 14, Wound Dressings, for further discussion of wound cleansing. The following substances are *not* advised for

TABLE 3-1 Questions to Include in a Subjective Interview of a Patient with a Wound

- When and how did the wound begin?
- Can any other precipitating event be associated with the onset of the wound?
  - A walk in bare foot
  - A fall
  - A new pair of shoes
  - An insect bite
  - A surgical or invasive procedure
- What kind of treatment has been used?
- Is the wound improving or regressing?
- What other signs and symptoms are present?
  - Fever
  - Itching
  - Pain
- Describe the pain. Quantify the pain. What alleviates the pain?
- What other disease processes are present?
- What medications (with dosages) are being taken?
  - Prescription
  - Herbal
  - Over the counter
- Are there any allergies relevant to the wound?
  - Analgesics
  - Antibiotics
  - Adhesives
  - Latex
- What is the nutritional status?
  - Are you a vegetarian or vegan?
  - What did you have for dinner last night? For breakfast this morning?
- What are the alcohol, tobacco, and drug habits?
- What is the physical activity level?
- What kind of assistive device is required for functional activities?
- What kind of shoes does the patient wear?

TABLE 3-2 Signs and Symptoms That Suggest a Patient Be Referred to a Primary Care Physician or an Emergency Care Facility

Sign or Symptom	Suspicious Condition
Erythema, edema, deep pain, hot skin	Necrotizing fasciitis Cellulitis
Shortness of breath Lower extremity edema	Congestive heart failure Renal failure
Chest pain	Acute MI
Rash, itching, edema, shortness of breath	Drug allergy, drug-induced hypersensitivity syndrome
Blisters and pain along a dermatome	Acute onset of herpes zoster
Dark mole with asymmetry, uneven borders, changing color, more than 1 cm in diameter, and evolving	Melanoma
Lower extremity pain that increases with activity or awakens the patient at night	Moderate to severe peripheral arterial disease
Syncope, dizziness	Hypotension, hypoglycemia
Decreased mental status	Hypoglycemia, sepsis, cerebral vascular event
Bleeding that is not controlled by pressure	Arterial leak, high INR, low platelet count
New onset of ecchymosis in a distal extremity	Peripheral arterial occlusion
Erythema, warm skin, pain with weight-bearing in patient with diabetes	Acute Charcot foot
Erythema more than 2 cm beyond the wound border of a diabetic foot ulcer	Wound infection
Probe to bone in an exposed wound	Osteomyelitis

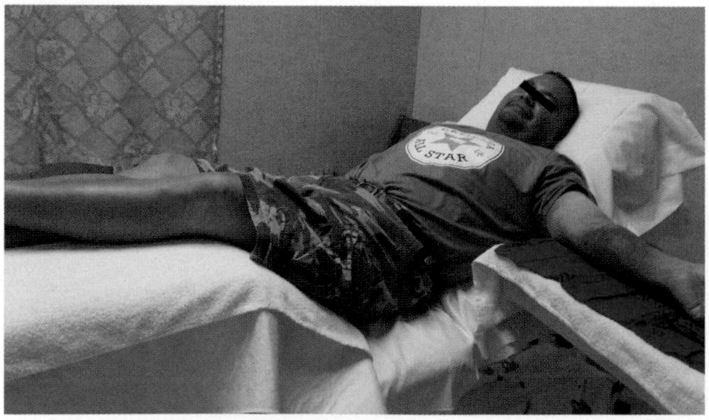

FIGURE 3-1 Patient position in out-patient setting. Patient with a left upper extremity wound is positioned with head slightly elevated and supported with pillows sufficient to accommodate any kyphosis; lower extremities elevated for edema reduction, access to wounds, and patient comfort; arm is supported on a table at a height that is comfortable for the shoulder. Having the hips and knees slightly bent is advised for older patients who may have low-back and leg pain due to spinal stenosis.

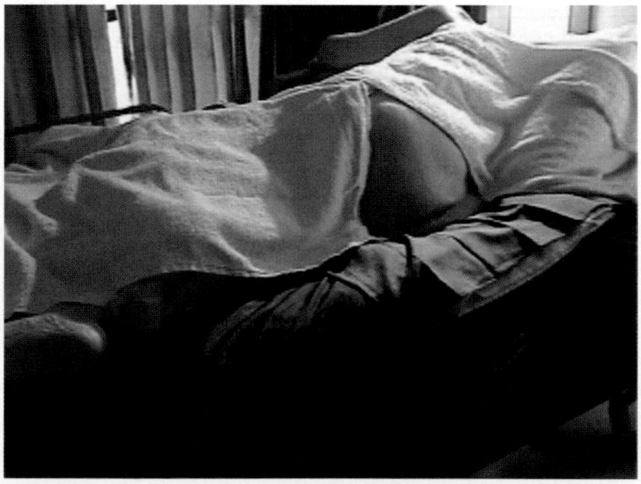

FIGURE 3-2 Patient position in in-patient setting. Patient is positioned on the side for access to a sacral wound. A pillow between the legs prevents medial knee pressure and aligns the sacrum/low back for comfort. The patient is draped for warmth and for modesty.

cleansing wounds, especially if there is exposed healthy tissue as in a traumatic injury:

- Hydrogen peroxide (H_2O_2): While diluted H_2O_2 may be useful for removing particulate debris, recent coagulum, and dried blood or debris at the wound edge, undiluted H_2O_2 may be cytotoxic to clean or granulating tissue by reducing fibroblast activity.[1]
- Ionic soaps and detergents: These cleansers (eg, pHisohex) can irritate tissue and increase the potential for infection if used on the wound surface.
- Iodine: 1% iodine is associated with decreased wound healing and has not been shown to decrease the risk of infection over normal saline (when cleansing a new, traumatic wound); concentrated iodine is cytotoxic.[2]

After cleansing, the wound and integumentary assessment includes location, size, tissue type, drainage, periwound skin color, edema, edges, odor, signs of infection, and pain. A standardized assessment tool such as the one developed by Barbara Bates-Jensen can be helpful in guiding the clinician through the assessment process and provides an objective total score and subsequent outcome measures as the wound healing progresses, or can give an indication that the wound is deteriorating (**TABLE 3-3**).[3]

The Pressure Ulcer Scale for Healing (PUSH©), developed by the National Pressure Injury Advisory Panel to measure progress or regression in pressure ulcers, grades a wound based on length, width, exudate amount, and tissue type.[4] These parameters are based on the Centers for Medicare and Medicaid Services (CMS) definition of wound progress: a decrease in area or volume, amount of exudate, and amount of necrotic tissue.[5] The study by Hon et al. found the PUSH© to be responsive to wound progress in pressure, venous, and diabetic ulcers; however, it is more sensitive in larger wounds than in smaller wounds in the last stages of healing.[5] The PUSH© tool has also been found to be responsive to burns and scalds, skin tears, surgical wounds, and traumatic wounds.[6]

TABLE 3-3 Bates-Jensen Wound Assessment Tool

Instructions for use

General Guidelines:

Fill out the attached rating sheet to assess a wound's status after reading the definitions and methods of assessment described below. Evaluate once a week and whenever a change occurs in the wound. Rate according to each item by picking the response that best describes the wound and entering that score in the item score column for the appropriate date. When you have rated the wound on all items, determine the total score by adding together the 13-item scores. The HIGHER the total score, the more severe the wound status. Plot total score on the Wound Status Continuum to determine progress. If the wound has healed/resolved, score items 1, 2, 3 and 4 as = 0.

Specific Instructions:

1. **Size**: Use ruler to measure the longest and widest aspect of the wound surface in centimeters; multiply length x width. Score as = 0 if wound healed/resolved.

2. **Depth**: Pick the depth, thickness, most appropriate to the wound using these additional descriptions, score as = 0 if wound healed/resolved:
   1 = tissues damaged but no break in skin surface.
   2 = superficial, abrasion, blister or shallow crater. Even with, &/or elevated above skin surface (e.g., hyperplasia).
   3 = deep crater with or without undermining of adjacent tissue.
   4 = visualization of tissue layers not possible due to necrosis.
   5 = supporting structures include tendon, joint capsule.

3. **Edges**: Score as = 0 if wound healed/resolved. Use this guide:

Indistinct, diffuse	=	unable to clearly distinguish wound outline.
Attached	=	even or flush with wound base, no sides or walls present; flat.
Not attached	=	sides or walls are present; floor or base of wound is deeper than edge.
Rolled under, thickened	=	soft to firm and flexible to touch.
Hyperkeratosis	=	callous-like tissue formation around wound & at edges.
Fibrotic, scarred	=	hard, rigid to touch.

4. **Undermining**: Score as = 0 if wound healed/resolved. Assess by inserting a cotton tipped applicator under the wound edge; advance it as far as it will go without using undue force; raise the tip of the applicator so it may be seen or felt on the surface of the skin; mark the surface with a pen; measure the distance from the mark on the skin to the edge of the wound. Continue process around the wound. Then use a transparent metric measuring guide with concentric circles divided into 4 (25%) pie-shaped quadrants to help determine percent of wound involved.

TABLE 3-3 Bates-Jensen Wound Assessment Tool (*Continued*)

5. **Necrotic Tissue Type**: Pick the type of necrotic tissue that is predominant in the wound according to color, consistency and adherence using this guide:

White/gray non-viable tissue	=	may appear prior to wound opening; skin surface is white or gray.
Non-adherent, yellow slough	=	thin, mucinous substance; scattered throughout wound bed; easily separated from wound tissue.
Loosely adherent, yellow slough	=	thick, stringy, clumps of debris; attached to wound tissue.
Adherent, soft, black eschar	=	soggy tissue; strongly attached to tissue in center or base of wound.
Firmly adherent, hard/black eschar	=	firm, crusty tissue; strongly attached to wound base and edges (like a hard scab).

6. **Necrotic Tissue Amount**: Use a transparent metric measuring guide with concentric circles divided into 4 (25%) pie-shaped quadrants to help determine percent of wound involved.

7. **Exudate Type**: Some dressings interact with wound drainage to produce a gel or trap liquid. Before assessing exudate type, gently cleanse wound with normal saline or water. Pick the exudate type that is predominant in the wound according to color and consistency, using this guide:

Bloody	=	thin, bright red
Serosanguineous	=	thin, watery pale red to pink
Serous	=	thin, watery, clear
Purulent	=	thin or thick, opaque tan to yellow or green may have offensive odor

8. **Exudate Amount**: Use a transparent metric measuring guide with concentric circles divided into 4 (25%) pie-shaped quadrants to determine percent of dressing involved with exudate. Use this guide:

None	=	wound tissues dry.
Scant	=	wound tissues moist; no measurable exudate.
Small	=	wound tissues wet; moisture evenly distributed in wound; drainage involves ≤25% dressing.
Moderate	=	wound tissues saturated; drainage may or may not be evenly distributed in wound; drainage involves >25% to ≤75% dressing.
Large	=	wound tissues bathed in fluid; drainage freely expressed; may or may not be evenly distributed in wound; drainage involves >75% of dressing.

9. **Skin Color Surrounding Wound**: Assess tissues within 4cm of wound edge. Dark-skinned persons show the colors "bright red" and "dark red" as a deepening of normal ethnic skin color or a purple hue. As healing occurs in dark-skinned persons, the new skin is pink and may never darken.

10. **Peripheral Tissue Edema & Induration**: Assess tissues within 4cm of wound edge. Non-pitting edema appears as skin that is shiny and taut. Identify pitting edema by firmly pressing a finger down into the tissues and waiting for 5 seconds, on release of pressure, tissues fail to resume previous position and an indentation appears. Induration is abnormal firmness of tissues with margins. Assess by gently pinching the tissues. Induration results in an inability to pinch the tissues. Use a transparent metric measuring guide to determine how far edema or induration extends beyond wound.

11. **Granulation Tissue**: Granulation tissue is the growth of small blood vessels and connective tissue to fill in full thickness wounds. Tissue is healthy when bright, beefy red, shiny and granular with a velvety appearance. Poor vascular supply appears as pale pink or blanched to dull, dusky red color.

12. **Epithelialization**: Epithelialization is the process of epidermal resurfacing and appears as pink or red skin. In partial thickness wounds it can occur throughout the wound bed as well as from the wound edges. In full thickness wounds it occurs from the edges only. Use a transparent metric measuring guide with concentric circles divided into 4 (25%) pie-shaped quadrants to help determine percent of wound involved and to measure the distance the epithelial tissue extends into the wound.

TABLE 3-3 Bates-Jensen Wound Assessment Tool (*Continued*)

BATES-JENSEN WOUND ASSESSMENT TOOL

NAME

Complete the rating sheet to assess wound status. Evaluate each item by picking the response that best describes the wound and entering the score in the item score column for the appropriate date. If the wound has healed/resolved, score items 1, 2, 3, & 4 as = 0.

Location: Anatomic site. Circle, identify right **(R)** or left **(L)** and use **"X"** to mark site on body diagrams:

___	Sacrum & coccyx	___	Lateral ankle
___	Trochanter	___	Medial ankle
___	Ischial tuberosity	___	Heel
___	Buttock	___	Other site: ______________.

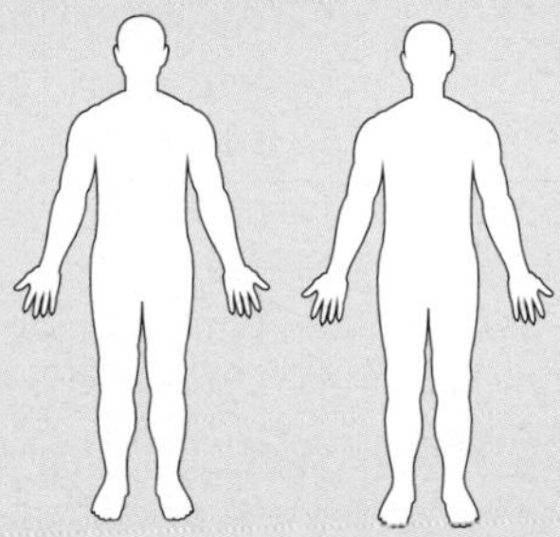

Shape: Overall wound pattern; assess by observing perimeter and depth.

Circle and date appropriate description:

___	Irregular	___	Linear or elongated	
___	Round/oval	___	Bowl/boat	
___	Square/rectangle	___	Butterfly	Other Shape

Item	Assessment	Date Score	Date Score	Date Score
1. Size*	*0 = Healed, resolved wound 1 = Length × width <4 sq cm 2 = Length × width 4 to ≤16 sq cm 3 = Length × width 16.1 to ≤36 sq cm 4 = Length × width 36.1 to ≤80 sq cm 5 = Length × width >80 sq cm			
2. Depth*	*0 = Healed, resolved wound 1 = Non-blanchable erythema on intact skin 2 = Partial thickness skin loss involving epidermis &/or dermis 3 = Full thickness skin loss involving damage or necrosis of subcutaneous tissue; may extend down to but not through underlying fascia; &/or mixed partial & full thickness &/or tissue layers obscured by granulation tissue 4 = Obscured by necrosis 5 = Full thickness skin loss with extensive destruction, tissue necrosis or damage to muscle, bone or supporting structures			
3. Edges*	*0 = Healed, resolved wound 1 = Indistinct, diffuse, none clearly visible 2 = Distinct, outline clearly visible, attached, even with wound base 3 = Well-defined, not attached to wound base 4 = Well-defined, not attached to base, rolled under, thickened 5 = Well-defined, fibrotic, scarred or hyperkeratotic			
4. Under-mining*	*0 = Healed, resolved wound 1 = None present 2 = Undermining <2 cm in any area 3 = Undermining 2–4 cm involving <50% wound margins 4 = Undermining 2–4 cm involving >50% wound margins 5 = Undermining >4 cm or Tunneling in any area			
5. Necrotic Tissue Type	1 = None visible 2 = White/gray non-viable tissue &/or non-adherent yellow slough 3 = Loosely adherent yellow slough 4 = Adherent, soft, black eschar 5 = Firmly adherent, hard, black eschar			
6. Necrotic Tissue Amount	1 = None visible 2 = <25% of wound bed covered 3 = 25% to 50% of wound covered 4 = >50% and <75% of wound covered 5 = 75% to 100% of wound covered			

TABLE 3-3 Bates-Jensen Wound Assessment Tool (*Continued*)

Item	Assessment	Date Score	Date Score	Date Score
7. Exudate Type	1 = None 2 = Bloody 3 = Serosanguineous: thin, watery, pale red/pink 4 = Serous: thin, watery, clear 5 = Purulent: thin or thick, opaque, tan/yellow, with or without odor			
8. Exudate Amount	1 = None, dry wound 2 = Scant, wound moist but no observable exudate 3 = Small 4 = Moderate 5 = Large			
9. Skin Color Surrounding Wound	1 = Pink or normal for ethnic group 2 = Bright red &/or blanches to touch 3 = White or gray pallor or hypopigmented 4 = Dark red or purple &/or non-blanchable 5 = Black or hyperpigmented			
10. Peripheral Tissue Edema	1 = No swelling or edema 2 = Non-pitting edema extends <4 cm around wound 3 = Non-pitting edema extends >4 cm around wound 4 = Pitting edema extends <4 cm around wound 5 = Crepitus and/or pitting edema extends >4 cm around wound			
11. Peripheral Tissue Induration	1 = None present 2 = Induration <2 cm around wound 3 = Induration 2–4 cm extending <50% around wound 4 = Induration 2–4 cm extending >50% around wound 5 = Induration >4 cm in any area around wound			
12. Granulation Tissue	1 = Skin intact or partial thickness wound 2 = Bright, beefy red; 75% to 100% of wound filled &/or tissue overgrowth 3 = Bright, beefy red; <75% & >25% of wound filled 4 = Pink, &/or dull, dusky red &/or fills ≤25% of wound 5 = No granulation tissue present			
13. Epithelialization	1 = 100% wound covered, surface intact 2 = 75% to <100% wound covered &/or epithelial tissue extends >0.5 cm into wound bed 3 = 50% to <75% wound covered &/or epithelial tissue extends to <0.5 cm into wound bed 4 = 25% to <50% wound covered 5 = <25% wound covered			
	TOTAL SCORE			
	SIGNATURE			

WOUND STATUS CONTINUUM

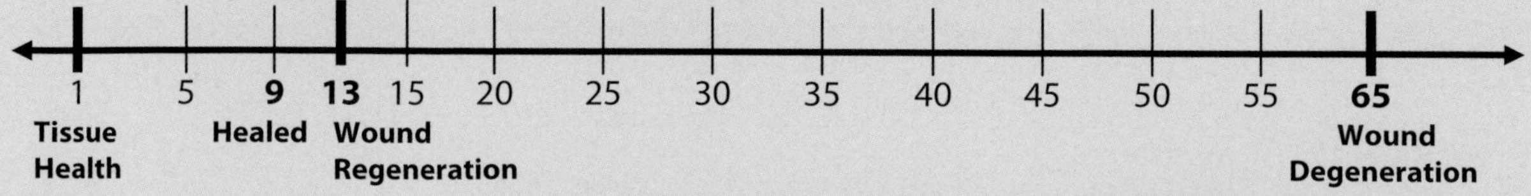

Plot the total score on the Wound Status Continuum by putting an **"X"** on the line and the date beneath the line. Plot multiple scores with their dates to see-at-a-glance regeneration or degeneration of the wound.

The Wound Healing Index (WHI) was developed to stratify patients with wounds according to the wound characteristics and underlying conditions that affect wound healing, and thus validly predict likelihood of wound healing.[7] The WHI can then be used to stratify patients for random controlled trials and to identify patients early in treatment who would benefit from advanced therapies. The variables that were identified as significant for patients with wounds of all types include the following: wound size, wound age, number of wounds of any etiology, evidence of bioburden, type of tissue exposed (eg, using Wagner scale or PU staging), being nonambulatory, and requiring hospitalization in the course of treatment.[7] Further studies have identified additional significant variables for diabetic foot ulcers (patient age, renal dialysis, and peripheral vascular disease[8]) and for pressure ulcers on any body area except the heel (PU Stage III or IV, patient age, having renal transplant, paralysis, malnutrition, and patient hospitalization for any reason[9]).

Chronic wounds are known to have a significant impact on the patient's quality of life,[10,11] and assessing that impact is an important part of the initial evaluation, not only for understanding the patient's emotional and functional status, but also for helping to set reasonable and meaningful goals. Several tools that have been developed to assess quality of life include the following: Freiburg Life Quality Assessment[12,13] (has a short version adapted for venous disease and lymphedema), Wound-QoL questionnaire,[14,15] the Cardiff Wound Impact Schedule,[16] and the Wurzburg Wound Score for lower extremity arterial and vascular wounds.[17]

TABLE 3-4 provides a list of assessment tools intended to help the evaluator (1) create an accurate picture of the wound status, (2) assess pain associated with the wound, (3) assess patient-reported quality of life issues, (4) develop an effective and appropriate care plan, and (5) document objectively the progression or regression of a wound. The

TABLE 3-4 Assessment Tools for Objective Wound Documentation

Name of Tool	Purpose of Tool	Electronic Access
WOUND ASSESSMENT		
Bates-Jensen Wound Assessment Tool (BWAT)	Assess wounds of all types, monitor wound healing	Copy may be obtained from mbatesjen@sonnet.ucla.edu
Braden Scale	Assess risk of pressure injury formation	https://www.in.gov/isdh/files/Braden_Scale.pdf
Glamorgan Pressure Injury Risk Assessment	Assess risk of pressure injury in pediatric patients	https://www.rch.org.au/uploadedFiles/Main/Content/rchcpg/Revised_Glamorgan_Reference_Guide.pdf
Gosnell Scale	Assess risk of pressure injury formation for patients in extended care or >65 years in age	https://answers.yahoo.com/question/index?qid=1006032101152
Healing Progression Rate Tool	Assess wound healing specifically for PUs, using the current NPUAP definitions and descriptions	Young DL, Estocado N, Feng D, Black J. The development and preliminary validity testing of the Healing Progression Rate Tool. *Ostomy Wound Manage.* 2017;63(9):32–44. Available at: doi:10.25270/owm.2017.09.3244.
Long Beach Wound Scores	Scores severity of wounds, especially DFUs, based on size, tissue appearance, depth, infection, and perfusion	https://scivisionpub.com/pdfs/an-algorithm-for-evaluation-and-management-of-diabetic-foot-ulcers-1572.pdf
Norton Scale	Assess risk of pressure injury formation	https://agedcare.royalcommission.gov.au/system/files/2020-06/RCD.9999.0096.0460.pdf
Photographic Wound Assessment Tool (PWAT) Revised; adapted from BWAT	Assess wounds by interpretation of photographs (eg, in telemedicine or electronic consultation)	https://www.southwesthealthline.ca/healthlibrary_docs/b.9.3b.pwatinstruc.pdf
Pressure Ulcer Scale for Healing (PUSH)	Assess pressure injury healing in long-term care settings; developed by the NPIAP	https://www.sralab.org/sites/default/files/2017-06/push3.pdf
SCI-Pressure Ulcer Monitoring Tool	Assess pressure injury healing in patients with spinal cord injury	https://www.researchgate.net/figure/Spinal-Cord-Impairment-Pressure-Ulcer-Monitoring-Tool-SCI-PUMT_fig2_260755697
Sessing Scale	Assess pressure injury healing or regression	http://www.ncbi.nlm.nih.gov/pubmed/7806737
Shieh Score	Assess risk for hospital-acquired pressure injuries (HAPI)	https://pubmed.ncbi.nlm.nih.gov/33587474/
Sussman Wound Healing Tool (SWHT)[3]	Assess pressure injury healing and efficacy of interventions; may be used for wounds of all types	https://woundeducators.com/tools-to-measure-wound-healing/ Bates-Jensen BM, Sussman C. Tools to measure wound healing. In: Bates-Jensen BM, Sussman C, eds. Wound Care: A Collaborative Practice Manual for Health Care Professionals. Baltimore, MD: Lippincott Williams & Wilkins; 2012:131–161.
Waterlow score	Assess risk of pressure ulcer formation	http://www.judy-waterlow.co.uk/downloads/intex.htm

TABLE 3-4 Assessment Tools for Objective Wound Documentation (*Continued*)

Name of Tool	Purpose of Tool	Electronic Access
Wound Healing Index	Identify patient and wound factors that affect likelihood of wound healing	Horn SD, Fife CE, Smout RJ, Barrett RS, Thomson B. Development of a wound healing index for patients with chronic wounds. *Wound Repair Regen*. 2013;21:823–832.
Wound Trend Scale	Assess lower leg wound management, includes screening for infection and cues for physician referral	Campbell NA, Campbell DL, Turner A. The Wound Trend Scale: A retrospective review of utility and predictive value in the assessment and documentation of lower leg ulcers. *Ostomy Wound Manage*. 2016;62(12):40–53.
PAIN ASSESSMENT		
Behavior Scale for Pain Management	Assess pain in patients in critical care units using facial expression, upper extremity movement, and ventilation compliance	Gomarverdi S, Sedighie L, Seifrabiei MA, Nikooseresht M. Comparison of two pain scales: Behavioral Pain Scale and Critical-care Pain Observation Tool during invasive and noninvasive procedures in intensive care unit-admitted patients. *Iran J Nurs Midwifery Res*. 2019;24(2):151–155.
Critical care Pain Observation Tool (CPOT)	Assess pain in patients in critical care units using facial expression, body movements, ventilator compliance (intubated), vocalization (nonintubated), muscle tension, and upper extremity tone with passive stretching	Gomarverdi S, Sedighie L, Seifrabiei MA, Nikooseresht M. Comparison of two pain scales: Behavioral Pain Scale and Critical-care Pain Observation Tool during invasive and noninvasive procedures in intensive care unit-admitted patients. *Iran J Nurs Midwifery Res*. 2019;24(2):151–155.
Faces Pain Scale (Wong Baker)	Assess pain intensity on a scale of 0–5 based on identification with facial expressions	http://www.pediatricnursing.net/interestarticles/1401_Wong.pdf
FLACC Behavior Pain Assessment Scale (Face, Legs, Activity, Cry, Consolability)	Assess pain in children from newborn to age 3	https://www1.health.gov.au/internet/publications/publishing.nsf/Content/triageqrg~triageqrg-pain~triageqrg-FLACC
McCaffrey Initial Pain Assessment Tool	Assess pain at initial evaluation; provides diagram of human body so patient can indicate location and questions to help patient describe pain and its effects on daily life. Gives permission for duplication and use in the clinic	https://nida.nih.gov/sites/default/files/McCaffreyInitialPainAssessmentTool.pdf
NOPPAIN (Non-communicative Patient's Pain Assessment Instrument)	Assess pain in non-communicative patients	https://prc.coh.org/PainNOA/NOPPAIN_B.pdf
PAINAD	Assess pain in patients unable to verbalize intensity (eg, advanced Alzheimer or comatose patients). Uses nonverbal behaviors in response to painful stimuli (breathing, negative vocalization, facial expression, body language, consolability)	http://dementiapathways.ie/_filecache/04a/ddd/98-painad.pdf
Visual Analog Pain Assessment Scale (VAS)	Assess pain intensity on a scale of 1–10	http://img.medscape.com/article/742/580/VAS.pdf
QUALITY OF LIFE ASSESSMENT		
Cardiff Wound Impact Questionnaire	Assess patient-reported impact of chronic wounds on quality of life and identify patient concerns	https://swrwoundcareprogram.ca/Uploads/ContentDocuments/CardiffTool.pdf
Freiburg Life Quality Assessment	Assess effect of chronic wounds on patient's quality of life; also adapted for patients with lymphedema, venous disease, burns, and other skin disorders	https://www.ncbi.nlm.nih.gov/pubmed/15197001 https://onlinelibrary.wiley.com/doi/10.1111/iwj.12803
Wound QoL Questionnaire	Assess the effect of chronic wounds on patient's quality of life	https://www.daemen.edu/sites/default/files/Wound-Outcome-Measure-Questionnaire.pdf
Wuerzburg Wound Score	Assess quality of life effects of lower extremity arterial and venous wounds	https://www.doi.1024/0301-1526/a000378

literature provides several comparisons of the various tools used to assess wounds and/or predict risk for pressure ulcer development and the clinician is advised to select one that is most appropriate for the patient population being served.[18–22] Use of these assessment tools as applicable to each patient is highly recommended for determining efficacy of interventions and reporting progress to third-party payers.

Location

Location is an important component of determining the wound etiology. **TABLE 3-5** provides a summary of the characteristics of the four typical wound etiologies (arterial, venous, pressure, and neuropathic) and the location differences that are a significant aspect of determining the wound etiology. Location is described by anatomical body part, using medical terms to define specifics (**FIGURES 3-3** to **3-6**).

TABLE 3-5 Characteristics of the Four Typical Wound Etiologies

WOUND EVALUATION BY ETIOLOGY					
	Location	**Tissue**	**Pain**	**Skin**	**Exudate**
Arterial	Distal digits (toes or fingers)	Dry, necrotic or slough, little or no granulation	Yes!!! May have dependent leg syndrome or rest pain	Dry, hairless, shiny, thin, positive rubor of dependency	None unless infected
Venous	Lower one-third of the leg (called the gaiter area)	Red or pink, bark-like texture, yellow slough Poor granulation	Generally not painful; if painful, either infection or another diagnosis needs to be considered	Hemosiderous (dark, brawny appearance) Atrophie blanche	Varies, may have copious serous drainage before compression therapy
Pressure	Over bony prominences	Varies from nonblanchable erythema to dark red to eschar	Varies depending on the structures involved	Discolored from erythematous to hypoxic; may be macerated or excoriated	Varies
Neuropathic	Weight-bearing surface of the foot or dorsal digits	Callus or blister, slough, may probe to bone, necrotic with PAD	None!!! Until infected, then deep throbbing	Dry, thick, scaly, hyperkeratotic	Varies, depending on infection

Developed by Rose Hamm; used with permission.

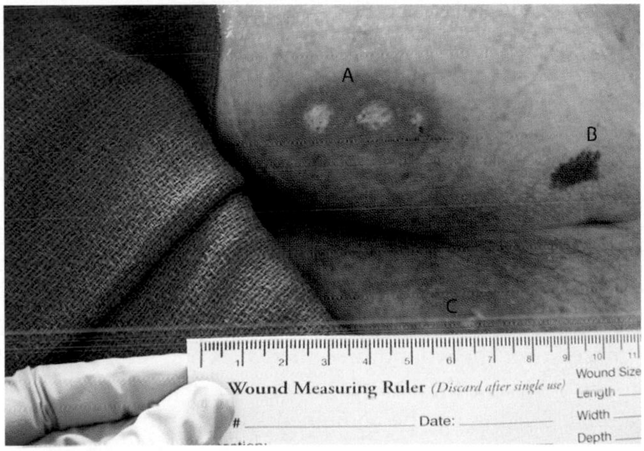

FIGURE 3-3 Location of wound on sacrum. Wounds are located on (**A**) left gluteal region, (**B**) left sacral area, and (**C**) right superior gluteal region.

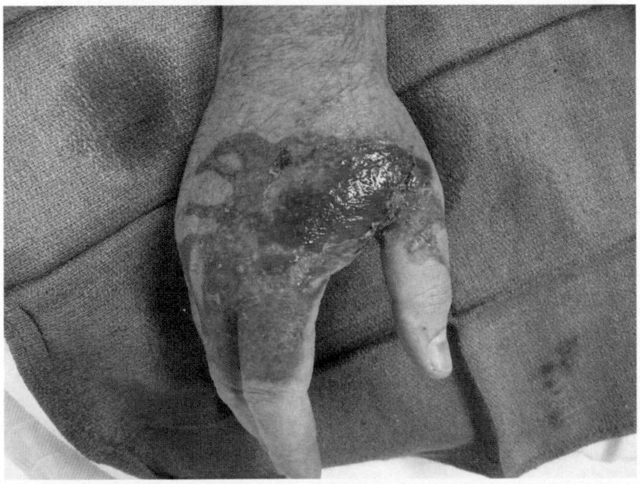

FIGURE 3-4 Location of wound on the hand. Wound located on the lateral dorsal aspect of the right hand, including the web space, second and third proximal phalanxes.

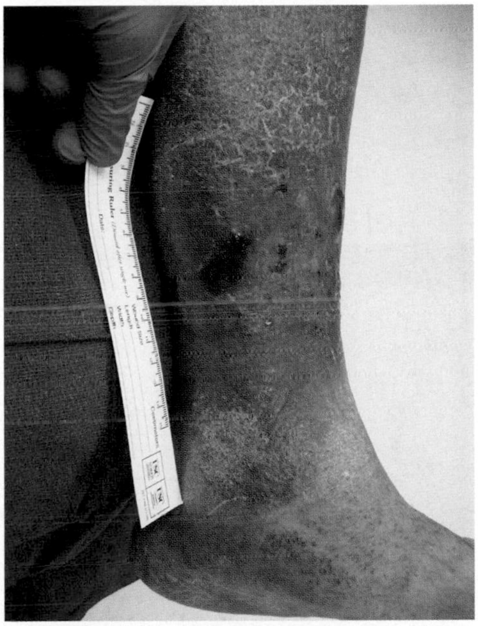

FIGURE 3-5 Location of wound on lower extremity. Wound located on the gaiter (or distal 1/3) area of the right lateral leg.

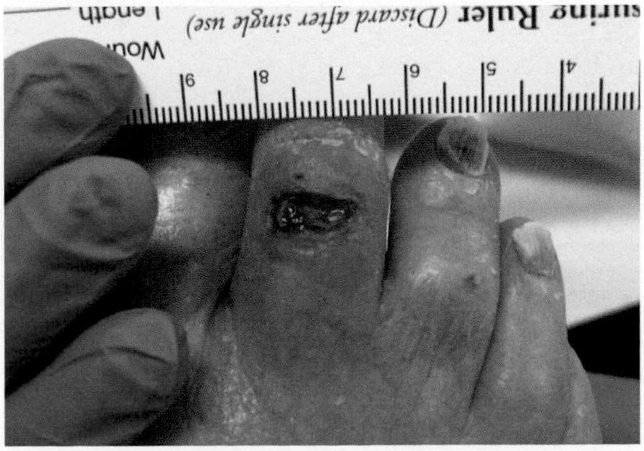

FIGURE 3-6 Location of wound on dorsal foot. Wound located on the dorsal proximal interphalangeal joint of the right second toe.

Dimensions

Wound size is a major outcome measurement and is used to document improvement or lack of response to interventions, or to predict healing potential.[22–25] For example, diabetic foot wounds that decrease in size during the first 4–6 weeks of healing are more likely to have full closure.[26] Periodic measurements give objective feedback about the efficacy of treatment and serve as indicators as to when interventions need to be changed due to lack of tissue response. Wound dimensions are also one of the primary indicators used by third-party payers to determine treatment efficacy. Wound surface area can be calculated in several different ways; however, electronic assessment is being used more frequently in conjunction with electronic medical records.

Perpendicular Method The perpendicular (or ruler) method measures the wound length at its longest dimension and the width at the longest dimension perpendicular to the length (**FIGURE 3-7**). Measurements are recorded in either centimeters (cm) or millimeters (mm), and can be multiplied for a surface area ($A = \text{length} \times \text{width}$), although it would be approximate because wounds are rarely shaped like a rectangle. Elliptical surface area can also be calculated [$A = (\pi \times \text{length} \times \text{width})/4$].[27] Volume can be calculated with the ruler method ($V = \text{length} \times \text{width} \times \text{depth}$); the depth is measured with a sterile applicator perpendicular from the deepest area to the wound surface. The perpendicular method has been shown to have good reliability in wounds <4 cm^2,[28] and it is quick, easy, and inexpensive; however, it has the disadvantage of overestimating wound surface area.[27–29]

Clock Method The clock method imagines a clock superimposed on the wound with 12:00 placed cephalically and 6:00 placed caudally. Measurements are then taken at any direction on the clock and documented (eg, 6 cm at 12–6:00 for length or 2 cm from 3–9:00 for undermining) (**FIGURE 3-8**). When using the clock method, which is beneficial for sacral ulcers, the position of the patient is also documented in order to have consistency of wound configuration between measurements. For example, if a patient is positioned in right side lying for measurements at the time of initial evaluation and in left side lying 1 week later for reassessment, the wound will have a different orientation and configuration, and comparison of measurements may not be as valid. The clock method is also helpful in describing wound landmarks (eg, undermining and sinuses) as illustrated in **FIGURE 3-9**.

Tracing Tracing uses a clear plastic measuring guide over the wound to trace the edges and is useful for wounds that have serpentine or uneven edges (**FIGURE 3-10A, B**). A clear film is placed over the wound first, then a second layer of film or measuring guide; the wound is traced with a permanent marking pen. Tracing can be combined with planimetry software

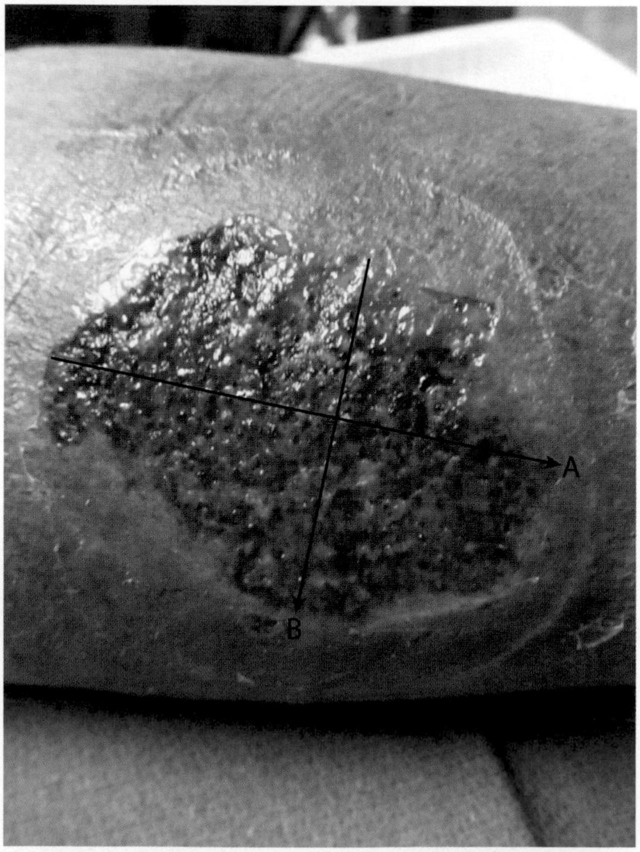

FIGURE 3-7 Perpendicular method. The perpendicular method measures the wound at the longest dimension (**A**) as the length, and the longest dimension perpendicular to the length (**B**) as the width. Measurements are recorded as length × width.

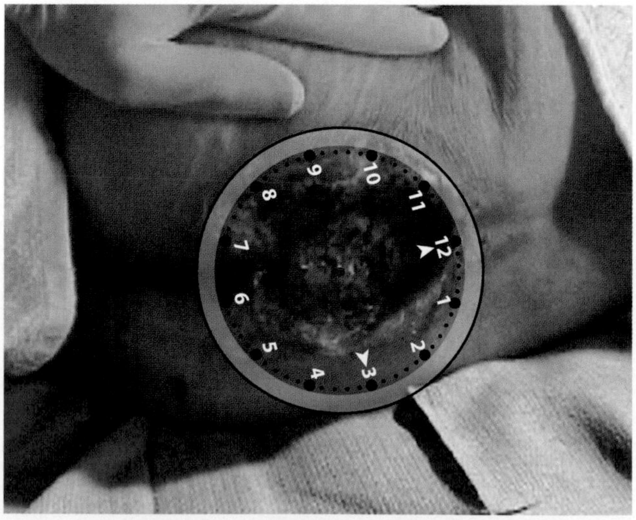

FIGURE 3-8 Clock method for wound surface area. The clock method is useful for aligning wounds with anatomical position in which 12:00 is cephalic and 6:00 is caudal, 3:00 is right lateral, and 9:00 is left lateral.

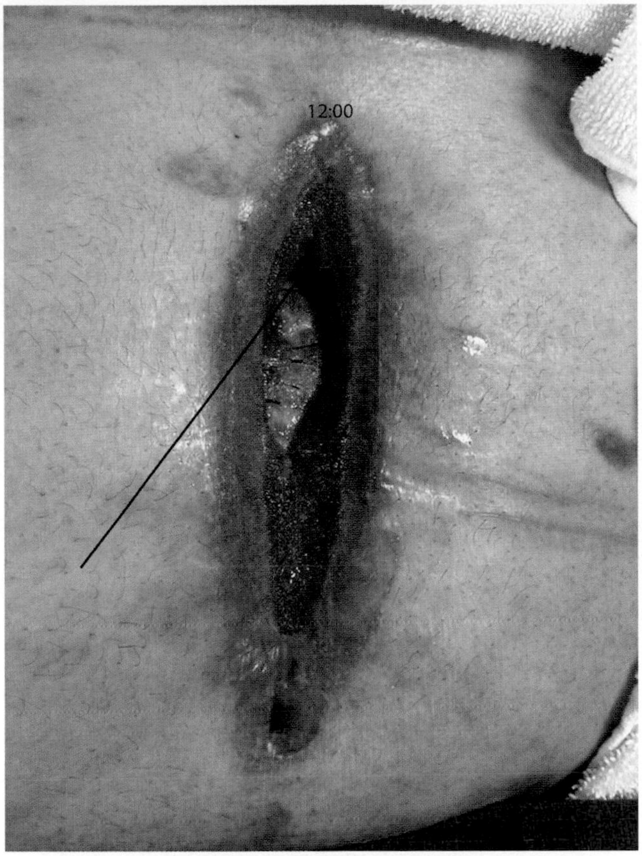

FIGURE 3-9 Clock method for location of sinus or undermining. This incisional abdominal wound has a sinus at 12:00 or the superior aspect.

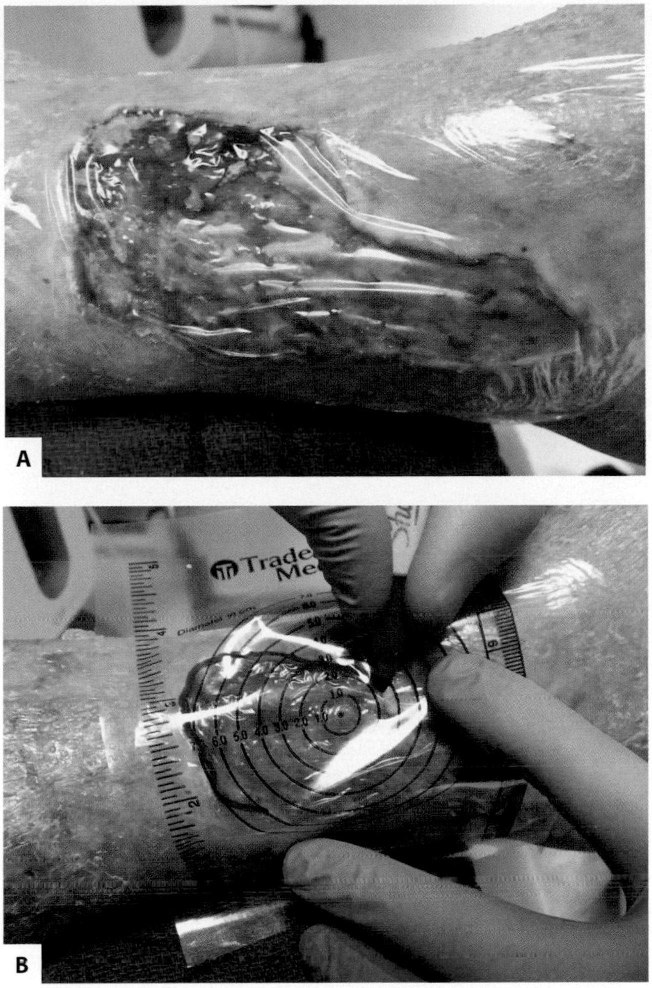

FIGURE 3-10 Tracing a wound. A. Before placing the tracing guide on the wound, a clear plastic film is placed on the wound to prevent wound fluids and possible infection from being transferred to the patient chart. **B.** The tracing guide is placed over the first layer of plastic film and the wound is traced with an indelible marking pen. Tracing is recommended for serpentine wounds that do not have well-defined lengths and widths to measure.

to determine the wound surface area: the wound is manually traced, scanned into computer software, and exact surface area calculated.[27] The disadvantages of wound tracing are the following: sinuses, undermining, and depth are not measured; discomfort to the patient with pressure on the wound; risk of contamination; and obscured edges if there is moisture under the film.[30] Although it is rarely used in modern clinics, tracing can still be of value in situations where other methods of measuring are not available.

Digital Planimetry Digital photography has become the standard for taking pictures of wounds due to its availability and its ability to be downloaded into electronic medical records. High resolution allows excellent visualization of wound characteristics. Four notable aspects of an ideal wound photograph are the setting, exposure and background, lighting, and camera position.[31,32] **TABLE 3-6** lists related recommendations for achieving optimal results when using digital cameras.

Planimetry uses software to calculate dimensions from digital photography. Results of surface area have been shown to be more accurate with planimetry, especially with wounds over 4 cm^2. Digital photographs are downloaded into the computer and software calculates dimensions, surface area,

TABLE 3-6 Guidelines for Obtaining Optimal Results When Using Digital Photographs and Planimetry

- Position the patient so that the wound can be easily visualized.
- Center the wound in the viewbox.
- Adjust the lighting for equal illumination in order to eliminate shadows.
- Use blue or green towels around the wound to eliminate busy backgrounds and other features that may identify the patient, and to absorb light and prevent reflecting light waves that may wash out the wound color.
- Close curtains or shades so that only fluorescent light exists in the room; this also minimizes glare.
- Position camera so it is not facing a light source and do not use flash.
- Place one or two disposable rulers at the edges of the wound to assess size.
- Hold the camera at a 90-degree angle to the wound bed to avoid distortion of the shape.

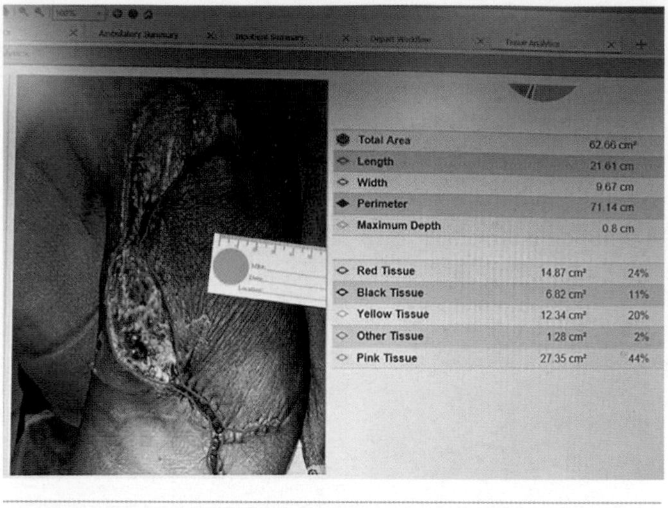

FIGURE 3-11 Screenshot showing the wound area, dimensions, perimeter, and maximum depth, as well as the area/percentages of tissue by color. The green dots are measurement references for the software.

estimated volume, and circumference. Some applications also include percentages of tissue type based on color analysis and graphs indicating change over time (**FIGURE 3-11**). Planimetry has been shown to be the most accurate method for calculating wound measurements[28,33–35]; however, consistency in recorded assessments requires diligent staff training to have adequate inter-reliability.[31]

Subcutaneous Extensions

Some wounds, especially pressure, diabetic foot, and surgical wounds, tend to have necrotic subcutaneous tissue that prevents the wound edge from adhering to the wound bed. The author terms these *subcutaneous extensions* because the actual wound extends beneath the visible epithelial edge. Examples include undermining, sinuses, tunnels, and fistulas. Because the presence of subcutaneous extensions may be an indication of underlying infection or lead to deeper abscesses, documentation of measurement (in depth) and location (using the clock method of anatomic position) is an essential part of the wound assessment.[4,36] Treatment plans need to include debridement, cleansing, and dressing application to subcutaneous extensions, as well as the visible wound bed.

Undermining is a result of necrotic hypodermal connective tissue that disrupts the attachment of the skin to the underlying structures. Dark discolored skin around the visible periphery of the wound may be an indication of undermining and is explored with a sterile instrument to determine the extent. Documentation includes the depth at the deepest point and the extent using the clock orientation (**FIGURE 3-12A, B**).

Sinuses are extensions that run along a fascial plane and may contain fluid trapped in the deeper area that can lead to abscess formation if not explored and thoroughly cleansed. Suspicion of a sinus is indicated by observation of a dark area at the edge of a wound. Depth is measured with a sterile alginate-tipped applicator and location recorded using the clock orientation (**FIGURE 3-13A, B**).

Tunneling occurs when two cutaneous wounds connect (**FIGURE 3-14**). The two cutaneous wounds may initially appear to be two separate wounds, but probing reveals that the subcutaneous tissue between the openings is necrotic and not connected to the under surface

CLINICAL CONSIDERATION

Probing is best accomplished with a calcium alginate-tipped applicator as fibers left in the wound are biodegradable and will not lead to granuloma formation. If these applicators are not available, cotton-tipped applicators may be used; moistening the tip with normal saline or sterile water will help prevent the loss of cotton fibers in the deeper wound bed. Sterile metal instruments are advised if the evaluator is probing for possible bone exposure.

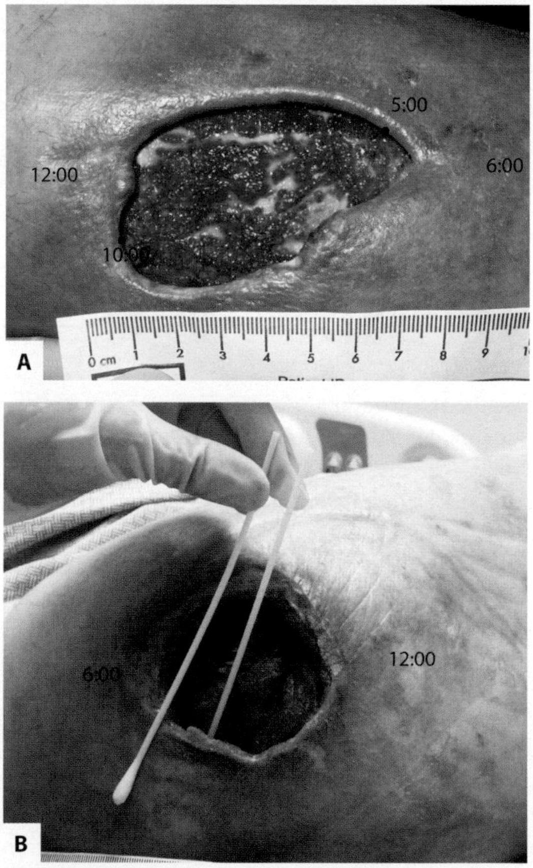

FIGURE 3-12 Undermining. A. The shadow that extends across the left and upper borders of the wound indicates undermining where the skin is detached from the underlying structure, usually a result of autolysis of the subcutaneous tissue. The depth of undermining would be recorded, for example, as 3–5 mm from 10:00 to 5:00. **B.** Undermining is being measured in the pressure wound on a greater trochanter. The applicator on the outside indicates the depth of the undermining, which would be documented, for example, as 3.5 cm at 4:00.

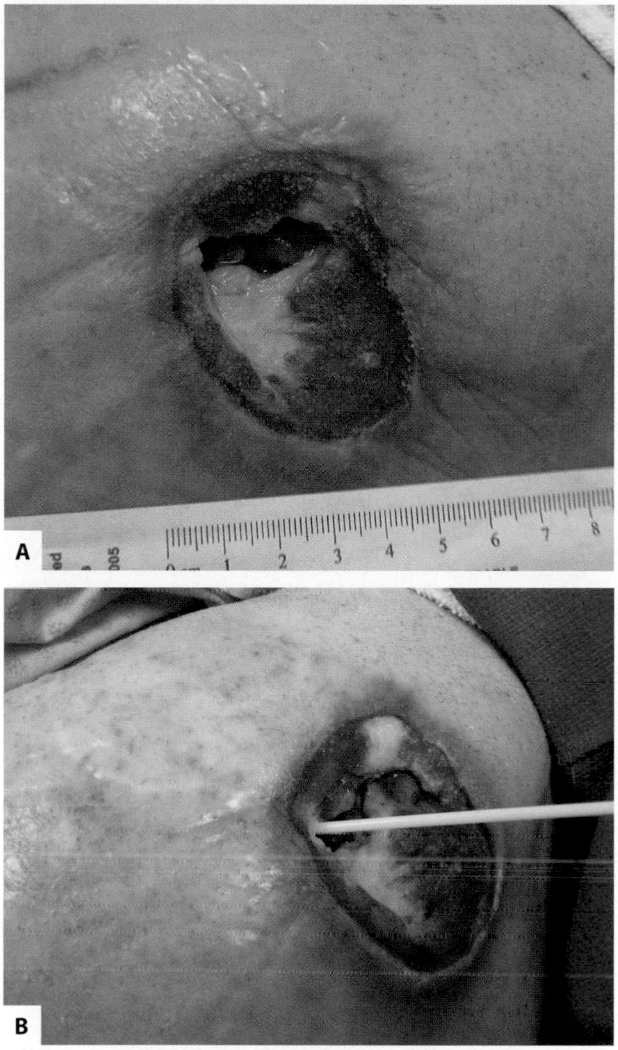

FIGURE 3-13 Sinus. A sinus or fascial track is indicated by the dark opening in the visible wound bed in photo **A**. In photo **B**, the sinus is being explored with a sterile applicator to determine the depth and possible pockets of fluid.

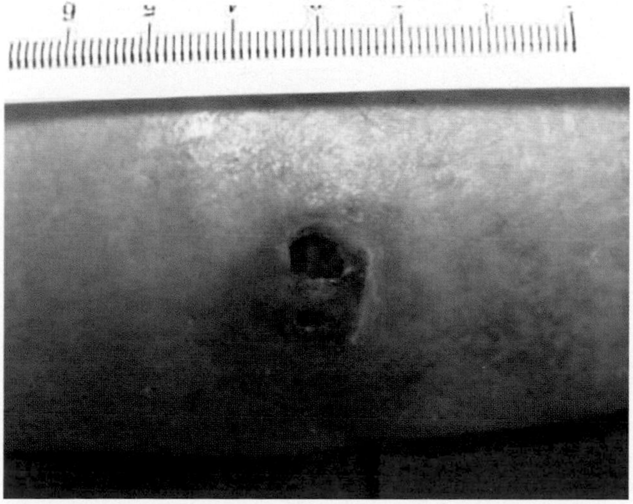

FIGURE 3-14 Tunneling. A tunneling wound has two openings that are connected beneath the skin.

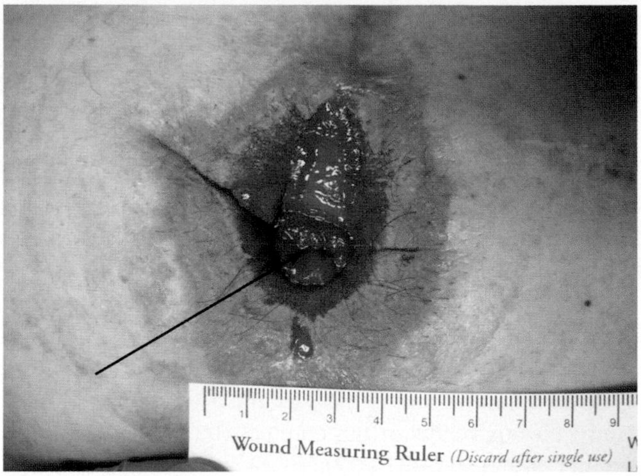

FIGURE 3-15 Fistula. An enterocutaneous fistula is a connection between some part of the gastric system and the skin, often occurring after intestinal resection or gastric surgery. In this photo, the fistula is surrounded by a full-thickness wound, and the drainage that comes from the fistula can be caustic to the skin. When the fistula is surgically created, the everted part of the bowel is termed a *stoma.*

of the skin. In this case, the sizes of the two openings and the length of the tissue loss between the openings are measured and documented.

A *fistula* is defined as an abnormal connection between two epithelium-lined structures where a connection does not usually exist. Sometimes it is created for medical purposes, for example, in the case of an arteriovenous fistula between an upper extremity artery and vein for hemodialysis access. The type most frequently encountered in wound care is an enterocutaneous or enteroatmospheric fistula that connects some part of the digestive system with the skin or wound surface (**FIGURE 3-15**). While the depth of the fistula is not appropriate to measure, the location is a component of the wound assessment. The type of drainage (eg, thin green, thick brown, or solid brown) can indicate the location of the digestive track where the fistula originates.

Tissue Type

Identification of the tissue type within a wound bed is necessary for understanding the phase of healing and for developing a plan of care, especially the optimal type of debridement and dressings. If one observes a structure that cannot be named or identified during the evaluation or treatment procedure, the procedure should be discontinued until research can help identify the tissue of concern. A documentation technique that is helpful in measuring outcomes is to assign a percentage of the total wound surface to each tissue type. While this is approximate at best, especially when using the perpendicular or ruler technique rather than sophisticated software, it does help document improvement in tissue quality as the wound progresses from inflammation to granulation to epithelialization. Normal structures (eg, skin, bone, muscle, tendon, and adipose) may be either viable or nonviable, healthy or not healthy, and are identified as such in the evaluation.

Eschar is nonviable or necrotic tissue that covers all or part of a wound base. It is composed of dead skin or subcutaneous cells and may vary in color (black, brown, gray, yellow, tan) and texture (hard, dry, rubbery, soft). Eschar is not synonymous with what is commonly called a "scab," which is a result of blood and serum hardening over a fresh wound (**FIGURE 3-16**).

Slough is nonviable subcutaneous tissue, often found under eschar, and is a result of the body's autolytic process to phagocytose dead cells. The usually soft and yellow substance has no real texture and is hard to grasp with forceps, unlike stringy, fibrous yellow or tan connective tissue that may also be under eschar (**FIGURE 3-17**).

Granulation tissue, the hallmark of the proliferative healing phase, is composed of extracellular matrix and capillaries. It is the tissue that the body produces to fill in a wound cavity and to support new epithelial growth, and has, as its name suggests, a granular appearance. Note that not all red tissue is granulation tissue; for example, immediately after surgery, muscle and subcutaneous tissue may also be red but have a different texture. For this reason, describing wounds by color only (as is sometimes discussed in the literature or used by some digital software) may be misleading in the documentation (**FIGURE 3-18A, B**).

Muscle is identified by its location, its striated appearance, and its ability to contract with voluntary movement. In addition, healthy muscle bleeds when cut, is sensate and thus painful with stimulation, and is red. Conversely, unhealthy muscle is gray or brown, is insensate and therefore painless, does not bleed when cut, and has no contractibility (**FIGURE 3-19**).

Bone is identified by its location and its hard texture when probed with a metal instrument. The color is tan when healthy,

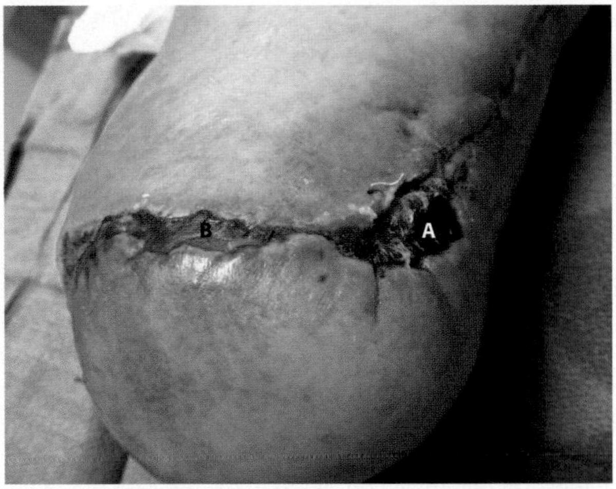

FIGURE 3-16 Eschar. The wound on the below-knee amputation site contains (**A**) hard dry black eschar and (**B**) softer brown eschar, both consisting of dead or necrotic tissue.

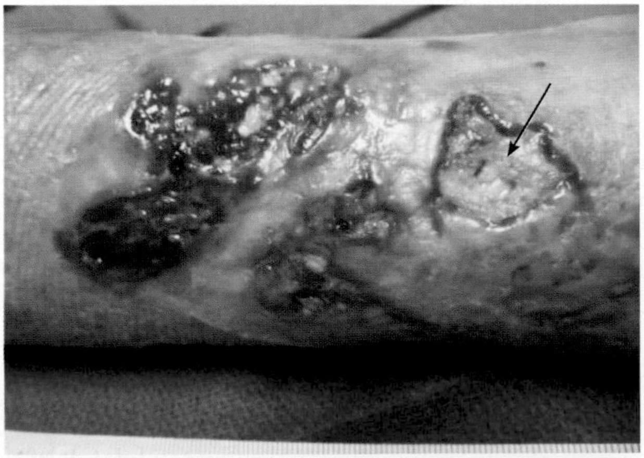

FIGURE 3-17 Slough. The soft yellow substance on the wound surface is a result of autolysis of subcutaneous or connective tissue. Slough has no texture and is best removed with a curette.

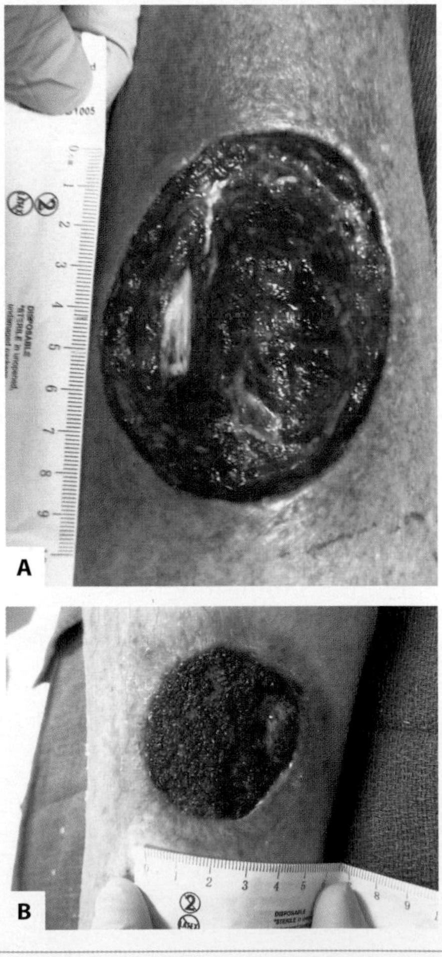

FIGURE 3-18 Granulation tissue. Granulation tissue is composed of new capillaries in an extracellular matrix and has a granular, beefy red appearance, as seen in photo **B**. The subcutaneous tissue in photo **A** is also red, but has a different texture, indicating that it is not fully granulated. Photo **A** is transitioning from inflammation to proliferation; photo **B** is in the proliferative phase.

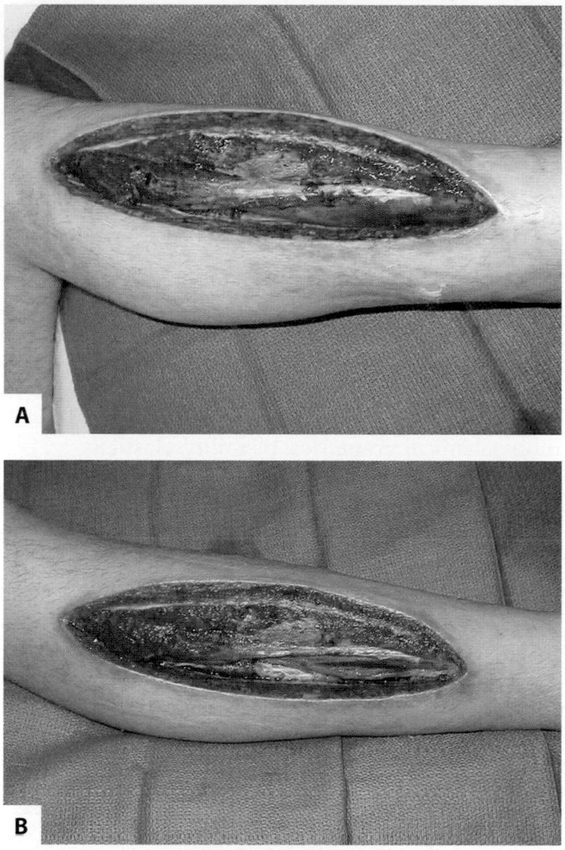

FIGURE 3-19 Unhealthy or nonviable muscle. A. Unhealthy or nonviable muscle is dull gray or brown, is insensate and therefore does not cause pain when touched, does not bleed when cut, and does not twitch or respond to tactile stimulation. In addition, if the patient is asked to perform a joint movement, the nonviable muscle will not contract. Surgical removal is usually required for wound healing to progress. Nonviable muscle is observed in this fasciotomy wound at the time of initial evaluation. **B.** Three days later, the wound has started to granulate; however, nonviable muscle is still visible and requires further surgical debridement.

and darker brown or black when necrotic. Usually bone is covered by periosteum, the bilayer covering (composed of collagen and fibroblasts) of almost all bone, which contributes to bone repair and nutrition (**FIGURE 3-20**).[37] Because of its importance in maintaining viability of the bone underneath, the periosteum should be kept moist and protected at all times. Necrotic bone usually requires surgical debridement; however, small, loose bone fragments may be removed during sharp debridement (**FIGURE 3-21**).

Tendons are readily observed in full-thickness wounds of the dorsal feet and hands where there is less subcutaneous tissue between the skin and the tendons. An important component of healthy tendons is paratenon, the fatty synovial fluid that fills the sheath around the tendon and thereby provides moisture, nutrients, and glidability. The healthy tendon sheath requires a moist dressing to prevent desiccation, defined as destruction by drying out (**FIGURE 3-22**). Nonviable tendon requires debridement for full wound healing to occur and is

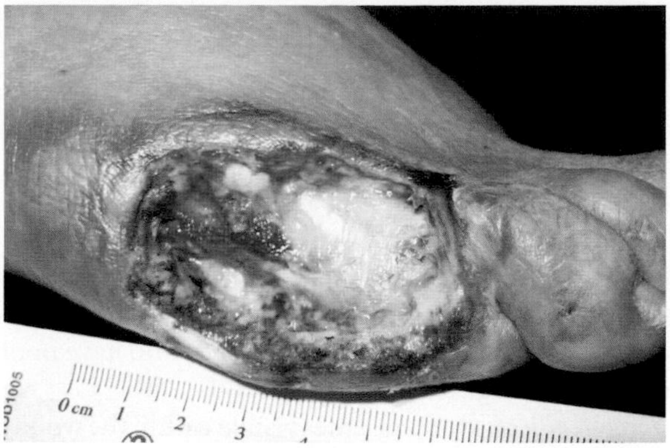

FIGURE 3-20 Viable bone. Viable bone covered with periosteum and fascia is observed in the foot where the great toe has been amputated, leaving the second metatarsal head exposed.

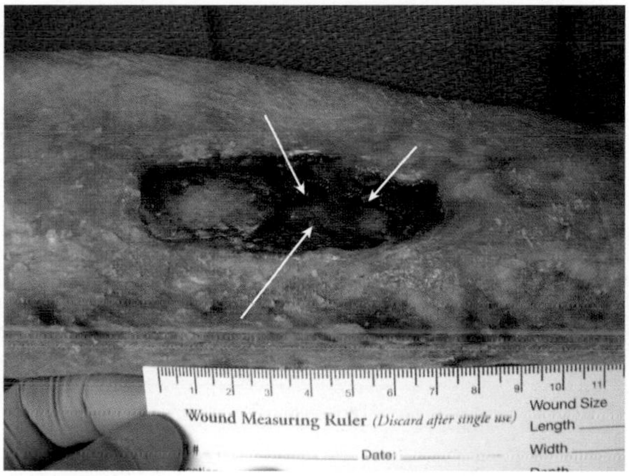

FIGURE 3-21 Nonviable bone. Nonviable bone in a lower leg that has been treated with radiation for a malignant tumor. Granulation tissue (seen at the tips of the white arrows) will sometimes push through the cortical bone from the underlying trabecular bone; however, the necrotic bone usually has to be resected for the wound to heal.

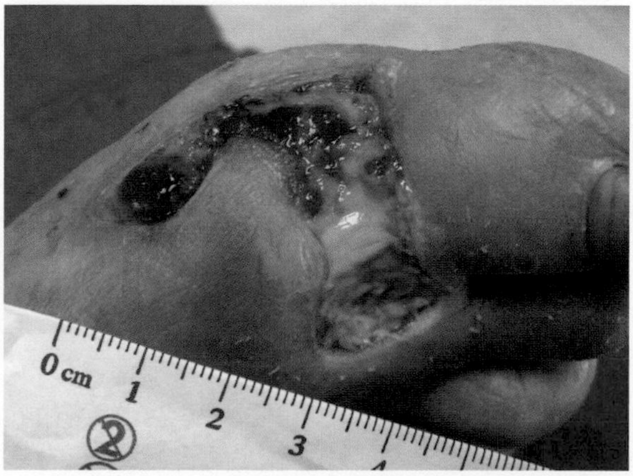

FIGURE 3-22 Viable tendon. The extensor tendon with an intact paratenon is observed in the great toe after a bunionectomy incision dehisced.

usually performed in surgery. However, sometimes fiber by fiber debridement in a chronic full-thickness wound is advisable. In this case, if the tissue surrounding the tendon is viable, granulation tissue will penetrate the tendon and support re-epithelialization (**FIGURE 3-23**).

Adipose (fat) tissue appears as shiny globules when viable, and shriveled darker yellow tissue when nonviable. Because of its poor vascularity, adipose easily becomes nonviable and infected and is very slow to vascularize and granulate. This can become very problematic in obese patients who have nonhealing abdominal surgical incisions (**FIGURE 3-24**).

Foreign objects are sometimes visible within the wound bed (eg, sutures, staples, dressing remnants, splinters, or shards of glass after trauma). If a foreign object remains in the subcutaneous tissue and the skin grows over it, a granuloma may form and cause a small reopening due to the exudate that develops as the body tries to autolyse the object. Persistent drainage from an otherwise closed wound is a red flag for a foreign object in the subcutaneous tissue. These objects are evaluated for the best method of removal (ie, sharp vs. surgical debridement), as well as for signs of infection (**FIGURE 3-25A, B**).

Scar tissue can be hard and stiff which can interfere with joint range of motion, functional activities, cosmesis, and quality of life (**FIGURE 3-26A–C**). Scar tissue is evaluated by the following characteristics:

- Color: erythema and pigmentation
- Dimensions: surface area, thickness, and volume
- Texture
- Biomechanical properties: pliability, elasticity
- Pathophysiologic disturbances: transcutaneous oxygen tension, transepidermal water loss, moisture content
- Tissue microstructure
- Pain and sensation[38]

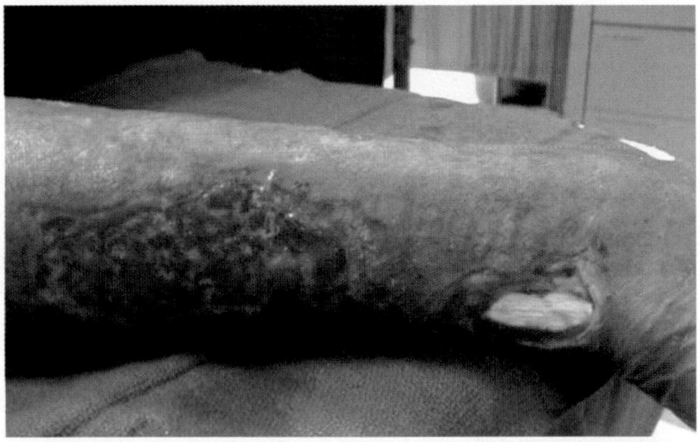

FIGURE 3-23 Nonviable tendon. The Achilles tendon in the heel has lost its paratenon sheath and thus is stringy and dull. Selective debridement of the nonviable fibers will allow the granulation tissue to advance over the wound and in some cases will allow the wound to re-epithelialize. Loss of function depends on the amount of tendon that is lost.

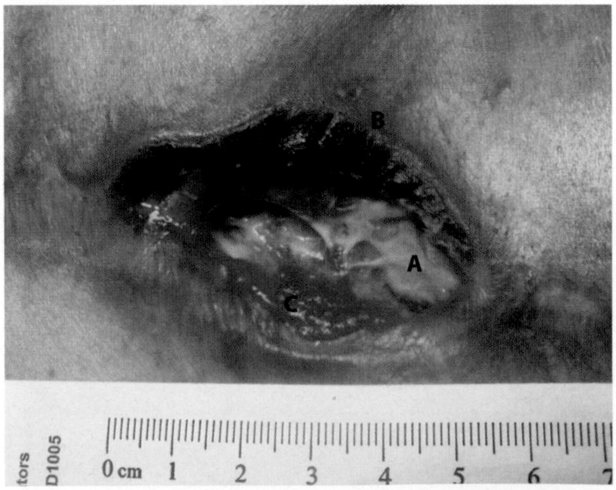

FIGURE 3-24 Adipose in an abdominal wound. Three distinct tissue types are observed in this abdominal wound: (**A**) shriveled yellow adipose, (**B**) dry black eschar, and (**C**) red granulation tissue.

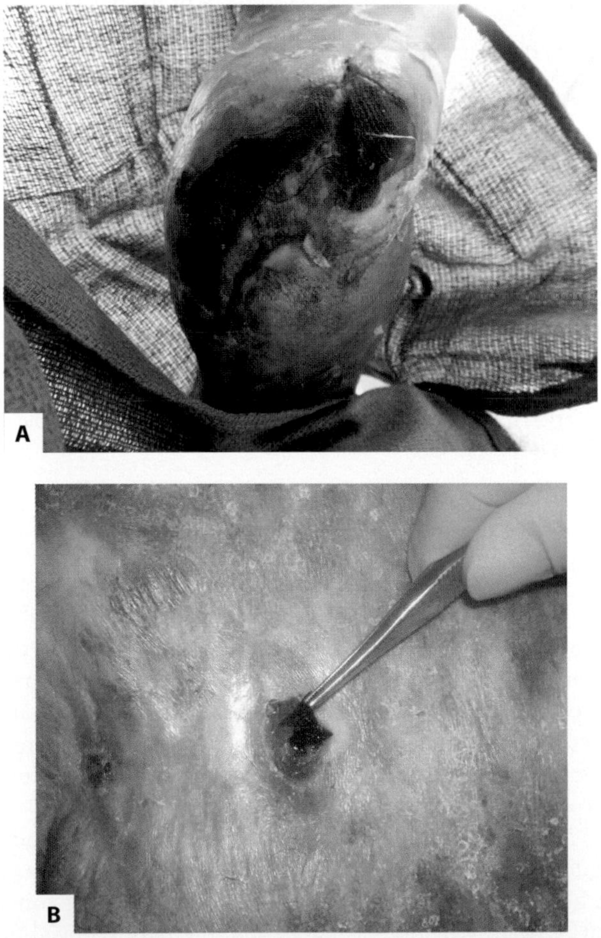

FIGURE 3-25 Foreign objects. A. Both the suture and the eschar on the heel wound are perceived as foreign objects by the body and need to be removed for the wound to progress. **B.** The deep suture extruding from the last area of a dehisced abdominal wound will keep the wound from fully re-epithelializing unless it is removed.

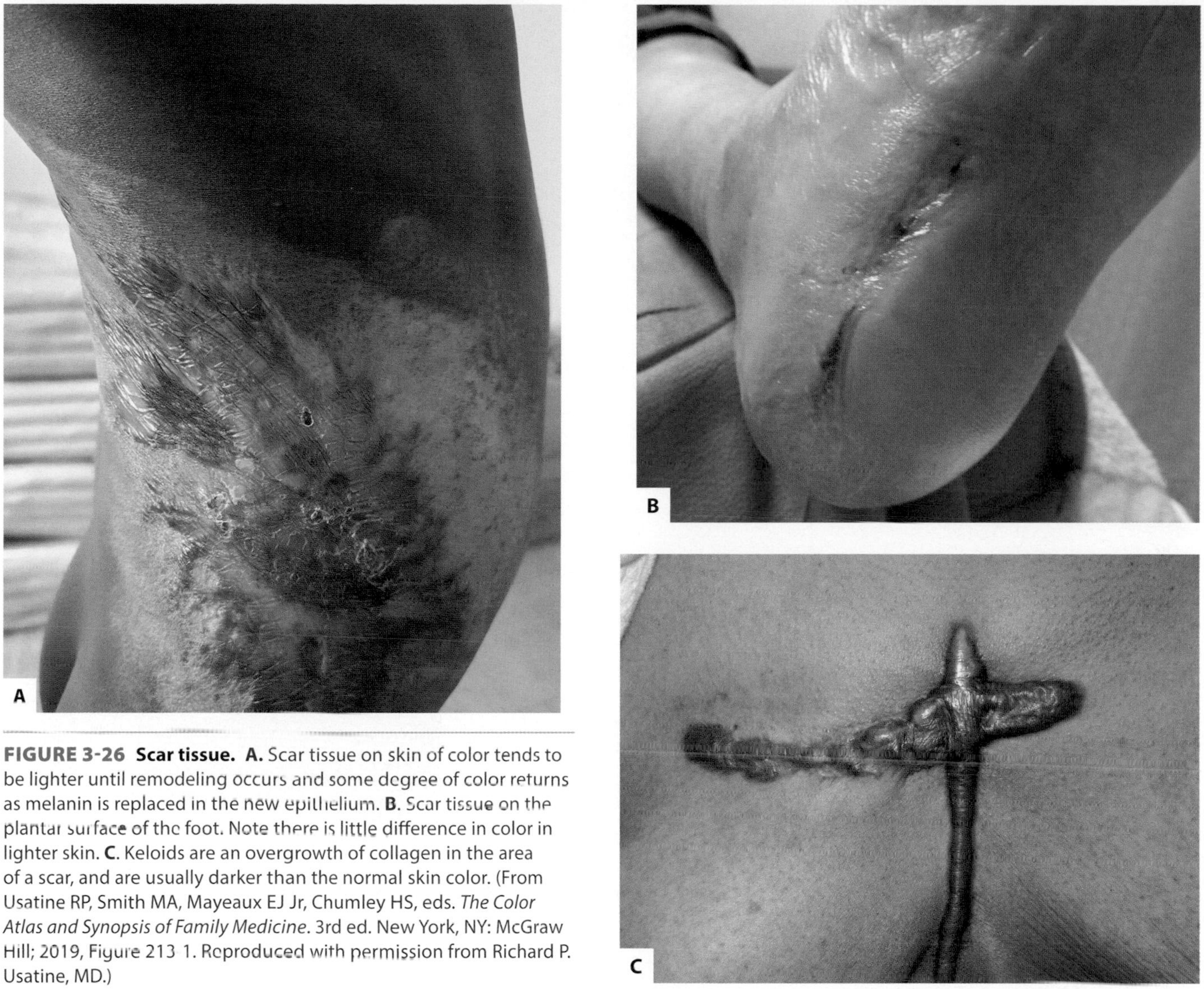

FIGURE 3-26 Scar tissue. A. Scar tissue on skin of color tends to be lighter until remodeling occurs and some degree of color returns as melanin is replaced in the new epithelium. **B.** Scar tissue on the plantar surface of the foot. Note there is little difference in color in lighter skin. **C.** Keloids are an overgrowth of collagen in the area of a scar, and are usually darker than the normal skin color. (From Usatine RP, Smith MA, Mayeaux EJ Jr, Chumley HS, eds. *The Color Atlas and Synopsis of Family Medicine*. 3rd ed. New York, NY: McGraw Hill; 2019, Figure 213-1. Reproduced with permission from Richard P. Usatine, MD.)

Imaging devices that are used to assess scars include reflectance spectroscopy (for color), laser imaging (for microcirculation), and computerized analysis of digital photographs (for two- and three-dimensional measurements).[38]

Several scar scales have been developed; however, the Vancouver Scar Scale is the most frequently used in the clinical setting, especially for burn patients (**TABLE 3-7**). Scar severity and impact on the patient's quality of life drive decisions on how best to treat scars, including exercise, compression garments, silicone dressings, stretching and massage, and in some cases, surgery.

Drainage

Drainage, or lack of it, provides valuable information about the wound status in terms of healing phase, infection, and other factors that may be inhibiting wound healing.[39,40] In addition to identification of the drainage type, the amount is also documented and becomes an outcome measure as it decreases in amount and improves in quality. While terms like *scant*, *minimum*, *moderate*, *heavy*, and *copious* have been used to describe the amount of drainage, no definitions have been established for these terms. The author suggests the definitions in **TABLE 3-8** that may be helpful for the clinician in describing the amount of drainage observed during the assessment.

Serous drainage is clear watery serum that normally appears during the inflammatory phase of acute wound healing and diminishes as healing progresses. It contains proteins but has no evident red blood cells or cellular debris to give it color. Common examples are the clear fluid in a blister or from an abrasion, and the drainage from an edematous extremity (**FIGURE 3-27A, B**).

Sanguineous drainage is thin blood that drains from a surgical or acute traumatic wound, or from the wound tissue (eg, subcutaneous or granulation) of a patient who is prone to bleeding because of medications (eg, anticoagulants) or low platelet count. Excessive bleeding slows down the healing process because of the loss of platelets, growth factors,

TABLE 3-7 Vancouver Scar Scale (VSS)

Scar Characteristic	Score
Vascularity	
Normal	0
Pink	1
Red	2
Purple	3
Pigmentation	
Normal	0
Hypopigmentation	1
Hyperpigmentation	2
Pliability	
Normal	0
Supple	1
Yielding	2
Firm	3
Ropes	4
Contracture	5
Height (mm)	
Flat	0
<2	1
2~5	2
>5	3
Total score	13

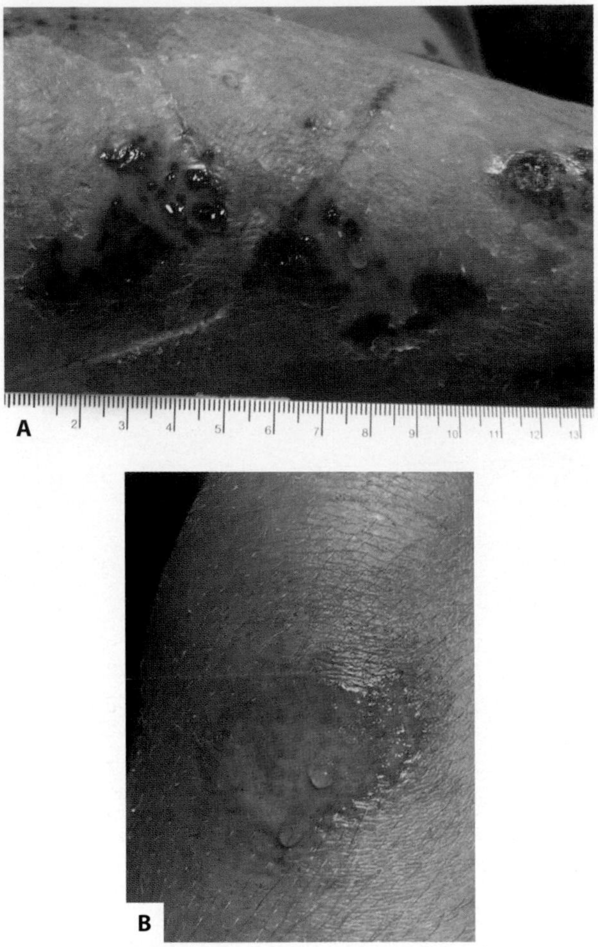

FIGURE 3-27 Serous drainage. A. Clear serous fluid draining from lower leg wounds, and **B.** from an acute knee abrasion.

TABLE 3-8 Definitions of Terms Used to Describe Amount of Drainage

Term	Description Based on Observation at Dressing Removal
Scant	Barely any drainage visible on the side of the dressing next to the wound; none visible after dressing removal.
Minimum	Drainage visible on the inner side of the dressing only; may be some visible on the wound bed after dressing removal; no new drainage expressed during treatment.
Moderate	Drainage visible on the inner side and small amount on the outer side of the dressing; some drainage visible on the wound bed after dressing removal; some drainage occurring during prolonged treatments.
Heavy	Drainage visible on both the inner side and outer side of the dressing; drainage visible immediately after dressing removal and after wound cleansing; may continue throughout the treatment.
Copious	Drainage not contained by a dressing deemed appropriate for the wound; drainage continues throughout the treatment requiring continuous cleansing, suctioning, or, in the case of bleeding, pressure or thrombotic applications.

and other cells required for the healing cascade to progress. Bleeding that clots within the wound bed is termed *coagulum* (**FIGURE 3-28A, B**).

Serosanguineous drainage is pink serous drainage because of the presence of a few red blood cells in the fluid (**FIGURE 3-29**).

Exudate is pale yellow drainage composed of serum, dead cells, and lysed debris with a high protein concentration (specific gravity > 1.015) (**FIGURE 3-30**).[41] It is usually present in the inflammatory phase as the body autolyses the dead cells that result from the injury. *Transudate* is serous drainage that has a low protein concentration (specific gravity < 1.015).

Purulence is thick, often odiferous, drainage that contains a large amount of lysed debris and bacteria. Commonly called *pus*, it indicates that a wound is locally infected (**FIGURE 3-31**). *Seropurulence* is cloudy yellow or tan drainage, a sign that the body is destroying bacteria that may be in the wound; intervention to prevent infection is indicated.

Lymphatic drainage is serous drainage that has a high concentration of protein and fat molecules that are too large to be resorbed by the capillaries; it is frequently seen in surgical wounds that are in close proximity to lymph nodes (eg, the

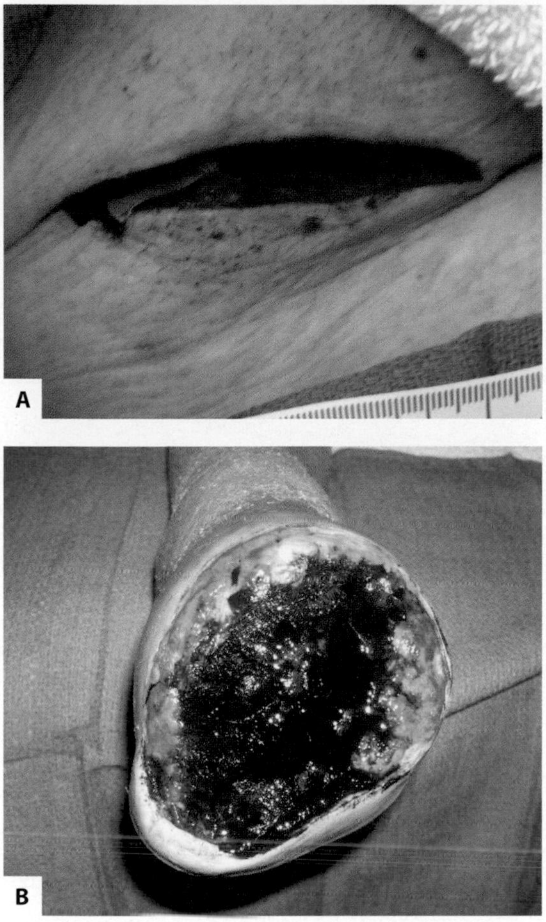

FIGURE 3-28 Sanguineous drainage. A. Sanguineous drainage is simply a medical term for bleeding, as is seen in the groin wound. It may be the result of a severed vessel, low platelets, or anticoagulation medication. **B.** A large amount of coagulum has collected in the base of the recent transmetatarsal amputation. Coagulum is removed cautiously as it may be serving as a clot to prevent further bleeding; if no new bleeding is occurring under the coagulum, it is removed to allow the healing process to progress.

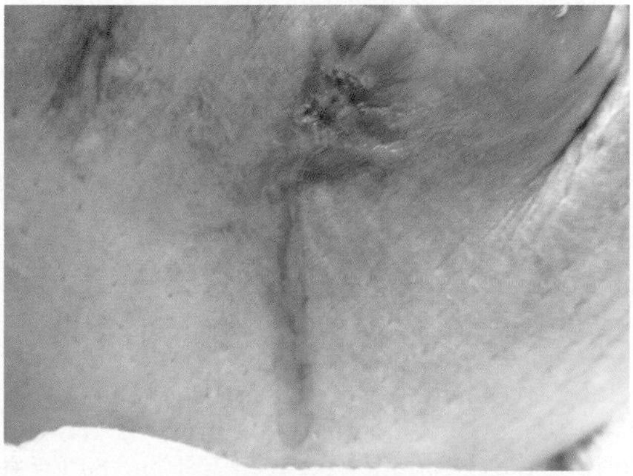

FIGURE 3-29 Serosanguineous drainage. Serosanguineous drainage is flowing from the pinpoint opening in an otherwise closed surgical incision, indicating a subcutaneous seroma or a small granuloma around an undissolved suture. Usually this type of wound needs to be opened, irrigated, and any foreign or necrotic tissue removed, a procedure termed *incision and drainage (I&D)*.

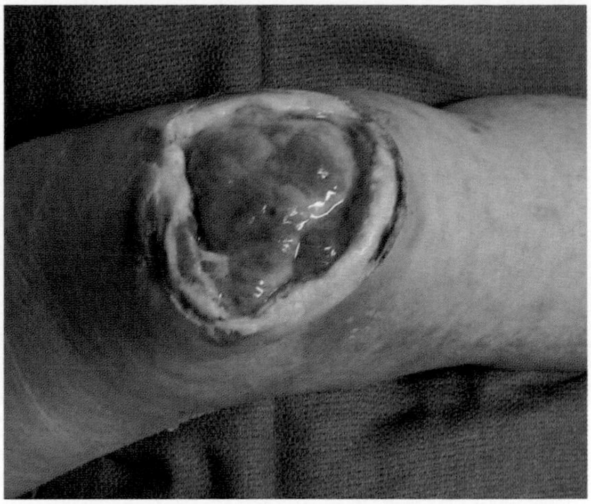

FIGURE 3-30 Exudate. The yellow drainage termed *exudate* can be seen on the right side of the heel wound. Because of the high protein content, the drainage sometimes coagulates on the surface of the wound and is referred to as *pseudoeschar* or *gelatinous edema*.

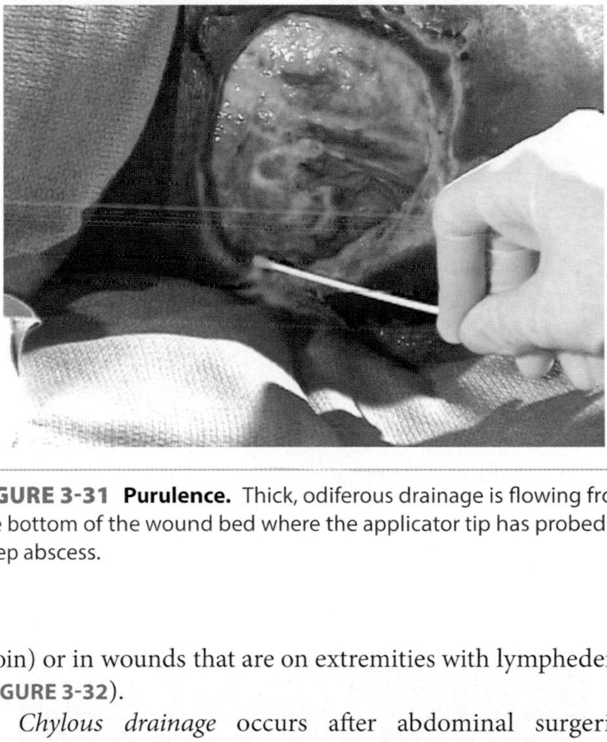

FIGURE 3-31 Purulence. Thick, odiferous drainage is flowing from the bottom of the wound bed where the applicator tip has probed a deep abscess.

groin) or in wounds that are on extremities with lymphedema (**FIGURE 3-32**).

Chylous drainage occurs after abdominal surgeries, especially retroperitoneal ones, where there is trauma to the cisterna chyli or adjacent lymphatic trunks. The lymphatic system carries fluid with fat and protein molecules too large to return via the venous system; therefore, the chylous drainage that leaks from the wound is rich in triglycerides, giving it a thick, white, milky consistency (**FIGURE 3-33**).[42] The lymphatic system, its functions, and disorders are discussed in detail in Chapter 5, Lymphedema.

Infected drainage, in addition to being thick and opaque, may have a greenish tint with a distinct odor, indicative of a *Pseudomonas* infection (**FIGURE 3-34**).

Enterocutaneous or *enteroatmospheric fistula drainage* can vary from thin and watery to thick and formed, from green

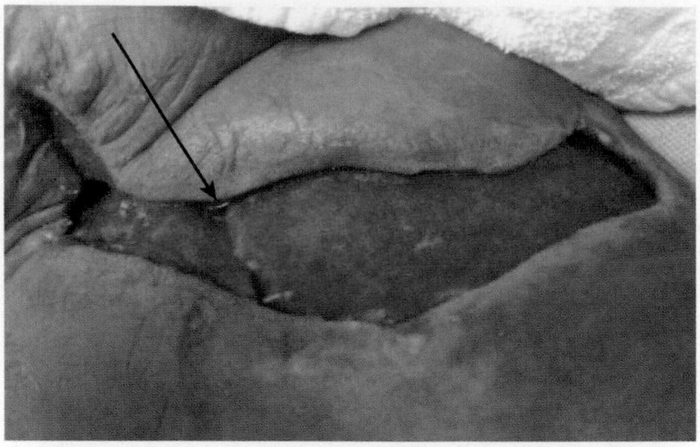

FIGURE 3-32 Lymphatic drainage. Clear lymphatic fluid is frequently seen in groin wounds when the lymph vessels have been severed and flow through the lymph nodes is interrupted. The fluid can be seen collecting at the upper edge of the wound.

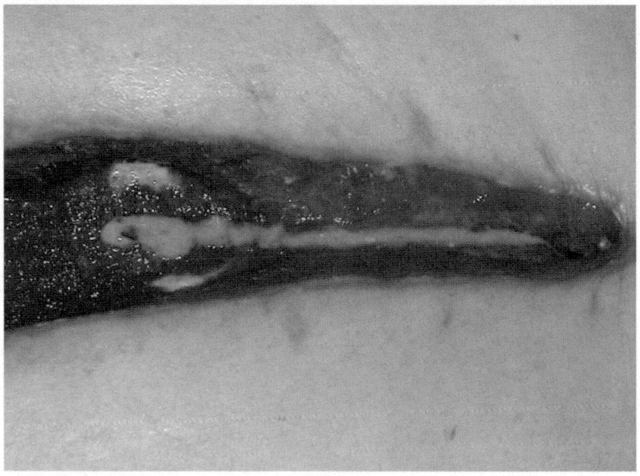

FIGURE 3-33 Chyle. Chylous fluid is draining from the abdominal wound of a patient who had gastric bypass surgery. The thick, milky white fluid may be mistaken for purulence; however, it is the high emulsified fat content in the abdominal lymphatic fluid that gives chyle its appearance.

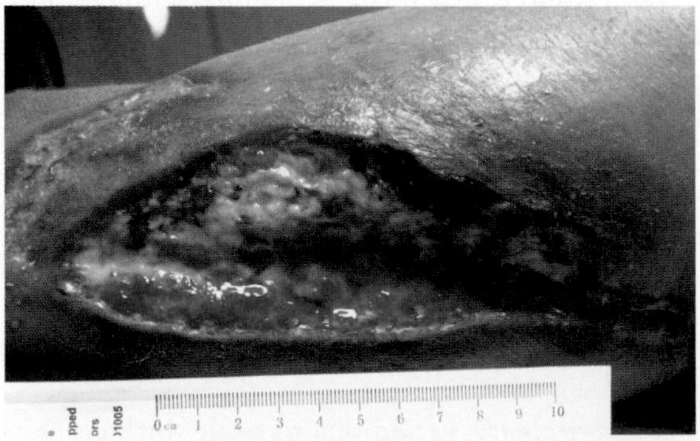

FIGURE 3-34 Drainage with *Pseudomonas* infection The green tint to the slough in this lower extremity wound indicates a high probability of the presence of *Pseudomonas*, either critical contamination or infection. It may also be accompanied by a sweet smell that is characteristic of the *Pseudomonas* microbe.

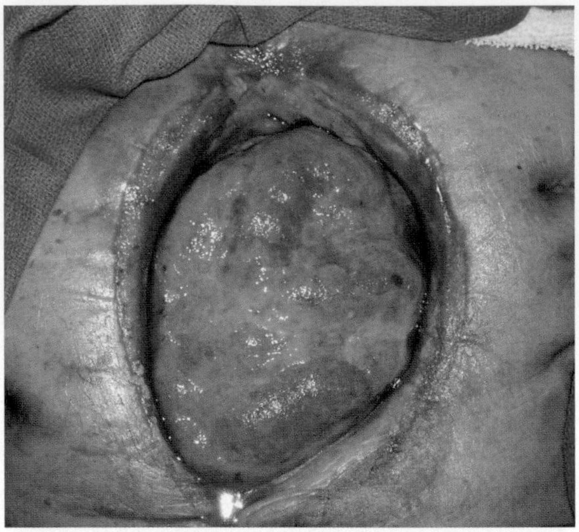

FIGURE 3-35 Fistula drainage. The thin watery brown drainage seen in the periphery of this abdominal wound is from a fistula located in the deep area at the wound periphery, termed *gutter*. Thin, sometimes green, drainage is usually from the more proximal intestine, whereas brown and thicker contents are usually from the more distal or large bowel.

bilious to brown fecal matter, and from no odor to strong odor, all depending on the location of the fistula. If drainage is suspected to be from a new fistula, the referring physician should be notified immediately (**FIGURE 3-35**).

Periwound Skin

Careful examination of the periwound skin may provide clues to the wound etiology, the extent of tissue damage, and tissue vascularity for healing. Characteristics that are notable include color, temperature, and texture. In Chapter 1, Anatomy and Physiology of the Integumentary System, some of the physiologic differences in skin of varying color are discussed and need to be considered when evaluating periwound skin. Changes in color can be harder to detect in hyperpigmented skin; therefore, it is essential to assess temperature and texture in such cases.[43] Comparison with an uninvolved area of the body is especially helpful in detecting individual changes in color.

Temperature Temperature differences can be palpable with the examiner's hand, or can be objectively measured with an infrared skin thermometer, thermistor, skin thermometer strips, infrared camera,[44] or thermogram.[23]

Normal skin temperature on the trunk is between 92°F and 96°F; on the extremities, between 75°F and 80°F.[23] Studies have indicated that 33°C is the critical level required for normal cellular activity.[45] A difference (increase) of 3°F or more indicates presence of pathology (eg, inflammation secondary to deep tissue injury, infection in the wound or periwound tissue, or acute Charcot foot fracture).[44–49] A decrease in skin temperature is usually suggestive of arterial insufficiency that has become ischemia. Possible diagnoses include severe peripheral vascular disease with arterial occlusion, embolic occlusion, compartment syndrome, or severe hypotension.

Color *Erythema* is defined as redness of the skin and can be caused by a multitude of conditions. It may be further defined as blanchable (meaning it turns lighter with pressure and recovers to its original color within seconds) or nonblanchable. Causes of blanchable skin include inflammation, infection, allergic reaction, sunburn, frostbite, or reactive hyperemia (increased blood supply to an area that occurs after the blood supply has been absent and is then restored, eg, after revascularization surgery) (**FIGURES 3-36** to **3-39**). Redness in areas

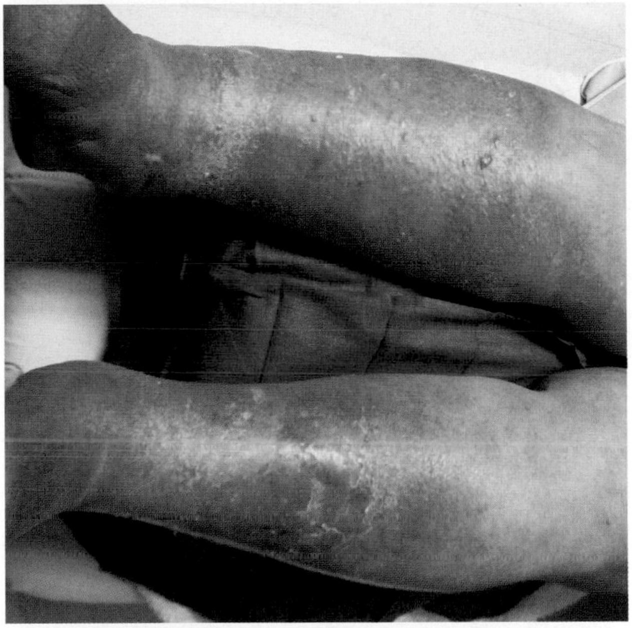

FIGURE 3-36 Cellulitis. The erythema on the bilateral lower extremities is a result of cellulitis, a frequent complication of chronic edema or lymphedema.

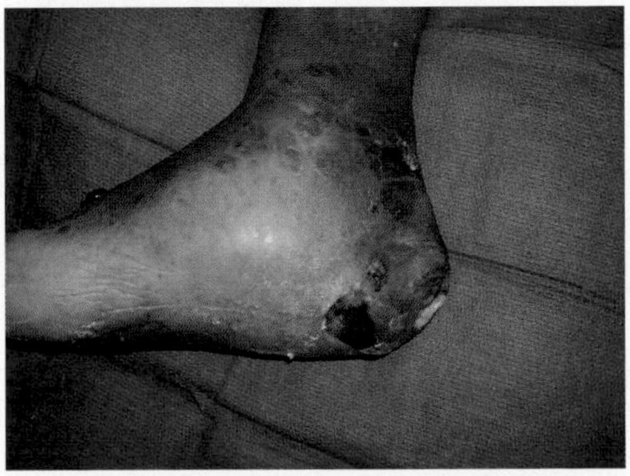

FIGURE 3-37 Infection. The erythema and edema surrounding the pressure ulcer on the heel indicate there is deep infection. Other signs to note are warmth, pain with weight-bearing, and drainage from the wound. For diabetic foot ulcers, erythema that extends more than 2 cm from the edge of the wound is highly correlated with infection. If the wound can be probed to bone, there is a strong probability of osteomyelitis, or infection of the underlying bone.[44]

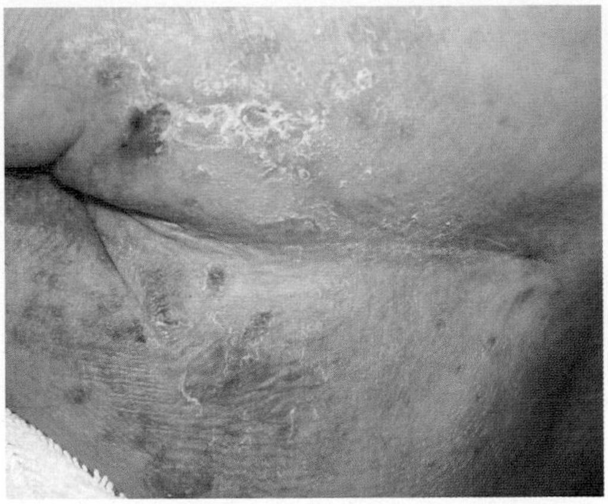

FIGURE 3-38 Excoriation. The erythema on the sacral/perianal skin is a result of excoriation, or loss of the epidermis, from moisture and friction.

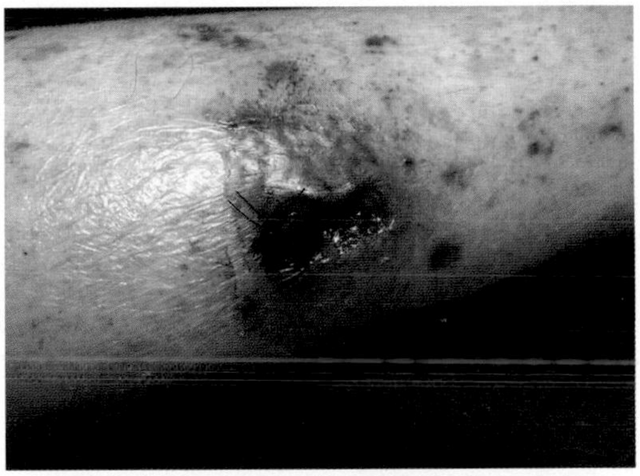

FIGURE 3-39 Inflammation. The erythema in this lower extremity wound is an inflammatory response to an acute injury, a pathogen, or a vasculitic disorder. A tissue biopsy has been performed (note the suture site) to help determine the underlying pathology.

that have nonblanchable erythema is related to altered blood perfusion.[50] As with all abnormal characteristics, determining the cause of erythema is a necessary precedent to treatment.

Cyanosis is a blue-to-purple discoloration indicating lack of blood flow to the area. Initially it may be termed *dusky*, a visible early sign of hypoxia. Cyanosis usually occurs in the distal extremities as a result of severe peripheral vascular disease, emboli, or Raynaud's syndrome (**FIGURE 3-40**).

Dark red discoloration is a result of capillary bleeding that occurs in the deep tissue as a result of bone shearing on the adjacent soft tissue. Suspected deep tissue injury (see Chapter 6, Pressure Injuries and Ulcers) and pre-ulcerative lesions on the diabetic foot are two examples where this type of discoloration is observed (**FIGURES 3-41** and **3-42**).

Hemosiderin staining is a brownish-purple discoloration most frequently seen in patients with chronic venous insufficiency. Red blood cells are trapped in the interstitial congestion, and when they die by apoptosis, the body lyses the dead cells and the hemoglobin attached to them. The by-products of this autolytic process migrate to the superficial cutaneous layers and cause the discoloration (**FIGURE 3-43**).

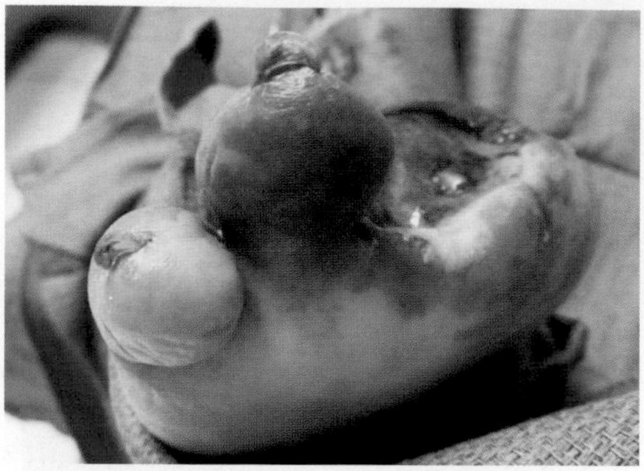

FIGURE 3-40 Cyanosis. Several degrees of hypoxia can be distinguished on the foot with severe peripheral arterial disease—the red mottled appearance on the plantar medial foot, the purple on the lateral aspect of the fourth toe, and the almost black area on the medial plantar surface of the fourth toe. The blanched white skin on the plantar foot is an additional indication of lack of blood flow to the foot.

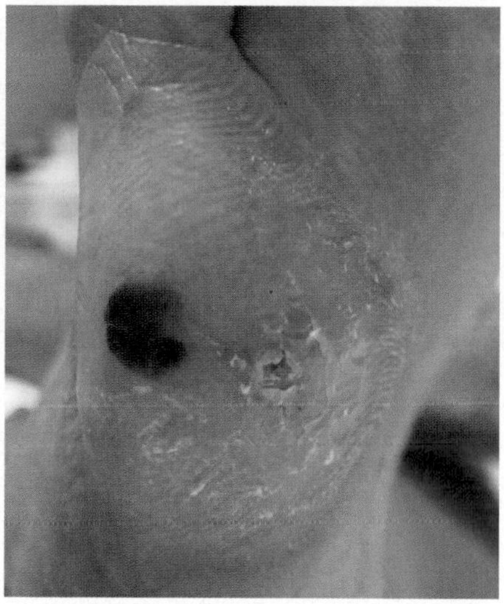

FIGURE 3-41 Dark red discoloration on plantar foot. The dark discoloration on the plantar surface of a diabetic foot, while not specifically termed deep tissue injury, is from the same mechanical force—shearing of the bone against the adjacent subcutaneous tissue causing capillary destruction and deposition of red blood cells in the epidermis. If the cause (usually poorly fitting shoes) is not removed, the tissue damage will lead to full-thickness ulceration.

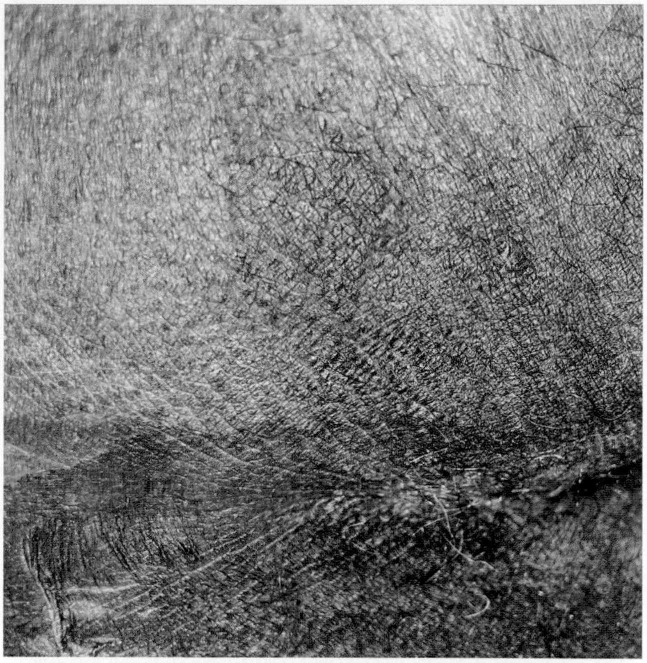

FIGURE 3-42 Deep tissue injury on a patient with darker skin. Changes in skin texture and temperature are also indications of deep tissue injury.

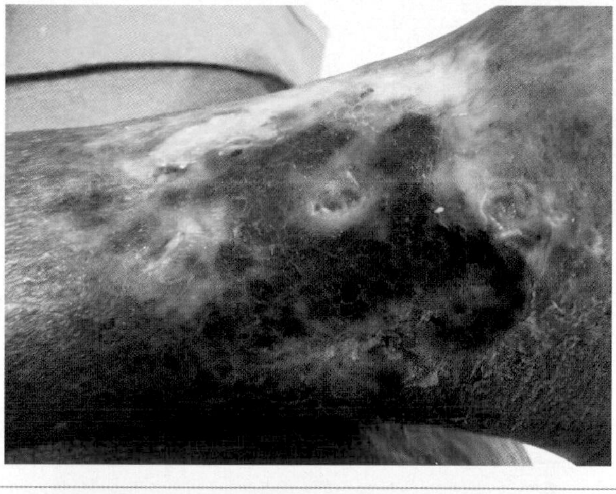

FIGURE 3-43 Hemosiderin staining. The dark staining in the skin of a patient with chronic venous insufficiency is a result of the autolysis of hemoglobin in the dead red blood cells that migrate to the dermis/epidermis. Other signs of venous insufficiency are the bark-like texture of the skin, the thick scaling of the epidermis, and the location of the wound above the ankle.

Ecchymosis or bruising is a result of deep tissue trauma that causes hemorrhaging of the blood vessels, resulting in dark-red-to-blue discoloration that goes through a sequence of colors (bluish-red to green to yellow) as it heals (**FIGURE 3-44**).

Blanched or lighter skin relative to the person's natural color can be the result of decreased blood supply to the skin, a sign of underlying infection, or a result of chronic venous insufficiency. In the latter case, it is termed *atrophie blanche* (**FIGURE 3-45A, B**).

Jaundice (or yellow skin, sclerae, mucous membranes, and excretions including wound drainage) is a result of hyperbilirubinemia and may be associated with a variety of disorders such as cirrhosis, hepatitis, obstruction of the bile duct, or hemolytic blood transfusion reaction (**FIGURE 3-46**).[51] Hyperbilirubinemia can also occur in infants who have either overproduction of bilirubin or a reduction in glucuronide conjugation in the liver.[52,53]

Texture Changes in skin texture include a thin, shiny appearance with no hair (a result of peripheral arterial disease);

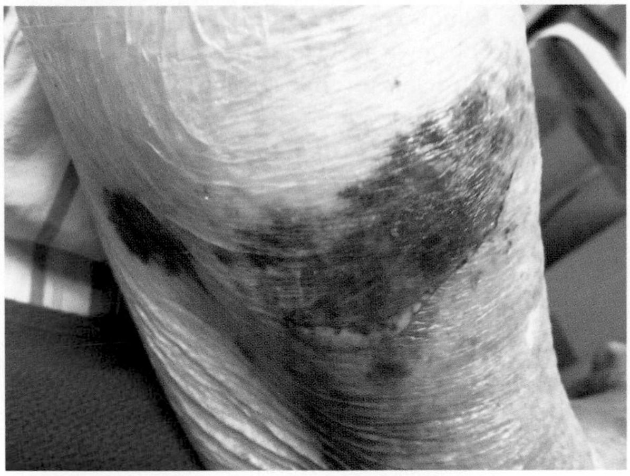

FIGURE 3-44 Ecchymosis Ecchymosis or bruising is visible around the skin tear on the lower extremity as a result of acute trauma.

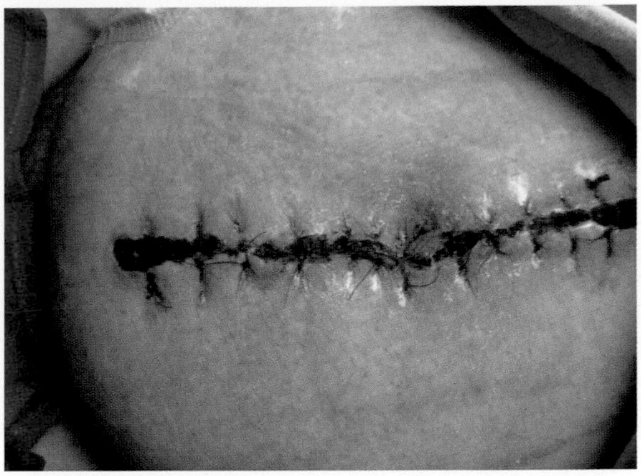

FIGURE 3-46 Jaundice. The yellow, or jaundiced, skin on this patient who has recently received a liver transplant is typical of hyperbilirubinemia associated with liver failure.

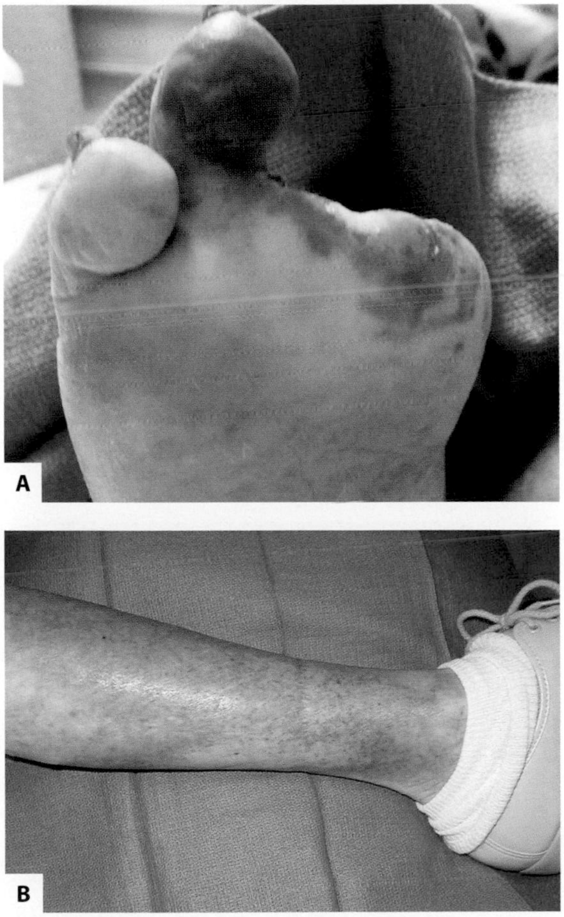

FIGURE 3-45 Blanched skin. A. The yellowish-white area over the second, third, and fourth plantar metatarsal heads is a common indication of underlying infection. The fluid may also cause the skin to be boggy, or there may be fluctuance in the subcutaneous tissue. **B.** Atrophie blanche, a sign of chronic venous insufficiency, is a result of decreased blood flow to the skin due to the venous interstitial congestion. The white area of atrophie blanche is visible on the posterior aspect of the lower extremity gaiter area.

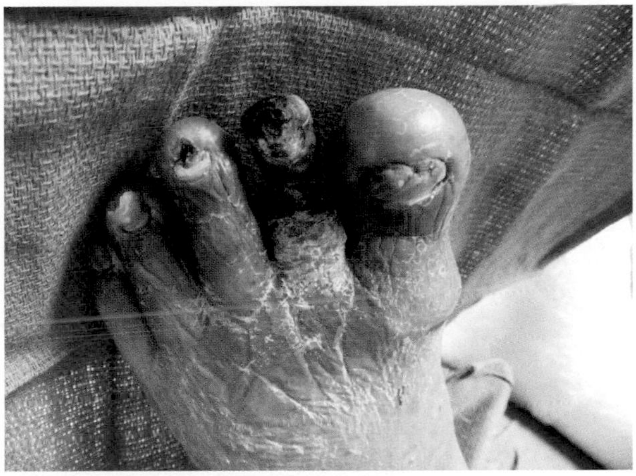

FIGURE 3-47 Skin changes with arterial disease. The foot on the patient with severe peripheral arterial disease shows several signs of poor circulation—no hair growth on the toes; thick nails with probable fungus, termed *onychomycosis*; dry gangrene of the second toe; and dry, cracking skin. Vascular screening would probably reveal nonpalpable pulses and weak or absent Doppler signals of the dorsalis pedis and posterior tibial arteries.

thick, rough with thick scales (a result of chronic venous insufficiency); or orange peel texture, also called *peau d'orange* (a result of chronic edema). The skin may also become indurated, meaning the subcutaneous tissue is hard and firm (also a result of chronic edema, eg, with lymphedema) with fibrosis of the underlying connective tissue (**FIGURES 3-47** to **3-50**).

Edema

Edema results from abnormal amounts of water in the subcutaneous or interstitial tissue. When observed during an evaluation, the cause of the edema is determined by further exploring patient history, systems review, medications, and other symptoms. Again, the question, *why?*, has to be answered. Causes, measurement, and diagnosis of edema are discussed at length

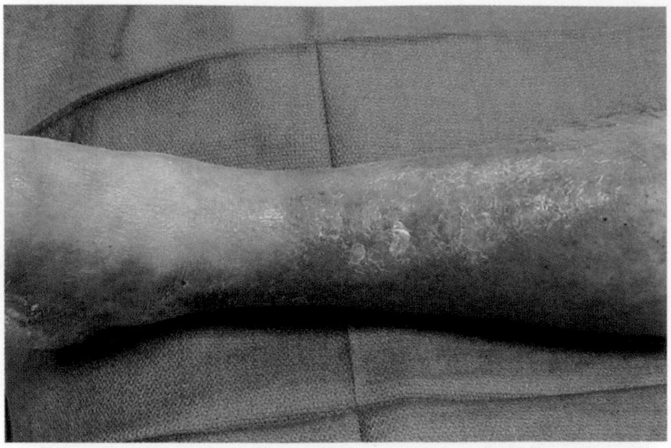

FIGURE 3-48 Venous scales. The thick epidermal scales on the lower leg are a common sign of chronic venous insufficiency.

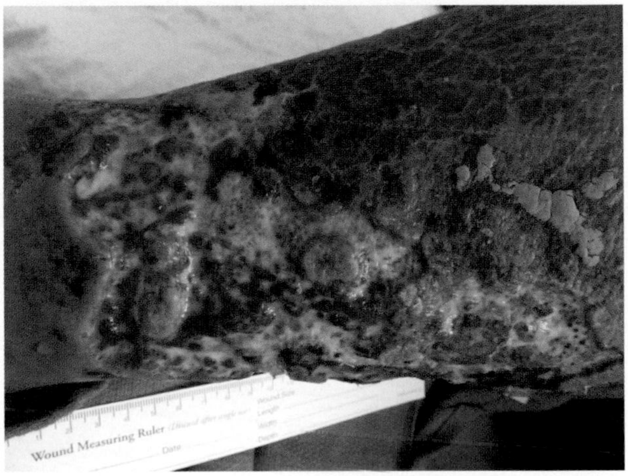

FIGURE 3-49 Texture changes. Several signs of chronic venous insufficiency (besides the typical serpentine wounds) are the orange peel texture of the skin, the hemosiderin stains, and the thick bark-like skin.

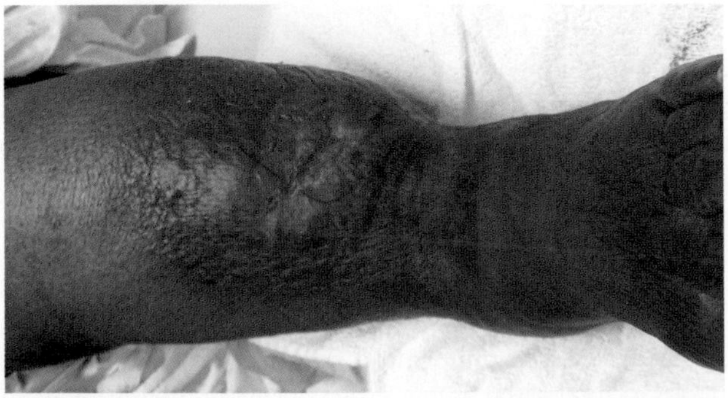

FIGURE 3-50 Induration. The hard, discolored area around the wound is termed *induration*, a sign of severe edema and fibrosis of the subcutaneous tissue. Again, note the orange peel texture and hemosiderosis.

in Chapter 5, Lymphedema. Examples of edema associated with wounds are shown in **FIGURES 3-51** to **3-54**. Note that sudden onset of edema in one extremity, edema associated with pain, or edema associated with any other cardiovascular symptoms require that the patient be seen by a medical specialist on an emergent basis.

Wound Edges

Observing what is happening at the wound edges can provide information on the cause of the wound as well as the healing potential. As the wound goes through the proliferative phase, careful attention to the edges will also facilitate wound re-epithelialization.

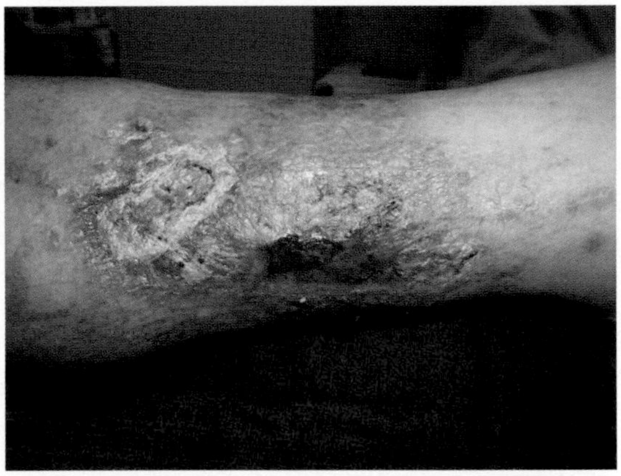

FIGURE 3-51 Edema due to chronic venous insufficiency. The most common cause of lower extremity edema is chronic venous insufficiency, and it is usually associated with other signs and symptoms such as hemosiderosis, thick scaly skin, open wounds, complaints of heavy aching feelings, and frequent cellulitis.

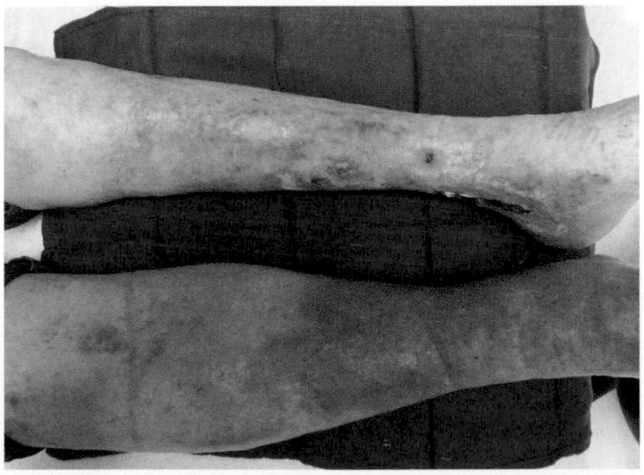

FIGURE 3-52 Edema due to obstruction. Sudden onset of edema that does not respond to standard therapy (ie, compression) is indicative of an obstruction proximal to the area that is edematous. This patient developed sudden onset of right lower extremity that extended to the groin, while she was being treated for the left lower extremity venous wound. The etiology of the right lower extremity edema was a rare malignancy that caused obstruction of the pelvic and abdominal lymph nodes.

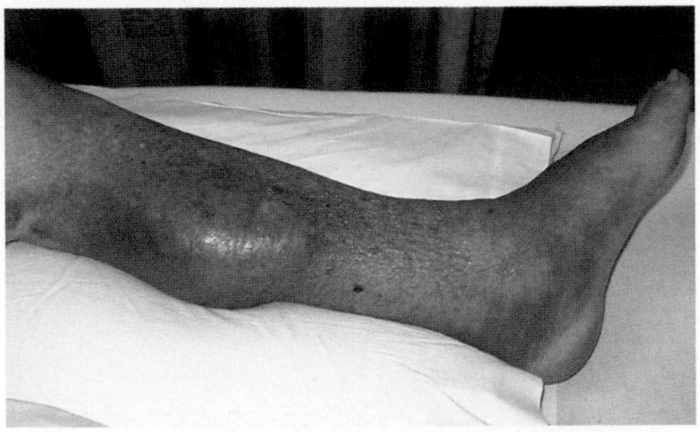

FIGURE 3-53 Edema due to trauma. A fall caused the severe hematoma and surrounding local edema on the calf as well as the distal pedal edema and ecchymosis.

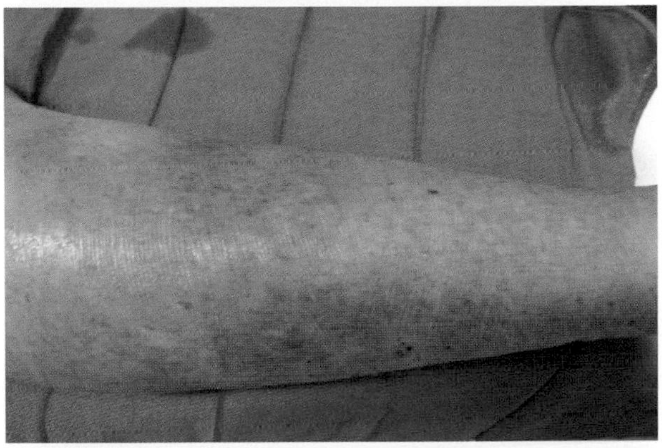

FIGURE 3-54 Edema due to systemic disorders. Edema secondary to systemic disease is usually bilateral and may not have the skin changes seen with chronic venous insufficiency. The ridges visible on the skin are commonly seen after removal of bandages as a result of the decrease in the fluid content of the subcutaneous tissue. It is a positive indication that the compression is effective.

Even edges are usually a result of ischemia to the skin, as in peripheral arterial disease, which causes the wound to have a "punched-out" appearance. Other causes of hypoxia that may result in even edges include poor cardiac output, anemia due to other underlying disorders (eg, a gastrointestinal bleed or sickle cell anemia), and high-dose hydroxyurea. In any of these cases, treatment of the underlying pathology is a must in order for wound healing to occur (**FIGURES 3-55** and **3-56**).

Uneven or serpentine edges are typically seen in wounds caused by chronic venous insufficiency (**FIGURE 3-57**).

Rolled edges occur when the epithelial cells at the edge are unable to migrate across the wound bed. This may be a result of an unhealthy wound bed, inability to produce the basement membrane that the epithelial cells adhere to, or a condition termed *epibole* in which the upper epidermal cells roll down over the lower epidermal cells and prevent epithelial migration across the wound bed. The exact mechanism for the inability of keratinocytes to respond to signaling pathways that stimulate them to migrate across the wound surface is not fully understood; however, the abnormal keratinocytes must

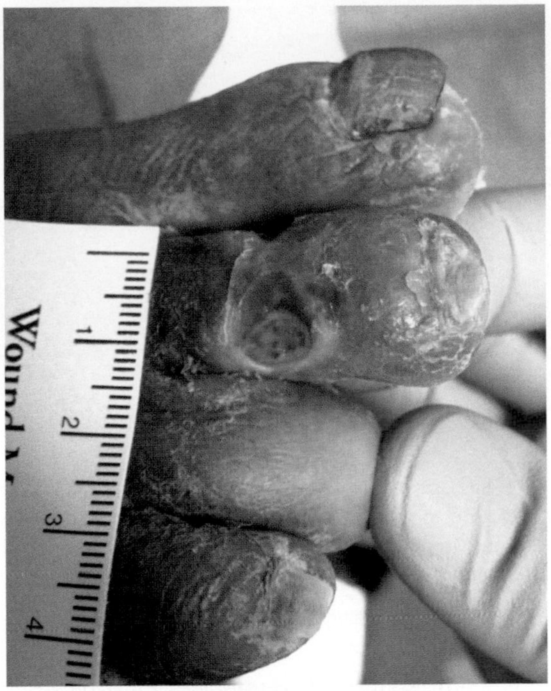

FIGURE 3-55 Even edges. Arterial wounds usually have even edges, giving them a punched-out effect. The granulation, if any, is of poor quality, and other signs of arterial insufficiency are usually present. A second wound is barely visible on the medial aspect of the second toe, illustrating the necessity of doing a good interdigital examination when assessing the foot.

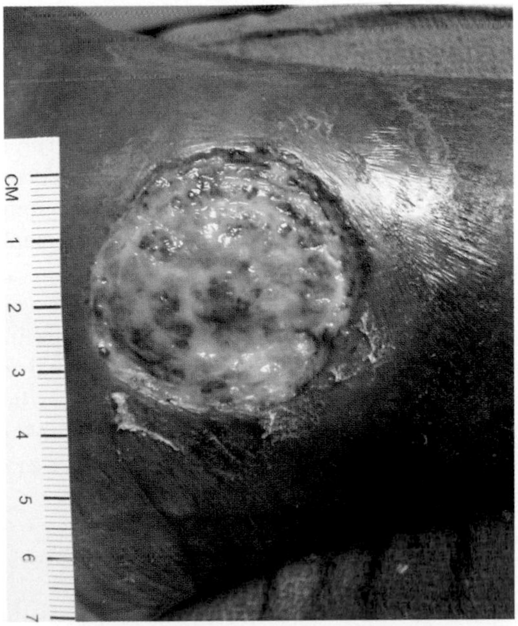

FIGURE 3-56 Even edges due to cardiac disease. Wounds on the lower extremity may appear to be arterial or venous and still not respond to standard care. The patient cardiac status, eg, output and ejection fraction, may be insufficient for good perfusion of the distal lower extremity, giving the wound arterial characteristics, even if it is at an unusual location, as seen in this patient with a wound on the malleolus. The cause of the wound is probably pressure, with failure to heal because of cardiac disease.

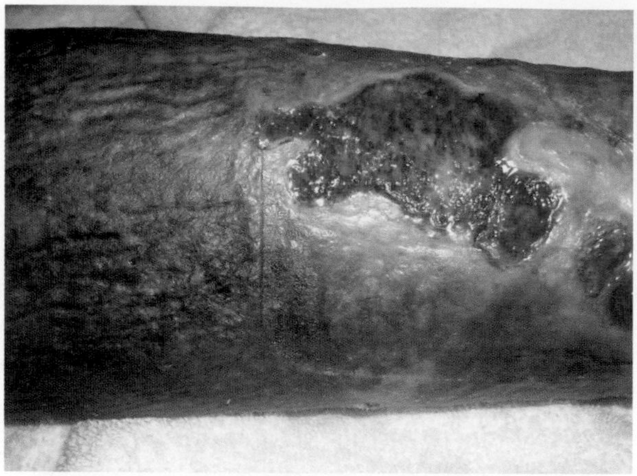

FIGURE 3-57 Uneven edges. Uneven or serpentine edges are typical of wounds caused by venous insufficiency. Other signs seen on this lower extremity wound that suggest venous disease include the hemosiderin stains and edema.

be removed, unresponsive keratinocytes must be stimulated, and/or exogenous keratinocytes must be provided to stimulate epithelial migration. Treatment interventions to stimulate re-epithelialization include advanced or biological dressings and biophysical agents (eg, electrical stimulation, therapeutic ultrasound, negative pressure wound therapy, and hyperbaric oxygen therapy) (**FIGURE 3-58A, B**).[54,55]

Detached edges are a sign of undermining, wound regression possibly due to bacteria load, or premature epithelial migration without a basement membrane adequate to keep the new epithelium attached to the underlying tissue. (**FIGURE 3-59**).

Hyperkeratosis, or *callus*, is a result of overproduction of the stratum corneum or outer layer of the epidermis, usually as a result of repeated friction from shoes or some other device. It is most frequently observed on the foot from poorly fitting shoes or on the hands from mechanical labor, especially on an insensate foot or hand (**FIGURE 3-60**).

Epithelialization, the goal of every wound care intervention, is a sign that the wound is entering the final stages of the proliferative healing phase. Sometimes the preceding basement membrane can be observed on the edge of the granulation tissue, appearing as a thin clear film (**FIGURE 3-61**). This is a fascinating process to observe!

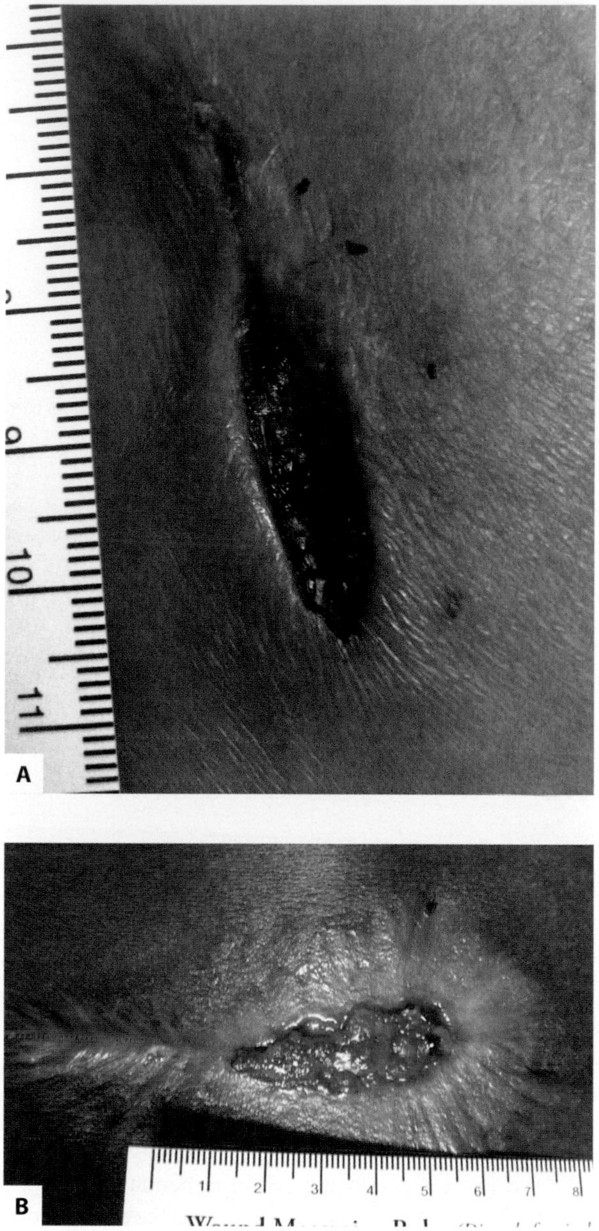

FIGURE 3-58 A. Rolled edges. Rolled edges are usually adhered to the adjacent tissue and must be debrided in order for the granulation tissue and healthy epithelial cells to progress to re-epithelialization of the wound bed. **B. Epibole.** Epibole occurs when the epidermal cells roll down over the lower epidermal cells, thereby preventing the progression of epithelial migration across the wound bed, as seen at the upper edge of this wound. Unlike the wound in **A**, where the rolled edges attach to necrotic tissue, the epidermal cells of epibole usually are adjacent to granulation tissue.

Wound Odor

Wound odor can be a detective signal and something the evaluator learns to recognize. Almost all wounds will have some odor with dressing removal as a result of the interaction between the drainage, the wound, and the dressing; however, the odor to be concerned about is that which persists after the wound has been thoroughly cleaned. Following are some verbal descriptions of common wound odors.

Pseudomonas has a distinctive sweet odor and usually accompanies drainage that has a greenish tint. *Infection* has a putrid smell, and *necrotic* tissue has a unique "dead" odor. *Malignant* tissue can have a musky odor similar to wet cardboard. Sometimes an odor will indicate what type of dressing or topical agent the patient has been putting on the wound (eg, Dakins solution will smell like bleach, acetic acid will smell like vinegar, and dressings with iodine will smell like just that—iodine). If odor is present, lack of odor can be an appropriate initial goal, especially for the patient receiving palliative care.

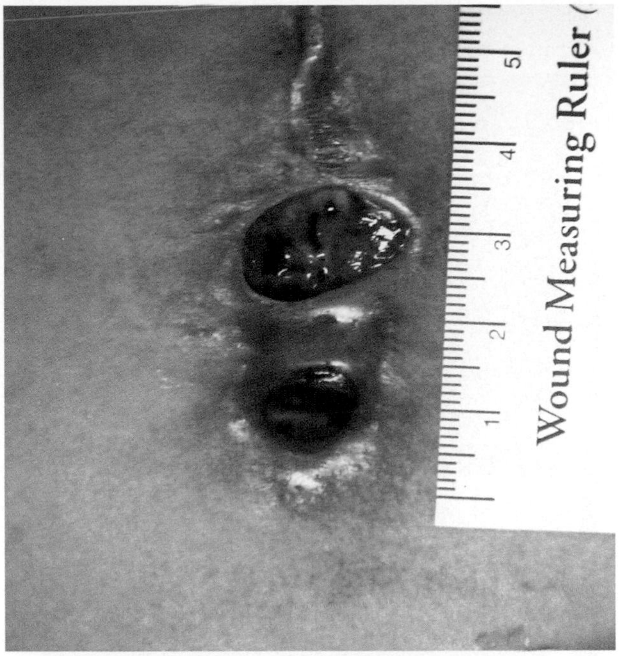

FIGURE 3-59 Detached edges. The dark shadowing at the wound edges indicates that the epithelium is detached from the underlying subcutaneous tissue.

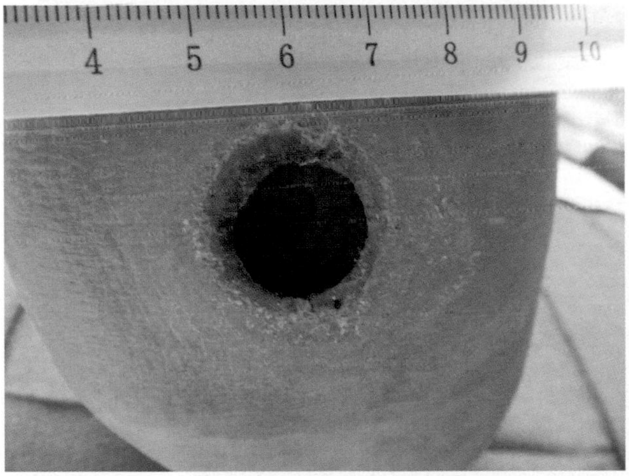

FIGURE 3-60 Hyperkeratosis. Hyperkeratosis, or overdevelopment of the stratum corneum, is common at wound edges where friction is a contributing factor, eg, on the plantar surface of the diabetic foot. It is composed of dead cells and must be debrided in order for healing to progress.

Infection

Signs of infection are listed in **TABLE 3-9**; however, some of the same signs are indicative of inflammation. One distinct difference is that inflammation does not usually have the same odor that accompanies infection because the number of bacteria is significantly less. If there are sufficient signs to suggest infection, and certainly if there are systemic signs of infection such as fever (more than 100.4°F that does not decrease 1–2 days after surgery), malaise, elevated white count, or altered mental status, referral to a medical specialist for antibiotic

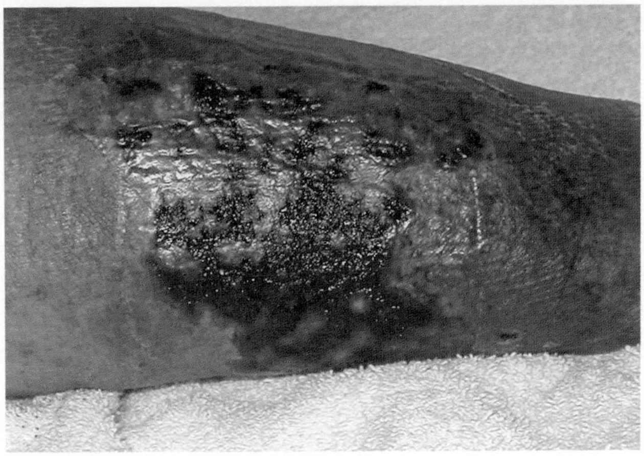

FIGURE 3-61 Epithelial migration. Migration of the epithelial cells across a healthy granulated wound bed is preceded by the formation of basement membrane or a thin layer of fibronectin that serves as the glue for the epithelial cells. Re-epithelialization occurs at the wound margins or at the hair follicles and sweat glands in partial-thickness wounds, as indicated by the islands of new skin growth seen scattered throughout the wound bed.

TABLE 3-9 Signs of Infection

Erythema—usually darker than erythema seen in inflammation, distinct borders, may streak away from the wound
Pain—usually deep and described as throbbing; increasing in intensity
Edema—usually diffuse borders and localized to the wound site rather than full extremity edema observed with chronic venous insufficiency or lymphedema
Heat—usually can be palpated as warm periwound skin; may be measured with an infrared skin thermometer; a difference of 3°F compared to the contralateral side is significant
Purulence—usually thick exudate that may or may not have an odor
Malaise—patient complains of feeling tired, lack of energy

therapy is indicated. Infection is best confirmed by biopsy or fluorescence imaging; surface swabs and purulent samples are considered inadequate for confirming tissue infection in most skin and soft tissue lesions.[56] Infection is discussed in more detail in Chapter 12.

Imaging for Wound Diagnostics

Technologic advances have resulted in the development of a number of noninvasive optical imaging modalities that can provide real-time assessment of the wound microenvironment.[57] The information provided by the imaging devices is both diagnostic and prognostic, thus helping to drive decision making about interventions throughout the course of treatment. In

CLINICAL CONSIDERATION

One consideration in differentiating infection from inflammation for a postsurgical patient is the time since the procedure. Surgical incisions will have some signs of inflammation for several days, including a slight ridge along the incision. If, however, the signs occur a week or more after the procedure, infection must be ruled out.

addition to digital planimetry, the following imaging technologies are being used more frequently in wound management:

Near-infrared spectroscopy (NIRS) is a technology that uses near-infrared light (650–1,100 nm) to measure the absorption of the light by hemoglobin and thus determine the oxygenation status of that tissue and provide information on the microcirculation.[58] NIRS can assess tissue oxygen saturation, oxyhemoglobin, deoxyhemoglobin, and total hemoglobin in large areas of tissue and a few centimeters in depth. Reflectance NIRS cameras then produce anatomical colored images of the region, providing digital oxygen saturation values at any number of selected sites on the image (**FIGURE 3-62A, B**). NIRS is beneficial in monitoring hypoperfusion, inflammation, infection, and venous congestion as treatment and wound healing progress, which assists in making clinical decisions. The information can also be used to monitor changes in tissue perfusion as treatment progresses.[59,60] Certain NIRS devices can also give an accurate temperature reading of the tissue (**FIGURE 3-63**).

Noncontact fluorescence imaging allows visualization of bacterial fluorescence at point of care without the use of contrast agents or patient contact (**FIGURE 3-64**). Moderate to heavy bacterial loads are detected by the imaging device which uses safe violet light illumination (406 nm) to detect red and cyan fluorescence signatures emitted from bacteria, with red indicating the presence of most common bacteria at 10^4 CFUs/g tissue and cyan pseudomonas at 10^4 CFUs/g tissue (**FIGURES 3-65** and **3-66**). The immediate results from fluorescence allow clinicians to provide timely care (eg, cleansing with appropriate agents and debridement) without waiting for the results of cultures or biopsies. Fluorescence imaging has been shown to detect

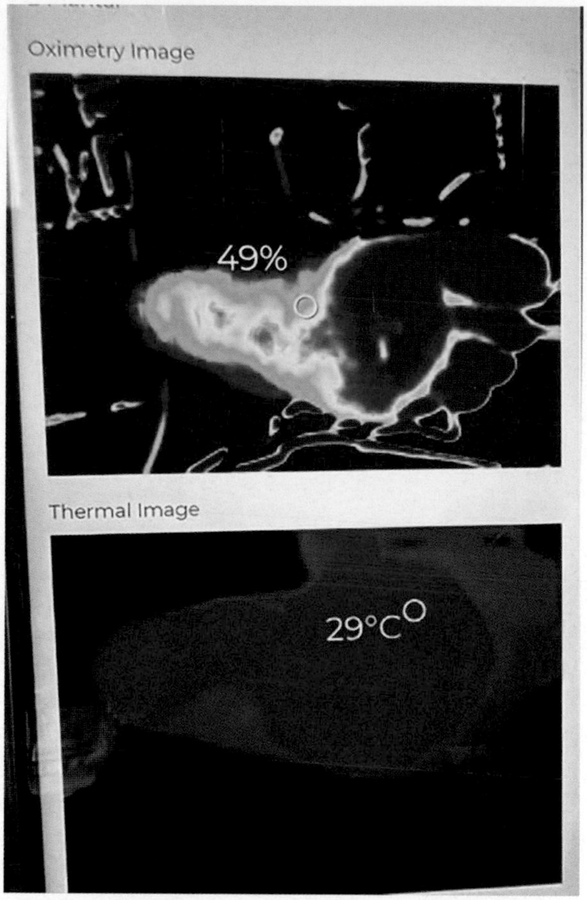

FIGURE 3-63 Images of the plantar foot showing tissue oxygenation as well as temperature.

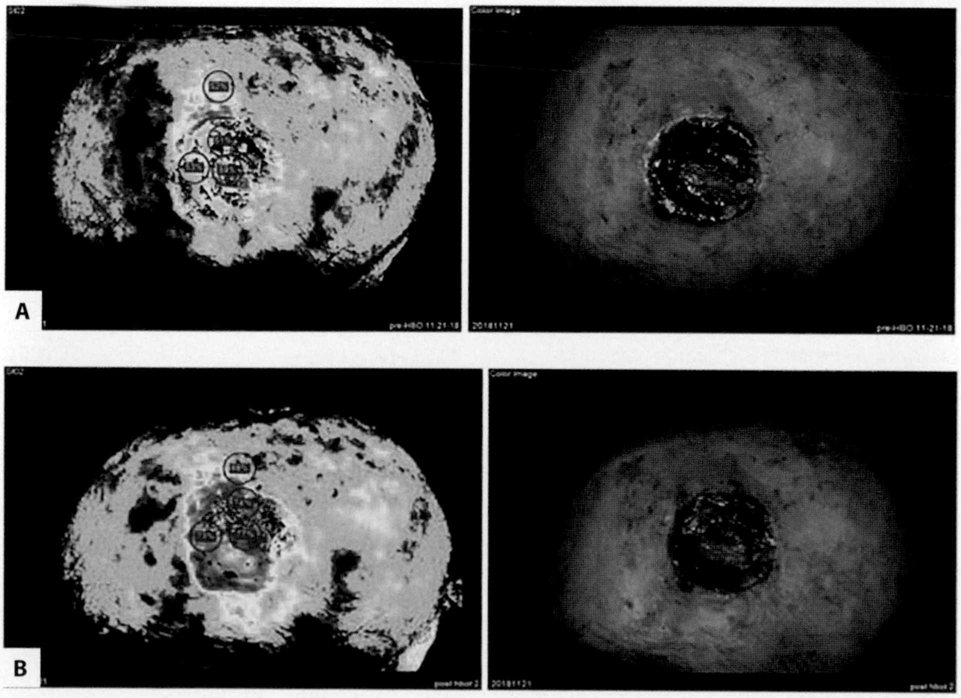

FIGURE 3-62 A. Images of tissue perfusion with near-infrared spectroscopy. The orange-red areas in the same vacinity as the wound indicate tissue oxygenation. Baseline image of a scalp wound with a necrotic graft before the 1st hyperbaric oxygen treatment. **B.** After the 1st hyperbaric oxygen treatment; note the increase of oxygenation in the wound indicated by the red-orange area of the image. (Photographs courtesy of Dr. Jeffrey Niezgoda. Used with permission.)

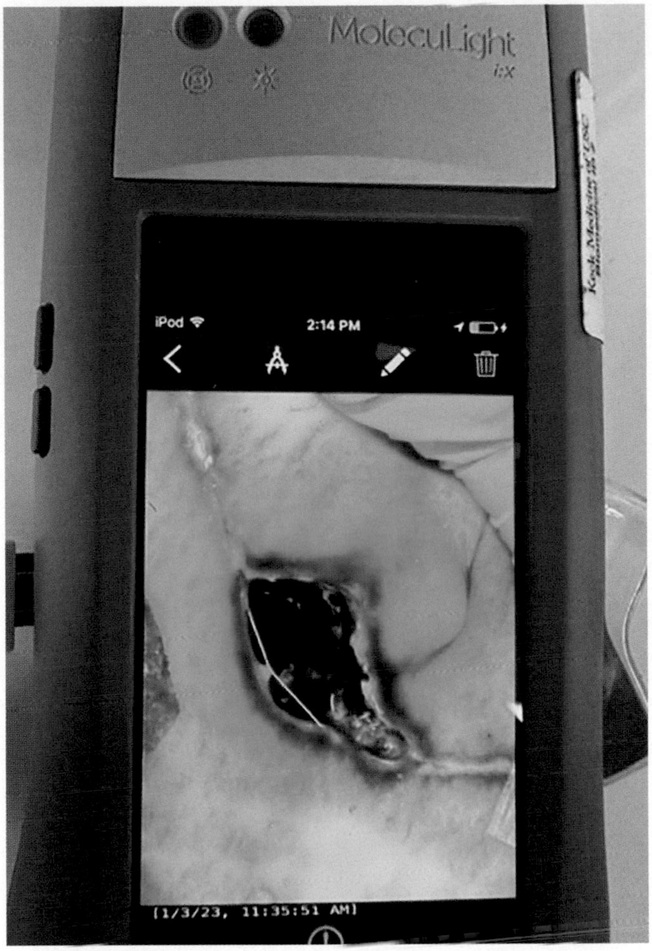

FIGURE 3-64 Fluorescence imaging device.

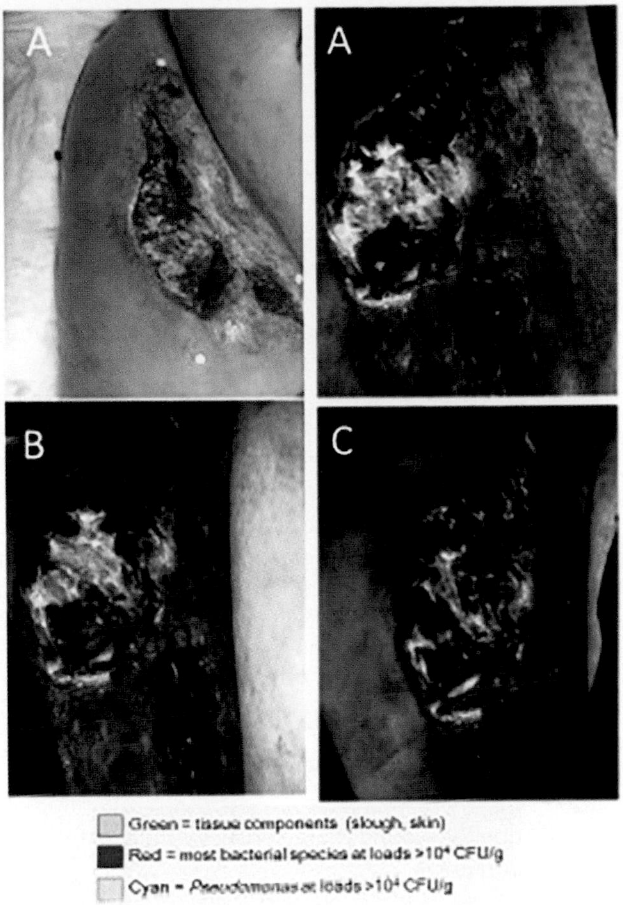

FIGURE 3-65 Fluorescence images. A. Left: An incisional wound after hip surgery. Right: Initial scan showing red fluorescence in the wound and periwound skin, indicative of bacterial presence. **B**. Wound and periwound skin after vigorous cleansing. **C**. Wound after debridement of necrotic tissue. The decrease in bacterial presence was sufficient to allow application of negative pressure after the same treatment session, without having to wait several days for the results of a culture or biopsy to confirm the presence of bacteria. (Used with permission. Photographs courtesy of MolecuLight, Inc.)

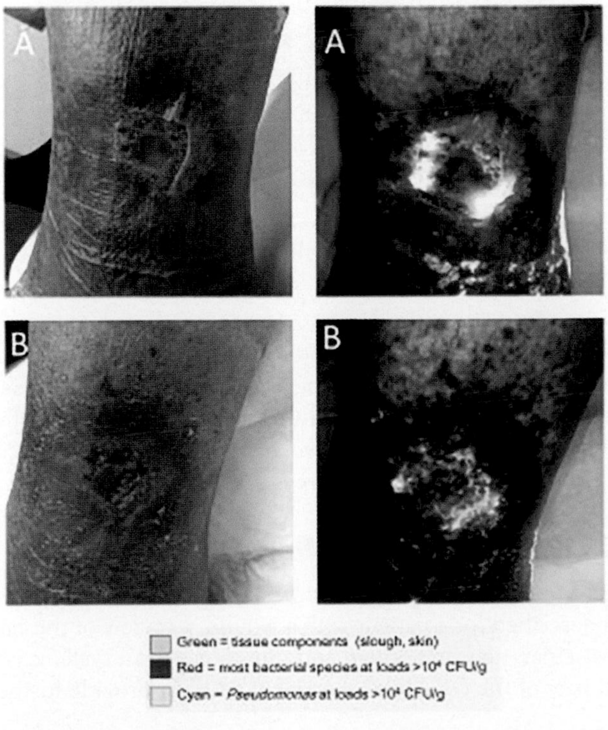

FIGURE 3-66 A. Left: Venous leg ulcer (VLU). Right: Fluorescence imaging of the VLU showing bright white/cyan fluorescence before debridement. **B.** Left: The VLU after debridement. Right: Fluorescence imaging after debridement showing a significant reduction in bacterial fluorescence. (Used with permission. Photographs courtesy of MolecuLight, Inc.)

CASE STUDY

INTRODUCTION

A 71-year-old male is referred to the out-patient clinic with two wounds on the right lower leg as a result of fasciotomies. Medical history includes bladder cancer for which he had a radical cystectomy and neobladder performed 10 weeks prior to referral. Two days after surgery he developed right lower extremity compartment syndrome that required surgical release of the pressure with medial and lateral fasciotomies (**FIGURES 3-67** to **3-69**). The medial wound is 18 cm × 3 cm; the lateral wound is 16 cm × 1 cm. There is a moderate amount of sanguineous drainage on the old dressing but no active bleeding with dressing removal. There is no odor noted with dressing removal.

Other medical history includes coronary artery disease with coronary artery bypass graft one year ago, Type 2 diabetes, hypertension, insomnia, and recurrence of infections during recovery period. He lives with his wife in a two-story home and works for the family business.

DISCUSSION QUESTIONS

1. What questions would be included in obtaining the subjective history?
2. Describe the wound characteristics visible in the photographs.
3. Using the information provided and the photos of the wounds, calculate the Bates-Jensen Wound Assessment Tool score for both the medial and lateral wounds.

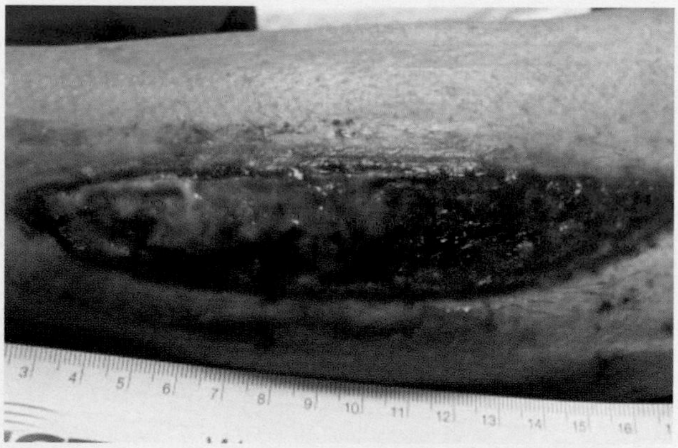

FIGURE 3-67 Right medial lower leg fasciotomy wound.

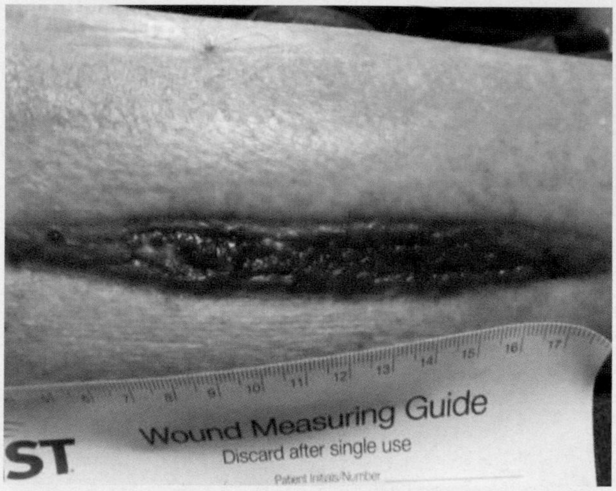

FIGURE 3-68 Close-up view of the distal medial wound.

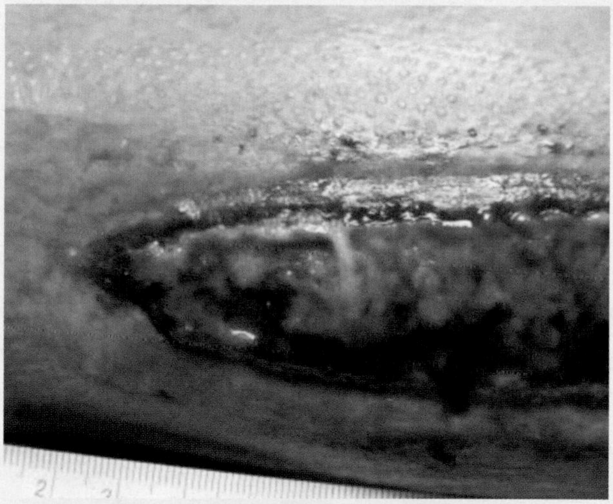

FIGURE 3-69 Right lateral lower leg fasciotomy wound.

bacteria in biofilm, thus providing more efficient detection of bacteria and facilitating earlier debridement, which in turn can reduce the need for antimicrobials and antibiotics.[61]

Pain

Pain is often referred to as the fifth vital sign and requires documentation with any procedure, medication, or wound intervention. There are several useful tools available to help patients quantify pain (**TABLE 3-10**). However, in addition to the presence and intensity, it is imperative that the evaluator determine the *cause* of the pain. For example, if a patient with a cast on the lower leg complains of pain, asking the patient to describe the pain and to indicate exactly where the pain is felt will help to rule out a poorly fitting cast that may be causing a wound on a bony prominence. **TABLE 3-11** provides some of the typical causes of different types of pain.

REVIEW OF SYSTEMS

In addition to the detailed review of the integumentary system described for a patient with a wound, a review of the cardiovascular, neuromuscular, and musculoskeletal systems is a vital part of the complete assessment and can provide further

TABLE 3-10 Visual Analog Scale

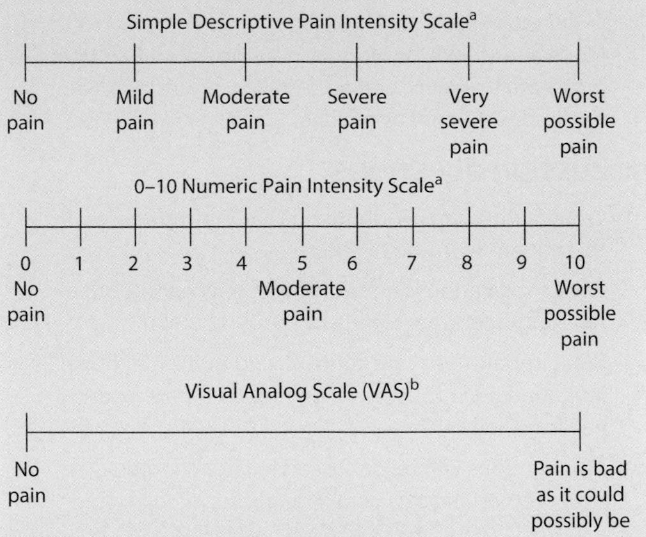

[a]If used as a graphic rating scale, a 10-cm baseline is recommended.
[b]A 10-cm baseline is recommended for VAS scales.

TABLE 3-11 Pain: Typical Descriptions and Causes

Pain Description	Possible Cause
Ache, heavy	Chronic venous insufficiency, edema
Burning	Friction, blisters, abrasion, neuropathy
Cramping	Intermittent claudication, hypoxia
Electric	Stimulation of exposed nerves
Sharp	Inflammation
Stinging	Reaction to topical dressing
Throbbing	Infection
Tingling	Neuropathy, too much pressure from compression

insight into contributing factors leading to wound formation or delayed healing.

The basic assessment for any patient will be discussed here, and details specific to particular diagnoses will be discussed in the diagnostic chapters.

Cardiovascular/Pulmonary System

If cardiac output or pulmonary function is compromised, less oxygen delivery to the wounded tissue will result in delayed healing responses. Critical levels may need to be addressed by changes in medication, surgical intervention, or activity levels in order to facilitate the healing. Cardiopulmonary tests and measures recommended for cardiovascular patients include blood pressure, oxygen saturation levels, and respirations (both quantity and quality). Vascular screening includes peripheral pulses, capillary refill, and ankle-brachial index (if arterial insufficiency is detected). Other signs of vascular insufficiency to observe are thick nails with onychomycosis, lack of hair on the digits and lower leg, and thin shiny skin. Refer to Chapter 4, Vascular Wounds, for more details on the vascular assessment.

Musculoskeletal System

The musculoskeletal assessment includes range of motion, especially of the foot and ankle for patients with diabetic or venous wounds, the spine and hips for patients with pressure injuries, and the upper extremities and hands for patients who need to use assistive devices for offloading or need to reposition for pressure redistribution. Strength measurements are

CASE STUDY

CONCLUSION

Cardiopulmonary review of Mr. MT revealed the following:

- *Vital signs:* blood pressure 135/70; heart rate 82; oxygen saturation 98% at rest.
- Shortness of breath with minimal exertion.
- Dorsalis pedis and posterior tibial pulses not palpable; positive Doppler signal.
- Capillary refill on the great toe: 4 seconds.
- Ankle-brachial index: 0.65.

Musculoskeletal review revealed the following:

- Range of motion within normal limits except for the right ankle (0- to 15-degree plantarflexion).
- Right ankle strength: 2/5, right knee and hip: 2+/5. Left lower extremity strength: grossly 3+/5; bilateral upper extremity strength: 4−/5.
- Edema in the right foot and lower leg, pitting in the foot only.
- Patient reports loss of weight (>30 pounds) during illness and daughter reports patient has poor appetite and does not want to eat.
- *Function:* Mod assist for bed mobility and supine to sit, min assist for transfers from wheelchair to bed.
- *Gait:* Ambulates 50 feet with front-wheel walker, close supervision; uses step-to gait sequence with poor awareness of right foot placement and partial weight-bearing on the right. Patient able to express his fear of falling.

CASE STUDY

Neurologic review reveals the following:

- Alert and oriented ×4.
- Follows two-step commands.
- No response to 6.65 monofilament on the right foot; positive response to 5.07 monofilament on the left.
- Impaired proprioception of the right great toe and ankle.

Other pertinent information:

- Blood sugars range from 100 to 130 (per patient report).
- Pain levels are 2–4/10 with any tactile stimulation to the wound bed.
- Lifting is restricted to 5 pounds.
- Medications include Norvasc, Lipitor, Amaryl, sodium bicarbonate, Plavix, aspirin, Miralax, oxycodone, Neurontin, and Tylenol as needed.

DISCUSSION QUESTIONS

1. What factors can be identified that may interfere with this patient's wound healing?
2. What medication is he taking that may contribute to the sanguineous drainage from his wounds?
3. What impairments are contributing to his functional limitations? Do these have an impact on his wound healing and how?
4. Interventions will be discussed in later chapters. However, what goals would be appropriate for this patient?

taken to ensure adequate ability to use devices, to reposition, and to ambulate with a normal gait cycle. Anatomical deformities that may contribute to diabetic foot or pressure ulcer formation need to be noted and adaptations included in the plan of care. Strength and/or stretching exercises may be indicated to redistribute pressure, improve gait dynamics, or improve blood flow to specific areas. Muscular atrophy that increases the risk of pressure injury formation is assessed and is a prerequisite for selection of support surfaces to both prevent and treat pressure injuries. Chapter 15, Exercise for the Patient with a Wound, provides more diagnosis-specific information on Exercise for Patients with Wounds.

In addition to individual muscles or muscle groups, overall muscle mass is observed for patients who may be either underweight or overweight, as both conditions can affect the ability to heal wounds. Body mass index (BMI) is the measurement used to assess muscle mass, and is defined by this equation:

$$\text{BMI} = \frac{\text{weight (in kg)}}{\text{height (in m}^2)} \quad \text{OR} \quad \frac{\text{weight (in pounds)}}{\text{height (in in.}^2)} \times 705$$

A BMI of less than 19 may indicate malnutrition with a risk for protein energy malnutrition, and a BMI of more than 30 indicates obesity, which can also affect wound healing.[62] Loss of lean body mass (LBM) has also been shown to have deleterious effects on the body and on wound healing, and the following guidelines have been established:

- 10% loss of LBM—impaired immune system, increased risk of infection, protein still available for wound healing.
- 15% loss of LBM—weakness, increased risk of infection, wound healing rate decreases, new wounds develop.
- 20% loss of LBM—wound healing ceases, new wounds develop, skin becomes thinner because of collagen depletion.[63]

Protein energy malnutrition and its effect on wound healing are discussed in more detail in Chapter 12.

Neurologic System

Neurologic testing includes both central and peripheral nervous systems. The ability to comprehend and follow instructions is necessary for compliance with home instructions (eg, off-loading, exercise programs, diet, dressing changes), and for learning new tasks (eg, gait training or repositioning). Peripheral testing (including sensation, vibration, proprioception, pressure, and reflexes) is an integral part of the assessment of a patient with a pressure injury or a diabetic foot ulcer in order to determine if the patient has protective sensation and ability to feel the consequences when pressures are causing tissue damage.

SUMMARY

Evaluation of a patient with a wound is necessarily a time-consuming, meticulous process in order to determine why the patient has a wound, why it is not healing, and what the optimal evidence-based care plan should be in order to facilitate healing. Only when the *why* has been answered can complete healing and long-term prevention of recurrence be achieved. Spending time and effort with the patient initially and being thorough in all aspects of the evaluation will facilitate faster healing rates, prevent further patient discomfort and disability, save professional provider time, foster better patient adherence and trust in the clinician, and promote wise use of precious medical supplies and dollars in the overall course of treatment.

STUDY QUESTIONS

1. Which of the following questions is inappropriate to ask as part of the subjective history?
   a. What did you have for dinner last night?
   b. What are your goals for therapy?
   c. How much will your insurance pay for treatment?
   d. What kind of assistive device do you use for walking?
2. Which of the following tools is recommended for assessing wound progression or regression?
   a. OPTIMAL
   b. BWAT
   c. Visual Analog Scale
   d. Braden Scale
3. Drainage that indicates the wound has not achieved hemostasis or that the patient is on anticoagulant medication is termed
   a. Sanguineous.
   b. Serous.
   c. Purulent.
   d. Transudate.
4. Pain associated with deep infection is usually described as
   a. Tingling.
   b. Burning.
   c. Stinging.
   d. Throbbing.
5. The subcutaneous extension that results from autolysis of subcutaneous tissue at the edge of the wound bed is termed
   a. Fistula.
   b. Sinus track.
   c. Tunneling.
   d. Undermining.
6. Greenish drainage on the dressing when removed from a chronic wound is indicative of local infection with which of the following microbes?
   a. *Methicillin-resistant Staphylococcus aureus*
   b. *Pseudomonas aeruginosa*
   c. *Vancomycin-resistant Enterococcus*
   d. *Carbapenem-resistant Klebsiella*
7. The dark discoloration seen in the lower leg of a patient with chronic venous insufficiency is a result of
   a. Arterial insufficiency.
   b. Inflammation as a result of the interstitial inflammation.
   c. Autolysis of dead red blood cells and hemoglobin.
   d. Medication that causes chronic edema.
8. Wounds located on the lower 1/3 of the leg, termed the *gaiter area*, are most likely to be associated with
   a. Arterial insufficiency.
   b. Diabetic neuropathy.
   c. Pressure.
   d. Chronic venous insufficiency.
9. A patient is being treated in an out-patient clinic for a hand wound that resulted from a spider bite. He comes to his appointment with the complaint of severe shortness of breath after walking from the garage to the clinic. The appropriate course of action is
   a. Have him lie down while you perform the routine wound care.
   b. Have him return home after his appointment with instructions to rest.
   c. Have him go to his primary care physician or emergency room as soon as possible.
   d. Recommend that he exercise more so that his endurance increases.
10. A patient who is being treated for a dehisced abdominal incision states that she used to weigh 150 pounds (about 6 weeks ago) but has lost weight and now only weighs 120 pounds. Will this impact the patient's healing and if so, how?
    a. This is normal after a surgery and she should heal just fine.
    b. This much weight loss will prevent healing from occurring and she should see a registered nutritionist for diet recommendations to build lean body mass.
    c. This is a significant amount of weight loss after surgery, but healing should progress normally if she uses a protein supplement.
    d. The patient should begin a light exercise program to help build lean body mass.
11. The cyan color in fluorescence imaging indicates the presence of
    a. *E. coli.*
    b. Methicillin-resistant *Staphylococcus aureus.*
    c. *Pseudomonas.*
    d. Vancomycin-resistant *Enterococcus.*

Answers: 1-c; 2-b; 3-a; 4-d; 5-d; 6-b; 7-c; 8-d; 9-c; 10-b;11-c

REFERENCES

1. Wilkins RG, Unverdorben M. Wound cleaning and wound healing: a concise review. *Adv Skin Wound Care*. 2012;26(4):160-163.
2. Jones TR. Wound care. In: Stone CK, Humphries RL, eds. *Current Diagnosis & Treatment Emergency Medicine*. 8th ed. New York, NY: McGraw-Hill; 2017. Available at: http://www.accessmedicine.com/content.aspx?aID=55752180. Accessed March 19, 2023.
3. Black JM. Pressure injuries. In: Halter JB, Ouslander JG, Studenski S, et al, eds. *Hazzard's Geriatric Medicine and Gerontology*. 8th ed. McGraw Hill; 2022. Available at: https://accessmedicine.mhmedical.com/content.aspx?bookid=3201&sectionid=266875297. Accessed March 19, 2023.
4. National Pressure Injury Advisory Panel. Pressure Ulcer Scale for Healing (PUSH). Available at: https://npiap.com/page/PUSHTool. Accessed March 15, 2023.
5. Hon J, Lagden K, McLaren AM, et al. A prospective, multicenter study to validate use of the Pressure Ulcer Scale for Healing (PUSH©) in patients with diabetic, venous, and pressure ulcers. *Ostomy Wound Manage*. 2010;56(2):26-36.
6. Choi PH, Chin WY, Wan EYF, Lam CLK. Evaluation of the internal and external responsiveness of the Pressure Ulcer Scale for Healing (PUSH) tool for assessing acute and chronic wounds. *J Adv Nurs*. 2016;72(5):1134-1143.
7. Horn SD, Fife CE, Smout RJ, Barrett RS, Thomson B. Development of a wound healing index for patients with chronic wounds. *Wound Repair Regen*. 2013;21:823-832.

8. Fife C, Horn S, Smout R, Barrett RS, Thomson B. A predictive model for diabetic foot ulcer outcome: The Wound Healing Index. *Adv Wound Care*. 2016;5(7):279-287.
9. Horn SD, Barrett RS, Fife CE, Thomson B. A predictive model for pressure ulcer outcome: the wound healing index. *Adv Skin Wound Care*. 2015:28(12):560-572.
10. Erfurt-Berge C, Renner R. Lebensqualität bei Patienten mit chronischen Wunden [Quality of life in patients with chronic wounds]. *Hautarzt*. 2020;71(11):863-869. German.
11. Dantas JS, Silva C, Nogueira WP, et al. Health related quality of life predictors in people with chronic wounds. *J Tissue Viability*. 2022;31(4):741-745.
12. Augustin M, Herberger K, Rusenbach SJ, Schafer I, Zschocke I, Blome C. Quality of life evaluation in wounds: validation of the Freiburg life quality assessment-wound module, a disease-specific instrument. *Int Wound J*. 2010;7(6):493-501.
13. Augustin M, Debus ES, Bruning G, et al. Development and validation of a short version of the Freiburg life quality assessment for chronic venous disease (FLQA-VS-10). *Wound Medicine*. 2015;8:31-35.
14. Augustin M, Montero EC, Zander N, et al. Validity and feasibility of the wound-QoL questionnaire on health-related quality of life in chronic wounds. *Wound Repair Regen*. 2017;25(5):852-857.
15. Blome C, Baade K, Debus ES, Price P, Augustin M. The "Wound-QoL": a short questionnaire measuring quality of life in patients with chronic wounds based on three established disease-specific instruments. *Wound Repair Regen*. 2014;22(4):504-514.
16. Cardiff Wound Impact Schedule. Available at: http://www.southwesthealthline.ca/healthlibrary_docs/B.4.2.CardiffWoundImpactQuest.pdf. Accessed March 16, 2023.
17. Engelhardt M, Spech L, Diener H, Faller H, Augustin M, Debus ES. Validation of the disease-specific quality of life Wuerzburg wound score in patients with chronic leg ulcer. *Vasa*. 2014;43(5):372-379.
18. Mortenson WB, Miller WC.; SCIRE Research Team. A review of scales for assessing the risk of developing a pressure ulcer in individuals with SCI. *Spinal Cord*. 2008;46:168-175.
19. Gunes UY. A prospective study evaluating the Pressure Ulcer Scale for Healing (PUSH Tool) to assess stage II, stage III, and stage IV pressure ulcers. *Ostomy Wound Manage*. 2009;55(5):48-52.
20. Mullins M, Thomason SS, Legro M. Monitoring pressure ulcer healing in persons with disabilities. *Rehabil Nurs*. 2005;30(3):92-99.
21. Greatrex-White S, Moxey H. Wound assessment tools and nurses' needs: an evaluation study. *Int Wound J*. 2015;12(3):293-301.
22. Moore ZE, Patton D. Risk assessment tools for the prevention of pressure ulcers. *Cochrane Database Syst Rev*. 2019;1(1):CD006471.
23. Romanelli M, Dini V, Bertone MS, Brilli C. Measuring wound outcomes. *Wounds*. 2007;19(11):294-298.
24. Toygar I, Simsir IY, Cetinkalp S. Evaluation of three different techniques for measuring wound area in diabetic foot ulcers: a reproducibility study. *J Wound Care*. 2020;29(9):518-524.
25. Foltynski P, Ciechanowska A, Ladyzynski P. Wound surface area measurement methods. *Biocybern Biomed Eng*. 2021;41(4):1454-1465.
26. Sheehan P, Jones P, Giurini JM, Caselli A, Veves A. Percent change in wound area of diabetic foot ulcers over a 4-week period is a robust predictor of complete healing in a 12-week prospective trial. *Plast Reconstr Surg*. 2006;117(7 suppl):239S-244S.
27. Wendland D, Taylor DWM. Wound measurement tools and techniques: a review. *J Acute Care Phys Ther*. 2017;8(2):42-57.
28. Wendelken ME, Berg WT, Lichtenstein P, Markowitz L, Comfort C, Alvarez OM. Wounds measured from digital photographs using photodigital planimetry software. *Wounds*. 2011;23(9):267-275.
29. Chang AC, Dearman B, Greenwood JE. A comparison of wound area measurement techniques: visitrak versus photography. *Eplasty*. 2011;11:e18.
30. Gabison S, McGillivray C, Hitzig SL, Nussbaum E. A study of the utility and equivalency of 2 methods of wound measurement: digitized tracing versus digital photography. *Adv Skin Wound Care*. 2015;28(6):252-258.
31. Onuh OC, Brydges HT, Nasr H, et al. Capturing essentials in wound photography past, present, and future: a proposed algorithm for standardization. *Adv Skin Wound Care*. 2022;35(9):483-492.
32. Foltynski P. Ways to increase precision and accuracy of wound area measurement using smart devices: advanced app planimator. *PLoS One*. 2018;13(3):e0192485.
33. Yesiloglu N, Yildiz K, Akpinar AC, Gorfulu T, Sirinoglu H, Ozcan A. Histogram planimetry method for the measurement of irregular wounds. *Wounds*. 2016;28(9):328-333.
34. Rogers LC, Bevilacqua NJ, Armstrong DG, Andros G. Digital planimetry results in more accurate wound measurements: a comparison to standard ruler measurements. *J Diabetes Sci Technol*. 2010;4(4):799-802.
35. Gethin G. The importance of continuous wound measuring. *Wounds*. 2006;2(2):60-68.
36. Lipsky BA, Berendt AR, Cornia PB, et al. Executive summary: 2012 infectious diseases society of america clinical practice guideline for the diagnosis and treatment of diabetic foot infections. *Clin Infect Dis*. 2012;54(12):1679-1684.
37. Mescher AL. Bone. In: Mescher AL, ed. *Junqueira's Basic Histology Text and Atlas*. 16th ed. McGraw Hill; 2021. Available at: https://accessmedicine.mhmedical.com/content.aspx?bookid=3047&sectionid=255120777. Accessed March 15, 2023.
38. Lee KC, Dretzke J, Grover L, Logan A, Moiemen N. A systematic review of objective burn scar measurements. *Burns Trauma*. 2016;4:14.
39. Gualtieri T, Bonomo P, Sottili M, et al. Biomarkers in wound drainage fluids of head and neck squamous cell carcinoma patients receiving neck dissection: a pilot study. *Clin Transl Radiat Oncol*. 2020;23:60-64.
40. Canbek U, Dibek E, Akgun U, et al. Analysis of the fluid biochemistry in patients with prolonged wound drainage after hip hemiarthroplasty. *Injury*. 2021;52(4):918-925.
41. Fantone JC, Ward PA. Inflammation. In: Rubin E, Farber JL, eds. *Essential Pathology*. Philadelphia, PA: JB Lippincott; 1995:26.
42. Davis CM, Goswami AK, Khaja M, et al. Post-operative chylous ascites: applications of interventional techniques. *J Radiol Nurs*. 2021;40(2):126-130.
43. Francis KF. Assessment and identification of skin disorders in skin of color: an integrative review. *J Wound Ostomy Continence Nurs*. 2023;50(2):107-114.
44. Dini V, Salvo P, Janowska A, Francesco FD, Barbini A, Romaelli M. Correlation between wound temperature obtained with an infrared camera and clinical wound bed score in venous leg ulcers. *Wounds*. 2015;27(10):274-278.
45. Armstrong DG, Lipsky BA, Polis AB, Abramson MA. Does dermal thermometry predict clinical outcome in diabetic foot infection? Analysis of data from the SIDESTEP trial. *Int Wound J*. 2006;3(4):302-307.
46. Sussman C. Assessment of the patient, skin, and wound. In: Sussman C, Bates-Jensen B, eds. *Wound Care: A Collaborative Practice Manual for Health Professionals*. 4th ed. Baltimore, MD: Lippincott Williams & Wilkins; 2012:53-109.

47. Mufti A, Somayaji R, Coutts P, Sibbald RG. Infrared skin thermometry: validating and comparing techniques to detect periwound skin infection. *Adv Skin Wound Care*. 2018;31(1):607-617.
48. Fierheller M, Sibbald RG. A clinical investigation into the relationship between increased periwound skin temperature and local wound infection in patients with chronic leg ulcers. *Adv Skin Wound Care*. 2010;23(8):367-379.
49. Houghton VJ, Bower VM, Chant DC. Is an increase in skin temperature predictive of neuropathic foot ulceration in people with diabetes? A systematic review and meta-analysis. *J Foot Ankle Res*. 2013;6(1):31.
50. Lindgren M, Malmqvist LA, Sjöberg F, Ek AC. Altered skin blood perfusion in areas with non blanchable erythema: an explorative study. *Int Wound J*. 2006;3(3):215-223.
51. Goodman CC. The hepatic, pancreatic, and biliary systems. In: Goodman CC, Fuller KS, Boisonnault WG, eds. *Pathology: Implications for the Physical Therapist*. Philadelphia, PA: Saunders; 2003:667-703.
52. Pace EJ, Brown CM, DeGeorge KC. Neonatal hyperbilirubinemia: an evidence-based approach. *J Fam Pract*. 2019;68(1):E4-E11.
53. Lee B, Piersante T, Calkins KL. Neonatal hyperbilirubinemia. *Pediatr Ann*. 2022;51(6):e219-e227.
54. Woo K, Ayello EA, Sibbald RG. The edge effect: current therapeutic options to advance the wound edge. *Adv Skin Wound Care*. 2007;20(2):99-117.
55. Luo S, Yufit T, Carson P, et al. Differential keratin expression during epiboly in a wound model of bioengineered skin and in human chronic wounds. *Int J Low Extrem Wounds*. 2011;10(3):122-129.
56. Miller JM, Binnicker MJ, Campbell S, et al. A guide to utilization of the microbiology laboratory for diagnosis of infectious diseases: 2018 update by the Infectious Diseases Society of America and the American Society for Microbiology. *Clin Infect Dis*. 2018;67(6):e1-e94.
57. Li S, Mohamedi AH, Senkowsky J, et al. Imaging in chronic wound diagnostics. *Adv Wound Care*. 2020;9(5):245-263.
58. Jayachandran M, Rodriguez S, Solis E, Lei J, Godavarty A. Critical review of noninvasive optical technologies for wound imaging. *Adv Wound Care (New Rochelle)*. 2016;5(8):349-359.
59. Lindelauf AAMA, Saelmans AG, van Kuijk SMJ, van der Hulst RRWJ, Schols RM. Near-infrared spectroscopy (NIRS) versus hyperspectral imaging (HSI) to detect flap failure in reconstructive surgery: a systematic review. *Life (Basel)*. 2022;12(1):65.
60. Chen M, Lin B, Su C, et al. The application of wireless near infrared spectroscopy on detecting peripheral circulation in patients with diabetes foot ulcer when doing Buerger's exercise. *Lasers Surg Med*. 2017;49(7):652-657.
61. Lopez AJ, Jones LM, Reynolds L, et al. Detection of bacterial fluorescence from in vivo wound biofilms using a point-of-care fluorescence imaging device. *Int Wound J*. 2021;18(5):626-638.
62. Posthauer ME, Dorner B, Collins N. Nutrition: a critical component of wound healing. *Adv Skin Wound Care*. 2010;23(12):560-572.
63. Litchford MD. Nutritional issues in the patient with diabetes and foot ulcers. In: Bowker JH, Pfeifer MA, eds. *Levin and O'Neal's The Diabetic Foot*. 7th ed. Philadelphia, MA: Mosby; 2008:199-217.

PART TWO
Wound Diagnosis

CHAPTER FOUR

Vascular Wounds

Stephanie Woelfel, PT, DPT, CWS; Alexander DiBartolomeo, MD; Christian Ochoa, MD; and Vincent L. Rowe, MD

CHAPTER OBJECTIVES

At the end of this chapter, the learner will be able to:

1. **Relate the pathological changes in the vascular anatomy to the formation of arterial and venous wounds.**
2. **Differentiate between arterial and venous wounds.**
3. **Perform a vascular screening and interpret noninvasive vascular studies for arterial and venous disorders.**
4. **Use the information obtained from vascular studies to develop a plan of care for arterial wounds (before and after surgery) and venous wounds.**
5. **Determine when and whether surgical intervention is needed for patients with arterial and venous wounds.**
6. **Select the appropriate compression therapy for patients with lower extremity vascular wounds based upon vascular studies.**

INTRODUCTION

The vascular system is an intricate system of arteries, veins, and lymphatic vessels designed to transport the blood from the heart to the tissues, providing oxygen and nutrients necessary to sustain life, then from the tissues back to the heart and lungs for gas exchange and recirculation (**FIGURE 4-1**). An interruption to blood flow in any one or more of the vessels can cause significant and critical pathologies that result in integumentary changes, wounds, or impaired healing. If pathology is present in the arterial system causing a wound to develop due to inadequate supply of oxygen and nutrients, the wound is termed *ischemic*; if the pathology is in the venous system, the wound is termed *venous*. Both types have very defining characteristics, and predictable vascular study results are used to determine the optimal plan of care for the individual patient. This chapter focuses on the pathophysiology, prevention, and treatment of arterial and venous wounds; lymphatic disorders are discussed in Chapter 5, Lymphedema.

Vascular diseases such as peripheral artery disease (PAD) and chronic venous insufficiency (CVI) are the cause of most lower extremity wounds. The clinical spectrum of PAD ranges from asymptomatic disease to mild claudication to tissue loss or gangrene. When patients with PAD have rest pain, gangrene, or ulceration of the lower extremity, it is termed "*chronic limb-threatening ischemia (CLTI).*" The presence of CLTI in a patient is significant not only for potential lower extremity wounds and limb loss, but also as an independent risk factor for cardiovascular morbidity and mortality. The major cause of CLTI is a reduction in distal tissue perfusion below the resting metabolic requirements usually associated with atherosclerosis; however, other conditions may cause wounds that appear to be arterial or ischemic (**TABLE 4-1**). Diabetes is one of the most serious and prevalent of these disorders. The combination of diabetes and PAD may lead to foot ulceration or gangrene, potentially resulting in amputation. The risk of amputation is more than four times higher for patients with diabetes and PAD than for patients with PAD alone and has been increasing over time.[1]

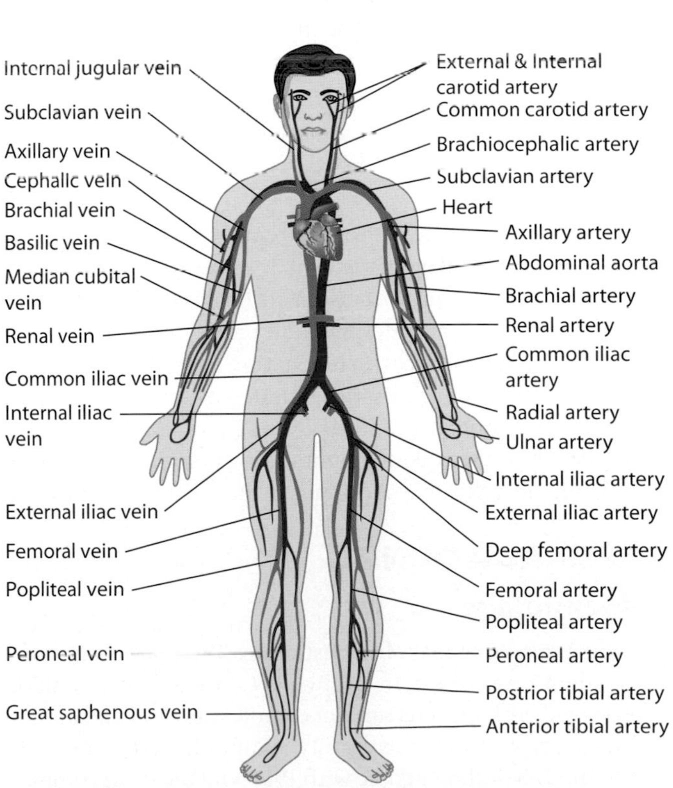

FIGURE 4-1 Anatomy of the arterial and venous circulatory systems. The circulatory system consists of the cardiac, arterial, venous, and lymphatic systems. The arterial system is further delineated into the macrocirculation (arteries large enough to be named) and microcirculation (capillaries and arterioles too small to be named). The lymphatic system is illustrated in Chapter 5.

TABLE 4-1 Differential Diagnosis of Lower Extremity Wounds

Inflammatory disorders
- Granuloma annulare
- Necrobiosis lipoidica
- Pyoderma gangrenosum
- Sweet's disease

Malignancy
- Malignant transformation of long-standing ulcer (Marjolin's)
- Metastatic malignancies
- Primary skin malignancies
- Ulcers associated with hematologic or internal malignancies

Pressure injuries

Infectious disorders
- Bacterial (*Pseudomonas*, staphylococcal scalded skin syndrome, streptococcal necrotizing fasciitis)
- Fungal (blastomycosis, chromomycosis, Madura foot)
- Mycobacterial (*M. leprae, M. tuberculosis, M. ulcerans*)
- Parasitic (Chagas disease, leishmaniasis)
- Viral (herpes simplex, herpes zoster)

Trauma (burns, postsurgical trauma)

Bites (eg, dog, snake, spider)

Medication-related ulcers
- Drug reactions leading to blisters and large-scale wounds (erythema multiforme, Stevens–Johnson syndrome, toxic epidermal necrolysis)

Autoimmune disorders
- Blistering (epidermolysis bullosa, pemphigoid, pemphigus)
- Non-blistering (dermatomyositis, lupus, rheumatoid arthritis, scleroderma)

Atherosclerotic arterial ischemic ulcers

Non-atherosclerotic ischemic ulcers
- Hypertensive ulcers (Martorel's)
- Sickle cell disease
- Thromboangiitis obliterans
- Vasculitis
  - Churg–Strauss syndrome
  - Henoch–Schönlein purpura
  - Leukocytoclastic vasculitis
  - Microscopic polyangiitis
  - Polyarteritis nodosa
  - Urticarial vasculitis
  - Wegener's granulomatosis
  - Embolic (cholesterol emboli, hyperoxaluria)
  - Thrombotic
- Antiphospholipid antibody syndrome
- Disseminated intravascular coagulation, purpura fulminans
- Heparin necrosis
- Homocystinuria
- Livedoid vasculitis
- Polycythemia vera
- Thrombotic thrombocytopenic purpura
- Vasospastic/Raynaud's disease
- Venous ulcers

Neuropathic disorders
- Diabetes
- Leprosy

The pathologies listed in this chart can cause wounds that appear similar to wounds caused by peripheral arterial disease. Making the correct differential diagnosis is imperative because treatment of the underlying disorder is the first step toward successful wound healing. Some of these disorders are discussed further in Chapter 9.

The presence of any lower extremity wound requires an evaluation of vascular status which determines the ability of the wound or surgical incision to heal. Healing of a foot wound may take months despite undergoing revascularization procedures. The goal of revascularization in patients with PAD is to ensure that the maximum amount of arterial perfusion is present to support wound healing. There is a high rate of recidivism and subsequent amputation when the treatment of the vascular insufficiency is not performed in a timely manner.

ARTERIAL WOUNDS

Epidemiology

The most recent global study estimates there are more than 200 million cases of PAD worldwide. Of these, 20–40 million cases will likely have intermittent claudication and 100 million will have atypical lower extremity symptoms. Forty-five million of the 200 million people with PAD will die from coronary or cerebrovascular disease during a 10-year period.[2] These are most likely underestimates, especially considering the trend of increasing prevalence of PAD each year and the need for an updated global estimate.[3]

The prevalence of PAD is typically higher in men, although women in lower socioeconomic groups are affected at double the rate of men.[4] The prevalence of PAD rises with age, increasing to over 20% in individuals over 80 years old.[5] Regardless of symptoms, PAD can significantly impact a patient's quality of life—even patients with asymptomatic PAD demonstrate impaired lower extremity function, greater mobility loss, and quicker functional decline than people without PAD.[2] The true incidence of CLTI is unknown; however, an estimate of the U.S. population suggested there are 3500 new cases of CLTI per million individuals per year.[6] In Europe this incidence is approximately 500 to 1000 new cases of CLTI per million individuals per year.[7] The majority of individuals who have CLTI with ulceration or gangrene also suffer from DM. It is estimated that up to 70% of all lower extremity amputations are diabetes related and most of those patients present with a foot ulcer that develops into an infected limb or gangrene.[8,9] Almost 50% of patients who undergo amputation for CLTI will require amputation of the opposite limb within 5 years.

The economic impact involved in the care of patients with chronic wounds is staggering. The annual Medicare spend in treating arterial ulcers is \$2–3 billion, venous ulcers \$0.7–1.5 billion, and diabetic foot ulcers \$6.2–18.7 billion.[10] Included in the estimates are physician visits, hospital admissions for wound debridement, or surgical revascularization, rehabilitation, and wound care supplies.

The prevalence of PAD with *intermittent claudication* (a clinical syndrome characterized by leg pain induced by exercise and relieved by rest) among males and females is between a ratio of 1:1 and 2:1. This ratio increases when an ulcer or gangrene is present to at least 3:1. The prevalence of CLTI increases substantially as the population ages.[7]

The natural progression of CLTI is largely unknown since most published studies include performance of some revascularization procedure. However, there are some patients for whom an operation is prohibitive due to multiple comorbidities or limited life expectancy. A study by Marston et al. followed a cohort of patients with CLTI who presented with uncomplicated limb ulcers.[11] Revascularization was not performed due to medical comorbidities or anatomic considerations that did not allow surgical intervention. A total of 142 patients were followed for 1 year with the primary endpoint being major limb amputation. During the study, the wounds were treated with a specific protocol that emphasized pressure redistribution, debridement, infection control, and moist wound healing. The limb loss or amputation rate for these patients was 19% at 6 months and 28% at 12 months. Interestingly, complete wound closure was achievable in 25% at 6 months and 52% at 12 months. The only significant factor that affected wound closure was the initial size of the wound.

Arterial insufficiency not only causes wounds, but also portends negatively on the patient's lifespan. The most common cause of death in patients with severe PAD or CLTI is coronary artery disease. Depending upon the severity of the CLTI, patients with rest pain, which is the presence of pain without any exertion usually in the foot and digits, have more than a 70% mortality rate at 5 years. Even though this patient population may have a high mortality rate and are often treated in a palliative manner, conservative care can help alleviate pain and/or heal wounds.

Pathophysiology

Risk Factors The most common cause of PAD is arteriosclerosis (**FIGURE 4-2**). Risk factors for the development of this pathology include age, smoking, diabetes, hypertension, hypercholesterolemia, air pollution, family history, and obesity. Prevention and treatment of arterial wounds depend upon adequate identification and management of risk factors.

Macro- and Microcirculation Occlusion of the arterial system can occur in either the *macrocirculation* (defined as those arteries large enough to be named or with a diameter more than 0.5 mm) or the *microcirculation* (defined as the arterioles and capillaries too small to be named or with a diameter less than 0.5 mm). Atherosclerosis tends to affect the larger vessels while reduced capillary flow (also called *small vessel disease*) is observed most frequently as a result of diabetes.

Critical Phases of Ischemia In the early stages of PAD, the circulatory system compensates by establishing collateral circulation around the occlusions to maintain peripheral blood flow. The *first critical phase* of the disease occurs when the collateral circulation is insufficient for the metabolic needs of the affected extremity; therefore, the limited blood supply is shunted to the muscles where flow resistance is low instead of to the skin where resistance is high. A wound caused by trauma (eg, a blister from poorly fitting shoes, a skin tear, or a cut from poor foot care) during this period of decreased skin perfusion is more likely to become infected and fail to heal. The nonhealing wound may be the first indication that a patient has PAD.

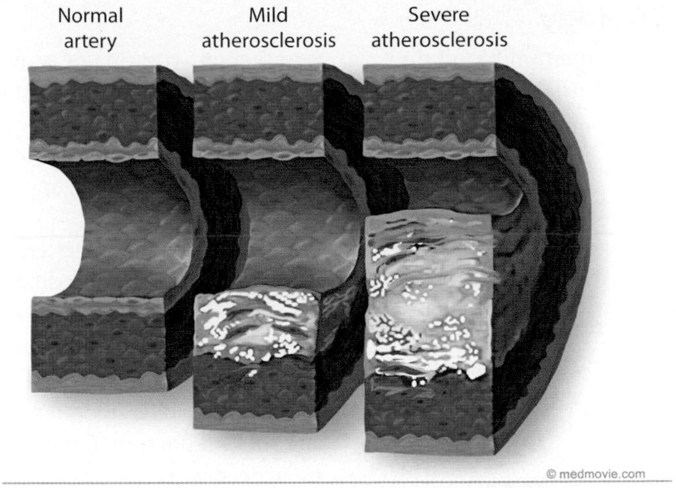

FIGURE 4-2 Atherosclerosis. Atherosclerosis is one type of arteriosclerosis in which fatty plaques composed of low-density fatty acids erode the artery wall with resulting deposition of macrophages and white blood cells. The plaque increases in size over time, causing a gradual decrease in the size of the arterial lumen and reduced blood flow to the distal tissues. The critical level is occlusion of more than 80% of the arterial lumen. In addition, particles of plaque can break away, migrate to smaller arteries or arterioles (termed *thromboemboli*), and cause tissue ischemia. (Reproduced with permission from Medmovie.com.)

Because exercise increases the muscle oxygen demand, and thereby its blood volume requirements, a *second critical phase* occurs when activity or exercise causes relative ischemia and pain. This onset of intermittent *claudication* is a second indication that the patient may have PAD.

When the PAD becomes severe, the *third critical phase*, the patient may experience rest pain, gangrene, or nonhealing wounds in the extremity below the occlusion. During this phase, the patient may prefer to have the leg in a dependent position, which allows gravity to assist blood flow to the distal extremity and thus alleviate some of the pain caused by ischemia. The patient frequently complains of rest pain during the night, a result of lower blood pressure and subsequent diminished flow to the most distal aspect of the lower extremity.

CLINICAL CONSIDERATION

Symptoms similar to PAD may be caused by lumbar spinal stenosis. A person with ischemic pain will feel pain relief with cessation of activity, whereas a person with spinal stenosis claudication will feel pain relief only with a change of position, for example, standing to sitting or sitting to lying. Determination of whether gluteal/lower extremity pain is due to spinal stenosis or due to ischemia and arterial insufficiency to the painful muscles is important for effective and appropriate medical management.

Etiology

Impairment of blood flow can occur acutely (trauma or acute thrombosis) or chronically (atherosclerosis). Both acute and chronic arterial insufficiency at any level (arteries, arterioles, capillaries) can lead to the formation of lower or upper extremity wounds.

Obstruction of arterial flow can also be classified as anatomic or functional. Anatomic causes of obstruction include thromboemboli and vasculitis (**FIGURES 4-3A–D** and **4-4**). Functional impairment occurs in conditions such as Raynaud's phenomenon in which abnormal vasomotor function leads to reversible obstruction (**FIGURE 4-5**). In severe cases this may result in ulceration. Other potential causes of impaired arterial flow include upper extremity arteriovenous fistulas and aneurysms (**FIGURES 4-6A** and **4-6B**).

CLINICAL CONSIDERATION

A wound that has the characteristics of arterial insufficiency on the foot of a young person is a red flag that the etiology is probably not arteriosclerosis. Other atypical disorders (eg, thromboangiitis obliterans or Buerger disease) need to be considered.

Non-atherosclerotic or vasculitic disorders need to be considered in patients who present with signs of tissue ischemia in the presence of normal or diminished pulses. For example, thromboangiitis obliterans, also known as Buerger disease, is a macrovascular disorder common in men who are heavy smokers. The pathology is an immune and inflammatory disease of the peripheral arteries accompanied by vasospasm and thrombi in the arterial segments to the feet and/or hands. Occlusion of the arteries causes tissue ischemia which results in thin, shiny skin and thickened malformed nails. Other symptoms include pain, tenderness, erythema caused

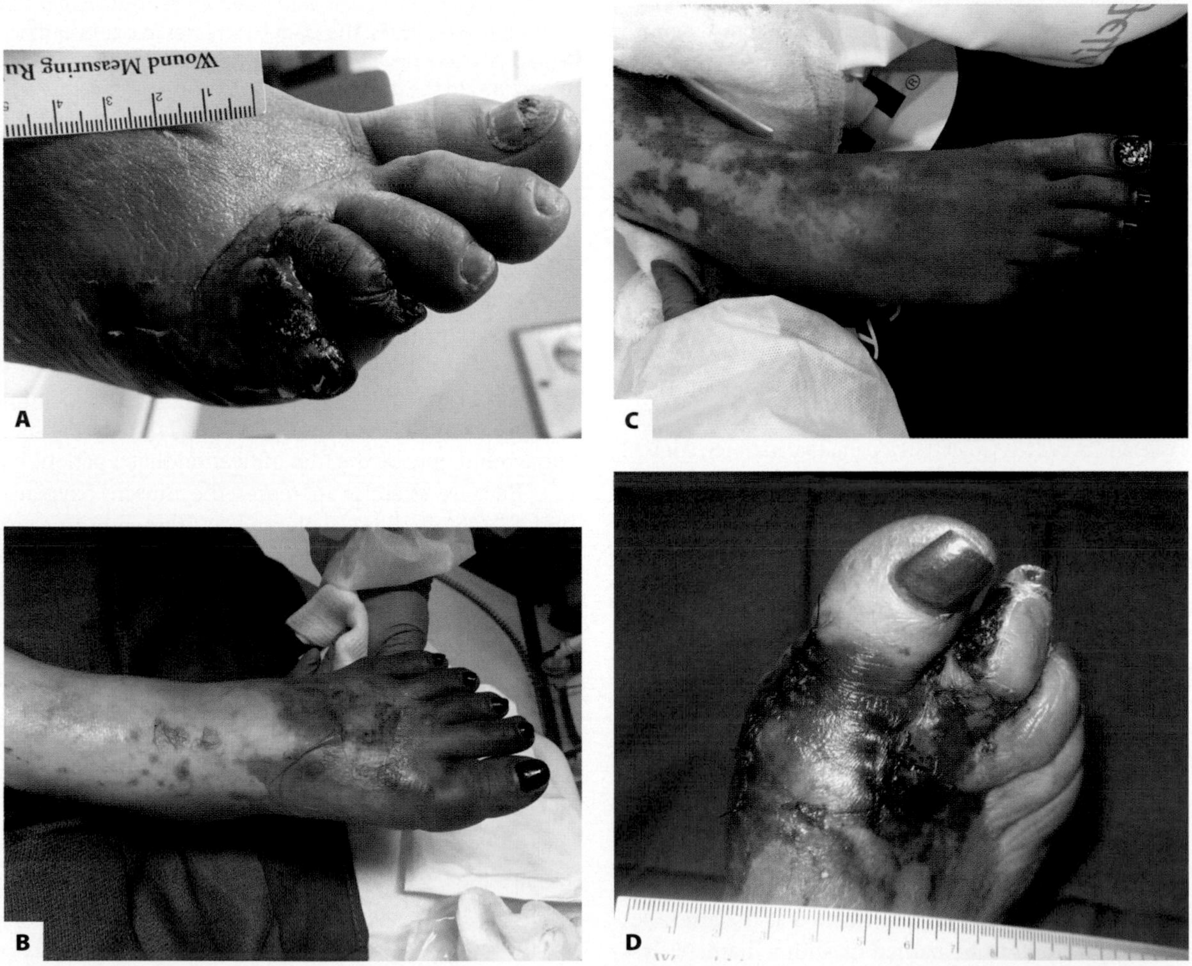

FIGURE 4-3 A–C. Arterial wounds due to thromboemboli. Arterial wounds that are caused by thromboemboli begin as dusky discoloration (as noted in the third toe of **A** and the foot of **B and C**) and progress to dry or wet gangrene (as noted in the fourth and fifth toes of **A**). If the tissue reperfuses as the medical condition improves, milder cases can resolve and healing can progress almost like a bruise healing. The tissue necrosis may become well-defined by a process termed *demarcation* (as noted in the second toe of **D**). Debridement is usually deferred until demarcation is complete unless there are signs of clinical infection; protective measures are recommended to prevent further tissue loss. Keeping the extremity warm using dressings or protective boots facilitates vasodilation, which can help maximize perfusion. The addition of external heat sources is not recommended as there is a high risk for burns in tissue with compromised perfusion. **D. Arterial wound due to trauma** Trauma from multiple causes, including surgery, can result in clotting and thrombi that occlude vessels of any size. Distal tissue will become necrotic unless flow is restored emergently.

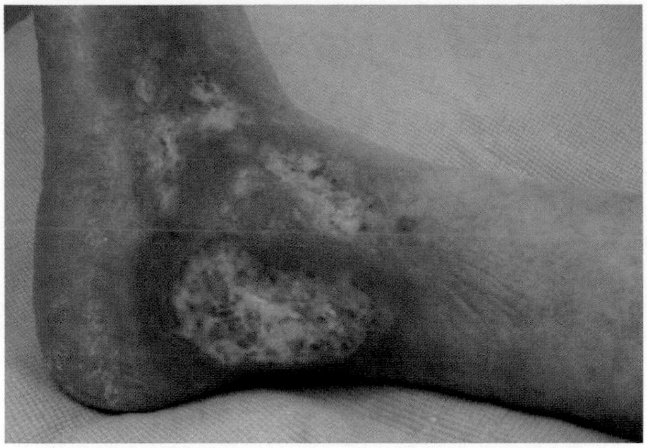

FIGURE 4-4 Ischemic wound due to vasculitis. Vasculitis, an inflammation of the vessels that results in edema and occlusion, most often occurs in patients who have autoimmune disorders (eg, systemic lupus erythematosus, rheumatoid arthritis, untreated hepatitis). The wounds are exquisitely painful, do not become necrotic like other arterial wounds, and may occur on any part of the body. (See Chapter 9, Atypical Wounds.)

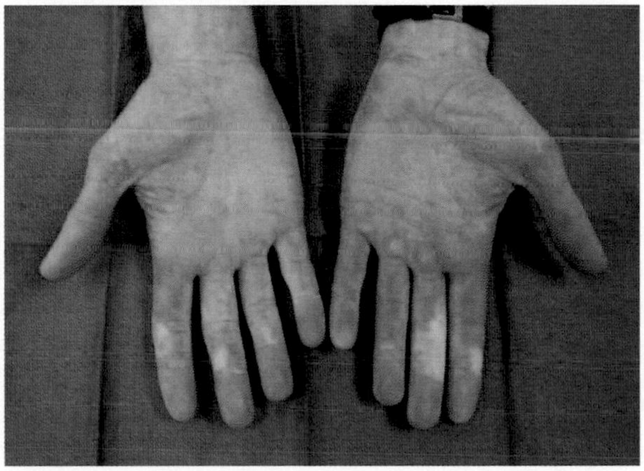

FIGURE 4-5 Raynaud's phenomenon. Raynaud's syndrome is caused by vasospasm of the small arteries and arterioles resulting in ischemic changes such as skin color, numbness, and cold sensations. The attacks can be triggered by cold exposure or emotional distress. Symptoms are bilateral, begin distal, and progress proximally, and in severe chronic cases can result in ulceration or gangrene.

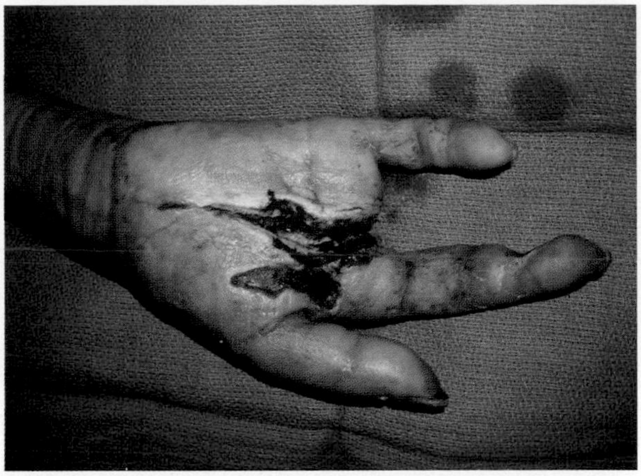

FIGURE 4-6A Arterial wound due to AV shunt for hemodialysis. Patients who are on long-term hemodialysis and have a history of clotted AV shunts may develop arterial wounds in the fingers due to decreased blood flow distal to the shunt.

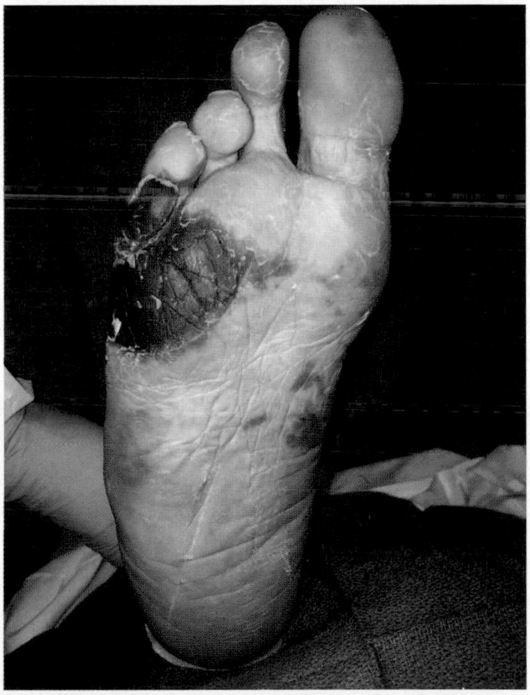

FIGURE 4-6B Arterial wound on the plantar foot due to ruptured aortic aneurysm. Proximal disruption of blood flow can result in distal manifestations.

by dilated capillaries, and cyanosis caused by deoxygenated blood cells in the interstitium. If the disease exacerbates, the patient is at risk for gangrene or ulceration. Successful treatment must include cessation of smoking (**FIGURES 4-7** and **4-8**).[12]

Patient Evaluation

The initial assessment of any wound begins with a thorough history and physical examination, a process necessary to establish a diagnosis of wound etiology. The history includes screening for risk factors of atherosclerosis—especially smoking, diabetes, hyperlipidemia, and hypertension. Patients who have these risk factors need aggressive education and the best medical therapy to modify these factors and encourage lifestyle changes. A vascular medical history of coronary artery disease (angina pectoris or myocardial infarction) and carotid disease (transient ischemic attacks or ischemic stroke) increases the likelihood of PAD because atherosclerosis is a systemic disease. Assessment of ambulation tolerance (by both

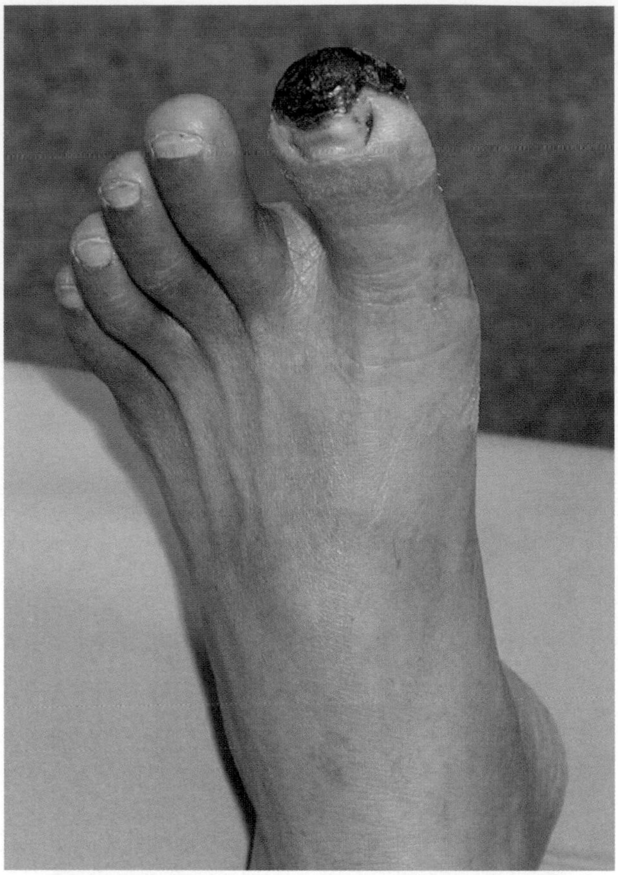

FIGURE 4-7 Buerger disease. Buerger disease, also known as *thromboangiitis obliterans*, is an immune inflammatory disease of the smaller peripheral arteries. Symptoms can vary from mild pain of the area distal to the inflamed arteries to severe vasospasm with cyanosis or occlusion with gangrene.

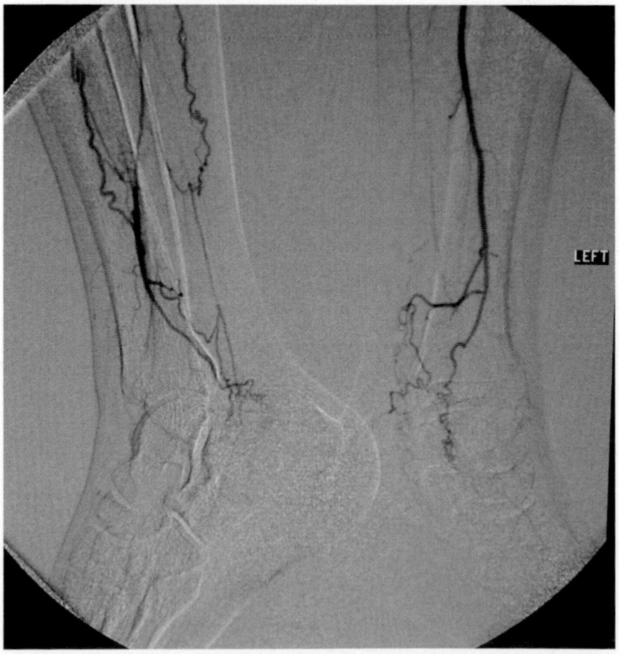

FIGURE 4-8 Radiograph of Buerger disease. Arterial radiograph of patient with Buerger disease shows the convoluted, distorted vessels in the distal lower extremity.

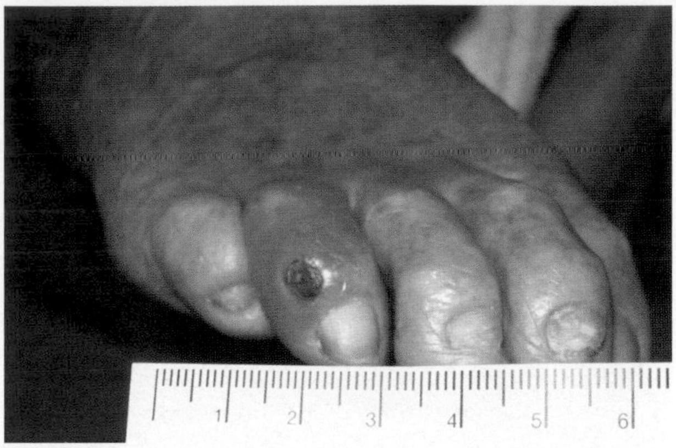

FIGURE 4-9 Typical arterial wound. The typical arterial wound due to PAD is located on the distal digit, has a round punched-out appearance, dry-to-necrotic wound bed, and little or no granulation tissue. The wounds tend to be painful with poor healing potential without restoration of blood supply.

patient report and treadmill testing) may uncover intermittent claudication. Other comorbidities, medications, and surgical history are obtained to determine any other contributing factors that may inhibit wound healing.

Clinical Presentation

A thorough wound assessment and information about how the wound began are important in determining the etiology. Refer to Chapter 3, Examination and Evaluation of the Patient with a Wound, for more details on obtaining a subjective history.

The location, size, and depth of the wound are defining characteristics of ischemic wounds, which tend to be small and round with smooth, well-demarcated borders. The wound base is typically pale (lack of arterial inflow), lacks granulation tissue, and may be shallow or deep (**FIGURE 4-9**). Wet or dry necrotic tissue may be present; *wet gangrene* is defined by gangrene with active infection and must be urgently debrided (**FIGURES 4-10** and **4-11**). Arterial wounds tend to occur at the distal digits, although wounds that occur from pressure on other parts of the foot (eg, the malleoli) may not heal due to arterial insufficiency (**FIGURE 4-12**). Because of the ischemia, arterial wounds are painful, especially at night. Pain that is reduced with leg dependence is indicative of rest pain.

Clinical signs of infection such as malodor, exudate, and erythema should lead to initiation of appropriate antibiotic treatment, proper debridement, and application of antimicrobial dressings. The presence of any exudate is characterized by the amount and color (refer to Chapter 3). If the wound can be probed to bone and osteomyelitis is suspected, referral to an infectious disease specialist is recommended for antibiotic consideration and to a surgeon for possible excision of the infected bone (**FIGURE 4-13**).

Other observations indicative of PAD include hair loss, atrophy of muscle and subcutaneous tissues, discoloration, dependent hyperemia, and dry, fissured skin (**FIGURE 4-14**).

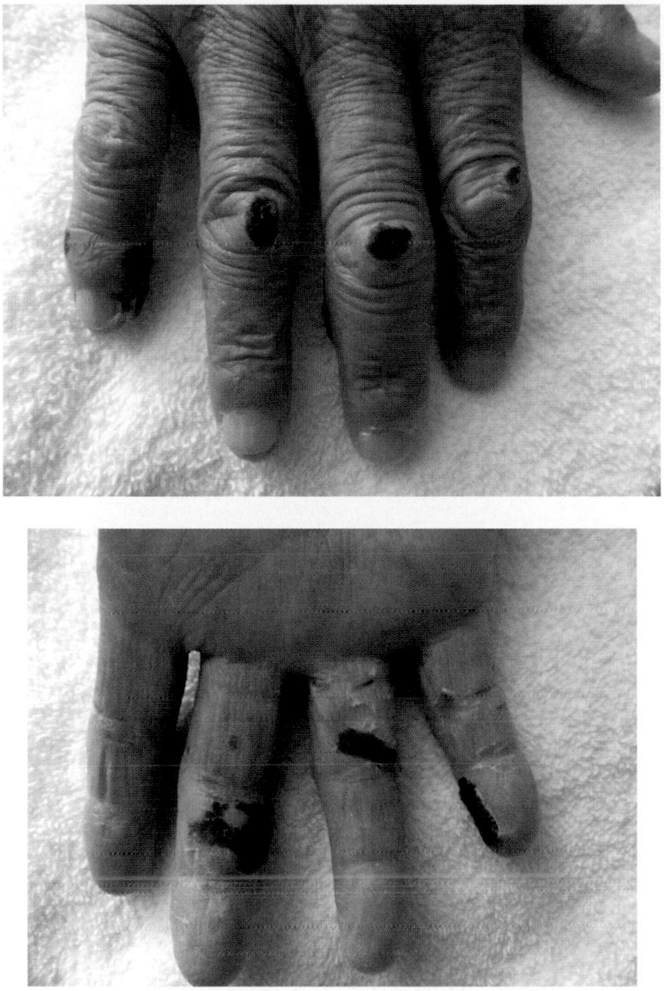

FIGURE 4-10 Dry gangrene. Arterial wounds with dry adhered eschar and no signs of infection are termed *dry gangrene*.

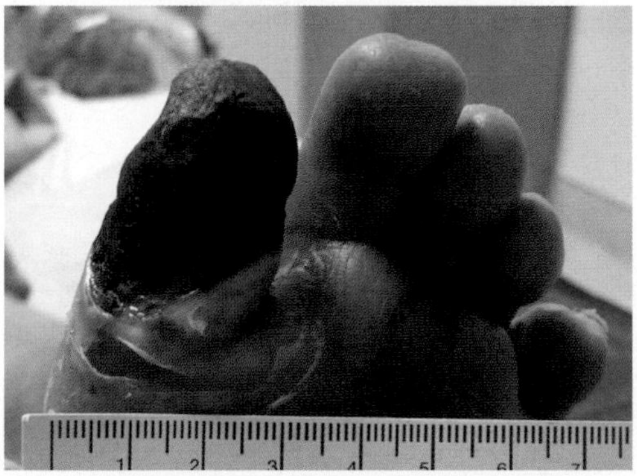

FIGURE 4-11 Wet gangrene. If the necrotic tissue becomes infected with drainage, detached edges, and wet periwound skin, it is termed *wet gangrene*.

Wound classification systems used to stratify the severity of the ulceration are based on the size, location, amount of tissue loss, presence of infection, and the status of the arterial blood flow. The following classification systems are specific to diabetic foot wounds: Wagner grading; the University of Texas (UT)

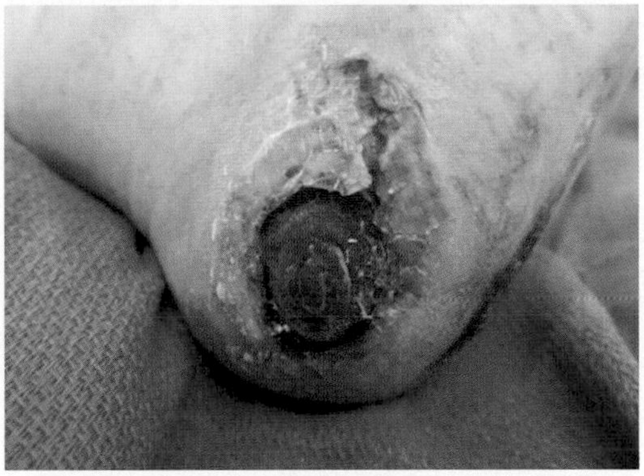

FIGURE 4-12 Nonhealing pressure injury secondary to arterial insufficiency. Wounds of other etiologies (eg, trauma, pressure, or venous insufficiency) that fail to heal may be one of the first signs that a person has PAD. If the edges stay adhered with no signs of infection, debridement is deferred or not recommended until perfusion is restored and signs of angiogenesis are visible at the edges. Loose detached edges, as seen in this heel pressure ulcer, may be removed to increase the oxygen perfusion of the periwound skin and decrease the risk of infection.

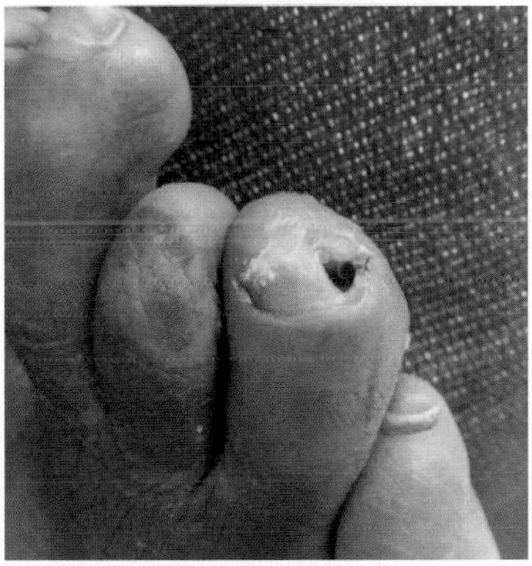

FIGURE 4-13 Osteomyelitis. Osteomyelitis is suspected in any arterial wound that can be probed to bone or that has an edematous "sausage-like" appearance.

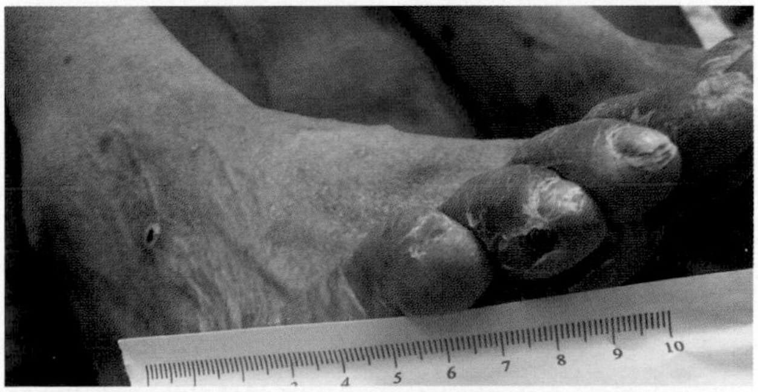

FIGURE 4-14 Typical appearance of extremity with PAD. Extremities that have PAD tend to have thin shiny skin, atrophied subcutaneous tissue and muscles, thick yellow nails, lack of hair, dry fissured skin, discoloration, and dependent hyperemia (termed *rubor of dependency*).

TABLE 4-2 Classification Systems for Diabetic Foot Wounds

System	Classification	System	Classification
Wagner	Grade 0: Impending skin lesion, presence of predisposing bony deformity, or healed ulcer Grade 1: Superficial skin ulcer that does not involve subcutaneous tissue Grade 2: Full-thickness ulcer that exposes bone, tendon, ligaments, or joint capsule Grade 3: Full-thickness ulcer with presence of osteitis, osteomyelitis, or abscess Grade 4: Gangrenous digit Grade 5: Gangrene severe enough to necessitate foot amputation	PEDIS Perfusion Extent/size Depth of tissue loss Infection Sensation or neuropathy	1. Wound lacking purulence or inflammation. Uninfected. 2. Presence of more than two manifestations of inflammation (purulence or erythema, pain, tenderness, warmth, or induration), but any cellulitis or erythema extends less than 2 cm around the ulcer, and infection is limited to the skin or superficial or subcutaneous tissues; no other local complications or systemic illness. Mild infection. 3. Infections as grade 2 in a patient who is systemically well and metabolically stable but who has one or more of the following: cellulitis extending >2 cm, lymphangitic streaking spread beneath the superficial fascia, deep-tissue abscess, gangrene, and involvement of muscle, tendon, joint, or bone. Moderate infection. 4. Infection in a patient with systemic toxicity or metabolic instability (eg, fever, chills, tachycardia, hypotension, confusion, vomiting, leukocytosis, acidosis, severe hyperglycemia, or azotemia).
UT Classification	Grade 0: No open lesions; may have deformity A: Without infection or ischemia B: With infection C: With ischemia D: With infection + ischemia Grade 1: Superficial wound not involving tendon, capsule, or bone A: Without infection or ischemia B: With infection C: With ischemia D: With infection + ischemia Grade 2: Wound penetrating to tendon or capsule A: Without infection or ischemia B: With infection C: With ischemia D: With infection + ischemia Grade 3: Wound penetrating to bone or joint A: Without infection or ischemia B: With infection C: With ischemia D: With infection + ischemia	SINBAD Site Ischemia Neuropathy Bacterial Infection Area Depth	0 = Forefoot 1 = Midfoot and hindfoot 0 = Pedal blood flow intact (at least one palpable pulse) 1 = Clinical evidence of reduced pedal flow 0 = Protective sensation intact 1 = Protective sensation lost 0 = None 1 = Present 0 = Ulcer < 1 cm^2 1 = Ulcer ≥ 1 cm^2 0 = Ulcer confined to skin and subcutaneous tissue 1 = Ulcer reaching muscle, tendon or deeper

Data from Brodsky JW. Classification of foot lesions in diabetic patients. In: Bowker JH, Pfeifer MA, eds. *Levin and O'Neal's The Diabetic Foot*. 7th ed. Philadelphia, PA: Mosby; 2008:227–239; Monteiro-Soares M, Russell D, Boyko EJ, et al; International Working Group on the Diabetic Foot (IWGDF). Guidelines on the classification of diabetic foot ulcers (IWGDF 2019). *Diab Metab Res Rev*. 2020;36(Suppl 1): e3273.

classification; PEDIS or Perfusion, Extent, Depth, Infection, Sensation; and SINBAD or Site, Ischemia, Neuropathy, Bacterial infection, Area and Depth (**TABLE 4-2**).[8] To incorporate wound classification with PAD and presence of infection, a classification system was created for the lower extremity threatened limb based on **W**ound, **I**schemia, and **f**oot **I**nfection (WIfI) (**FIGURE 4-15**).[13] The wound, ischemia, and infection are each graded and a total WIfI score is calculated to determine the patient's clinical staging, placing patients into one of four classes from *very low* to *high* risk of amputation at 1 year. The WIfI classification system has been validated for (1) risk stratification of amputation at 1 year and (2) need for limb revascularization. Recently a functional ambulatory scoring component was added to the WIfI classification system to address patient-oriented functional outcome and amputation risk (**TABLE 4-3**).[14]

Noninvasive Vascular Studies

Pulses The initial step of a vascular examination is palpation of pulses in the involved extremity that are compared with pulses of the contralateral limb in order to determine the extent of diminished flow. The palpation of peripheral pulses is subjective and affected by both the skill of the examiner and the room temperature. Patience is sometimes needed to feel pedal

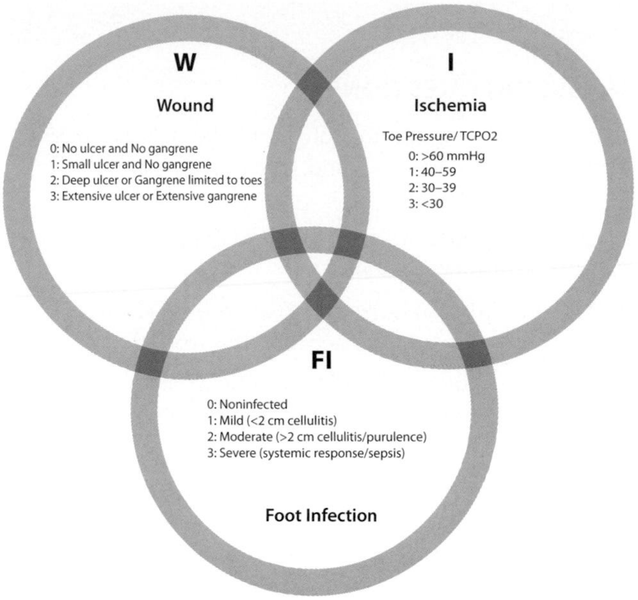

FIGURE 4-15 The WIfI lower extremity threatened limb classification. The Society for Vascular Surgery developed the Wound, Ischemia and foot Infection (WIFI) classification system to "permit more meaningful analysis of outcomes for various forms of therapy" in patients who have critical limb ischemia.[13] The system takes into consideration the extent of the wound, the degree of perfusion, and the presence of infection. (Courtesy of Dr. David G. Armstrong.)

TABLE 4-3 The Functional Ambulatory Score Adjunct to WIfI

Grade	Baseline Functional Level
0	Able to ambulate outside the home with or without an assistive device
1	Ambulates only within the household with or without an assistive device
2	Limb is used for transferring only
3	Bed bound

The functional ambulatory score in WIfI is to guide clinicians toward more patient-focused outcomes.

Reproduced with permission from Khan T, Plotkin A, Magee GA, et al. Functional ambulatory status as a potential adjunctive decision-making tool following wound, level of ischemia, and severity of foot infection assessment. *J Vasc Surg.* 2020;72(2):738-746.

pulses and the examiner may be misled by "feeling" one's own pulse, especially when using the thumb which has a strong digital pulse. Strength and interpretation of pulses have two different commonly used grades; thus, consistency among team members is needed for accurate communication (**TABLE 4-4**).

The character of the pulse refers to the upstroke, downstroke, and presence of thrills. In stiffened vessels or in vessels with high outflow resistance, the upstroke or radial expansion of the vessel may be slowed. In the presence of low outflow resistance, such as proximal to a traumatic arteriovenous fistula, downstroke may be significantly reduced. The absence of pulses suggests a proximal critical stenosis or occlusion. After palpation

CASE STUDY

A 74-year-old male is admitted to acute care with a nonhealing wound on the right lateral heel of more than 6 months' duration (**FIGURE 4-16**). Medical history includes type 2 diabetes, end-stage renal disease requiring hemodialysis three times a week, and hypertension. He has been admitted for further vascular studies, pain management, and possible revascularization of the lower extremity. A popliteal artery angioplasty and stent failed to establish blood flow sufficient for healing to occur.

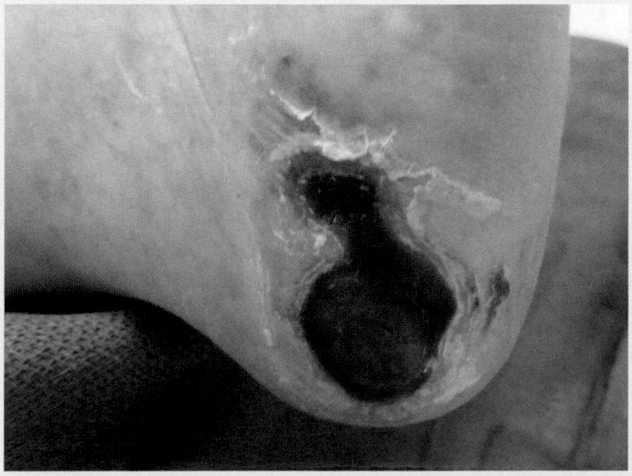

FIGURE 4-16 Case study. Right heel pressure injury that was first evidence of PAD; size 5.5 cm × 3.3 cm.

Daily medications include the following:

- Aspirin 81 mg daily
- Clopidogrel (Plavix) 75 mg daily
- Furosemide 40 mg daily
- Isoniazid 300 mg daily
- Sevelamer (Renvela) 800 mg daily
- Sitagliptin (Januvia) 25 mg
- Fish oil
- Vitamin B6
- Vital signs: normal for age

Laboratory values include the following:

- Hematocrit—31.3%
- Hemoglobin—10.4 g/dL

Continued next page—

CASE STUDY (Continued)

- Platelets—140,000/mm^3
- Albumin—3.8 g/dL
- HbA1C—8.7
- INR—1
- Prothrombin time (PT)—13.3 seconds
- Partial thromboplastin time (PTT)—30.4
- BUN—50 mg/dL
- Creatinine—8.33 mg/dL

When you enter the room, the patient is sitting in bed with the right leg dangling over the side.

DISCUSSION QUESTIONS

1. Based upon the information in Chapter 3 on evaluation of the patient with a wound, describe the patient's wounds and foot.
2. Classify the patient's wounds using the Wagner, UT, and WIfI classification systems.
3. What information is needed to use the PEDIS and SINBAD classification systems for this wound?
4. Using the information in Chapter 12, what are the factors that might impede this patient's ability to heal?

CLINICAL CONSIDERATION

Suggestions for palpating pulses include the following:

Test in a warm room that optimizes arterial dilation, not constriction.

Position the patient in supine with access from both sides of the bed.

Avoid the use of the thumb, which has less discriminating sensation.

Palpate pulses on the contralateral side for an indication of anatomical location of the artery.

Encourage the patient to relax so as not to be confused by moving tendons, etc.[15]

of the pulses, auscultation of the pulses by the examiner permits the detection of bruits, which is the sound of turbulent flow usually due to a nearby stenotic lesion or high velocity flow. The pulse examination, when correlated with clinical symptoms, helps identify the site and severity of arterial occlusive lesions and indicates when further vascular testing is necessary.

Audible Handheld Doppler (AHHD) Examination If pulses are faint or not palpable, a hand-held Doppler can detect flow within the vessel by utilizing reflected ultrasound waves. Although the Doppler may be able to detect flow that is not palpable, the presence of a signal is not an indication of normal flow (**FIGURE 4-17**). A peripheral artery without significant disease will generally have a triphasic or biphasic signal, while stenotic or occlusive disease and changes in velocity waveforms will cause the signal to be monophasic. The AHHD examination is usually begun distally and is not indicated at the more proximal locations if a pulse is palpable or audible. Use of an AHHD has the benefit of not being impacted by vascular calcifications. In a study of 379 limbs in 200 patients comparing AHHD to sequential lower-leg Doppler readings, AHHD demonstrated good specificity for excluding arterial disease (98.6% posterior tibial and 97.8% dorsalis pedis) but poor sensitivity for *diagnosing* arterial disease (37.5% posterior tibial and 30.2% dorsalis pedis).[16] Patients with known or suspected angiosomal deficits require a full vascular work-up regardless of AHHD results.

TABLE 4-4 Grading Scales for Pulse Examination

1. Scale of 0 to 3+	2. Scale of 0 to 4+
0: Absent pulse	0: No palpable pulse
1+: Diminished pulse	1+: Faint but detectable pulse
2+: Normal pulse	2+: Diminished pulse
3+: Pathologically prominent pulse, such as the water-hammer pulse of severe aortic insufficiency or if the artery is aneurysmal	3+: Normal pulse
	4+: Bounding pulse

Data from Hill DR, Smith RB. Examination of the extremities: pulses, bruits, and phlebitis. In: Walker HK, Hall WD, Hurst JW, eds. *Clinical Methods: The History, Physical, and Laboratory Examinations*. 3rd ed. Boston, MA: Butterworths; 1990. Available at: http://www.ncbi.nlm.nih.gov/books/NBK350. Accessed October 20, 2013.

Capillary Refill Time The severity of microvascular disease (eg, with patients who have diabetes or Raynaud's phenomenon) can be estimated by counting capillary refill time (CRT). CRT is measured by pressing the end of the toe or the skin just proximal to the wound until the color disappears and by measuring the time for recovery to the original color (**FIGURE 4-18**). Normal CRT is less than 3 seconds; however, it is prolonged in extremities with microvascular disease and may vary greatly among patients. Thus, CRT is only a screening test and an indicator that more precise vascular testing may be indicated.

Rubor of Dependency Rubor of dependency test is a screening procedure for ischemia that can be performed at bedside; thus, it is not definitive but indicative of PAD. The extremity is elevated to 30 degrees and observed for pallor. When the foot with normal circulation is placed into a dependent position, it will become a healthy pink color in approximately 15 seconds. If the reperfusion takes 30 seconds or longer and causes a dark-red or rubor appearance, the test is positive for severe ischemic disease.[17] The faster the pallor appears in the elevated position or the longer it takes for the rubor to appear in the dependent position, the more severe the PAD.

Ankle-Brachial Index The ankle-brachial index (ABI), a ratio of the ankle systolic blood pressure to the brachial systolic blood pressure, indicates the severity of peripheral arterial disease present in the lower extremity. To perform the test a 10–12 cm sphygmomanometer cuff is placed just above the ankle and

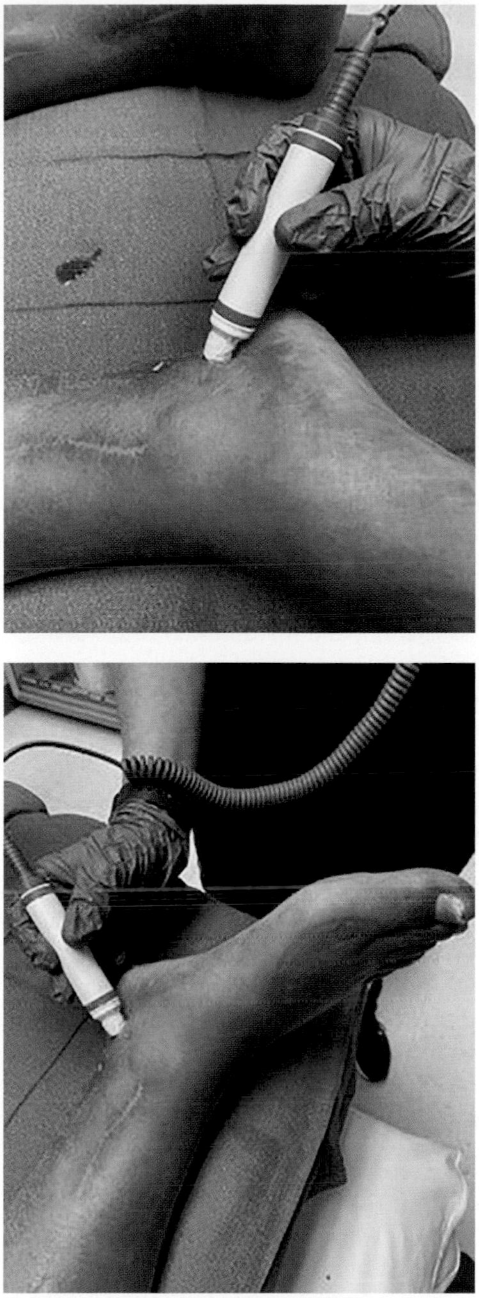

FIGURE 4-17 Hand-held Doppler. A hand-held Doppler is used to detect blood flow if pulses are not palpable. Doppler sounds can be described as triphasic, biphasic, monophasic, or absent.

inflated. A hand-held Doppler is used to measure the systolic pressure of the posterior tibial and the dorsalis pedis arteries of each leg by noting the pressure at which the pulse returns as the cuff is deflated. Then, the pressures are divided by the higher of the brachial pressures. The equations for the ABI are as follows:

Right ABI

$$\frac{\text{Higher of the right ankle systolic pressure (posterior tibial or dorsalis pedis)}}{\text{Higher brachial systolic pressure (left or right arm)}}$$

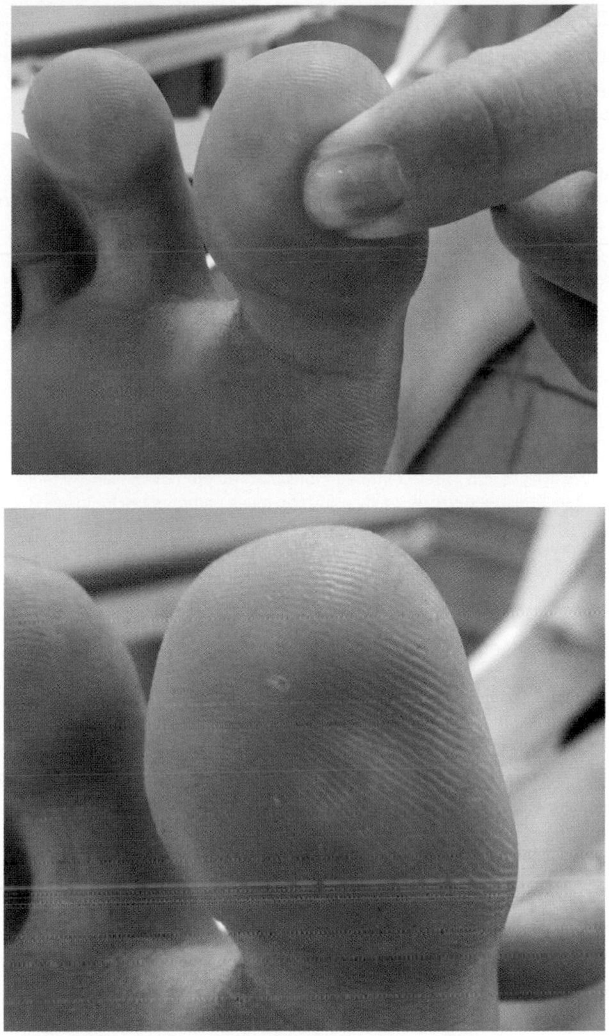

FIGURE 4-18 Capillary refill time. Capillary refill time is measured by pressing the skin until it blanches, releasing, and counting the seconds it takes to return to normal color. Normal capillary refill time is 2 seconds; more than 3 seconds is indicative of microcirculation abnormality or small vessel disease.

Left ABI

$$\frac{\text{Higher of the left ankle systolic pressure (posterior tibial or dorsalis pedis)}}{\text{Higher brachial systolic pressure (left or right arm)}}$$

The only contraindication for performing the ABI examination is the presence of an ulcer near the ankle since compression of the ulcer with the sphygmomanometer cuff may cause significant pain to the patient. Interpretations of ABI values are listed in **TABLE 4-5**. In some patients with diabetes, severe chronic kidney disease (CKD), or other diseases that cause vascular calcification, the pedal vessels at the ankle become noncompressible. This leads to an elevation of the ankle pressure which can present as an ABI > 1.30, or produce an ABI that seems to be normal, when the lower extremity circulation is, in fact, inadequate.[18] In these patients it is preferable to

TABLE 4-5 Interpretation of Ankle-Brachial Index

1.0–1.2: Normal
0.8–1.0: Minimal peripheral arterial disease. Compression for edema control is safe to use.
0.5–0.8: Moderate peripheral arterial disease, often accompanied by intermittent claudication. Referral to a vascular specialist is advised. Compression therapy is contraindicated if <0.6; modified compression is indicated if 0.6–0.8.
<0.5: Severe ischemia with resting pain. Compression therapy is always contraindicated.
<0.2: Tissue death will occur.
1–1.3: May occur with venous hypertension.
>1.3: Non-reliable in patients with diabetes or other calcification of the arteries. Recommend additional vascular testing.

Ankle-brachial index (ABI) is used to determine the severity of peripheral arterial occlusive disease and to select interventions that will promote healing without causing more tissue necrosis, eg, by using too much compression for lower extremity edema or by debriding a poorly perfused wound with eschar. The test can be easily performed in any clinical setting with a blood pressure cuff and hand-held Doppler.

measure a toe pressure rather than the ankle pressure. Another scenario when the ABI may be inaccurate and unreliable is for patients who have heel pressure injuries; the anterior tibial artery may be compressible when the posterior tibial artery is not compressible, making the calculated ABI a misleading indicator of adequate perfusion for wound healing.[19]

Toe Pressures Toe pressures are used for patients with calcified vessels and abnormally high ABIs or noncompressible vessels, typical of patients with diabetes, severe CKD, and the elderly. A toe pressure should always be used for patients with diabetes. A pneumatic cuff, about 1.2 times the diameter of the digit, is wrapped around the proximal phalanx and a flow sensor is applied distally to the digit. Following the WIfI classification, toe pressure ≥60 mmHg is normal, 40–59 mmHg is grade 1, 30–39 mmHg is grade 2, and <30 mmHg is grade 3. Most patients with foot wounds caused by PAD have a toe pressure less than 30 mmHg. Healing usually occurs on nondiabetic patients with a toe pressure greater than 30 mmHg, and on diabetic patients, greater than 55 mmHg.[20] The normal toe-brachial index (TBI), also considered a reliable indicator of lower extremity vascular status, is 0.8–0.99.[21] A toe pressure <30 mmHg or a TBI ≤0.2 infers a diagnosis of severe ischemia or critical limb ischemia.[22]

Segmental Pressures Segmental limb pressure is measured by combining Doppler ultrasound or plethysmography with blood pressure measurements at various locations on the arms and legs. Segmental pressures are a useful adjunct to the physical examination and ABI because they can illustrate differences in blood pressure at specific sites in the extremities and identify gradients that indicate the presence of disease.

A normal variation in the pressures between limb segments is 20–30 mmHg. A difference of 30 mmHg or greater indicates significant obstruction. Similarly, variations of pressure between symmetric limb segments do not differ by more than 20 mmHg unless there is an abnormality. Although they are strong indicators, limb pressure measurements are far less sensitive and specific than duplex imaging in the accurate diagnosis of arterial disease (**FIGURE 4-19**).[23]

Pedal Acceleration Time A recently introduced noninvasive test for patients with calcific tibial disease or extensive tissue loss is the pedal acceleration time. Acceleration time is obtained via duplex ultrasound by measuring the time over slope from the start of systole to the peak of systole. Based on the values obtained, patients can be placed into one of the following four classes of ischemia: Class 1, no ischemia; Class 2, mild ischemia; Class 3, moderate ischemia; and Class 4, severe ischemia. The pedal acceleration time has been correlated with ABIs and shown to be an independent predictor for limb salvage.[24]

Transcutaneous Oxygen Perfusion ($TcPO_2$) Another important tool in evaluating the patient with the chronic wound is measurement of transcutaneous oxygen measurements ($TcPO_2$), defined as skin oxygenation. The measurement of $TcPO_2$ depends on the cutaneous blood flow, the oxyhemoglobin dissociation, and the diffusion of oxygen through the tissues. As such, it reflects the metabolic state of the target tissues. The measurements are usually taken on the dorsum of the foot, anteromedial calf approximately 10 cm below the patella, and in the thigh approximately 10 cm above the patella, with the limb in a dependent position to help increase blood flow (**FIGURE 4-20**). The reference site is usually on the chest in the infraclavicular area.

Normal $TcPO_2$ is between 60 and 90 mmHg. On the WIfI classification, $TcPO_2$ ≥ 60 mmHg is grade 0, 40–59 mmHg is grade 1, 30–39 mmHg is grade 2, and <30 mmHg is grade 3. If the tissue surrounding an ulcer has a $TcPO_2$ less than 20 mmHg, the wound likely will not heal. In addition, patients with a $TcPO_2$ less than 20 mmHg will typically experience rest pain (**TABLE 4-6**). **TABLE 4-7** lists vascular assessments that have been discussed with the value that indicates wound healing is possible.

Exercise Stress Test The exercise stress test (EST) assesses PAD in patients with borderline ABIs (0.92–1.0) and symptoms of claudication. A resting ABI is performed first, after which the patient walks on a treadmill (typically at 2 miles per hour with an incline of 10–12%) for 5 minutes or until symptoms of claudication cause the patient to cease the activity. An

TABLE 4-6 Interpretation of $TcPO_2$

<20 mmHg: Unlikely for healing to occur.
20–30 mmHg: Healing can be expected, but may be delayed.
<30 mmHg: Proximal to the toes: wound should not be debrided until revascularization is accomplished.
>30 mmHg: Proximal to the toes: wound can be debrided.
>40 mmHg: Desired for healing of minor amputation site.
60–90 mmHg: Normal.

Transcutaneous oxygen tension ($TcPO_2$) is a measure of oxygen tension in the skin and is used to determine severity of microvascular disease. The readings also serve as indicators for wound healing potential and safe debridement of necrotic tissue.

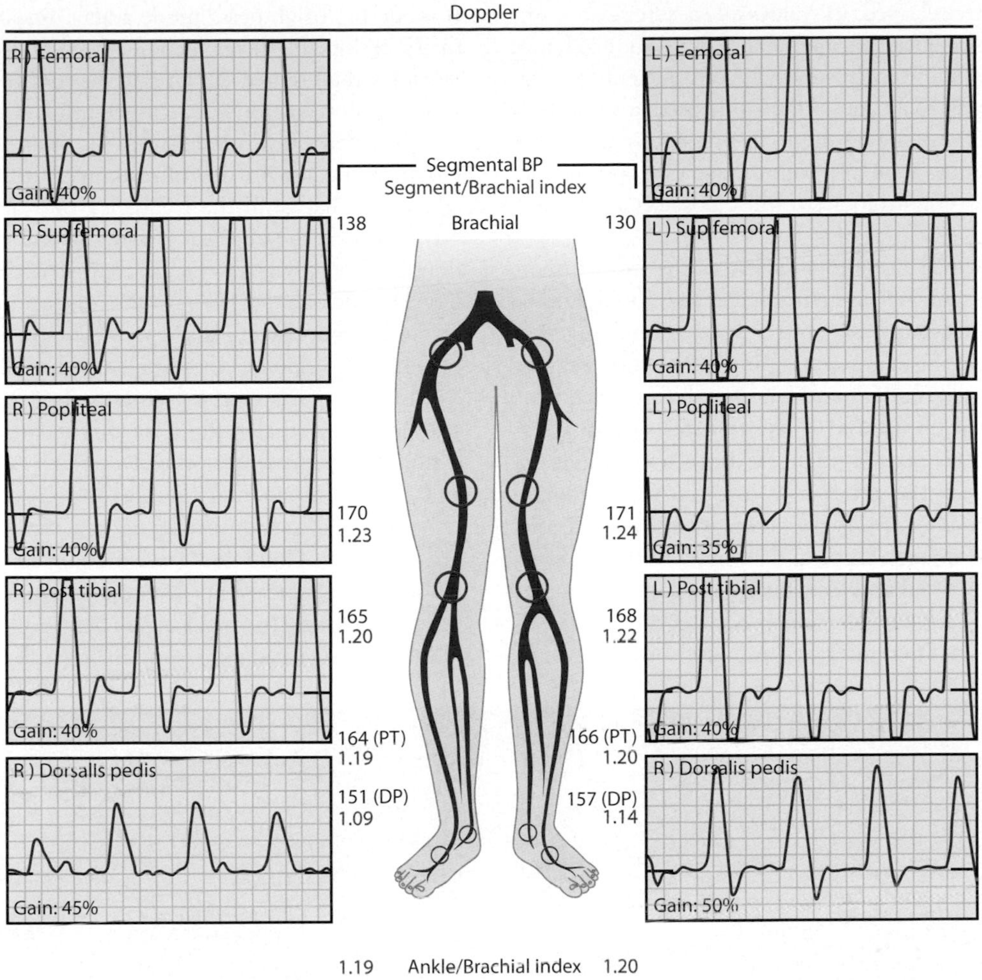

FIGURE 4-19 Arterial profile including segmental pressures. This study shows arterial waveforms from the femoral artery through the toes. Pressures and waveforms analyses are evaluated at each arterial segment. Triphasic arterial waveforms are identified throughout all segments except the right dorsalis pedis artery where the waveform displays a biphasic pattern. Comparison to the brachial artery pressure allows calculation of the ankle-brachial index.

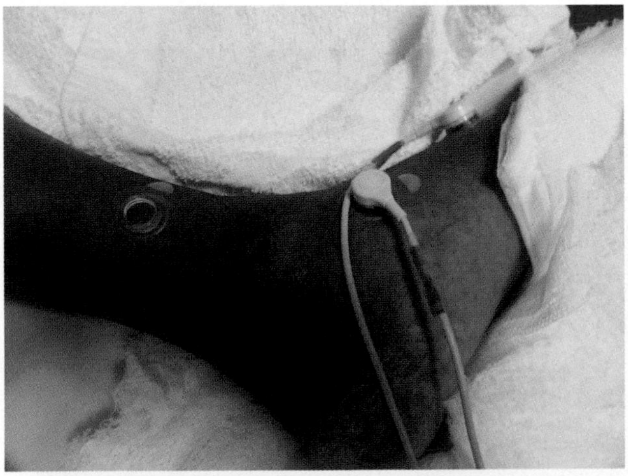

FIGURE 4-20 Measuring transcutaneous oxygen tension. Transcutaneous oxygen tension, measured on the foot of a patient with arterial wounds on the toes, is a good indicator of healing potential.

TABLE 4-7 Vascular Assessments and Wound Healing

Assessment	Value Indicative of Healing Potential
Palpable pulse—dorsalis pedis, posterior tibialis	>80 mmHg
Ankle-brachial index	>0.6 and <1.4
Transcutaneous oxygen tension ($TcPO_2$)	>30 mmHg
Toe pressure	>30–55 mmHg
Audible hand-held Doppler	Triphasic or biphasic sound

Reproduced with permission from Sibbald RG, Elliott JA, Persaud-Jaimangal R, et al. Wound Bed Preparation 2021. *Adv Skin Wound Care.* 2021;34(4):183-195.

alternative exercise activity is performance of 50 heel raises in the standing position. The duration of exercise and the nature of the symptoms are recorded. The patient is placed in a supine position and the ankle pressure measurements are recorded every 30 seconds until (1) the BP has returned to baseline or (2) 10 minutes have elapsed. BP values after exercise are compared to pre-exercise values. Normally, there is little or no change in the ankle or brachial BPs; however, PAD sufficient to cause claudication will result in a drop in the ankle pressure of at least 25 mmHg, 25% decline of the resting ankle pressure, or a decrease in the ABI > 0.15. A negative EST with the same symptoms suggests cardiorespiratory, neurologic, or musculoskeletal disease.[25]

Arterial Duplex Ultrasonography is one of the most important diagnostic tools for the vascular system. Many of the terms associated with ultrasound are often used interchangeably and/or incorrectly. A basic understanding of how the technology is applied will help understand when each test is needed.

The principle of ultrasound is the transmission of ultrasound signals from the ultrasound probe that echo from the tissues and are received by the same probe. The time that the sound wave takes to return after it was emitted is measured and used to create ultrasound images. Time and strength of the returned sound waves are amplified and transformed into a visual representation described as A-mode or B-mode. A-mode or "amplitude" mode represents the signal as an amplitude (**FIGURE 4-21**). B-mode or "brightness" mode adds a linear array of scanners that scan a plane through the body to create a 2D image with densities represented as varying degrees of "brightness." This creates a more anatomical representation (**FIGURE 4-22**).

Doppler ultrasound builds on this by combining the Doppler effect with the ultrasound (**FIGURE 4-23**). Doppler effect is a change in the frequency of a detected wave when the source or the detector is moving and can measure blood flow. Differences in flow can be represented as changes in color flow Doppler. In addition, Doppler ultrasound can be continuous or pulsed waves. Pulsed wave Doppler has the advantage of detecting velocities in a small area very accurately, whereas continuous wave can measure higher velocity flows over a larger area. Finally, the term *duplex ultrasound* refers to a simultaneous presentation of Doppler (usually pulsed wave) and 2D or B-mode imaging (**FIGURE 4-24**).

Duplex ultrasound imaging provides both anatomic and hemodynamic blood flow assessment in a noninvasive manner. Duplex ultrasound can provide spectral analysis, which shows the complete spectrum of frequencies (ie, blood flow velocities) found in the arterial waveform during a single cardiac cycle.

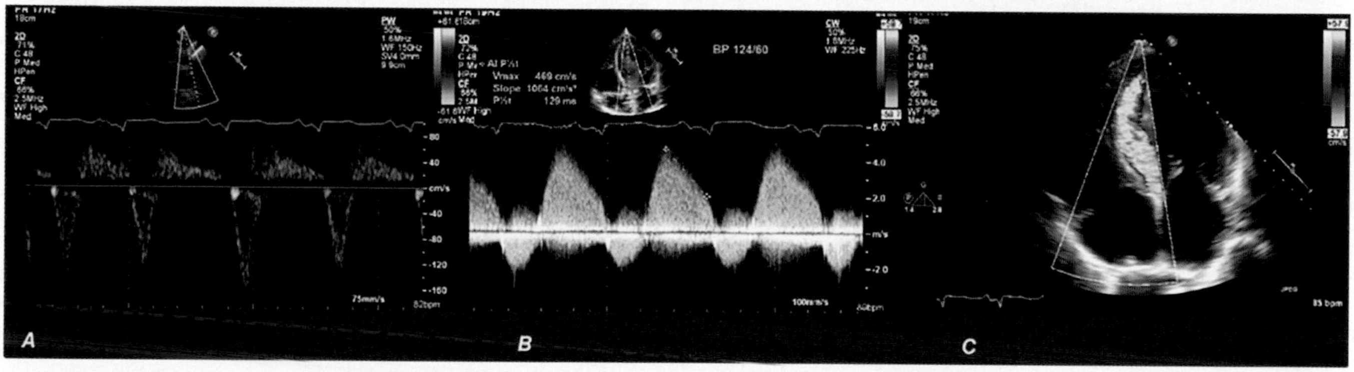

FIGURE 4-21 Three types of Doppler ultrasound. A and B. Pulsed and continuous wave Doppler waveforms with time on horizontal axis and velocity of blood flow on vertical axis. **C.** Color flow Doppler, where velocities are encoded by colors according to scale on right side of screen and superimposed on a two-dimensional grayscale image. (Reproduced with permission from Joseph Loscalzo, Anthony Fauci, Denis Kasper, Stephen Hauser, Dan Longo, J. Larry Jameson: *Harrison's Principles of Internal Medicine*, 21e; McGraw Hill LLC 2022.)

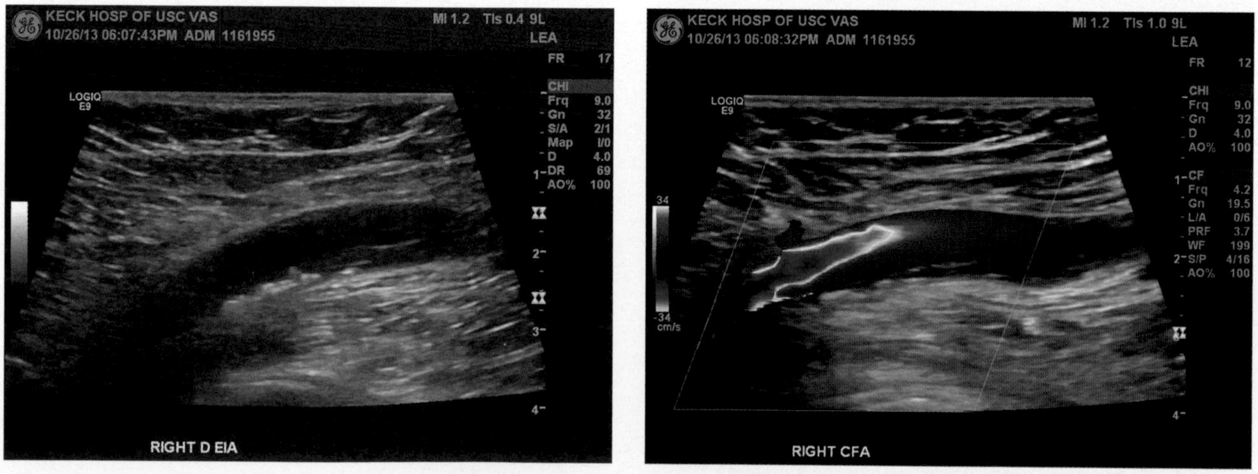

FIGURE 4-22 Ultrasound, B-mode. B-mode ultrasound is the reflected sound waves plotted on an oscilloscope to create a two-dimensional image of the anatomical structure. Figure **A** is the external iliac artery without color (the artery is the dark area in the middle of the image), and figure **B** is the right common femoral artery with color added to show direction of flow. Red is typically flow away from the heart and blue is flow toward the heart. A mosaic of color is interpreted as a stenosis, a point at which flow is scattered in both directions.

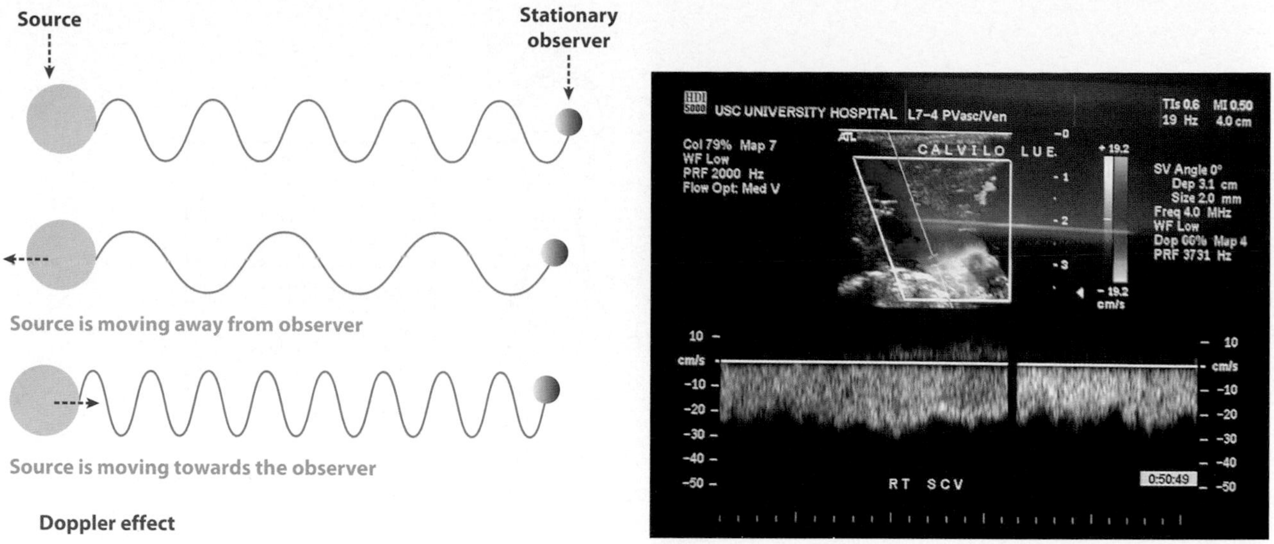

FIGURE 4-23 Doppler with color flow imaging. The Doppler effect is used to measure the velocity of blood flow in a vessel and is based upon the principle that flow toward the receiver creates shorter waves than flow away from the receiver. The velocity of flow in the vessel (in this case a vein) is shown on the bottom of the screen in the color flow imaging.

The normal waveform, termed triphasic, is made up of three components that correspond to different phases of arterial flow: (1) rapid antegrade flow reaching a peak during systole due to left ventricle contraction, (2) transient reversal of flow during early diastole due to reflection caused by peripheral resistance, and (3) slow antegrade flow during late diastole after closure of the aortic valve generated by large and medium compliant arteries. Lesions are identified by a change in waveform characteristics or an increase in peak systolic velocity (PSV) followed by a low velocity (**FIGURE 4-25A, B**). Certain ratios of the PSV within an area of stenosis to the PSV of the proximal normal segment correlate with the degree of stenosis.

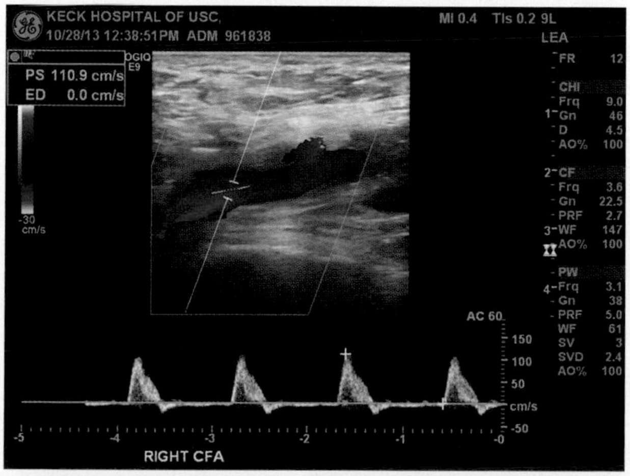

FIGURE 4-24 Arterial duplex with color flow imaging Arterial duplex scan of the common femoral artery. The flow pattern is laminar in nature (as identified by the homogeneous color of the moving blood through the vessel imaged). The waveform is a triphasic waveform with a peak systolic velocity of 110.9 cm/s. Signs of a stenotic lesion would show a more mosaic flow color and higher velocities (over 250 cm/s).

Computerized Tomographic Arteriography Accurate evaluation of the arterial blood supply is paramount for successful revascularization of the ischemic extremity for patients with or without diabetes. Arterial imaging is challenging for patients with ischemic complications because they frequently have underlying renal insufficiency, a condition that limits the amount of iodinated contrast that can be injected.

Computerized tomographic arteriography (CTA) involves injection of contrast medium into a vein followed by CT scan of the diseased arteries. CTA is a safe, noninvasive procedure that provides high-quality imaging of the arteries; however, significant arterial disease can impede the transit of contrast in the distal segments of the extremity, in which case more images and higher radiation doses are required. Consideration of the patient's renal function is necessary, given the use of contrast. Depending on the location and disease type being evaluated, CTA is just one of the diagnostic tools needed for proper surgical planning.

Magnetic Resonance Angiography Magnetic resonance angiography (MRA) can be performed with a contrast agent injected intravenously, termed *flow dependent*, because the presence of the contrast in the diseased arteries depends upon the blood flow getting to that area. The MRA can also be done without contrast, termed *flow independent*. MRA images are not obscured by arterial calcification; however, the disadvantages are motion artifact, long acquisition times, anxiety in patients who are claustrophobic, and possible nephrogenic systemic fibrosis in the patient with renal insufficiency.

For patients who require revascularization, arteriography using digital subtraction techniques is preferred to determine

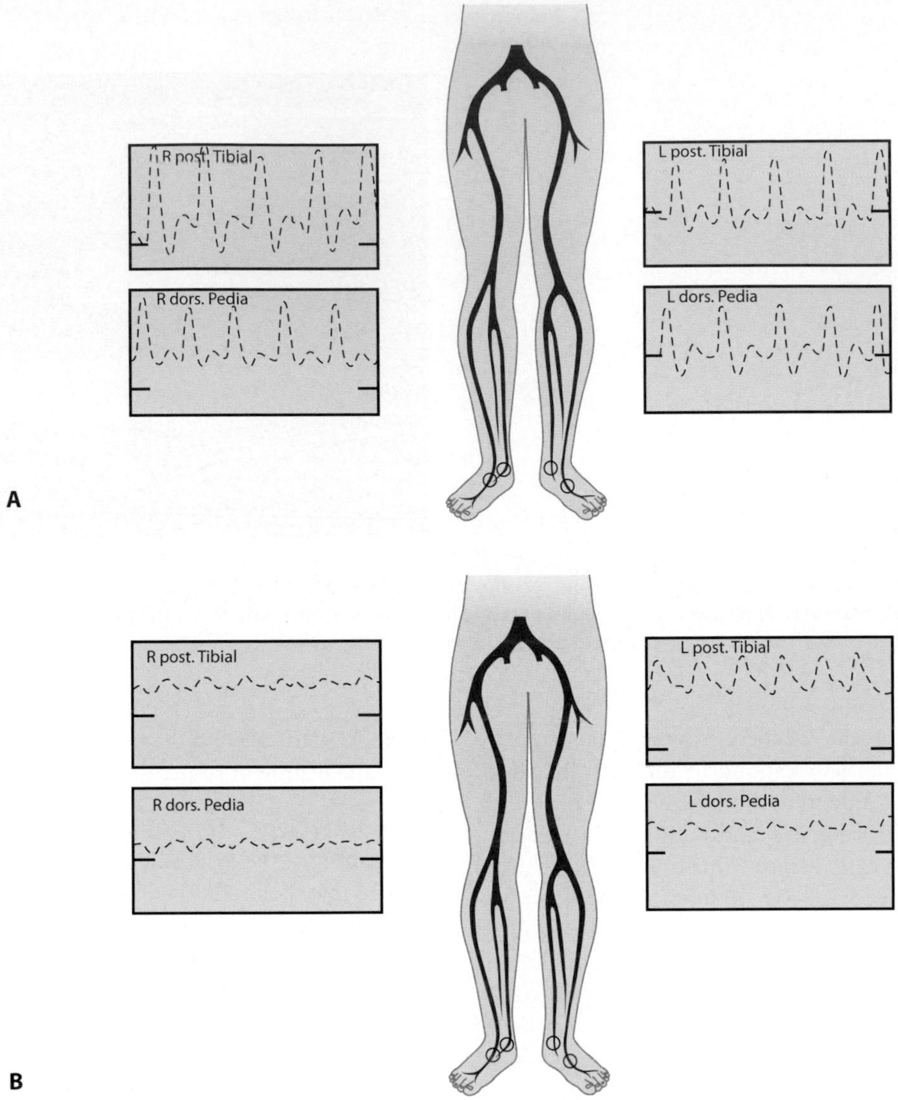

FIGURE 4-25 Arterial waveforms A. Normal arterial waveforms are triphasic and correspond to phases of arterial flow. **B.** Abnormal waveforms occur with macrovascular occlusion and vary from moderate (biphasic) to severe (monophasic and flat), depending on the extent of the occlusion.

appropriateness for endovascular revascularization versus surgical bypass (**FIGURES 4-26** and **4-27**).

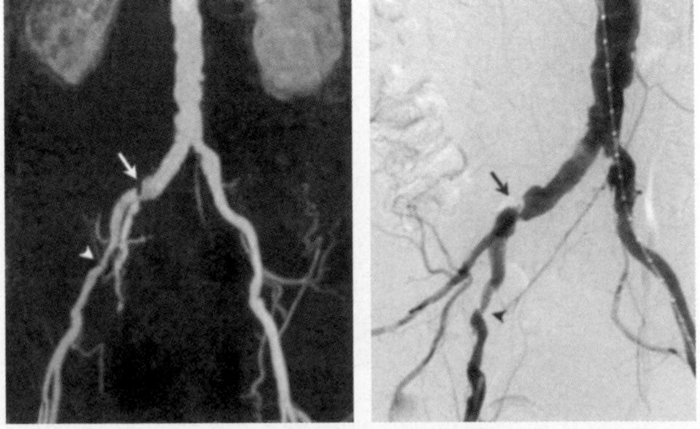

FIGURE 4-26 Magnetic resonance arteriography. Magnetic resonance arteriography of a male with intermittent claudication. The arrows point to the stenoses in the right common iliac artery and external iliac artery.

Invasive Tests

Arteriogram Angiography (or arteriography when referring specifically to the arterial system) is radiographic imaging of a contrast-filled blood vessel (**FIGURE 4-28**). Despite advances in the quality and availability of the previously described modalities, arteriography remains the gold standard for presurgical evaluation of the diseased arteries. There are clinical scenarios in which angiography is not the first choice because of its invasiveness; however, when addressing arterial disease of the lower extremities, it is usually the preferred diagnostic modality. In addition, it can be an efficient approach since after the diagnostic information has been collected, endovascular treatment can be completed in the same procedure.

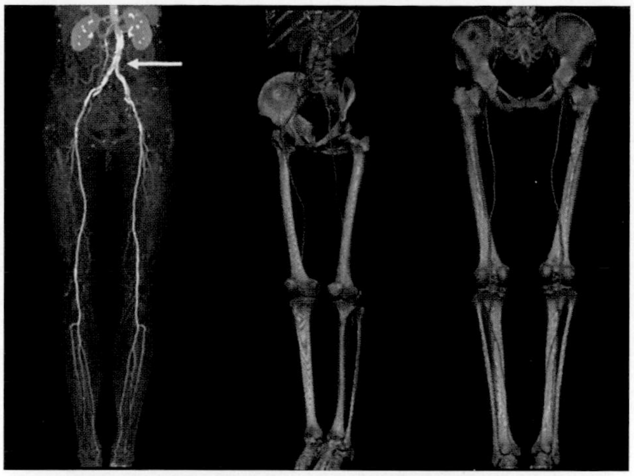

FIGURE 4-27 Computerized tomography arteriography. CTA image of a male with calcifications in the abdominal aorta. The peripheral vessels are patent in both lower extremities.

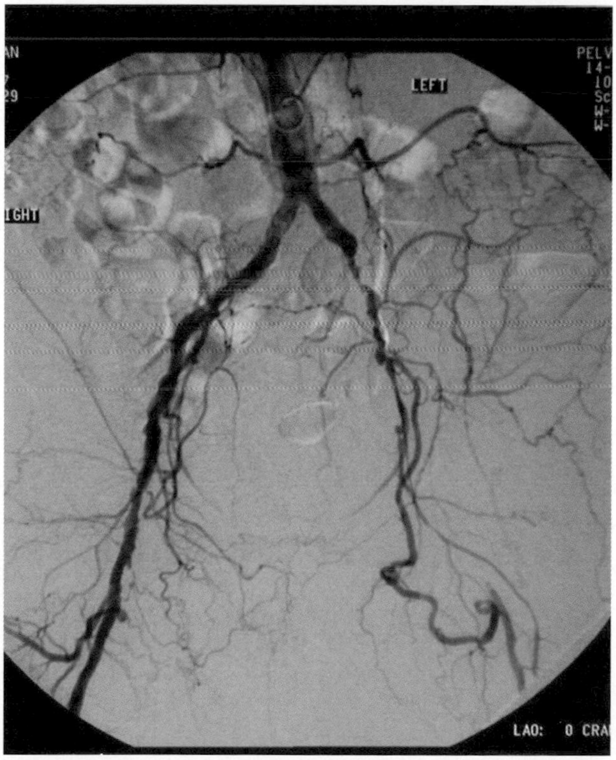

FIGURE 4-28 Arteriogram of lower extremity vessels. Arteriogram of the aortoiliac segment of the arterial circulation. Extensive disease is seen in the left distal common iliac and the external iliac is occluded. The vessel seen traversing through the pelvis is the internal iliac artery, which is the main collateral vessel for the occluded external iliac artery on the left.

Arteriography is performed in a procedure room or operating room with a generator, X-ray unit, detector, c-arm, and display monitors. The contrast agent is injected manually or via a power injector into the vasculature. An alternative to use of iodinated contrast is CO_2 arteriography, in which CO_2 gas is injected to transiently displace blood in the vessel and thereby create an image. CO_2 as a contrast agent is preferable in circumstances where systemic or renal toxicity from iodinated contrast is contraindicated or risky for the patient.

Digital subtraction refers to enhancement of the imaging prior to interpretation. The fluoroscopic image is processed, digitized, and amplified to create an easier-to-visualize image with static radiopaque structures removed. Arteriography is done through single injection with staged or stepped technique (the contrast is injected and images are taken either at various points along the extremity to follow the contrast load or via a rotational method). This technique can create a 3D image of the contrast outline using a detector that rotates between two points as the contrast is injected.

The limitations of arteriography are operator dependence, contrast and radiation exposure, and the inability of the image to effectively characterize the surrounding anatomy or vessel wall.

Prevention

Prevention of arterial wounds is predicated on identifying risk factors and reducing their impact on the integrity of both macro- and microcirculation. Important strategies include the following:

- Instruct and encourage the patient who smokes to stop by participation in smoking cessation programs.
- Educate the patient about blood glucose controls to minimize the risk of PAD.
- Educate the patient on the need to control hypertension, hyperlipidemia, and hypercholesterolemia through diet, exercise, and medication.
- Encourage the patient to initiate supervised exercise therapy to develop collateral circulation in the lower extremity, especially in the case of intermittent claudication.[26–29] See Chapter 15, Exercise for the Patient with a Wound, for additional details on supervised exercise therapy for intermittent claudication.

All patients who have any of the risk factors for atherosclerosis should be medically optimized.[28] Control of hypertension is measured with a goal of systolic pressures less than 130 mmHg and diastolic pressures less than 80 mmHg. Antiplatelet therapy (eg, aspirin or clopidogrel) has been shown to reduce myocardial infarction, stroke, or death in patients with symptomatic lower extremity ischemia. Statin medications are used in all patients with PAD to reduce cardiovascular risk and mortality.[30] Smoking cessation is critical in halting the progression of atherosclerosis and in reducing bypass graft failure after revascularization.

Treatment

Presurgical Wound Care Wound care before a patient has revascularization is based on protection of the wounded tissue and areas at risk for developing additional wounds (eg, heels and malleoli). Suggested strategies include the following, with the understanding that care is based on the individual patient's presentation, pain, and wound location:

- Debridement of an arterial wound without adequate perfusion for wound healing will make the wound larger. Therefore, intact dry eschar is not debrided. Infected tissue, termed *wet gangrene*, is debrided either with sharp or surgical techniques.
- The skin and necrotic tissue are kept dry and protected with sterile gauze or absorbent, wicking dressings between the toes. Swabbing the wound margins daily with alcohol or iodine solution helps minimize the risk of infection. Dry antimicrobial dressings may also be used to prevent maceration and infection while waiting for revascularization and reperfusion (**FIGURE 4-29**).
- The heels are protected from pressure by placing a pillow under the calf and thigh or by using an off-loading boot (**FIGURE 4-30**).
- A foot cradle on the bed helps to keep the weight of bed linens off affected distal digits.
- Post-op shoes help protect the toes from extra pressure, and assistive devices can help further off-load the involved foot.
- In severe cases, the patient is advised to avoid exercise, or limit exercise to functional tasks, in order to decrease the oxygen consumption of surrounding muscles and optimize perfusion to the ischemic areas.
- Elevating the head of the bed allows gravity to assist in increasing the blood flow to the foot. Discourage limb elevation that may further reduce blood flow to the distal extremity.
- Keeping the affected extremity warm with dressings or protective boots helps prevent further vasoconstriction due to cold exposure.
- Hot soaks, hot water bottles, or heating pads are discouraged because the diabetic foot is often insensate and cannot feel burning sensations. Also, because of autonomic neuropathy, the vessels cannot vasodilate to dissipate the heat, resulting in the accumulation of heat in the tissue and subsequent blistering, ulceration, or infection.
- Adjunctive therapies may be indicated for increased microcirculation (eg, electrical stimulation, low-frequency noncontact ultrasound, and growth factors).[31]
- Cellular and tissue-based products or biological dressings are NOT appropriate for use at this time because the wound environment is not yet optimized.

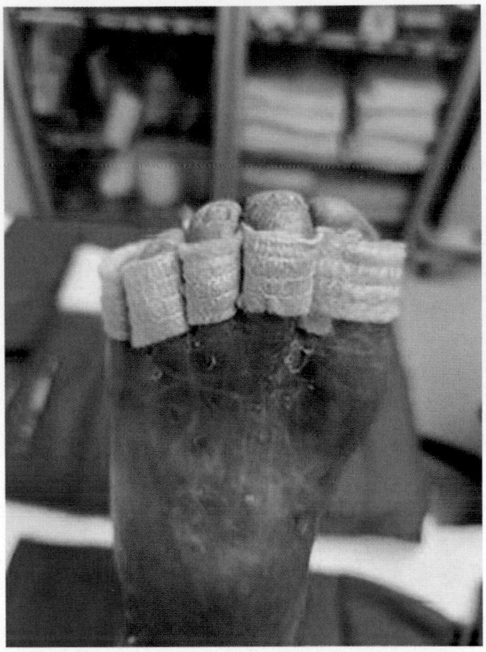

FIGURE 4-29 Presurgical protection of ischemic digits. Absorbent dressings are placed between the toes of an ischemic foot to prevent friction and maceration of the interdigital spaces.

CASE STUDY *(Continued)*

Vascular screening of the patient during the initial evaluation reveals the following:

Left: dorsalis pedis 2+; posterior tibialis 1+ and confirmed by strong Doppler

Right: dorsalis pedis—no palpable pulse, monophasic Doppler; posterior tibialis—no Doppler

Left capillary refill—4 seconds

Right capillary refill—6 seconds

Rubor of dependence is noted on both LEs; patient prefers dependent position of right LE.

Temperature of the right forefoot is cool as compared to the left.

The heel wound is 5.5 cm × 3.3 cm; the toe wound is 6.5 cm × 2 cm. There is scant drainage from either wound, no odor, ischemic mottling of the periwound skin, and 8–10/10 pain with any tactile stimulation.

DISCUSSION QUESTIONS

1. What is the appropriate treatment care plan for the patient?
2. What further diagnostic tests are indicated to determine the best revascularization technique?
3. Using the UT classification, what would be the type of lesion on both the heel and the forefoot?
4. Using the WIfI scale, what is the prognosis of this patient?

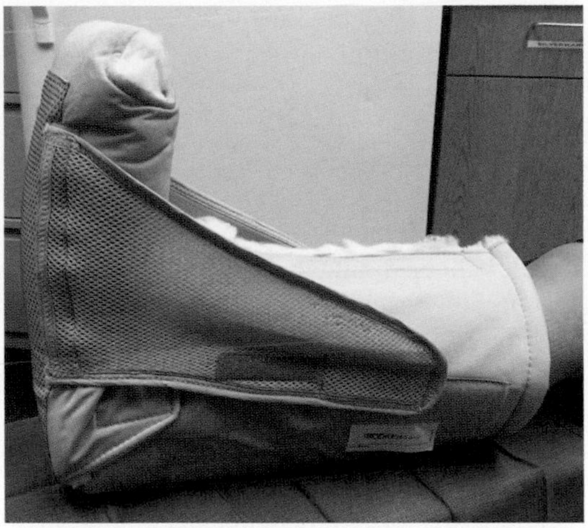

FIGURE 4-30 Use of protective boots for the ischemic limb. Soft boots provide protection for the heels and certain devices can also increase local tissue perfusion. The heels are floated inside the device with no contact on the bed. Nonrigid devices are advised especially if the patient has a plantarflexion contracture.

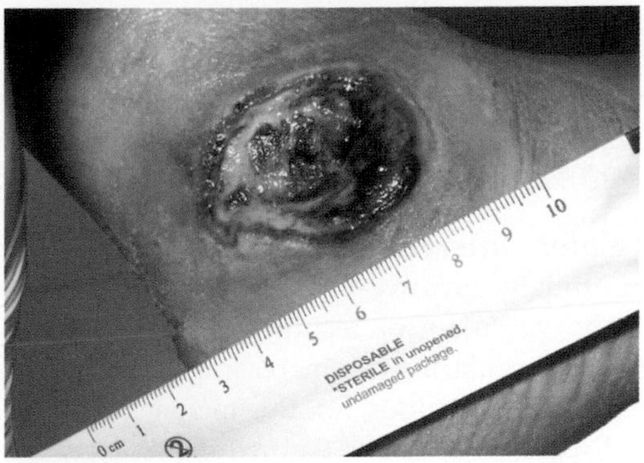

FIGURE 4-32 Appropriate wound for postsurgical debridement. After revascularization, debridement is performed when signs of angiogenesis (ie, granulation at the periphery of the wound) are visible.

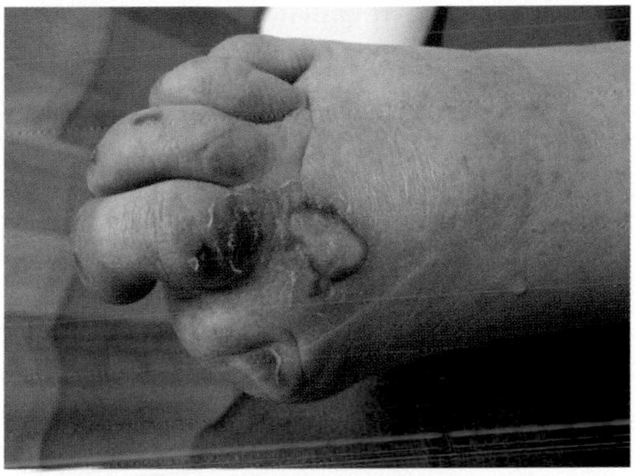

FIGURE 4-33 Should this wound be debrided? Two wounds are visible on this foot—dry eschar on the toes and yellow rubbery eschar at the base of the second toe. Debridement would be determined by patient history of revascularization or by $TcPO_2$ measurements. The dry eschar on the toes would best be left in place and removed as the epithelium migrates under the edges. Enzymatic debridement of the yellow eschar would be indicated, especially if the eschar feels adherent to the underlying tendons.

Surgical Interventions If wet gangrene or *infected tissue* is present on the extremity wound, urgent sharp or surgical debridement of the devitalized tissue is performed. (Refer to Chapter 13, Wound Debridement.) Infection both impedes wound healing and causes pain. If there is inadequate blood flow for healing, debridement of *noninfected tissue* is deferred until after revascularization is performed. After successful revascularization, the exact timing for debridement has not been determined, but often sharp debridement is performed after signs of angiogenesis (ie, granulation) are visible at the wound edges. If the patient is not a candidate for revascularization, dry eschar should be left intact (**FIGURES 4-31** to **4-33**). Debridement of intact eschar on an extremity with poor healing potential exposes the underlying tissue to possible contamination and infection. Debridement into viable tissue causes further tissue damage, which can lead to extension of the necrosis if severe ischemia is present. The eschar is best kept dry and protected.

Selective debridement is performed with a scalpel, curette, or hydrosurgery using a device called Versajet (Smith & Nephew, London, UK), or low-frequency contact ultrasound. After the necrotic tissue is removed, principles of moist wound healing are used to facilitate wound closure.

Several adjunct therapies are indicated for debrided wounds, including electrical stimulation, low-frequency noncontact ultrasound, ultraviolet light (for infection), pulsed lavage with suction (for removal of coagulum after surgical debridement or minor amputations), and negative pressure wound therapy (NPWT) for wound contraction and stimulation of granulation tissue. The benefits of NPWT include increased granulation tissue, exudate management, removal of infectious material, promotion of angiogenesis and perfusion, and a decrease in wound size. Precautions

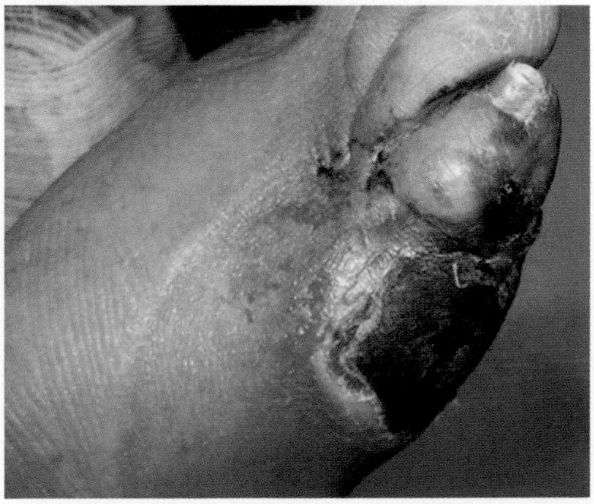

FIGURE 4-31 Eschar on ischemic foot. Dry, attached eschar on an ischemic foot should not be debrided until after revascularization. Removal of necrotic tissue without adequate blood flow results in a larger wound and more tissue loss. The exception is presence of infection that puts the patient or the extremity at risk.

are indicated, however, prior to the formation of collateral circulation and signs of angiogenesis in the wound bed or if hemostasis is not achieved. Use of NPWT in these conditions may cause the wound to deteriorate and form new eschar (**FIGURE 4-34**).

Endovascular Interventions Advances in endovascular (ie, minimally invasive procedures performed by access through the vasculature) techniques have made decision making in revascularization increasingly complex. To consolidate recommendations for the management of atherosclerotic disease, The Trans-Atlantic Inter-Society Consensus (TASC) on Management of Peripheral Arterial Disease was first written and published in 2000; it was revised in 2007 as TASC II with a supplement added in 2015 to include infrapopliteal arteries.[7,32] TASC guidelines categorize aortoiliac, femoropopliteal, and infrapopliteal disease by severity and base intervention recommendations on the extent of the disease. A new staging system for CLTI, the Global Limb Anatomic Staging System (GLASS), was published in 2020 with an aim to improve revascularization decision making by providing evidence-based revascularization recommendations.[33] Although there are multiple decision-making tools and progress in the evidence surrounding revascularization techniques, there is still not a one-size-fits-all algorithm for revascularization.

Options for endovascular therapy are multiple; however, the essential goal is to open the occluded segment with an instrument on a guidewire/catheter as opposed to performing an open incision. Balloon angioplasty is a technique by which an expandable balloon mounted on a wire is positioned deflated within the occluded/stenotic segment and then inflated to stretch the lumen to a larger diameter. For some arteries, stents (small expandable tubes) are placed in the occluded segment to help maintain vessel patency (**FIGURE 4-35**).

Another technique for more challenging occlusions where a wire cannot be passed through the occlusion is subintimal angioplasty, an endovascular technique in which a wire is used to create a "controlled dissection" at the occluded segment. The wire is traversed through a newly created false lumen and reenters the true lumen past the blockage. Once an opening has been made, the false lumen is expanded and stented.

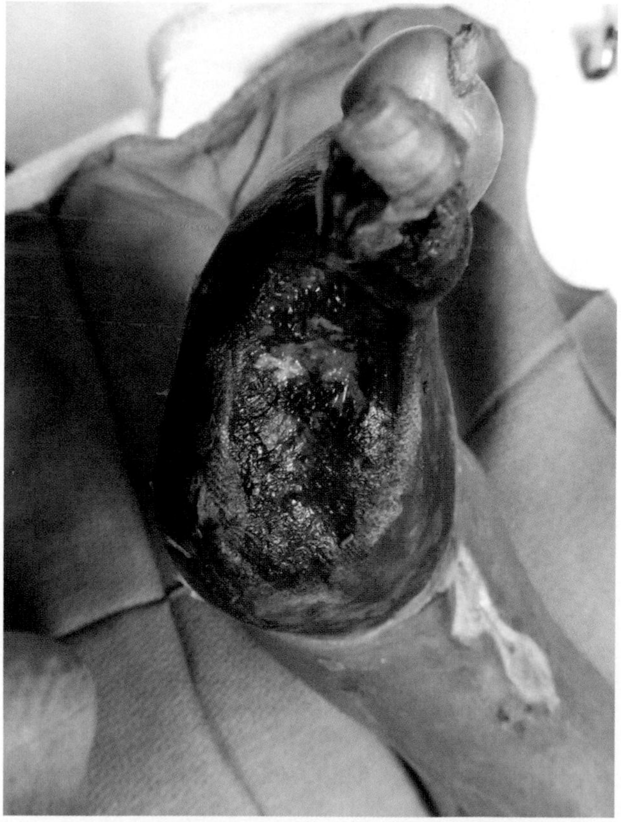

FIGURE 4-34 Amputation site not appropriate for NPWT. Negative pressure on an amputation site before reperfusion occurs can result in necrosis of the wound bed. Likewise, placing negative pressure on the amputation site before hemostasis is achieved will result in the loss of growth factors and cellular components that are needed for wound healing to progress.

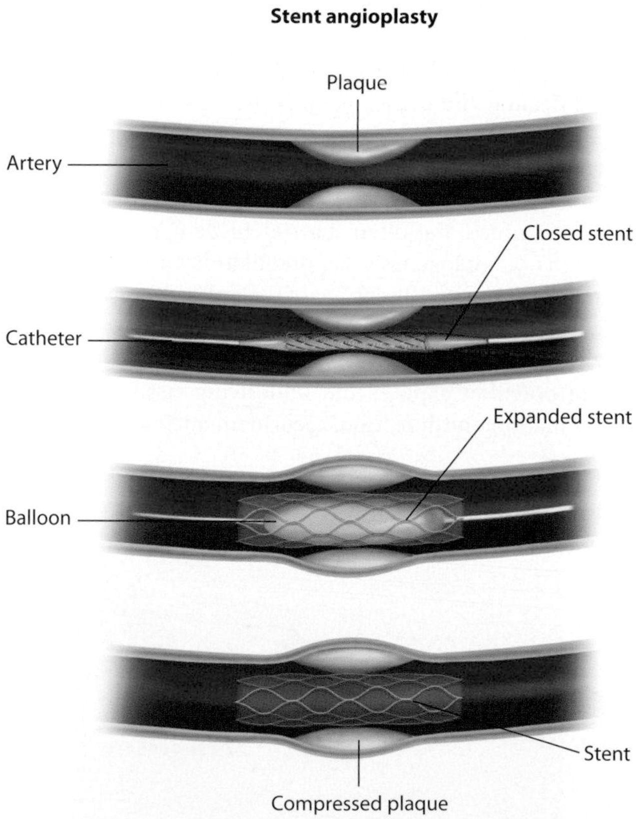

FIGURE 4-35 Endovascular angioplasty for a stenotic artery. A catheter is used to pass a closed stent through the artery to the area of stenosis, a balloon is used to expand the stent, and the balloon and catheter are removed. The stent remains in the artery, compressing the plaque against the arterial wall and increasing the size of the arterial lumen. This procedure is used for patients who are not candidates for bypass surgery and can reperfuse tissue sufficiently for wound healing to progress, albeit slowly.

CLINICAL CONSIDERATION

When using NPWT on a debrided arterial wound, reducing the pressure to 40–50 mmHg will prevent compression of superficial capillaries and subsequent tissue necrosis. If the superficial tissue shows signs of necrosis at the time of a dressing change, NPWT should be discontinued.

Revascularization Surgery Surgical intervention for PAD has many indications and options, and is dictated by the location and character of the occlusion.

Aortoiliac disease is increasingly managed with endovascular stenting. For lesions not amenable to endovascular treatment, revascularization is accomplished by a surgical bypass of the occluded segment from healthy proximal vessel (inflow) to healthy distal vessel (outflow) using a prosthetic tube graft. The bypass typically extends from the aorta to the femoral arteries via a transperitoneal or retroperitoneal approach (**FIGURE 4-36**). If the aorta is diseased and is a poor source of inflow or other contraindications are present, the thoracic aorta, axillary artery, and contralateral femoral artery may be used as the proximal in-flow vessel.

When disease involves the common femoral and profunda femoral artery, the standard of care remains open groin exploration, with endarterectomy, profundaplasty, or bypass procedures. The most commonly used graft conduit for bypasses of the lower extremity is the greater saphenous vein (GSV) as it has the best long-term patency.[34] Evaluation of the GSV as part of the work-up for revascularization is critical, as the initial results of the BEST-CLI trial demonstrated that for patients with CLTI who are appropriate candidates for open surgical and endovascular revascularization, patients with an adequate GSV who undergo open surgical revascularization have lower rates of major adverse limb events and death.[35] Although surgical bypass with GSV was superior to endovascular revascularization, it is important to note that patients in the trial who required an alternative conduit to GSV still had equivalent outcomes to those who underwent an endovascular reintervention. Femoropopliteal bypasses are commonly done for occlusions in the superficial femoral artery (SFA) and/or popliteal arteries with good distal outflow. In addition, femoral to infrapopliteal or tibial bypasses are performed for lesions of the distal popliteal or proximal tibial arteries.

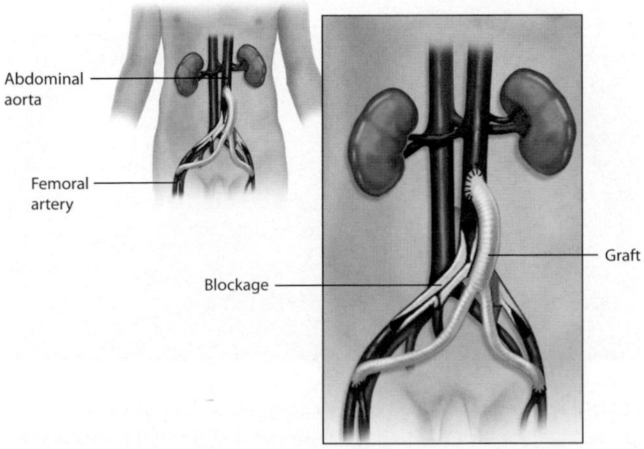

FIGURE 4-36 Illustration of aortofemoral vascular bypass. For patients with peripheral vascular disease of the aortoiliac region, a bypass graft from the aorta to both femoral arteries is indicated.

Postsurgical Treatment Postsurgical care of a patient with revascularization focuses on prevention of edema that can lead to dehiscence of the incision, prevention of infection, and meticulous wound care. Edema is managed by elevation, active ankle exercises, and wrapping with short stretch bandages in a spiral technique, especially when the patient begins to ambulate.

Control of medical conditions (eg, diabetes) is an important part of preventing infection, as well as standard precautions on the part of all clinicians caring for the patient. A dry antimicrobial dressing under the wrap may help with high-risk patients, and a recent addition to postoperative care is the disposable negative pressure incisional units that both manage any drainage and prevent shear of the incisional tissue.

Any separation (defined as <1 cm) or dehiscence (defined as >1 cm) of the incision is treated immediately with selective debridement (with meticulous care to avoid the graft), absorbent antimicrobial occlusive dressings, and edema management (**FIGURE 4-37**). After the wound is clean and there is no concern for graft erosion, negative pressure may be used to facilitate wound closure. Using negative pressure can also improve patient function due to the secure and occlusive dressings.

The groin incision also needs protection with dry sterile dressings because of the friction and moisture that can accumulate in that area and result in dehiscence.

If the surgery includes a digit, ray, or transmetatarsal amputation, wound care includes the following:

- Removal of any residual coagulum by either soft debridement with sterile gauze or pulsed lavage with suction (**FIGURE 4-38**)
- Selective debridement of devitalized tissue with care to preserve any viable tissue
- Moist wound dressings which may include biological materials on appropriately debrided, noninfected, and granulating wounds (refer to Chapter 14, Wound Dressings)
- Protective footwear to prevent pressure on the amputation site (**FIGURES 4-39** and **4-40**)
- Gait training with the appropriate assistive device

If the amputation is transtibial (TTA) or transfemoral (TFA), application of a residual limb wrap with short stretch bandages

CLINICAL CONSIDERATION

If a groin incision dehisces, there can be significant lymph drainage that impedes wound healing even with the use of NPWT. Hemostatic agents packed into the area of flow will stop the lymphatic drainage and allow faster wound closure.

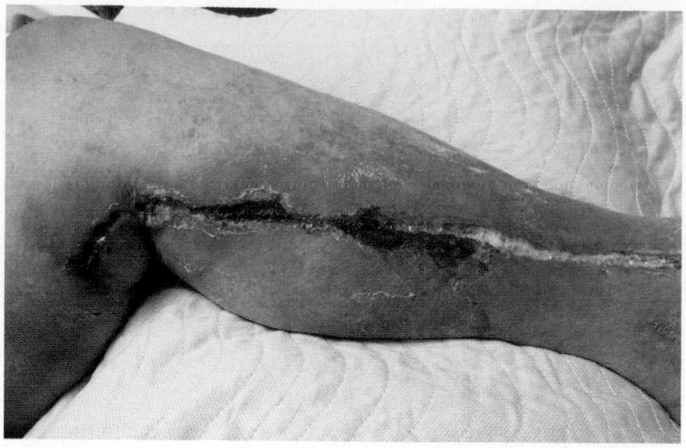

FIGURE 4-37 Incisional dehiscence. Incisional dehiscence occurs more in patients who are at risk for infection, such as those who have diabetes, protein-energy malnutrition, or obesity. Edema to the area or other external distraction forces on the incision can also lead to dehiscence.

is initiated postoperatively. In the case of TTA, the extremity may also be fitted with a special boot or cast to prevent knee flexion contractures from developing in the early rehab period (FIGURE 4-41). When using any type of wrap on an ischemic extremity, daily inspection is recommended to avoid development of soft tissue ischemia or pressure areas on bony prominences. Shrinker socks are typically deferred until *after* incisional healing has occurred and sutures/staples have been removed due to the distraction force on the incision line from donning and doffing these garments.

Finally, there are some patients with critical limb ischemia and wounds who are not candidates for revascularization or

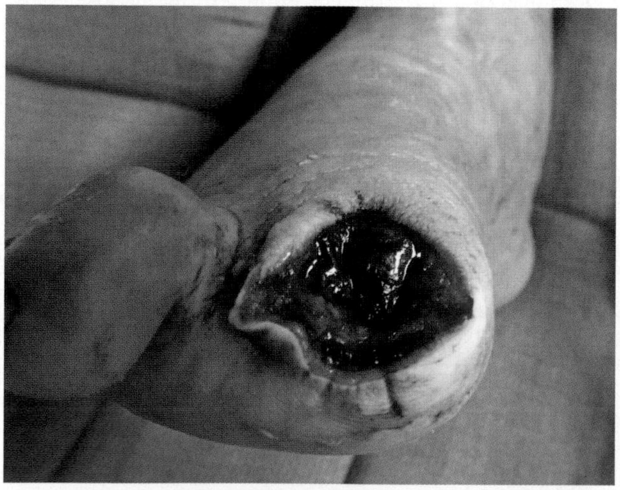

FIGURE 4-38 Coagulum in a post-amputation site. Coagulum in a post-amputation site needs to be removed by selective debridement using pulsed lavage with suction or another means to facilitate wound contraction, decrease the risk of infection, and decrease the amount of nonviable tissue the body has to autolyse. After the wound is clean, negative pressure wound therapy is indicated.

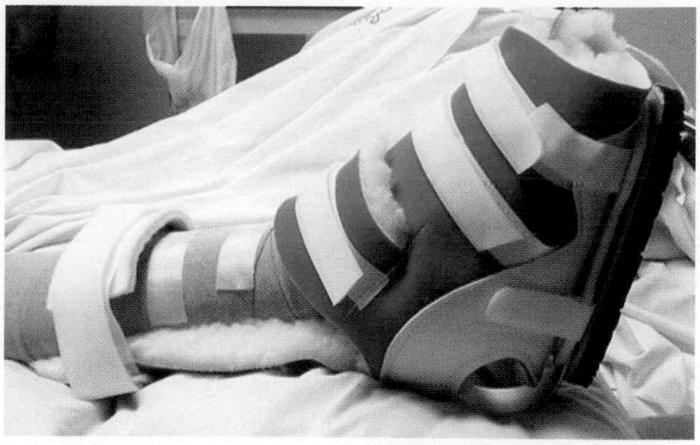

FIGURE 4-39 Rigid ankle-foot orthotic for the postsurgical ischemic foot. Ankle-foot orthoses may be helpful in protecting amputation sites and at-risk heels; however, frequent observation of the Achilles is recommended to ensure pressure relief.

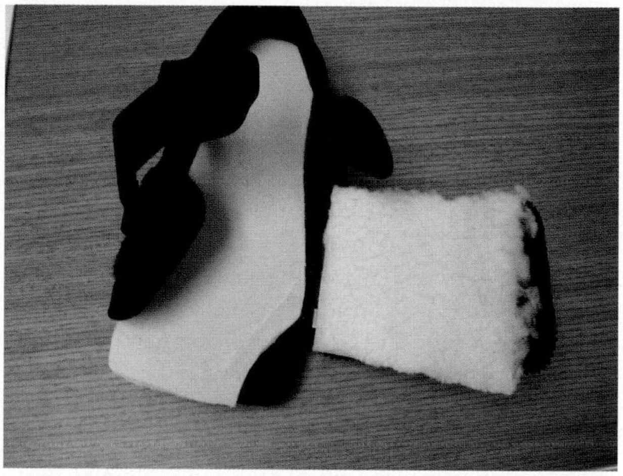

FIGURE 4-40 Postoperative shoes. The shoes can be padded with plastazote or dense foam for the plantar foot and lambswool for the dorsal foot. Early ambulation is an important part of the care plan for any revascularized patient.

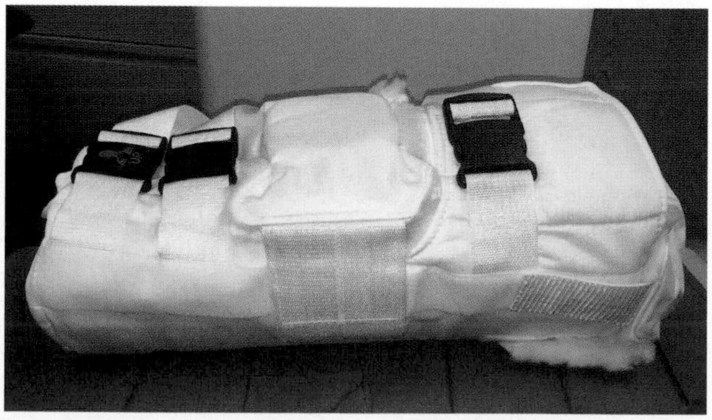

FIGURE 4-41 Protective boot for transtibial amputation. A protective boot for the transtibial amputation provides protection for the incision, maintains knee extension to prevent flexion contractures, provides cushion to prevent pressure points along the limb, and promotes vasodilation for wound healing by keeping the tissue warm.

CASE STUDY

CONCLUSION

The patient received a right popliteal to posterior tibial bypass graft with the right GSV. Four weeks later he had an amputation of the third toe, which had become well-demarcated at the edges with detached eschar, putting the foot at risk for infection. Subsequently, as is sometimes the case, the adjacent second toe became necrotic and required amputation (**FIGURE 4-43**). After removal of both toes, healthy granulation tissue formed, and NPWT was initiated on the amputation site (**FIGURE 4-44**).

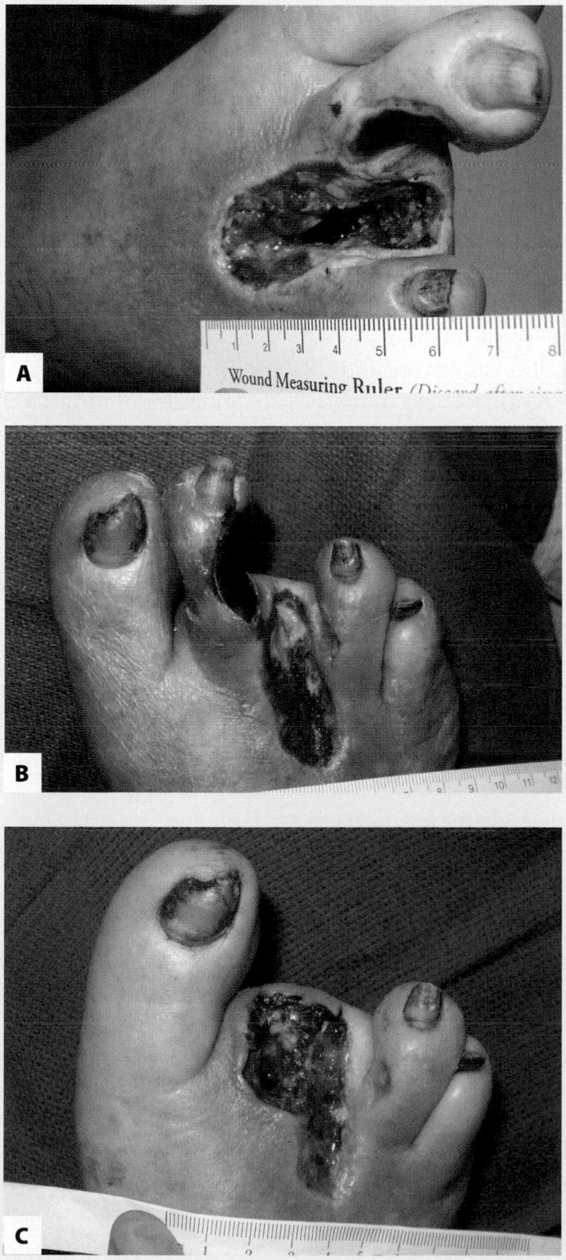

FIGURE 4-43 A–C. Post-amputation of the toes.

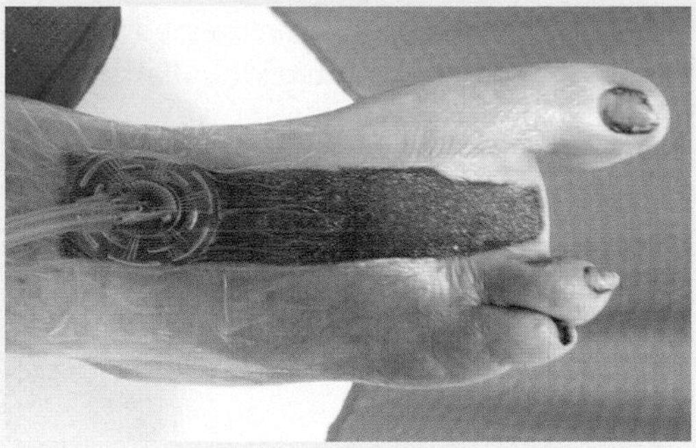

FIGURE 4-44 Treatment with NPWT.

The heel wound was off-loaded with a foam dressing and protective boots, and the edges were trimmed as the eschar lifted away from new epithelium (**FIGURE 4-45**). When the entire eschar was loose, an escharotomy was performed and the wound treated with collagen matrix and silicone-

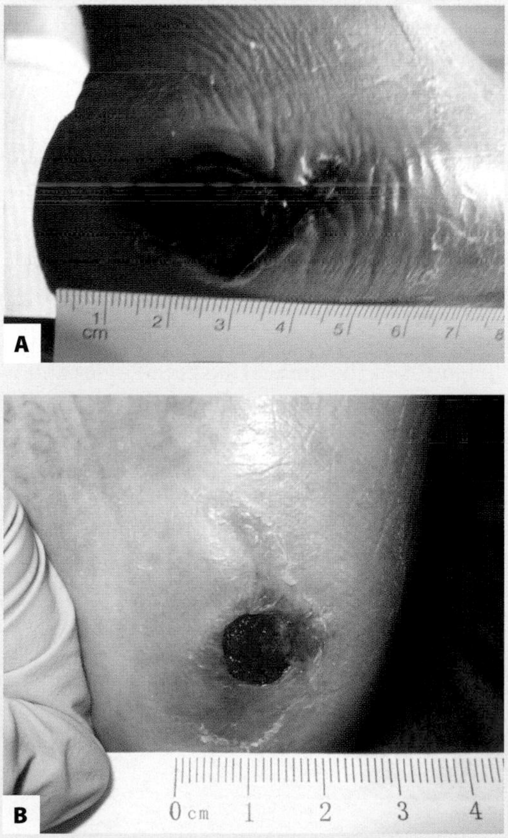

FIGURE 4-45 Heel wound case study A. The eschar on the patient's heel is becoming detached at the edges, a sign of adequate perfusion for healing. The eschar was trimmed on a weekly basis and was fully debrided when granulation was visible. Healing was slow, but the wound fully closed. **B.** The heel wound after 4 weeks of conservative debridement, moist wound healing, and off-loading.

Continued next page—

CASE STUDY *(Continued)*

backed dressings. Both wounds progressed steadily to full closure and the patient was fitted with diabetic shoes and custom-molded inserts (**FIGURE 4-46**).

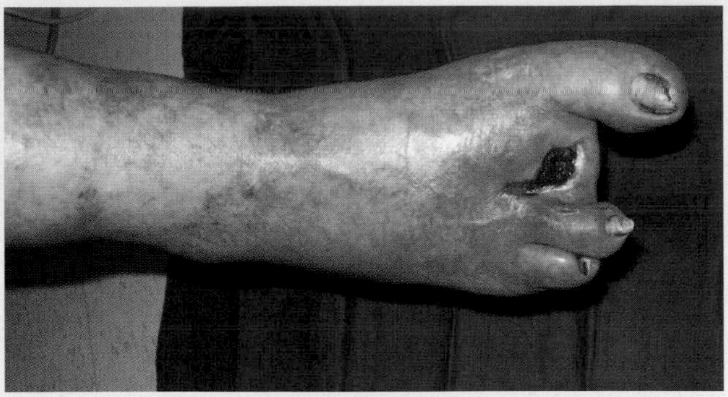

FIGURE 4-46 Wound almost closed.

who do not have positive outcomes with revascularization procedures. If there are no signs of infection and the edges of the wound remain adhered, conservative care, including meticulous skin care and cleansing of the edges daily with alcohol or iodine solution, can allow the patient to function at a baseline level. Over time, healing can occur by migration of the skin under the eschar. As the edges loosen, they are trimmed with sterile instruments, and with patience and protection, the wounds may heal (**FIGURE 4-42**). Pain management is an integral part of caring for these patients.

Summary

Arterial wounds can be slow and difficult to heal, involving careful management of all aspects of the patient's medical care. Accurate diagnosis of the underlying pathologies and patient-centered decisions on the most appropriate interventions to optimize perfusion are paramount to successful wound healing. Each phase of patient management requires different wound care and changing goals to ensure that the patient achieves not just wound closure, but optimal function and quality of life.

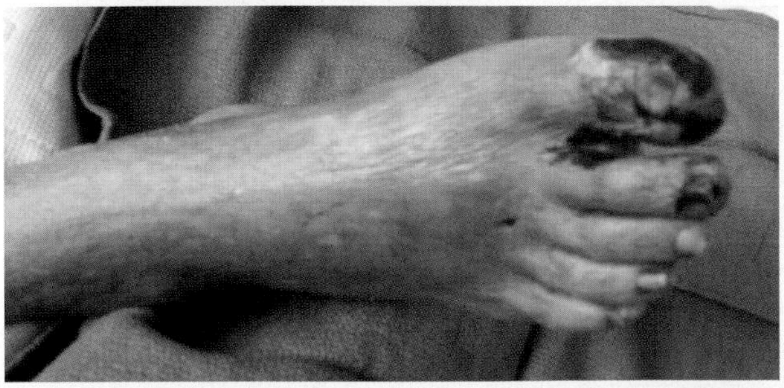

FIGURE 4-42 Wound on patient not a candidate for surgery. Ischemic wounds that are not or cannot be reperfused with vascular surgery are protected with alcohol or betadine cleansing at the edges, dry dressings, and footwear that does not put pressure on the wound.

VENOUS WOUNDS

Epidemiology

Venous wounds are a consequence of several disease mechanisms, but ultimately result from chronic venous insufficiency (CVI). An estimated 7 million people worldwide have some degree of CVI, and about 3 million of these develop venous wounds.[36] Varying prevalence rates may be due to differences in the classification or definition used, the methods of evaluation to determine wound etiology, and the geographic differences of the regions studied. Some of the better-known risk factors for first-time development of a venous wound include family history, physical activity (typically prolonged standing), history of ankle injury or immobility, and history of deep venous thrombosis (DVT).[37] Venous function is also affected by changes in estrogen and progesterone.[38]

CVI is a common illness and its most severe complications, namely venous ulcers, are often debilitating and slow healing. An annual economic burden of illness estimate for the United States totals $4.9 billion for deep venous disease–related venous leg ulcers.[39]

Anatomy

A review of lower extremity venous anatomy is essential for understanding the pathophysiology and treatment of venous disease. The venous system of the leg comprises two parallel and connected channels: the deep and superficial systems (**FIGURE 4-1**).

The *superficial* veins of the leg originate at the dorsal and deep plantar veins of the foot. The dorsal veins empty into the dorsal venous arch, which is continuous with the great and small saphenous veins. The GSV, which runs anterior to the medial malleolus and medial to the knee, is located in the superficial compartment and connects with the common femoral vein at the saphenofemoral junction (SPJ). Before the SPJ, the GSV receives medial and lateral accessory saphenous veins, as well as tributaries from the groin and anterior abdominal wall.

The small saphenous vein originates from the dorsal venous arch at the lateral foot and runs posterior to the lateral malleolus and into the posterior calf. It then penetrates the superficial fascia of the calf and empties into the popliteal vein.

The *deep* system originates with the digital veins that empty into metatarsal veins comprising the deep venous arch. This continues into the medial and lateral plantar veins, which then empty into the posterior tibial veins. The dorsalis pedis veins on the dorsum of the foot become the anterior tibial veins at the ankle. The paired posterior tibial veins run under the fascia of the deep posterior compartment, join with the paired peroneal and anterior tibial veins, and then join the popliteal vein. There are large venous sinuses within the soleus muscle that empty into the posterior tibial and peroneal veins. The popliteal vein enters a window in the adductor magnus, at which point it becomes the femoral vein (formerly superficial femoral vein). The femoral vein receives venous drainage from the profunda femoris vein, or deep femoral vein, after which it becomes the common femoral vein. At the inguinal ligament, the common femoral vein becomes the external iliac vein.

The superficial venous system connects to the deep system via perforating veins that cross through (perforate) the fascial layers. These perforators run perpendicular to the superficial and deep axial veins. The perforators vary in their anatomy and can enter the veins at various points the foot, medial and lateral calf, and mid- and distal thigh. The valves in the perforator veins aid in preventing reflux from the deep to

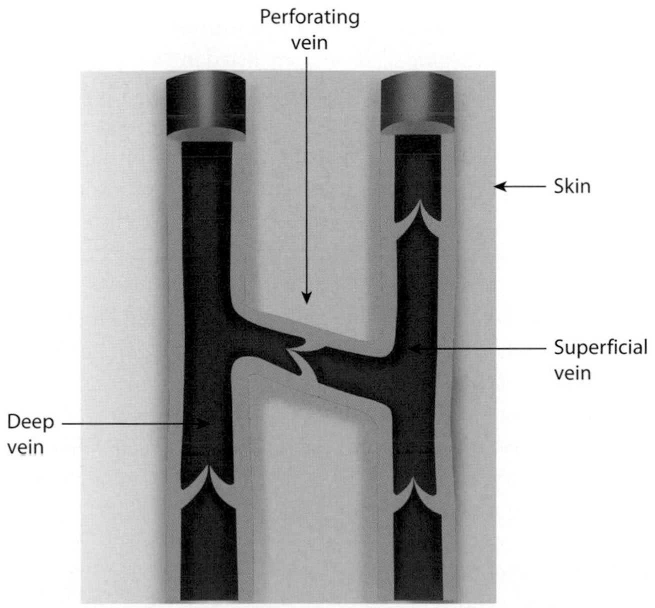

FIGURE 4-47 Anatomy of the veins. Venous flow is from the interstitial tissue into the venous capillaries, the venules, and the superficial veins, through the perforators into the deep veins. Retrograde flow is prevented by valves located in all three components of the peripheral venous system.

the superficial system, particularly during periods of standing and ambulation.

Normal Venous Physiology

The wall of a vein is made up of three layers: the intima, media, and adventitia. Vein walls have less smooth muscle and elastin than arteries. The adventitia of the venous wall contains adrenergic nerve fibers, especially in cutaneous veins. Sympathetic discharge, thermoregulatory centers in the brain, temperature changes, pain, emotional stimuli, and volume changes can alter venous tone. Venous valves prevent retrograde flow (**FIGURE 4-47**); valvular incompetence, or failure, leads to reflux and its associated symptoms. Venous valves are most prevalent in the distal lower extremity and decrease moving proximally. The superior vena cava (SVC) and inferior vena cava (IVC) do not have valves. Because veins do not have significant amounts of elastin, they can withstand large volume shifts with small changes in pressure. Therefore, most of the capacitance of the vasculature is in the venous system. The return of the blood to the heart from the leg is facilitated by the muscle pump function of the calf; when the calf muscle compresses the gastrocnemius and soleus sinuses, blood is propelled toward the heart.

Etiology

Venous insufficiency is due to failure of normal venous return that occurs through several mechanisms classified as primary, secondary, or congenital. Ultimately, CVI causes the higher pressure in the deep venous system to be transmitted to the superficial veins (termed *venous hypertension*),[40] resulting in impaired return of venous blood flow to the heart. The underlying pathology is most commonly due to incompetence of the valves of the deep or superficial venous system (**FIGURE 4-48**). In the scenario of venous valvular incompetence, there is inadequate coaptation of the valves; therefore, the valves do not prevent retrograde flow of blood. Other contributing factors include dysfunction of the gastrocsoleus muscle that works as a venous pump to push blood flow from the superficial veins to the deep veins (**FIGURE 4-49**), inherent vessel factors associated with genetic predisposition, and venous obstruction (ie, DVT). Patients who have Factor V Leiden are at

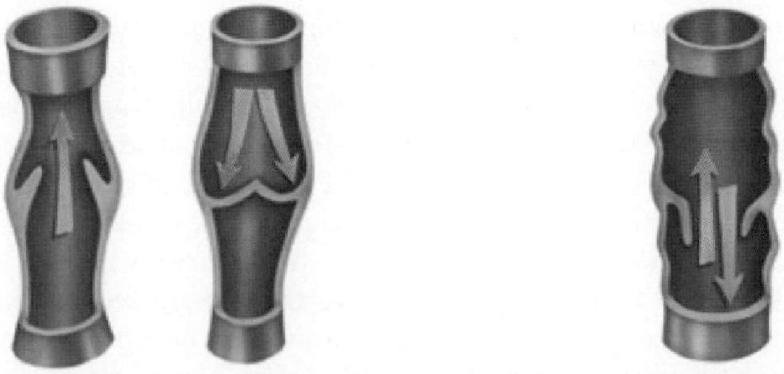

FIGURE 4-48 Incompetent valves. Normal venous flow is maintained by a series of valves that function to prevent backwash. With vein distention (eg, with age) the valves do not close completely, termed *incompetent valves*, and chronic venous insufficiency results.

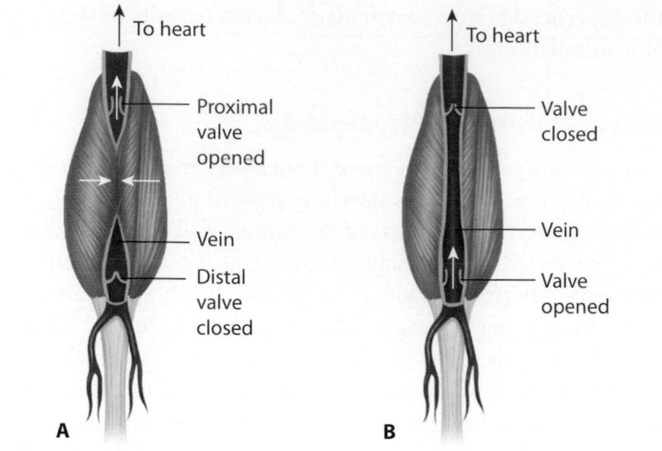

FIGURE 4-49 Venous pump. The gastrocsoleus muscle group works as a venous pump to facilitate the movement of fluid in the distal lower extremity back toward the heart. The pump is activated during any activity that involves gastrocsoleus contraction, especially during ambulation if the ankle range of motion and muscle strength is sufficient to cause compression of the deep veins. The pump action results in compression of the deep vein during push-off, creating a pressure on the vein sufficient to push the blood out of the vein. **A.** The pressure drops to 15–30 mmHg when the muscle relaxes (during swing, loading response, and midstance phases of gait). **B.** This gradient between the deep veins and the superficial veins allows the blood to flow through the perforators and into the deep veins until the next gastrocsoleus contraction, at which point the blood is again forced proximally toward the heart. During the muscle contraction, the proximal valve is open to allow flow of the fluid, and the distal valve is closed to prevent reflux. During the relaxed period, the proximal valve is closed and the distal valve is open, allowing flow through the vein without reflux when the vein is at its largest. If the gastrocsoleus does not function, either from muscle weakness or ankle joint hypomobility, the fluid pools in the deep veins, then in the perforators and superficial veins, and leads to interstitial edema and venous hypertension.

higher risk for developing DVTs, especially in conjunction with pregnancy or long-term hormone replacement therapy. **TABLE 4-8** lists the risk factors for acquiring venous insufficiency.

TABLE 4-8 Risk Factors for Chronic Venous Insufficiency

- Varicose veins
- Deep vein thrombosis
- Previous vein surgery
- Multiple pregnancies
- Congestive heart failure
- Coronary artery bypass surgery with saphenous vein harvesting
- Hip, knee, or ankle trauma
- Ankle immobility
- Prolonged standing or sitting
- Family history
- Age over 50
- Obesity
- Female sex
- Smoking

Data from Ortega MA, Fraile-Martinez O, Garcia-Montero C, et al. Understanding chronic venous disease: a critical overview of its pathophysiology and medical management. *J Clin Med*. 2021;10(15):3239.

Pathophysiology

In the normal peripheral circulation, blood volume is pumped out of the extremity, and the veins refill from the arterial flow. However, with CVI the veins fill from both arterial flow and retrograde venous flow due to dysfunctional valves, resulting in venous hypertension. *Congenital* CVI results from venous angiodysplasias, such as Klippel–Trenaunay syndrome and vascular malformations as seen in Parkes Weber syndrome.[41] *Primary* CVI occurs when valve failure is the result of weakness in the vessel wall or valve leaflets. *Secondary* CVI occurs in response to a previous event and is further categorized as *intravenous* or *extravenous*. Secondary intravenous occurs when the vein wall and valves are adversely affected. In secondary extravenous cases, there is no evidence of vein damage but local or systemic venous hemodynamics are hindered by external causes.[41]

The most common manifestation of CVI caused by reflux is varicose veins, or veins that are tortuous and distended (**FIGURE 4-50A–C**). When the incompetent valves are located at junctions of the deep and superficial systems, the high pressure in the deep system is transmitted to the superficial veins. For this reason, varicose veins often start at the saphenofemoral and saphenopopliteal junctions and in the perforating system.

Obstruction of the deep veins can also limit the outflow of blood and cause increased venous pressure. The obstruction may occur because of a secondary intravenous cause, for example, DVT or venous stenosis. Vascular and integumentary changes occur after a DVT and can lead to *postthrombotic syndrome*. The DVT results in valve destruction, which in turn leads to incompetence and persistent venous hypertension both at rest and during ambulation. Signs and symptoms of postthrombotic syndrome, also termed *postphlebitic syndrome*, are listed in **TABLE 4-9** and are illustrated in **FIGURE 4-51**. The obstruction can also result from a secondary extravenous cause, for example, in May–Thurner syndrome, a condition in which the right common iliac artery compresses the left common iliac vein. The compression causes chronic thickening of the vein wall and webbing within the vein that prevents flow from the left lower extremity and results in higher risk for thrombosis and edema.

Normal contraction of the calf muscles during ambulation assists in return of blood to the heart by functioning as a mechanical pump (**FIGURE 4-49**). Insufficient contraction of the muscle due to muscle weakness or paralysis, joint hypomobility, joint fusion, or gait impairment contributes to ineffective venous emptying and increased venous pressure.

The ineffective emptying and increased pressure in large vessel hemodynamics are thought to cause venous microangiopathy, defined as

CLINICAL CONSIDERATION

Evaluating for pitting in areas with minimal soft tissue (eg, the ankle and gaiter area) will help determine if edema is truly present. However, edema may be camouflaged in patients with gastrocsoleus atrophy because the leg presents with a fairly normal size as compared to the contralateral extremity.

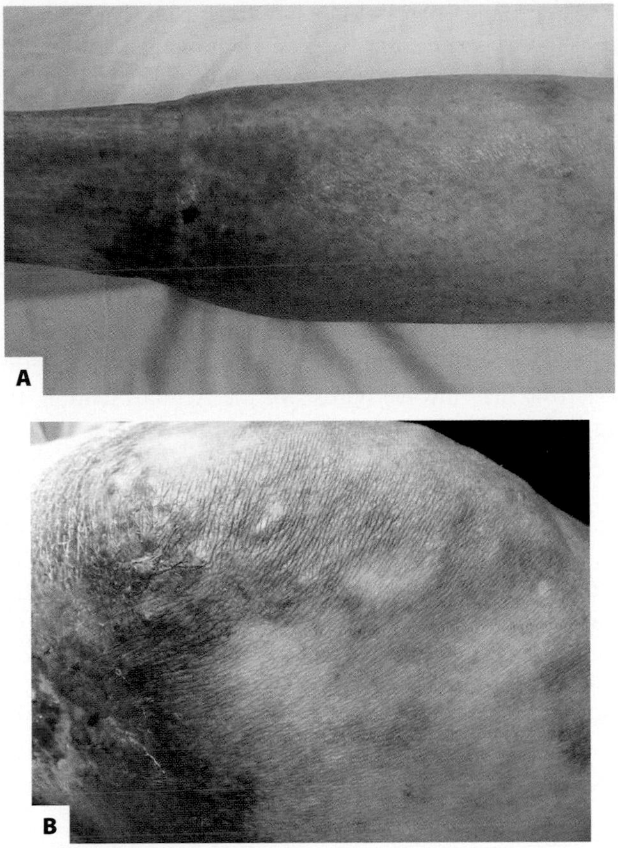

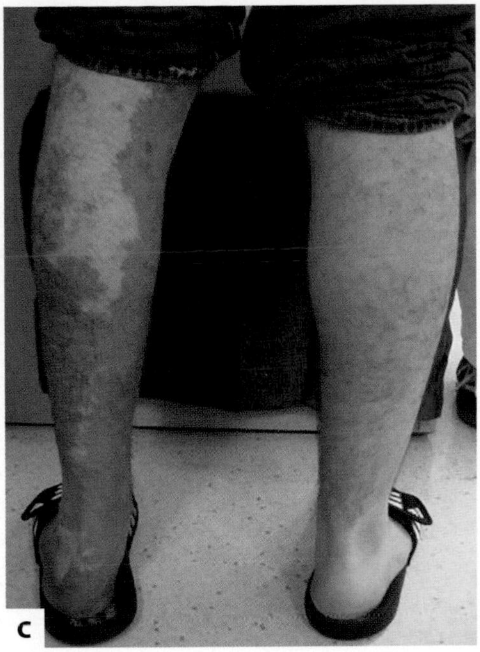

FIGURE 4-50 Varicose veins. Varicose veins are enlarged tortuous veins, the result of chronic fluid back-flow from incompetent valves. Varicosities in the superficial veins are visible through the skin. Patient **A** has a healed venous ulcer with hemosiderin staining of the gaiter area and varicose veins in the proximal calf. The constriction seen in the lower leg is the result of socks with elastic at the top, which the patient has been wearing instead of the recommended compression garments. Patient **B** has a congenital condition, Klippel–Trenaunay–Weber syndrome, with visible varicose veins in the lower thigh. Panel **C** shows the patient with Klippel–Trenaunay–Weber syndrome. Atrophy of the calf muscles is seen on the left leg as compared with the right and contributed to his chronic edema. In addition, he developed a significant leg length discrepancy that affected his gait.

derangements in venous function at the cellular level. As venous pressure is elevated, the microscopic anatomy of the vessel breaks down to allow spillage of serum proteins and red blood cells (RBCs) into the interstitial areas where they are trapped by the interstitial edema. When the RBCs die, the hemoglobin is released into the extracellular spaces where it is phagocytosed by macrophages. The by-products of lysed hemoglobin cause the dark, brawny discoloration termed *hemosiderin staining* (**FIGURE 4-52**).[42]

The predominant theories of CVI pathophysiology are (1) fibrin cuff formation, (2) growth factor trapping, and (3) white blood cell trapping. The original theory of the fibrin cuff proposed by Browse and Burnand[43] involves leaking of fibrinogen into the pericapillary space, thus creating a "cuff" that forms around the venous capillary. This was speculated to increase the diffusion barrier, restrict the diffusion of oxygen into the subcutaneous tissue and skin, and thereby maintain an inflammatory state. This theory has largely been supplanted by other findings but is still thought to play a role in CVI pathology.

TABLE 4-9 Signs and Symptoms of Postthrombotic Syndrome

- Aching or cramping in the extremity
- Feeling that the leg is heavy or tired
- Itching or tingling
- Chronic edema
- Varicose veins
- Hemosiderin staining of the skin
- Ulceration

Postthrombotic syndrome is a collection of signs and symptoms that occur long-term after a patient has a deep vein thrombosis, which, if untreated, increases a patient's risk of developing a venous wound. Preventive strategies include compression therapy, meticulous skin care, and exercise.

The leukocyte-trapping theory involves the sequestering or trapping of leukocytes in the capillaries or postcapillary venules. Venous hypertension results in decreased flow, which in turn causes the accumulation of white cells in the capillaries. The adhesion of activated white blood cells releases inflammatory mediators and proteolytic enzymes that cause endothelial damage. This process may also increase permeability and contribute to protein leak.[44] As this inflammatory reaction progresses, the endothelial glycocalyx and endothelial cells are altered which leads to progressive endothelial dysfunction. The severity of this dysfunction is associated with the clinical severity of CVI.[41]

Finally, trapping of growth factors by fibrin and other macromolecules is thought to occur via the same mechanism as the trapping of white blood cells. When the growth factors are bound, they are unavailable to facilitate healing.[45]

Clinical Presentation

As the varicose veins dilate and become tortuous, they may become painful because of distention. Patients describe the

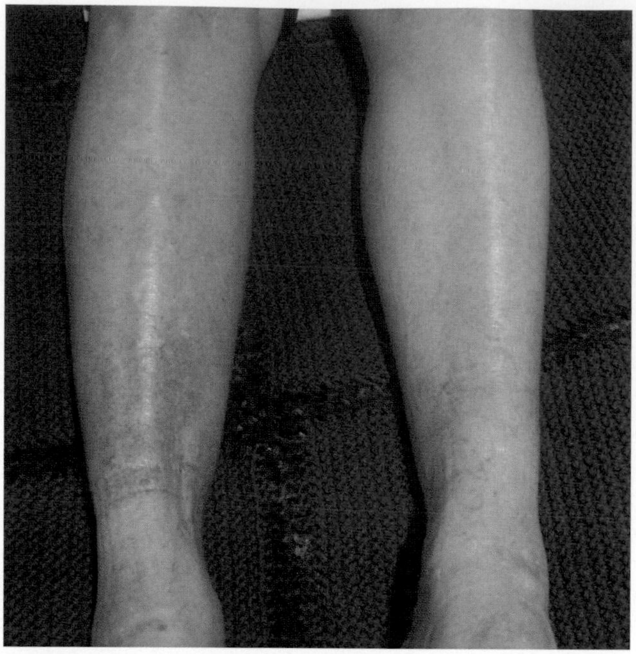

FIGURE 4-51 Postthrombotic syndrome. Patients who have a deep vein thrombosis are at risk for CVI with ulceration. Postthrombotic syndrome is characterized by the symptoms listed in **TABLE 4-7** and visualized in the right lower extremity of this patient who had a femoral DVT. Initial symptoms included pain distal to the thrombosis, severe edema, and erythema of the lower leg.

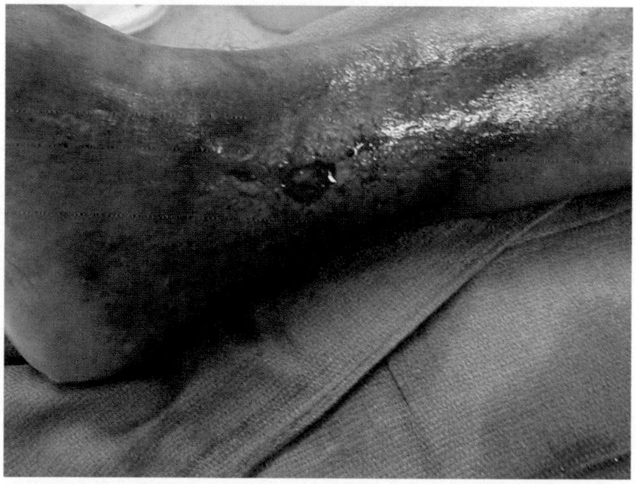

FIGURE 4-52 Hemosiderin deposition in the skin. The dark staining in the lower leg of a patient with CVI is a result of the autolysis of entrapped red blood cells and the attached hemoglobin molecules. The by-products of autolysis migrate into the epidermis and produce the discoloration.

pain or discomfort in the leg as heaviness, aching, or limb fatigue that is worsened by prolonged standing and relieved by elevation of the extremity. Edema begins in the foot and ankle and extends up the leg with progressive worsening during the day as the legs are dependent and fluid accumulates. These veins are also prone to superficial thrombophlebitis, as well as occasional bleeding and thinning of the overlying skin.

Skin changes that may also develop include hyperpigmentation in the perimalleolar region from hemosiderin deposition; lipodermatosclerosis with scarring and thickening of the skin secondary to fibrosis in the dermis and subcutaneous fatty tissue; and atrophie blanche, circular whitish and atrophic skin surrounded by dilated capillaries and hyperpigmentation. Brawny edema of the distal calf, fibrotic and hypertrophic skin, and hyperpigmentation are also visible signs of CVI. The constellation of these findings is sometimes referred to as "champagne bottle leg," due to the resemblance of the lower leg to an inverted champagne bottle. These are further described and illustrated in **FIGURES 4-52** to **4-57**. Advanced lipodermatosclerosis may involve fibrosis of the Achilles tendon, thus impairing motor function of the extremity. Patients may also develop eczematous dermatitis, cellulitis, and lymphangitis.

When evaluating the etiology of edema and ulcerations in CVI, a comprehensive medical and surgical history is crucial, with special attention to family history of varicosities, leg ulceration, thrombotic disorders, previous history of deep venous thrombosis or phlebitis, use of anticoagulation, abnormal clotting factors, unexplained transient unilateral edema, or previous venous-related interventions. The interconnectedness of the venous, lymph, and integumentary systems cannot be overstated. All edema, at its core, is lymphedema[46] and evidence shows that lymphatic anatomy and contractility decline

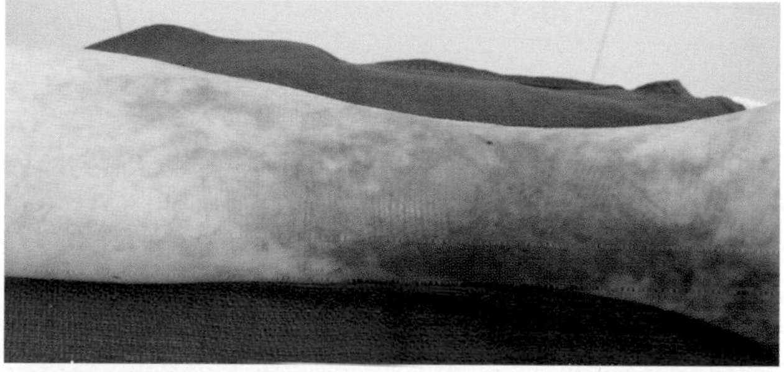

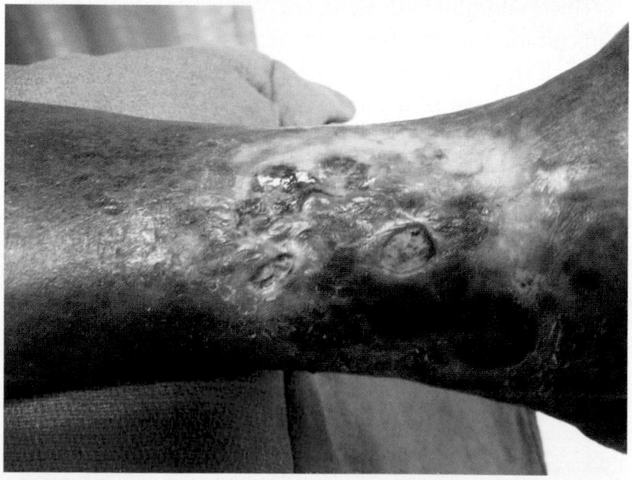

FIGURE 4-53 Lipodermatosclerosis. Lipodermatosclerosis, defined as scarring of the skin and fat, is the result of fibrin leaking into the subcutaneous tissue, causing fat necrosis, thickened smooth skin, subcutaneous immotility, and in severe cases, ulceration. Both lower extremities also have extensive hemosiderosis.

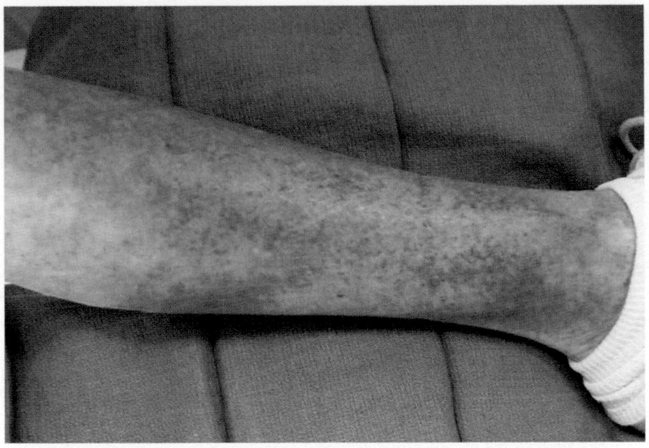

FIGURE 4-54 Atrophie blanche. Obstruction of the small vessels to the skin results in atrophie blanche, literally *white skin*, and may be a precursor to ulceration. Wounds that have adjacent atrophie blanche will frequently extend into the white area before full healing can occur.

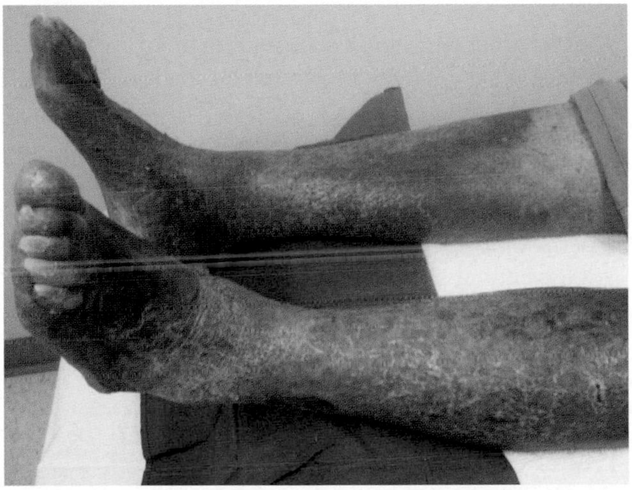

FIGURE 4-55 Brawny edema. Brawny, ordinarily defined as strong and firm, in this case refers to the discoloration from hemosiderin. Brawny edema is characterized by firm, discolored skin with non-pitting edema due to the underlying fibrosis of subcutaneous tissue.

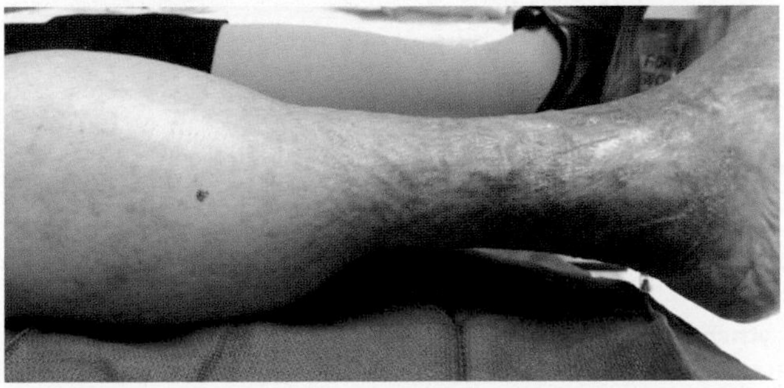

FIGURE 4-56 Champagne-bottle leg. Lipodermatosclerosis of the ankle and gaiter area can prevent flow into that part, resulting in excessive collection of fluid in the calf and the champagne-bottle shape of the leg.

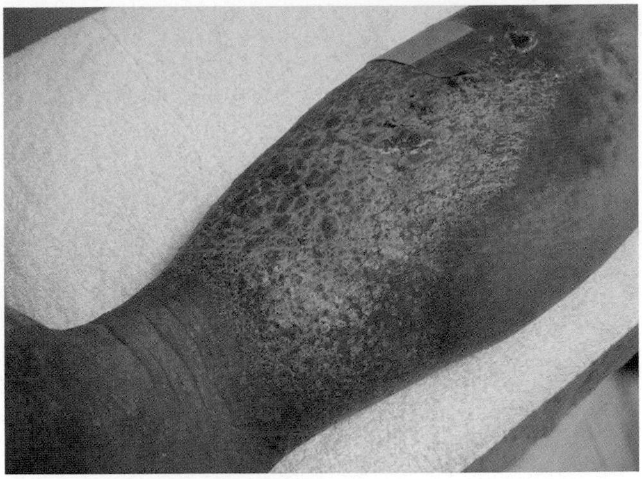

FIGURE 4-57 Fibrotic, hypertrophic skin. In addition to the fibrosis of the subcutaneous tissue, the epidermis can become thick and scaly. If not managed adequately, the skin under the scales can ulcerate or bacteria can collect and cause cellulitis. The erythema seen in this photo is suggestive of cellulitis.

with the progression of CVI, potentially leading to venous wounds.[47] Although unilateral edema may suggest venous pathology, a variety of other illnesses with a similar presentation need to be excluded.

Unilateral edema is more likely to be caused by CVI, whereas bilateral edema is usually caused by some systemic disorder (eg, renal failure, kidney failure, congestive heart failure) or by medications. Edema that has a sudden onset, is hard and indurated, and does not respond to compression should raise concern for obstruction of the pelvic or abdominal lymph nodes by malignancy (**FIGURE 4-58**). The correct differential diagnosis is imperative for effective interventions.

Additional signs and symptoms that are typical of venous wounds include the following:

- *Location:* Venous wounds occur above the medial and lateral malleoli in the distal third of the lower leg, termed the *gaiter area* (**FIGURE 4-59**). If the wound is outside of this area (eg, directly on the malleolus, on the postmalleolar skin, on the calf, or on the proximal leg), an etiology other than venous should be considered even with the presence of edema.
- *History of wound formation:* Venous wounds tend to be preceded and surrounded by changes in color and texture of the skin and have a more insidious development. If there are no skin changes and the wound onset was sudden, even in the presence of edema, other causes need to be considered. For example, a traumatic wound, a wound secondary to sickle cell disease, or a surgical incision may cause edema that then impedes wound healing; however, it would not be diagnosed as a venous wound.
- *Wound appearance:* Venous wounds tend to have uneven edges (termed *serpentine*), shallow depth, and a fibrotic or granular wound base (**FIGURE 4-60**). If the wound

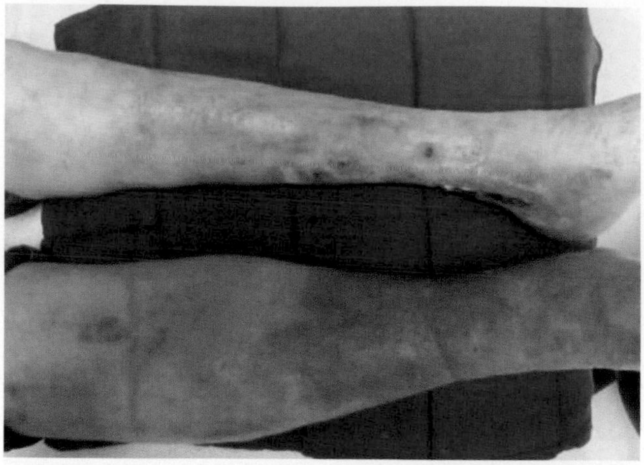

FIGURE 4-58 Lower extremity edema due to lymph node obstruction. Sudden onset of hard, indurating edema that does not respond to compression is suggestive of abdominal or groin lymph node obstruction, frequently related to metastatic disease. Urgent medical referral is imperative for timely diagnosis and treatment.

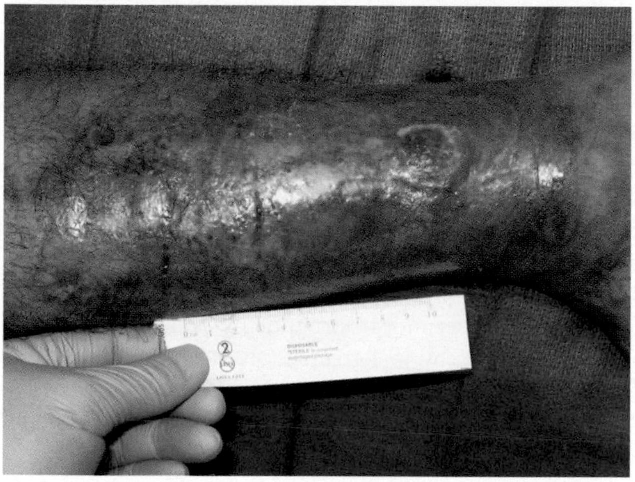

FIGURE 4-59 Location of a venous wound. Venous wounds occur in the medial or lateral gaiter area, defined as the distal third of the lower leg. Wounds outside this area, including over or distal to the ankle, on the calf, or on the anterior shin, are usually caused by some other etiology although chronic edema may impede the healing.

has been present for a long period, the edges may be senescent or rolled. There is usually little if any eschar.

- *Periwound skin:* Changes in the periwound skin include increased dermal thickness (eg, >1.985 mm measured with high-frequency ultrasound), hemosiderin staining, crusting or scaling, lipodermatosclerosis, varicosities, or atrophie blanche.[48]
- *Drainage:* Just as water flows from a hole in a hose or water pipe, fluid flows from a wound on an edematous extremity. Drainage from a venous wound is usually serous; however, if infection is present, it may be thick, purulent, and odiferous. If a wound appears venous in all respects but tends to have little or no drainage, there is concern for concomitant arterial insufficiency.
- *Pain:* Venous wound pain can be due to multiple reasons including manipulation of the wound itself, neuropathy and nerve damage, edema, lipodermatosclerosis, superficial and deep vein phlebitis, infection, contact dermatitis, and atrophie blanche. Pain-reducing interventions should take into account severity, predisposing factors (wound cleansing, debridement, prolonged standing, etc.) and type of pain (nociceptive, neuropathic, or a combination). Wounds that are exquisitely painful to any tactile stimulation are more likely to be vasculitic or arterial (**FIGURE 4-61**).

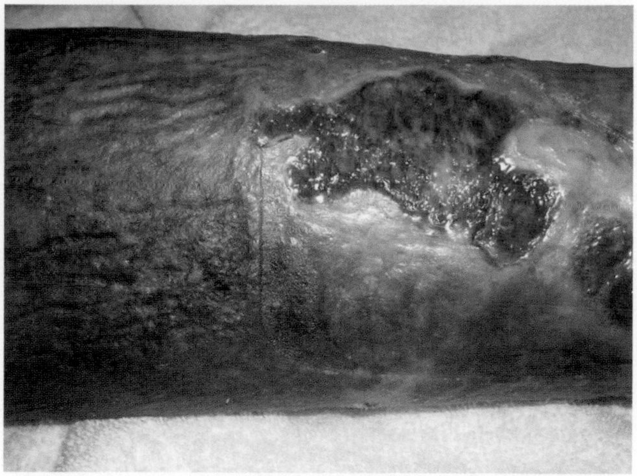

FIGURE 4-60 Typical appearance of a venous wound. A venous wound typically has serpentine, or uneven, edges; striated granulation or yellow fibrous tissue; serous or serosanguineous drainage; and rolled edges. Wounds with even, punched-out edges should be evaluated for an arterial component.

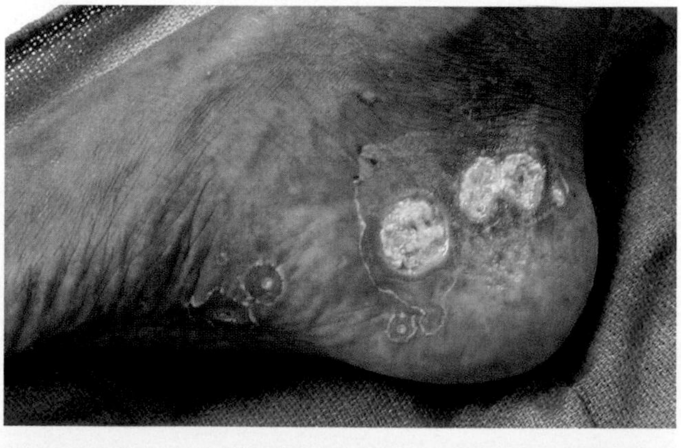

FIGURE 4-61 Vasculitic wounds on patient with systemic lupus erythematosus. Vasculitic wounds may be close to the typical location of venous wounds, but as in this photo, can be anywhere on the extremity. If they appear on or distal to the ankle, the wounds are probably not venous in origin, although the vasculitic inflammation may cause edema. In addition, vasculitic wounds are very painful, are usually smaller than most venous wounds, and require treatment of the underlying vasculitis in addition to wound care.

CASE STUDY

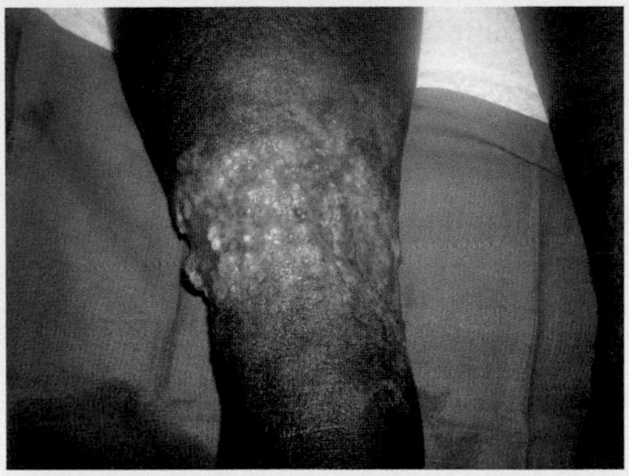

FIGURE 4-62 Right lower extremity of case study

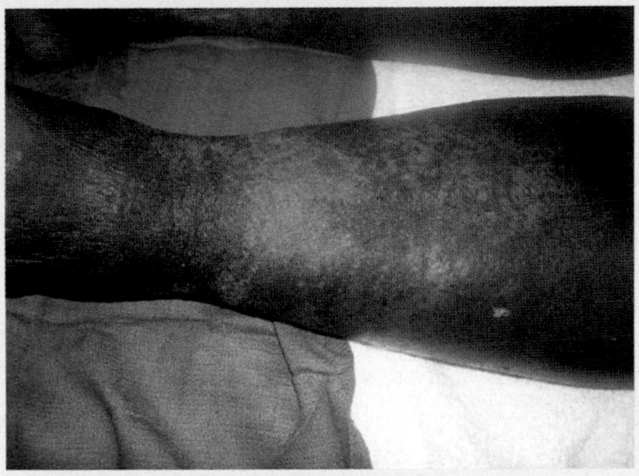

FIGURE 4-63 Left lower extremity of case study

A 52-year-old female presents with a history of nonhealing wounds on the right medial and lateral lower extremity in the gaiter area, of more than 1-year duration (**FIGURES 4-62** and **4-63**).

SUBJECTIVE INFORMATION

- Patient works as a manager for a department store and wants to continue to work while she is being treated.
- Pain levels are 6–8/10 almost constantly and 10/10 with any tactile stimulation to the wound bed.
- Patient is currently applying Silvadene to the wounds daily and covers them with cotton gauze and pads, anchored with tape.
- Patient lives in a one-story home with her husband and two dogs.
- Patient reports copious drainage that interferes with her social and professional life, as well as keeping her awake at night.

MEDICAL HISTORY

- History of hypertension
- History of hysterectomy about 5 years previously; no pregnancies reported
- History of obesity
- History of DVT in the right femoral vein
- Negative for diabetes, cardiac disease, and peripheral arterial disease

VASCULAR EXAMINATION

- Pulses—right posterior tibial not palpable because of the wound, strong Doppler signal; right dorsalis pedis 2+; left pedal pulses 3+

DISCUSSION QUESTIONS

1. What skin changes are observed in the lower extremity?
2. Describe the tissue in the wound bed.
3. What other information is needed to determine the cause of the patient's wounds?
4. Classify the patient's venous disease and wounds using the CEAP system.
5. Which noninvasive tests are indicated for this patient and why? What would you expect to learn about the patient to make a diagnosis?
6. Which invasive tests are indicated and why?

Skin temperature elevated more than 1.1°C or 3°F is suggestive of infection, along with erythema of the periwound skin, increased drainage with odor, friable granulation tissue, and pain.[49] Wounds that fail to improve within 6 weeks after initiation of treatment are very likely not a result of CVI and should be investigated for other diagnoses (**TABLE 4-10**). Studies have also indicated that wounds that decrease by 40% in the first 3 weeks of treatment have higher healing rate.[42]

Classification of Venous Wounds

The International Consensus Committee on Chronic Venous Disease has developed a classification of CVI, designed to standardize parameters for medical and surgical research. In the CEAP classification, each letter stands for a particular dimension of the disease: ***C*** represents the clinical signs, ***E*** stands for the etiology, ***A*** is for the anatomy involved, and ***P*** is the pathophysiology.[50,51] Since its introduction in 1993 the CEAP classification has undergone multiple updates, with the

TABLE 4-10 Differential Diagnosis of Venous Wounds

Wounds that fail to heal after 6 weeks of evidence-based care (compression, moist wound healing, exercise) should be studied further for diagnoses that may appear as venous wounds but are indeed caused by other pathologies[36]:

- Malignancies
- Vasculitis
- Polyarteritis nodosum
- Vasculopathy
- Pyoderma gangrenosum
- Mycobacterial or fungal infections
- Necrobiosis lipoidica diabeticorum
- Systemic lupus erythematosus wounds
- Cryoglobulinemia

most recent rendition in 2020 adding additional substratification to the classes.[52] Refer to **TABLE 4-11** for a complete outline of the CEAP classification with illustrations.

With the CEAP classification in mind, there are four questions to be addressed during the process of evaluating a patient with a venous wound.

1. What are the clinical signs present in the lower extremity?
2. What is the etiology of the venous stasis disease?
3. Where is the anatomic disease process occurring?
4. Is the pathology at that anatomical location obstruction or incompetent valves resulting in reflux, or a combination of the two?

TABLE 4-11 CEAP Classification of Venous Wounds

C represents the clinical signs, **E** stands for the etiology, **A** is for the anatomy involved, and **P** is the pathophysiology.

Clinical signs are identified from the following list, then designated symptomatic or asymptomatic:

0 = No visible or palpable signs of venous disease

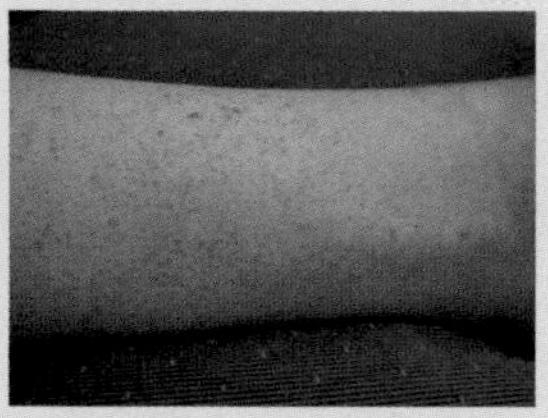

1 = Telangiectasia or reticular veins—small dilated veins (0.5–1 mm in diameter) that develop in the superficial skin as a result of venous hypertension

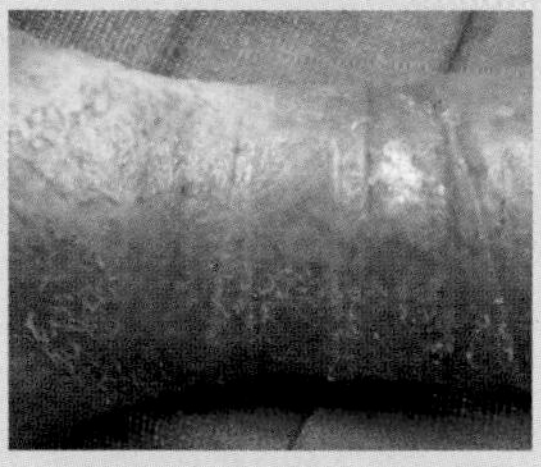

2 = Varicose veins—dilated, tortuous veins in the lower leg that signify the progression of CVI due to venous hypertension

2r = Recurrent varicose veins

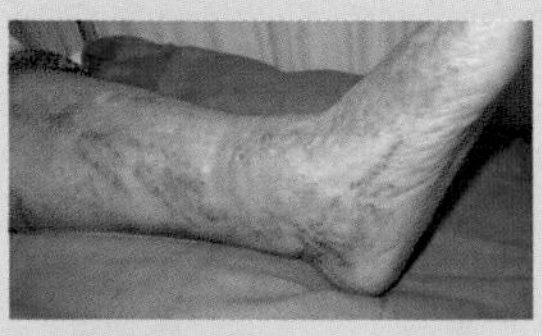

3 = Edema without ulceration

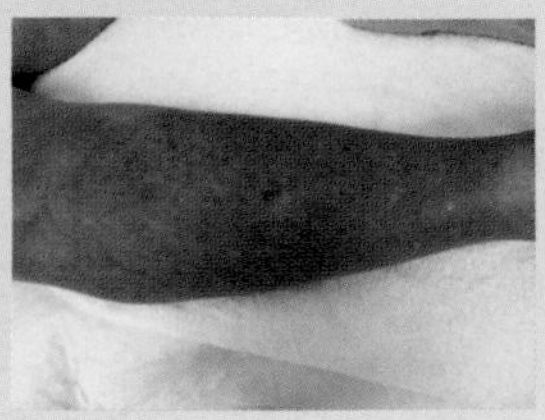

4 = Skin and subcutaneous changes ascribed to venous disease

4a = Pigmentation or eczema

4b = Lipodermatosclerosis or atrophie blanche

4c = Corona phlebectatica

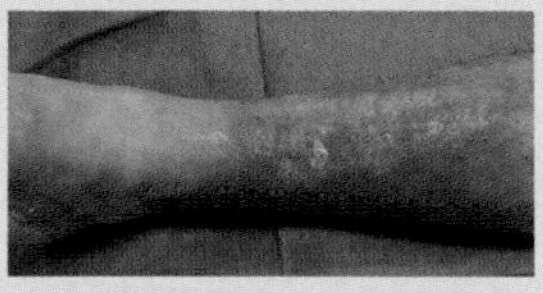

5 = Skin changes as defined above with healed ulceration

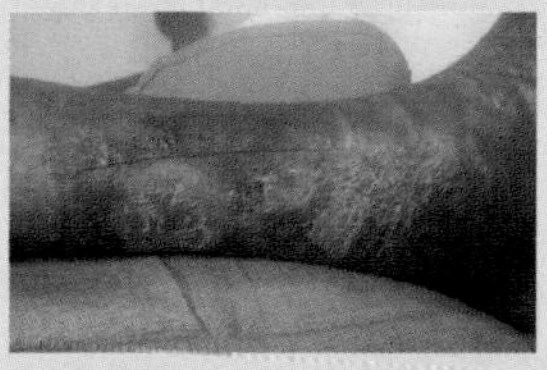

6 = Skin changes as defined above with active ulceration

6r = Recurrent venous ulceration

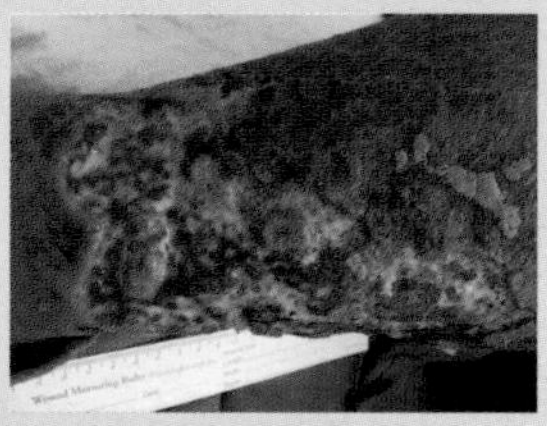

S: symptomatic, including ache, pain, tightness, skin irritation, heaviness, muscle cramps, and other complaints attributable to venous dysfunction

A: asymptomatic

Etiology is defined as one of the following:

Ep: Primary, in which venous insufficiency is the primary disease process observed

Es: Secondary, in which another disease process occurs first (for example, acquired lymphatic insufficiency)

Esi: Secondary—intravenous (vein wall and valves are adversely affected)

Ese: Secondary—extravenous (no evidence of vein damage, but local or systemic venous hemodynamic is impaired)

Ec: Congenital (for example, congenital valvular dysfunction)

En: No venous cause identified

(Continued)

TABLE 4-11 CEAP Classification of Venous Wounds (*Continued*)

Anatomical class is divided into the following: As: Superficial veins Ad: Deep veins Ap: Perforating veins An: No venous location identified Superficial veins: 1. Tel = Telangiectasia 2. Ret = Reticular veins 3. GSVa = Great saphenous vein, above knee 4. GSVb = Great saphenous vein, below knee 5. SSV = Small saphenous vein 6. AASV = Anterior accessory saphenous vein 7. NSV = Non-saphenous vein Deep veins: 8. IVC = Inferior vena cava 9. CIV = Common iliac vein 10. IIV = Internal iliac vein 11. EIV = External iliac vein 12. PELV = Pelvic vein 13. CFV = Common femoral vein	14. DFV = Deep femoral vein 15. FV = Femoral vein 16. POPV = Popliteal vein 17. TIBV = Crural (Tibial) vein 18. PRV = Peroneal vein 19. ATV = Anterior tibial vein 20. PTV = Posterior tibial vein 21. MUSC = Muscular veins 22. GAV = Gastrocnemius vein 23. SOV = Soleal vein Perforating veins: 24. TPV = Thigh perforator vein 25. CPV = Calf perforator vein **P**athophysiology is classified as follows: Pr: Reflux, usually from incompetent valves Po: Obstruction, usually from DVT; refers to a total occlusion of one of the veins at any point *or* more than 50% narrowing of at least half of a vein segment Pr,o: Reflux and obstruction Pn: No venous pathophysiology identifiable

Data from Lurie F, Passman M, Meisner M, et al. The 2020 update of the CEAP classification system and reporting standards. *J Vasc Surg Venous Lymphat Disord*. 2020;8:342e52.

In addition, the clinician needs to identify other disease processes, assess for infection, and identify contributing factors that can be addressed in the care plan.

Patient Examination

A comprehensive examination of any patient with a wound below the knee, including a venous wound, begins with an assessment of the arterial circulation, as discussed in the section on arterial wounds. A notable sign that arterial insufficiency may be impeding the wound healing is lack of hair growth in the lower half of the leg and foot.[42] An ankle-brachial index is indicated if there is any sign of diminished flow, and results less than 0.8 suggest that the patient should be referred to a vascular specialist.[53]

The venous system is assessed with the patient in both standing and supine positions. Standing increases venous hypertension and dilates the veins, thereby facilitating the examination. Patients with superficial valvular incompetence commonly exhibit palpable GSVs. Palpable cords may also be present (**FIGURE 4-64**). CVI dermatitis at the distal ankle can mimic eczema or dermatitis of another cause. For this reason, history and physical findings must be weighed alongside focused vascular studies, both invasive and noninvasive.

A thorough wound assessment includes all the components discussed in Chapter 3. The clinical findings are used to select interventions, determine outcomes, and measure progress.

Noninvasive Vascular Studies

Venous Duplex Examination Duplex ultrasound for superficial/deep/perforating vein assessment has largely replaced the Brodie–Trendelenburg and Perthes tests. There are different types of venous ultrasonography, including compression ultrasound (B-mode imaging only), duplex ultrasound (B-mode imaging and Doppler waveform analysis), and color Doppler imaging. Different lower extremity veins are best evaluated with different techniques. Compression ultrasound is typically performed on the proximal deep veins (the common femoral, femoral, and popliteal veins), whereas a combination of duplex ultrasound and color Doppler imaging is used to evaluate the calf and iliac veins.[54]

Valve reflux is identified with distal augmentation of flow and release, normal deep breathing, and performance of a Valsalva maneuver. Augmentation of flow is achieved by compressing the leg distal to the ultrasound probe to exaggerate the natural calf-pump mechanism and increase fluid return. The probe is used to obtain sample volumes from the femoral and saphenous veins. Sudden release of augmentation allows the assessment of reflux and valvular competence. Reflux is defined by the presence of reversed flow for >500 ms in the superficial veins and >1000 ms for the

CLINICAL CONSIDERATION

Approximation of central venous pressure is a screening test to determine if an element of congestive heart failure (CHF) is contributing to lower extremity edema. The hand is held below the heart until the veins are visibly filled. When the hand is elevated slightly above heart level, the veins flatten if there is minimal risk of CHF being present because the fluid can return to the central vascular system. If, however, the veins remain distended, referral to the physician for further medical care is advised before any compression therapy is initiated. Prominent jugular venous distention is another visible sign of increased central venous pressure with CHF.

deep veins. The small saphenous vein and popliteal veins are then examined. Perforator veins can also be assessed this way.[54]

In addition, assessment of microcirculation by transcutaneous oxygen tension can predict wound healing potential as discussed in the section on arterial wounds. Values of more than 30 mmHg in the periwound skin suggest sufficient oxygenation for healing to occur.

Invasive Testing

Invasive vascular studies include phlebography or venography, ambulatory venous pressure, and intravenous ultrasound. Phlebography uses intravenous contrast and radiography to help distinguish saphenofemoral anatomy and reflux. Although its routine use has largely been replaced by venous duplex imaging, phlebography is occasionally performed before deep vein reconstruction or in patients with inconclusive duplex results before other venous surgery.

Ambulatory venous pressure is considered the hemodynamic gold standard for the assessment of CVI[55]; however, it is seldom used in clinical practice because of its invasive nature, concern about its accuracy, and availability of numerous alternative diagnostic modalities. A needle is inserted into the pedal vein and connected to a pressure transducer; pressure is measured at rest and after exercise, as well as before and after placement of an ankle cuff to distinguish deep from superficial venous disease.

Intravascular ultrasound has gained acceptance in the management of venous disease and is increasingly being used to help guide interventions. A catheter-based ultrasound probe is used to visualize periluminal vessel anatomy to assess for obstructive disease. Intravascular ultrasound may be superior to venography in estimating the morphology and severity of central venous stenosis, especially in the pelvis, and in visualizing the details of intraluminal anatomy.[56]

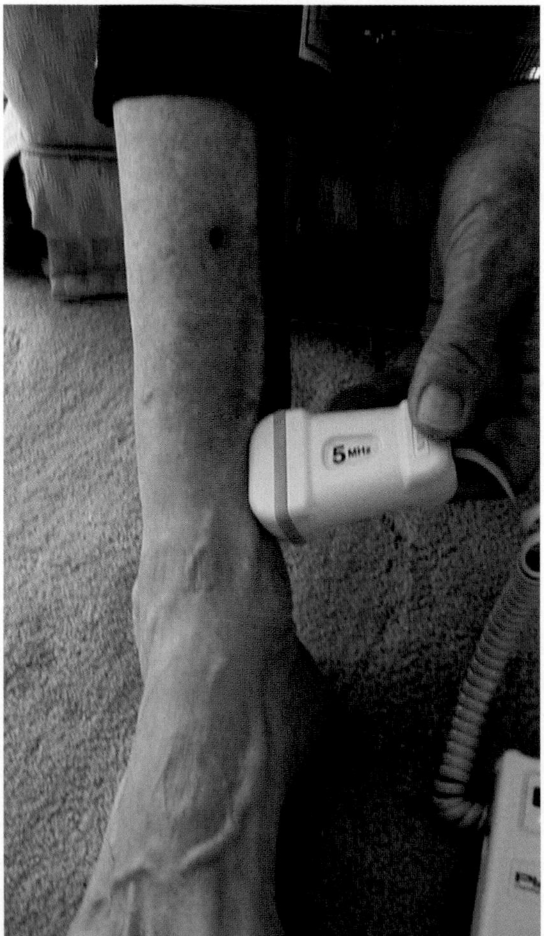

FIGURE 4-64 Distended saphenous vein. Distended veins are visible in the lower leg due to superficial valvular incompetence or with compression of the blood pressure cuff around the calf when testing for augmented venous flow.

Prevention

Guidelines have been published by various societies for the management of venous leg ulcers.

The Wound Healing Society established their guidelines in 2006 and published updated guidelines in 2012 and 2015.[57] The Society for Vascular Surgery and the American Venous Forum published their guidelines for the management of venous leg ulcers in 2014.[58] The guidelines published by these organizations are the basis of this discussion on prevention and treatment.

Prevention is predicated on first determining the risk factors of any individual, then providing the education needed to effect lifestyle changes, including causes of skin breakdown, principles of good skin care, smoking cessation, how and why to use compression, and appropriate exercise.[42] See Chapter 15 for additional information regarding exercise for patients with venous insufficiency and/or wounds. Additional strategies are to avoid prolonged standing and sitting, avoid crossing the legs, and wear light compression garments, especially for flying and for prolonged standing or sitting. Elevation with the leg higher than the heart is supported for prevention and treatment; however, it is not sufficient in and of itself. Elevation is only a principle to use when sitting or supine and is not a substitute for compression and exercise.

Nonsurgical Treatment

Selection of treatment strategies is guided by the disease severity using the CEAP classification system in a stepwise fashion. The mainstay of initial treatment for CVI is nonsurgical measures to reduce symptoms, prevent the development of secondary complications, and halt disease progression. The four basic components of wound treatment include compression, treatment of infection, moist wound healing, and exercise to activate and strengthen the venous pump.

Compression Two questions drive the selection of compression for the patient with a lower extremity wound: (1) What is the wound etiology? and (2) What materials and wrapping technique are best for the patient?

An algorithm for the first question is presented in **FIGURE 4-65**. Bilateral edema *can* be present because of reflux

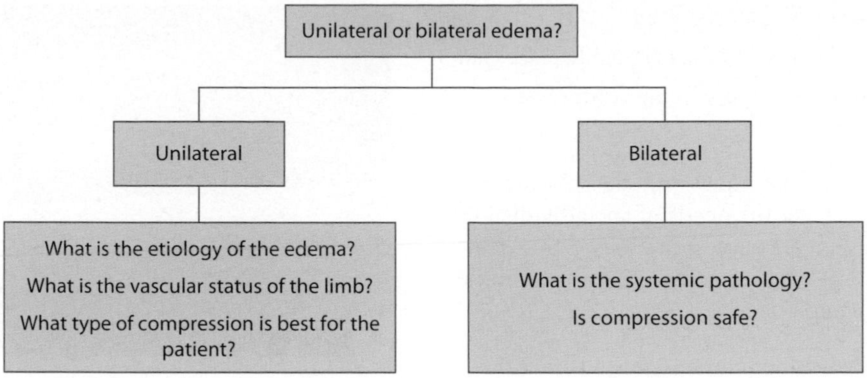

FIGURE 4-65 Algorithm for addressing lower extremity edema. Compression selection begins with a careful assessment of the edema. If the patient has bilateral lower extremity edema, systemic disorders such as congestive heart failure, kidney failure, or liver disease must be ruled out, as well as carefully reviewing medications. (See Chapter 5, Lymphedema.) If the patient has severe heart failure (New York Heart Association [NYHA] Class IV), compression may need to be modified or deferred until the underlying issue is corrected.[59] Any systemic issue must be addressed for local treatment to be effective. All edema has a lymph component to it and would benefit from manual lymphatic drainage, exercise, and compression. Vascular status must be evaluated to determine the type of compression that is best for the individual patient.

CLINICAL CONSIDERATION

An engaging way for a patient to perform ankle exercises is to "write" the alphabet with the big toe while sitting on the edge of a chair. This activates the lower leg muscles in all the compartments and mobilizes the ankle joint in all directions.

or obstruction; however, systemic diseases that cause edema need to be ruled out and treated. In some cases of severe heart failure (New York Heart Association [NYHA] Class IV), compression may be deferred until the patient is stabilized.[59]

An algorithm for selection of materials and wrapping technique based on the lower extremity ABI is presented in **FIGURE 4-66**. Materials are classified as elastic or inelastic and can be applied as a single-layer or multilayer, and wrapping can be performed in a spiral or a Figure-8 pattern. The principles of compression are based on the following: (1) there must be a gradient between the pressure at the ankle and at the calf in order to push the fluid cephalad, and the usual differential for a limb with no arterial disease is 40 mmHg at the ankle and 18 mmHg at the calf,[60] and (2) Laplace's law, which has been modified to determine the sub-bandage pressure by using the following equation:

$$\text{Pressure} = \frac{T \times N \times 4630}{C \times W}$$

Pressure = the sub-bandage pressure, also termed the *compression force*

T = the tension of the material, determined by the material and how much it is stretched

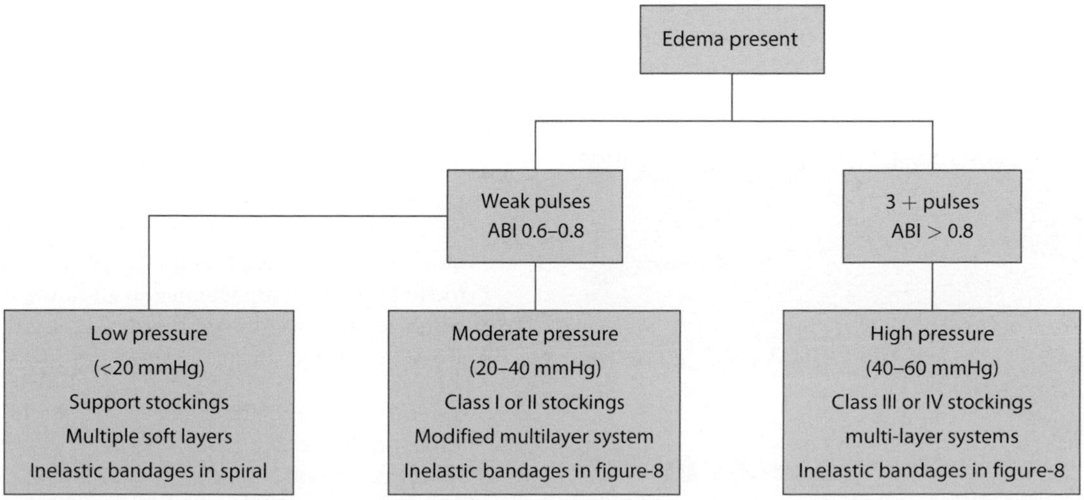

FIGURE 4-66 Algorithm for selection of appropriate compression therapy. Selection of the appropriate compression therapy is based on vascular examination and patient comfort and tolerance. Every garment, compression system, elastic or inelastic wrap has a tension that determines the amount of pressure when properly applied. Manufacturer's guidelines should be followed carefully to avoid complications that can occur with inappropriate compression therapy. Compression of any type is generally contraindicated if the ABI is less than 0.5; however, if the patient can tolerate multiple layers of soft gauze wrapping, it may be beneficial in activating the lymphatics as well as anchoring the appropriate primary dressing.

N = the number of layers of material used

4630 = a constant calculated using the original Laplace's law

C = circumference of the extremity being compressed

W = width of the bandage

Using the principles in the equation, the sub-bandage pressure can be altered to meet the needs of an individual by changing any of the components of the equations. Some of the more common applications of these principles in the clinical setting include the following:

- Tension is varied by the kind of material used and how much it is stretched. Stiffer materials provide more pressure, and elastic materials provide more compression as they are stretched. Appropriate pressure with elastic materials is usually calculated on a 50% stretch (eg, the elastic component of a multilayer compression system). Consistent tension, regardless of the material used, is needed for consistency and to avoid high/low-pressure areas along the extremity.
- The number of layers provided by a wrap depends upon the technique used (eg, a spiral wrap with a 50% overlap will result in two layers; a spiral wrap with 66% overlap, three layers; and figure-8 wrap, four layers). If all other factors are equal, a figure-8 wrap will produce two times the compression force of a spiral wrap (**FIGURES 4-67** and **4-68**). A multilayer wrap is recommended when wrapping for edema management.
- If the extremity has no contour, the compression will be the same throughout the entire length, if the other factors are equivalent. To obtain a pressure gradient between the ankle and calf, there must be a circumference differential. If the limb is shaped like a pencil (ie, with no difference in size between the ankle and the calf), extra padding can be placed around the calf to create a cone shape that results in the ankle/calf differential. Also, if the limb is shaped like a champagne bottle, padding can be placed around the ankle to even out the shape and reduce the gradient to 40/18 mmHg (**FIGURES 4-69** and **4-70**).
- Wide bandages provide less compression than narrow ones; thus using narrow bandages distally can help create greater pressure around the ankle, and using wider bandages around the calf can help reduce the proximal pressure. This principle is used especially when wrapping toe to thigh for lymphedema. In addition, narrow bandages are easier to apply around the ankle without creating wrinkles that can cause high-pressure spots.

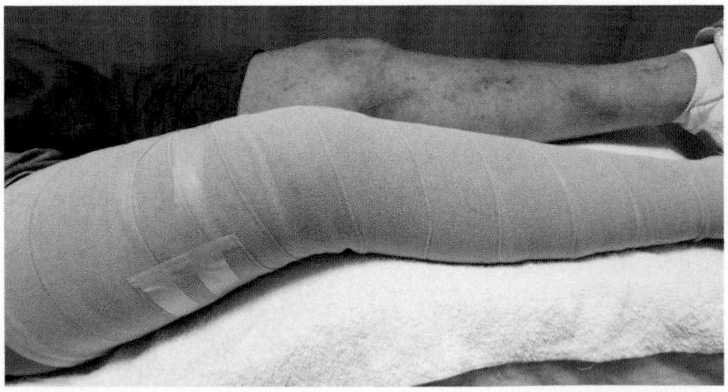

FIGURE 4-67 Spiral wrap of the lower extremity. A spiral wrap is performed with the bandage kept at a 30–45-degree angle and can have a 50% overlap (providing two layers of compression) or 66% overlap (providing three layers of compression). Consistency of overlap and tension is essential for optimal therapy and requires practice, practice, and more practice for any clinician.

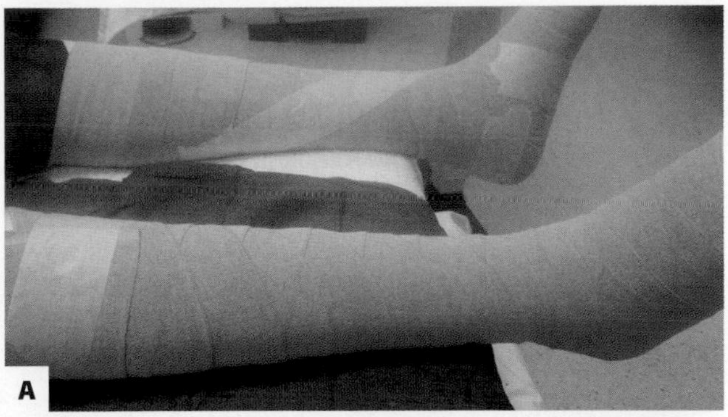

A

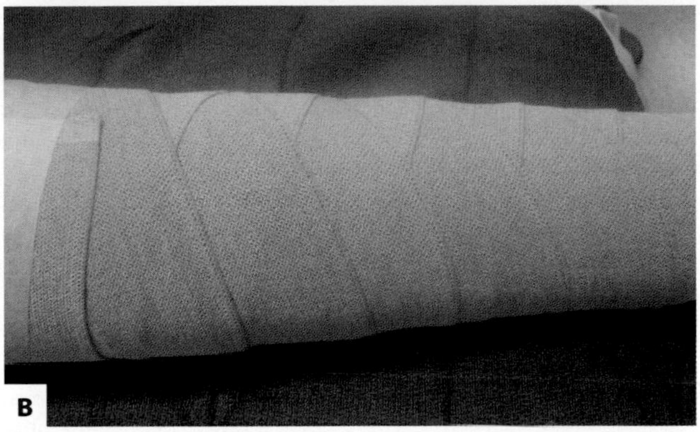

B

FIGURE 4-68 Figure-8 wrap. A. Compression of the lower extremity must include the foot and ankle. Two or three wraps around the foot and figure-8 around the ankle are the best techniques to anchor the bandages and prevent wrinkles that can abrade and blister the skin. Tape over the "seams" of the wrap prevent loosening and slippage of the bandages. **B.** Figure-8 wrap provides four layers of compression and is performed with consistent 50% overlap and a 45-degree angle of the bandages. A consistent chevron appearance on the anterior leg provides feedback to the clinician about the quality of the wrap.

Several compression garments or systems are available, including graded elastic compressive stockings, zinc oxide paste and gauze boots, multilayered compression systems, layered bandaging using either inelastic or elastic bandages, and garments with adjustable elastic or nonelastic Velcro straps (**FIGURES 4-71** to **4-76**). Compression stockings are classified according to the amount of pressure provided at the ankle and are prescribed according to symptoms and history of ulceration (**TABLE 4-12**).

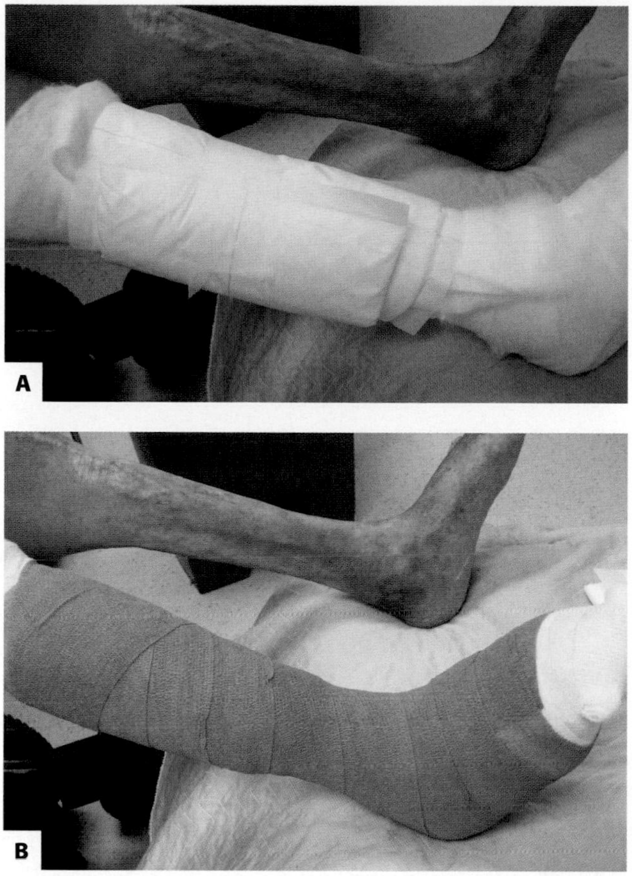

FIGURE 4-69 Adding padding to a straight leg. The ideal shape of the lower extremity to achieve the pressure differential for fluid return is a cone. **A.** If the leg is straight, or a "pencil leg," padding around the calf helps to increase the calf circumference and thereby create an ankle/calf pressure gradient. **B.** The completed compression wrap illustrates the desired shape.

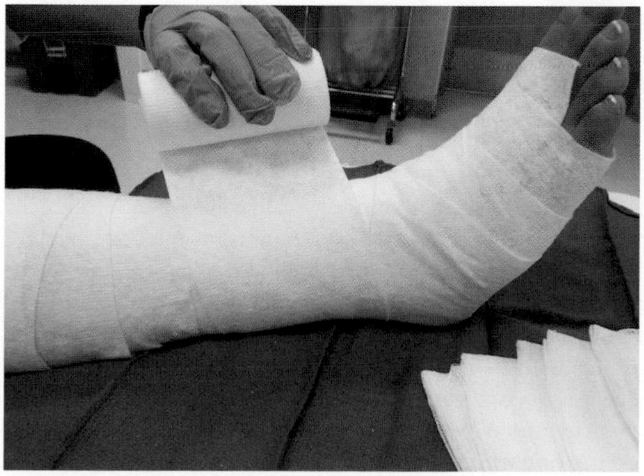

FIGURE 4-70 Adding padding to a "champagne-bottle" ankle. Similarly, if the ankle is atrophied and the calf enlarged, like the champagne bottle, padding around the ankle will decrease the pressure gradient so that it is closer to the ideal 40/18 mmHg. This can be accomplished by adding gauze padding, cast padding, or any soft conformable material around the ankle to create the ideal conical shape before applying the compression layer(s).

A review of the evidence and the above-mentioned guidelines provide direction on which compression is the most efficacious in promoting wound healing. For example, elastic compression is more effective than inelastic.[42] This may be explained by findings by Partsch, who measured sub-bandage pressure of zinc paste bandages immediately and 24 hours after application. They found that the pressure of zinc paste bandages *during dorsiflexion* dropped from 130–140 mmHg to 40–50 mmHg, suggesting that the effectiveness of a rigid system decreases because the leg reduces in size but the bandage does not.[61] Multilayer systems, on the other hand, "give" as the limb reduces in size and sub-bandage pressure remains high. Another difference is that inelastic bandages are more effective if the gastrocsoleus muscle is functioning—the

CLINICAL CONSIDERATION

While Laplace's law supplies the science of compression, the art is in the hands of the clinician who is applying the bandages. Absolute and consistent tension on the bandages, meticulous placement for appropriate overlap, and avoidance of wrinkles are necessary for patient comfort and optimal outcomes.

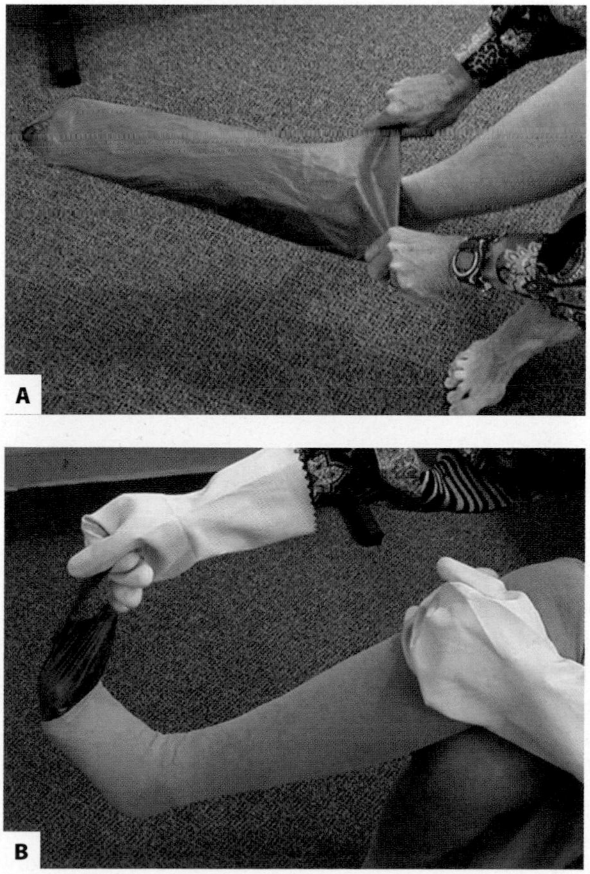

FIGURE 4-71 Graded compression garments. A. Slippery toe sock. **B.** Graded compression garments for the lower extremities are available in knee high thigh high, and panty style There are also several types of donning aides, including the slippery toe sock seen in **A** and **B**, as well as a wire cage that is useful for patients who have difficulty reaching the foot.

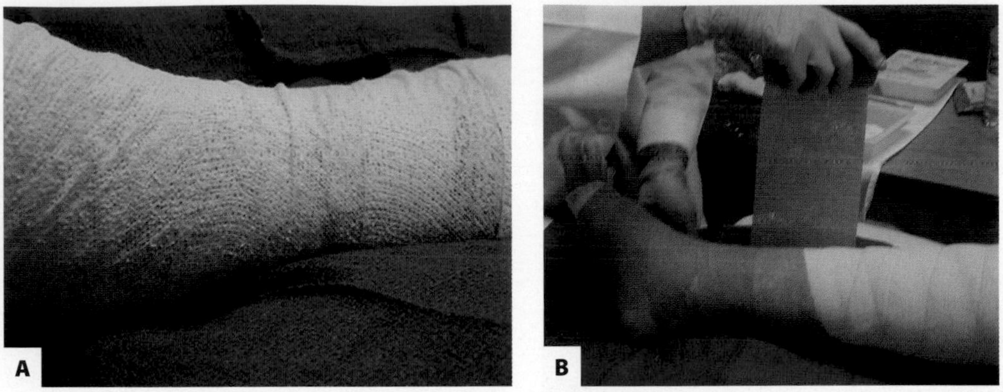

FIGURE 4-72 Zinc oxide paste and gauze boots. For many years, the zinc oxide paste and gauze boots (commonly called the Unna boot) were the mainstay of compression for venous insufficiency. The gauze is impregnated with a zinc oxide paste that hardens after application, much like a cast, and forms a rigid compression bandage. **A.** The boot has been adapted in several ways, including using a hydrocolloid primary dressing over the wound and a self-adhering bandage on the outside (termed the *Duke boot*). **B.** The disadvantage of the zinc paste boots is the inability to contract as the extremity becomes smaller, thus providing less pressure and allowing the leg to telescope inside the bandage.

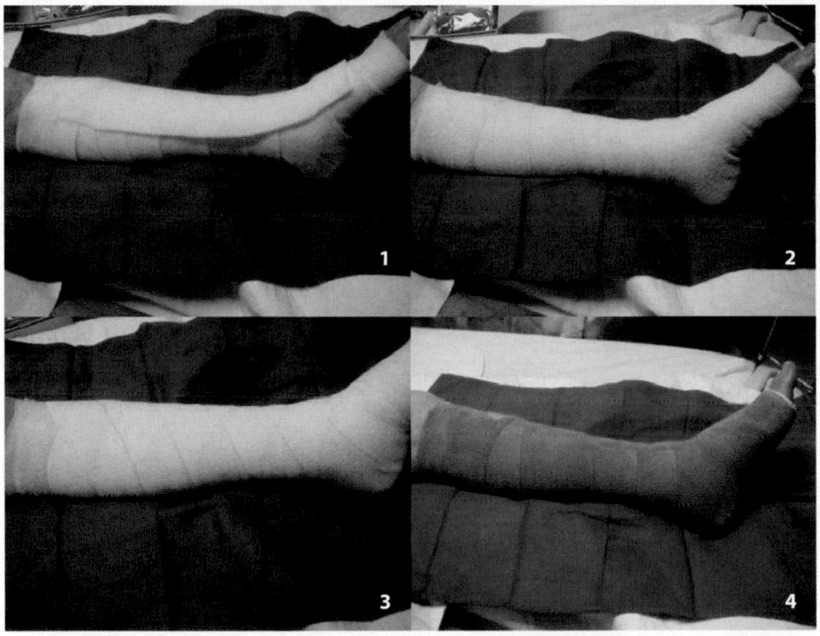

FIGURE 4-73 Multilayer compression systems. Multilayer compression systems vary from two to four layers and include a combination of soft padding, inelastic bandages, elastic bandages, and self-adhering bandages. Additional layers of the soft padding can be placed over bony prominences (eg, the shin or ankles) to prevent pressure areas or around the calf or ankle to help shape the extremity. A four-layer system is pictured here showing (1) Soft padding layer wrapped in spiral. (2) Inelastic layer that is wrapped in a spiral and provides the first layer of pressure. (3) Elastic layer that is wrapped in a figure-8 and provides the majority of the pressure. (4) A self-adhering bandage that anchors the system and prevents slippage. Depending on the system, layers can be omitted or application technique can be adjusted for modified compression if the ABI is between 0.6 and 0.8. The compression systems are changed every 3–7 days, depending on the amount of drainage from the wound and patient tolerance.

muscle pushes against the rigid bandage with contraction and thereby produces pressure on the veins.[62] Elastic bandages provide compression both at rest and during ambulation, regardless of the muscle action, and are thus more effective for patients with a hypomobile or fused ankle or with paralysis. *Elastic bandages are not recommended for patients with arterial insufficiency with ABI 0.5 or less or if absolute ankle pressure is less than 60 mmHg, as the compression could compromise arterial perfusion.*[63]

An extensive Cochrane review concluded that wounds treated with compression heal faster than those treated without compression; multilayer systems facilitate faster healing than single-layer bandages; and multilayer systems with an elastic component were more effective than those without.[64]

Intermittent pneumatic compression pumps are useful in reducing edema at a first visit before applying a compression bandage, or for patients who do not tolerate other types of compression to use at home, especially after wound healing has occurred.[65] More discussion on pumps is included in Chapter 5.

The benefits of compression therapy have been well-defined, with significant improvement in pain, swelling, skin pigmentation, activity, and well-being if a high level of compliance with therapy is maintained. In fact, with a structured regimen of compression therapy, patients with venous ulcers can achieve a 67% healing rate at 12 weeks and up to an 81% healing rate within 24 weeks.[66]

Treatment of Infection Evaluating and treating a venous wound for infection or for periwound cellulitis is an integral part of caring for the patient and facilitating wound healing. Edema fluid neutralizes the fatty acids of sebum and inactivates the bactericidal properties of the skin, making venous wounds extremely susceptible to developing infection.[57]

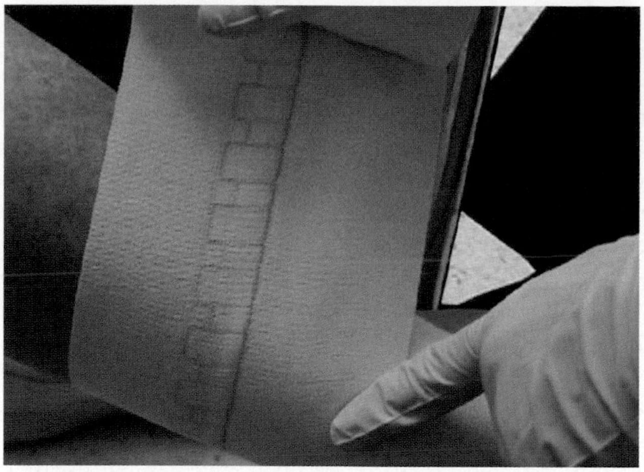

FIGURE 4-74 Single-layer elastic bandages. Single-layer elastic bandages need to be used with caution because they maintain a high resting pressure at all times. Application with consistent and even compression takes practice. Some brands have guides woven into the bandage to help the clinician monitor the amount of stretch, or tension, that is placed on the bandage. Studies have shown that single-layer bandages are not as effective in facilitating wound healing; they may, however, be helpful in reducing edema on extremities without wounds while compression garments are being obtained, provided the patient has adequate arterial flow.

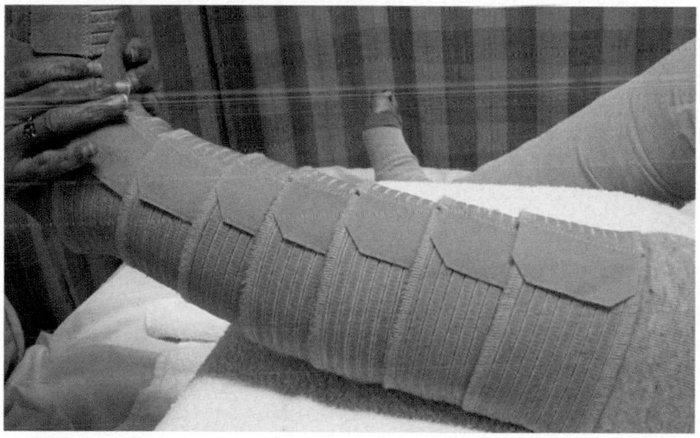

FIGURE 4-75 Compression garments. The FarrowWrap (FarrowMed, Bryan, Texas) is a compression garment consisting of a foot piece and a series of Velcro bands that extend from the ankle to the upper calf, providing low resting and high working pressures like a short-stretch bandage system. The amount of tension can vary by the amount of stretch placed on each band. The system is beneficial for patients who have difficulty donning elastic garments. (Used with permission from Rose Hamm.)

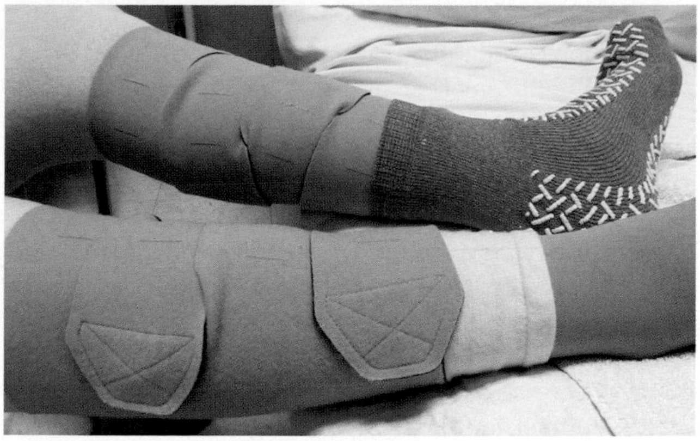

FIGURE 4-76 CircAid. CircAid (CircAid Medical Products, Whitsett, NC) consists of adjustable nonelastic Velcro bands that provide compression at recommended pressures for long-term edema management. These garments are custom fit to each patient.

TABLE 4-12 Classification of Compression Stockings

Description	Amount of Pressure at the Ankle	Indications for Use
Support	15–20 mmHg	Early signs of CVI without ulceration, prophylaxis for high-risk factors
Class I	20–30 mmHg	Signs of CVI without ulceration, post-sclerotherapy, prophylaxis for high-risk factors, post-healing with inability to don/doff or tolerate higher compression, mild lymphedema
Class II	30–40 mmHg	Post-ulceration, pronounced varicose disease, moderate lymphedema, posttraumatic edema, burn scar management
Class III	40–50 mmHg	Severe lymphedema, severe CVI, with venous wounds and no arterial disease
Class IV	60+ mmHg	Severe lymphedema, elephantiasis, severe postthrombotic disease

The following are based on guidelines for infection control in the treatment of venous ulcers:

- Debridement of necrotic tissue on a venous wound reduces the bacteria and the risk of infection. Debridement is an integral part of wound bed preparation and facilitates the healing process.
- If the wound edges do not begin to epithelialize within 2 weeks of initiation of therapy, infection should be ruled out by fluorescence imaging and if indicated, either a tissue biopsy or quantitative swab culture for both aerobic and anaerobic bacteria.
- Clinical infection has traditionally been defined as $\geq 1 \times 10^6$ colony forming units (CFUs) per gram of tissue; however, clinical signs and symptoms are essential to initial diagnosis.
- Topical antimicrobial dressings may be considered for any wound with signs of local infection; however, they should be discontinued when bacterial balance is achieved.
- Systemically administered antibiotics are recommended for venous leg ulcers with the above levels of bacteria and clinical evidence of infection. Debridement and

antibiotic therapy are most useful for eradicating infection. Antibiotic treatment should be limited to 2 weeks unless persistent infection is present.[58]

Dressings The amount of drainage and the presence of bacteria are the primary factors to consider when selecting a dressing. Initially, absorbent dressings such as alginates, hydrofibers, hydroactives, and foams are recommended to manage exudate and protect the periwound skin from maceration. Application of skin protectants under compression bandages is also helpful for periwound skin. As the wound granulates and drainage decreases, advanced dressings such as collagens may facilitate epithelial migration at the edges. Biological dressings or cellular/acellular matrix products (CAMPs) may facilitate closure once the wound bed is clean and granulated,[67] and can be helpful for hard-to-heal wounds that have not shown signs of healing after 4–6 weeks of standard therapy. An extensive Cochrane review concluded that the dressing was not a factor in wound healing, and that indeed compression is the determinant intervention.[68]

Medications Some oral agents (eg, diosmin and rutoside) used in Europe have been reported to improve the feeling of heaviness, fatigue, and even edema of CVI, but these agents are not available in the United States. Pentoxifylline, an oral medication that improves the microcirculation and thereby improves healing rates, is supported by both guidelines and a Cochrane review.[69] Its benefit may be most noticeable in patients who have combined arterial and venous insufficiency. Oral supplementation with micronized purified flavonoid fraction may also be a useful adjunct when combined with compression therapy.[41,57] In addition, if the wound is failing to show progress, a careful review of the patient's medications for drugs that may impede wound healing (eg, NSAIDs) is recommended.

Dysfunction in the calf muscle pump plays a significant role in the pathophysiology of CVI, and supervised graded exercise programs are recommended to rehabilitate the muscle pump and improve symptoms.[57] See Chapter 15 for additional details.

Adjunctive Therapy Wounds that decrease in size by 20–40% in 4 weeks are likely to heal completely by week 12.[70] Wounds that do not progress with standard treatment may benefit from adjunctive therapies, including electrical stimulation, noncontact low-frequency ultrasound, bi-layered living cellular dressings (eg, Apligraf, Organogenesis, Inc., Canton, MA), ultraviolet C, and NPWT (for extensive wounds with some depth). Therapies that have not been shown to have statistically significant effects on venous wound healing include hyperbaric oxygen, laser, phototherapy, and whirlpool.[48,57]

Invasive Therapy When CVI is refractory to medical and/or local treatment, invasive options are used to both reduce edema and facilitate wound healing. Removal of the saphenous vein with high ligation of the SPJ is the classical standard procedure for superficial saphenous insufficiency in more severe CEAP classes.[71] This procedure, plus stripping of the great saphenous vein, results in significant improvement in venous hemodynamics, provides symptomatic relief, and assists in ulcer healing.[72] Although this treatment is effective, the morbidity of the procedure has made it second choice of treatment to current endovascular therapies.

Advances in endovascular surgery have led to successful closure of incompetent veins using radiofrequency ablation (RFA), endovenous laser ablation, and medical glue. These procedures are percutaneous, do not require general anesthesia, and are performed on an outpatient basis. All three endovenous methods have been shown to be effective.[73] Both ablation therapies are recommended as the initial treatment for saphenous vein insufficiency. As medical glue is a newer therapy it is not yet recommended by major societies as a first-line therapy, but is commonly used as an initial therapy in practice.

Surgical Interventions

The decision to recommend surgical intervention is based on the degree of disease according to CEAP classification and the success or failure of nonoperative management. Listed below are the predominant surgical interventions and their indications.

Sclerotherapy Sclerotherapy is a treatment for obliterating telangiectases, reticular veins, and varicose veins. Rather than remove the diseased vessel surgically, sclerotherapy obliterates and seals the vessel in situ. Sclerosing, a procedure in which agents are injected into the venous segments by direct visualization or ultrasound guidance, can be used as primary treatment or in conjunction with surgical procedures for the correction of CVI.

Foam sclerotherapy combines traditional liquid sclerosing agents with gas to create a foam that has more surface area and expands to reach greater areas of the vessel. Data suggests that it is safe and has equivalent healing and success rates with conventional surgery.[74]

The use of medical glue for treatment of venous insufficiency is termed *cyanoacrylate embolization*, which uses the endovenous application of *n*-butyl cyanoacrylate to close the incompetent vein. The compound rapidly solidifies within the vein lumen and triggers an inflammatory reaction on the vein wall to induce closure. The advantage of this technique is that it does not require tumescent anesthesia to be administered.[73] This technique has demonstrated similar closure rates and quality-of-life improvement as with RFA over a 24-month study period and is now commonly used in place of radiofrequency and laser ablation.[75]

Endovenous Radiofrequency and Laser Ablation Thermal energy in the form of radiofrequency or laser treatment is used to obliterate veins. This technique is used for saphenous vein reflux as the recommended initial therapy. Both methods use an ultrasound-guided percutaneous access to the great or small saphenous vein. A tumescent anesthesia formula is administered along the course of the vein to be treated. These catheters generate heat, which causes thermal injury to the vein wall, leading to thrombosis and eventually fibrosis. Several studies comparing endovenous ablation with conventional ligation and stripping found that the short-term efficacy and safety of ablation and surgery are comparable, although the surgical group had increased postoperative pain and bruising.[76]

Endovascular Therapy Historically, iliac vein stenosis and obstruction causing CVI were treated with surgical procedures such as cross-femoral venous bypass or iliac vein reconstructions with prosthetic material. Endovenous stenting has replaced the traditional bypass. Iliac vein stenting results in clinical improvement with high levels of complete pain relief, complete resolution of edema, and venous ulcer healing.[55]

Open surgical procedures are reserved for patients who do not respond to less invasive treatment (usually with anatomic abnormalities) and form the basis for the endovascular therapies that are becoming widely used as a first-line intervention.

Ligation and Stripping and Venous Phlebectomy Removal of the saphenous vein with high ligation of the SPJ was one of the first treatments developed, going back to the mid-1800s or earlier.[77] This procedure was the surgical standard for superficial saphenous insufficiency in CEAP clinical classes 2 to 6. Varicose clusters that communicate with the saphenous vein are often avulsed during the same procedure by phlebectomy.

In a study evaluating patients with venous ulcers and reflux of the superficial and deep venous systems, randomization to surgery (only on the superficial venous segments) plus compression therapy led to a reduction in ulcer recurrence at 12 months when compared with compression alone (12% vs. 28%). This supported an additional benefit of correcting the incompetent superficial venous system for prevention of ulcer recurrence.[78]

Valve Reconstruction Venous valve reconstruction of the deep vein valves has a success rate of >70% at 5 years of follow-up. Internal valvuloplasty demonstrated better results than external valvuloplasty when considering ulcer recurrence and competence of repaired valves.[79] A percutaneous valve has also been studied with moderate success, and the creation of a neovalve from the intima and media of the thickened venous wall to fashion a new monocuspid or bicuspid valve has also been undertaken with moderate success in select patients.[80]

In summary, current research suggests that endovenous therapy, RFA, and laser ablation are the gold standards. Cyanoacrylate embolization is gaining popularity and has shown to be as effective as thermal ablation. There is a select role for stripping and ligation but many of the historically used surgical techniques have been discontinued in favor of less invasive, less morbid endovascular techniques that offer equivalent benefit.

Post-Closure Care

Full re-epithelialization does not mean the wound is fully healed, only that it has entered the remodeling phase, and during this phase the skin is fragile and the wound is

CASE STUDY

CONCLUSION

The patient responded to standard care of compression, nonadherent dressings, and noncontact low-frequency ultrasound. The small wound on the left leg healed and the patient transitioned to a compression garment on that side. No vascular procedures were indicated due to her initial progress, including a decrease in pain levels to 5–6/10 with treatment.

Ankle exercises were included to increase range of motion and facilitate heel/toe gait sequence with good outcomes; the patient was able to ambulate without gait impairments; however, her work did require prolonged standing.

After 3 months of therapy, the wounds stalled (FIGURE 4-77). There were no signs of infection but because of the chronicity of the wounds, cultures were obtained and were negative. NPWT was added to the standard care of

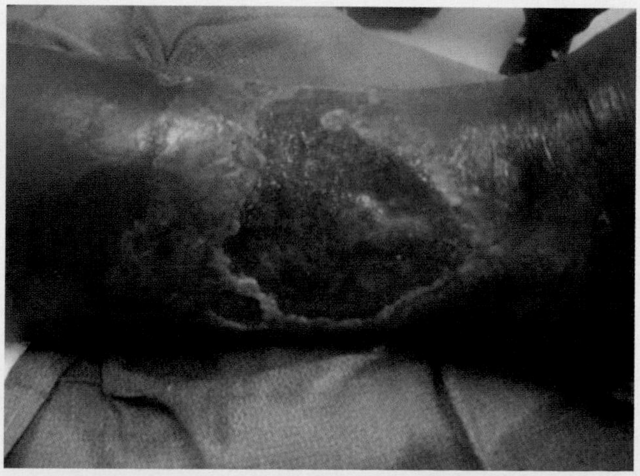

FIGURE 4-77 Right lateral lower extremity before use of negative pressure.

CASE STUDY *(Continued)*

selective debridement, absorbent dressings, and multilayer compression. The patient took a 3-week leave of absence from work with little improvement in both tissue quality and wound size. The patient had poor tolerance for negative pressure and requested that it be discontinued after a 3-week trial. The wounds did respond with increased granulation, flatter edges, and less epibole (**FIGURES 4-78** and **4-79**).

Collagen matrix dressings were added to the plan of care with slight increase in epithelial migration at the edges. At this point, the clinician reviewed again with the patient all of her recent laboratory values and medications. The patient admitted to taking 800 mg of Motrin a day, which she had been advised to take for pain. After consulting with her physician, medications were adjusted to a different pain medication given transdermally, and the patient discontinued Motrin with no need for alternative pain meds. She was also started on pentoxifylline. Within 1 week new epidermis was visible at the edges, and the patient made significant and rapid improvement with full closure within 3 months.

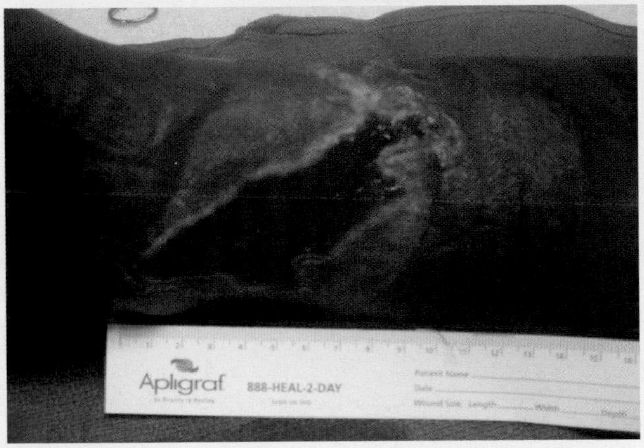

FIGURE 4-78 Right medial lower extremity after use of negative pressure.

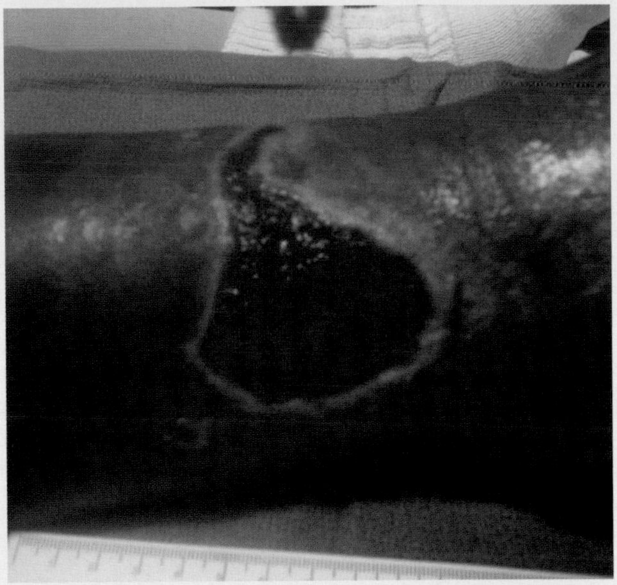

FIGURE 4-79 Right lateral lower extremity after use of negative pressure.

vulnerable to recurrence. Post-closure care to prevent recurrence includes consistent wearing of compression garments, continued exercise, and meticulous skin care. If a patient has a history of ulceration, at least Class II garments are recommended unless the patient is unable to don them or has confirmed PAD that has not been treated by a vascular specialist. There are several donning aids available for patients with other impairments (eg, arthritic hands or total hip replacement), and the patient needs to demonstrate competency in donning and doffing the garments before being discharged from therapy. For patients who require extensive compression therapy to achieve wound closure, transitioning to the garments may involve alternating use of the garments with weekly application of compression systems. This allows the skin to remodel and progress toward final healing, so there is less risk for abrasion or skin tearing with the use of garments, and it provides the clinician with the opportunity to monitor the patient adherence and response to the garments. Compression garments consisting of either elastic or nonelastic Velcro straps are available for patients who have difficulty donning stockings. A recommended wearing schedule is to don the garments in the morning immediately upon awakening and before the limb swells, and to remove them at night before showering and providing skin care. The importance of adherence to post-healing protocols cannot be overemphasized to patients who have closed venous wounds.

SUMMARY

Venous wounds result from CVI and are a common and difficult condition to manage. Venous insufficiency can be primary, secondary, or congenital. Mechanisms for the failure of the venous system are valve incompetence, obstruction or postthrombotic syndrome, inherent vessel wall factors, and impaired calf-pump mechanism. Venous disease causes integumentary changes visible on physical examination; it is usually diagnosed with noninvasive means and classified according to universal consensus guidelines. Compression therapy is the main component of treatment, with topical/local wound care, exercise, and adjunctive therapies used to facilitate healing. Endovascular and/or surgical treatment may be required in the most severe cases.

STUDY QUESTIONS

1. The most common cause of peripheral artery disease is
   a. Trauma.
   b. Hypertension.
   c. Arteriosclerosis.
   d. Smoking.
2. Where are arterial wounds usually located?
   a. On bony prominences of the lower extremity
   b. On the plantar foot
   c. On the malleoli
   d. On the distal digits
3. A 79-year-old male with a nonhealing wound on the lateral heel is referred for wound care. Which of the following characteristics is a criterion for urgent debridement?
   a. 2+ dorsalis pedis and 1+ posterior tibialis pulses
   b. Blanching of the periwound skin
   c. Ankle-brachial index of 0.6
   d. Detached edges with seropurulent drainage and mild odor
4. During an assessment of a patient with a nonhealing wound on the great toe, it is noted that the capillary refill is 6 seconds. Which of the following tests would be most appropriate to determine if the patient has adequate perfusion for healing?
   a. Ankle-brachial index
   b. Transcutaneous oxygen tension
   c. Exercise stress test
   d. Duplex with color flow imaging
5. Which clinical sign is associated with a $TcPO_2$ less than 20 mmHg?
   a. Rest pain
   b. Mild rubor of dependency
   c. Delayed but adequate wound healing
   d. Impaired sensation
6. Which of the following does *not* modify risk or contribute to venous ulcers?
   a. Family history
   b. Hormonal changes during pregnancy
   c. Diabetes
   d. Prior DVT
7. Symptoms of venous insufficiency include
   a. Ulcers of the distal toes.
   b. Pain relieved by standing.
   c. Diminished pulses.
   d. Feelings of aching heaviness in the lower extremity.
8. The thickened, brawny edema and skin discoloration caused by backup and leakage of fibrin and hemosiderin is called
   a. Telangiectasia.
   b. Lipodermatosclerosis.
   c. May–Thurner syndrome.
   d. Dermatomyofibrosis.
9. The diagnostic method of choice for venous insufficiency is
   a. The Brodie–Trendelenburg test.
   b. MRI.
   c. Venography.
   d. Doppler ultrasound.
10. Most venous ulcers will respond fully to compression therapy.
    a. True
    b. False

Answers: 1-c; 2-d; 3-d; 4-b; 5-a; 6-c; 7-d; 8-b; 9-d; 10-a

REFERENCES

1. Humphries MD, Brunson A, Li CS, et al. Amputation trends for patients with lower extremity ulcers due to diabetes and peripheral artery disease using statewide data. *J Vasc Surg*. 2016;64(6):1747-1755.
2. Fowkes FG, Rudan D, Rudan I, et al. Comparison of global estimates of prevalence and risk factors for peripheral artery disease in 2000 and 2010: a systematic review and analysis. *Lancet*. 2013;382:1329-1340.
3. Conte MS, Bradbury AW, Kolh P, et al. Global vascular guidelines on the management of chronic limb-threatening ischemia. *Eur J Vasc Endovasc Surg*. 2019;58(1S):S1-S109.
4. Eid MA, Mehta KS, Goodney PP. Epidemiology of peripheral artery disease. *Semin Vasc Surg*. 2021;34(1):38-46.
5. Shu J, Santulli G. Update on peripheral artery disease: epidemiology and evidence-based facts. *Atherosclerosis*. 2018;275:379-381.
6. Nehler MR, Duval S, Diao L, et al. Epidemiology of peripheral arterial disease and critical limb ischemia in an insured national population. *J Vasc Surg*. 2014;60(3):686-695.
7. Norgren L, Hiatt WR, Dormandy JA, et al. Inter-Society Consensus for the Management of Peripheral Arterial Disease (TASC II). *J Vasc Surg*. 2007;45(Suppl S):S5-S67
8. Monteiro-Soares M, Russell D, Boyko EJ, et al.; International Working Group on the Diabetic Foot (IWGDF). Guidelines on the classification of diabetic foot ulcers (IWGDF 2019). *Diab Metab Res Rev*. 2020;36(Suppl 1):e3273.
9. Boulton AJ, Vileikyte L, Ragnarson-Tennvall G, Apelqvist J. The global burden of diabetic foot disease. *Lancet*. 2005;366(9498):1719-1724.
10. Nussbaum SR, Carter MJ, Fife CE, et al. An economic evaluation of the impact, cost, and Medicare policy implications of chronic nonhealing wounds. *Value Health*. 2018;21(1): 27-32.
11. Marston WA, Davies SW, Armstrong D, et al. Natural history of limbs with arterial insufficiency and chronic ulceration treated without revascularization. *J Vasc Surg*. 2006;44(1):108-114.
12. Brashers VL. Alterations of cardiovascular function. In: Huether SE, McCone KL, eds. *Understanding Pathophysiology*. 4th ed. St. Louis, MO: Mosby; 2008:606-675.
13. Mills JL, Conte MS, Armstrong DG, et al. The society for vascular surgery lower extremity threatened limb classification system: risk stratification based on wound, ischemia, and foot infection (WIFI). *J Vasc Surg*. 2014;59:220-234.
14. Khan T, Plotkin A, Magee GA, et al. Functional ambulatory status as a potential adjunctive decision-making tool following wound, level of ischemia, and severity of foot infections assessment. *J Vasc Surg*. 2020;72(2):738-746.
15. Hill DR, Smith RB. Examination of the extremities: pulses, bruits, and phlebitis. In: Walker HK, Hall WD, Hurst JW, eds. *Clinical Methods: The History, Physical, and Laboratory Examinations*. 3rd ed. Boston, MA: Butterworths; 1990.
16. Alavi A, Sibbald RG, Nabavizadeh R, Valaei F, Coutts P, Mayer D. Audible handheld Doppler ultrasound determines reliable and inexpensive exclusion of significant peripheral arterial disease. *Vascular*. 2015;23(6):622-629.

17. Lampe KE. The general evaluation. In: Kloth LC, McCullough JM, eds. *Wound Healing: Alternatives in Management.* 4th ed. Philadelphia, PA: FA Davis; 2010:65-93.
18. AbuRahma AF, Adams E, AbuRahma J, et al. Critical analysis and limitations of resting ankle-brachial index in the diagnosis of symptomatic peripheral arterial disease patients and the role of diabetes mellitus and chronic kidney disease. *J Vasc Surg.* 2020;71(3):937-945.
19. Crowell A, Meyr AJ. Accuracy of the ankle-brachial index in the assessment of arterial perfusion of heel pressure injuries. *Wounds.* 2017;29(2):51-55.
20. Carter SA. The relationship of distal systolic pressures to healing of skin lesions in limbs with arterial occlusive disease, with special reference to diabetes mellitus. *Scand J Clin Lab Invest Suppl.* 1973;128:239-243.
21. Siegal A. Noninvasive vascular testing. In: Sussman C, Bates-Jensen BM, eds. *Wound Care: A Collaborative Practice Manual for Physical Therapists and Nurses.* Gaithersburg, MD: Aspen; 1998:125-135.
22. Suzuki K. How to diagnose peripheral arterial disease. *Podiatry Today.* 2007;20(4):54-65.
23. Kupinski AM. Segmental pressure measurement and plethysmography. *J Vasc Technol.* 2002;26(1):32-38.
24. Teso D, Sommerset J, Dally M, Feliciano B, Vea Y, Jones RK. Pedal Acceleration Time (PAT): a novel predictor of limb salvage. *Ann Vasc Surg.* 2021;75:189-193.
25. Rose S. Noninvasive vascular laboratory for evaluation of peripheral arterial occlusive disease: part II: clinical applications: chronic, usually atherosclerotic, lower extremity ischemia. *J Vasc Interv Radiol.* 2000;11(10):1257-1275.
26. Jewell DV, Shishehbor MH, Walsworth MK. Centers for Medicare and Medicaid Services policy regarding supervised exercise for patients with intermittent claudication: the good, the bad, and the ugly. *J Orthop Sports Phys Ther.* 2017;47(12):892-894.
27. Jansen SCP, Abaraogu UO, Lauret GJ, Fakhry F, Fokkenrood HJP, Teijink JAW. Modes of exercise training for intermittent claudication. *Cochrane Database Syst Rev.* 2020;8(8):CD009638.
28. Society for Vascular Surgery Lower Extremity Guidelines Writing Group; Conte MS, Pomposelli FB, Clair DG, et al. Society for Vascular Surgery practice guidelines for atherosclerotic occlusive disease of the lower extremities: management of asymptomatic disease and claudication. *J Vasc Surg.* 2015;61(3 suppl):2S-41S.
29. Woo K, Siracuse JJ, Klingbeil K, et al. Society for Vascular Surgery appropriate use criteria for management of intermittent claudication. *J Vasc Surg.* 2022;76(1):3-22.e1.
30. Harris SK, Roos MG, Landry GJ. Statin use in patients with peripheral arterial disease. *J Vasc Surg.* 2016;64(6):1881-1888.
31. Ennis WJ, Borhani M, Meneses P. Management and diagnosis of vascular ulcers. In: Sussman C, Bates-Jenson BM, eds. *Wound Care: A Collaborative Practice Manual for Health Care Professionals.* Baltimore, MD: Aspen; 2012:309-324.
32. TASC Steering Committee, Jaff MR, White CJ, Hiatt WR, et al. An update on methods for revasculatization and expansion of the TASC lesion classification to include below-the-knee arteries: a supplement to the inter-society consensus for the management of peripheral arterial disease (TASC II). *Vasc Med.* 2015;20(5): 465-478.
33. Wijnand JGJ, Zarowsky D, Wu B, et al. The Global Limb Anatomic Staging System (GLASS) for SLTI: improving inter-observer agreement. *J Clin Med.* 2021;10(16):3454.
34. Ambler GK, Twine CP. Graft type for femoro-popliteal bypass surgery. *Cochrane Database Syst Rev.* 2018;2(2):CD001487.
35. Farber A, Menard MT, Conte MS, et al. Surgery or endovascular therapy for chronic limb-threatening ischemia. *N Engl J Med.* 2022;387(25):2305-2316.
36. Johnson J, Yates S, Burgess J. Venous insufficiency, venous ulcers, and lymphedema. In: Doughty D, McNichol L, eds. *Wound, Ostomy and Continence Nurse's Society Core Curriculum: Wound Management.* Philadelphia, PA: Wolters Kluwer; 2016.
37. Etufugh CN, Phillips TJ. Venous ulcers. *Clin Dermatol.* 2007;25(1):121-130.
38. Perrot-Applanat M, Cohen-Solal K, Milgrom E, Finet M. Progesterone receptor expression in human saphenous veins. *Circulation.* 1995;92(10):2975-2983.
39. Kolluri R, Lugli M, Villalba L, et al. An estimate of the economic burden of venous leg ulcers associated with deep venous disease. *Vasc Med.* 2022;27(1):63-72.
40. Pieper B, Kirsner R, Templin TN. Novel mechanisms on the pathophysiology of venous ulcers. In: Sen CH, ed. *Advances in Wound Care.* New Rochelle, NY: Mary Ann Liebert; 2010:190-196.
41. Ortega MA, Fraile-Martinez O, Garcia-Montero C, et al. Understanding chronic venous disease: a critical overview of its pathophysiology and medical management. *J Clin Med.* 2021;10(15):3239.
42. Eberhardt RT, Raffetto JD. Chronic venous insufficiency. *Circulation.* 2005;111:2398-2409.
43. Browse N, Burnand K. The cause of venous ulceration. *Lancet.* 1982;2:243-245.
44. McCulloch JM. Venous insufficiency and ulceration. In: McCulloch JM, Kloth LC, eds. Wound Healing: Evidence-Based Management. 4th ed. Philadelphia, PA: FA Davis; 2010:248-255.
45. Falanga V, Eaglstein WH. The trap hypothesis of venous ulceration. *Lancet.* 1993;341:1006-1008.
46. Hettrick H, Aviles F. All edema is lymphedema: progressing lymphedema and wound management to an integrated model of care. *Wound Manag Prev.* 2022;68(1):8-15.
47. Rasmussen JC, Zhu B, Morrow JR, et al. Degradation of lymphatic anatomy and function in early venous insufficiency. *J Vasc Surg Venous Lymphat Disord.* 2021;9(3): 720-730.
48. *Association for the Advancement of Wound Care (AAWC) Venous Ulcer Guidelines.* Malvern, PA: Association for the Advancement of Wound Care (AAWC). December 2015. Available at: appendix c guideline icvug-textformatrecommendations-final v42 changessaved18aug17. pdf (memberclicks.net). Accessed March 5, 2023.
49. Sibbald RG, Woo K, Ayello EA. Increased bacterial burden and infection: the story of NERDS and STONES. *Adv Skin and Wound Care.* 2006;19(8):447-461.
50. Porter JM, Moneta GL. Reporting standards in venous disease: an update. International Consensus Committee on Chronic Venous Disease. *J Vasc Surg.* 1995;21:635-645.
51. Classification and grading of chronic venous disease in the lower limbs. A consensus statement. Ad Hoc Committee, American Venous Forum. *J Cardiovasc Surg.* 1997;38(5):437-441.
52. Lurie F, Passman M, Meisner M, et al. The 2020 update of the CEAP classification system and reporting standards. *J Vasc Surg Venous Lymphat Disord.* 2020;8(3):342-352.
53. Barrows C, Miller R, Townsend D, et al. Best practice recommendations for the prevention and treatment of venous leg ulcers: update 2006. *Adv Skin Wound Care.* 2007;20:611-621.
54. Zierler BK. Ultrasonography and diagnosis of venous thromboembolism. *Circulation.* 2004;109(12 suppl 1):19-14.
55. Sidway AP, Perler BA, eds. *Rutherford's Vascular Surgery.* 10th ed. Philadelphia, PA: Elsevier Health Sciences; 2023.

56. Neglen P, Raju S. Intravascular ultrasound scan evaluation of the obstructed vein. *J Vasc Surg*. 2002;35(4):694-700.
57. Marston W, Tang J, Kirsner RS, Ennis W. Wound Healing 2015 update on guidelines for venous ulcers. *Wound Repair Regen*. 2016;24(1):136-144.
58. O'Donnell TFJr, Passman MA, Marston WA, et al. Management of venous leg ulcers: clinical practice guidelines of the Society for Vascular Surgery and the American Venous Forum. *J Vasc Surg*. 2014;60(2 Suppl):3S-59S.
59. Rabe E, Partch H, Morrison N, et al. Risks and contraindications of medical compression treatment—a critical reappraisal. An international consensus statement. *Phlebology*. 2020;35(7): 447-460.
60. Partsch H. Compression therapy: clinical and experimental evidence. *Ann Vasc Dis*. 2012;5(4):416-422.
61. Mosti G, Partsch H. Comparison of three portable instruments to measure compression pressure. *Int Angiol*. 2010;29:426-430.
62. Mosti G, Partsch H. Inelastic bandages maintain their hemodynamic effectiveness over time despite significant pressure loss. *J Vasc Surg*. 2010;52(4):925-931.
63. Luri F, Bittar S, Kasper G. Optimal compression therapy and wound care for venous ulcers. *Surg Clin N Am*. 2018;98:349-360.
64. Shi C, Dumville JC, Cullum N, Connaughton E, Norman G. Compression bandages or stockings versus no compression for treating venous leg ulcers. *Cochrane Database Syst Rev*. 2021;7(7):CD013397.
65. Partsch H. Intermittent pneumatic compression in immobile patients. *Int Wound J*. 2008;5(3):389-397.
66. Mościcka P, Szewczyk MT, Cwajda-Białasik J, Jawień A. The role of compression therapy in the treatment of venous leg ulcers. *Adv Clin Exp Med*. 2019;28(6):847-852.
67. Alvarez OM, Makowitz L, Patel M. Venous ulcers treated with a hyaluronic acid extracellular matrix and compression therapy: interim analysis of a randomized controlled trial. *Wounds*. 2017;29(7):E51-E54.
68. Palfreyman SJ, Nelson EA, Lochiel R, Michaels JA. Dressings for healing venous leg ulcers. *Cochrane Database Syst Rev*. 2006;3:CD001103.
69. Jull AB, Arroll B, Parag V, Watera J. Pentoxifylline for treating venous leg ulcers. *Cochrane Database Syst Rev*. 2012;12: CD001733.
70. Sibbald RG, Elliott JA, Persaud-Jaimangal R, et al. Wound bed preparation 2021. *Adv Skin Wound Care*. 2021;34(4):183-195.
71. Sarin S, Scurr JH, Coleridge Smith PD. Stripping of the long saphenous vein in the treatment of primary varicose veins. *Br J Surg*. 1992;79(9):889-893.
72. Lafrati MD, O'Donnell TF. Surgical interventions: varicose veins. In: Cronenwett JL, Johnston W, eds. *Rutherfords Vascular Surgery*. 7th ed. Philadelphia, PA: Saunders; 2010:855-871.
73. Amshar M, Nugraha RA, Butabara EAD, Siddiq T, Indriani S, Adiarto S. Cyanoacrylate Embolization versus endovenous laser ablation in treating saphenous vein insufficiency: s systematic review and meta-analysis. *Ann Vasc Surg*. 2022;80:313-324.
74. Kulkarni SR, Slim FJ, Emerson LG, et al. Effect of foam sclerotherapy on healing and long-term recurrence in chronic venous leg ulcers. *Phlebology*. 2013;28(3):140-146.
75. Gibson K, Morrison N, Kolluri R, et al. Twenty-four month results from a randomized trial of cyanoacrylate closure versus radiofrequency ablation for the treatment of incompetent great saphenous veins. *J Vasc Surg Venous Lymphat Disord*. 2018;6(5): 606-613.
76. Rasmussen LH, Bjoern L, Lawaetz M, et al. Randomized trial comparing endovenous laser ablation of the great saphenous vein with high ligation and stripping in patients with varicose veins: short-term results. *J Vasc Surg*. 2007;46:308-315.
77. van den Bremer J, Moll FL. Historical overview of varicose vein surgery. *Ann Vasc Surg*. 2010;24(3):426-432.
78. Barwell JR, Davies CE, Deacon J, et al. Comparison of surgery and compression with compression alone in chronic venous ulceration (ESCHAR study): randomized controlled trial. *Lancet*. 2004; 363:1854-1859.
79. Maleti O, Lugli M, Tripathi RK. Deep venous reconstructive surgery. *Semin Vasc Surg*. 2015;28(1):39-46.
80. Maleti O, Lugli M. Neovalve construction in post-thrombotic syndrome. *J Vasc Surg*. 2006;43:794-799.

CHAPTER FIVE

Lymphedema

Marisa Perdomo, PT, DPT, CLT-Foldi, CES and
Rose L. Hamm, PT, DPT, FACCWS

CHAPTER OBJECTIVES

At the end of this chapter, the learner will be able to:

1. **Differentiate between the components of the lymphatic and the venous system.**
2. **Relate the function of each lymph system component to the formation of lymphedema.**
3. **Diagnose lymphedema according to cause, pathophysiology, and stage.**
4. **Differentiate between lymphedema and chronic venous insufficiency.**
5. **Define the components of Starling's Law and describe their role in lymphatic flow.**
6. **Select the appropriate compression therapy for a patient with peripheral lymphedema.**
7. **Design an exercise program for a patient with lymphedema.**
8. **Discuss the principles of manual lymphatic mobilization, as well as the indications and contraindications.**
9. **Educate patients on skin care and strategies to prevent recurrent lymphedema complications.**

INTRODUCTION

Lymphedema is a chronic inflammatory condition that develops as a result of lymphatic insufficiency. Lymphatic insufficiency occurs from a decrease in reabsorption or transportation capacity of the lymphatic system. It can be primary malformation of the lymph system or an acquired condition due to obstruction or damage to the system (**TABLE 5-1**).

The lymphatic system is interrelated with all other systems of the body. Its primary functions include conducting immune system surveillance, assisting the cardiovascular system to maintain fluid homeostasis, and aiding digestive system in the breakdown of long-chain fatty acids. The immunological functions involve both the immediate response to pathogens and the long-term resistance to repeated exposure to pathogens.

ANATOMY OF THE LYMPH SYSTEM

The body's immunological function is performed by the lymphoid organs, including the spleen, thymus, tonsils, Peyer's patches located in the small intestine, bone marrow, and lymph nodes (**FIGURE 5-1**).

The lymphatic system is a body-wide network of superficial and deep vessels connected by perforating vessels, similar to the venous system. It is comprised of lymph capillaries, lymphatic precollectors, collectors, trunks, and ducts (**FIGURE 5-2**). The superficial vessels, located directly under the skin and above the fascia, drain the dermis and subcutaneous tissues. The deep vessels are located below the fascia and drain all the tissues deep into the fascia. There are connecting vessels that perforate the fascia to transport the fluid from the deep vessel system to the superficial vessel system, which is the opposite of how the venous system functions. The lymphatic vessels are similar to arteries in that the larger collecting vessels have smooth muscle in their walls, and they are similar to the veins in that the collecting vessels contain valves that allow for unidirectional flow of the fluids.

The superficial system begins with the lymphatic *capillaries* that appear much like a fishnet underneath all of the skin (**FIGURE 5-3**). The capillaries are the smallest-diameter vessels and thus have the largest numbers. As the diameter of the more proximal lymphatic vessels increases, the number of lymphatic vessels decreases. Lymph capillaries have anchoring filaments that attach to the basement membrane between the dermis and epidermis (**FIGURE 5-4**). The lymph capillaries are more permeable than the vascular capillaries and therefore can absorb larger molecules of protein and fat. Each lymph capillary is composed of a single layer of overlapping flat endothelial cells, and the overlapping junction is called the *inlet junction*. The capillary does not contain valves, thus allowing the fluid to move in any direction within the capillary system.

The capillaries merge and become *precollectors* that have a larger diameter and therefore a lower pressure, thus facilitating the movement of the fluid from the capillary to the precollector. The precollectors also have an overlapping endothelial anatomy that allows them to absorb interstitial fluid, and they have both a limited number of valves and a limited smooth muscle structure that allows them to initiate transportation of the collected fluids.

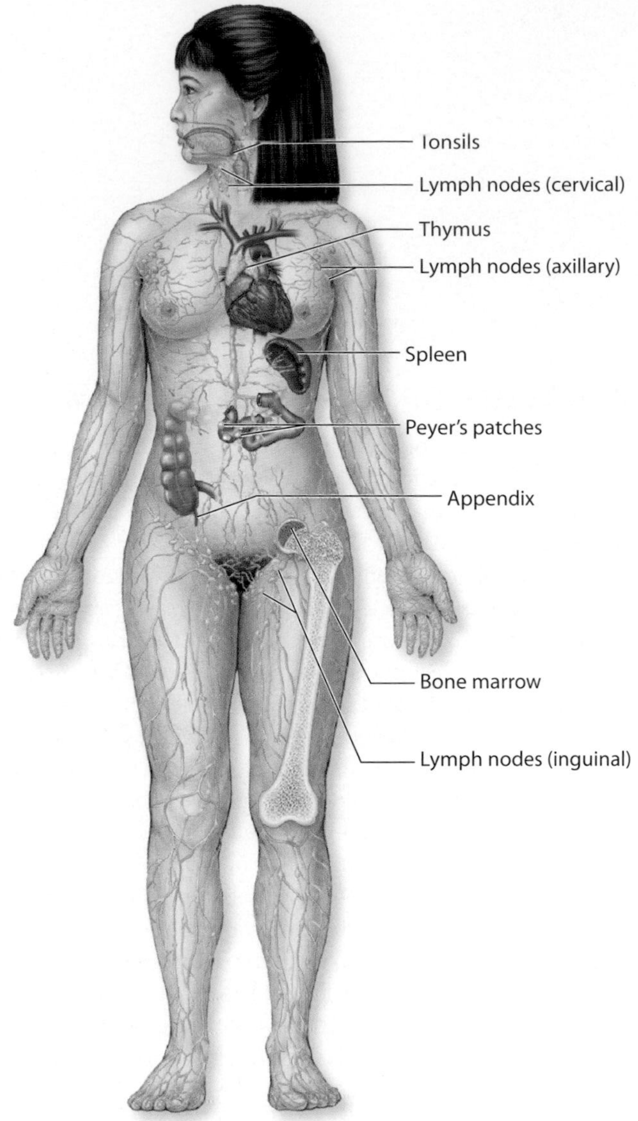

FIGURE 5-1 Anatomy of the immune system.

Spleen provides lymphocyte proliferation, immune surveillance, and immune response; removes old or damage platelets and blood cells from the blood; removes debris and foreign matter from the blood. It has other functions not related to the lymph system that are not discussed here.

Thymus secretes thymosin and thymopoietin, hormones that enable T-lymphocytes to become activated against specific pathogens; it does not directly fight the antigens.

Tonsils capture and remove pathogens in the airway during inhalation.

Peyer's patches, structurally similar to tonsils, are located in small intestines. They destroy bacteria in the intestines and generate "memory lymphocytes" for long-term immunity.

Bone marrow, also called myeloid tissue, is responsible for production of all the cells of the immune system through the process of hemopoiesis. The stem cells become common myeloid stem cells or common lymphoid stem cells that further differentiate into red blood cells, platelets, and white blood cells.

Lymph nodes are the biological filter station for antigens present in lymph fluid; responsible for purifying and draining lymph fluid.

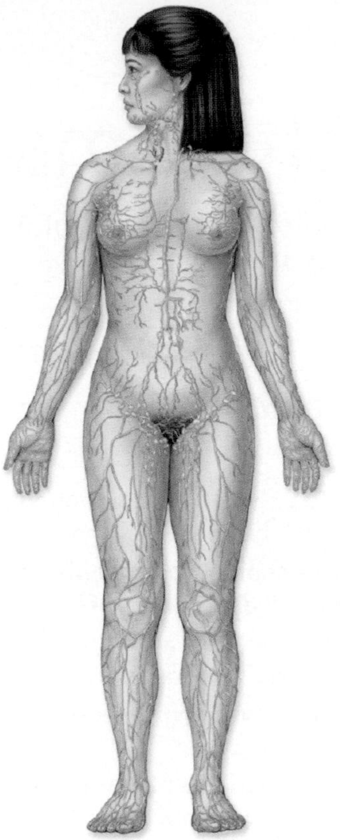

FIGURE 5-2 Full-body lymphatic system. The superficial network of lymphatic vessels has specific drainage routes to regional lymph nodes.

All of the precollectors merge to become larger diameter vessels, termed *collectors.* The collectors first bring the lymph fluid to the lymph nodes and then carry the remaining fluid to the larger *lymphatic trunks.* The anatomical structure of the collectors is similar to the construction of the veins in that they have three distinct layers (intima, media, and adventitia) and well-defined valves that permit flow to go in only one direction—toward the heart. Within the lymph collector, the vessel segment between two valves is termed the *lymphangion* (**FIGURE 5-5**). Each lymphangion has an autonomic-driven resting contraction rate of approximately 10 to 12 contractions per minute.[1] (This is further discussed in the section "Physiology of Lymphatic Flow".) The superficial lymphatic collectors are located in the subcutaneous fatty hypodermis and follow a direct route toward the regional lymph nodes. The deep lymphatic collectors follow the pathway of larger blood vessels. Lymph collectors drain lymph fluid from specific areas of the body, creating lymphatic

CLINICAL CONSIDERATION

The removal of any regional lymph nodes results in a reduced transportation rate of lymph fluid through the nodes, thus increasing the possibility of lymph fluid accumulation distally, as well as resulting in a compromised immune system response to foreign pathogens, which increases the risk of developing infection.

TABLE 5-1 Primary and Secondary Lymphedema: Causes, Onset, and Characteristics

Primary Lymphedema Causes	Onset	Secondary Lymphedema Causes	Onset
Inherited genetic mutations resulting in abnormal development of lymph vessels: ▪ Hypoplasia ▪ Hyperplasia ▪ Aplasia ▪ Kinmonth syndrome (inguinal lymph node fibrosis) Genetic mutations with autosomal dominant pattern: ▪ Chromosome 5q34-q35 ▪ FLT4 ▪ FOXC2 ▪ VEGFR3 ▪ SOX18	Variable age onset depending on the gene involved[a]	Damage to lymph nodes and/or lymph vessels that results in decreased lymphatic reabsorption and transportation (mechanical insufficiency) Trauma Radiation therapy Tumor obstruction Infection CVI	Any time after damage to lymph nodes and vessels: either soon after lymph node dissection *or* months, years, *or* decades later Dependent on patient medical history, comorbidities (number of lymph nodes removed, radiation therapy, chemotherapy, venous pathologies, and obesity), and general health
Milroy's disease (congenital lymphedema) FOXC2 VEGFR3 SOX18[a]	Onset during infancy[a]	Surgery Trauma Radiation therapy Tumor obstruction (cancer) Infection CVI	Dependent on patient medical history, comorbidities, and general health
Meige's disease (lymphedema praecox) MIM153200[a]	Onset in childhood or around puberty; may begin in early 20s or 30s		
Lymphedema tarda	Onset at 35 years or later		

[a]Primary and secondary lymphedema differ in causes and onset, which are used to make a differential diagnosis; however, the characteristics are very similar—an edematous limb, skin changes, loss of joint spaces. There are some characteristics of hereditary lymphedema, however, that distinguish it from secondary lymphedema. These include but are not limited to hypoparathyroidism, microcephaly, intestinal lymphangiectasia, ptosis, yellow nails, pleural effusions, cerebral arteriovenous anomalies, distichiasis, congenital heart defects, and webbing of the neck.

Data from Connell F, Brice G, Jeffery S, Keeley V, Mortimer P, Mansour S. A new classification system for primary lymphatic dysplasias based on phenotype. *Clin Genet.* 2010;77:438–452; Levinson KL, et al. Age of onset in hereditary lymphedema. *J Pediatr.* 2003;142:704–708; Rizzo C. Lymphedema praecox. *Derm Online J.* 2009;15(8):7.

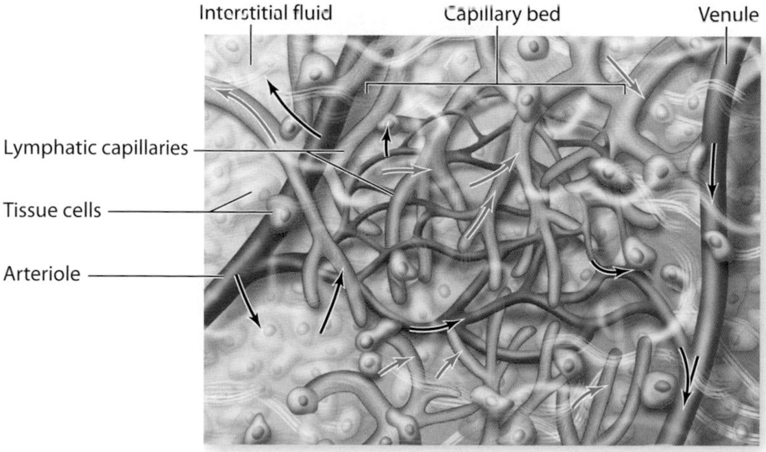

FIGURE 5-3 Lymphatic capillaries that intertwine with the arterial and venous capillary bed. Molecules and fluid flow from the arterial capillary bed into the tissue spaces (black arrows) and from the interstitial spaces into the initial lymphatic capillary, termed *reabsorption* (green arrows). Lymph fluid then flows from the initial lymph capillaries into slightly larger vessels, termed *precollectors*. Fat and protein molecules that are too large to enter the venous capillaries must be reabsorbed by the initial lymphatics or initial lymph capillaries.

"territories" that drain to specific regional lymph nodes. These lymphatic territories are defined by lymphatic watersheds that delineate the body into specific collection and drainage patterns (**FIGURE 5-6**). Although there is some cross-connection between the territories via the watersheds, most of the fluid flows directly to its own regional lymph nodes. If there is fluid overload in one area, some of the fluid can be diverted to another region via the watershed connections.

The lymph nodes (estimated to be about 700) are located in clusters throughout the body (**FIGURE 5-7**). Each lymph

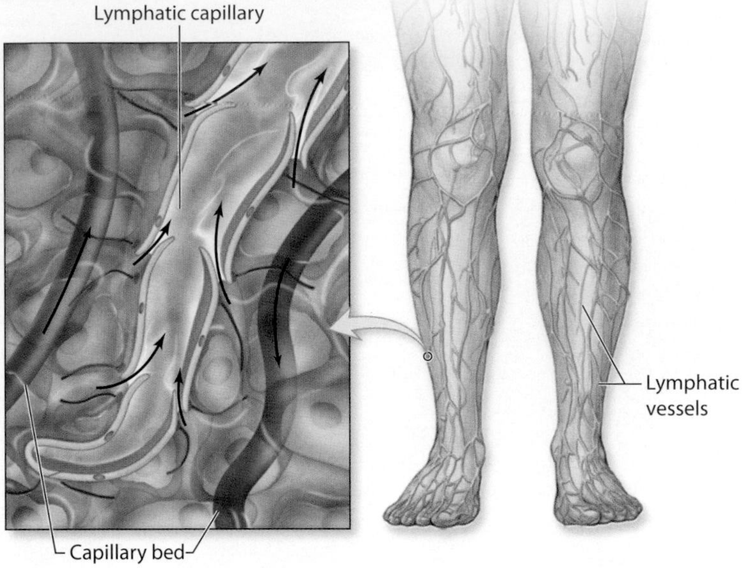

FIGURE 5-4 Anchoring filaments of the lymphatic capillaries. The initial lymphatic capillary is connected to the basement membrane by anchoring filaments. When the interstitial pressure gradient (ie, concentration of protein molecules) is high, tension is exerted on the anchoring filaments, which results in pulling the single layer of overlapping endothelial cells. This tension opens the filament and allows the fluid to enter the initial lymphatic capillary where the pressure is low.

node is bean-shaped and surrounded by a dense fibrous capsule (**FIGURE 5-8**). The collectors converge at the convex side of the lymph nodes where they are termed *afferent lymph vessels*. The fluid moves through the cortex of the node, into the medulla, and exits on the concave side via *efferent vessels* that then become trunks. The number of efferent vessels is less than the number of afferent vessels, resulting in a decreased transportation rate through the lymph nodes, and thus allowing the immune system cells time to phagocytose the pathogens that are in the lymphatic fluid.

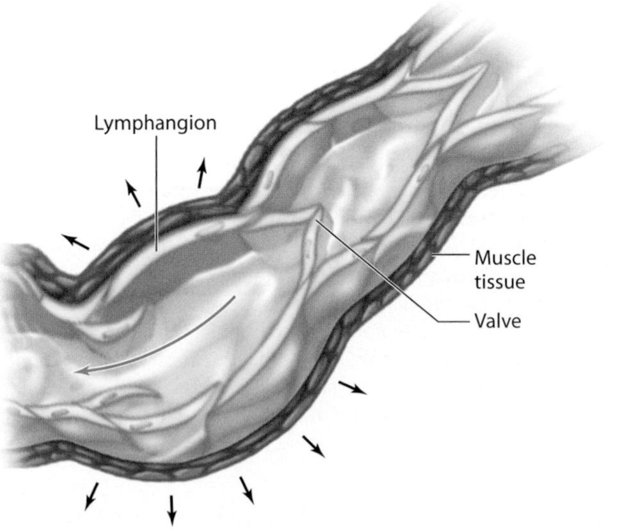

FIGURE 5-5 Lymphangion. The lymph vessels containing lymphangions are adjacent to the muscle; thus, when the muscle contracts the lymph flow is increased. Valves and smooth muscle in the angion promote directional flow of the fluid and prevent reflux, much like the valves in veins.

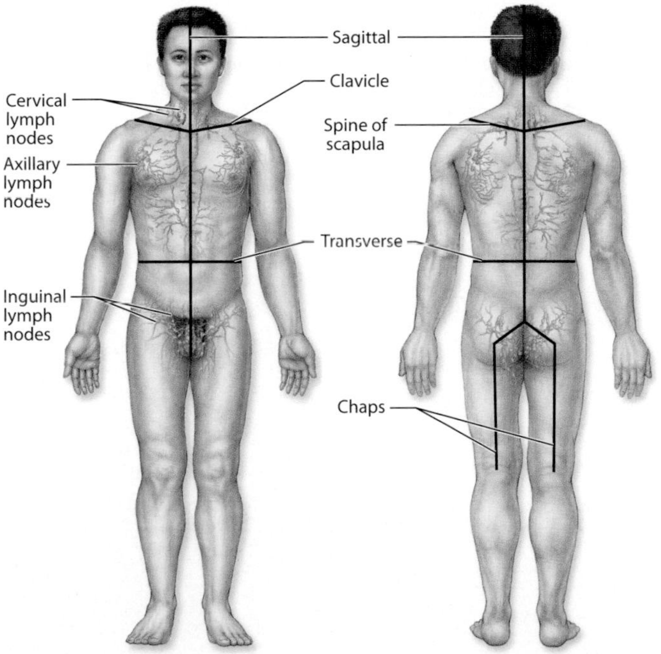

FIGURE 5-6 Lymphatic watersheds. The body is divided into lymph territories that allow drainage of the lymph flow from specific body regions to specific regional lymph nodes. The deep vessels do not cross between watersheds (areas of collection); however, there are some superficial vessels that cross the watershed boundaries and thereby divert lymph fluid from one quadrant to another when there are conditions of overload. The superficial pathways that cross between watersheds can be encouraged with manual lymphatic mobilization to direct more flow to open areas; however, it is usually inadequate to remove the majority of the fluid in the affected quadrant.

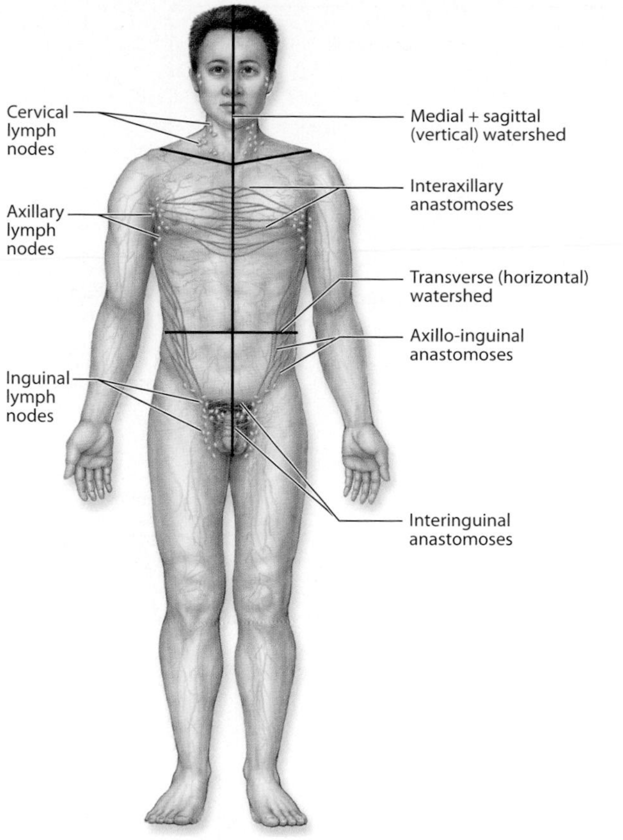

FIGURE 5-7 Clusters of lymph nodes throughout the body. Lymph nodes are located strategically throughout the body, in conjunction with the superficial anastomoses that allow fluid to cross the watershed boundaries. The lymph system naturally diverts fluid across the watershed during times of overload; however, in lymphedema, it is insufficient to manage the total volume of fluid needing to be transported. Manual lymphatic mobilization stimulates these anastomoses to increase the rate of flow.

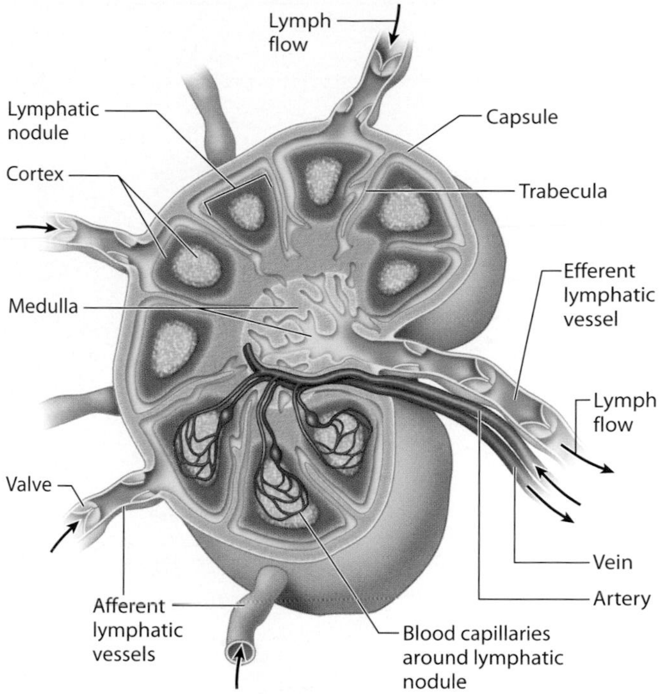

FIGURE 5-8 Lymph node anatomy. A greater number of afferent vessels bring fluid to a lymph node and a lesser number of efferent vessels leave the lymph node. This anatomical arrangement permits a slower rate of lymph transport through the lymph nodes and thus allows time for the immune system to phagocytose bacteria, waste products, and dead cells. For individuals with cancer who undergo a lymph node dissection, the rate of flow through the regional lymph node is automatically decreased. This sets the stage for potential lymphatic congestion in the affected quadrant and may lead to lymphedema.

When the superficial and deep collectors converge, the vessels are termed *trunks*. The trunks are similar in construction to the collectors except they are larger in diameter and contain more smooth muscle in the vessel wall (**FIGURE 5-9**). The trunks are named as follows: right and left lumbar trunks, gastrointestinal trunk, jugular trunk, supraclavicular trunk, subclavian trunk, parasternal trunk, and bronchomediastinal trunk. The right and left trunks and the gastrointestinal trunk converge in the anterior area of T-11-L2 to form the *cisterna chyli*, which is the beginning of the thoracic duct. The thoracic duct ascends cephalically along the anterior vertebral column and perforates the diaphragm.

CLINICAL CONSIDERATION

Lymph nodes become enlarged when they try to contain and destroy pathogens such as bacteria or cancer cells. These enlarged nodes are an indication of an underlying pathology that needs to be diagnosed and treated.

The only direct connection between the lymphatic system and the venous system occurs where the thoracic duct (on the left) and the right lymphatic duct enter the venous angles. The venous angle is formed by the convergence of the internal jugular and subclavian veins (**FIGURE 5-10**). This is the anatomical termination of what is described as the lymphatic system.

CLINICAL CONSIDERATION

Diaphragmatic breathing provides a force to promote lymphatic drainage from the thoracic duct into the venous angle. This results in a negative pressure gradient within the thoracic duct, therefore promoting distal-to-proximal lymph transport.

PHYSIOLOGY OF LYMPHATIC FLOW

The purpose of the lymphatic capillaries is to absorb interstitial fluid and molecules, and when the fluid enters the capillaries, it is termed *lymphatic fluid*. The endothelial cell junctions overlap, creating inlet valves, so that when the interstitial protein concentration increases, tension on the anchoring filaments causes the inlet valves to open and allows absorption of the larger fat and protein molecules. These inlet valves remain open as long as the interstitial pressure (a result of plasma protein concentration) remains higher than the pressure within the lymph capillary.

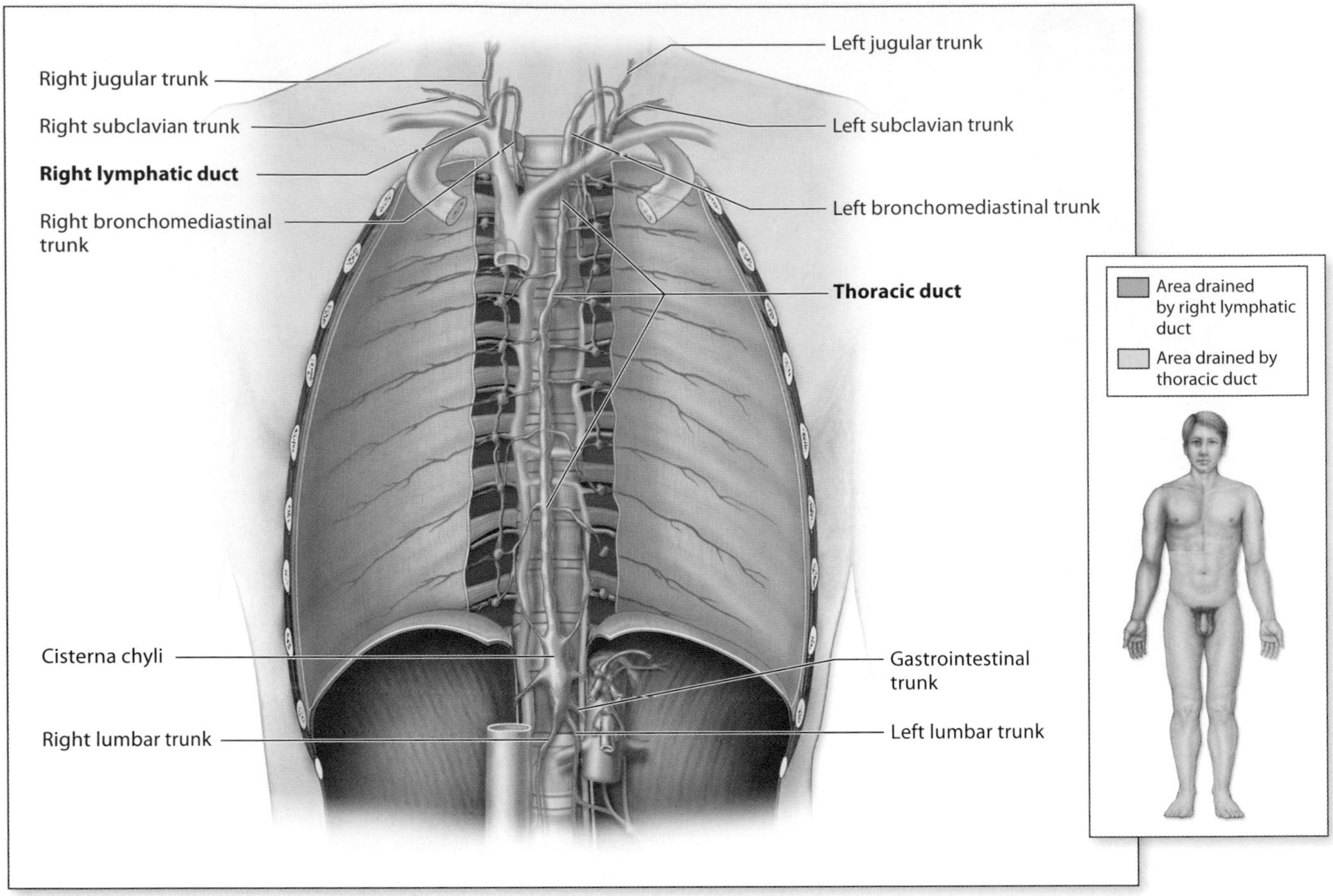

FIGURE 5-9 Lymphatic trunks and the territories that drain into the trunks. The collecting vessels merge to form lymphatic trunks.

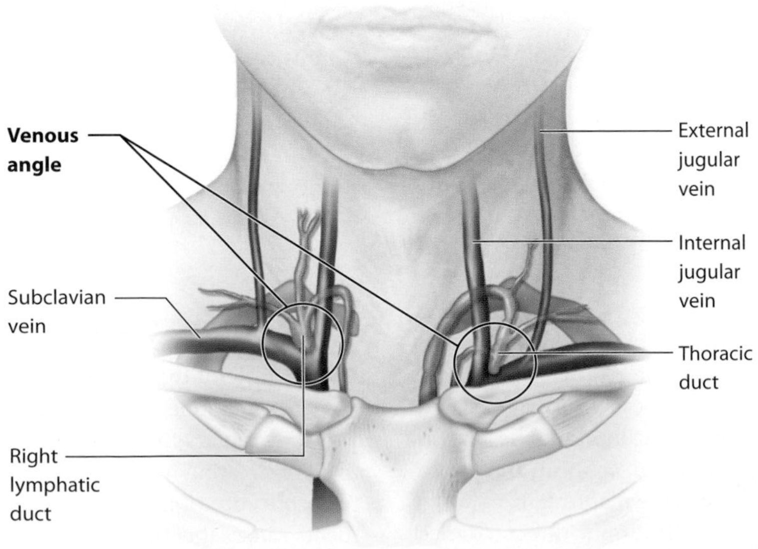

FIGURE 5-10 Venous angle. The venous angle is formed by the junction of the internal jugular vein and the subclavian vein. The thoracic duct on the left and the right lymphatic duct insert directly into this junction, which is termed the ***venous angle***. The venous angle flows into the brachiocephalic vein.

CASE STUDY

INTRODUCTION

An 80-year-old male presents with bilateral lower extremity edema (left greater than right) that has recently worsened and is preventing him from playing golf. Past medical history includes the history of myocardial infarct with residual cardiomyopathy (15 years ago), chronic renal insufficiency, Type 2 diabetes for which the patient takes oral medications, history of gout in the left great toe, and history of prostate cancer that was diagnosed 6 years ago and is being treated by "watchful waiting," meaning there is no treatment except yearly monitoring of PSA levels (**FIGURE 5-11A, B**).

DISCUSSION QUESTIONS

1. What questions are appropriate to ask the patient in order to obtain the subjective history?
2. What additional objective information is needed to determine the cause of the edema?
3. What tests and measures are indicated to determine the plan of care for this patient?

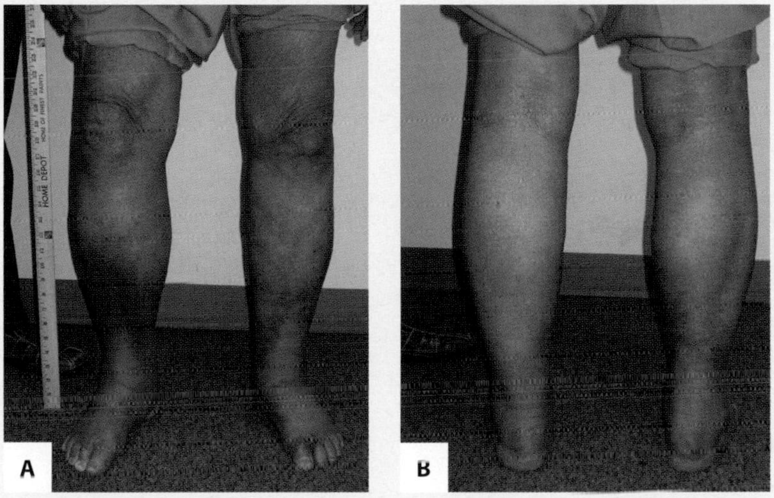

FIGURE 5-11 A, B. Case study photographs. The case study patient presents with bilateral arterial, venous, and lymphatic insufficiency.

Fluid movement between the capillaries (arterial, venous, and lymphatic) and the interstitial spaces is governed by Starling's Law of Equilibrium. This law describes how the osmotic and hydrostatic pressures in the capillaries and interstitial tissue determine the direction of fluid movement. The irony of this equation is that equilibrium is never really achieved because of the dynamic nature of the human body, which does not allow the pressure gradient to equal zero; therefore, fluid is always moving, or in physiologic terms, fluid is constantly being filtrated and reabsorbed at the capillary bed (**FIGURE 5-12**).[2,3] Recent research by Levick and Michel examined microvascular fluid movement at the capillary bed. These researchers discovered a lining in the capillary wall called the endothelial glycocalyx that impedes fluid reabsorption back into the venule. Therefore, interstitial fluid must be reabsorbed into the initial lymphatic vessels. Revision of Starling's Law of Equilibrium emphasizes the role of oncotic pressure in the interstitium and its effect on tissue fluid balance. This finding does not negate Starling's Law of Equilibrium. Rather, it emphasizes the importance of the function of the lymphatic system in prevention of edema and therefore the necessity of interventions to promote

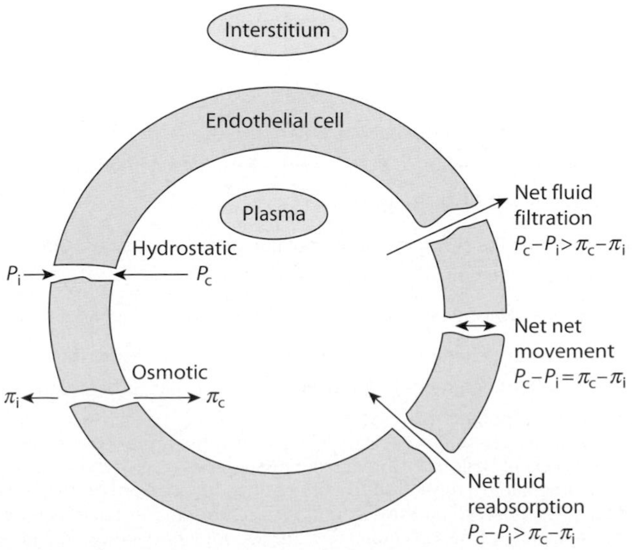

FIGURE 5-12 Starling's Law of Equilibrium.

lymphatic reabsorption and transportation and thereby prevent peripheral edema such as lymphedema.[4,5]

The difference between the net hydrostatic pressure and the net osmotic pressure is the force that determines the direction of fluid flow (TABLE 5-2). When the fluid flows from the interstitial space into the capillaries, it is termed *reabsorption* and can occur at both the venule and the lymphatic capillaries. When the fluid flows from the capillaries into the interstitial space, it is termed *filtration*. Equilibrium occurs when an equal amount of fluid moves from the arterial capillaries into the

TABLE 5-2 Definitions for the Physiological Components of Starling's Law of Equilibrium

Capillary bed forces—Forces responsible for direction of fluid movement at the capillary bed membrane. There are four forces: two hydrostatic and two oncotic pressures that affect transcapillary fluid exchange at the capillary bed.
Hydrostatic pressure (HP)—Pressure exerted on the vessel wall by the fluid (water).
Capillary hydrostatic pressure (HP_c)—Pressure from water that drives fluid out of the capillary (ie, filtration); is highest at the arteriolar end of the capillary and lowest at the venule end.
Interstitial hydrostatic pressure (HP_i)—Pressure generated by the volume of water in the interstitial spaces. As more fluid filters into the interstitium, both the volume of the interstitial space and the hydrostatic pressure within that space increase.
Net hydrostatic pressure (net HP)—Difference between the capillary HP (HP_c) and the interstitial HP (HP_{if}).
Osmotic pressure (OP)—Pressure exerted by plasma protein molecule concentration that is required to prevent the flow of water across a semipermeable membrane via osmosis.
Capillary osmotic pressure (OP_c)—Pressure that drives fluid into the capillary bed. The capillary membrane is readily permeable to ions; therefore, the osmotic pressure within the capillary is determined by the presence of plasma proteins (that are relatively impermeable to the capillary membrane). This pressure is referred to as the "oncotic" pressure or "colloid osmotic" pressure because it is generated by colloids. Albumin generates about 70% of the oncotic pressure, which is typically 25–30 mmHg.
Interstitial osmotic pressure (OP_i)—Pressure of the interstitial fluid that depends on the interstitial plasma protein concentration and the reflection coefficient of the capillary wall. The more permeable the capillary barrier is to proteins, the higher the interstitial oncotic pressure. This pressure is also determined by the amount of fluid filtration into the interstitium.
Reabsorption—Process by which fluid moves from the interstitial spaces into the capillary bed.
Filtration—Process by which fluid moves from the capillary bed into the interstitial spaces. Starling's hypothesis states that "the fluid movement due to filtration across the wall of a capillary is dependent on the balance between the hydrostatic pressure gradient and the oncotic pressure gradient across the capillary." The four Starling's forces are: 1. Hydrostatic pressure in the capillary (Pc) 2. Hydrostatic pressure in the interstitium (Pi) 3. Oncotic pressure in the capillary (pc) 4. Oncotic pressure in the interstitium (pi) The balance of these forces allows calculation of the net driving pressure for filtration. Under normal physiological conditions at the capillary bed, the exchange of fluids, nutrients, cellular debris, and waste products is primarily due to diffusion and filtration between the blood and tissues. Net filtration of fluid across the capillary membrane is governed by the balance of filtration forces and reabsorption forces. The direction of fluid movement is dependent on the difference between hydrostatic pressure (HP) and osmotic pressure (OP). HP is the same as capillary blood pressure, which varies along the length of capillary, and under normal circumstances that pressure is lower in the venous end and higher in the capillary end.
Fluid is forced OUT of arterial end of capillary bed when: Net hydrostatic pressure (net HP) = $HP_c - HP_{if}$ > Net osmotic pressure (net OP)$OP_c - OP_{if}$ FLUID IS FORCED OUT = FILTRATION
Fluid is forced INTO the venous end of the capillary when: Net hydrostatic pressure (net HP) = $HP_c - HP_{if}$ < Net osmotic pressure (net OP)$OP_c - OP_{if}$ FLUID IS FORCED IN = REABSORPTION To determine the ***resultant*** amount of fluid movement across the entire capillary bed: Net filtration pressure = difference between: Net HP – Net OP (arterial end) and NET HP – NET OP (venous end) If the resultant difference is **positive**, the fluid is moved into the interstitial spaces. If the resultant difference is **negative**, the fluid is reabsorbed into the capillary bed. The one component missing from Starling's Law of Equilibrium is the lymphatic capillary. If the lymphatic capillary is healthy and functioning normally, the lymphatic capillary will reabsorb the protein molecules that escape at the arterial end of the capillary bed. If this process is functioning, there is no net buildup of interstitial pressure. However, if there is lymphatic insufficiency or overload, the normally negative pressure gradient within the initial lymphatic becomes positive (overload of protein molecules), at which point the initial lymphatics can no longer absorb the protein molecules. The result is the accumulation of protein molecules within the interstitial spaces. This will alter both the HP_{if} and OP_{if} pressure gradients of the capillary bed. Protein molecules attract water and are too large to enter the venous capillary. With a positive pressure in the lymphatic capillary preventing reabsorption into the lymphatic system, the protein molecules plus water accumulate in the interstitial spaces and eventually cause the skin to stretch, resulting in visible edema. Filtration is normally not affected.

interstitial space and out of the interstitial space into the venous and lymphatic capillaries. Hydrostatic pressure is the pressure exerted by the blood on the capillary walls. Because the pressure is higher on the arterial side than on the venule side, fluid is pushed out of the capillary bed into the interstitial space. Osmotic pressure is the force created by large molecules such as plasma proteins, and it opposes hydrostatic pressure. Plasma protein molecules attract water so that in a normal system they facilitate reabsorption of the fluids back into the venule.[6]

The capillary wall is a semipermeable membrane, thus a force is required to move the larger protein molecules in and out of the capillary bed. At the arterial end where the net hydrostatic pressure is higher than the net osmotic pressure, the molecules are forced out of the capillary bed and into the interstitium. However, at the venule end, the net osmotic pressure is higher than the net hydrostatic pressure so the pressure is not sufficient to move the molecules from the interstitium into the capillary bed. Therefore, the molecules are reabsorbed into the lymphatic capillary at the overlapping endothelial junction. When this process is in balance so that fluids are adequately moved, no edema occurs. When there is an imbalance, for a variety of reasons and in either direction, edema develops. All edema pathology can be related to a problem with either filtration or reabsorption. When this happens, there is a transportation dysfunction—the freeway is clogged. The challenge to the clinician is to determine the pathology that prevents adequate flow of the fluid back into the central vascular system.

PATHOPHYSIOLOGY OF LYMPHEDEMA

Primary lymphedema is a result of congenital malformations of the lymphatic system, although the consequences may not be observed in the early years (**FIGURES 5-13** and **5-14A** and **B**).

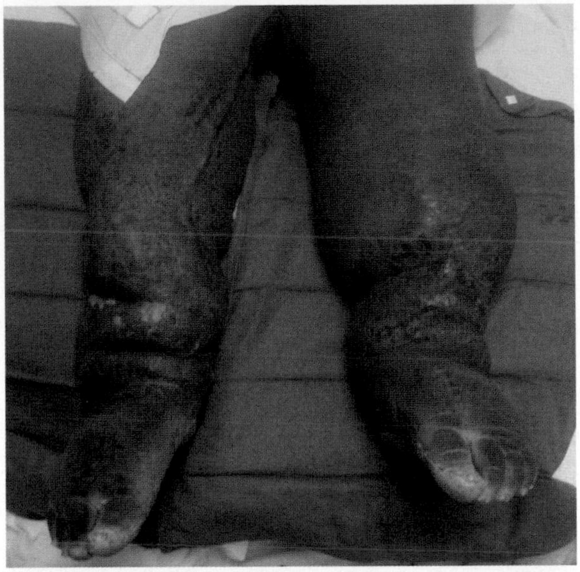

FIGURE 5-13 Primary lymphedema. Primary lymphedema in an Advanced Stage II progressing to Stage III; presents with significant skin changes and open wounds on L leg.

Secondary lymphedema is a result of acquired damage to the lymph vessels or nodes and subsequent impaired reabsorption and/or transportation of lymphatic fluid (**FIGURE 5-15**). Refer to **TABLE 5-1** for more details of both types.

A frequent cause of secondary lymphedema is chronic venous insufficiency (**FIGURE 5-16**).[7,8] The sequence of events is as follows: the venous system becomes compromised and cannot accommodate the normal amount of venous flow.

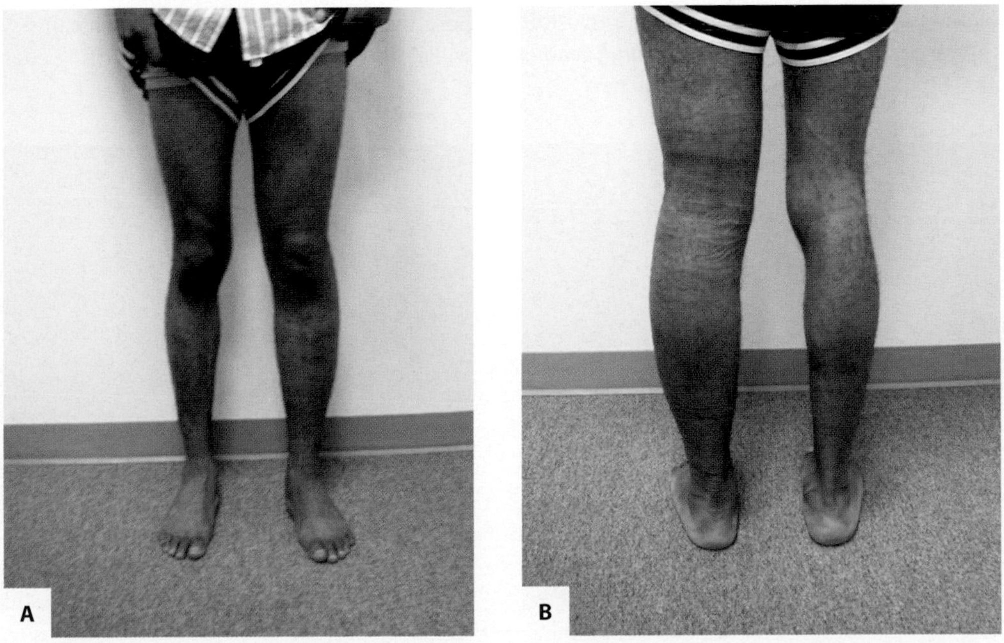

FIGURE 5-14 A. Lymphedema praecox (anterior view). B. Lymphedema praecox (posterior view). Anterior and posterior views of Stage II primary lymphedema as a result of cancer and its treatment. Note that the contour of the left lower extremity is proportionate even though the size discrepancy is obvious.

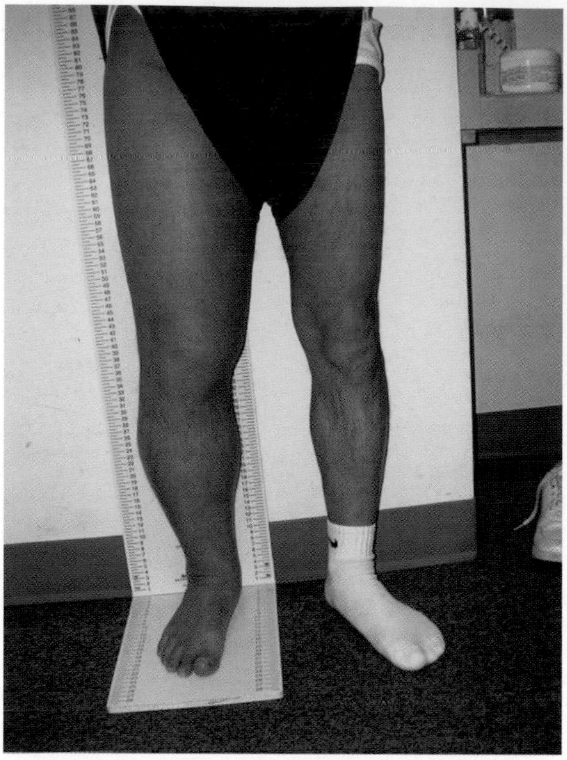

FIGURE 5-15 Secondary lymphedema. Stage II secondary lymphedema as a result of cancer treatment that resulted in clogged lymph nodes.

The lymphatic system, when healthy, can compensate because it can increase its rate of lymphangion contraction up to 10 times its resting volume and transport the fluid normally carried by the venous system.[1] For edema to develop in patients with chronic venous insufficiency, either one of the two following scenarios must occur: (1) *the lymphatic and venous load exceeds the maximum transport capacity of the lymphatic system* or (2) *the lymphatic system becomes impaired and cannot transport the usual fluid load.* The lymphatic impairment may be caused by incompetent lymphatic valves due to distended vessels.[9,10]

In the United States, the most recognized cause of lymphedema is related to cancer and its treatment (**FIGURE 5-17**).[11] The location and the severity of oncology-related lymphedema are influenced by the area affected, the location and total dosage of radiation, the extent of lymph node dissection, obesity, and the presence of comorbidities.[12,13] Clinical presentation can vary drastically and the treatment has to be individualized. Other causes of secondary lymphedema include trauma, infection, surgery in which the lymphatic vessels are severed or damaged, and systemic disorders (eg, liver, kidney, or cardiac disease) (**FIGURES 5-18** to **5-20**). However, any pathology that results in damage to the lymphatic system with decreased transport capacity will result in chronic secondary lymphedema, and clinical presentation will be essentially the same with variations only in relation to the severity of the damage.

Lipedema (**FIGURE 5-21**) is a chronic disease of lipid metabolism that is often misdiagnosed as lymphedema.[14] Although the clinical presentation is similar, there are distinct differences that aid in making a differential diagnosis. For example, there is no edema in the feet, the edema is either bilateral or quadrilateral, the texture is soft and non-pitting, the skin temperature may be cooler than the trunk, and the skin may be hypersensitive to light touch. The underlying pathology is thought to be due to an abnormal deposition of adipose cells in the subcutaneous tissue, as well as a possible inheritance of genetic X-linked abnormalities.[15] Over time, however, if the superficial lymphatic system becomes compressed by the adipose tissue, secondary lymphedema can develop and the feet will also become edematous and pitting edema can occur.[16]

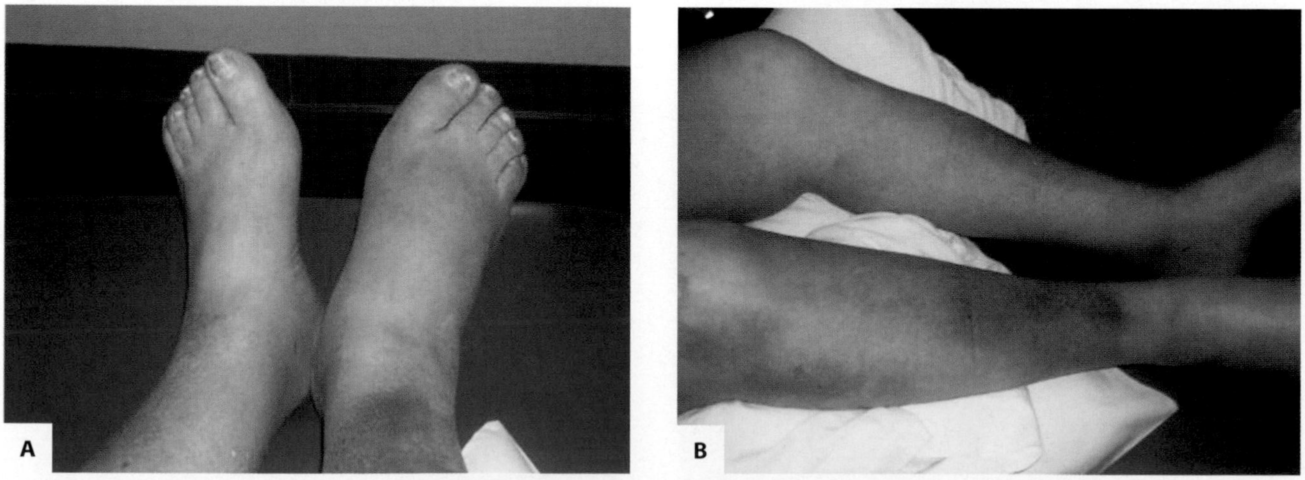

FIGURE 5-16 Chronic venous insufficiency with secondary lymphedema. Secondary lymphedema is frequently a consequence of chronic venous insufficiency. The hemosiderin stains (a byproduct of autolysis of hemoglobin released from red blood cells trapped in the interstitial tissue) are characteristic of chronic venous insufficiency. The pedal edema on the dorsum of the foot is also characteristic of secondary lymphedema.

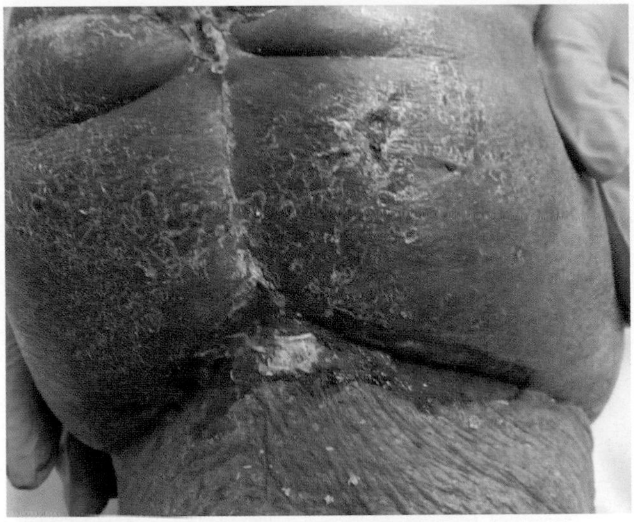

FIGURE 5-17 Lymphedema as a result of cancer and radiation (head and neck cancer). Lymphedema as a result of radiation can occur in any body part where the lymphatic vessels are damaged and the flow is interrupted. Note the changes in the skin, termed *dry desquamation*, in which the epidermal layer is sloughing much like superficial sunburn.

Stages of Lymphedema

The International Society of Lymphology has identified and defined the stages of lymphedema, as described in TABLE 5-3.[17] Lymphedema is a chronic inflammatory condition; therefore, over time there is deposition of collagen fibers and adipose cells in the interstitial tissue of the affected region. Once the diagnosis of lymphedema is established, the severity is used to determine the stage of the disease. The extent of fibrosis and adipose is defined in the stages and is used to determine the patient's prognosis.

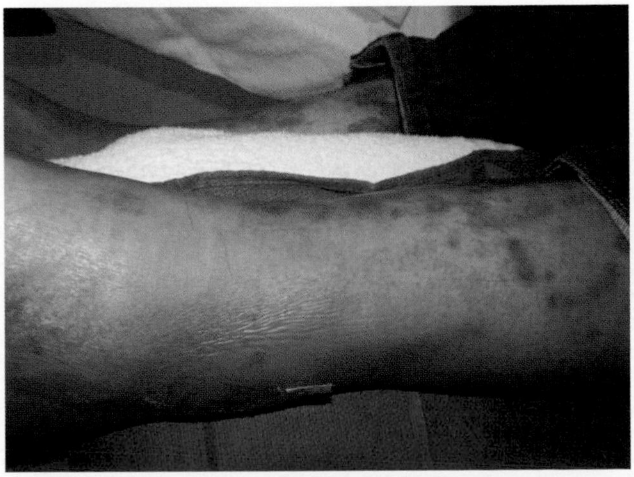

FIGURE 5-18 Secondary lymphedema due to trauma. The tight, orange-peel texture of the lower leg skin is a result of lymphedema that has developed after a lateral ankle injury. Any trauma that disrupts the lymphatic flow, limits joint range of motion, and alters gait cycle can result in lymphedema formation.

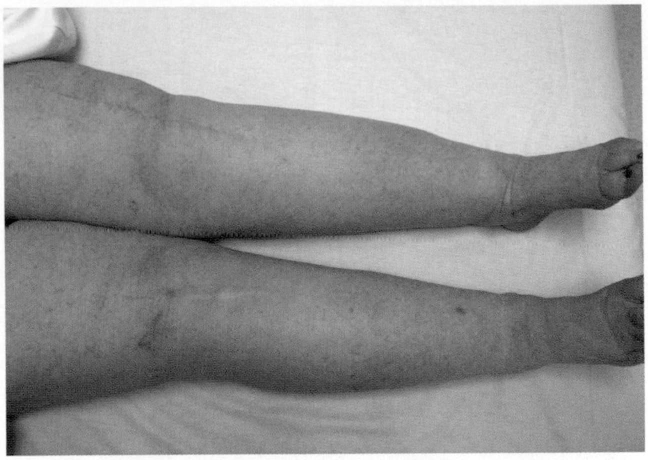

FIGURE 5-19 Secondary lymphedema due to orthopedic surgery. Secondary lymphedema is common after lower extremity surgeries that interfere with lymphatic flow through the popliteal or inguinal lymph nodes, such as total knee or total hip replacements. Early mobilization, isometric exercises, and compression with short stretch bandages are recommended to prevent or treat this type of edema. Reduction of the edema through these strategies will subsequently result in better functional outcomes.

Risk Factors for Lymphedema

Risk factors for lymphedema formation that have been identified are listed in TABLE 5-4. In addition, recent research suggests that certain individuals may have a genetic predisposition to lymphedema development; this is especially important for the oncology population.[18] Evaluation of a patient with peripheral edema needs to include investigation of any comorbidities that may impair the lymphatic and venous systems. The development of secondary lymphedema is typically a result of multiple

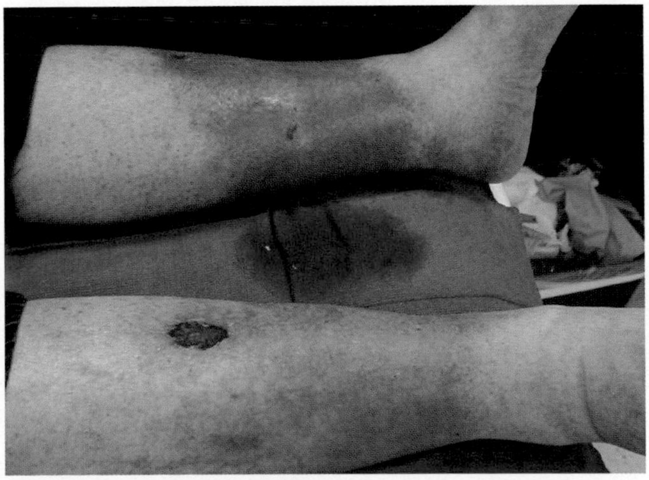

FIGURE 5-20 Secondary lymphedema due to systemic disorder. Bilateral lymphedema may be indicative of a systemic disorder (eg, congestive heart failure as in the case of this patient). The erythema of both lower legs is suggestive of cellulitis, which would be treated with antibiotics. Compression with short stretch bandages is recommended after both the congestive heart failure and the cellulitis have been treated.

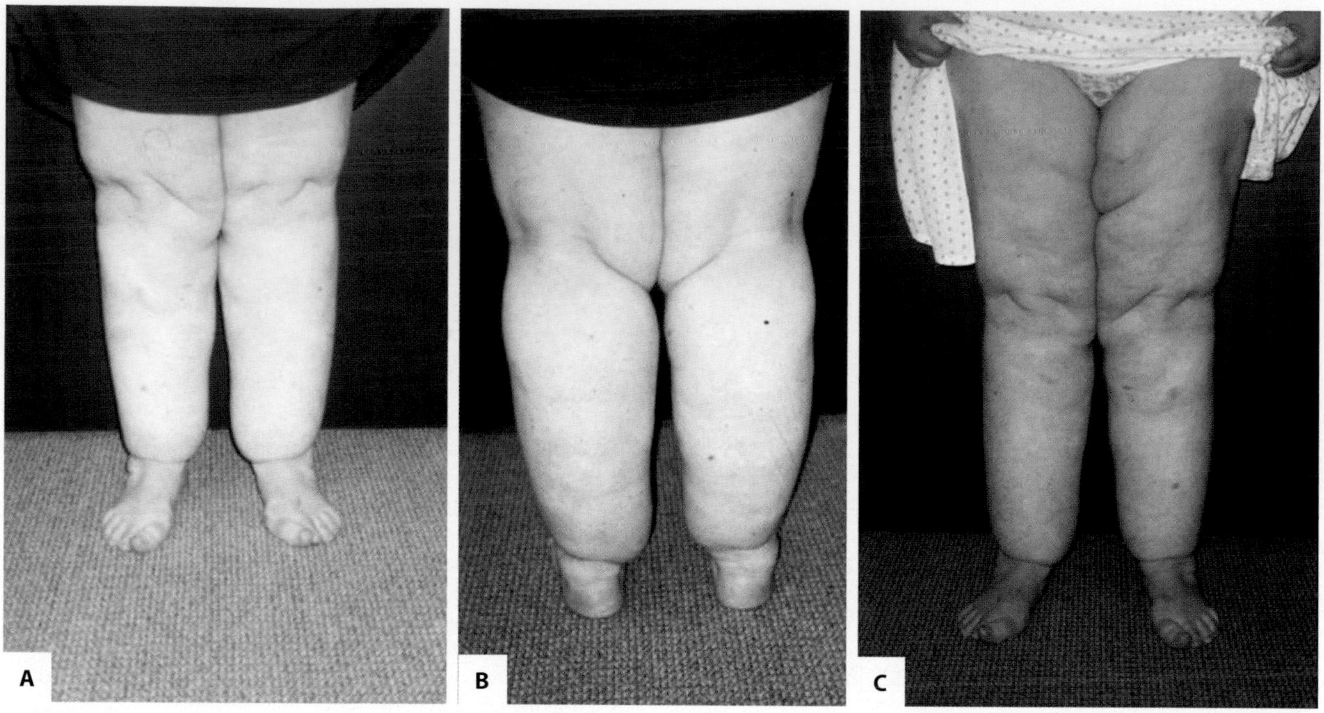

FIGURE 5-21 Lipedema A and **B** at the time of initial evaluation and **C** is after 4 months of treatment. Lipedema is often mistaken for lymphedema. Note the columnar shape of the legs, sparing of the feet and ankles, and the significant skin folds above the ankles. Lipedema is a hereditary disorder and ***not*** a result of obesity.

risk factors and/or insults to the lymphatic system; therefore, a complete systems review is required for any patient who presents with peripheral edema.

Clinical Presentation of Lymphedema

Evaluation of the clinical presentation of lymphedema includes both the volume of the involved extremity and the degree of fibrosis in the interstitial tissue. In the early stages, the edema is soft and pitting (**FIGURE 5-22A** and **B**); however, as more collagen fibers are deposited, the tissue becomes more firm and less compressible. As the fibrosis becomes more severe, the tissue becomes non-pitting. Both pitting and non-pitting edema are often present in the same extremity. Infection is one of the primary causes of the progression of lymphedema to a more severe stage.

TABLE 5-3 Stages of Lymphedema

Stage 0	Stage 1	Stage 2	Stage 3
Subclinical stage: Lymph transport is Impaired; however, lymphatic load has not yet exceeded the transport capacity. Swelling is not evident. Clinical symptoms: Patients may report heaviness, tightness, or sensory changes in the affected limbs. This stage may persist for months or years before edema is detectable.	Edema may be variable, ie, decrease with rest or sleep and increase with activity. Edema is very soft, easily pits with little to no fibrosis. Elevation of the limb results in dissipation of the edema. Patient may report heaviness, tightness, sensory changes, or pain in the limb.	Edema no longer dissipates with elevation of the limb. Palpation is positive for fibrosis and results in indentation of the skin. Fibrosis ranges from soft and pitting (early stage II) to hard and non-pitting (late stage II). Both are commonly present in various locations along the involved limb. Skin mobility may be decreased and texture may be brawny. Positive Stemmer sign ▪ UE: may be present in the dorsum of the fingers. ▪ LE is commonly present in the dorsum of the toes. Increased likelihood of skin infection.	Palpation: The fibrotic changes of the skin and subcutaneous tissues continue to increase in severity. Fat deposits in the subcutaneous tissues lead to the following clinical signs and symptoms. Little to no skin mobility is present. Hair follicles may be coarse or absent. Subcutaneous fat deposits and worsening of fibrosis result in increased skin folds, loss of joint spaces, papillomas, skin hyperpigmentation, hyperkeratosis, cysts, and fistulas. Pitting is absent or minimally present with significant pressure and, if present, dissipates rapidly. Palpation of the limb is hard. Stemmer sign intensifies. Patient has history of recurrent bacterial infections/fungal infections. Volume of lymphedema significantly increases resulting in loss of joint spaces and bony prominences, and limb shape is unrecognizable.

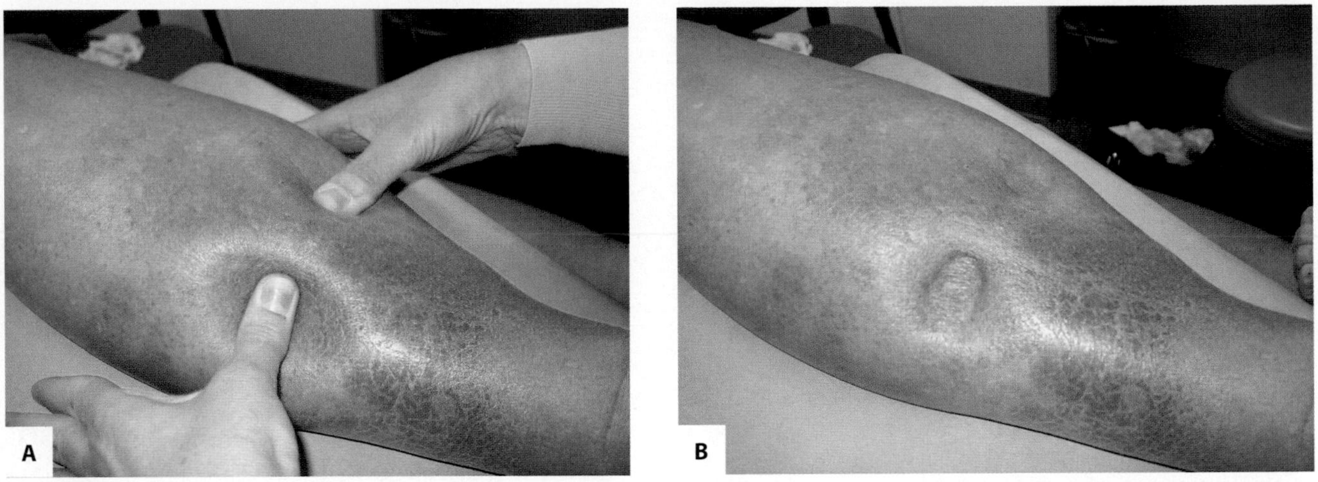

FIGURE 5-22 A, B. Pitting edema. Failure of the tissue to rebound after pressure with a finger is termed *pitting edema* and occurs during the early stages of lymphedema. As a result of chronic lymphedema, the subcutaneous tissue becomes fibrotic and does not pit; this is a characteristic of later stages of lymphedema. During the earlier stages, the deeper the pitting and the longer the rebound time, the better the prognosis for resolution of the symptoms. If the tissue is very thick and hard, there will be little to no pitting and a fast refill time, both indicating that longer treatment time and more compression therapy will be needed to remodel the fibrosis.

Patient complaints in the early stages of lymphedema include heaviness, tightness, aching, and sensory changes.[19,20] Corresponding to these complaints, the evaluator will note a loss of skin mobility; as the lymphedema progresses, the skin becomes tighter and less mobile. The difficulty or inability to mobilize or "tent" the skin over the dorsum of the foot (metatarsals) is termed the *Stemmer sign* (**FIGURE 5-23**).[7,21,22] This tightness of the skin and underlying tissue may result in loss of range of motion and subsequent functional impairments, especially with limited ankle dorsiflexion which subsequently results in altered gait and increased fall risk.

TABLE 5-4 Risk Factors for Secondary Lymphedema

UE Lymphedema	LE Lymphedema
History of UE venous pathologies	History of LE venous pathologies
Surgical damage or removal of axillary lymph nodes/vessels	Surgical damage or removal of pelvic, abdominal, or inguinal lymph nodes/vessels
Mastectomy	Multiple pregnancies
Chemotherapy	Abdominal surgery
Metastatic lymph nodes	Kidney, liver, cardiac dysfunction, or failure
Radiation therapy, fibrosis	Hypertension
Genetic predisposition	Radiation therapy, fibrosis
Lack of adherence to exercise program	Genetic predisposition/Factor 5 Leiden
Comorbidities: autoimmune diseases, obesity	Comorbidities: autoimmune diseases, HTN, obesity, DM
Infections, seroma, wounds	Infections, seroma, wounds
Smoking	Smoking
Scar tissue	Scar tissue

Any pathology that compromises lymphatic reabsorption and transportation is a risk factor. Usually a combination of risk factors is the cause of lymphatic insufficiency and secondary lymphedema. The most commonly overlooked risk factor is chronic venous pathologies; the most recognized cause is oncology-related secondary lymphedema (ie, with breast cancer). In oncology-related secondary lymphedema, surgery and radiation therapy can either independently or combined result in secondary lymphedema.

Data from Asdourian MS, Swaroop MN, Sayegh HE, et al. Association between precautionary behaviors and breast cancer-related lymphedema in patients undergoing bilateral surgery. *J Clin Oncol*. 2017;35(35):3934-3941 and Stuiver MM, Ten Tusscher MR, McNeely ML. Which are the best conservative interventions for lymphedema after breast cancer surgery? *BMJ*. 2017;357:j2330.

The clinical presentation of lymphedema associated with malignancy, radiation, or surgical interventions may involve any affected body part (eg, breast, head and neck, tongue, genitals). Lymph node dissection or radiation scarring may cause decreased lymphatic transport to the regional lymph nodes and subsequent fluid accumulation (edema) in the quadrant or territory distal to the injured nodes. For

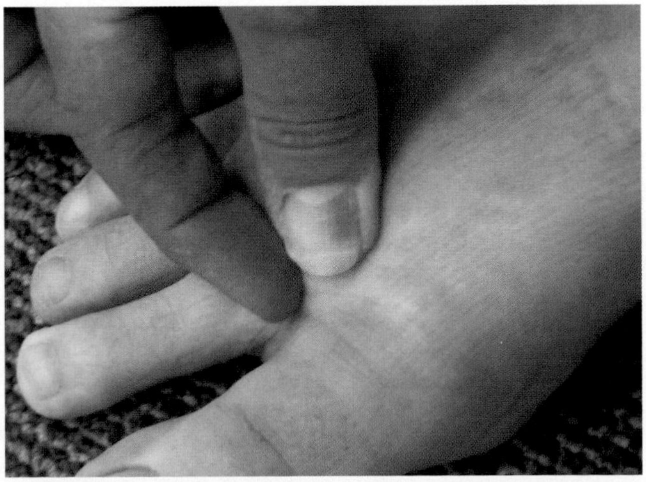

FIGURE 5-23 Stemmer sign. Inability to tent or pinch the skin at the distal foot is termed a positive Stemmer sign and is indicative of decreased skin mobility and elasticity as a result of chronic lymphedema.

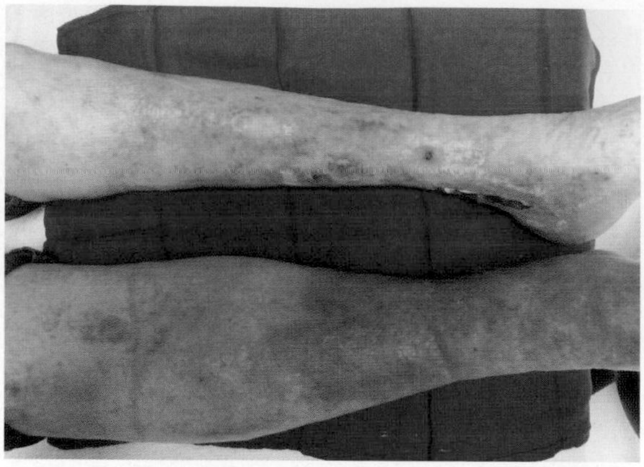

FIGURE 5-24 Lymphedema as a result of occlusion to the abdominal lymph nodes. Sudden onset of unilateral edema that is hard and does not respond to compression is suggestive of pelvic or abdominal lymph node obstruction. This patient was being seen for wounds on the left lower extremity; however, the severe, sudden-onset edema of the right leg was the result of a rare abdominal malignancy that caused node obstruction.

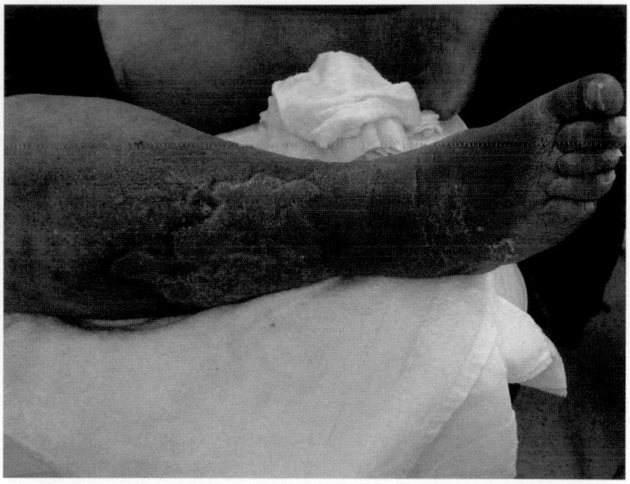

FIGURE 5-26 Skin changes as a result of lymphedema. Changes in the skin color and texture occur with chronic lymphedema, including thick skin, discoloration, papillomatosis, and in this case, scarring from recurrent wounds on the lateral leg. Note the fungus, termed *onychomycosis*, on the toe nails.

example, if there is an obstruction to the pelvic and abdominal lymph nodes and vessels, genital and/or lower extremity edema may develop (FIGURE 5-24). As the stages progress, the fat and fibrosis lead to loss of anatomical landmarks such as joint lines and skin folds (FIGURE 5-25). Skin changes that may occur include hyperkeratosis, papillomatosis, and lymphocoeles (FIGURE 5-26).

Differential Diagnosis of Lymphedema

The presence of any edema is a symptom of some underlying pathology that has to be identified in order to have an effective plan of care. Diagnosis is based on the patient history, physical examination, and laboratory tests to confirm or rule out

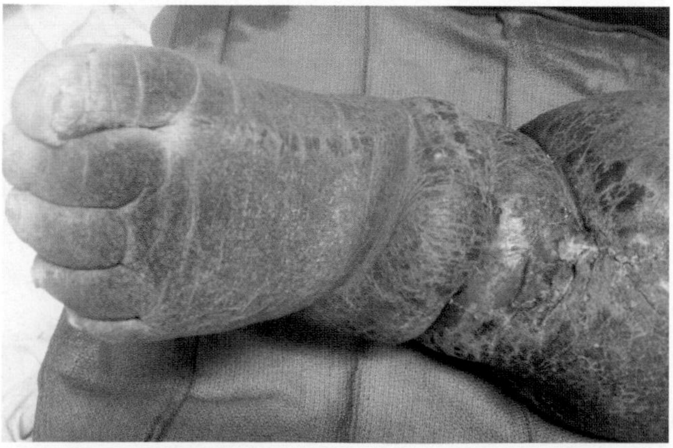

FIGURE 5-25 Anatomic changes in late stages of lymphedema. Anatomic changes as a result of lymphedema include the loss of joint spaces, toe deformities, hyperkeratosis, papillomas, and color variations in the skin.

systemic pathologies (eg, endocrine, cardiopulmonary, renal, or hepatic diseases) or vascular pathologies (eg, deep vein thrombosis). Some of the questions that can help with the differential diagnosis process include the following:

- Is the edema unilateral or bilateral?
- Was the onset sudden or gradual?
- Is the edema local or widespread?
- What are the patient comorbidities?
- Is there a history of cancer?
- Is there a history of venous disorders?
- What are the medications? (see TABLE 5-5)
- What are the psychosocial behaviors?
- What is the pain pattern?

Clinical guidelines for diagnoses of upper quadrant lymphedema secondary to cancer were developed by the Oncology Academy of the American Physical Therapy Association.[23,24] Specific guidelines include the following recommended assessment tools: self -report of symptoms, bioimpedance analysis, volume measurements calculated from circumferential measurements, and/or water displacement (FIGURES 5-27 and 5-28).[25] Circumferential measurements are converted to a volume using the formula for a truncated cone (FIGURE 5-29).[26] This process, which can also be used for lower extremity lymphedema, is essential for ensuring accurate diagnosis and for measuring outcomes. Recommendations were developed based on the stage of the lymphedema and the body part involved.[23]

Several imaging techniques to assist in diagnosis, treatment planning, outcome measurements, and research have been discussed in the literature. *Radionuclide lymphoscintigraphy* involves subcutaneous or intradermal injection of a radiotracer

TABLE 5-5 Medications That May Contribute to Peripheral Edema

Antiarrhythmics (amiodarone, Norpace, Flecainide)
Anticoagulants (Plavix, Crestor, Lipitor, Arixtra, Cilostazol)
Antidepressants
Antifungals (Amphotericin)
Antihypertensive (nitrates, hydralazine, minoxidil)
Antineoplastic (Xeloda, Aromasin, Herceptin, Zometa)
Antiosteoporotic agents (Actonel, Bisphosphates)
Antisympathetics (reserpine, guanethidine)
Beta-blockers (Tenormin, Coreg, Labetalol, Toprol)
Calcium channel blockers (Verapamil, Nifedipine)
Chemotherapy agents (docetaxel, cisplatin, tretinoin)
Centrally acting agents (clonidine, methyldopa)
Corticosteroids
Direct vasodilators (hydralazine, minoxidil, diazoxide)
Glitazones, Actos, Avandia (DM)
Hormones (estrogens/progesterones/testosterone)
Nonsteroidal anti-inflammatory agents
Nonselective cyclooxygenase inhibitors
Selective cyclooxygenase-2 inhibitors
Troglitazone
Phenylbutazone
Parkinson agents (Mirapex, pramipexole)
Valproic acid

Reproduced with permission from Cho S, Atwood JE. Peripheral edema. *Am J Med.* 2002; 113(7):580-586.

(usually Tc-filtered sulfur colloid with a particle size < 100 nm) into the involved and the uninvolved extremities (for control data), followed by nuclear imaging.[27,28] Qualitative and quantitative readings can be used to confirm a differential diagnosis of lymphedema, assess the efficacy of therapeutic interventions, and predict the risk of post-operative lymphedema.

Near-infrared (NIR) fluorescence imaging with indocyanine green is a "non-invasive assessment of both lymphatic architecture and function as well as potential disease markers of lymphatic function."[29] Clinical applications include intraoperative assessment of lymphatic vessel patency, delineation of tumors, and assessment of lymphatic flow both during and after therapeutic interventions.[30]

Ultrasonography is used to evaluate the amount and quality of dermal thickening and fibrosis present in edematous tissue, which can help differentiate between lymphedema and lipedema in the lower extremity.[31,32] The ultrasonic measurement of a limb's soft tissue cross-sectional area can help evaluate tissue stiffness. Clinically, these measurements may assist in selection of materials for compression therapy.[33]

Tissue dielectric devices provide a measurement of localized tissue water content by sending an electromagnetic wave into the tissue and measuring the time for wave reflection back to the sensor. The measurement is used to calculate the tissue dielectric constant (TDC), which is determined by the amount of bound and free water in the tissue. The higher TDC value reflects higher water content which in turn has the potential to help detect earlier development of lymphedema. Recent research suggests that TDC has diagnostic potential for lymphedema of the arm, leg, trunk, and venous-related edema.[34–36]

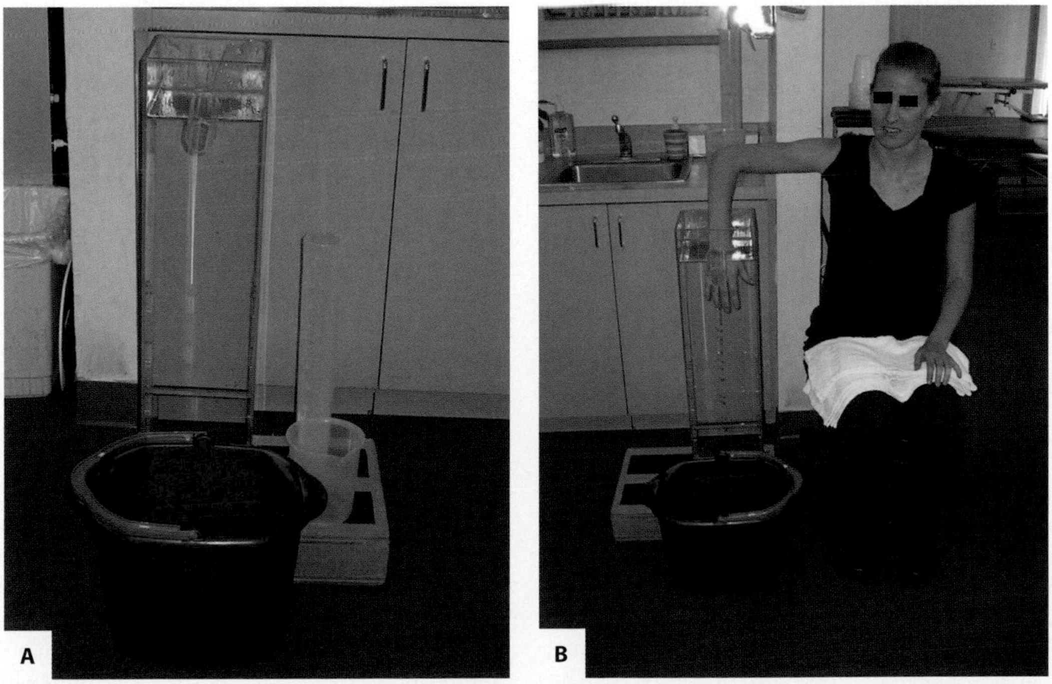

FIGURE 5-27 A, B. Volumetric measurement: water displacement technique. A. Equipment set-up to perform displacement volumetric measurements. When the extremity is inserted into the tank of water, the displaced water flows into the blue container; when the extremity is extracted, the amount of water displaced is measured (**B**).

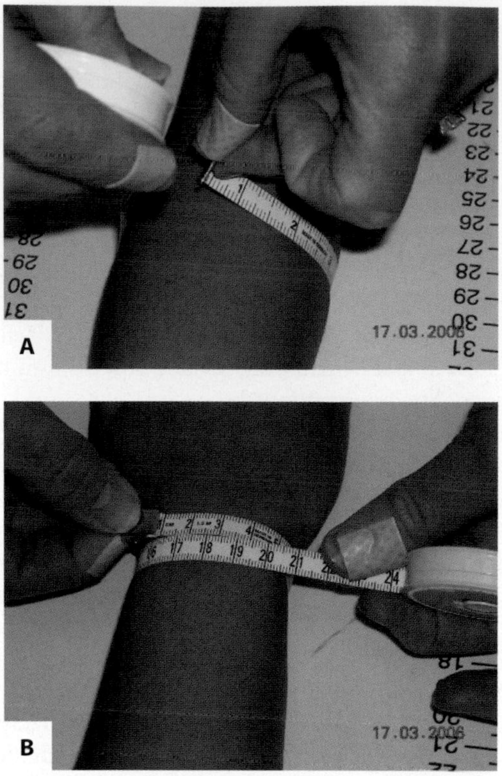

FIGURE 5-28 A, B. Volumetric measurement: tape measure technique. **A** and **B** demonstrate the upper extremity circumferential measurement technique. The tape is placed perpendicular to the arm, proper "tautness" is ensured by applying enough tension to take up the slack but not wrinkle the skin, and measurements are recorded at least two times and averaged for the results. (Photographs used with permission of Marisa Perdomo.)

Summed Truncated Cone
$V = (h)(C^2 + Cc + c^2)/12\pi$
The arm is divided into "segments" with the "h" being constant either 4 cm or 10 cm for the arm and typically 10 cm for the leg. Each of the segments is considered a "mini" cone and all of the segments are summed to determine the volume of the limb.

h = height of cone; C = proximal circumferential;
c = distal circumference

FIGURE 5-29 Summed truncated Cone for the upper extremity.

An additional aspect of patient evaluation is the effect of the lymphedema on *quality of life*. Tools that have been validated to measure the quality of life are described in **TABLE 5-6**. A systemic review of patient-reported outcome instruments regarding the quality of life among breast cancer patients with lymphedema was reported by Pusic et al.; they recommended the *Upper Limb Lymphedema 27 (ULL-27)* as it demonstrated strong psychometric properties.[37] The Functional Assessment of Cancer Therapy—Breast with or without the arm subscale (FACT-B; FACT-B+4), Disability of Arm, Shoulder, and Hand (DASH) Questionnaire, and Lymphedema Quality of Life (LYQOL) questionnaire have also been validated for measuring the quality of life.

The *Lymph-ICF-LL* for patients with lower extremity lymphedema consists of 28 questions for the following domains: physical function, mental function, general tasks/household activities, mobility activities, and life/social domain. Psychometric properties and test–retest reliability are both reported as acceptable to good range.[38] The *Patient Benefit Index (PBI)* allows patients to rate the extent to which their goals have been met and consists of the following two parts: (1) the Patient Needs Questionnaire in which patients rate the importance of 23 patient-relevant goals on a scale of 1–5 ("not at all" to "very") and (2) the Patient Benefit Questionnaire in which patients rate the extent of their goal achievement on the same 1–5 scale.[39] The Freiburg Life Quality Assessment for Lymphedema (FLQA-L) initially consisted of 92 items; however, it has been shortened and adapted for a variety of skin conditions, including wounds, chronic venous insufficiency, and other specific skin conditions.[40–42] Regardless of the tool used, assessing health-related quality of life is an integral part of the total evaluation of patients with lymphedema.

CLINICAL CONSIDERATION

A cardiovascular exercise routine is beneficial for both systems; however, the 24-hour response needs to be monitored and assessed if lymphedema increases, in which case the intensity or duration of exercise is decreased.

TREATMENT OF LYMPHEDEMA

Treatment of any disorder begins with effective risk assessment and reduction, and the best strategy for secondary lymphedema is to optimize lymphatic flow so that if the lymphatic system is overloaded (eg, with CVI) or damaged (eg, with surgery, trauma, or radiation), the transport capacity remains sufficient to manage the lymphatic load. This is especially important for patients who have chronic venous insufficiency in whom the lymphatic system must compensate for the venous insufficiency by increasing its transportation capacity (eg, by increasing lymphangion contraction rate) over a long period of time. The chronic high demand placed on the lymphatic system leads to valvular distention and a lower lymphangion contraction rate, resulting in secondary lymphedema.[43] See **TABLE 5-7** for strategies to optimize both venous and lymphatic flow.

The development of surgical interventions and advancements in microsurgery have increased treatment options for those individuals who have not responded well with standard treatment (CDT). *Lymphovenous anastomosis* (LVA) may reduce lymphedema by restoring lymphatic drainage and transportation. *Vascularized lymph node transplantation* can increase the number of functional lymph nodes following lymph node dissection and thereby improve lymphatic flow. *Liposuction* techniques can be beneficial for removing adipose tissue and fibrosis. Proper evaluation of the lymphatic system via imaging techniques such as MRI, lymphoscintigraphy,

TABLE 5-6 Tools to Measure Quality of Life in Patients with Lymphedema

Name of Tool	Primary Measurement	Patient Population	Reference
Upper Limb Lymphatic-27	Physical function Mental function Daily activities Hobbies and job Mobility Social activities	Patients with breast cancer	Pusic AL, Cemal Y, Albornoz C, et al. Quality of life among breast cancer patients with lymphedema: a systematic review of patient-reported outcomes instruments and outcomes. *J Cancer Surviv.* 2013;7(1):83-92.
Functional Assessment of Cancer Therapy with or without the arm subscale (Fact-B or Fact-B+4	Domains: Physical, social, emotional, and functional well-being Breast cancer subscale Arm subscale	Patients with upper extremity lymphedema and history of cancer treatment	Hahn EA, Segawa E, Kaiser K, Cella D, Smith B. Validation of the Functional Assessment of Cancer Therapy-Breast (FACT-B) quality of life instrument. *J Clin Oncol*. 2015;33(suppl e1):7753.
Disability of Arm, Shoulder, and Hand (DASH) Short form and 30 item questionnaire	Upper extremity musculoskeletal function, disability and monitor change/function over time	Patients with upper extremity lymphedema of any etiology	Gummesson C, Atroshi I, EKdahl C. The disabilities of arm, shoulder and hand (DASH) outcome questionnaire: longitudinal construct validity and measuring self-rated health change after surgery. *BMC Musculoskelet Disord*. 2003;4:11.
Lymphedema Quality of Life for upper limbs (LYMQOL_UL)	Physical Function Mental Function Daily activities Hobbies and Job Mobility Social activities	Individuals with breast cancer	Keeley VL, Veigas D, Crooks S, et al. The development of a condition-specific quality of life measure for lymphoedema (LYMQOL). *Eur J Lymphol*. 2004;12(41):36. Keeley V, Crooks S, Locke J, et al. A quality of life measure for limb lymphoedema (LYMQOL). *J Lymphoedema*. 2010;5:26–37.
Lymph ICF-LL/UE	Physical function, mental function, general tasks/household activities, mobility activities, and life/social domain	Patients with lower extremity lymphedema and breast cancer	Cornelissen AJM, Kool M, Keuter XHA, Jeuts EM, et al. Quality of Life Questionnaires in Breast Cancer-Related Lymphedema Patients: Review of the Literature. *Lymphat Res Biol*. 2018;16(2):134-139. Devoogdt N, De Broef A, Hendrickx A, Damstra R, et. al, Lymphoedema Functioning, Disability and Health Questionnaire for Lower Limb Lymphoedema (Lymph-ICF-LL): Reliability and Validity. *PTJ*. 2014;94(5):705-721.
Patient Benefit Index (2 parts)	Patient perception of met goals	Patients with lymphedema, lipedema, and lipolymphedema	Blome C, Augustin M, Heyer K, et al. Evaluation of patient-relevant outcomes of lymphedema and lipedema treatment: development and validation of a new benefit tool. *Eur J Vasc Endovasc Surg*. 2014;47(1):100–107. Duygu E, Bakar Y, Keser I. An Important Tool in Lymphedema Management: Validation of Turkish Version of the Patient Benefit Index-Lymphedema. *Lymphat Res Biol*. 2020;18(1):49-55.
Freiburg Life Quality Assessment for lymphedema (FLQA-L)	Psychometrics vary depending on the adaptation for a specific diagnosis, but may include the following: Physical complaints Everyday life Social life Emotional status Therapy Satisfaction with treatment Occupation	Patients with lymphedema, wounds, chronic venous insufficiency, and other skin conditions	Augustin M, Conde Montero E, Hagenström K, Herberger K, Blome C. Validation of a short-form of the Freiburg Life Quality Assessment for lymphoedema (FLQA-LS) instrument. *Br J Dermatol*. 2018;179(6):1329-1333.

and/or indocyanine green fluorescent lymphography is necessary to determine which surgical approach is indicated. These surgical interventions may also be combined in certain cases to improve physiologic lymph flow and reduce fibrosis.[44,45]

Establishing patient eligibility for one of these surgical interventions varies across medical centers and may be dependent on the stage of lymphedema and availability of normal functioning lymph nodes and vessels.

The first step in treating any peripheral edema is determining and treating any underlying pathologies that are contributing to the edema formation. Whereas compression has traditionally been recognized as the primary intervention for

CASE STUDY

CONTINUED

Subjective information obtained from the patient:

- Reports a mild heart attack and takes the following medications:
  - Lipitor, 20 mg
  - Coreg (beta-blocker), 6.25 mg
  - Metoprolol, 100 mg daily
  - Coumadin, varies with INR, from 2 to 4 mg daily
  - Lasix, 40 mg daily
  - Metformin hydrochloride, extended release, 1000 mg daily,
  - ASA, 81 mg
- Reports his last ejection fraction was 45%; the patient is seen by his cardiologist two times a year.
- Reports being careful regarding high-fat, high-cholesterol foods, but admits to liking ice cream daily.
- Works as the owner of a moving van company and goes to office daily.
- Uses a rolling walker with a seat in all environments except at work.
- Lives with his wife in a one-story house with a daily housekeeper.

Objective information obtained from tests and measures:

- Unable to sit or stand without upper extremity (UE) assist; with UE assist, able to do 3 in 30 seconds.
- Six-minute walk test with the walker, 390 yards.
- Bilateral Trendelenburg gait with the rolling walker has little or no heel/toe sequence during gait cycle.
- ABI: left is 0.65, right is 0.7.
- Pulses: left DP 1+, PT 2+; right DP 2+, PT 2+.
- Auscultation of lungs—negative for crackles or congestion, decreased breath sounds in bilateral lower lobes.
- Auscultation of heart—negative for S3 heart sounds.
- Monofilament testing—+ response to 5.07 monofilament on both plantar feet, all points.
- Range of motion—hip extension bilaterally to neutral, lacks 5 degrees of knee extension bilaterally (5- to 120-degree knee flexion), 5-degree DF, 20-degree PF.
- Strength (bilaterally)—gluteus medius 3–/5, hip extensors 3–/5, ankle 2+/5.
- The patient reports glucose levels ranging from 120 to 200 fasting and last HbA1C (per lab results) was 7.5.

DISCUSSION QUESTIONS

1. What are the patient's risk factors for lymphedema?
2. What is the physiological rationale for his lymphedema?
3. What other information is needed before treatment can be initiated?

edema, evidence demonstrates that compression therapy and exercise are the two most efficacious interventions; manual lymphatic mobilization is an effective adjunct therapy. Skin hygiene is important for reducing the risk of infection.[46,47] The combination and sequence of therapies depend on the etiology and the individual presentation.

Before compression can be applied or prescribed, a complete vascular screening is needed to avoid compromise of

TABLE 5-7 Strategies to Optimize Venous and Lymphatic Flow

Exercise	Compression Therapy	Precautions
FOR LYMPHEDEMA:		
Diaphragmatic breathing. Range proximal joints first and move distally; begin with active and gradually add resistance. Aerobic exercise. End exercise session with diaphragmatic breathing.	Multilayer compression bandages with short-stretch bandages. Intermittent compression pumps. Garments to assist in maintaining reduction of lymphedema. Best used after physical therapy reduces the lymphedema.	Maintain healthy skin. Wear nonrestrictive clothing. Avoid excessive weight gain.
FOR VENOUS INSUFFICIENCY WITHOUT LYMPHEDEMA:		
Ankle mobilizations and stretches. Ankle pumps. Heel/toe raises, sitting and progress to standing. Walking with exaggerated heel/toe sequence.	Multilayer compression systems. Semi-rigid compression with short stretch bandages. Compression stockings measured to fit the individual. Garments essential for prevention of venous dysfunction after DVT to prevent CVI. Intermittent compression pump as adjunct to self-management program.	Avoid prolonged sitting with legs crossed. Avoid prolonged standing. Wear nonrestrictive clothing. Avoid smoking.

CLINICAL CONSIDERATION

In addition to the specific strategies for CVI and lymphedema, the plan of care should address all of the impairments that negatively impact joint ROM and muscle strength. In both venous and lymphatic dysfunction, muscle contraction plays a critical role in assisting fluid transportation.

blood flow and skin complications from existing arterial insufficiency. This is especially important for patients who have a history of smoking, diabetes, or age over 60, all of whom are at higher risk for arterial insufficiency. See Chapter 4, Vascular Wounds, for information on vascular screening and guidelines for lower extremity compression.

All of the interventions are designed to increase reabsorption at the venous/lymphatic capillaries, decrease the rate of capillary filtration, facilitate movement of the fluid from the distal superficial veins to the deep veins via the perforators, and assist lymphangion contraction. The interventions work together to increase the negative pressure gradient within the lymphatic and vascular vessels, thus promoting fluid movement from distal to proximal. It is the gradient, or difference in distal and proximal pressures, that forces the fluid flow in a specific direction. In the venous system, the venous pump creates 0 mmHg pressure in the deep veins so that fluid in the superficial veins moves to the deep veins, then proximally to the central system via the vena cava (see **TABLE 5-8**).

Lymph transport is dependent on a negative pressure gradient within all of the lymphatic vessels. In the lymphatic system, the negative pressure in the thoracic duct and right lymphatic duct allows the *fluid* to move from distal to proximal (**FIGURE 5-30**). In order to accomplish this, treatment has to begin centrally and proximally and progress distally as each lymphatic component reaches a state of negative pressure. The negative pressure in the lymphatic capillaries facilitates the movement of fluid from the interstitial tissue into the lymphatic system (deep to superficial). Lymph transport is dependent on a negative pressure gradient within all of the lymphatic vessels. Therefore, treatment is predicated upon creating a negative pressure gradient in the proximal vessels (ie, the thoracic duct and right lymphatic duct) first, and then creating a negative pressure gradient in the sequential vessels, proximal to distal.

Manual Lymphatic Drainage Mobilization

For patients with lymphedema, manual lymphatic drainage (MLD) mobilization directs the fluid to an unaffected lymph node region. MLD is a specialized massage technique that stretches the skin which then stimulates lymphangion contractions in the superficial lymph vessels. The technique requires just enough pressure to stretch the skin (termed the "on phase") and then a smooth release of the skin (termed the "off phase") without the clinician pushing the skin back to its original starting point. The direction of the skin stretch governs the direction of lymph flow. The strokes are smooth and rhythmical in nature (**FIGURE 5-31**). Seven to ten repetitions of each stroke are performed in each location, beginning with stimulation of the central vessels, and then progressing sequentially, proximal to distal, along the extremity while maintaining the skin stretch toward the desired endpoint of fluid flow. MLD is followed by compression to help prevent return of fluid to the previous state of congestion.[48,49]

Compression Therapy

In addition to mobilizing the fluid, compression is used to restore Starling's Law of Equilibrium to normal, and thereby reduce the visible edema. This is accomplished by reducing the capillary filtration rate, increasing the reabsorption rate, and providing support to lymph transportation. **TABLE 5-9** lists the different types of bandage and compression systems available and the indications for each type of compression.[49–51] Compression devices using Velcro straps are options for patients who have difficulty applying compression wraps and are discussed in the venous section of Chapter 4.

For lymphedema management, bandages are worn 20 out of 24 hours, thus allowing time out of the bandages each day for skin care, skin inspection, and laundering of the bandages (see **FIGURES 5-32** to **5-34**). The most effective plan of care involves reapplying the bandages daily until the fibrosis is

TABLE 5-8 Common Edema Diagnoses and Recommended Interventions

	AROM/ Joint Mobs	Compression Garments or Bandages	Muscle Strengthening	Gait Training	MLD/ Mobilization	Breathing Exercises	Aerobic Exercises	Skin Care	Patient Education
CVI	x	x	x	x				x	x
Secondary lymphedema	x	x	x	x	x	x	x	x	x
Lipedema		x	x	x	x	x		x	x
Orthopedic conditions with edema	x	x	x	x[a]	x	x		x	x
CVI/ lymphedema	x	x	x	x	x	x	x	x	x

[a]Gait training is conditional, depending on the injury and weight-bearing status.

The selection of intervention(s) is individualized based on the evaluation of the patients' activities and participation restrictions and not just the edema diagnosis.

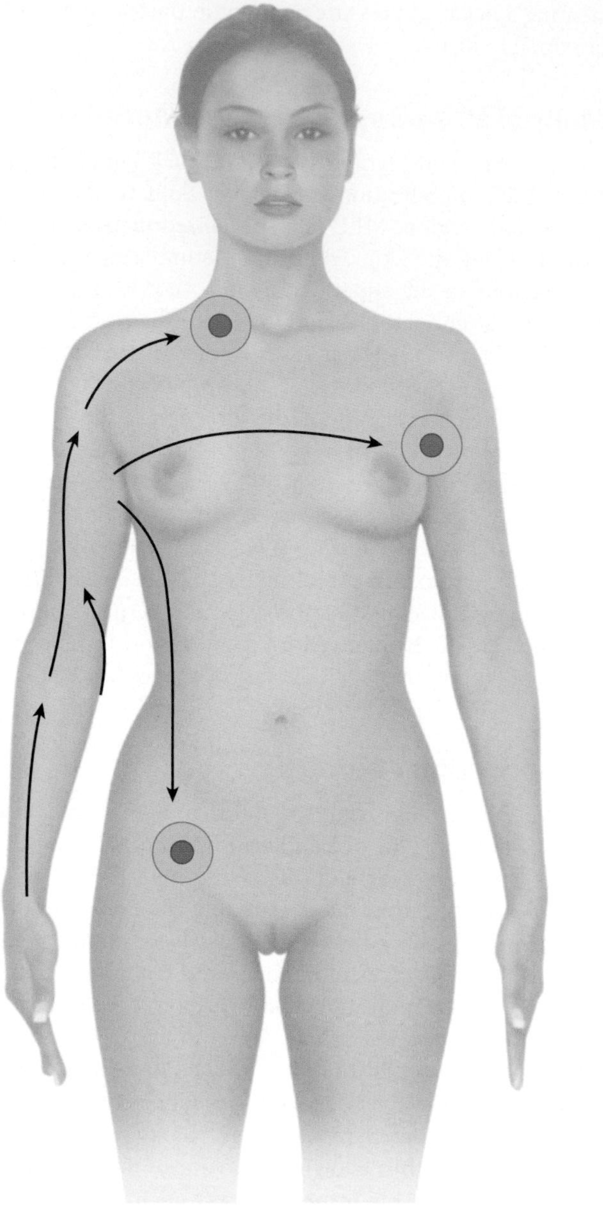

FIGURE 5-30 Flow of lymphatic fluid during manual lymphatic mobilization. Lymphatic fluid flows from deep to superficial, distal to proximal as a result of negative pressure created by manual lymphatic mobilization. The circles represent lymph node regions: supraclavicular, axillary, and inguinal. The arrows demonstrate potential lymph drainage pathways for an individual with right upper extremity lymphedema secondary to breast cancer. The therapist must decide if there are any contraindications to mobilizing lymph fluid to these alternate lymph node regions.

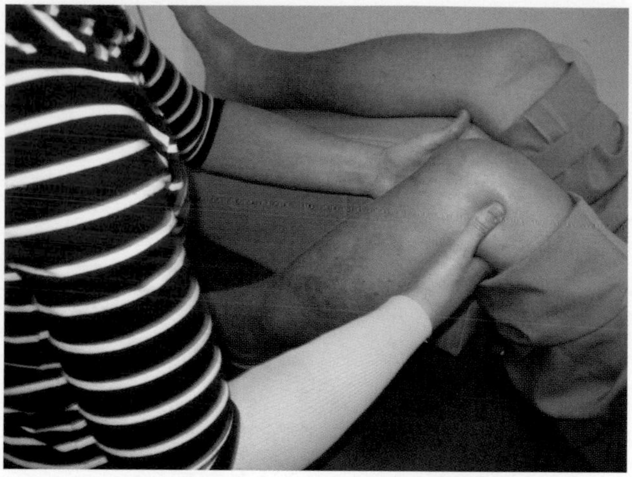

FIGURE 5-31 Manual lymphatic drainage mobilization. MLD mob requires specialized training and practice to be effective in moving lymphatic fluid from distal to proximal by first creating negative pressure in the proximal lymphatic structures, as well as moving the fluid from the deep tissue to the superficial lymphatic capillaries. In order for MLD to be effective, a negative pressure gradient is generated with diaphragmatic breathing and stimulation of the abdominal, supraclavicular, and cervical lymph node chains. The trunk is treated next, followed by the affected extremity proximal to distal. At the end of the treatment, the affected limb can be treated distal to proximal. MLD should be repeated with stimulation of cervical and supraclavicular lymph nodes and diaphragmatic breathing exercises. As with any intervention, the therapist must determine if any contraindications are present.

remodeled and the volume reduction has stabilized, at which point the patient is transitioned to a compression garment. Criteria for stabilized edema reduction include pliable tissue with no induration and no further decrease in girth for 7 to 10 days.

Selection and measurement for optimal garments are individualized to facilitate adherence to daily wear. Garments may be custom fit or over the counter; however, proper fit is of utmost importance. Generally, the larger and more fibrotic extremity requires a heavier garment with more coarse fabric and potentially a higher class of compression, provided the patient can tolerate the pressure (refer Table 4-11 for information about the classes of compression). **FIGURES 5-35** and **5-36** illustrate the flat-knit and circular-knit construction used for compression garments. Length of the garment is dependent on the extent of the edema (eg, if the edema is limited to below the knee, then a knee-high garment is appropriate; if the edema extends into or above the knee, a thigh-high or pantyhose garment is advised). Garments have a limited shelf-life of effective compression, ranging from 3 to 6 months, and need to be reordered according to the manufacturer's guidelines (**FIGURES 5-37** and **5-38**). Remeasurement and reassessment of the extremity are advised prior to reordering

CLINICAL CONSIDERATION

When performing manual lymphatic mobilization on a patient who has congestive heart failure, the clinician must be cautious not to overload the heart with fluid that is being moved from the periphery into the central vascular system. Evidence of overload can be assessed using the Borg Scale of Perceived Exertion, monitoring urinary output, and observing for signs of acute congestive heart failure. Caution may involve using limited interventions (eg, mild exercise and modified compression therapy) until the patient's response to treatment is evaluated.[52]

TABLE 5-9 Types of Bandage Systems and Indications

Long stretch bandages: provide high pressure at rest and low pressure with activity. Goal is to move fluid into the deep venous system. *Indications*: component of multilayer compression for CVI *Contraindications*: ABI < 0.8, vasculitis, lymphedema
Short stretch bandages: provide high pressure with activity and low pressure at rest. Goal is to decrease filtration and increase reabsorption and transportation of lymphatic fluid. *Indications:* lymphedema, lipedema, CVI with arterial compromise (ABI 0.5–0.8), traumatic edema, post-surgical swelling *Contraindications/precautions:* ABI < 0.5, insensate extremity, uncompensated congested heart failure, cellulitis (unless being treated)

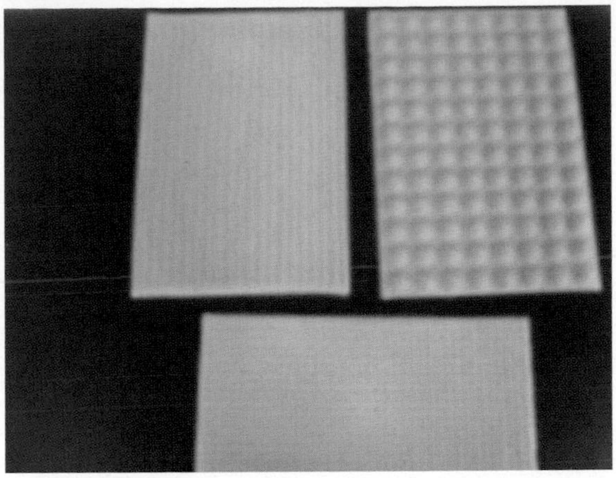

FIGURE 5-33 Foam used with compression. Convoluted foam is used under compression bandages to help soften the hard fibrotic subcutaneous tissue that can develop with prolonged chronic edema. The firmer the fibrosis, the denser the foam needs to be.

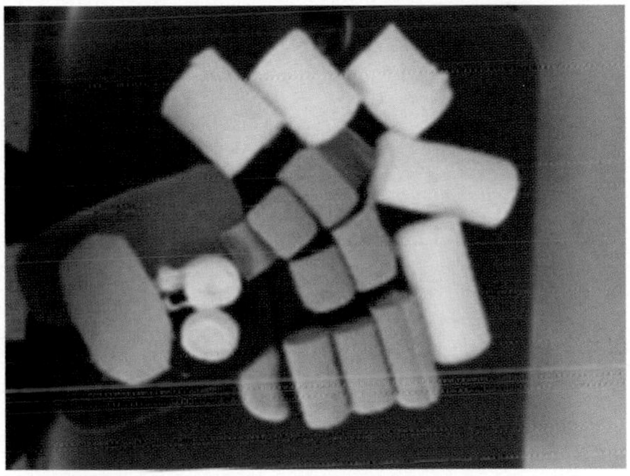

FIGURE 5-32 Components of a compression bandage kit. A compression bandage kit includes foam, narrow gauze rolls for the fingers or toes, soft cotton padding for the first layer against the skin, and short stretch bandages of various widths. Narrow bandages are used distally, and progressively wider bandages used as the application progresses proximally.

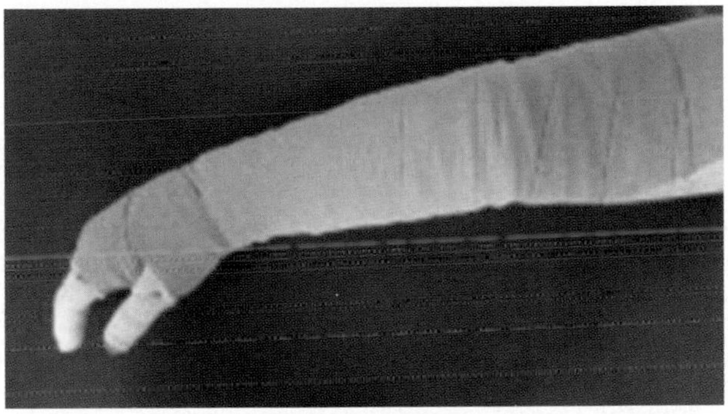

FIGURE 5-34 Compression bandages on an upper extremity. Upper extremity compression begins with wrapping the fingers with narrow gauze in multiple layers, then the hand in narrow short stretch bandages, and then the forearm and arm, using a figure-8 or chevron pattern with wider bandages.

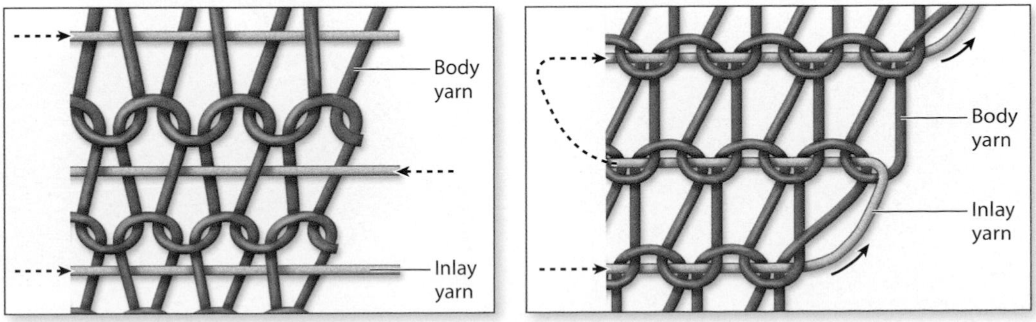

FIGURE 5-35 Flat-knit construction of compression garments. Flat-knit fabric is composed of the body yarn and the inlay yarn, and the tightness of the knit determines the coarseness of the fabric. Garments made of flat-knit fabric need to be stitched and are usually custom fit for better shape conformity. The total number of needles can be increased or decreased to produce variation in width and shape. The garments are generally coarser, less cosmetic, and stiffer; however, they are also better at bridging skin folds and less likely to cut the skin or cause a tourniquet effect.

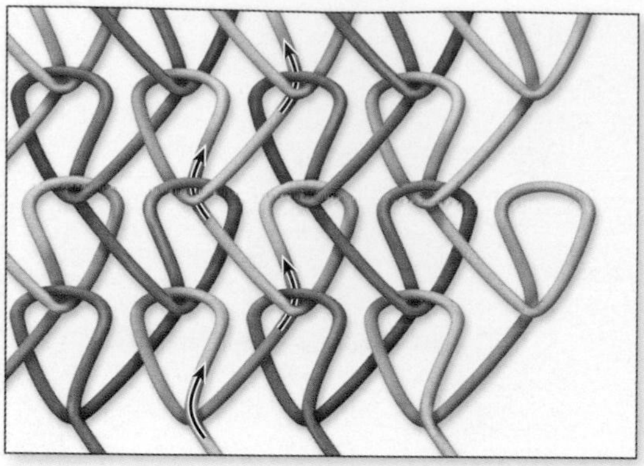

FIGURE 5-36 Circular knit of compression garments. Circular knit uses a fixed number of needles to produce a thinner fabric that is more cosmetically acceptable. It reduces the range of distortion but also increases the risk of creating a tourniquet effect if not properly fitted or donned.

garments in order to assure the optimal fit. Daily washing of the garment is recommended for skin integrity and for maintaining the proper pressure gradient.

Pumps

Compression pumps may be used as a complement to treatment of both venous and lymphatic pathologies (**FIGURE 5-39**). Venous pumps were designed based on the physiology of the venous system (intended to increase the venous return by generating high pressure in mmHg to promote reabsorption into the venous capillaries and facilitate flow through the superficial and deep veins), whereas the lymphatic pumps were designed based on the physiology of the lymphatic system (intended to increase the lymphatic circulation, central first and progressing sequentially proximal to distal). The lymphatic compression pump creates a negative pressure gradient within the thoracic duct, which then allows lymph fluid to move from an area of high pressure to low pressure. In other words, the proximal anatomical structures of the lymphatic system have to be emptied before the distal structures will drain. Studies have not demonstrated return of protein molecules with either of the pump systems[53]; however, research has demonstrated that the lymphatic pumps are more effective in reducing lymphedema than the venous pumps.[48,49,51]

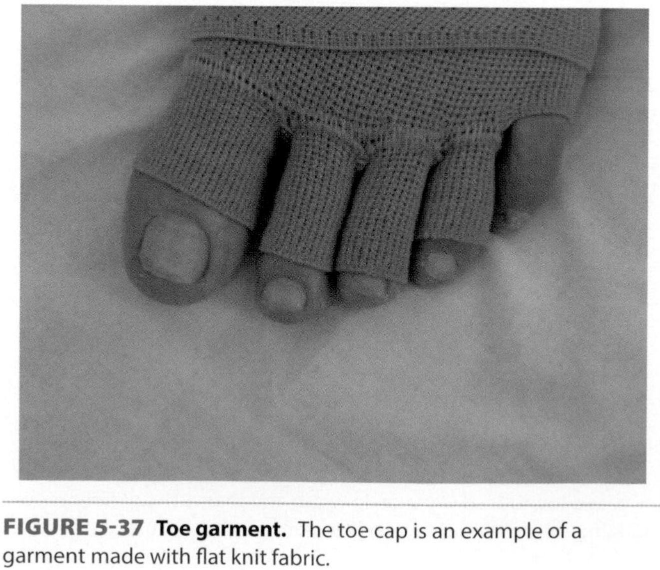

FIGURE 5-37 Toe garment. The toe cap is an example of a garment made with flat knit fabric.

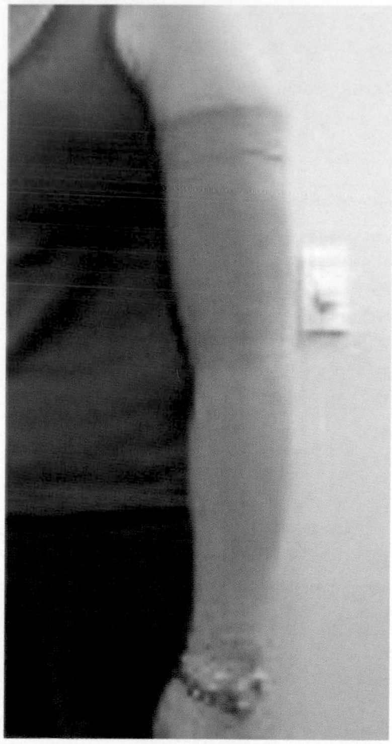

FIGURE 5-38 Upper extremity compression garment. The upper extremity garment is an example of construction with circular knit fabric.

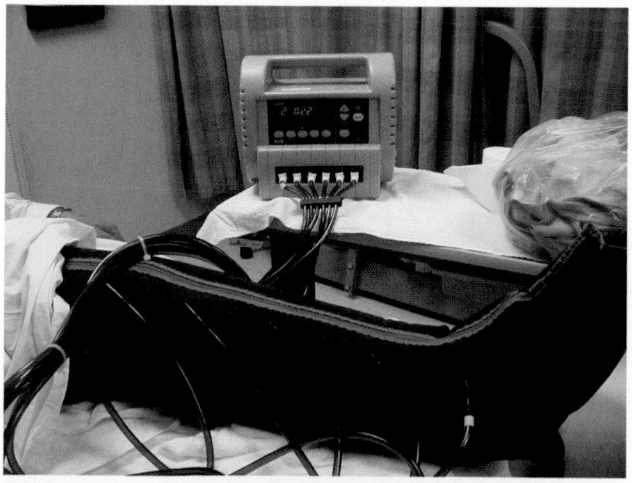

FIGURE 5-39 Intermittent compression pump for chronic venous insufficiency. The intermittent compression pump is an adjunct therapy for peripheral edema. It is beneficial initially for decreasing edema before applying compression, and after resolution, for long-term edema management for those patients who cannot don/doff any type of garment.

TABLE 5-10 Exercise Programs for the Upper and Lower Extremities

Upper extremity:	Lower extremity:
Diaphragmatic breathing	Diaphragmatic breathing
Abdominal exercises	Abdominal exercises
Neck rotations	Neck rotations
Shoulder circles	Shoulder circles
Shoulder to hand	Gluteal exercises (bridging)
Pectoralis major ex (PNF diagonal D1, horizontal humeral adduction)	Inguinal lymph node stimulation (knee to chest)
Scapular adduction (rowing, scapular retraction)	Anterior/posterior/lateral/medial thigh extension (open chain SLR in all four planes)
Latissimus (modified pull-down)	Knee flexion/extension
Internal/external rotation	Ankle (ankle pumps, circumduction)
Forward flexion to 90 degrees	Progress to closed chain exercises:
Elbow flexion/extension	Marching in place
Wrist flexion/extension/circles	Modified squats
Finger flexion/extension/abduction/adduction	Heel/toe raises
Begin the exercises for the upper extremity by working from the shoulder to the hand, and then work distal to proximal with emphasis on shoulder rotation, circles, and breathing.	Modified lunges
	Side-stepping
	Grapevine side to side
	Walking backward
	End with inguinal node stimulation and diaphragmatic breathing.

There are several different compression pumps for the management of lymphedema. Clinicians and patients need to carefully follow the manufacturer's recommendations regarding pressure gradients and on/off times. Not all compression pumps are designed to stimulate the thoracic duct prior to stimulating the involved extremity. Exercise and diaphragmatic breathing techniques can be performed prior to utilization of a compression pump when needed. Further research is needed to determine which compression pumps are most effective as well as determining what pressure gradients are most appropriate.

CLINICAL CONSIDERATION

Aquatherapy is contraindicated for any patient with an open wound, fragile skin, or insensate feet. Water exercises are beneficial for patients with very heavy limbs; however, meticulous skin care is required because of the effects of chlorine. Aqua shoes are recommended for patients with lower extremity lymphedema in order to reduce the risk of repetitive trauma to the plantar surface of the foot and subsequent viral, fungal, or bacterial infection. Any bony deformities of the feet and the interdigital spaces need to be inspected before and after every exercise session.

Exercise

Muscle contraction assists in lymphatic flow. The exercise sequence is based on the physiological flow of lymphatic fluid; therefore, a lymph drainage exercise program begins with central exercises to stimulate the thoracic duct, cisterna chyli, and right lymphatic duct. Diaphragmatic breathing and/or aerobic exercises are the best exercises to achieve a negative pressure gradient in these central vessels. The affected limb exercises begin proximally and progress distally, and then are performed distal to proximal, followed by stimulation of the central vessels. Exercises are individualized according to each patient's edema presentation and level of physical fitness. Resistive exercises can be safely incorporated into the sequence in order to strengthen the muscles and thereby increase the effectiveness of the muscle pump.[24]

Examples of exercise progression for the upper and lower extremity are listed in **TABLE 5-10**.[54]

Frequency, intensity, repetitions, and rest periods are based on the patient's level of physical fitness and exercise tolerance in order to prevent overloading the lymphatic system. All patients are advised to participate in a cardiovascular exercise program to stimulate the thoracic duct and cisterna chyli and to improve overall conditioning. Increased numbers of repetitions and weights, as well as shorter rest periods, may be added as the patient improves and the lymphedema decreases.

There are no special diets or restrictions for upper and lower extremity lymphedema; however, maintaining a normal BMI is strongly encouraged.

Skin Care

Consequences of poor skin hygiene can be cellulitis or erysipelas (defined as an infection of the upper dermis and superficial lymphatics). With lymphedema the skin becomes dry, flaky, and cracking, which may provide a portal for bacteria to enter the skin. The first line of defense is the hydrolipid layer in the epidermis. When the tissue is congested with lymph fluid, the white blood cells may not reach the pathogens to phagocytose the bacteria. In addition, the decrease in transport capacity does not allow for adequate removal of bacterial debris that is present. If the skin is weeping, the moisture accentuates the risk for bacterial colonization and possible infection. Following are recommendations for lymphedema skin care[55]:

- Moisturize with low pH, fragrant-free, hypoallergenic lotion, eg, a ceramide-containing emollient.
- Inspect the skin, interdigital spaces, and skin folds for cracks, blisters, and skin tears.
- Wash the skin daily with a mild hypoallergenic soap or moisturizing soap substitute; dry thoroughly with a clean towel, including the interdigital spaces.
- Seek podiatric care if the patient cannot reach the toenails.
- Do not cut cuticles (may cause skin openings that become infected); keep moisturized and pushed back.
- Wear protective gloves and shoes during activities that may cause minor trauma (eg, gardening, cooking); use an electric razor for shaving.
- Avoid overexposure to the sun because of the tendency to sun burn and blister.

CASE STUDY

CONCLUSION

DISCUSSION QUESTIONS

1. What are the preferred interventions for this patient?
2. What are the parameters for each of the interventions?
3. What are the patient-centered outcome measures?

The patient had CVI with secondary lymphedema. There was concern for arterial insufficiency due to his comorbidities; however, the ABI was sufficient for short stretch compression bandages (**FIGURE 5-40**). Compression was indicated only to the knee because the diagnosis was CVI with secondary lymphedema (note that the edema stops at the knee). The patient was on Lasix, which was a concern for fluid overload of the kidneys. After consultation with the MD regarding his medication, Lasix was increased and the patient and his family were trained to monitor body weight, orthostatic hypotension, and increased need to void.

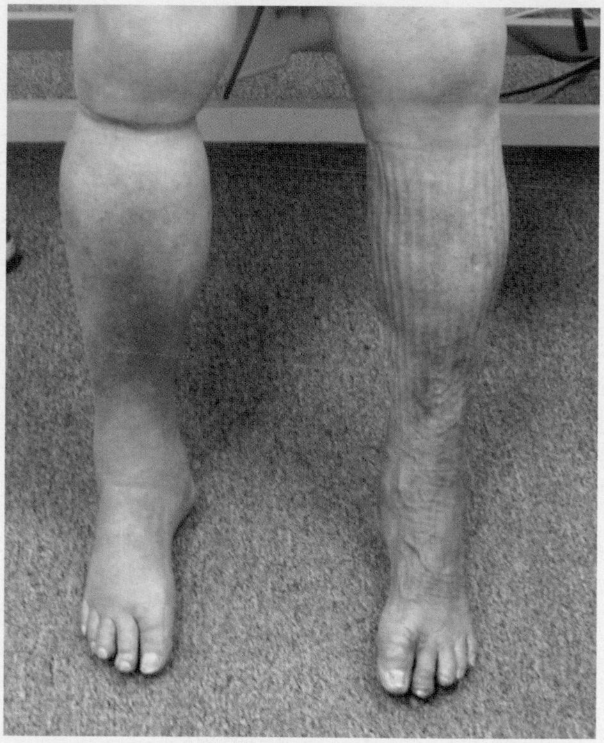

FIGURE 5-40 Case study after treatment. After treatment with MLD and compression therapy, the patient was transitioned to compression stockings. Note the indentation in the soft tissue on the right lower leg just below the knee. Such indentations are a result of inappropriate donning of the garment, resulting in restriction of lymphatic and venous return in places where there is high compression. This in turn causes a tourniquet effect with resulting increased edema below the constriction. This is observed in the larger size of the right calf as compared to the left.

Treatment goals:

Decrease edema by 50–75%.

Increase hip and ankle ROM.

Increase gluteal muscle strength to alleviate the Trendelenburg gait.

Functional goals:

Patient will be able to ambulate with heel/toe sequence sufficient to activate venous pump.

Patients will be able to play golf.

Interventions:

MLD.

Short stretch bandages to knee.

Exercise:

Supine ROM exercises proximal to distal with progression to weight bearing as strength and balance improved.

Patient was seen for 32 visits over a 4-month period.

Outcomes:

Improved 6-minute walk to 500 yards.

Performed 7 sit-to-stands in 30 seconds with UE assist.

Ambulated with rolling walker using heel-toe gait.

Managed edema with knee-high garments.

Practiced putting with stand-by assist of one person for safety.

SUMMARY

Peripheral edema is a symptom of an underlying pathology that must be identified in order to develop an effective plan of care for the patient. Differential diagnosis requires information on all of the body systems and information from all of the medical specialists involved in the patient's care. The goal is to determine if the edema is caused by lymphatic dysfunction, venous insufficiency, organ failure, or medications. An effective care plan requires treatment of the underlying disorders and sometimes changes in medication. Although there are overlaps in the treatment of lymphedema and CVI (eg, exercise and compression therapy), there are specific differences; thus, management of the specific system (lymphatic versus venous) is essential in order to have the optimal outcomes.

STUDY QUESTIONS

1. Lymphatic flow in the lower extremity is
   a. Deep to superficial.
   b. Superficial to deep.
   c. Anterior to posterior.
   d. Posterior to anterior.
2. Which of the following mechanisms is not effective in assisting lymphatic flow?
   a. Diaphragmatic breathing
   b. Positive pressure gradient within the lymphatic system
   c. Muscle contractions
   d. Smooth muscle in the walls of the collecting vessels
3. Which of the following characteristics are associated with Stage III lymphedema?
   a. Hard non-pitting edema and presence of skin folds
   b. Mild fibrosis and pitting edema
   c. Normal joint range of motion and strength
   d. Negative Stemmer test and loss of skin mobility
4. A 62-year-old retired postal worker presents with the following symptoms: heaviness and aching in both lower extremities, hemosiderin stains on the lower 1/3 of the legs, bilateral edema from the dorsum of the foot to below the knee, positive Stemmer sign bilaterally, mild to moderate fibrosis in the lower leg, and 3+ distal pulses. Medical history is negative for diabetes. What is the most likely diagnosis for this patient?
   a. Kidney insufficiency
   b. Cardiac insufficiency
   c. Primary lymphedema
   d. CVI with secondary lymphedema
5. The most effective intervention for Stage II lymphedema is
   a. Education, garments, and MLD.
   b. Diuretics, garment, and exercise.
   c. MLD, compression therapy, and exercise.
   d. Education, compression pump, and diuretics.

Answers: 1-a; 2-b; 3-a; 4-d; 5-c

REFERENCES

1. Foldi M, StroBenreuther R. Lymph formation and lymph flow: physiological lymph drainage. In: Foldi M, StroBenreuther R, eds. *Foundations of Manual Lymph Drainage*. 3rd ed. St. Louis, MO: Elsevier Mosby; 2005:28-38.
2. Marieb EN. *Human Anatomy & Physiology*. 6th ed. London: Pearson; 2004:736-738, 773.
3. Rockson SG. Current concepts and future directions in the diagnosis and management of lymphatic vascular disease. *Vasc Med*. 2010; 15(3):223-231.
4. Levick JR, Michel CC. Microvascular fluid exchange and the revised Starling principle. *Cardiovasc Res*. 2010;87(2):198-210.
5. Michel CC, Woodcock TE, Curry Fitz-Roy E. Understanding and extending the Starling principle. *ACTA*. 2020;64:1032-1037.
6. Little RC, Ginsburg JM. The physiologic basis for clinical edema. *Arch Intern Med*. 1984;144:1661-1664.
7. Tiwari A, Cheng K, Button M, Myint F, Hamilton G. Differential diagnosis, investigation, and current treatment of lower limb Lymphedema. *Arch Surg*. 2003;138(2):152-161.
8. Sontheimer DL. Peripheral vascular disease: diagnosis and treatment. *Am Fam Physician*. 2006;73(11):1971-1976.
9. Zuther JE, Norton S. *Lymphedema Management: The Comprehensive Guide for Practitioners*. 4th ed. New York, NY: Thieme Medical Publishers; 2018.
10. Foldi E, Foldi E. Physiology and pathophysiology of the lymphatic system. In: Foldi E, Foldi M, eds. *Foldi Textbook of Lymphology*. 2nd ed. Munich: Elsevier; 2006:179-222.
11. Cormier JN, Askew RL, Mungovan KS, Xing Y, Ross MI, Armer JM. Lymphedema beyond breast cancer: a systematic review and meta-analysis of cancer-related secondary lymphedema. *Cancer*. 2010;116(22):5138-5149.
12. Norman SA, Localio AR, Potashnick SL, et al. Lymphedema in breast cancer survivors: incidence, degree, time course, treatment and symptoms. *J Clin Oncol*. 2009;27(3):390-397.
13. Lucci A, McCall LM, Beitsch PD, et al. Surgical complications associated with sentinel lymph node dissection (SLND) plus axillary lymph node dissection compared with SLND alone in the American college of Surgeons Oncology Group Trial Z0011. *J Clin Oncol*. 2007; 25:3657-3663.
14. Shin BW, Sim YJ, Jeong HJ, Kim GC. Lipedema, a rare disease. *Ann Rehabil Med*. 2011;35:922-927.
15. Child AH, Gordon KD, Sharpe P, et al. Lipedema: an inherited condition. *Am J Med Genet A*. 2010;152A:970-976.
16. Warren AG, Janz BA, Borud LJ, Stavin SA. Evaluation and management of fat leg syndrome. *Plast Reconstr Surg*. 2007;119:9e-15e.
17. International Society of Lymphology. The diagnosis and treatment of peripheral lymphedema: consensus document of the International Society of Lymphology. *Lymphology*. 2003(36):84-91.
18. Newman B, Lose F, Kedda MA, et al. Possible genetic predispostion to lymphedema after breast cancer. *Lymphat Res Bio*. 2012;10(1):2-13.
19. Armer JM, Stewart BR. A comparison of four diagnostic criteria for lymphedema in a post-breast cancer population. *Lymphat Res Biol*. 2005;3:208-217.
20. Gartner R, Jensen MB, Kronborg L, et al. Self-reported arm lymphedema and functional impairment after breast cancer treatment: a nationwide study of prevalence and associated factors. *Breast*. 2010;19:506-515.
21. Mortimer PS. Managing lymphedema. *Clin Dermatol*. 1995;13:499-505.

22. Ely JW, Osheroff JA, Chambliss ML, Ebell MH. Approach to leg edema of unclear etiology. *J Am Board Fam Med*. 2006;19:148-160.
23. Levenhagen K, Davies C, Perdomo M, Ryans K, Gilchrist L. Diagnosis of upper quadrant lymphedema secondary to cancer: clinical practice guidelines from the Oncology Section of the American Physical Therapy Association. *Phys Ther*. 2017;97(7):729-745.
24. Davies C, Levenhagen K, Ryans K, Perdomo M, Gilchrist L. Interventions for breast cancer-related lymphedema: clinical practice guideline from the Academy of Oncologic Physical Therapy of APTA. *Phys Ther*. 2020;100 (7):1163-1179.
25. Perdomo M, Davies C, Levenhagen K, Ryans K. Breast cancer edge task force outcomes: assessment measures of secondary lymphedema in breast cancer survivors. *Rehabil Oncol*. 2014;32(1):22-35.
26. Megens AM, Harris SR, Kim-Sing C, McKenzie DC. Measurement of upper extremity volume in women after axillary dissection for breast cancer. *Arch Phys Med Rehabil*. 2001;82:1639-1644.
27. Szuba A, Shin WS, Strauss HW, Rockson S. The third circulation: radionuclide lymphoscintigraphy in the evaluation of lymphedema. *J Nucl Med*. 2003;44:43-57.
28. Partsch H. Assessment of abnormal lymph drainage for the diagnosis of lymphedema by isotopic lymphangiography and by indirect lymphography. *Clin Dermatol*. 1995;13(5):445-450.
29. Rasmussen JC, Tan I, Marshall MV, Fife CE, Sevick-Muraca EM. Lymphatic imaging in humans with near-infrared fluorescence. *Curr Opin Biotechnol*. 2009;20(1):74-82.
30. Marshall MV, Rasmussen JC, Tan I, et al. Near-infrared fluorescence imagin in humans with indocyanin green: a review and update. *Open Surg Oncol J*. 2010;2(2):12-25.
31. Rockson SG. A Role for US in the diagnostic evaluation of lymphedema. *Lymphat Res Biol*. 2021;19(4):321.
32. Erdinç Gündüz N, Dilek B, Şahin E, Ellidokuz H, Akalın E. Diagnostic contribution of ultrasonography in breast cancer-related lymphedema. *Lymphat Res Biol*. 2021;19(6):517-523.
33. Kim SY, Lee CH, Heo SJ, Moon MH. The clinical usefulness of lymphedema measurement technique using ultrasound. *Lymphat Res Biol*. 2021;19(4):340-346.
34. Koehler LA, Mayrovitz HN. Tissue dielectric constant measures in women with and without clinical trunk lymphedema following breast cancer surgery: a 78-week longitudinal study. *Phys Ther*. 2020;100(8):1384-1392.
35. Liu Y, Long X, Guan J. Tissue dielectric constant combined with arm volume measurement as complementary methods in detection and assessment of breast cancer-related lymphedema. *Lymphat Res Biol*. 2022;20(1):26-32.
36. Mayrovitz HN. Tissue dielectric constant of the lower leg as an index of skin water: temporal variations. *Cureus*. 2022;14(7):e26506.
37. Pusic AL, Cemal Y, Albornoz C, et al. Quality of life among breast cancer patients with lymphedema: a systematic review of patient-reported outcome instruments and outcomes. *J Cancer Surviv*. 2013;7(1):83-92.
38. Devoogdt N, DeGroef A, Hendrickx A, et al. Lymphoedema functioning, disability and health questionnaire for lower limb lymphoedema (Lymph-ICF-LL): reliability and validity. *Phys Ther*. 2014;94(5):705-721.
39. Blome C, Augustin M, Heyer K, et al. Evaluation of patient-relevant outcomes of lymphedema and lipedema treatment: development and validation of a new benefit tool. *Eur J Vasc Endovasc Surg*. 2014;47(1):100-107.
40. Augustin M, Condo Montero E, Hagenstrom K, Herberger K, Blome C. Validation of a short form FLQA-LS quality of life instrument for lymphedema. *Br J Dermatol*. 2018;179(6):1329-1333.
41. Klein TM, Bal B, Newi AL, et al. Psychometric properties of the short version of the Freiburg life quality assessment for chronic venous disease. *J Vasc Surg Venous Lymphat Disord*. 2022;10(1):139-145.e1.
42. Augustin M, Herberger K, Rustenbach SJ, Schäfer I, Zschocke I, Blome C. Quality of life evaluation in wounds: validation of the Freiburg life quality assessment-wound module, a disease-specific instrument. *Int Wound J*. 2010;7:493-501.
43. Bunke N, Brown K, Bergan J. Phlebolymphemeda: usually unrecognized, often poorly treated. *Perspect Vasc Surg Endovasc Ther*. 2009;21(2):65-68.
44. Schaverien MV, Coroneos CJ. Surgical treatment of lymphedema. *Plast Reconstr Surg*. 2019;144(3):738-758.
45. Park KE, Chandler L, Mozzafari MA, Ly C, Lu X, Persing JA. Surgical management of lymphedema: a review of current literature. *Gland Surg*. 2022;9(2):503-511.
46. Mayrovitz HN. The standard of care for lymphedema: current concepts and physiological considerations. *Lymphat Res Biol*. 2009;7(2):101-108.
47. Oremus M, Walker K, Dayes I, Raina P. *Diagnosis and Treatment of Secondary Lymphedema*. AHRQ Technology Assessment Report Project ID: LYMTO9O8; 2010.
48. Huang TW, Tseng SH, Lin CC, et al. Effects of manual lymphatic drainage on breast cancer-related lymphedema: a systematic review and meta-analysis of randomized controlled trials. *World J Surg Oncol*. 2013;11:15.
49. Kerchner K, Fleischer A, Yosipovitch G. Lower extremity lymphedema update: pathophysiology, diagnosis, and treatment guidelines. *J Am Acad Dermatol*. 2008;59:324-331.
50. Preston N, Seers K, Mortimer P. Physical therapies for reducing and controlling lymphedema of the limbs. *Cochrane Database Syst Rev*. 2008(4):CD003141.
51. Rabe E, Partsch H, Hafner J, et al. Indications for medical compression stockings in venous and lymphatic disorders: an evidence-based consensus statement. *Phlebology*. 2018;33(3):163-184.
52. Vaassen MM. Manual lymph drainage in a patient with congestive heart failure: a case study. *Ostomy Wound Manage*. 2015;61(10): 38-45.
53. Feldman JL, Stout NL, Wanchai A, Stewart BR, Cormier JN, Armer JM. Intermittent pneumatic compressin therapy: a systematic review. *Lymphology*. 2012;45:13-25.
54. Chang CJ, Cormier JN. Lymphedema interventions: exercise, surgery and compression devices. *Semin Oncol Nurs*. 2013;29(1):28-40.
55. Fife C, Farrow W, Hevert AA, et al. Skin and wound care in lymphedema patients: a taxonomy, primer, and literature review. *Adv Skin Wound Care*. 2017;30(7):305-318.

Pressure Injuries and Ulcers

Aimée D. Garcia, MD, CWS, FACCWS

CHAPTER OBJECTIVES

At the end of this chapter, the learner will be able to:

1. **Understand the impact of pressure injuries on the healthcare system**
2. **Identify the factors leading to pressure injury and ulcer development.**
3. **List strategies for prevention of pressure injuries.**
4. **Complete a risk assessment scale to determine pressure injury risk.**
5. **Effectively implement strategies for pressure load management.**
6. **List and define the categories of bed types.**
7. **Describe proper wheelchair positioning to prevent tissue injury.**
8. **Define the National Pressure Injury Advisory Panel pressure injury and ulcer stages.**
9. **Discuss the elements of proper pressure ulcer treatment.**

INTRODUCTION

The National Pressure Injury Advisory Panel (NPIAP) defines a pressure injury as "**localized damage to the skin and/or underlying tissue, as a result of pressure or pressure in combination with shear. Pressure injuries usually occur over a bony prominence but may also be related to a medical or other object.**"[1] Despite the advances in technology in the last 10 years, pressure injuries continue to be a major healthcare issue. US Agency for Healthcare Research and Quality reports an increased pressure injury rate of 6% between 2014 and 2017. It is the only hospital-acquired condition rate that continues to increase nationwide.[2] Pressure injuries are noted to be the second most common diagnosis in US Healthcare system billing records and account for 60,000 deaths per year.[3] The incidence of pressure injuries is ~5–15% in the acute care setting, with higher rates reported in the ICU setting.[4] In long-term care, incidence can be ~25%. The highest risk populations continue to be spinal cord injury patients and the elderly. In a study by Margolis et al., it was determined that as compared to those 65 to 70 years of age, those over 80 years of age were 4 to 20 times more likely to develop a pressure ulcer.[5,6]

The cost of hospital-acquired pressure injuries is a significant burden to the healthcare system. A study by Padula and Delarmente showed that based on 2016 dollars, the cost of pressure injuries in the United States would exceed 26.8 billion dollars, with 56% of these pressure injuries being stage 3 or 4.[3] In the United Kingdom, the cost has been estimated at £2.2 billion annually which consumes 4% of the healthcare budget.[7] Given that the population continues to age and the majority of pressure injuries occur in individuals over the age of 70, it can be expected that the burden on the healthcare system will continue to increase unless we can significantly improve the development or worsening of pressure injuries.[8]

PATHOPHYSIOLOGY

Pressure injuries and ulcers occur primarily due to immobility; however, other factors such as moisture, friction, and shear also impact the formation of tissue damage and skin breakdown.* Moisture, as a risk factor for skin breakdown, can be defined as excess fluid against the skin (**FIGURE 6-1**). This can occur secondary to incontinence, wound drainage, or excessive perspiration. Excess moisture causes maceration of the skin, which makes it more vulnerable to friction and shear forces. Friction is the force caused by two surfaces rubbing against each other (**FIGURE 6-2**). These forces abrade the epidermis and lead to a decrease in strength and skin integrity, as well as a possible increase in shear in the deeper layers of tissue. The heels are the most common site of friction forces, and damage commonly presents as a blister, which can be filled with either serous fluid or blood, depending on the depth of the tissue injury (and appropriately termed as pressure injury).[9]

Shear forces occur when parallel forces move in opposite directions, such as a patient sliding down in the bed. The force damages capillaries with bleeding into the interstitial tissue which in turn leads to tissue anoxia and tissue necrosis. Shear forces causing deep tissue necrosis can lead to undermining and sinus tracts in pressure injuries. (**FIGURE 6-3**).

The most common sites for the development of pressure injuries are the sacrum, ischial tuberosities, trochanters, and heels; however, they can occur on any part of the body where

* Editor's note: Because of the recent discussion about definitions of pressure damage, in this chapter *injury* refers specifically to any deep tissue damage with the skin intact and *ulcer* refers to any tissue loss that involves the skin. Specific terms used in references are also used in the text; otherwise, in some cases, the terms may be used interchangeably.

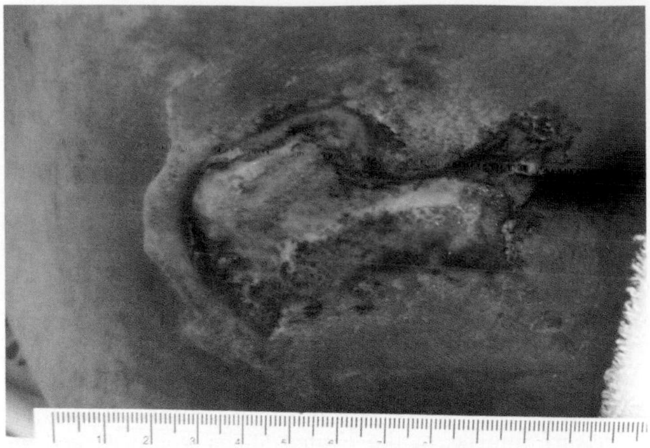

FIGURE 6-1 Moisture on skin. Moisture is one of the contributing factors to pressure ulcers, especially in the perineal and perianal areas. The changes in skin as a result of prolonged exposure include maceration, blanched color, and a papillary-like texture, as seen on the area around this sacral pressure ulcer. The drainage can be fecal, urinary, or wound moisture. In addition, the moisture can cause changes in the skin pH, especially in the case of fecal incontinence, which further weakens the skin and increases the risk of tissue damage.

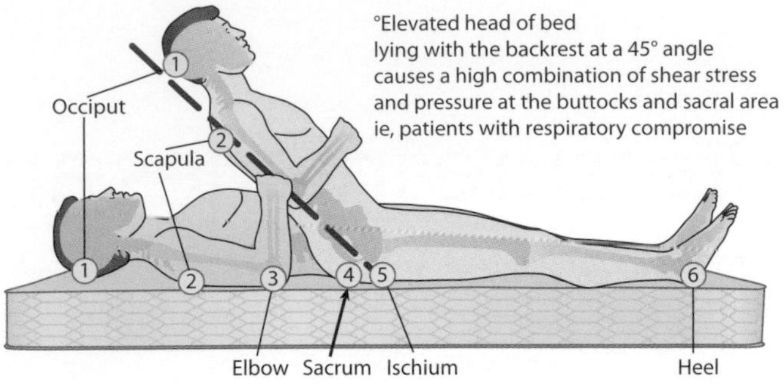

FIGURE 6-3 Shear.

there is unrelieved pressure between an external surface and a bony prominence for a prolonged period of time.[10] The location of pressure injury risk changes whether the patient is lying supine or sitting. If the patient is supine, the most common sites will be the sacrum and heels, but in a seated position, the greatest pressure will be on the ischial tuberosities (**FIGURE 6-4**). The amount of time leading to destruction varies as described in **TABLE 6-1**. Reversal of tissue necrosis may or may not occur depending on the patient's clinical comorbidities, the healing potential, and adequate pressure redistribution. Skin ulceration is an open wound that occurs within 2 weeks of tissue necrosis.[11] There is an inverse time/pressure curve to skin necrosis, meaning the higher the amount of sustained, unrelieved pressure, the shorter the time frame in which tissue death can occur (**FIGURE 6-5**).[12,13]

Given that the highest rates of pressure injuries occur on the sacrum, trochanters, and heels, it is estimated that 70% of pressure injuries occur from the waist down. Healthcare professionals have an obligation to monitor patient skin and to implement a care plan to prevent pressure injuries from occurring or to facilitate healing of any pressure ulcers a patient may develop. The purpose of this chapter is to educate the healthcare professional on prevention, assessment, and treatment of pressure injuries and ulcers.

PREVENTION

The prevention of pressure injury begins with a thorough assessment of the patient's skin. Once this is complete, *any lesions* (or lack of) of any etiology are documented in the medical record by the evaluating clinician who documents and photographs the existing wounds; however, the MD must

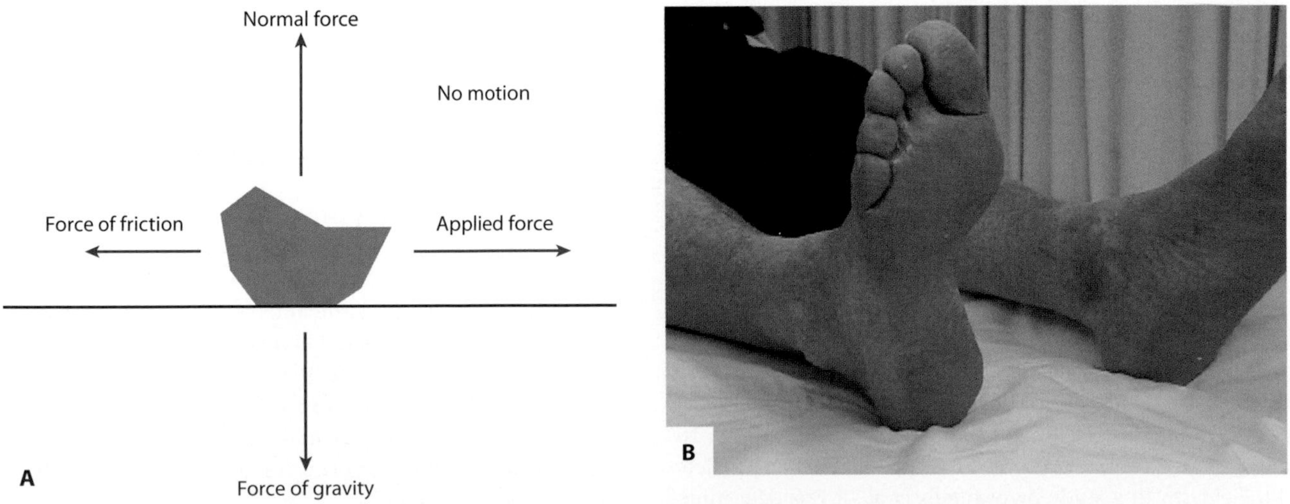

FIGURE 6-2 A, B. Friction is defined as the force that results when two objects rub against each other. When skin moves back and forth over a surface (eg, heels on the bed linens), friction occurs and causes erosion of the epidermis and/or blistering between the epidermis and dermis. The schematic demonstrates the small surface area of the heel that becomes the surface area in contact with the bed surface, and the photograph illustrates the most common source of friction, heels rubbing on the bed linen.

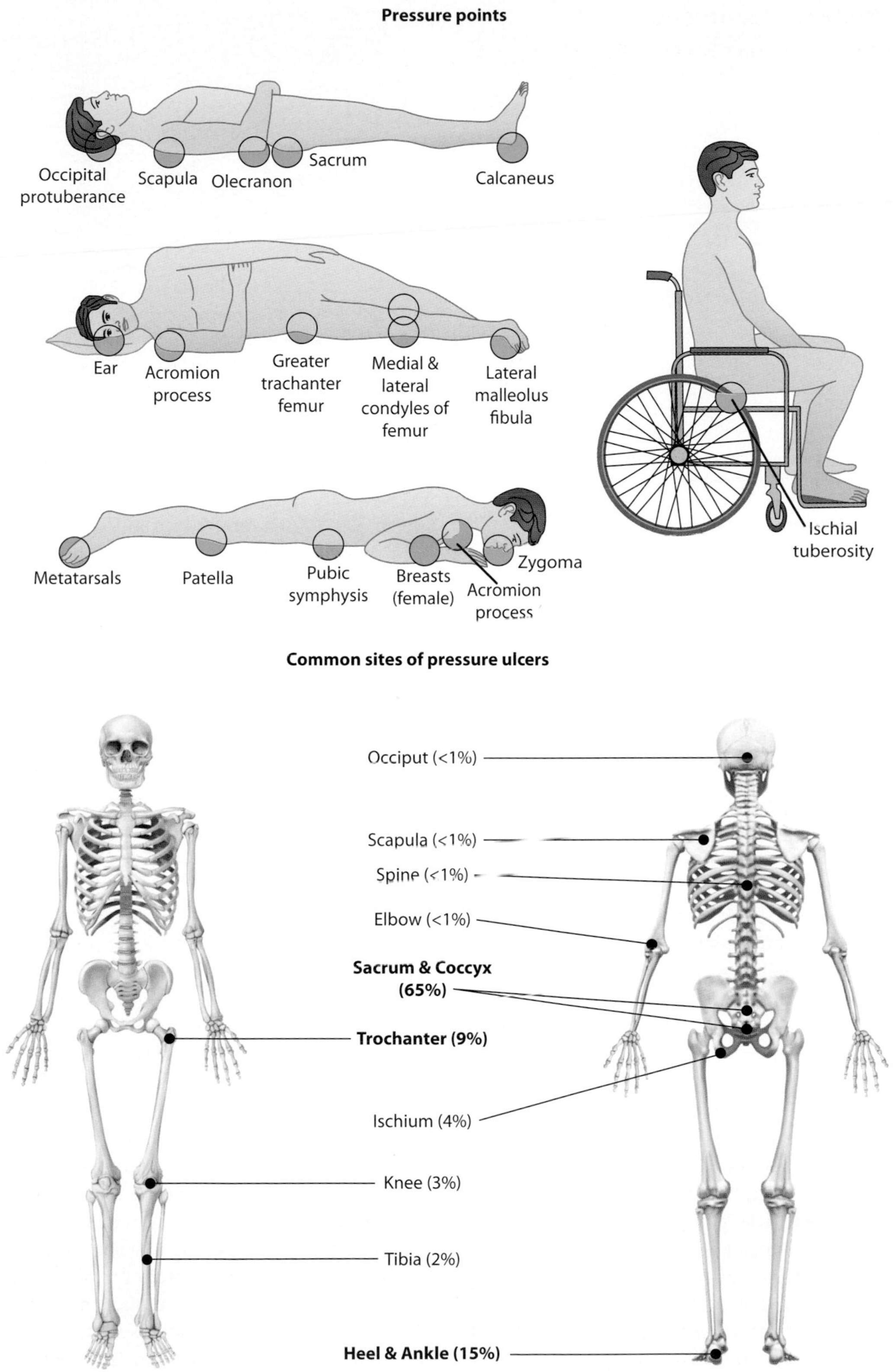

FIGURE 6-4 Areas of the body at risk for pressure injuries. By definition, pressure injuries and ulcers develop from mechanical forces applied over bony prominences where there is little or no soft tissue to dissipate the forces (friction, shear, or direct pressure). The most vulnerable areas depend upon the individual's body build.

TABLE 6-1 Time to Tissue Destruction

Tissue Damage	Definition	Time Frame	Time to Recovery
Tissue hyperemia	Blanchable erythema or redness	30 minutes	1 hour if pressure is relieved
Tissue ischemia	Deeper redness with damage of the underlying tissue	2–6 hours of unrelieved pressure	36 hours if pressure is relieved
Necrosis	Destruction of tissue	>6 hours of unrelieved pressure	Reversal of tissue necrosis may or may not occur depending on the patient's clinical comorbidities and their healing potential

Tissue damage is dependent on the time and intensity of exposure to the mechanical forces, and recovery without ulceration varies according to the patient's healing potential.[10]

Adapted from Bates-Jensen BM. Pressure ulcers: pathophysiology, detection, and prevention. In: Sussman C, Bates-Jensen BM, eds. *Wound Care: A Collaborative Practice Manual for Health Professionals*. Baltimore, MD: Lippincott Williams & Wilkins; 2012:230-277.

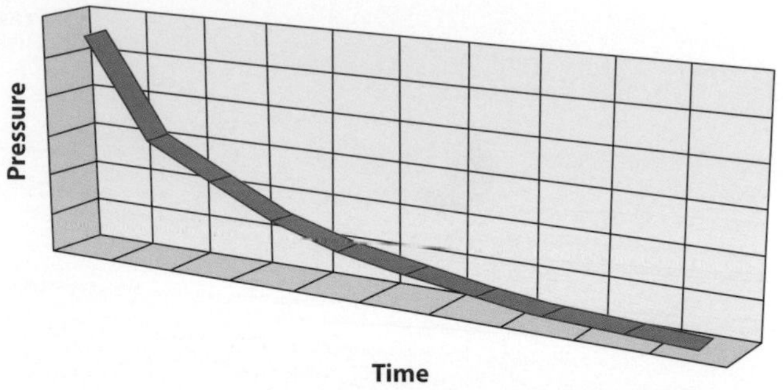

FIGURE 6-5 Time/pressure curve for pressure ulcer formation. Tissue damage can occur with prolonged exposure to low pressures or short exposure to high forces, depending on the body morphology, the surface, and the underlying comorbidities. Thus, care plans need to be individualized to the patient's medical status, body type, and risk factors.

sign the documentation within 48 hours of admission. Not only is this good clinical practice, but as of October 2008, the Center for Medicare and Medicaid Services (CMS) has linked payment of the higher Diagnostic Related Group (DRG) associated with pressure ulcers to this documentation.[14] An assessment tool for the risk of skin breakdown is advised both on admission and periodically thereafter. The most common and most validated scale used in the United States is the Braden scale (**TABLE 6-2**).[15,16]

This tool assesses six parameters, including activity, mobility, nutrition, sensory perception, moisture, and friction/shear. The highest possible score on examination is 23; any score less than 18 is considered at risk. This scale, however, is not meant to replace clinical judgment. The assessment is also subject to change depending on the patient's medical condition; therefore, it needs to be rescored if changes in the clinical assessment occur. For example, when admitted to the hospital for an elective knee surgery, the patient is usually alert and oriented, able to toilet independently, has limited activity and mobility due to knee pain, but is eating well and has no issues with friction or shear. That patient would have a Braden score of 21 and would be considered at low risk for pressure ulcer development. If the patient has complications during surgery and cannot be weaned off of the ventilator, the medical status changes. The patient is now in an ICU setting, intubated, sedated, and incontinent, and therefore at moderate risk for friction/shear when being turned and repositioned. The nutrition is adequate because parenteral nutrition is initiated. This patient now has a Braden score of 10 and is considered at high risk for pressure ulcer formation.

Once risk is assessed, prevention strategies are implemented to minimize the risk of skin breakdown. The first of these strategies is turning and repositioning, which will be discussed in detail. Use of pressure redistribution surfaces for both the bed and the wheelchair will help reduce pressure on bony prominences. Another aspect of prevention is management of the medical factors that can put patients at higher risk for skin breakdown. Containment of urinary or fecal incontinence, protection of the skin with a moisture barrier or silicone-backed foam dressing,[13] assessment and maximization of the patient's nutrition, improved mobility, and proper management of underlying medical conditions such as diabetes and hypertension are several strategies that decrease the risk of skin breakdown.

INTERVENTIONS TO MANAGE TISSUE LOADING

As described above, both the magnitude and duration of tissue loading are important in the prevention of tissue damage. When a pressure injury or ulcer is present, managing the duration and magnitude of loading requires a greater level of attention and is accomplished by using bed support surfaces and wheelchair cushions. These devices are designed to redistribute pressures away from the primary load-bearing parts of the body that are the areas at the highest risk for skin and subcutaneous tissue damage. Clinically, managing the *duration* of loading is accomplished with postural changes that redistribute loads away from tissues for periods of time (eg, with turning schedules for persons in bed and with weight-shifting activities for persons sitting in wheelchairs). In addition, some cushions and support surfaces can actively change their load redistribution properties to reduce the duration of loading.

Research has not defined a specific threshold for an acceptable magnitude of pressure on tissues. Without a clear mandate of acceptable loading on the tissues, clinicians are challenged to manage loads through interventions that must take into account ever-changing technology and the physiology and anatomical structure of any particular patient. Decisions about appropriate interventions can be facilitated by a working knowledge of support surfaces and positioning technologies, as well as the benefits and deficiencies of different designs.

TABLE 6-2 Braden Scale for Predicting Pressure Sore Risk

PATIENT'S NAME ______	EVALUATOR'S NAME ______			DATE OF ASSESSMENT				
SENSORY PERCEPTION Ability to respond meaningfully to pressure-related discomfort	**1. Completely Limited** Unresponsive (does not moan, flinch, or grasp) to painful stimuli, due to diminished level of consciousness or sedation. OR Limited ability to feel pain over most of body.	**2. Very Limited** Responds only to painful stimuli. Cannot communicate discomfort except by moaning or restlessness. OR Has a sensory impairment, which limits the ability to feel pain or discomfort over half of body.	**3. Slightly Limited** Responds to verbal commands, but cannot always communicate discomfort or the need to be turned. OR Has some sensory impairment, which limits ability to feel pain or discomfort in one or two extremities.	**4. No Impairment** Responds to verbal commands. Has no sensory deficit, which would limit ability to feel or voice pain or discomfort.				
MOISTURE Degree to which skin is exposed to moisture	**1. Constantly Moist** Skin is kept moist almost constantly by perspiration, urine, etc. Dampness is detected every time patient is moved or turned.	**2. Very Moist** Skin is often, but not always, moist. Linen must be changed at least once a shift.	**3. Occasionally Moist** Skin is occasionally moist, requiring an extra linen change approximately once a day.	**4. Rarely Moist** Skin is usually dry, linen only requires changing at routine intervals.				
ACTIVITY Degree of physical activity	**1. Bedfast** Confined to bed.	**2. Chairfast** Ability to walk severely limited or nonexistent. Cannot bear own weight and/or must be assisted into chair or wheelchair.	**3. Walks Occasionally** Walks occasionally during day, but for very short distances, with or without assistance. Spends majority of each shift in bed or chair.	**4. Walks Frequently** Walks outside room at least twice a day and inside room at least once every 2 hours during waking hours.				
MOBILITY Ability to change and control body position	**1. Completely Immobile** Does not make even slight changes in body or extremity position without assistance.	**2. Very Limited** Makes occasional slight changes in body or extremity position but unable to make frequent or significant changes independently.	**3. Slightly Limited** Makes frequent though slight changes in body or extremity position independently.	**4. No Limitation** Makes major and frequent changes in position without assistance.				
NUTRITION *Usual* food intake pattern	**1. Very Poor** Never eats a complete meal. Rarely eats more than one-third of any food offered. Eats two servings or less of protein (meat or dairy products) per day. Takes fluids poorly. Does not take a liquid dietary supplement. OR Is NPO and/or maintained on clear liquids or IV's for more than 5 days.	**2. Probably Inadequate** Rarely eats a complete meal and generally eats only about half of any food offered. Protein intake includes only three servings of meat or dairy products per day. Occasionally will take a dietary supplement. OR Receives less than optimum amount of liquid diet or tube feeding.	**3. Adequate** Eats over half of most meals. Eats a total of four servings of protein (meat, dairy products) per day. Occasionally will refuse a meal, but will usually take a supplement when offered. OR Is on a tube feeding or TPN regimen, which probably meets most of nutritional needs.	**4. Excellent** Eats most of every meal. Never refuses a meal. Usually eats a total of four or more servings of meat and dairy products. Occasionally eats between meals. Does not require supplementation.				
FRICTION AND SHEAR	**1. Problem** Requires moderate to maximum assistance in moving. Complete lifting without sliding against sheets is impossible. Frequently slides down in bed or chair, requiring frequent repositioning with maximum assistance. Spasticity, contractures, or agitation leads to almost constant friction.	**2. Potential Problem** Moves feebly or requires minimum assistance. During a move skin probably slides to some extent against sheets, chair, restraints, or other devices. Maintains relatively good position in chair or bed most of the time but occasionally slides down.	**3. No Apparent Problem** Moves in bed and in chair independently and has sufficient muscle strength to lift up completely during move. Maintains good position in bed or chair.					
				Total Score				

CASE STUDY

INTRODUCTION

An 82-year-old frail female is admitted to acute care with a history of Type 2 diabetes (last hemoglobin A1c-8.0), hypertension, congestive heart failure with an ejection fraction of 35–40%, chronic kidney disease with a baseline creatinine of 2.1, atrial fibrillation (on Coumadin therapy), and osteoporosis. She lives alone in her own home and is able to do most of her activities of daily living without assistance. She is sometimes incontinent of urine, but is continent of bowels. She ambulates with a rolling walker. She was in her usual state of health until she sustained a fall in her home. She was able to call 911 and when paramedics arrived, she complained of right hip pain. She was taken to the ER for evaluation where hip X-rays revealed a right intertrochanteric fracture. The patient was evaluated by the orthopedic surgeon, but will require risk stratification prior to surgery due to her multiple comorbidities.

DISCUSSION QUESTIONS

1. What factors place this patient at risk for pressure injury development?
2. She is being admitted to the hospital. What strategies can be implemented to minimize her risk of skin breakdown?

CONTINUATION

The patient was admitted to the surgical floor and placed in Buck's traction until she could be cleared for surgery. She was placed on oxycodone/acetaminophen pain medication by the attending physician to help control her pain. She also has a zolpidem prescription for sleep. On day 2 of hospitalization, the patient is noted by her family to be confused. Because of the traction, she is now incontinent of bowel and bladder. The patient is noted to have non-blanching redness on the right heel.

DISCUSSION QUESTIONS

1. What was the patient's Braden score on admission? What risk level did that make her?
2. What is the patient's Braden score at this point in the clinical history?
3. What additional factors have put this patient at higher risk for pressure injury formation?

Support Surfaces: Beds, Mattresses, and Overlays

Horizontal support surfaces (such as bed systems, mattresses, and overlays) play a large role in managing tissue loads, especially in the many environments where people are in bed for extended periods, are potentially immobile, and have comorbidities and/or injuries that weaken the body. Being comfortable with the terminology used to characterize and describe horizontal support surfaces is important for any clinician when reading research about this technology and when communicating with other professionals about appropriate interventions. The NPIAP has developed a list of common terms and definitions for such purposes.[17] **TABLE 6-3** lists several categories and features of support surfaces and their respective definitions, and **FIGURES 6-6** to **6-9** illustrate some of the designs.

TABLE 6-3 Categories and Features of Support Surfaces

CATEGORIES OF SUPPORT SURFACES	
Reactive support surface	A powered or nonpowered support surface with the capability to change its load distribution properties only in response to applied load
Active support surface	A powered support surface with the capability to change its load distribution properties, with or without applied load
Nonpowered	Any support surface not requiring or using external sources of energy for operation
Powered	Any support surface requiring or using external sources of energy for operation
Integrated bed system	A bed frame and support surface that are combined into a single unit whereby the surface is unable to function separately
Mattress	A support surface designed to be placed directly on the existing bed frame
Overlay	An additional support surface designed to be placed directly on top of an existing surface
FEATURES OF SUPPORT SURFACES	
Air fluidized	A feature of a support surface that provides pressure redistribution via a fluid-like medium created by forcing air through beads as characterized by immersion and envelopment
Alternating pressure	A feature of a support surface that provides pressure redistribution via cyclic changes in loading and unloading as characterized by frequency, duration, amplitude, and rate of change parameters
Lateral rotation	A feature of a support surface that provides rotation about a longitudinal axis as characterized by degree of patient turn, duration, and frequency
Low air loss	A feature of a support surface that provides a flow of air to assist in managing the heat and humidity (microclimate) of the skin

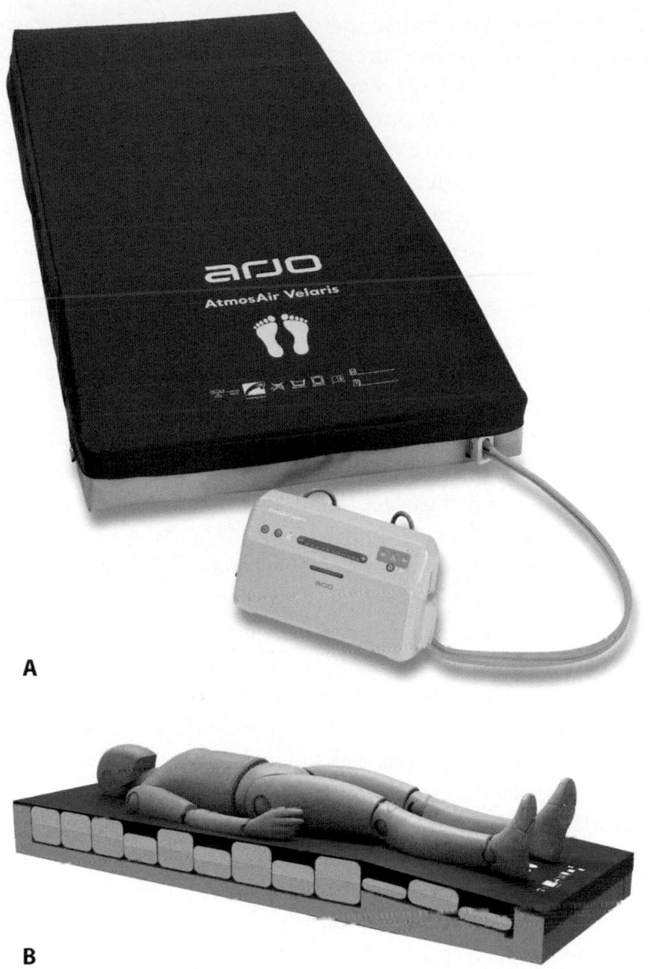

FIGURE 6-6 A. Reactive pressure and treatment surface. An air/foam hybrid mattress with nine cells that allow air to move and redistribute pressure as the patient moves in the bed. Also has the ability to convert to an active system by connecting a pump that alternates air in the A/B cells, thereby offloading tissue six times an hour. Therapy can be individualized as the patient conditions changes. (Photo used with permission of Arjo, Inc. All rights reserved.) **B.** Cross-section of the active therapy mattress showing the alternating cells. (Photo used with permission of Arjo, Inc. All rights reserved.)

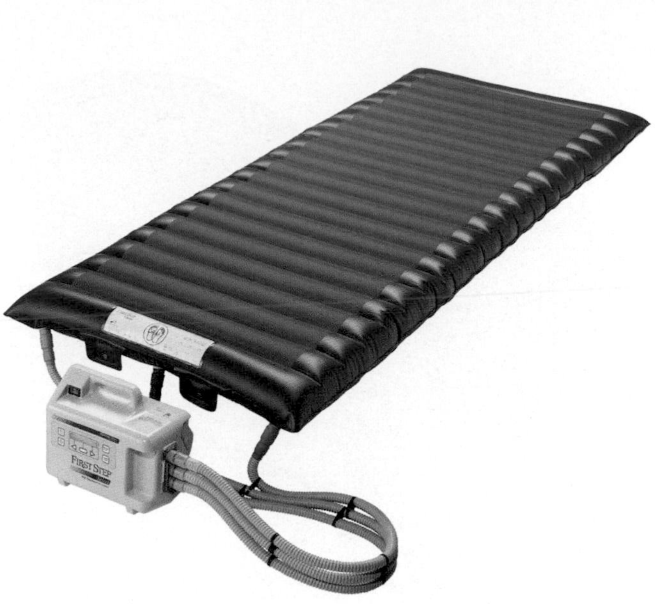

FIGURE 6-7 Reactive air mattress. Reactive air mattress overlay with a low air loss (LAL) feature that aids in microclimate management. (Photo used with permission of Arjo, Inc. All rights reserved.)

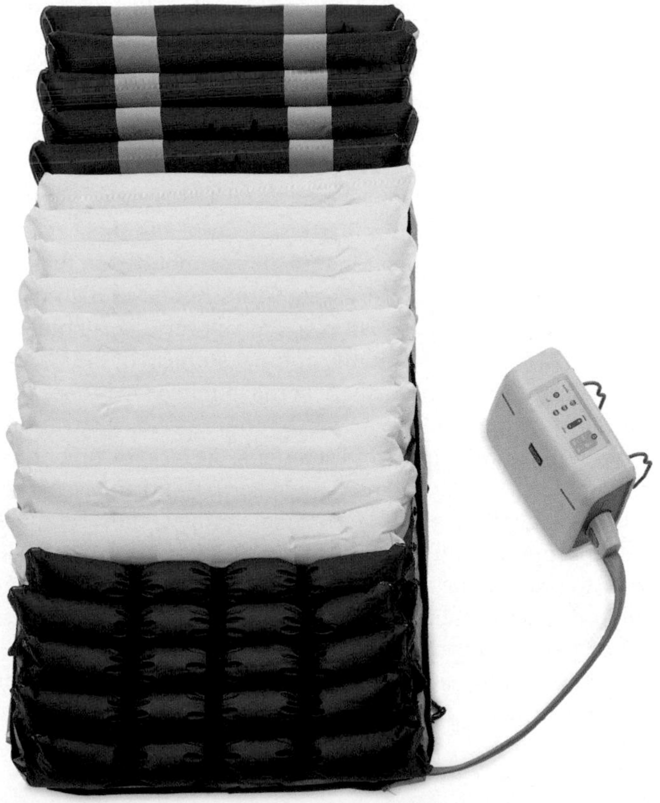

FIGURE 6-8 Active mattress replacement system. Full air active system with alternating pressure in which every other cell inflates and deflates every 10 minutes, thereby providing pressure redistribution for immobile patients. Can be deflated to make transfers or procedures easier to perform. (Photo used with permission of Arjo, Inc. All rights reserved.)

Selection of the most appropriate support surface for the patient might be constrained by the hospital or care environment, but generally multiple options are available. Informed decisions, of course, begin with an evaluation of the patient or client, but also must include basic knowledge of products.

Pressure injury risk evaluation combined with assessment of function, including the patient's ability to reposition in bed and the ability to transfer into and out of bed, is the first step in deciding on a support surface. Differences in product features and design form the basis of an informed clinical decision that is best made by the multidisciplinary team involved in the patient's care. Some support surface characteristics are technical in nature, such as the quality of parts, warranty, expected lifespan, and maintenance requirements. For example, a

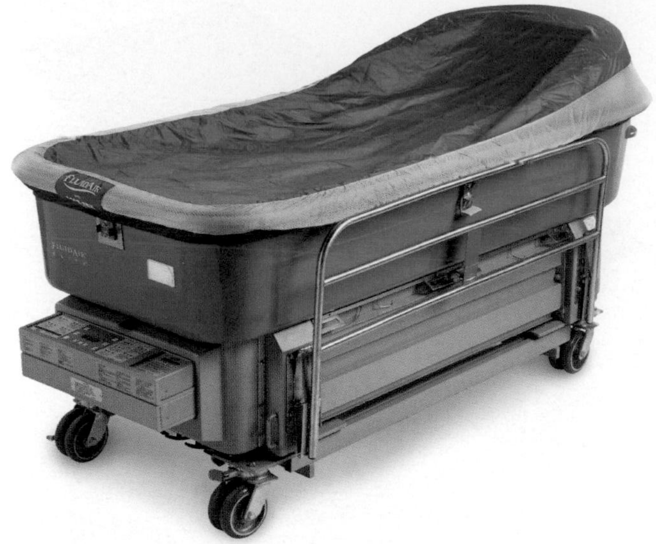

FIGURE 6-9 Fluid air bed. Full body air fluidized therapy. Considered reactive, it is also referred to as a sand or bead bed. (Photo used with permission of Arjo, Inc. All rights reserved.)

support surface that requires periodic adjustment and maintenance may be appropriate in a facility with the capacity to handle those tasks, whereas it might not be a good choice in certain homecare environments, unless the patient and/or caregivers are comfortable in making those adjustments.

Support surfaces are designed to protect the skin and underlying tissues by allowing the patient to immerse or sink into the surface. *Immersion* redistributes pressures and *envelops* the body in an attempt to equalize external forces as much as possible. A support surface must be soft enough to allow immersion without bottoming out. Compliant support surfaces can deflect only so far before they cannot deflect further. This defines a "bottomed-out" state and results in high pressures on tissues. Because achieving an appropriate amount of immersion is so important, the optimal stiffness of the surface must take into account the patient morphology. A surface that is too firm will not allow the person to immerse, whereas one that is too soft might not afford a stable surface for functional mobility (eg, turning and moving in bed). Foam and gel materials generally have a fixed functional stiffness; thus, a surface with appropriate stiffness and thickness needs to be selected in order to provide the requisite support. Surfaces using air typically offer adjustability, thereby allowing functional stiffness to be appropriately adapted for each patient. In both cases, reevaluation after selection must be done to ensure that the support surface is properly configured to protect tissues and support the body.

Evaluating the Effectiveness of Support Surfaces

A large amount of research has focused on the effectiveness of support surfaces. Some use direct measures of clinical outcomes such as pressure injury incidence or time for pressure ulcers to heal. Others use indirect measures, including variables such as interface pressure, blood flow, and temperature. Both approaches have merit but report quite different information about support surface performance. An effective review of the literature requires an assessment of methodologies and devices with respect to how they apply to a particular situation. The patient population (eg, orthopedic neurological, geriatric), care environments (eg, ICU, homecare long-term care), and types of support surfaces may impact how results influence care decisions. Notably, treatment studies—in which subjects already have tissue damage—are fundamentally different from prevention studies. For the purpose of this chapter, a select number of comparisons are highlighted as a means to illustrate how studies are configured to investigate effectiveness. Several recent articles and documents have provided an overview of support surface research and can be referred to for more detailed information.[18–22]

Most studies compare different classes of products as defined in **TABLE 6-3** rather than compare similarly designed products. For example, many more studies compare a standard hospital mattress to a specialty mattress instead of comparing two different types of low-air-loss beds. Moreover, studies tend to focus on a specific model from one manufacturer. Any study involving technology has the potential to become outdated simply because technology changes. This does not mean that historical studies have no value; instead, it acknowledges the challenge of focusing solely on published literature to make clinical decisions and highlights the need to keep abreast of this ever-changing body of knowledge.

The most common research comparison is against a "standard" hospital bed or mattress. Even though there are differences in what constitutes a standard hospital mattress, the results are clear: standard mattresses are not effective in prevention or treatment of pressure injuries and ulcers. Nonpowered, constant-low-pressure support surfaces (foam, air, gel, and combinations of these materials) are more effective in preventing pressure injuries than a standard mattress.[18–20] In fact, standards of practice recognize this by mandating the use of alternative surfaces in the care plans for persons who are at risk for or already have pressure damage.

Studies comparing advanced active technologies including low-air-loss, alternating-pressure, and fluidized surfaces tend to find them to be equivocal in effectiveness.[23–25] Evidence shows that these types of advanced support surfaces have roles to play in both prevention and treatment of pressure injuries. Equivocal results should also motivate clinicians to read the literature in order to better understand the results and how the lack of significant results can also be clinically useful.

Protecting the Heels and Lower Extremities

For patients in bed, heels are particularly prone to pressure injury, considering the anatomy of the posterior heel, the portion in contact with the support surface, and the amount of both direct pressure and friction that occurs at the heel (**FIGURE 6-2**).[26,27] The calcaneus forms a small, narrow prominence that must bear the weight of the foot and part of the leg when the patient is supine. The foot is a small mass, and the small surface area results in damaging pressure. In addition, the lower extremity is more prone to peripheral arterial disease, peripheral neuropathy, and edema which makes the heel more at risk for pressure injury development.[28]

Many commercial devices and approaches are available to reduce or eliminate pressure on the heels. Mattresses and overlays are often designed to support the heels using softer materials or different designs than those used to support the rest of the body. Two additional types of devices are available: (1) user-worn boots or heel protectors, and (2) positioners to elevate the heels.[29,30]

The user-worn approach consists of a boot or pad that encases the foot and heel and attaches directly to the person (FIGURES 6-10 to 6-12). These can be made from air bladders, foam, gel, or sheepskin materials. These devices remain in place during changes in position and as the legs move in bed; therefore, the fit and securement must be assessed. Most user-worn devices help prevent the ankle from plantar flexing (aka, foot drop) and some are designed to keep the ankle and foot aligned even in the presence of tone or spasm via the use of a rigid shell. If, however, the patient already has a plantar flexion contraction, the rigid support is contraindicated because peak pressures will occur at the plantar metatarsal heads and the Achilles tendons, causing pressure injury in these areas (FIGURE 6-13). The exception is the rigid ankle-foot-orthosis that has an adjustable ankle joint to accommodate plantarflexion contractures. Ambulation while wearing heel boots and pads is typically contraindicated (unless there is an ambulation sole attached); thus, these devices are not recommended when encouraging patients to transfer out of bed independently.

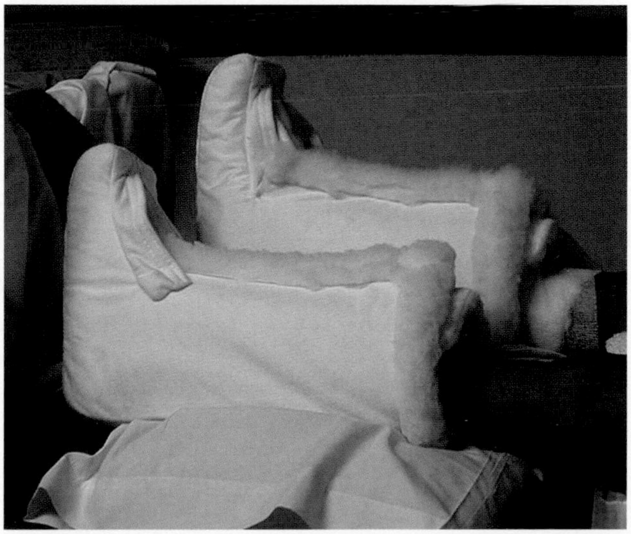

FIGURE 6-10 User-worn heel protector. The Rooke boot is made of pliable sheepskin-like material that can be worn in bed and for limited ambulation. It is available with either a rigid frame to maintain ankle range of motion and without a frame to accommodate plantar flexion contractures.

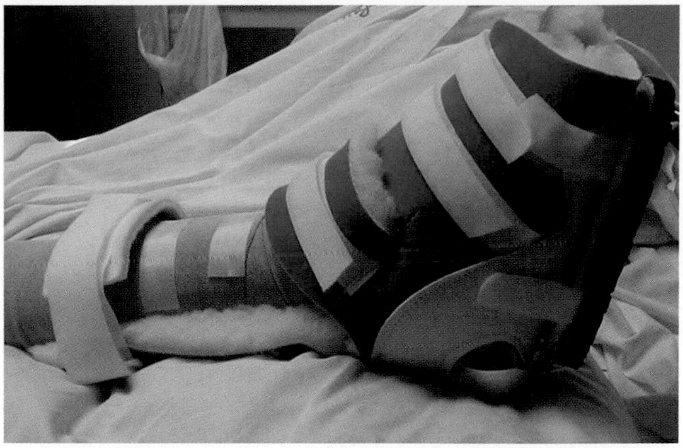

FIGURE 6-11 Rigid ankle-foot orthosis with heel relieved of any contact, both in supine and standing positions. Many of these orthoses come with ambulating soles for safe weight bearing activities.

The other category of heel protection is achieved by elevating (or floating) the heels completely off the surface by placing a positioning pad or pillows under the calf. Although some may extend to the knee, caution is advised with orthopedic patients when support under the knee may lead to knee flexion contractures (eg, after a total knee replacement). Several products can be purchased to provide heel elevation function (FIGURE 6-14) and are made from inflatable bladders or foam. Regular bed pillows can be used to elevate the heels; however, they have been shown to be less effective because they compress and get out of position more easily (FIGURE 6-15).[31,32] Heel elevation devices do not necessarily accommodate changes in position and therefore must be assessed whenever a person returns to a supine posture or moves the legs. In addition, care must be taken not to elevate the foot in a manner that induces hyperextension at the knee, which will become uncomfortable. Any lower extremity positioning approach should be done after assessing ranges of motion at the hip, knees, and ankle to ensure that external positioners maintain appropriate joint positions.

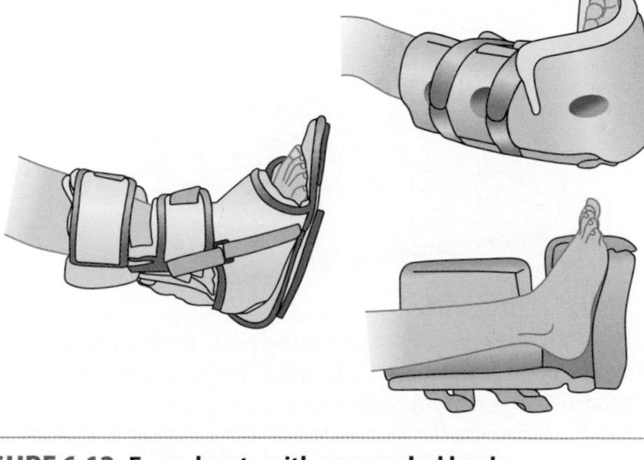

FIGURE 6-12 Foam boots with suspended heels.

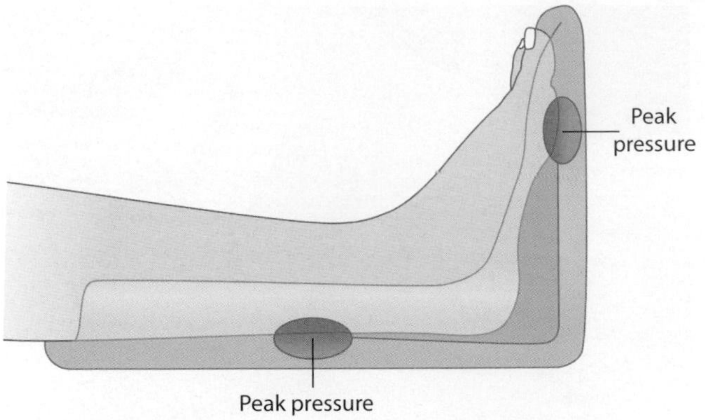

FIGURE 6-13 Plantar flexed ankle. A plantar flexed ankle that cannot be passively stretched to neutral will have peak pressures at the metatarsal heads and the Achilles tendon when placed in a rigid AFO, thus putting these tissues at risk for pressure injury formation. Some AFOs have adjustable ankle joints to adapt to plantar flexion contractures.

Positioning people in varying degrees of side-lying requires padding and positioners to ensure bony prominences are adequately protected (**FIGURE 6-16**). The malleoli and knees can be subjected to high pressures when side-lying. These issues are discussed in the section "Recumbent Postures."

Wheelchairs and Wheelchair Cushions

People who use wheelchairs are as varied as people who ambulate. They exhibit a wide range of medical diagnoses, but share the functional limitation of being nonambulatory or unable to ambulate functionally or safely. Because many wheelchair users sit throughout the day, many are at risk of developing pressure damage. Wheelchair users are assessed with respect to two common risk factors—immobility and sensation. Persons who are unable to recognize pain or discomfort while sitting are naturally at high risk for developing ulcers. Similarly,

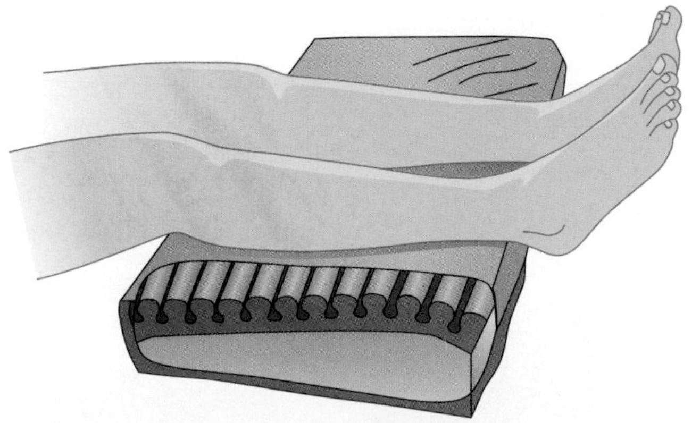

FIGURE 6-14 Heel and foot elevating pad. Pads under the calves are effective in off-loading or floating the heels; however, they may be displaced as the patient repositions. Care must be taken to avoid prolonged pressure on the posterior calf if the patient is insensate or atrophied (eg, a patient with spinal cord injury).

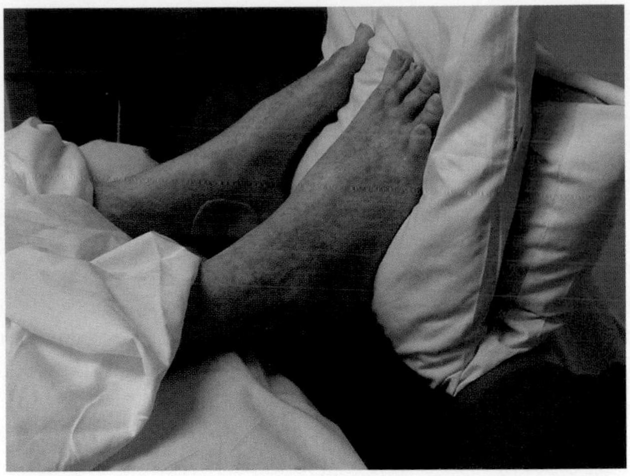

FIGURE 6-15 Pillows used to off-load the heels. When commercial devices are not available or not adaptable to a patient, pillows can be used creatively to accomplish pressure redistribution. This patient has bilateral foot drop and also tends to slide down in bed, putting the plantar metatarsal heads at risk. A pillow under the calves floats the heels and a folded pillow between the feet and the end of the bed off-loads the plantar surfaces. While improvisations may not be ideal, they can be effective for short-term care when combined with frequent repositioning and skin inspection.

persons unable to move in their seat or to shift weight and self-correct posture are also at heightened risk. In both cases, these wheelchair users will be unable to recognize when damaging loads are placed on their skin and subcutaneous tissues.

Sitting-acquired pressure injuries typically present at the load-bearing parts of the pelvis, specifically the ischial tuberosities and sacrum/coccyx (**FIGURE 6-17**). However, pressure injuries can arise in other anatomical locations if the magnitude and duration of loading exceed levels that the tissue can withstand. Other sites can be at risk in response to poor positioning within the wheelchair, including the scapular region, head, lateral trunk, knees, and feet. Therefore, proper positioning and body support are important in the prevention and management of tissue damage.

Wheelchair Positioning and Fitting

Wheelchairs are not a one-size-fits-all piece of equipment. Because wheelchairs are functional devices, wheelchair users

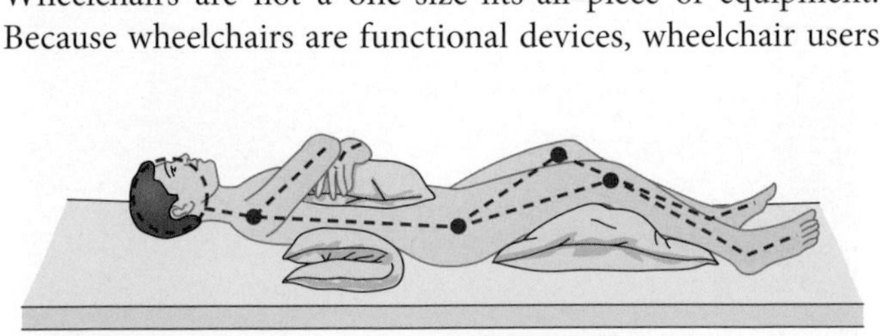

FIGURE 6-16 Thirty-degree side-lying posture. Thirty-degree side-lying posture uses a foam wedge for positioning and pillows under the arms and legs and between the knees to protect bony prominences of all extremities and the sacrum. Folded pillows may be used behind the back and sacrum if foam wedge is not available. (Used with permission of Stephen Sprigle PT, PhD.)

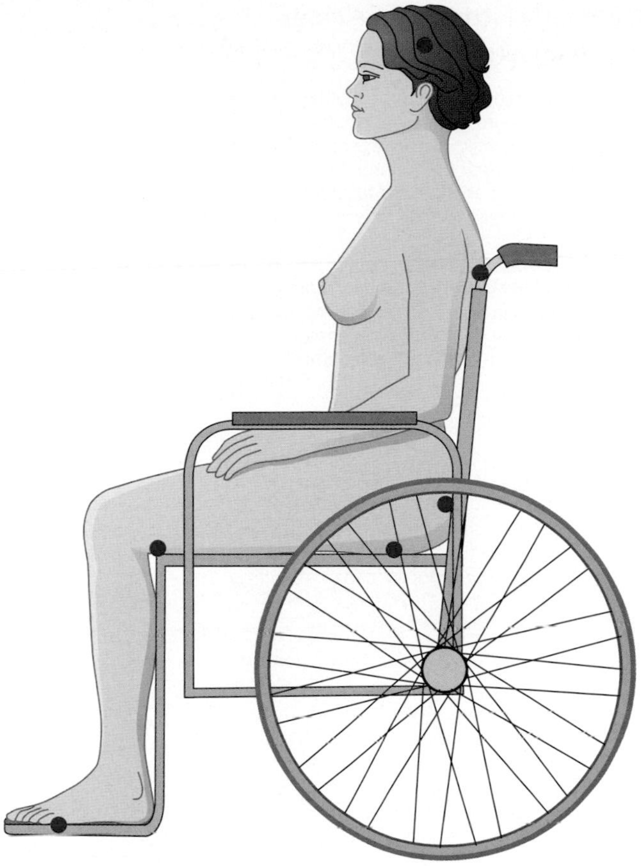

FIGURE 6-17 Vulnerable areas when patient is sitting in wheelchair. The most vulnerable areas for skin breakdown when a patient is sitting in a wheelchair include the ischial tuberosities, sacrum, coccyx, scapula, head (when using high-back chairs), lateral trunk, knees, and feet. (Adapted from *Preventing Pressure Ulcers: A Patient's Guide*. Washington, DC: US Department of Health and Human Services, USGPO 617-025/68298; 1992.)

are assessed from both functional and medical perspectives. Proper fit of the wheelchair to the individual is of utmost importance.

Several common problems arise when a wheelchair is poorly fitted to the wheelchair user. These include:

- Sliding out of chair
- Poor sitting tolerance
- Lateral trunk instability
- Poor thigh/foot stability
- Inability to reach the ground to propel
- Inability to hand propel effectively

These problems result in an increased risk of skin breakdown because postural problems due to inadequate body support result in high pressures at areas of bony prominences. For example, a poorly fitted wheelchair seat can encourage a person to slide forward on the seat. This results in the pelvis rotating posteriorly and exposes the sacrum and coccyx to

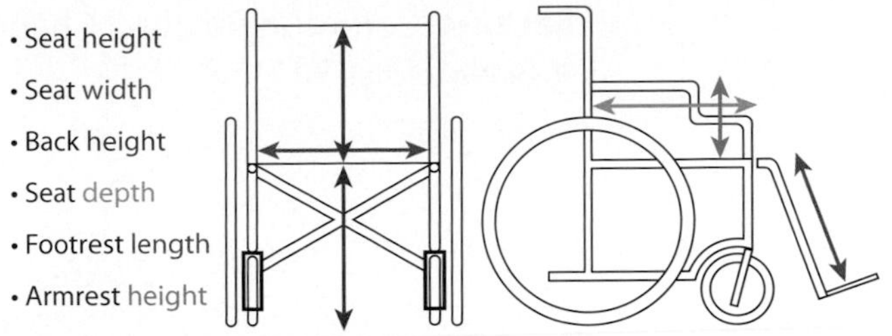

FIGURE 6-18 Wheelchair dimensions to consider when fitting a chair for an individual. (From WoundZoom, Inc. Used with permission from Stephen Sprigle, PT, PhD.)

unnecessary loading. Lateral trunk instability can result in a person leaning against the backrest upright, which results in a pelvic obliquity that elevates pressure on one ischial tuberosity and can cause high localized pressure on the lateral trunk.

Six wheelchair measurements are considered when configuring a wheelchair to a person: seat height, seat width, seat depth, backrest height, footrest height, and armrest height (**FIGURE 6-18**). Seat height, seat width, seat depth, and backrest height are dimensions that are usually selected when ordering a wheelchair. Conversely, footrest height can be adjusted on nearly all wheelchairs, and most chairs permit armrest height adjustment. These features can, therefore, be matched to the individual during the fitting process.

A poorly fitting wheelchair has a detrimental impact on posture, thereby resulting in decreased function and increased loading on the buttocks. A slouched kyphotic posture is the most common poor posture resulting from an inadequate wheelchair and seating system. This posture is characterized by a posterior pelvic tilt and kyphotic spine. A slouched posture elevates pressure at the sacrum and coccyx, and the resulting increased forward sliding tendency exposes the tissues to friction and shear strain. **TABLE 6-4** lists some common postural impacts of a poorly fitted wheelchair.

Wheelchair Cushions

Wheelchair cushions are required for all wheelchair users because wheelchair seat upholstery is simply not designed or intended to offer adequate support. The selection of wheelchair cushions for persons identified to be at risk of pressure ulcers is obviously more involved and requires more attention than the selection of a cushion for a person with intact sensation and adequate mobility who uses a wheelchair for only short durations of time. Many wheelchair users sit in their wheelchairs throughout the day, sometimes for 12 hours or more.

Hundreds of cushions are commercially available, so many options exist for both full-time and part-time wheelchair users. A basic understanding of materials, design, and performance can assist the clinician in selecting appropriate cushions for wheelchair users. The two most important things to remember are: (1) no one cushion is best for all people, and (2) cushion selection must reflect the needs, function, and activities of the wheelchair user. The second point highlights the fact that cushions serve other roles besides managing loads

TABLE 6-4 Common Postural Changes in a Poorly Fitting Wheelchair

Poor Wheelchair Fit		Postural Impact
Seat too high	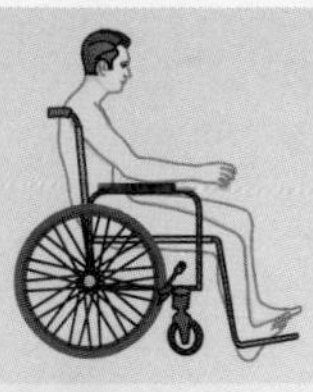	For someone who propels with one or both feet, a high seat height will encourage sliding forward on the seat in order to reach the ground. This results in a slouched posture and further increases the tendency to slide forward.
Seat too low or footrest too high	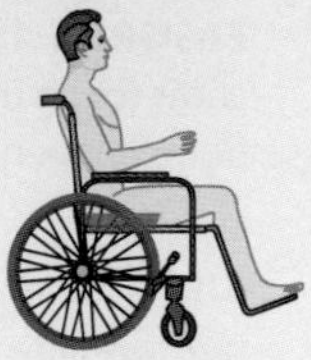	Knees are elevated and thighs rise off seat surface, leading to increased loading on the buttocks and ischial tuberosities and poor lower limb stability.
Seat too wide	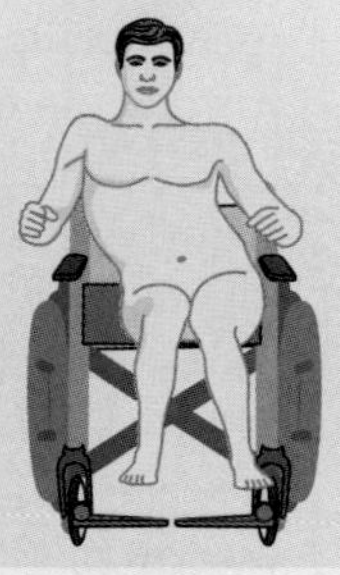	Leaning to use armrests induces a pelvic obliquity and increases pressure on the ischial tuberosity; an unnecessarily wide wheelchair leads to poor access to handrims and reduced maneuverability.
Seat too narrow	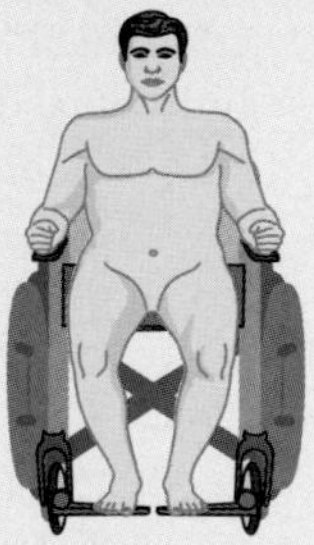	The chair is difficult to transfer into; contact with armrests or clothing guards increases pressures on lateral tissues.
Seat depth too long	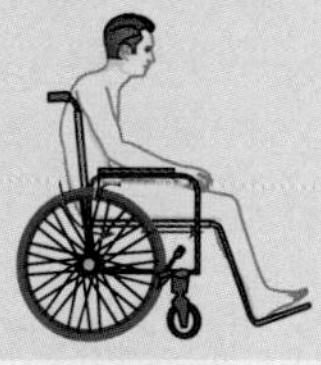	Contact at popliteal region encourages a person to slide forward into a slouched posture that thereby increases sliding tendency and elevates sacral/coccyx pressure.
Seat depth too short	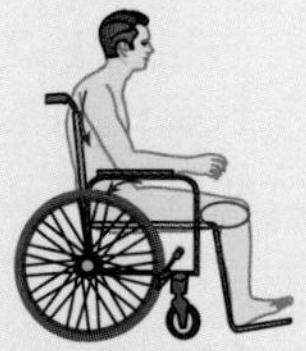	Inadequate thigh contact decreases postural stability, resulting in sliding forward into a slouched posture; poor lower limb stability can lead to external or internal rotation at the hips.
Backrest height too low	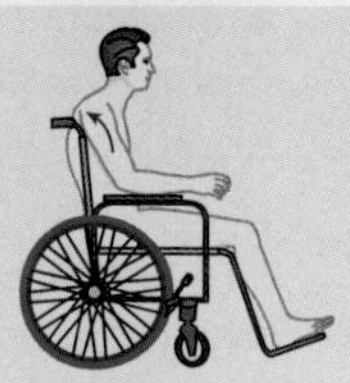	Inadequate trunk stability can result in a person seeking support by leaning to one side, which results in pelvic obliquity or sliding forward into a slouched, kyphotic posture.
Backrest height too high	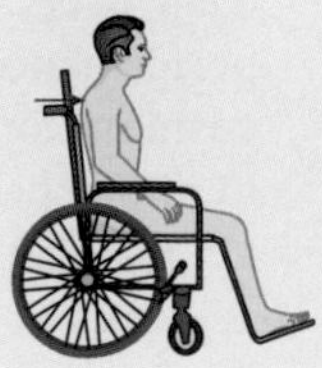	A backrest that is too high increases loading at the scapula and pushes the upper trunk forward; this can lead to a person sliding into a kyphotic, slouched posture; a high backrest can also hinder upper extremity reach.

Used with permission from Stephen Sprigle, PT, PhD.

TABLE 6-5 Common Materials Used in Cushion Construction

Material	Benefits and Reasons for Use	Drawbacks
Foam	Inexpensive; comes in many stiffnesses, can be carved, cut, and molded easily; lightweight; good resilience and damping properties.	Heat insulator, so entraps body heat; needs to be protected from light and moisture; can have short lifespan.
Air	Lightweight; offers adjustability; good impact, damping, and resilience.	Impermeable bladder impacts cushion mass, can hinder effectiveness and heat management; inflation needs to be checked regularly; can be punctured.
Viscous fluid	Displaces in response to load to envelop the buttocks; some fluids provide heat transmissibility.	Can be heavy; poor resilience and impact damping; creep over time can reduce performance; its impermeable bladder can hinder effectiveness and heat management; nonadjustable.
Elastomer	Used as a top layer to envelop the buttocks and dissipate heat.	Can be heavy and expensive; incompressible, so must be used with other materials to fully envelop; poor impact damping; can creep over time.

on tissues. Cushions impact many aspects of functioning during everyday activities, including posture, comfort, transfers, heat and moisture of the cushion interface, and a host of other factors. In addition, the environment of use, amount of use, and activity level of the user influence cushion selection. A person who sits in a wheelchair for 16 hours a day and travels outdoors over a variety of surfaces has different needs than a person who sits in a wheelchair for 2 hours per day because he or she transfers into other chairs and surfaces. Clinicians use their skills to evaluate their clients and patients in order to select an appropriate cushion. Therefore, combining the functional impact of cushions with requirements to promote skin health is the appropriate approach.

Using the terminology in **TABLE 6-3**, most wheelchair cushions can be described as reactive and nonpowered. Although a few powered, active cushions do exist, they are not commonly used except in complex situations (eg, a person with a history of multiple pressure ulcers). Cushions can be flat or contoured and are designed to deform and deflect to accommodate the buttocks.

Wheelchair cushions are made from a variety of materials and reflect many designs, although four materials dominate: foam, air, viscous fluid, and elastomers. Foam cushions are the most common; however, most advanced cushion designs use a combination of materials with the intent of maximizing cushion performance by managing the good and poor features of each material. **TABLE 6-5** lists these common materials, some of their beneficial features, and their limitations. **FIGURE 6-19** illustrates the myriad cushions fabricated with different materials.

In the spinal cord injury population, air cushions have been shown to be more effective in reducing the interface pressure than gel and foam cushions.[33–35]

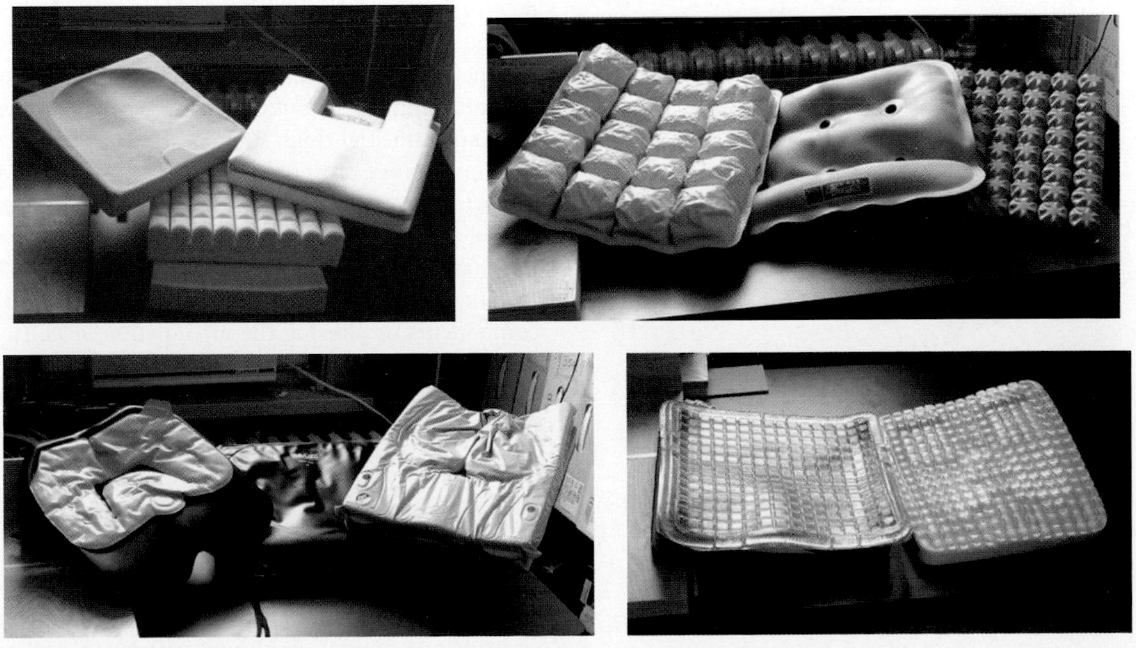

FIGURE 6-19 Wheelchair cushions. Designs of wheelchair cushions highlighting various materials of construction. (Used with permission, Stephen Sprigle, PT, PhD.)

Functionally, cushions can be categorized by their skin protection and positioning capabilities. Although many cushions are designed to provide both functionalities, the following sections discuss the rationale behind these general categories.

Skin Protection Cushions

Cushions designed for skin protection target loading on the skin, as well as adequately managing temperature and moisture at the buttock–cushion interface. In addition, they offer a stable base of support. In the seated posture, loading on the buttocks represents the greatest risk for tissue damage. Cushions attempt to redistribute pressures away from bony prominences such as the ischial tuberosities and sacrum/coccyx by the following techniques: (1) envelopment and (2) redirection or off-loading.

Envelopment is defined as the capability of a support surface in deforming around and encompassing the contour of the human body.[36] In order to properly envelop, cushions must deflect and deform to immerse the buttocks in the material. Due to the design of the pelvis, about 4 cm of *immersion* is needed to adequately encompass the buttocks. This is based on the inferior position of the ischial tuberosities during sitting (**FIGURE 6-20**). As a result, cushions need adequate thickness to permit that amount of immersion. Foam cushions that are only 5 cm (2") thick will probably not suffice as skin protection cushions.

Some cushions are designed to purposely redirect forces away from bony prominences using cutouts or contours in the cushion surface (**FIGURE 6-21**). As a result, cushions with cutouts and contours require the person to sit on the cushion in a specific location; therefore, proper training and instruction should be an integral part of any cushion fitting session.

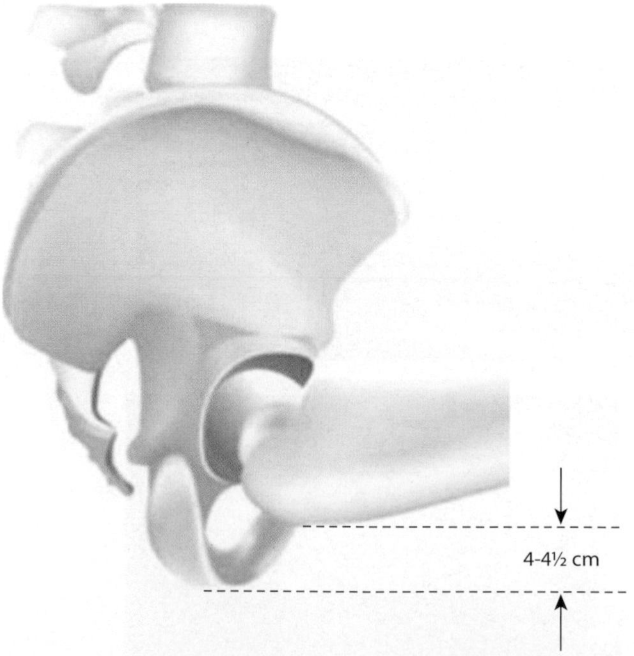

FIGURE 6-20 Anatomic relationship between the inferior aspects of the ischial tuberosity and greater trochanter. (Used with permission, Stephen Sprigle, PT, PhD.)

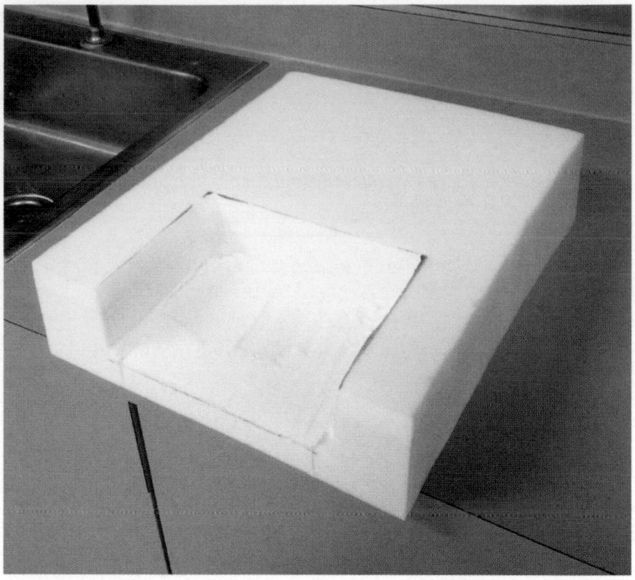

FIGURE 6-21 Cushions with cutout or reliefs to redirect loading. Cushions with cutouts are frequently custom-made to fit the patient's anatomical dimensions. Because shifting weight in the cushions will change the pressure points, appropriate training and use are required for optimal efficacy.

Positioning Cushions

Postural support is an important factor in cushion selection, just as it is in wheelchair fitting, because cushions are important in facilitating seated functional activities. Positioning can be grossly categorized as alignment, accommodation, or correction. In order to properly *align* the body in an erect and symmetric posture, cushions may include certain features such as contouring for the buttocks, lateral pelvic supports, and lateral and/or medial thigh supports (**FIGURE 6-22**). Appropriate cushions do not promote a slouched posture and prevent the buttocks from sliding forward in the seat. Clients who sit with a fixed asymmetry (such as a pelvic obliquity) require a cushion that can *accommodate* a deformity. These cushions often include some adjustable feature, such as adding or removing components or altering the air inflation level. Conversely, if an asymmetry is *correctable*, a cushion can be used to position a client into a symmetric posture by the same means and thereby correct the faulty posture. Evaluation (including range of motion, tone, and functional assessment) is needed to determine which type of positioning is optimal for the patient.

Positioning features of cushions typically result in a cushion surface that is site specific, meaning that the user must sit on the cushion correctly. For example, sitting too forward on a cushion may result in the person sitting on the medial thigh support or pommel. Cushions with deep contours or pronounced positioning features are designed to provide a very stable sitting surface; however, these characteristics may also

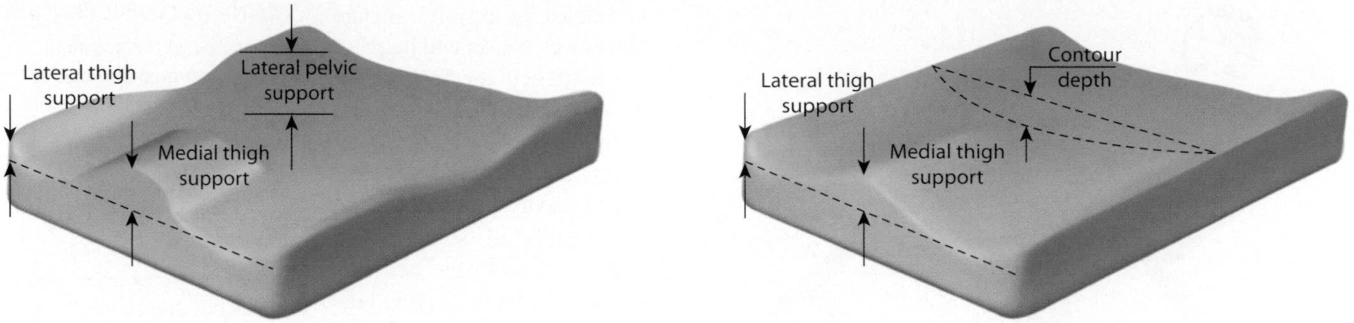

FIGURE 6-22 Flat (A) and contoured (B) cushions with positioning features. (Used with permission from Stephen Sprigle, PT, PhD, © Georgia Tech Research Corporation, Atlanta, GA.)

impede function. For example, a contoured cushion with a pommel may be needed to position the lower extremities, but it can also impede transfers if the person cannot overcome this positioning feature. This again underscores the importance of a proper assessment because all cushions will have benefits and deficiencies that must be reconciled for each individual user.

In summary, many wheelchair cushions are commercially available. Having myriad choices can empower clinicians and clients, but selection can also be confusing. By reflecting on the seating goals for the patient or client and the various cushion materials and designs available, an informed decision can be made.

INTERVENTIONS TO REDUCE THE DURATION OF LOADING

The motor and sensory systems are responsible for ensuring that the body can move periodically to change posture. An individual responds to discomfort, often subconsciously, with small movements, postural shifts, or fidgeting. Research on sitting and comfort[37–40] has led to the understanding that sitting is a dynamic activity. Many people at risk of developing pressure injuries either are unable to effectively reposition themselves or do not have the sensory feedback to elicit movement. Therefore, the losses of mobility and sensation are identified as risk factors within every pressure ulcer risk assessment scale. This information is used to target movement as a means to redistribute pressure and alter the duration of loading on tissues via turning schedules while in bed and weight-shifting strategies while seated.

Recumbent Postures

Positioning in bed has significant influence on tissue health. Because some people spend long continuous hours in bed, tissues can be exposed to pressures, temperatures, and humidity that can lead to tissue necrosis or prevent tissues from healing properly. The first clinical objective of recumbent positioning is to support the body in a safe, stable, and functional manner. This requires an assessment of body alignment, joint angles, and weight-bearing surfaces in various postures that are commonly adopted by patients in bed. No single recumbent posture can be maintained for long durations. As noted below, each posture has both benefits and drawbacks, so, typically, though not always, patients are sequenced through postures over time.

Supine

The supine position can be considered the default recumbent posture, and for good reasons. Supine positioning offers the patient an opportunity to interact with other people and the environment, to perform in-bed functional tasks, and to be accessible for and participate in clinical care. However, supine positioning also exposes certain anatomical sites to potentially harmful tissue loading. The sacrum and the heels are the two most common sites for pressure ulcer development and both sites are loaded in supine. Other posterior structures such as the occiput, scapula, and iliac crests can also be exposed to elevated pressures in the supine position.

Pillows, positioning devices, articulating bed frames, and support surfaces are used in combination to support and position the body. Therefore, these factors are considered when assessing the supine positioning of a patient.

Pillows are used to support the head; however, in excess they can put the cervical and thoracic vertebrae into too much flexion and result in discomfort. If the patient is on a ventilator or has a nasogastric feeding tube, pillows under the head and neck need careful monitoring so that function of the equipment is not interrupted. Bed articulation can be used to slightly raise the head and trunk as a substitute for using multiple pillows; however, elevating the head of the bed has potential detriments, which are discussed below.

The bed and supporting surface should accommodate the patient's asymmetries and postural deformities, not the other way around. Assessing ranges of motion of the trunk, hips, and lower extremities provides information needed to select positioning devices to accommodate fixed deformities and promote stable posture. For example, the presence of a knee flexion contracture can be accommodated by proper placement of a foam positioner, pillow, or bed frame adjustment fitted to the knee range of motion.

Because the supine position exposes several anatomical sites to potentially harmful pressures, changes in position are necessary. Semireclined and side-lying postures are two

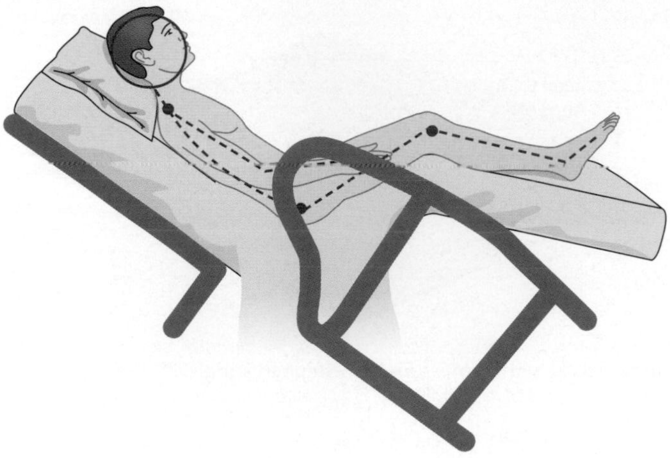

FIGURE 6-23 Semireclined or Fowler's position. Raising the knee portion of the bed frame will counteract sliding tendency but can expose the sacrum to higher loading.

common alternative postures, but each has drawbacks from a pressure-loading perspective. Nonetheless, these drawbacks can be minimized by following certain guidelines and understanding the biomechanics of these postures.

Reclined Positions

A semireclined position, sometimes referred to as Fowler's position, results from elevating the head of the bed (**FIGURE 6-23**). Elevating the head is done to facilitate eating, reading, interacting with visitors, and many other functional activities. This posture, however, also changes the loading on the body, which has resulted in the common practice of limiting head of bed elevation to 30 degrees or less in order to prevent friction and shear. Principles of physics dictate that any elevation will increase the tendency for the patient to slide down in the bed (**FIGURE 6-18**). Upper-body weight is projected downward due to gravity and the inclined bed results in some forces being normal to the bed surface and some projecting tangentially. This tangential force results in a tendency to slide downward and may produce friction on the skin. As noted above, friction can be damaging to the tissues by causing abrasion and blistering

CLINICAL CONSIDERATION

Pressures on the popliteal fossa must be minimized to prevent compression of the neurovascular structures that can lead to pain, paresthesia, and circulation impingement. Pillows under the knees of a patient who has had a total knee replacement may result in a slight knee flexion contracture and alter the gait pattern.

If the body weight moves downward and the skin remains in place on the bed surface, shear forces occur between the sacrum and the adjacent soft tissue, resulting in capillary damage, bleeding into the tissues, and a resulting inflammatory response and tissue necrosis. This shear strain and subsequent tissue loss is the pathophysiology of deep sinus and undermining formation, deep tissue injury, and eventual Stage III and IV sacral pressure ulcers (see **FIGURE 6-3**).

Despite the common practice of limiting head of bed elevation to 30 degrees, there is no minimum threshold for this tangential force. The greater the angle of the bed, the greater the sliding tendency. Therefore, the impact of head of bed elevation must be evaluated for each patient. If a patient continually slides downward and must be moved back into position, then elevation is too great. Strategies to counteract the sliding tendency include gatching the bedframe at the hips by elevating the knee portion of the bed frame (**FIGURE 6-24**). Before elevating or gatching the head and knee portions of

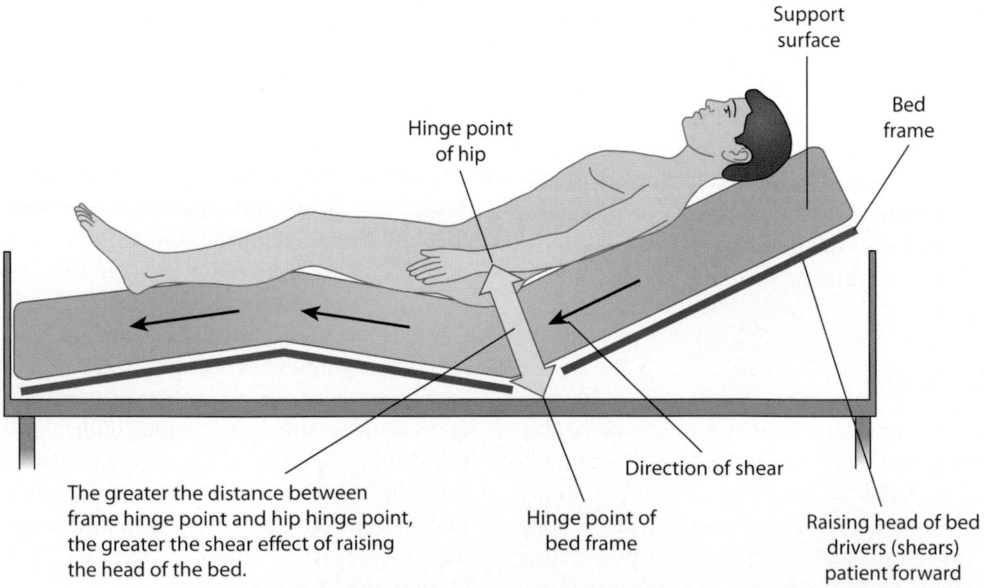

FIGURE 6-24 Position of patient in bed to prevent sliding. Aligning the hips with the joint angle of the bed assists in preventing sliding, which causes both friction and shear forces at the sacral area. Note the slight gatching of the bed at the knees as well. When repositioning the patient in bed, gatching the knees *before* raising the head is another strategy to prevent sliding.

CLINICAL CONSIDERATION

Note that while keeping the head of the bed less than 30 degrees is advisable for prevention of pressure ulcers, certain medical conditions require the head to be elevated 30 degrees or more (eg, if the patient has a nasogastric tube), and in those situations, the medical concern must take precedence.

the bed, the hips must be in line with the hinge of the bedframe to allow the body to flex appropriately.

This position, however, raises the second issue of a semireclined position. A valley is created when the head and knee are raised, which results in greater body weight being borne at the lower back and sacrum. Therefore, just like any position, a semireclined position should not be maintained for long durations. The key to proper bed positioning is to vary the postures so that loading is continually redistributed to different parts of the body.

Side-Lying Positions

The need to relieve pressure from the sacrum, scapula, and other posterior bony prominences requires the use of varying degrees of side-lying. The most common side-lying posture rotates the trunk and pelvis 30 degrees with respect to the horizontal support surface. This posture can eliminate pressures on the sacrum while avoiding the high pressures on the trochanters and iliac crests that tend to occur in a full 90-degree side-lying posture. External supports are needed to maintain the body in a 30-degree side-lying posture. Foam wedges are typically more effective than pillows because they provide more stable support (**FIGURE 6-16**). The wedge is positioned to support the trunk and shoulders and can be placed to totally relieve pressure on the sacrum. In addition, the knees and ankles must be separated with pillows or padding to protect the bony prominences. Finally, a pillow under the upper arm helps maintain the shoulder in a comfortable and stable position.

Turning Frequency

Manual repositioning has been cited as the most commonly used turning strategy and also as the most expensive.[41] The need for repositioning has been cited in literature and textbooks since 1800s,[42] and evidence that some repositioning is necessary can be found across decades of literature.

In the United States, common practice requires that at-risk patients are repositioned at least every 2 hours "if consistent with overall patient goals."[43] The origins of this practice remain unclear and it has been adopted despite the lack of strong scientific evidence.[39,44–46] Nonetheless, the need for repositioning is corroborated by all the research that identifies duration of loading as a causative factor in pressure ulcer occurrence.

The vast differences in patients, amount and type of tissues overlying bony prominences, and performance of support surfaces demand that the required frequency of turning is not the same for every individual. The clinical challenge lies in the fact that not turning frequently enough has worse consequences compared to turning too frequently. Some research has investigated the influence of the support surface in determining the optimal turning schedule. Defloor et al. showed pressure ulcer outcomes of patients lying on a standard mattress with 2- and 3-hour turning schedules were similar to the outcomes of patients lying on a viscoelastic mattress with a 6-hour turning schedule. These researchers also found that turning every 4 hours when using a viscoelastic mattress significantly reduced Stage II pressure ulcer incidence.[47]

CLINICAL CONSIDERATION

Turning schedules are not the same for every patient. Small, cachectic, hypotensive patients require turning more frequently than every 2 hours. Turning schedules need to be individualized based on risk factors for pressure injury formation, body type, and support surface.

Other research suggests that turning may need to occur more frequently than every 2 hours, and that sufficient pressure reduction surfaces are needed in addition to turning.[44,47–49] A recent study by Vanderwee et al.[49] found no differences in pressure ulcer occurrences between patients repositioned every 4 hours and those positioned for 2 hours in side-lying and 4 hours in supine. Furthermore, these authors confirmed a readily accepted clinical situation—patients who are able to reposition in bed will do so. On the one hand, functional movement in bed should be promoted because it sequences the person through different postures. However, if independent repositioning involves a return to supine with no subsequent changes in position, additional intervention may be needed to ensure adequate turning frequency.

Wheelchair Weight Shifts and Pressure Reliefs

The need to reduce the duration of loading is just as important in sitting as it is when lying in bed. Thus, during rehabilitation, wheelchair users are taught preventative weight shifts or pressure reliefs in order to relieve pressure from the buttocks and thereby minimize the potential for skin breakdown. Guidelines have been published recommending frequency of weight-shift activities,[39,40] with a primary focus on persons with spinal cord injury;[50] however, these principles can be applied to all wheelchair users. The guidelines vary considerably and recommend that persons perform pressure reliefs every 15, 30, or 60 minutes. They also suggest that the duration of the pressure relief should last 15–30 seconds up to a full minute.[51–53] Based on the wide range of these guidelines, one can infer that they were based on a combination of clinical experience, clinical insight, and research findings. Therefore, clinicians need to work with their clients to define a routine to which the patient will adhere.

Weight shifting will be more easily adopted as a routine if taught as a relatively frequent activity as opposed to a less-frequent one. One compromise might be to train wheelchair users to perform weight shifts every 30 minutes with 30-second duration. However, the most important goal should be to devise a plan that is attainable for the individual. Research also suggests that functional movements tend to be more preventative than scheduled, routine pressure reliefs.[54]

Three common weight-shift options are a lift, forward lean, and side-to-side weight shift. A lift has the benefit of completely off-loading the buttocks, but it is also the hardest to perform from a functional standpoint (**FIGURE 6-25**). Not all persons can generate the forces or have the postural control necessary to perform this maneuver. A forward lean is performed by shifting the trunk as far forward as possible (**FIGURE 6-26**). Although some people have the flexibility to flex the trunk all the way to the thighs, this is not possible for many wheelchair users, so a lesser lean can also be used. By resting the elbows on the knees, buttocks loading can be reduced (**FIGURE 6-27**). Proper training is imperative because a small forward lean will not be sufficient. Side leans can also be effective, and wheelchair users can be taught to hook around the armrest or grab the drive wheels to maintain balance (**FIGURE 6-28**). Naturally, a side lean to one side must be followed by one to the opposite side to ensure the entire buttock surface is unweighted.

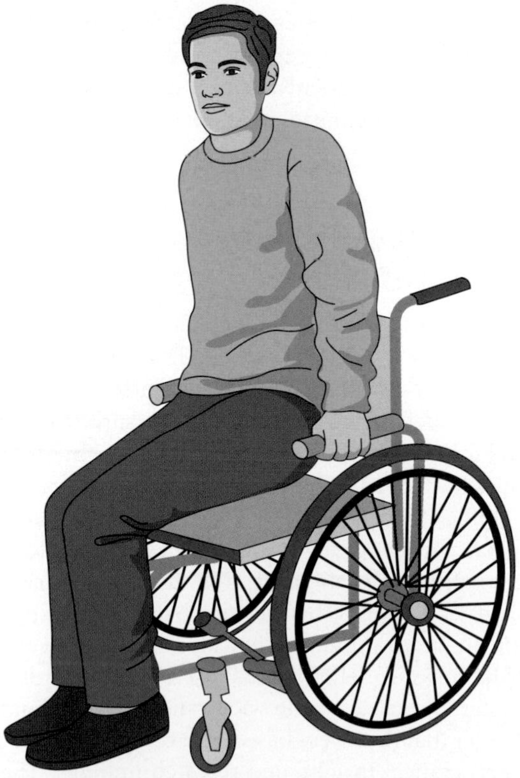

FIGURE 6-25 Lift pressure relief. It requires that the individual have sufficient upper extremity strength to lift the buttocks off the chair and maintain the position for at least 30 seconds. This not only relieves the pressure but also allows reperfusion of any tissue that has been compressed.

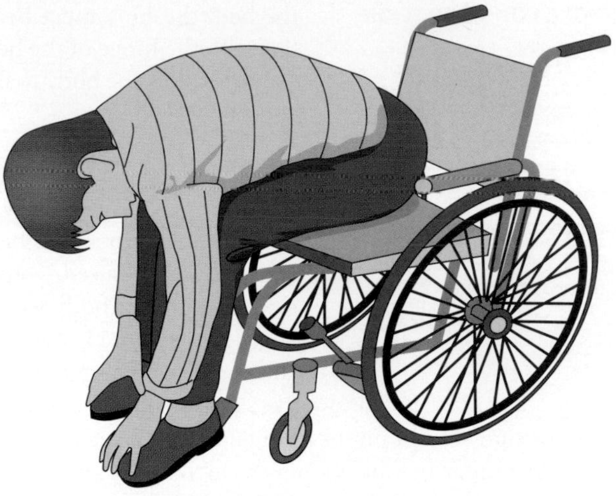

FIGURE 6-26 Full-forward lean to accomplish weight shift.

DOCUMENTATION

Despite the interventions put in place to prevent pressure injury and ulcer development, skin breakdown can occur. As with any other organ system, documentation of a normal or abnormal examination of the skin is a routine part of the physical examination. If skin breakdown is present, thorough documentation requires a number of components, including anatomic location, pressure ulcer stage, size (length × width × depth in cm), character of the tissue in the wound, description of the periwound skin, type and amount of drainage, and finally, the presence of undermining or tunneling. (Refer to Chapter 3, Examination and Evaluation of the Patient with a Wound, for a more detailed discussion of wound assessment and description.) **TABLES 6-6** and **6-7** are provided to aid in the visual assessment of pressure injuries. The elements of this documentation can create a

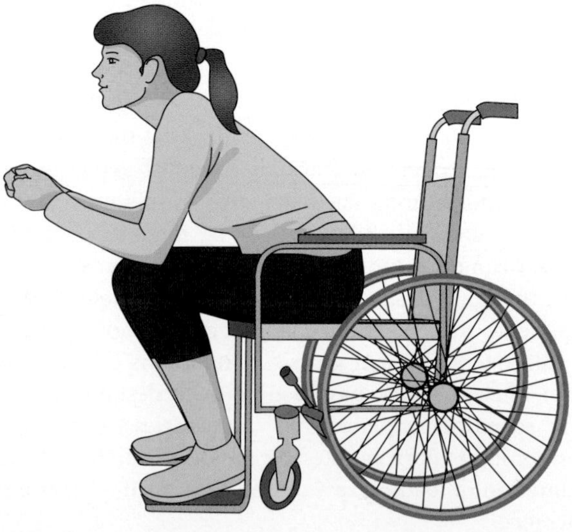

FIGURE 6-27 Partial forward lean. Some weight reduction is achieved by leaning forward with the elbows on the knees, thereby taking some of the weight off the sacrum and ischial tuberosities. (Used with permission from Stephen Sprigle, PT, PhD.)

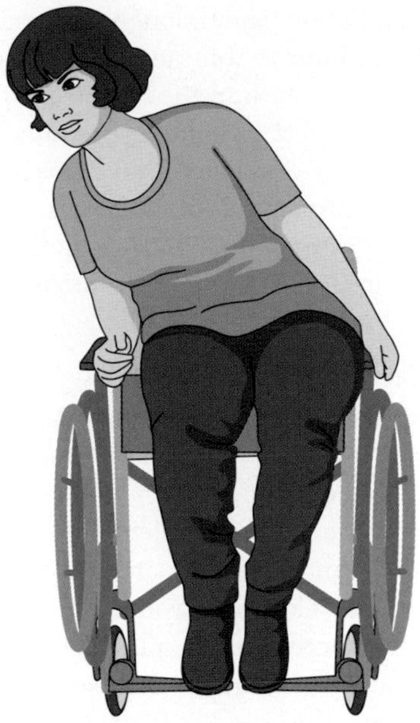

FIGURE 6-28 Partial weight shifts. Simply leaning from one side relieves some pressure on the contralateral buttock.

clinical picture of the wound appearance; however, a photograph is also required in most settings. The documentation serves as a means of communication with the healthcare team and allows the provider to determine whether the wound is improving. Additionally, as per CMS guidelines, the ability to obtain certain specialty surfaces or treatments is linked to the stage of the pressure ulcer present.

The anatomic location of the wound needs to be very specific. A common mistake with documentation of location is the intermingling of terms for different anatomic areas. Although one healthcare provider may document the patient as having a wound on the sacrum, the next may describe it as the lower back, buttocks, or coccyx. These areas are anatomically different and only one of these descriptions would be correct. The documentation needs to be accurate and consistent between healthcare professionals. An anatomic chart is provided that outlines common areas of pressure ulcer development (**FIGURE 6-29**).

The next step of assessment is determination of what is termed the *pressure ulcer stage*, which is based on the depth of tissue damage. The current National Pressure Injury Advisory Panel (NPIAP) staging system was last revised by the NPIAP in 2016 in which the term *injury* replaces the term *ulcer*.[55] The definitions are as follows, and **TABLE 6-8** is provided to aid in determination of staging:

- **Stage I—Pressure Injury: Nonblanchable erythema of intact skin**

  Intact skin with a localized area of nonblanchable erythema, which may appear differently in darkly pigmented skin. The presence of blanchable erythema or changes in sensation, temperature, or

TABLE 6-6 Pressure Ulcer Tissue Characteristics

Photo	Type of Tissue and Characteristics
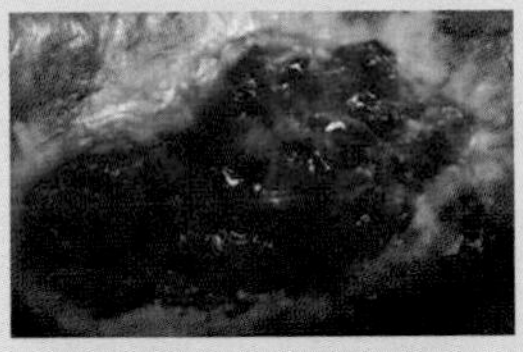	**Granulation Tissue** Highly vascularized tissue that replaces the initial fibrin clot in a wound. Vascularization is by ingrowth of capillary endothelium from the surrounding vasculature. The tissue is also rich in fibroblasts (that will eventually produce the fibrous tissue) and leucocytes. (Used with permission from Aimée Garcia, MD.)
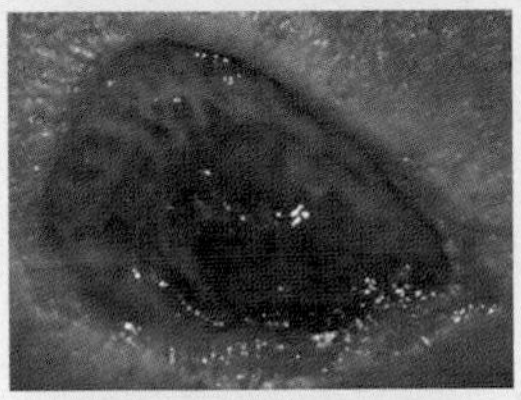	**Fibrinous Slough** Fibrinous tissue that has separated from the surrounding or underlying tissue. Slough is yellow and interspersed with the red granulation tissue in the wound bed, and is very difficult to remove with sharp debridement. (Used with permission from Aimée Garcia, MD.)
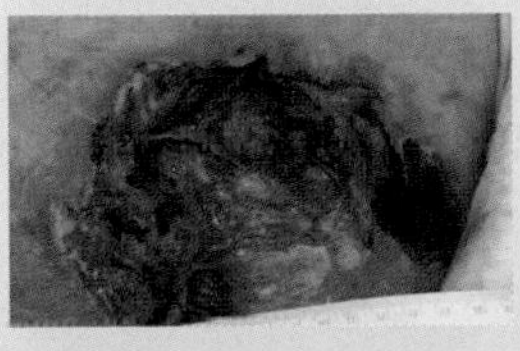	**Necrotic Tissue** Tissue that has died. Although the tissue is dead, it can still support bacterial growth, thereby leading to higher bacteria load or infection of a wound. (Used with permission from Aimée Garcia, MD.)
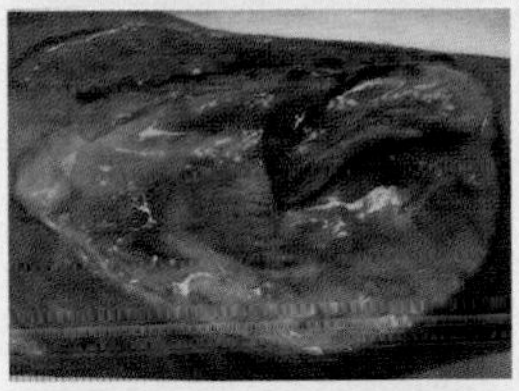	**Necrotic Slough** A layer or mass of dead tissue separated from surrounding living tissue. Necrotic slough can appear in a wound or an inflamed area and has to be debrided. (Used with permission from Aimée Garcia, MD.)
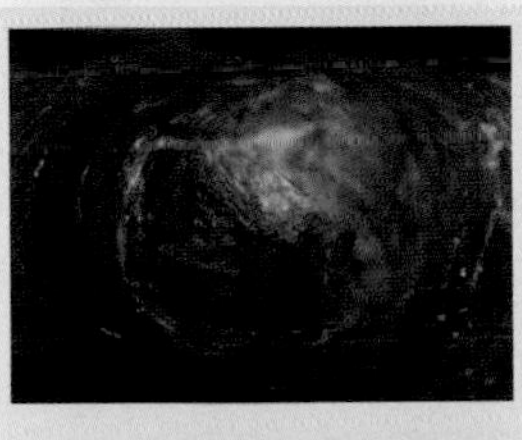	**Stable Eschar** Thick, leathery necrotic tissue; devitalized tissue. Stable eschar is hard leathery covering with no surrounding erythema, drainage, or odor. Because the tissue is dry, it will present as a hard covering. (Used with permission from Aimée Garcia, MD.)
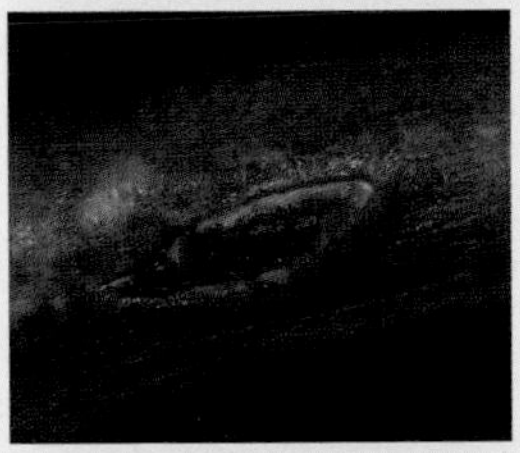	**Unstable Eschar** Thick, leathery necrotic tissue; devitalized tissue. Unstable eschar is a soft leathery covering of dead tissue with evidence of drainage, surrounding erythema, fluctuance, or odor. This tissue is wet in appearance with lifting of the eschar along the edges. Drainage is usually present with an unstable eschar. (Used with permission from Aimée Garcia, MD.)
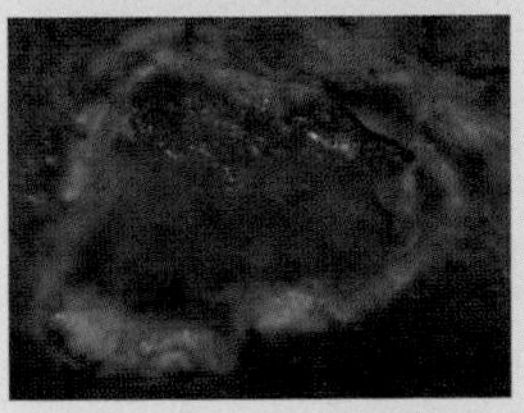	**Biofilm** A complex aggregation of microorganisms marked by the excretion of a protective and adhesive matrix. Biofilm appears as a gelatinous covering of the wound bed, but the microorganisms also invade deeper tissue and can only be seen by electron microscopy. The gelatinous covering is an indication of the bacterial colonies in the wound bed. (Used with permission from Aimée Garcia, MD.)

TABLE 6-7 Pressure Ulcer Periwound Characteristics

Photo	Tissue Characteristics
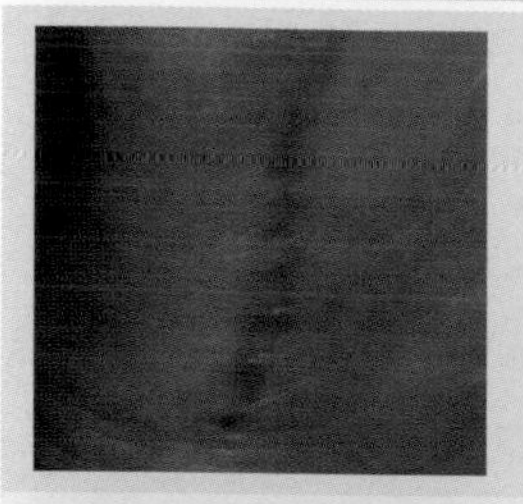	**Viable** Healthy tissue at the edges of the wound that will sustain healing. (Used with permission from Aimée Garcia, MD.)
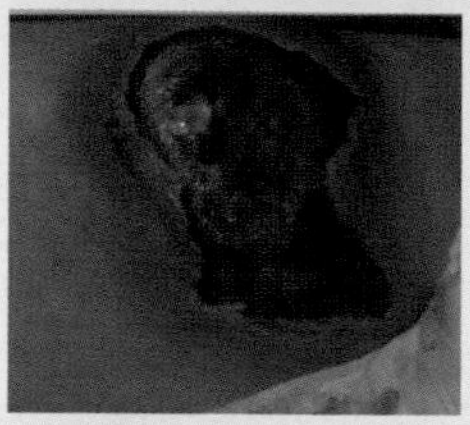	**Erythematous** Bright redness that indicates the presence of inflammation and/or infection in the surrounding tissue. (Used with permission from Aimée Garcia, MD.)
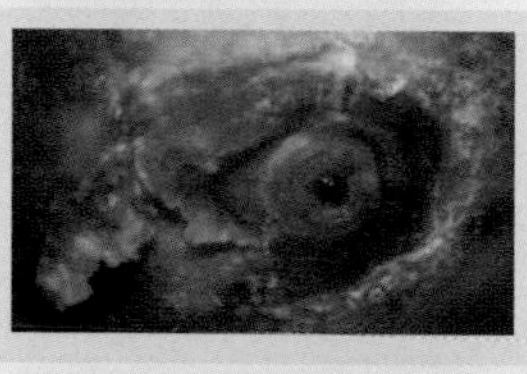	**Hyperkeratosis** Thick accumulation of the outer layer of epidermis at periwound that is nonviable. (Used with permission from Aimée Garcia, MD.)
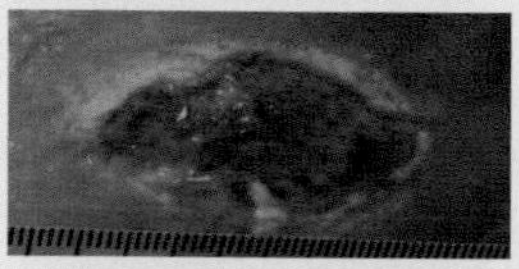	**Maceration** Accumulation of fluid in the soft tissue surrounding the wound bed, causing it to be white and boggy. (Used with permission from Aimée Garcia, MD.)
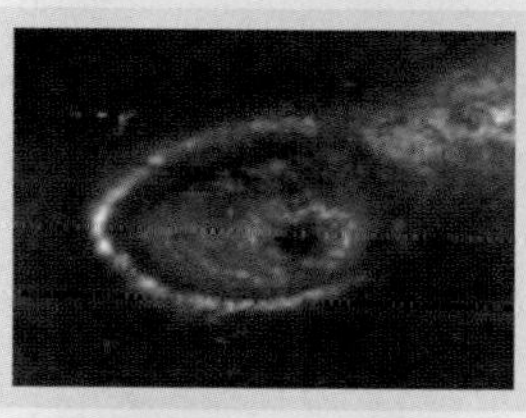	**Rolled Edge/Epibole** Rolled wound edges that can impede wound healing by limiting migration of keratinocytes. (Used with permission from Aimée Garcia, MD.)
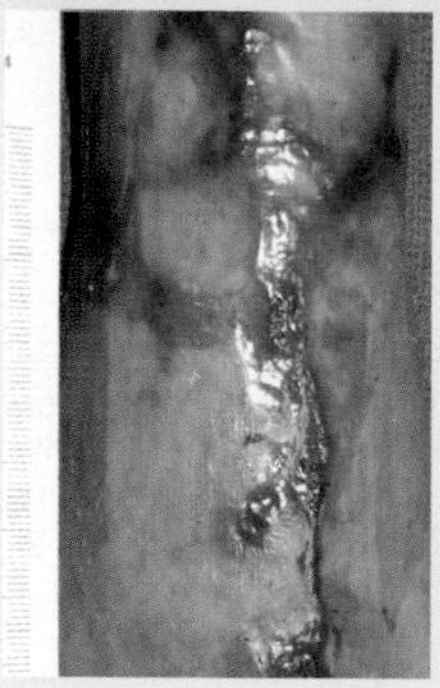	**Epithelialization** Migration of a layer of keratinocytes over the surface of the wound with maturation of the stratum corneum. Note the edges of this wound that are covered with new skin. (Used with permission from Dr. Foy White-Chu.)

firmness may precede visual changes. Color changes do not include purple or maroon discoloration; these may indicate deep tissue pressure injury.

- **Stage II—Pressure Injury: Partial-thickness skin loss with exposed dermis**

  Partial-thickness loss of skin with exposed dermis. The wound bed is viable, pink or red, moist, and may also present as an intact or ruptured serum-filled blister. Adipose (fat) is not visible and deeper tissues are not visible. Granulation tissue, slough, and eschar are not present. These injuries commonly result from adverse microclimate and shear in the skin over the pelvis and shear in the heel. This stage should not be used to describe moisture-associated skin damage (MASD) including incontinence-associated dermatitis (IAD), intertriginous dermatitis (ITD), medical adhesive–related skin injury (MARSI), or traumatic wounds (skin tears, burns, abrasions).

- **Stage III—Full-thickness tissue loss**

  Full-thickness loss of skin, in which adipose (fat) is visible in the ulcer and granulation tissue and epibole (rolled wound edges) are often present. Slough and/or eschar may be visible. The depth of tissue damage varies by anatomical location; areas of significant adiposity can develop deep wounds. Undermining and tunneling may occur. Fascia, muscle, tendon, ligament, cartilage, and/or bone are not exposed. If slough or eschar obscures the extent of tissue loss, this is an Unstageable Pressure Injury.

- **Stage IV—Full-thickness skin and tissue loss**

  Full-thickness skin and tissue loss with exposed or directly palpable fascia, muscle, tendon, ligament, cartilage, or bone in the ulcer. Slough and/or eschar may be visible. Epibole (rolled edges), undermining, and/or tunneling often occur. Depth varies by anatomical location. If slough or eschar obscures the extent of tissue loss this is an Unstageable Pressure Injury.

  Category/Stage IV ulcers can extend into muscle and/or supporting structures (eg, fascia, tendon, or joint capsule), making osteomyelitis or osteitis likely to occur. Exposed bone/muscle is visible or directly palpable.

- **Deep Tissue Pressure Injury: Persistent nonblanchable deep red, maroon, or purple discoloration**

  Intact or nonintact skin with localized area of persistent nonblanchable deep red, maroon, or purple discoloration or epidermal separation revealing a dark wound bed or blood-filled blister. Pain and temperature change often precedes skin color changes. Discoloration may appear differently in darkly pigmented skin. This injury results from intense and/or prolonged pressure and shear forces at the bone–muscle interface. The wound may evolve rapidly to reveal the actual extent of tissue injury or may resolve without tissue loss. If necrotic tissue, subcutaneous tissue, granulation tissue, fascia, muscle, or other underlying structures are visible, this indicates a full-thickness pressure injury (Unstageable, Stage III or Stage IV). Do not use DTPI to describe vascular, traumatic, neuropathic, or dermatologic conditions.

- **Unstageable Pressure Injury—Obscured full-thickness skin and tissue loss**

  Full-thickness skin and tissue loss in which the extent of tissue damage within the ulcer cannot be confirmed because it is obscured by slough or eschar. If slough

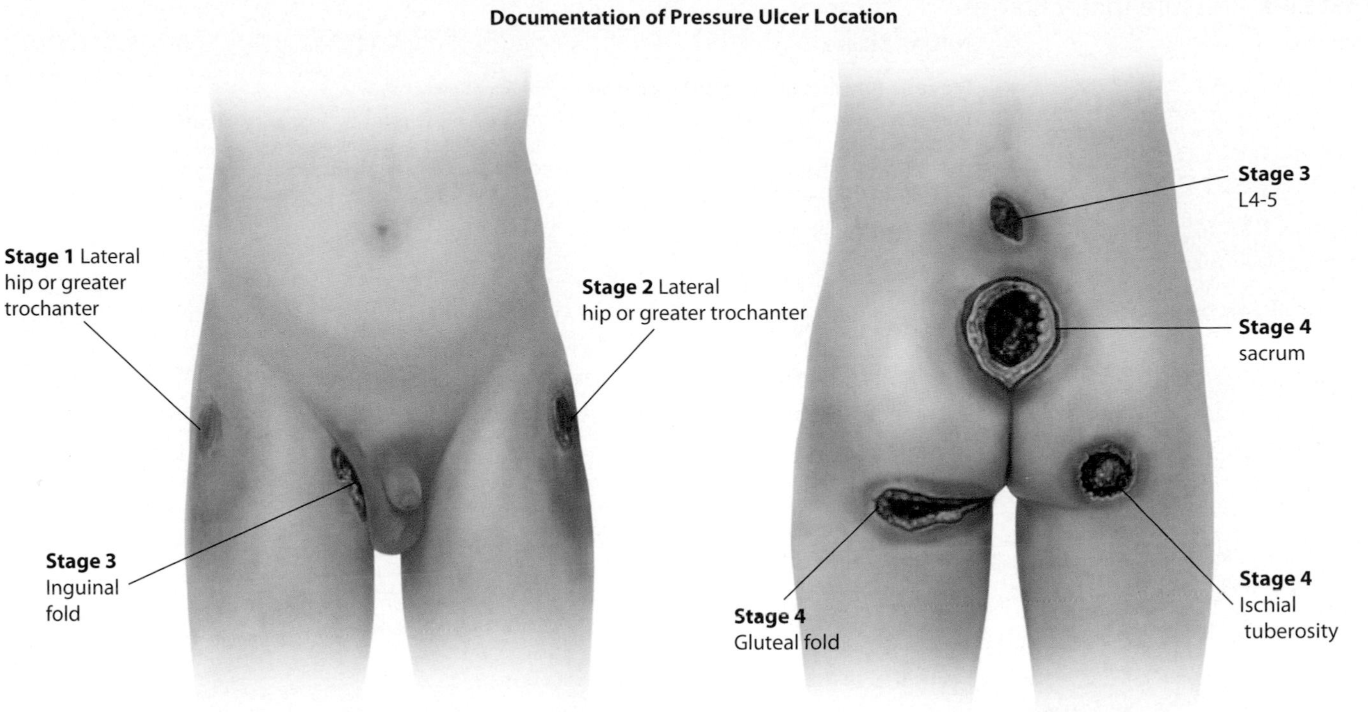

FIGURE 6-29 Anatomic nomenclature of sacral area. Accurate documentation of the pressure injury location is imperative. This schematic illustrates the correct anatomic position of the low back, sacrum, coccyx, buttock, ischial tuberosity, gluteal fold, and (lateral) greater trochanter.

or eschar is removed, a Stage III or Stage IV pressure injury will be revealed. Stable eschar (ie, dry, adherent, intact without erythema or fluctuance) on the heel or ischemic limb should not be softened or removed.

Two additional definitions provided in the 2016 revision include the following:

Medical Device–Related Pressure Injury: Medical device–related pressure injuries result from the use of devices designed and applied for diagnostic or therapeutic purposes. The resultant pressure injury generally conforms to the pattern or shape of the device. The injury should be staged using the staging system (**TABLE 6-9**).

Mucosal Membrane Pressure Injury: Mucosal membrane pressure injury is found on mucous membranes with a history of a medical device in use at the location of the injury. Due to the anatomy of the tissue, these injuries cannot be staged.

While it is natural to stage pressure injuries that are progressing to the next level, pressure injuries that are healing are *not* staged in reverse. For instance, if a Stage IV is granulating so that the exposed muscle is no longer visible, it is termed as Stage IV in the proliferative healing phase; it is not termed as Stage III. If that same Stage IV is closed with a surgical flap, it is termed as Stage IV in the remodeling phase even after the surgical incision is closed. Proper description of both stage and healing phase is important for DRGs, reimbursement, and other legal considerations.

What Is *Not* a Pressure Injury or Ulcer?

All too frequently during assessment of patients with wounds, different types of wounds that are *not* pressure injuries are labeled as pressure injuries. The NPIAP staging system that was described above is only to be used for the staging of pressure injuries and ulcers. All other wounds should be described by their etiology and level of tissue damage (eg, abrasion, partial thickness, or full thickness). **TABLE 6-10** outlines different wounds that may be misdiagnosed as pressure-related wounds, including incontinence-associated dermatitis, abscesses, burns, skin tears, inflammatory wounds, and malignancies. The clinical history of the wound development provides a clear understanding of the etiology. If, for example, the patient has been experiencing significant bowel incontinence due to diarrhea, the superficial skin breakdown on the buttocks region is probably incontinence-associated dermatitis; the primary cause is the contact of the stool against the skin and not pressure. An abscess may initially look like a pressure ulcer; however, after it has ruptured or been lanced, the wound does not resemble a pressure ulcer. If the patient with the wound presented in **TABLE 6-9** as an abscess, presented to the hospital from a nursing home with the wound shown and no clinical history were known about how the wound developed, this wound would likely be misdiagnosed as a pressure ulcer. If, however, it were documented or reported that the patient had developed an area of induration with associated pain, redness, and swelling, and the site had opened with copious amounts of purulent drainage, the clinical picture would be significantly different.

TABLE 6-8 Pressure Injury Stages

<table>
<tr><th>Photo</th><th>NPUAP Stages</th></tr>
<tr><td>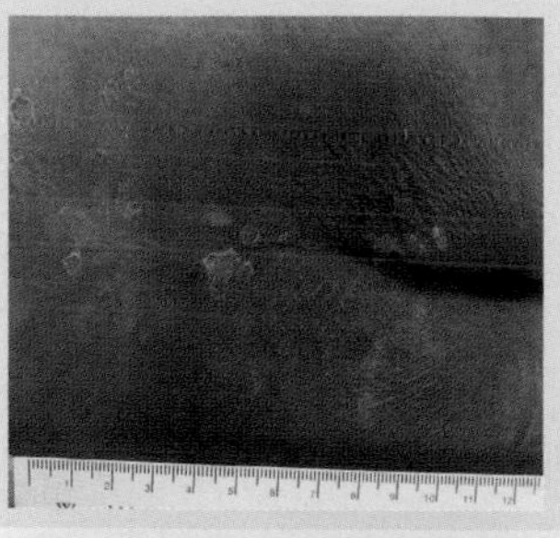</td><td>Stage I—Pressure Injury: Nonblanchable erythema of intact skin
Intact skin with a localized area of nonblanchable erythema, which may appear differently in darkly pigmented skin. Presence of blanchable erythema or changes in sensation, temperature, or firmness may precede visual changes. Color changes do not include purple or maroon discoloration; these may indicate deep tissue pressure injury.
(Used with permission from Dr. Foy White-Chu.)</td></tr>
<tr><td>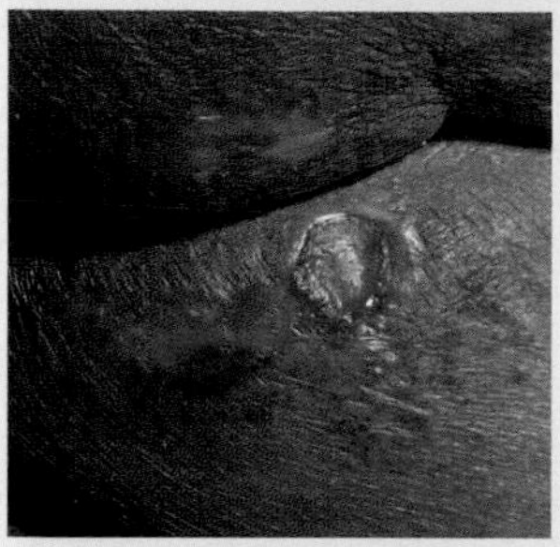</td><td>Stage II—Pressure Injury: Partial-thickness skin loss with exposed dermis
Partial-thickness loss of skin with exposed dermis. The wound bed is viable, pink or red, moist, and may also present as an intact or ruptured serum-filled blister. Adipose (fat) is not visible and deeper tissues are not visible. Granulation tissue, slough and eschar are not present. These injuries commonly result from adverse microclimate and shear in the skin over the pelvis and shear in the heel. This stage should not be used to describe moisture-associated skin damage (MASD) including incontinence-associated dermatitis (IAD), intertriginous dermatitis (ITD), medical adhesive–related skin injury (MARSI), or traumatic wounds (skin tears, burns, abrasions).
(Used with permission from Dr. Foy White-Chu.)</td></tr>
<tr><td>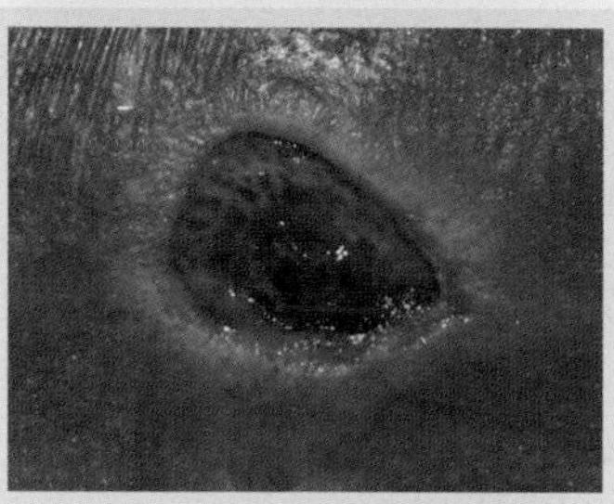</td><td>Stage III—Pressure Injury: Full-thickness skin loss
Full-thickness loss of skin, in which adipose (fat) is visible in the ulcer and granulation tissue and epibole (rolled wound edges) are often present. Slough and/or eschar may be visible. The depth of tissue damage varies by anatomical location; areas of significant adiposity can develop deep wounds. Undermining and tunneling may occur. Fascia, muscle, tendon, ligament, cartilage, and/or bone are not exposed. If slough or eschar obscures the extent of tissue loss, this is an Unstageable Pressure Injury.
(Used with permission from Aimée Garcia, MD.)</td></tr>
<tr><td>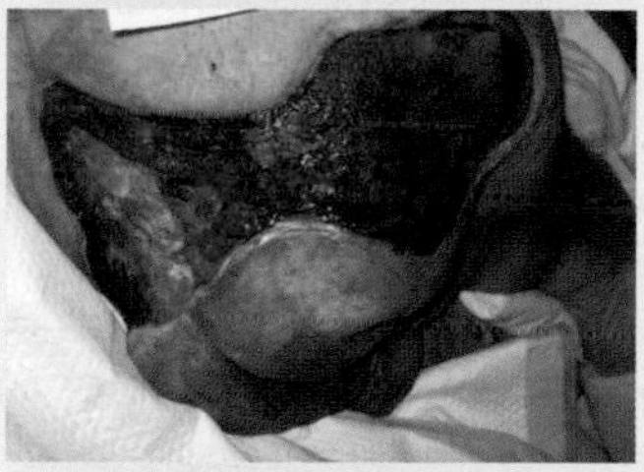</td><td>Stage IV—Pressure Injury: Full-thickness skin and tissue loss
Full-thickness skin and tissue loss with exposed or directly palpable fascia, muscle, tendon, ligament, cartilage, or bone in the ulcer. Slough and/or eschar may be visible. Epibole (rolled edges), undermining and/or tunneling often occur. Depth varies by anatomical location. If slough or eschar obscures the extent of tissue loss this is an Unstageable Pressure Injury.
(Used with permission from Aimée Garcia, MD.)</td></tr>
<tr><td>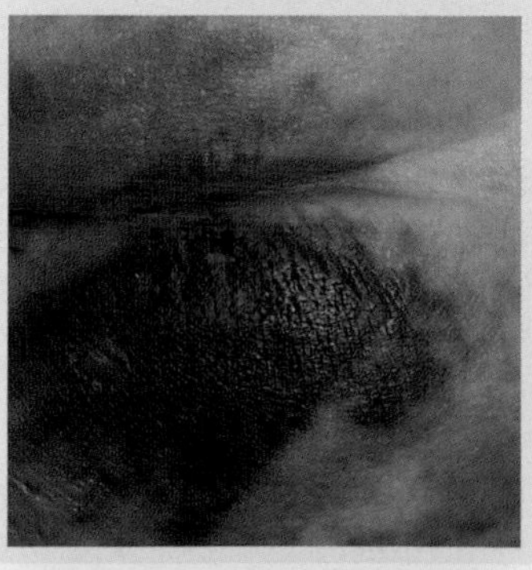</td><td>Deep Tissue Injury: Persistent nonblanchable deep red, maroon, or purple discoloration
Intact or nonintact skin with localized area of persistent nonblanchable deep red, maroon, purple discoloration or epidermal separation revealing a dark wound bed or blood filled blister. Pain and temperature change often precede skin color changes. Discoloration may appear differently in darkly pigmented skin. This injury results from intense and/or prolonged pressure and shear forces at the bone–muscle interface. The wound may evolve rapidly to reveal the actual extent of tissue injury, or may resolve without tissue loss. If necrotic tissue, subcutaneous tissue, granulation tissue, fascia, muscle, or other underlying structures are visible, this indicates a full thickness pressure injury (Unstageable, Stage III or Stage IV). Do not use DTPI to describe vascular, traumatic, neuropathic, or dermatologic conditions.
(Used with permission from Aimée Garcia, MD.)</td></tr>
<tr><td>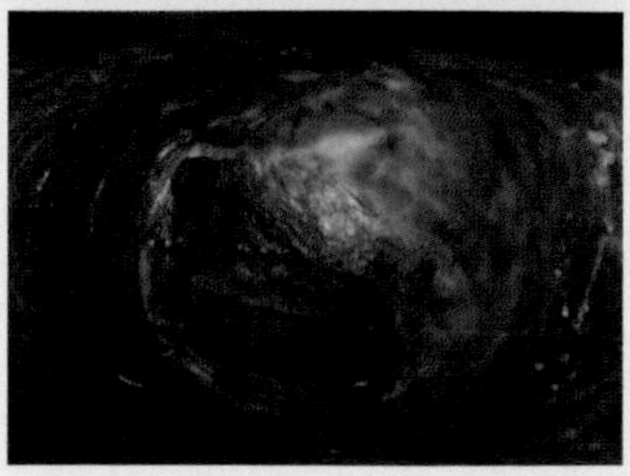</td><td>Unstageable Pressure Injury: Obscured full-thickness skin and tissue loss
Full-thickness skin and tissue loss in which the extent of tissue damage within the ulcer cannot be confirmed because it is obscured by slough or eschar. If slough or eschar is removed, a Stage III or Stage IV pressure injury will be revealed. Stable eschar (ie, dry, adherent, intact without erythema or fluctuance) on the heel or ischemic limb should not be softened or removed.
(Used with permission from Aimée Garcia, MD.)</td></tr>
</table>

Data from definitions as per NPUAP guidelines: www.npuap.org. Accessed December 1, 2018.

TABLE 6-9 Device-Associated Pressure Ulcers

Photo	What Is It?
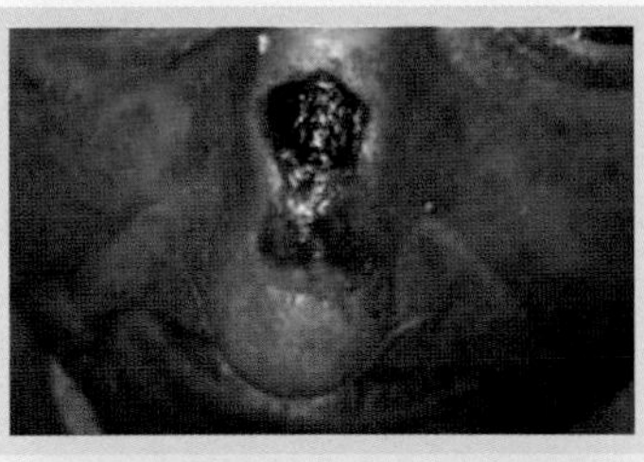	Necrosis on the bridge of the nose caused by pressure from a CPAP machine (Used with permission from Joyce Black, RN, PhD.)
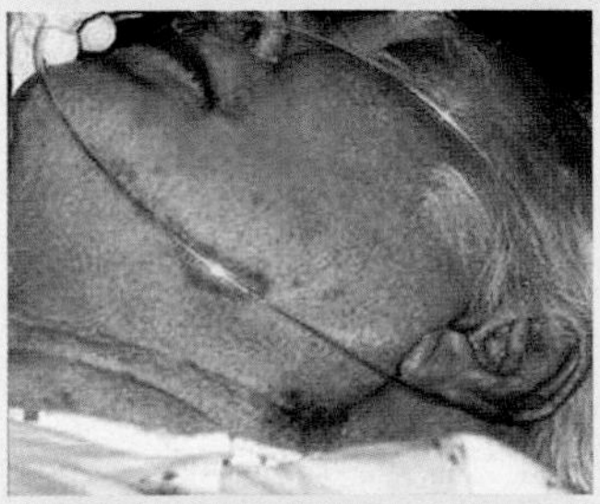	Necrosis due to oxygen tubing (Used with permission from Joyce Black, RN, PhD.)
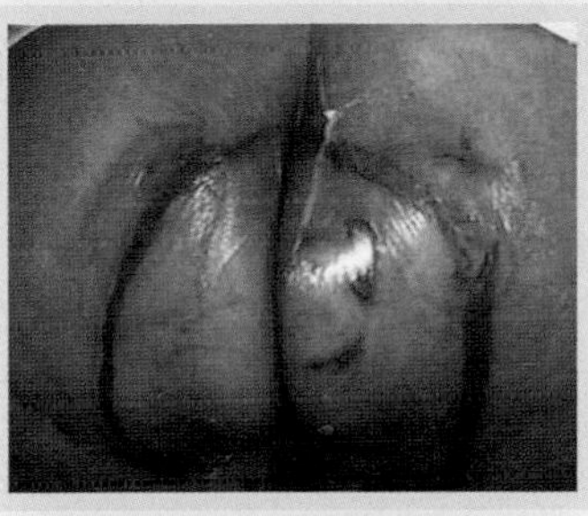	Necrosis due to a patient sitting on a bedside commode for a prolonged period of time (Used with permission from Rose Hamm, DPT.)
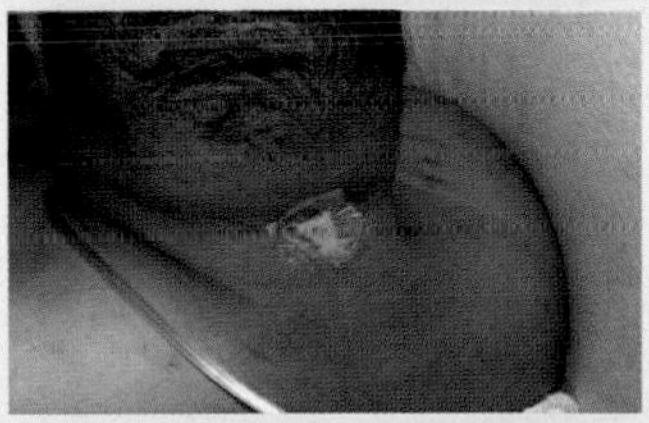	Necrosis of posterior neck due to taping of ET tube while the patient was intubated (Used with permission from Aimée Garcia, MD.)
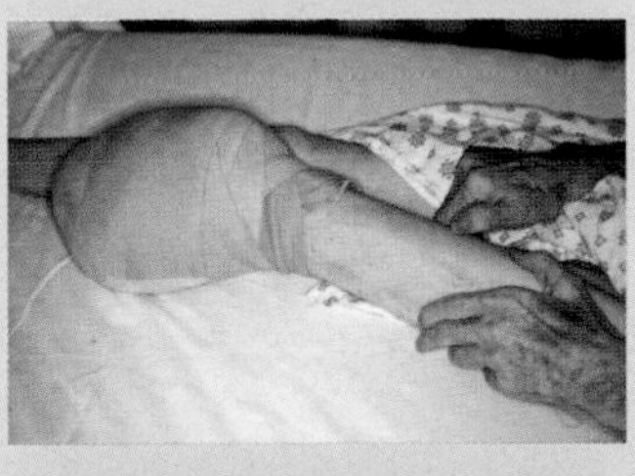 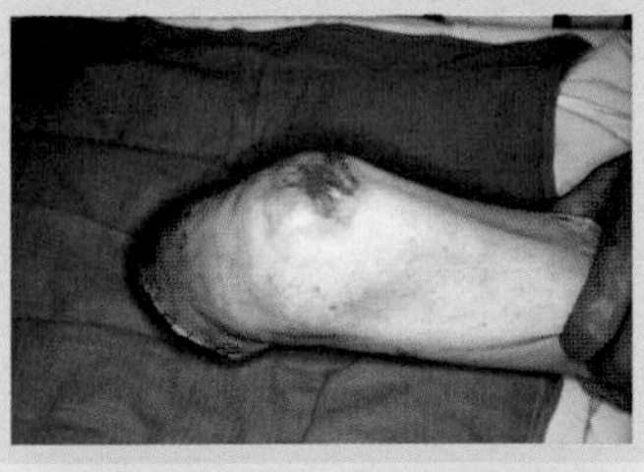	Necrosis on the knee due to a compression wrap being placed too tightly (Used with permission from Mary Sieggreen, NP.)
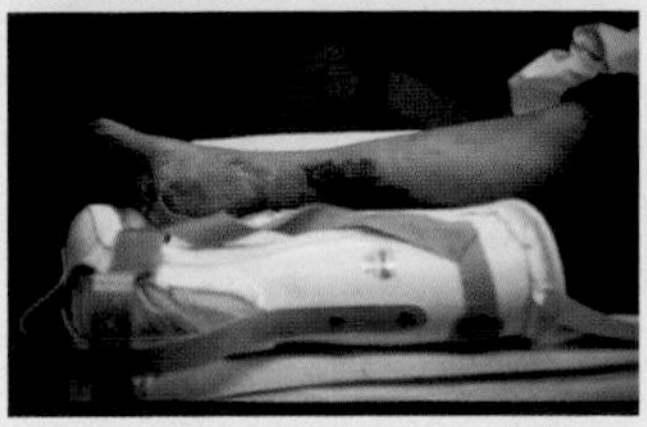	Necrosis due to a poorly fitting brace (Used with permission from Mary Sieggreen, NP.)

CASE STUDY *(Continued)*

The patient undergoes surgical intervention to repair the hip fracture. She receives a total hip arthroplasty and postoperatively is allowed to be full weight-bearing status. At postoperative day #5, she is found by the nursing staff to have a blood-filled blister on the right heel and a superficial area of skin breakdown on the sacrum. The sacral wound is partial thickness and there is no evidence of necrotic tissue. She is scheduled to start physical therapy; however, there is concern about the heel breakdown. As a result of the patient's immobility and the pain medication she is receiving, she has been having issues with constipation which has caused her to have decreased appetite.

DISCUSSION QUESTIONS

1. How would the patient's heel pressure injury be staged?
2. How would the patient's sacral pressure injury be staged?
3. What elements of the wound examination would be used to thoroughly document this wound?

DETECTION OF PRESSURE INJURIES

Skin and tissue assessment (STA) of any patient is a key component of pressure injury prevention. The NPIAP has eight recommendations for conducting an assessment (**TABLE 6-11**). STA routinely consists of skin color, blanchability, temperature, hardness, and other visible or palpable indicators of injury.[56] Visible changes may be especially difficult to discern in skin of color, more so on the trunk than on the heel where there are fewer melanocytes.[57] Technology advancements in detecting skin changes that are proving to be significant include subepidermal moisture measurements, other biomarkers, and continuous pressure mapping.

Subepidermal moisture detection uses a hand-held device to measure electrical biocapacitance of tissue in order to detect increases in subepidermal moisture (SEM). The measurement reflects the presence of edema in tissue below the stratum corneum, an early indication of the inflammatory response that occurs with pressure injury.[58] The device has been shown to detect positive findings 4.74 days +/− 2.39 days earlier than the diagnosis of pressure injury with STA.[56] This is especially significant in detection of pressure injury in skin of color, and has also been studied in persons with spinal cord injury; in nursing homes; and on the sacrum, buttocks, and heels.[57]

Other biomarkers that have been studied for early detection of pressure injury include serum albumin, serum hemoglobin, and C-reactive protein (CRP). A meta-analysis by Wang et al. suggests that the combination of hemoglobin, CRP, albumin, age, and gender is superior to any of the biomarkers alone.[59]

TABLE 6-10 What Is Not a Pressure Injury?

Photo	What Is It?
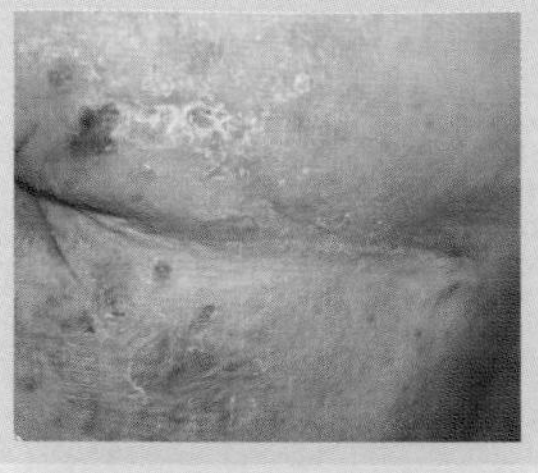	**Incontinence-Associated Dermatitis** Breakdown of the skin due to contact with moisture, which leads to superficial desquamation; can be associated with secondary candidiasis. (Used with permission from Dr. Foy White-Chu.)
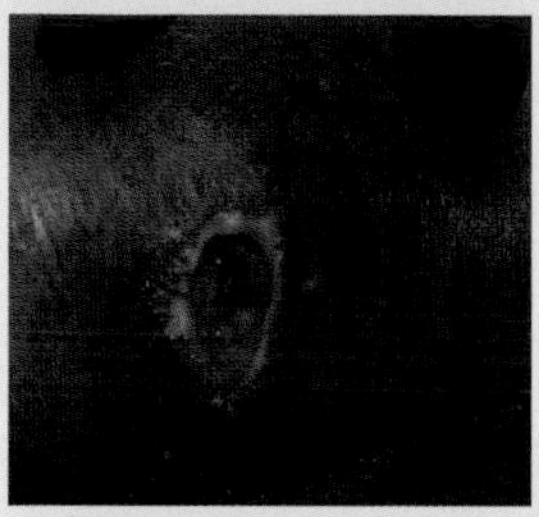	**Abscess** Deep necrotic autolysed tissue, often infected, with hard, warm, indurated skin. Abscesses either spontaneously open or need to be opened and drained, leaving a defect. The wound would be defined as full thickness, but is not staged. (Used with permission from Aimée Garcia, MD.)
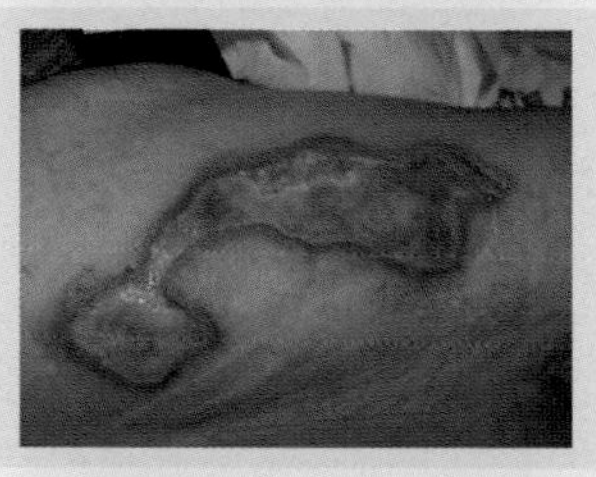	**Burn** The irregular shape of this wound and the location (not over a bony prominence) indicate another process. In this case, the patient spilled hot liquid over the leg, causing a full thickness burn. (Used with permission from Aimée Garcia, MD.)
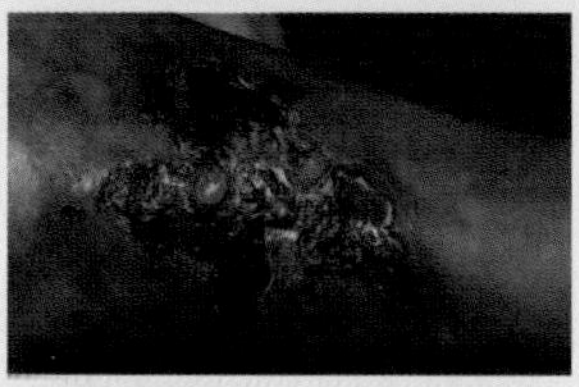	**Infection** This wound in the anterior leg is secondary to infection, which led to skin necrosis. The location of necrosis indicates that pressure was not the wound etiology. (Used with permission from Aimée Garcia, MD.)
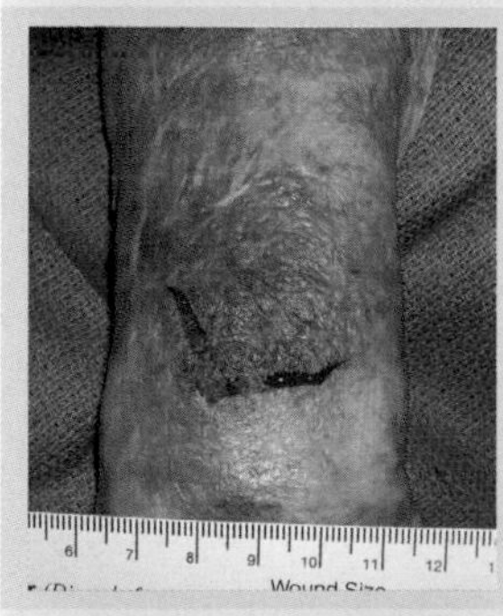	**Skin Tear** The skin in elderly individuals can be very thin, leading to superficial tears involving the epidermis and dermis. Frequently, a flap of skin is seen where the skin peeled back and may or may not survive the healing process. (Used with permission from Dr. Foy White-Chu.)
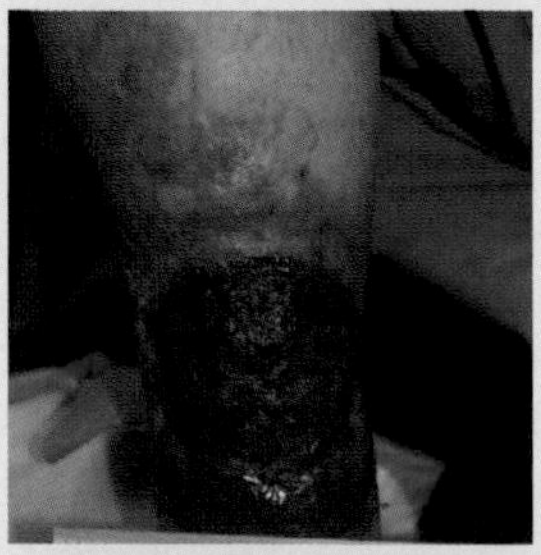	**Inflammatory Wounds** This wound is atypical in appearance, has a violaceous border, and is located on an area not typically associated with pressure. The diagnosis in this case is pyoderma gangrenosum. (Used with permission from Aimée Garcia, MD.)
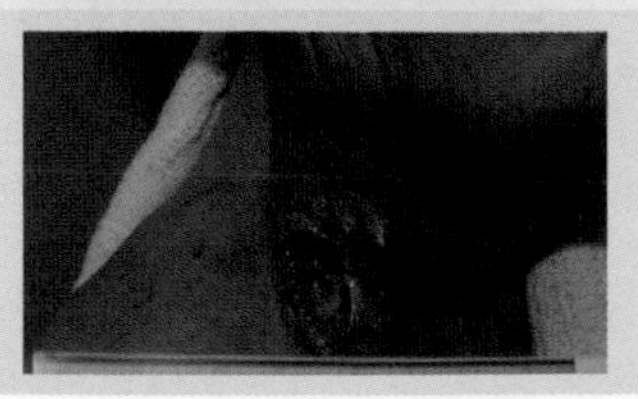	**Malignancy** This patient has an ulcerative lesion in the neck. This wound is secondary to squamous cell carcinoma of the head and neck. (Used with permission from Aimée Garcia, MD.)

TABLE 6-11 NPIAP Recommendations for Skin and Tissue Assessment

- Conduct a comprehensive skin and tissue assessment of any patient at risk of a pressure injury at admission to any healthcare facility, as part of every risk assessment, periodically after admission as risk changes, and prior to discharge from the care service.
- Identify presence of erythema.
- Differentiate blanchable from nonblanchable erythema with finger pressure or with transparent disk.
- Assess the temperature of skin and soft tissue by palpation or with infrared thermography.
- Consider using subepidermal moisture/edema measurement device as adjunct to routine assessment.
- Assess skin temperature and subepidermal moisture in patients with darkly pigmented skin.
- Evaluate the relevance of performing an objective skin assessment with a color chart when conducting a skin assessment.

Adapted from the EPUAP, NPIAP, and PPPIA. *Prevention and Treatment of Pressure Ulcers/Injuries: Clinical Practice Guidelines*. The International Guideline 2019:73-83.

A study by Krishnan et al. found that an increase in the concentration of the interferon-γ-induced protein of 10kd/CXCL10 in plasma and a decrease in the concentration of the cytokine interferon-α in urine (both inflammatory mediators) were observed about 4 days prior to the occurrence of a first pressure injury.[60]

Although these technologies are not readily available in every setting, the research shows that there are physiological changes that occur in the subcutaneous tissue, and indeed even systemically, prior to the outwardly visible signs of pressure injury.

TREATMENT OF PRESSURE INJURIES AND ULCERS

Treatment of pressure injuries and ulcers depends on the clinical presentation of the wound. The mainstays of treatment are debridement, maintaining a moist wound environment, decreasing bacterial load, and pressure redistribution. Necrotic tissue in the wound is removed by debridement unless the patient's clinical picture or goals of care preclude this course of care. Debridement of a wound has the following goals: removal of necrotic tissue which is a harbor for bacteria, determination of the depth of tissue damage, accurate staging of the pressure injury, and conversion of a chronic wound to an acute wound. The five main types of debridement used to remove necrotic tissue are sharp, enzymatic, mechanical, autolytic, and biologic. In addition, laser debridement and ultrasonic debridement are being utilized more frequently in the wound care field.[61] (A thorough discussion of debridement is presented in Chapter 13, Wound Debridement.) In addition to the standard of care as described, adjunct therapies have been shown to be beneficial in facilitating wound healing, including pressure injuries and ulcers (**TABLE 6-12**). Specific parameters for treatment are found in the chapters on adjunct therapies in Part Four of this book.

CASE STUDY *(Continued)*

The patient's heel developed soft necrotic tissue with surrounding erythema, light serous drainage with associated odor, and pain. She is limited in her ability to do physical therapy by the pain in her foot. The patient's sacral pressure ulcer now has a thin layer of yellow slough, but no evidence of periwound erythema. There are no signs or symptoms of infection. The attending physician wants to transfer the patient to a skilled nursing facility for ongoing physical therapy and wound care, but they need recommendations on how to treat the wounds on the heel and the sacrum.

DISCUSSION QUESTIONS

1. What debridement techniques are optimal for the patient's heel given her clinical picture? For her sacrum?
2. What is the best type of footwear for the patient to be able to ambulate?
3. What is the optimal sitting position for this patient, and how is it best achieved and maintained?
4. What are the possible complications that can occur due to the deterioration of the heel?

TABLE 6-12 Use of Biophysical Technologies for Treating Pressure Injuries

Technology	Indication
Electrical stimulation	Stage II, III, or IV that has not made significant improvement after 30 days of standard treatment (CMS regulation)
Negative pressure wound therapy	Stage III or IV that is cavernous and has been debrided; recommended to have <30% necrotic tissue in the wound bed
Noncontact, low-frequency ultrasound	Deep tissue injury
Pulsed lavage with suction	Stage III or IV that is necrotic and/or draining, in conjunction with sharp debridement
Hyperbaric oxygen therapy	Pressure-related ulcers on the foot of a patient who has diabetes
Ultraviolet	Stage II, III, or IV that is suspected to have bioburden
Low-level laser therapy	No evidence supporting the use for pressure ulcers

COMPLICATIONS OF PRESSURE ULCERS

Pressure ulcers can lead to multiple clinical complications, including wound infection, abscess formation, osteomyelitis, sepsis, and death. Infected pressure ulcers are one of the leading causes of infection in long-term care facilities and can lead to sepsis.[62–64] Because of the cellular changes that occur as a result of the disease process, patients with diabetes have a tenfold increase in developing and being hospitalized for a soft tissue or bone infection of the foot.[65] The level of bacteria in the wound bed includes colonization, local infection or critical colonization, and deep infection.

If the pressure ulcer has extensive necrosis or is close to the anus, thus increasing the risk for contamination with stool, surgical procedures such as debridement, diverting colostomies, and flaps or skin grafts may be required to effectively close the wound. Patients who develop larger or more complicated pressure ulcers need to be referred to specialists (eg, plastic surgeons, infectious disease physicians, wound care specialists) for comprehensive care and faster resolution. In addition to treating the wound and providing effective pressure redistribution, the overall medical condition of the patient is critical to wound healing, especially as it applies to nutrition, medications, and psychosocial factors. These issues are discussed in Chapter 12, Factors That Impede Wound Healing, and apply to both prevention and treatment of pressure ulcers.

SUMMARY

In summary, the goals of healthcare providers are early assessment for risk of pressure injury and ulcer development, implementation of preventive strategies, and if a pressure injury should develop, comprehensive assessment of the wound and early aggressive treatment to prevent further deterioration. Through education of healthcare providers, a decrease in the impact of pressure injuries and ulcers on the healthcare system are achievable outcomes for the multidisciplinary medical team, in addition to improvement in the patient's quality of life.

STUDY QUESTIONS

1. What is the force that occurs between the skin and linen when the head of the bed is elevated?
   a. Normal force
   b. Shear
   c. Friction
   d. Pressure
2. What are the two most common sites for pressure injury occurrence on a bedridden patient?
   a. Heel and sacrum
   b. Ischial tuberosity and sacrum
   c. Ischial tuberosity and greater trochanter
   d. Greater trochanter and scapula
3. The overall stiffness of a support surface directly impacts the ____________ of a person lying upon it.
   a. Posture
   b. Immersion
   c. Friction
   d. Safety
4. A pressure injury that extends to the fascia, but not through the fascia, is staged at what level?
   a. Stage I
   b. Stage II
   c. Stage III
   d. Stage IV
5. Which contributing factor is most likely to cause a deep sinus to form as part of the pressure ulcer?
   a. Friction
   b. Moisture
   c. Pressure
   d. Shear
6. A patient is bedridden with complications after open heart surgery and has a 20-degree dorsiflexion contracture on the right foot. What is the best pressure-redistribution device for the patient's heel in order to prevent a pressure injury?
   a. Rigid ankle-foot orthotic device
   b. Foam boot with suspended heel and adjustable ankle joint
   c. Pillows under the calves
   d. Heel and foot elevating pad
7. A patient who is confined to a wheelchair is most vulnerable for tissue injury at
   a. The heel.
   b. The thoracic spine.
   c. The posterior thigh.
   d. The coccyx.
8. Which wheelchair cushions offer the best pressure relief for a person at high risk of developing a pressure injury?
   a. Air
   b. Foam
   c. Gel
   d. Silicone
9. Ordering a wheelchair that is too wide for a patient is a good preventive strategy because he/she will probably grow into it.
   a. True
   b. False
10. All individuals need to be turned in bed every 2 hours to prevent pressure injury.
   a. True
   b. False

Answers: 1-c; 2-a; 3-b; 4-c; 5-d; 6-b; 7-d; 8-a; 9-b; 10-b

REFERENCES

1. National Pressure Injury Advisory Panel, European Pressure Ulcer Advisory Panel, and Pan Pacific Pressure Injury Alliance. Prevention and Treatment of Pressure Ulcers/Injuries: Clinical Practice Guideline. 2019: 16.
2. US Agency for Healthcare Research and Quality. Available at: www.ahrq.gov/news/newsroom/press-releases/hac-rates-declined.html.
3. Padula W, Delarmente BA. The national cost of hospital-acquired pressure injuries in the US. *Int Wound J.* 2019;16(3):634-640.
4. Marvis JS, Phillips TJ. Pressure ulcers: pathophysiology, epidemiology, risk factors, and presentation. *J Am Acad Dermatol.* 2019;81(4):881-890.
5. Caliri MH. Spinal cord injury and pressure ulcers. *Nurs Clin North Am.* 2005;40(2):337-347.
6. Margolis DJ, et al. The incidence and prevalence of pressure ulcers among elderly patients in general medicine practice. *Ann Epidemiol.* 2002;12:321-325.
7. Large J. A cost-effective pressure damage prevention strategy. *Br J Nurs.* 2011;20(6):S22-S25.

8. US Census Bureau. *Population Projection Program, Population Division*. Washington, DC: US Census Bureau; 2000.
9. Brienza D, Antokal S, Herbe L, et al. Friction-induced skin injuries-are they pressure ulcers? An updated NPUAP white paper. *J Wound Ostomy Continence Nurs*. 2015;42(1):62-64.
10. Takahashi Y, Isogai Z, Mizokami F, et al. Location-dependent depth and undermining formation of pressure ulcers. *J Tissue Viability*. 2013;22(3):63-67.
11. Bates-Jensen BM. Pressure ulcers: pathophysiology, detection, and prevention. In: Sussman C, Bates-Jensen BM, eds. *Wound Care: A Collaborative Practice Manual for Health Professionals*. Baltimore, MD: Lippincott Williams & Wilkins; 2012:230-277.
12. Kosiak M. Etiology of decubitus ulcers. *Arch Phys Med Rehabil*. 1961; 42:19-29.
13. Gefen A. Reswick and Rogers pressure-time curve for pressure ulcer risk. Part 1. *Nurs Stand*. 2009;23(45):64, 66, 68 passim.
14. Centers for Medicare and Medicaid. Available at: https://www.cms.gov/Medicare/Medicare-Fee-for-Service-Payment/HospitalAcqCond/Hospital-Acquired_Conditions. Accessed April 27, 2023.
15. Tescher AN, Branda ME, Byrne TJ, Naessens JM. All at-risk patients are not created equal: analysis of Braden pressure ulcer risk scores to identify specific risks. *J Wound Ostomy Continence Nurs*. 2012;39(3):282-291.
16. National Pressure Injury Advisory Panel, European Pressure Ulcer Advisory Panel, and Pan Pacific Pressure Injury Alliance. *Prevention and Treatment of Pressure Ulcers/Injuries: Clinical Practice Guideline*. 2019: 63.
17. National Pressure Injury Advisory Panel, European Pressure Ulcer Advisory Panel, and Pan Pacific Pressure Injury Alliance. Support surfaces. *Prevention and Treatment of Pressure Ulcers/Injuries: Clinical Practice Guideline*. 2019: 155-180.
18. Colin D, Rochet JM, Ribinik P. What is the best support surface in prevention and treatment, as of 2012, for a patient at risk and/or suffering from pressure ulcer sore? Developing French guidelines for clinical practice. *Ann Phys Rehabil Med*. 2012;55(7):466-481.
19. McInnes E, Asmara J, Bell-Syer S. Preventing pressure ulcers: are pressure-redistributing support surfaces effective? A Cochrane systematic review and meta-analysis. *Int J Nurs Stud*. 2012;49(3): 345-359.
20. McInnes E, Asmara J, Cullum N. Support surfaces for treating pressure injury: a Cochrane systematic review. *Int J Nurs Stud*. 2013; 50(3):419-430.
21. Shi C, Dumville JC, Cullum N. Support surfaces for pressure ulcer prevention: a network meta-analysis. *PLoS One*. 2018; 13(2):e0192707.
22. Serraes B, van Leen M, Schols J, Van Hecke A, Verhaeghe S, Beeckman D. Prevention of pressure ulcers with a static air support surface: a systematic review. *Int Wound J*. 2018;15(3):333-343.
23. Finnegan MJ, Gazzerro L, Finnegan JO, Lo P. Comparing the effectiveness of a specialized alternating air pressure mattress replacement system and an air-fluidized integrated bed in the management of post-operative flap patients: a randomized controlled pilot study. *J Tissue Viability*. 2008;17(1):2-9.
24. Russell L, Reynolds T, Carr J, Evans A, Holmes M. A comparison of healing rates on two pressure-relieving systems. *Br J Nurs*. 2000; 9(22):2270-2280.
25. Theaker C, Kuper M, Soni N. Pressure ulcer prevention in intensive care—a randomised control trial of two pressure-relieving devices. *Anaesthesia*. 2005;60(4):395-399.
26. Greenwood C. Heel pressure ulcers: understanding why they develop and how to prevent them. *Nurs Stand*. 2022;37(2):60-66.
27. Davies P. Preventing the development of heel pressure ulcers. *Nurs Stand*. 2018;33(7):69-76.
28. McGinnis E, Greenwood DC, Nelson EA, Nixon J. A prospective cohort study of prognostic factors for the healing of heel pressure ulcers. *Age Ageing*. 2014;43:267-271.
29. Junkin J, Gray M. Are pressure redistribution surfaces or heel protection devices effective for preventing heel pressure ulcers? *J Wound Ostomy Continence Nurs*. 2009;36(6):602-608.
30. Greenwood C, Nelson EA, Nixon J, Vargas-Palacios A, McGinnis E. Comparative effectiveness of heel-specific medical devices for the prevention of heel pressure ulcers: a systematic review. *J Tissue Viability*. 2022;31(4):579-592.
31. Heyneman A, Grypdonck VK, Defloor T. Effectiveness of two cushions in the prevention of heel pressure ulcers. *Worldviews Evid Based Nurs*. 2009;6(2):114-120.
32. Clegg R, Palfreyman S. Elevation devices for the prevention of heel pressure ulcers: a review. *Br J Nurs*. 2014;23(Suppl 20)S4-S11.
33. He C, Shi P. Interface pressure reduction effects of wheelchair cushions in individuals with spinal cord injury: a rapid review. *Disabil Rehabil*. 2022;44(6):827-834.
34. Peko Cohen L, Gefen A. Deep tissue loads in the seated buttocks on an off-loading wheelchair cushion versus air-cell-based and foam cushions: finite element studies. *Int Wound J*. 2017;14(6): 1327-1334.
35. Meaume S, Marty M, Colin D. Prospective observational study of single- or multi-compartment pressure ulcer prevention cushions: PRESCAROH project. *J Wound Care*. 2017;26(9):537-544.
36. Sprigle S, Press L, Davis K. Development of uniform terminology and procedures to describe wheelchair cushion characteristics. *J Rehabil Res Dev*. 2001;38(4):449-461.
37. de Looze MP, Kuijt-Evers LF, van Dieen J. Sitting comfort and discomfort and the relationships with objective measures. *Ergonomics*. 2003;46(10):985-997.
38. Fenety PA, Putnam C, Walker JM. In chair movement: validity, reliability and implications for measuring sitting discomfort. *Appl Ergon*. 2000;31(4):383-393.
39. Grandjean E. Sitting posture of car drivers from the point of view of ergonomics. In: Oborne DJ, Levis JA, eds. *Human Factors in Transport Research*. New York, NY: Academic Press; 1980:240-248.
40. Reenalda J, VanGeffen P, Nederhand M, Jannink M. Analysis of healthy sitting behavior: interface pressure distribution and subcutaneous tissue oxygenation. *J Rehab Res Devel*. 2009:46(5):577-586.
41. Richardson GM, Gardner S, Frantz RA. Nursing assessment: impact on type and cost of interventions to prevent pressure ulcers. *J Wound Ostomy Continence Nurs*. 1998;25(6):273-280.
42. Hagisawa S, Ferguson-Pell M. Evidence supporting the use of two-hourly turning for pressure ulcer prevention. *J Tissue Viability*. 2008;17(3):76-81.
43. Agency for Health Care Policy and Research. Pressure ulcers in adults: prediction and prevention. *Clin Pract Guide Quick Ref Guide Clin*. 1992;3:1-15.
44. Clark M. Repositioning to prevent pressure sores: what is the evidence? *Nurs Stand*. 1998;13(3):58-60, 62, 64.
45. Krapfl LA, Gray M. Does regular repositioning prevent pressure ulcers? *J Wound Ostomy Continence Nurs*. 2008;35(6):571-577.
46. Jocelyn Chew HS, Thiara E, Lopez V, Shorey S. Turning frequency in adult bedridden patients to prevent hospital-acquired pressure ulcer: a scoping review. *Int Wound J*. 2018;15(2):225-236.
47. Defloor T, De Bacquer D, Grypdonck MH. The effect of various combinations of turning and pressure reducing devices on the incidence of pressure ulcers. *Int J Nurs Stud*. 2005;42(1):37-46.

48. Gefen A. How much time does it take to get a pressure ulcer? Integrated evidence from human, animal, and in vitro studies. *Ostomy Wound Manage*. 2008;54(10):26-28, 30–35.
49. Vanderwee K, Grypdonck MH, DeBacquer D, Defloor T. Effectiveness of turning with unequal time intervals on the incidence of pressure ulcer lesions. *J Adv Nurs*. 2007;57(1):59-68.
50. Sprigle S, Sonenblum SE, Feng C. Pressure redistributing in-seat movement activities by persons with spinal cord injury over multiple epochs. *PLoS One*. 2019;14(2):e0210978.
51. Coggrave MJ, Rose LS. A specialist seating assessment clinic: changing pressure relief practice. *Spinal Cord*. 2003;41(12):692-695.
52. Nawoczenski DA. Pressure sores: prevention and management. In: Buchanan LE, Nawoczenski DA, eds. *Spinal Cord Injury: Concepts and Management Approaches*. Baltimore, MD: Williams &Wilkins; 1987.
53. Sliwinski MM, Druin E. Intervention principles and position change. In: Sisto SA, Druin E, Sliwinski MM, eds. *Spinal Cord Injuries: Management and Rehabilitation*. Maryland Heights, MO: Mosby; 2009.
54. Sonenblum SE, Feng C, Sprigle S. The relationship between in-seat movement and pressure ulcers in wheelchair users with SCI/D. *J Spinal Cord Med*. 2022:1-9.
55. National Pressure Ulcer Advisory Panel (NPUAP) announces a change in terminology from pressure ulcer to pressure injury and updates the stages of pressure injury. Available at: www.npuap.org/national-pressure-ulcer-advisory-panel-npuap-announces-a-change-in-terminology-from-pressure-ulcer-to-pressure-injury-and-updates-the-stages-of-pressure-injury. Accessed September 4, 2018.
56. Okonkwo H, Bryant R, Milne J, et al. A blinded clinical study using a subepidermal moisture biocapacitance measurement device for early detection of pressure injuries. *Wound Rep Reg*. 2020;28:364-374.
57. Bates-Jensen BM, McCreath HE, Nakagami G, Patlan A. Subepidermal moisture detection of heel pressure injury: the pressure ulcer detection study outcomes. *Int Wound J*. 2018;15(2):297-309.
58. Gefen A, Ross G. The subepidermal moisture scanner: the technology explained. *J Wound Care*. 2020;29(Sup2c):S10-S16.
59. Wang N, Lv L, Yan F, et al. Biomarkers for the early detection of pressure injury: a systematic review and meta-analysis. *J Tissue Viability*. 2022;31(2):259-267.
60. Krishnan S, Karg PE, Boninger ML, et al. Early detection of pressure ulcer development following traumatic spinal cord injury using inflammatory mediators. *Arch Phys Med Rehabil*. 2016;97(10): 1656-1662.
61. Emhoff TA, Ferro SA. Wound debridement. In: Sheffield PJ, Fife CE, eds. *Wound Care Practice*. 2nd ed. Flagstaff, AZ: Best Publishing; 2007.
62. Madhuri R, Sudeep SG, Wei W, Sunila RK, Rochon PA. Does this patient have infection of a chronic wound? *JAMA*. 2012;307(6):605-611.
63. Redelings MD, Lee NE, Sorvillo F. Pressure ulcers: more lethal than we thought? *Adv Skin Wound Care*. 2005;18(7):367-372.
64. Smith PW, Black JM, Black SB. Infected pressure ulcers in the long-term-care facility. *Infect Control Hosp Epidemiol*. 1999;20(5):358-361.
65. Boykoe EJ, Lipsky BA. Infection and diabetes mellitus. In: Harris MI, ed. *Diabetes in America*. 2nd ed. Bethesda, MD: National Institutes of Health; 1995:485-496.

CHAPTER SEVEN

Diabetes and the Diabetic Foot

Pamela Scarborough, PT, DPT, MS, CWS, FAAWC and James McGuire, DPM, PT, CPed, FAPWHc

CHAPTER OBJECTIVES

At the end of this chapter, the learner will be able to:

1. **Discuss the types and trends related to diabetes.**
2. **Recognize the effects of diabetes on all wound etiologies.**
3. **Identify risk factors leading to diabetic foot ulcers.**
4. **Compare and contrast different interventions appropriate for treatment of diabetic foot ulcers.**
5. **Develop a comprehensive plan of care for a patient with a diabetic foot ulcer.**
6. **Select the proper footwear to prevent and treat a diabetic foot ulcer.**

INTRODUCTION

The classic model of the neuropathic foot is most frequently associated with the disease of diabetes, a commonly encountered comorbidity in the population of patients with wounds. While many comorbidities have the potential to impact wound healing, this is especially true in people with diabetes. Therefore, healthcare professionals need to understand the diabetes disease process, its implications on the general health of the patient, and its impact specifically on wound healing. The wound care clinician does not manage the individual's diabetes—this responsibility belongs to a primary care physician or an endocrinologist who coordinates the overall diabetes plan of care.

However, it is the responsibility of the wound care clinician to (1) review the patient's blood glucose values to ensure there is adequate control of the disease to support effective wound healing and (2) recognize when the disease may be negatively affecting a patient's wound healing potential.

This chapter provides an overview of the epidemiology of diabetes, its effects on wound healing, clinical challenges that the comorbidity of diabetes poses to the form and function of the foot, and considerations for clinical interventions when a diabetic foot ulcer (DFU) is present. For comprehensive information on the pathophysiology and treatment of diabetes, the reader is referred to other sources, including the standards of care from the American Diabetes Association[1] and American Association of Clinical Endocrinologists' comprehensive diabetes management algorithm—2020.[2] This chapter also provides an overview of treatment strategies necessary for patients to control their diabetes in order to support wound management interventions. Blood glucose control is necessary to assist in attaining optimal outcomes for all hard-to-heal wounds, including diabetic or neuropathic foot ulcers.

CLINICAL CONSIDERATION

The disease state of diabetes is managed by a team of specialists. In the absence of a team, the primary care physician or endocrinologist will direct the medical management of this complicated disease.

DIABETES

Epidemiology and Healthcare Implications

The prevalence of diabetes has risen steadily and dramatically over the past several decades. Diabetes negatively impacts every organ and system of the body and is currently considered to be at epidemic proportions worldwide.[1,4] Recent estimates of the global prevalence for diabetes is 536.6 million individuals, projecting growth to 783.2 million in 2045.[4] The Centers for Disease Control and Prevention (CDC) estimates that as of 2019 the United States had 37.3 million people diagnosed with diabetes, or roughly 11.3% of the population, plus another 8.5 million who are undiagnosed with type 2 diabetes.[5] In addition to this number, over 96 million people have the condition of prediabetes, adding up to over 100 million people living with diabetes or prediabetes in the United States. More statistics are presented in **TABLE 7-1**.

The number of people at risk for or with diabetes continues to increase despite significant efforts to screen and educate the public. The major controllable risk factors associated with acquiring type 2 diabetes include obesity, lack of exercise and physical activity, lack of knowledge regarding good nutrition, lack of access to nutritional food, and poor dietary choices. Many people have a strong genetic predisposition for type 2 diabetes. When type 2 diabetes is a hereditary component, people should begin prevention strategies as part of their lifestyle as early in life as possible, learning the interventions to delay and, in some cases, prevent this potentially devastating disease.

CLINICAL CONSIDERATION

Diabetes is the most costly chronic illness in the United States. One in four healthcare dollars is spent on someone with a diabetes diagnosis.[3]

TABLE 7-1 Diabetes Report Card—What's New?

- The incidence of newly diagnosed cases of diabetes in the United States, which had been increasing continually for almost two decades, decreased from 9.3 per 1000 adults in 2009 to 5.9 per 1000 adults in 2019.
- Although the prevalence of prediabetes among U.S. adults remained steady from 2005–2008 to 2017–2020, the notification of prediabetes status increased nearly threefold (from 6.5% to 17.4%).
- American Indian or Alaska Native, non-Hispanic Black, Hispanic, and non-Hispanic Asian individuals are more likely to be diagnosed with diabetes than non-Hispanic White individuals (14.5%, 12.1%, 11.8%, 9.5%, and 7.4%, respectively).
- During the COVID-19 pandemic, diabetes emerged as an underlying condition that increases the risk of severe illness. Almost 4 in 10 adults who died from COVID-19 in the United States also had diabetes.

Data from Centers for Disease Control and Prevention. National Diabetes Statistics Report. https://www.cdc.gov/diabetes/data/statistics-report/index.html. Accessed April 26, 2023; Gold JA, Wong KK, Szablewski CM, et al. Characteristics and clinical outcomes of adult patients hospitalized with COVID-19—Georgia, March 2020. *MMWR Morb Mortal Wkly Rep*. 2020;69(18):545–550.

The burden of diabetes has profound implications for public health and healthcare systems nationally and internationally. The number of people with diabetes in the United States is growing so rapidly that the U.S. healthcare system is severely challenged financially by this one disease (**FIGURE 7-1**).[5] Currently, one in four healthcare dollars is spent on the management of diabetes and its associated complications.[3,6]

Classifications of Diabetes

Diabetes is classified into the following four categories:

1. **Type 1 diabetes** is due to autoimmune β-cell destruction of the pancreas, usually leading to absolute insulin deficiency, including latent autoimmune diabetes of adulthood.
2. **Type 2 diabetes** is caused by a non-autoimmune progressive loss of adequate β-cell insulin secretion from the pancreas, frequently with a background of insulin resistance and metabolic syndrome.
3. **Specific types of diabetes due to other causes**, eg, monogenic diabetes syndromes (such as neonatal diabetes and maturity-onset diabetes of the young), are diseases of the exocrine pancreas (such as cystic fibrosis and pancreatitis), and drug- or chemical-induced diabetes (such as with glucocorticoid use for the treatment of HIV/AIDS or after organ transplantation).
4. **Gestational diabetes mellitus** is diagnosed in the second or third trimester of pregnancy that was not clearly overt diabetes prior to gestation.[1]

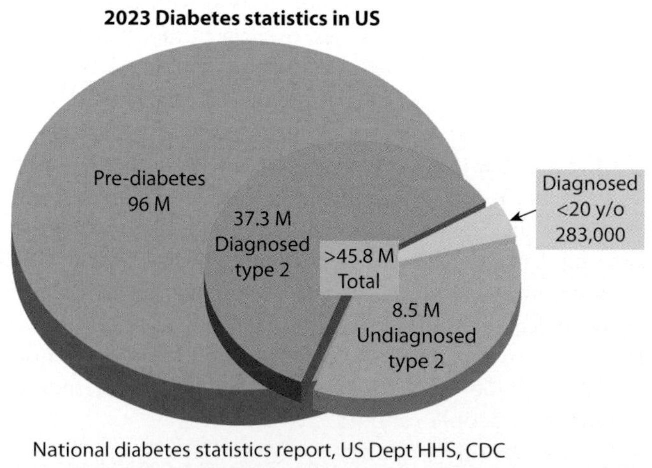

FIGURE 7-1 Diabetes statistics in the United States. Statistics on the prevalence of diabetes in the United States show evidence that it is an epidemic disease that accounts for over 30% of the Medicare budget for healthcare.[5] In addition, the estimated annual cost of caring for patients with diabetes is $327 billion.

Type 1 diabetes and type 2 diabetes are complex medical conditions characterized by varied clinical presentations and disease progression. Proper classification of the disease etiology is crucial for determining the appropriate diabetes management therapy; however, some individuals cannot be easily classified as having type 1 or type 2 diabetes at the time of diagnosis. The traditional concept that type 2 diabetes only occurs in adults and type 1 diabetes only in children is no longer accurate, as both diseases now occur in all age groups. Children with type 1 diabetes commonly present with hallmark symptoms of excessive thirst and urination, and nearly half of them present with diabetic ketoacidosis (DKA).[1]

Diabetes has a profound impact on health as a result of secondary complications such as heart disease, kidney disease, retinopathy, neuropathy, hard-to-heal wounds, and lower-limb amputation. In addition, people are acquiring type 2 diabetes at younger ages than ever before in the United States.[5] Therefore, type 2 diabetes is no longer a disease for only the over 40-year age group. Accordingly, providers are seeing younger people with diabetes-related complications, including issues related to foot pathology and wound healing challenges. It is estimated that 1 in 20 individuals with diabetes will develop a foot ulcer.[7] Furthermore, the older population is being affected the most from a number of perspectives, with the largest prevalence of diabetes in the over 65-year age group (**TABLE 7-2**).[5]

Healthcare professionals who care for people with diabetes who have chronic wounds are challenged to achieve wound closure and optimal wound healing outcomes. Unfortunately, wound healing rates in people with diabetes are reported to be as low as 60% after 1 year despite optimal treatment.[7]

Diabetes management strategies to achieve optimal blood glucose levels in conjunction with current evidence-based wound or foot care are necessary to provide an environment in which wound closure can occur.

Effects of Diabetes on Wound Healing

Faulty wound healing is a well-recognized complication of diabetes.[8] Current evidence confirms that diabetes inhibits all four phases of wound healing via the impaired function of the primary cells responsible for wound repair (ie, neutrophils,

TABLE 7-2 Prevalence of Diabetes in Three Age Groups

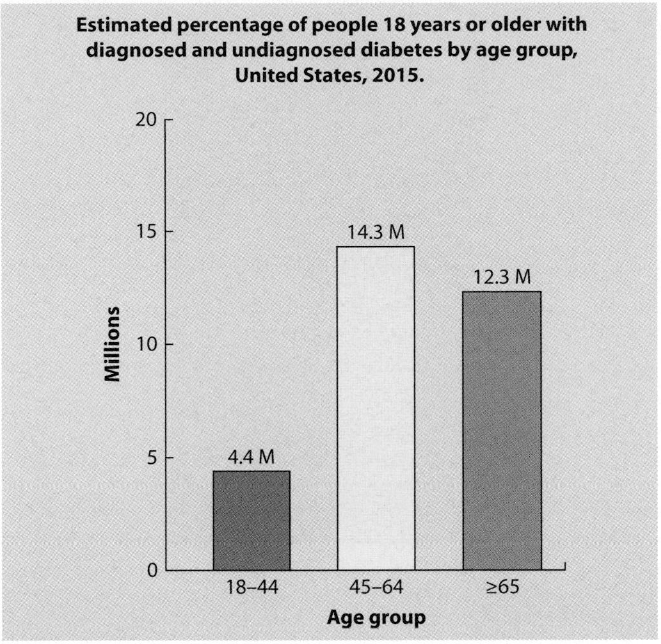

Most of the people in the two older age groups with diabetes are being treated for wounds. The startling rise in the number of cases of diabetes, particularly type 2 diabetes, is having a profound effect on the entire healthcare system. The incidence of diabetes in the United States has doubled in the last 15 years, with the highest prevalence among adults 65–79 years.[3] The national impact will intensify as the population continues to age.

TABLE 7-3 Mechanisms by Which Hyperglycemia Impairs Wound Healing

▪ Impaired function of • Neutrophils • Macrophages • Fibroblasts	▪ Decreased function of • Cytokines • Growth factors	▪ Accumulation of AGEs ▪ Nitric oxide dysfunction ▪ Decreased insulin availability ▪ Increased insulin resistance ▪ Altered homocysteine levels ▪ Macrovascular and microvascular impairments ▪ Neuropathy ▪ Immune function impairments ▪ Biochemical and hormone impairments

macrophages, and fibroblasts), frequently resulting in delayed healing, worsening, or non-healing wounds. In addition, there is decreased efficacy of cytokines and growth factors in people with diabetes and accompanying hyperglycemia. The accumulation of advanced glycosylation end products (AGEs, also referred to as advanced glycated end products), nitric oxide dysfunction, decreased insulin availability or increased insulin resistance, and altered homocysteine levels also contribute to the complex healing impairments for people with diabetes. Micro- and macrovascular disease, neuropathy, immune dysfunction, and biochemical and hormonal abnormalities all contribute to the altered tissue repair processes in people with diabetes in the presence of hyperglycemia (**TABLE 7-3**).[9,10]

One example of a diabetes-mediated impairment in wound healing is susceptibility to infection. Under normal conditions, during the hemostasis healing phase, there is immediate fibrin plug formation as platelets aggregate at the wound site. The platelets release growth factors and cytokines, which then recruit inflammatory cells; however, in a hyperglycemic environment, there is a delay in fibrin plug formation, leaving the wound open to contaminants. In addition, there is a delay (or decrease) in the release of growth factors and cytokines, causing impaired recruitment of the inflammatory cells. With this delay, the individual is at higher risk for wound infection. In fact, people with diabetes have more frequent infections than patients without diabetes.[9] The hyperglycemic environment supports the formation of *biofilms* which impede wound healing (see Chapter 12, Factors That Impede Wound Healing, for more information on biofilms). Recent studies have advanced the understanding of the pathophysiology of wound healing impairments in the presence of diabetes and hyperglycemia. Diabetes, with accompanying elevated blood glucose, causes impaired angiogenesis, neuropathies, sub-optimal chronic inflammatory response, barrier disruption, and subsequent polymicrobial infections. In addition, infection will increase the stress-related hormones needed to fight illness, which in turn increases blood glucose levels. Therefore, hyperglycemia in an individual whose blood glucose is usually well-controlled may be a sign of an acute infection.[10,11]

CLINICAL CONSIDERATION

The A1C test provides a measure of overall blood glucose for the previous 2–3 months. **TABLE 7-6** depicts A1C measurements and how they correlate to blood glucose levels. Note normal and high ranges for A1C. This test is important to help clinicians and patients understand how the diabetes management plan is working for the individual.[17]

Extensive research has focused on the causes of and interventions for diabetic (also termed *neuropathic*) foot wounds; however, the impairments related to diabetes are much more far-reaching than just the foot, affecting healing of all types of wounds regardless of etiology (eg, pressure ulcers, vascular and surgical wounds, burns). In summary, diabetes profoundly impairs the four overlapping phases of wound healing. The underlying mechanisms of the effects of diabetes on wound healing have been extensively investigated; however, a complete understanding of the complex and multifaceted pathophysiologic relationship between diabetes and defective healing continues to elude the scientific community.

CLINICAL CONSIDERATION

People with diabetes are at higher risk for infection because of delays in cellular function at both the hemostasis and inflammatory phases of healing. In addition, the maturation phase of wound healing is negatively impacted, causing decreased collagen synthesis which in turn makes the newly closed wound vulnerable for recurrence.[8]

CASE STUDY

INTRODUCTION

A 60-year-old male with a 15-year history of type 2 diabetes presents with a full-thickness neuropathic ulcer on the first metatarsal head of the right foot that has been present for 4 weeks (FIGURE 7-2). Past medical history includes hypertension, coronary artery disease, and peripheral arterial disease. His fasting blood glucose (FBG) reported by the patient is usually 120 mg/dL. During the subjective interview, the patient was unable to verbalize the importance of his A1C test results and had no knowledge of what this test meant to the overall management of his diabetes. He was given a diabetes management pamphlet from his physician and had some education from the pharmacist about his diabetes medications. He has had no formal diabetes self-management education. TABLE 7-4 contains the patient history and laboratory tests that were ordered. TABLE 7-5 contains the findings from the patient and foot examination.

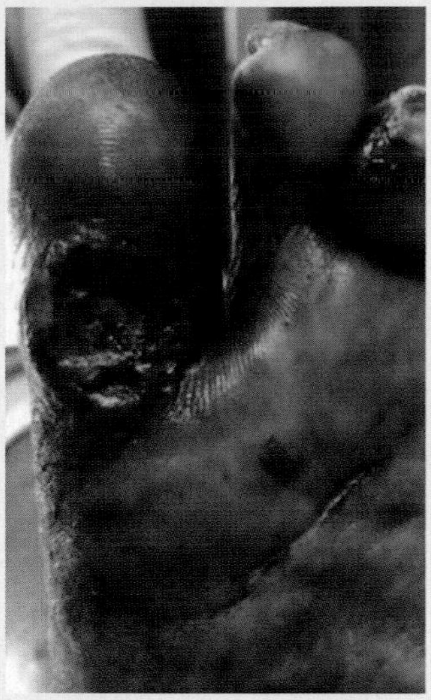

FIGURE 7-2 Case study. Full-thickness diabetic foot ulcer on the first metatarsal head.

CASE STUDY PLAN OF CARE

Diabetes Management Strategies The patient has poor blood glucose control as demonstrated by the high A1C of 9.0%, as well as the fasting blood glucose of 395 mg/dL (TABLE 7-6). His initial care involves getting the blood glucose under control. He is referred back to his primary care physician for a review of his overall diabetes management strategies, with a close look at the current medications to see if updates are needed to assist with glucose control. With blood glucose levels this high, the patient may need to begin insulin injections in addition to his current or updated oral medications. In addition, the patient's lipid panel shows that his cholesterol and triglycerides are high, which may contribute to coronary and peripheral arterial disease. Overall diabetes self-management education is critical for this patient with an emphasis on medical nutrition therapy to assist with nutrition choices that will help manage blood glucose, cholesterol, triglycerides, and weight.

TABLE 7-4 Case Study Information

Medical Diagnoses	
▪ 15-year history of type 2 DM ▪ Hypertension ▪ Depression ▪ Peripheral arterial disease • ABI = 1.3 intimal calcification • TBI = 0.5 (Normal 0.75)	▪ Osteoarthritis knees ▪ Nonproliferative retinopathy ▪ No known medication or dietary allergies ▪ Full-thickness ulceration on the submetatarsal head of the right foot; unable to probe to bone

Laboratory test results		Medications/Medical Indication
▪ Albumin: 3.9 g/dL (normal)	▪ Complete blood cell count	Glyburide: diabetes
▪ Cholesterol: 260 mg/dL (high)	▪ White blood cells: 7.0 × 10^9/L (normal)	Furosemide: CHF
▪ Triglycerides: 160 mg/dL (high)	▪ Red blood cells: 4.0 × 10^{12}/L (normal)	Lisinopril: HTN
▪ HDL cholesterol: 25 mg/dL (low)	▪ Hemoglobin: 12.0 g/dL (normal)	Sertraline t: depression
▪ LDL cholesterol: 130 mg/dL (high)	▪ Hematocrit: 40% (normal)	Apixaban: anticoagulation
▪ Total protein: 6.0 g/dL (normal)	▪ Neutrophils: 60% (normal)	Eye drops: glaucoma
▪ Fasting glucose: 395 mg/dL (high)	• Lymphocytes: 30% (normal)	Ibuprofen: joint pain
▪ Hemoglobin HbA1C: 9.0% (high)	• Platelets: 270 × 10^9/L (normal)	Gabapentin: neuropathic pain
▪ BUN: 16 mg/dL (normal)		
▪ Creatinine: 1.9 mg/dL (high)		

Vital signs: HR: 84, BP: 155/94, Resp.: 16, Temperature: 99.2.
Pain assessment—0/10 (peripheral neuropathy present).

TABLE 7-5 Foot Examination for the Case Study

Weight-Bearing Assessment	Non-Weight-Bearing Assessment
▪ Stance position—pronated ▪ LMI (lateral malleolar index)—(–)6 mm ▪ Calcaneal eversion—4 degrees everted ▪ Too many toes sign—B/L (**FIGURE 7-3A,B**) ▪ Hubscher maneuver—negative (no arch elevation with dorsiflexion of the hallux indicating hallux limitus—Note dorsal exostosis on the first metatarsal head) (**FIGURE 7-4**) ▪ Genu valgum absent ▪ Genu recurvatum noted (compensation for equinus) ▪ Contraction of the digits 2–5 noted B/L—minimal digital purchase in stance (**FIGURE 7-5**)	▪ Silfverskiold test 0 degree dorsiflexion knee bent and knee straight (**FIGURE 7-6**) ▪ Knee hyperextension noted ▪ Calcaneal inversion 8 degrees ▪ Calcaneal eversion 4 degrees ▪ Midtarsal joint hypermobility noted (high axis orientation as evidenced by transverse plane motion greater than frontal plane motion) ▪ Hallux ROM limited to 30-degree dorsiflexion (65 degrees needed for unrestricted ambulation) ▪ Hallux interphalangeal joint hypermobile secondary to force transfer to the IPJ because of the hallux limitus ▪ Fixed flexion contracture noted at the IP joints with subluxation and dorsal contracture of the metatarsophalangeal joints 2–4 (inability of either joint to extend and flex to 0 degree) ▪ Adductovarus fifth toe B/L ▪ Hallux abductovalgus deformity with moderate bunion B/L ▪ Plantar calluses at the hallux IPJ and under the first and fifth met heads B/L (**FIGURE 7-7**) ▪ Dorsal corns (heloma) second and fifth digits B/L

Vascular Assessment	Neurologic Assessment	Gait Analysis
▪ Dorsalis pedis pulses ¼ B/L ▪ Posterior tibial pulses nonpalpable B/L ▪ ABI 1.2, TBI 0.5 ▪ Biphasic Doppler Waveforms DP and PT B/L ▪ Hair absent from the toes and dorsal foot B/L ▪ Capillary refill time with feet horizontal 4 seconds (normal $\leq$ 2 seconds) ▪ Digital temperature warm to warm B/L ▪ Plantar rubor noted B/L ▪ No ankle or limb edema noted ▪ No varicosity noted ▪ Nails dystrophic with evidence of onychomycosis on all 10 toes	▪ Loss of protective sensation—LOPS hallux, third and fifth toes, first, third, and fifth metatarsal heads and dorsal first interspace B/L. Able to feel the 5.07 monofilament midfoot and heels B/L (**FIGURE 7-8**) ▪ Pinprick same as above ▪ Light touch absent below the ankle B/L ▪ Position sense absent DIPJs and MPJs B/L but WNL ankle and MTJs ▪ Manuel muscle test WNL with 4+/5-5/5 strength in all muscles tested ▪ Negative Babinski, negative clonus	▪ Observe barefoot and with shoes ▪ Look for abnormalities at heel strike early and late midstance and propulsion ▪ Observe postural changes during the swing phase ▪ Note step and stride length, cadence, foot placement and balance, apropulsive tendencies ▪ Check for early heel off, midfoot break, and abductory twist at heel off

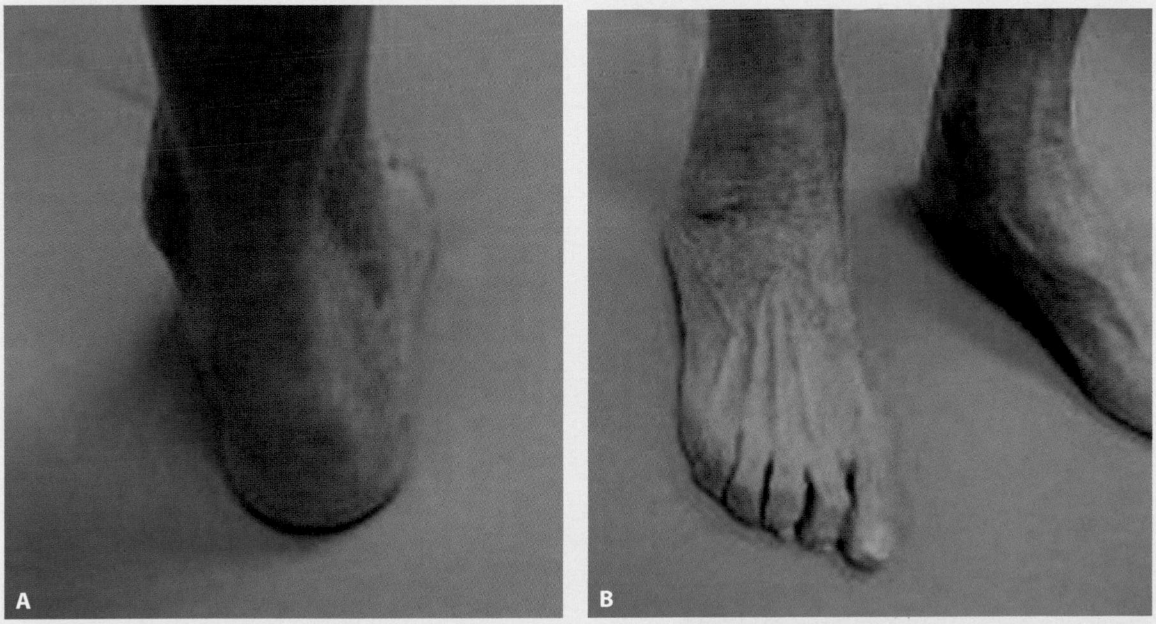

FIGURE 7-3 A, B. Calcaneal eversion and too many toes. The posterior view of the foot illustrates calcaneal eversion resulting in two toes visible on the lateral side, whereas if the ankle is in neutral no toes are visible on the lateral side.

TABLE 7-6 Critical Values for Hemoglobin HbA1C and Glucose

HbA1C%	Average Glucose
12.5%	312 mg/dL
12%	298 mg/dL
11.5%	283 mg/dL
11%	269 mg/dL
10.5%	255 mg/dL
10%	240 mg/dL
9.5%	226 mg/dL
9%	212 mg/dL
8.5%	197 mg/dL
8%	183 mg/dL
7.5%	169 mg/dL
7%	154 mg/dL
6.5%	140 mg/dL
6%	125 mg/dL
5.5%	111 mg/dL
5.0%	97 mg/dL

The numbers in green indicate normal values, and as the numbers progress to the top of the chart, they become more critical.

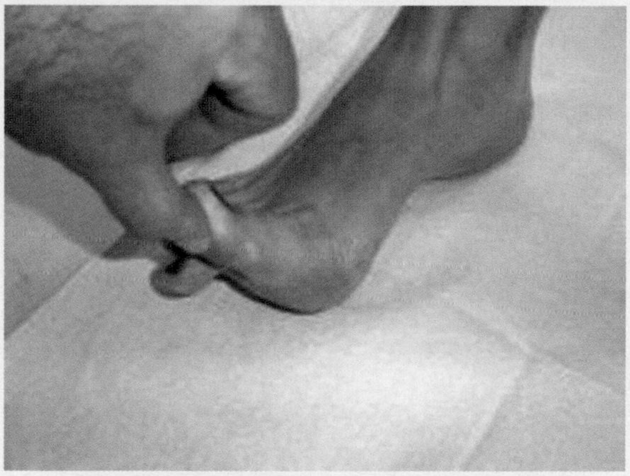

FIGURE 7-4 Hubscher maneuver.

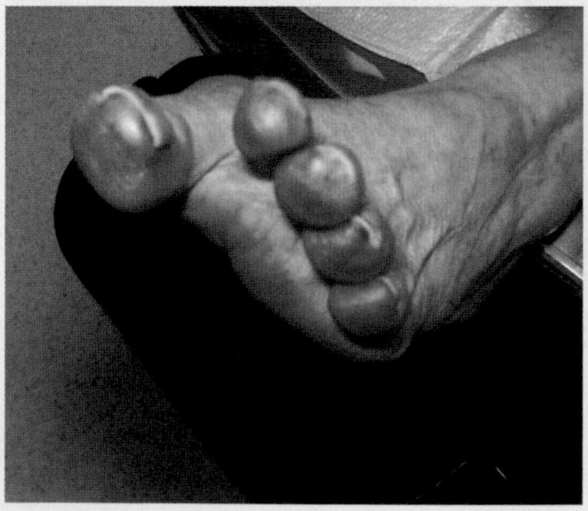

FIGURE 7-5 Intrinsic muscle wasting with retraction of the digits.

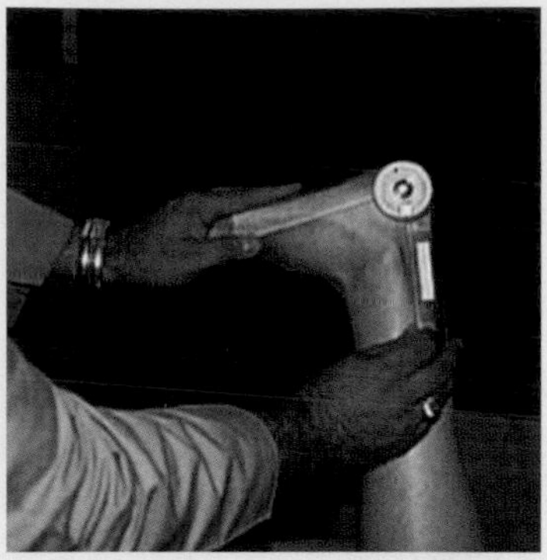

FIGURE 7-6 Silfverskiold test.

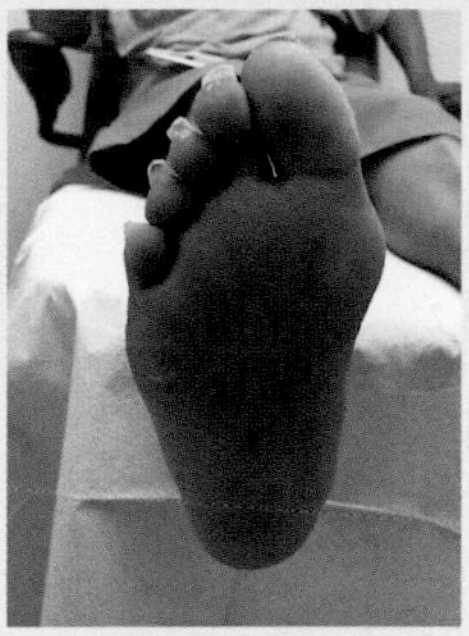

FIGURE 7-7 Plantar foot with calluses on first and fifth metatarsal heads.

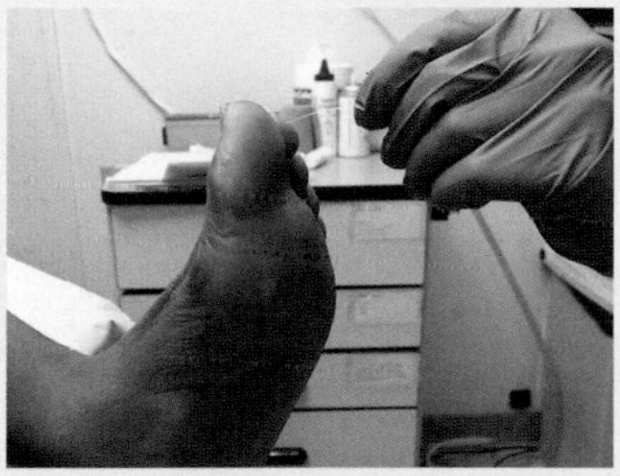

FIGURE 7-8 Semmes–Weinstein monofilament testing. Semmes–Weinstein monofilament testing is used to determine the loss of pressure sensation. The filament is placed on the test spot and pressed until the filament bends. The patient responds as to whether or not the pressure is felt. Inability to feel the 5.07 monofilament (which exerts 10 g of pressure) is termed *loss of protective sensation*.

DISCUSSION QUESTIONS

1. Based on the findings in TABLE 7-5, what tests and measures are indicated?
2. What findings indicate that the patient may have impaired healing potential?
3. What other medical disciplines would be helpful in treating this patient, other than specific wound care?

Medical Management and Team Care of Diabetes

Diabetes care is complex and multifaceted, requiring a team approach to patient-centered care, with the patient being an integral member of the team (**FIGURE 7-9**). While the medical team leader is the physician or nurse practitioner (who uses input, education services, and treatments from other healthcare providers), the management that occurs daily is provided by the patient (or by caregivers when the patient is too impaired to perform adequate self-management).[12] The ability of the patient to successfully manage the disease state of diabetes depends on extensive and ongoing training, education, and feedback from the healthcare team.

Effective wound management includes a review of the patient's diabetes management strategies. Glucose control is a primary intervention for initial wound closure, infection avoidance, and to help prevent the recurrence of these wounds.

The Association of Diabetes Care & Education Specialists (ADCES) is an interprofessional membership organization dedicated to improving prediabetes, diabetes and cardiometabolic care through innovative education, management and support.[13] This multidisciplinary professional organization has developed ADCES7, a series of behaviors to form the foundation for diabetes care and education specialists to use in teaching patients informed decision-making. The National Standards for Diabetes Self-Management Education and Support (DSMES) curriculum includes the same behaviors in its curriculum for diabetes self-management education[14] (see **TABLE 7-7**). The curriculum provides patients the education they need to change their lifestyle and habits to delay or avert the acute and chronic complications that occur with uncontrolled diabetes.

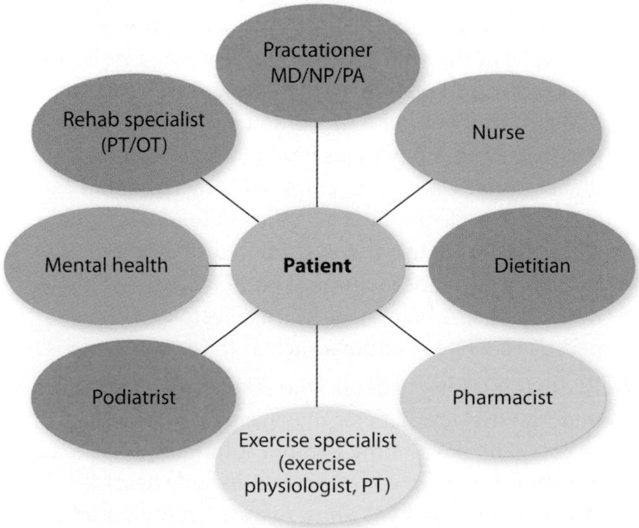

FIGURE 7-9 The diabetes care team. The team that cares for the patient with diabetes includes these healthcare specialists, each with an important role in caring for the total patient, with the patient being at the center of the team. The team must have the patient take responsibility for the overall day-to-day management of the disease.

TABLE 7-7 ADCES7 Self-Care Behaviors

- Describe the *DM disease process and treatment options.*
- Incorporate *healthy eating* into lifestyle.
- Incorporate *physical activity* into lifestyle.
- Use *medication(s) and devices safely* and for maximum therapeutic effectiveness.
- *Monitor blood glucose* and other parameters; interpret and use the results for self-management decision making.
- Prevent, detect, and treat *acute complications* (ie, hyperglycemia and hypoglycemia).
- Prevent, detect, and treat *chronic complications* (eg, heart and kidney disease, retinopathy, Charcot foot disease).
- Healthy coping to address psychosocial issues and concerns.
- Develop personal strategies (problem solving) to promote health and behavior change.

DSMES has been shown to be cost-effective by reducing hospital admissions and readmission, as well as reducing lifetime healthcare costs related to a lower risk for complications from this disease. This in turn improves the quality of life and longevity of people with diabetes.

Basic Elements of Diabetes Education

- **Healthy Coping:** Increased stress in one's life increases blood glucose levels. There are the daily types of stress (eg, traffic and getting the kids off to school), and the more serious issues such as divorce or money problems. Adding life stresses to the strain that diabetes causes can be overwhelming for some patients. When there are high levels of stress in the patient's life, healthy coping methods are critical to good health rather than harmful habits such as smoking, overeating, and excessive alcohol consumption. Some of the recommendations for handling stress for people with diabetes include the following: having a support system with people the patient trusts, performing physical activity which increases brain endorphins and in turn softens the stress response, thinking positive, and being good to one's self. Depression is a common issue for people with diabetes, and they may exhibit some of the following signs: lack of interest or pleasure in personal or social activities, not wanting to discuss their diabetes issues with family or friends, sleeping for long periods each day, and not providing daily self-care from a personal and/or diabetes perspective. Some people get so depressed they decide to give up on themselves and stop their good diabetes management. Recognizing patient depression is a healthcare assessment activity that should be done for all people with diabetes, both those with and without complications from their disease.[14]
- **Healthy Eating:** Patients are taught which foods assist with blood glucose control. The different types of macronutrients are described including carbohydrates, protein, and fats. Many people with diabetes think the diet issue is related to ingesting sugar, not understanding

that every type of carbohydrate influences blood glucose and that not all carbohydrates are created equal, meaning some cause the glucose to go high, while others have less effect on the overall blood glucose levels. Diabetes educators teach the person how to count carbohydrates, read food labels, measure each serving, develop an eating plan, prevent high or low blood glucose levels, and set goals for healthy eating.[14]

- **Being Active:** Being active is part of being healthy in general and is a necessary component for optimal health when a person has diabetes. Physical activity (including exercise) is a powerful modality for the person with diabetes and must be coordinated with the individual's medication and nutrition regimes. The effects of physical activity include lowering blood glucose, lowering cholesterol, improving blood pressure, lowering stress and anxiety, and improving mood. Depending on the associated complications (eg, diabetic retinopathy, diabetic neuropathy, and diabetic nephropathy), certain precautions and contraindications may be implemented to avoid physical activity-induced damage to already-compromised tissues and organs. For example, patients who have severe foot deformities or a history of DFUs need to be instructed in an activity program that does not cause friction and shear to the plantar foot structures. A referral to a physical therapist knowledgeable about exercises and diabetes is recommended for establishing an appropriate exercise program. Individuals will adhere to activity programs more readily when doing activities they enjoy such as dancing, bike riding, or walking the dog. The activity plan must be customized and embraced by the patient for long-term adherence to take place.[14]

CLINICAL CONSIDERATION

Exercises in a standing position that result in the foot being planted while the body moves (eg, squats, the elliptical, rowing) will produce shear between the subcutaneous tissue and the bony prominences of the plantar foot. Bicycling or using an upper extremity cycle ergometer is advised for cardiopulmonary conditioning if the individual has any risk factors for (or a history of) foot ulceration.

- **Glucose Monitoring:** Glucose monitoring helps patients determine the day-to-day control of their disease. Monitoring gives patients a tool to objectively determine if their blood glucose is too high or too low. This information helps them with day-to-day decisions related to food choices, amounts and types of activities they can do, and when and whether they need to see a medical professional. The patient who monitors consistently will discover abnormal glucose excursions and can get help as soon as possible to remedy the higher glucose levels.
- **Medications:** The drug armamentarium for glycemic control for people with diabetes is large and growing as the impairments related to diabetes are better understood. The different drugs and combination therapies address different pathophysiological mechanisms and different organs involved in blood glucose control. The management of type 1 diabetes and type 2 diabetes is completely different, as these are different diseases with the similar outcome of hyperglycemia.[12] Medications can be oral and/or injectable for type 2 diabetes; however, type 1 diabetes requires injectable insulin. Inhaled insulin, a new insulin delivery method, was approved by the FDA in June 2014 for use in both type 1 and type 2 diabetes. Inhaled insulin may take the place of short-acting insulins, but does not replace the intermediate and long-acting forms of insulin.[14] More information on medications are available at https://www.diabeteseducatorscalgary.ca/medications/complete-medication-table.html
- **Problem-Solving:** Preparation and planning are critical components of a well-designed diabetes management program. Patients should monitor their blood glucose levels, looking for too high (hyperglycemia) and too low (hypoglycemia) numbers. However, even the patient who is trying the best to plan well for managing the disease will sometimes find it difficult. Life has all kinds of ups and downs, and no matter how well patients plan, blood glucose can and will go in the wrong direction at some point. An example would be the patient whose blood glucose has been running 180–230 mg/dL for several days, when the random glucose readings are usually between 125 and 145 mg/dL. The patient knows these are higher than normal readings, but may not know why. This person needs professional help to determine if the diabetes management program is still working. There are several reasons the readings may be increasing, eg, illness, a wound infection (if a wound is present), failing beta cells in the pancreas requiring adding insulin to the medication regime, or the glucose strips are out of date. On the other hand, blood glucose can go low, particularly when patients are on oral or injectable diabetes medications. Examples of situations that cause glucose to go low is lack of sufficient food when diabetes medications are taken, too strenuous of an exercise or activity session, or the most common cause—diabetes medications. A bit of healthcare detective work is necessary when situations such as these arise.[14]
- **Reducing Risks:** Patients who take responsibility for their day-to-day diabetes management can prevent or delay the devastating complications of this disease. Some of the major complications include heart disease, stroke, nephropathy (kidney disease), retinopathy (eye disease), neuropathy, foot abnormalities, and non-healing wounds. In addition to controlling their blood glucose levels, patients with diabetes can reduce other risk factors that work in tandem with diabetes and cause the complications to be more severe. Healthy habits to

help prevent complications from diabetes include not smoking; seeing the healthcare practitioner who helps manage the diabetes on a regular basis; and having annual eye examinations, dental care, foot screens, and proper foot and nail care.[9]

Challenges in Caring for the Patients with Diabetes

Education There are many challenges in providing care for individuals with diabetes. Education is required not only for self-management of diabetes but also to positively affect wound closure and subsequent healing. Many people with hard-to-heal wounds and diabetes do not have the necessary information to adequately manage the disease, especially in the presence of a chronic wound that causes both psychological and physiological stress. The standard of care for individuals with diabetes is a referral to a comprehensive diabetes education program upon diagnosis of the disease[12]; however, many do not have access to a diabetes education center. Such individuals thus present to the wound management team with a critical deficiency in their ability to manage their disease. This deficiency itself could be a contributing factor to both the development of the wound and the impaired wound healing.

CLINICAL CONSIDERATION

The wound care clinician *must* review the patient's blood glucose values (both capillary or plasma glucose and the hemoglobin A1C) to determine if the patient needs to see a physician to adjust the medications in order to control their blood glucose.

CLINICAL CONSIDERATION

Many people with diabetes, especially type 2, do *not* receive adequate education for successful self-management, yet they are blamed for being non-adherent to their diabetes management program. Also, almost everyone backslides at times—some more frequently than others—on their diabetes management program. However, such lapses can simply represent the understandable difficulty of completely changing and constantly monitoring major aspects of one's daily life, including nutrition, physical activity, and often complex medication regimes. Thus, people with diabetes need both extensive initial education and ongoing support and encouragement from people familiar with the management strategies of this disease, including wound care professionals.

Depression and Burnout As mentioned previously, many people with diabetes have varying levels of depression,[12] which can mildly or severely compromise self-management, depending on their coping abilities. If the individual's diabetes management strategies are compromised by depression, the provider can expect more challenges for wound healing. Diabetes alone conveys psychological, social, and financial burdens on the affected individual; a wound creates additional psychological, social, and financial stress.

Burnout is a potential problem for everyone concerned—the patient can become burned out from living with diabetes and its associated complications continuously, with no respite, and the wound care team can become burned out by the impact of diabetes on wound healing and the perception that the patient is not optimally self-managing the disease or the wound, thereby "sabotaging" the wound care plan. The psychosocial impact of diabetes is life-altering, especially with the addition of chronic complications that frequently accompany diabetes, including unsightly, odiferous, and difficult-to-manage wounds. There are no easy answers or rote formulas for these challenges; providers must do their best to provide comprehensive support to these patients and their families.[12]

Adherence The patient's adherence to the overall disease management plan is critical. However, before placing the term *noncompliant* or *nonadherent* on the person with diabetes, the wound care clinician should assess (1) whether the patient has the best diabetes management plan individualized to their needs and (2) the patient's ability to self-manage the diabetes, and then provide an appropriate referral to address deficiencies if they exist. The status of the patient's diabetes control is prerequisite knowledge in order for the wound management team to help the patient create an environment for wound closure and healing. **TABLE 7-8** lists helpful strategies for the clinician who is working with a patient who is having difficulty with adherence.

CLINICAL CONSIDERATION

A person with type 2 diabetes may be further along in the disease process of β-cell failure than when they first started diabetes management treatment. Because type 2 diabetes is a progressive disease of β-cells function decline, the oral medications may no longer provide the control which they once did; that is, the β-cells are not able to respond to the insulin-secreting mechanism of the medications, or the patient's insulin resistance has increased and the medications that address insulin resistance are not able to function well enough to lower blood glucose. The wound care clinician may be the healthcare provider who recognizes or suspects a diabetes treatment regime needs updating to provide optimal blood glucose levels.

TABLE 7-8 Strategies to Help a Patient Develop Adherence to a Comprehensive Diabetes Management Program

1. Provide a referral for diabetes self-management education, if necessary.
2. Provide ongoing monitoring and encouragement.
3. Emphasize that DM self-management is a lifelong process.
4. Help the patient understand the health benefits, including wound healing, that make his or her hard work worthwhile.
5. Address relapse management by expressing understanding of the difficulty of adhering to the diabetes management program day in and day out.
6. Help the person realize that one instance of nonadherence should be seen in the context of just one lapse and not taken as proof that he or she is unable to be successful. Such an approach promotes rapport and sends the message that the clinician and the patient are on the same team.

The Wound Care Clinician's Role

The initial examination of the patient with a wound includes a basic assessment of the patient's diabetes management plan to ensure that the disease is under control. **TABLE 7-9** provides a list of intake components to consider, and **TABLE 7-10** lists the diagnostic criteria for diabetes.

A typical case scenario may present as follows: a patient with diabetes presents with a wound with signs and symptoms of infection. The blood glucose level is 345 mg/dL. The clinician needs to determine which came first: chronic hyperglycemia, which made the patient more susceptible to infection, or the existing infection which caused the blood glucose levels to increase. A comparison of the capillary or plasma blood glucose levels with a current A1C test can help make this determination. If the A1C value is high, the blood glucose has been out of control for several months, in which case diabetes management strategies are of paramount importance to lower the hyperglycemia, enhance infection control, and optimize wound healing. If the A1C shows adequate control, then the diabetes has been well managed, and an acute infection has caused the hyperglycemia. At this point, the patient may require the addition of insulin to the diabetes medication regime—at least temporarily—to help control the infection-instigated elevated blood glucose. The wound management team clinician can make this recommendation to the provider who manages the patient's diabetes. Thus, object glycemic tests can be used to help manage wound healing, remembering that diabetes is ever present and must be managed at all times to help create the best wound closure and healing outcomes.

CLINICAL CONSIDERATION

People who are on fixed or low incomes may take their medications sporadically to make them last longer. Another scenario is when older persons are confused about the medication regime altogether and embarrassed to tell someone that they need help with a functional method to adhere to the medication plan of care. Also, the wound management team members may be the first to recognize acute mental status changes or potential abuse and neglect issues that are impacting the patient's diabetes self-management and wound healing goals. Adherence or nonadherence to the diabetes and wound management program is often a complex issue reflecting other, underlying areas of concern.

TABLE 7-9 Important Questions to Ask a Person with Diabetes When Performing the Wound Evaluation

- Have you had a series of diabetes self-management classes?
  - Yes: How long ago? _____ months _____ years
- What medications do you take for DM? List the names and dose of each medication.
- How often do you monitor your blood glucose? What were they this morning when you awakened?
- Do you take your diabetes medications regularly without fail?
  - Yes
  - No: How often do you take your medications?

TABLE 7-10 Type 2 Diabetes Diagnostic Criteria for Adults

	TESTS		
Stage	**Fasting Plasma Glucose[a] Test**	**Casual Glucose[b] Test[c]**	**Oral Glucose Tolerance Test[d]**
Normal	<100 mg/dL	—	2-hour PPG <140 mg/dL
Prediabetes (increased risk for diabetes; also known as impaired glucose tolerance)	100–125 mg/dL	A1C = 5.7–6.4%	2-hour PPG 140–199 mg/dL
Diabetes	≥126 mg/dL	≥200 mg/dL (plus signs and symptoms)	2-hour PPG ≥200 mg/dL
		A1C ≥6.5%	

Abbreviation: PPG, postprandial glucose.

[a]Fasting means no calorie intake for 8 hours.

[b]Casual means testing any time of day without regard to time since last meal; signs and symptoms are the classic ones of polyuria, polydipsia, and unexplained weight loss.

[c]The A1C should be performed in a laboratory using a method that is NGSP certified and standardized to the Diabetes Control and Complications Trial assay.

[d]2-hour PPG indicates 2-hour postload glucose.

Data from American Diabetes Association. Standards of medical care in diabetes. *Diabetes Care.* 2018; 41 (suppl 1):S1–S2.

Conclusion (Diabetes)

The wound management team should have a working knowledge of the diagnosis of diabetes, diabetes management strategies (including the most commonly associated complications and the effects of diabetes on wound healing), as well as proficiency in performing a thorough assessment of the patient and the wound. While it is not the responsibility of the wound management team to oversee the person's diabetes—that duty belongs to the patient and the provider responsible for the medical management—the wound care team should assess if the disease is being managed as successfully as possible and recognize when other diabetes interventions and counseling need to be considered for optimal wound closure and healing outcomes.[15,16]

CLINICAL CONSIDERATION

The wound care clinician *must* review the patient's blood glucose values, both the capillary blood glucose and the hemoglobin A1C, to determine if the patient needs to see the primary care physician or endocrinologist to adjust the diabetes medications and determine if diabetes self-management education is required.

THE DIABETIC FOOT

The diabetic foot is a complicated pathological entity suffering from varying degrees of physiological and biomechanical imbalances. Prolonged exposure to slowly elevating blood glucose leads to glycosylation of multiple organ systems and progressively advancing neurovascular crises triggered by the loss of system homeostasis. The "perfect storm" of intrinsic and extrinsic stressors associated with diabetes causes a system collapse that results in a breakdown of the foot's ability to manage the combination of individual stressors, thereby leading to a breakdown sufficient to cause ulceration and/or neuroarthropathy of the diabetic foot.[17]

Once the skin has broken and exposed the underlying tissues to the risk of infection, the patient and the practitioner have a relatively short period of time within which to address the component problems and restore balance to the system, otherwise complications such as osteomyelitis or amputation may ensue. (**FIGURE 7-10**). The International Working Group on the Diabetic Foot (IWGDF) has worked since 1999 to develop practical guidelines for the prevention and treatment of diabetic foot disease including prevention, off-loading, peripheral artery disease, infection, wound healing interventions, and classification of DFUs.[18,19] These guidelines provide evidence-based recommendations to prevent and treat DFUs and their complications.

From the onset of the wound, there are approximately 30 days or 4 weeks to restore homeostasis and thereby prevent further tissue breakdown, possible infection, and progression to amputation. Standard of care must be initiated as soon as possible and continued for the first 4 weeks of care; advanced therapies to heal the wound can then be initiated at that time if 50% wound closure has not occurred. Dr. Peter Sheehan conducted a large, prospective, multicenter trial of 203 diabetic patients that assessed the ability of the *4-week healing rate* to predict complete healing at 12 weeks. He concluded that "patients in whom ulcer size fails to reduce by half over the first 4 weeks of treatment are unlikely to achieve wound healing over a reasonable period."[20] There is a fivefold increase in the risk of infection in wounds that progress beyond 4 weeks of therapy and a 155 times greater risk of amputation once an infection develops.[21]

A panel created for the American Diabetes Association Consensus Development Conference on Diabetic Foot Wound Care in April 1999 concluded, "Any wound that remains unhealed after 4 weeks is cause for concern, as it is associated with worse outcomes, including amputations."[22] It is evident from these studies that a wound on a diabetic foot is a very serious event and must be treated as such from day one. Early interventions such as risk assessment, educational initiatives, and aggressive treatment interventions can literally be life-saving for many patients with diabetes.

CLINICAL CONSIDERATION

After a thorough history, the physical examination assesses the dermatological, musculoskeletal, neurological, and vascular systems of the lower extremity. Skin conditions and lesions are noted and recorded in addition to the measurements of the wound or wounds on the foot.

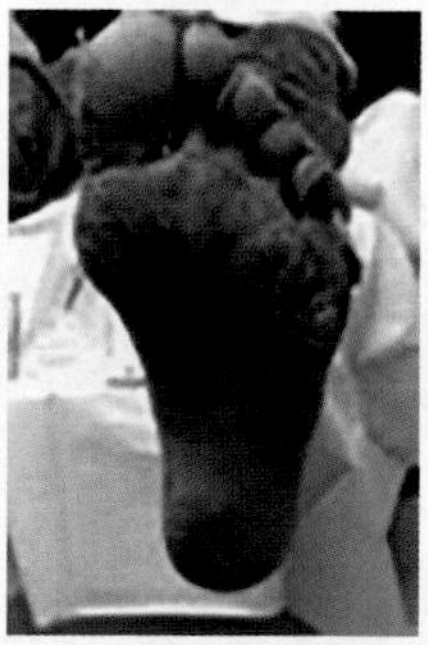

FIGURE 7-10 Submetatarsal five ulcer. The plantar wound under the fifth metatarsal is a result of a lateral column cavus deformity and an anterior lateral imbalance. These wounds would have a relatively short period of time for treatment before the risk of infection or osteomyelitis is greatly increased. Note the severe hyperkeratosis on the entire plantar foot surface.

Diabetes and the Effects on the Systems of the Foot

Foot problems are common in patients with diabetes and 25% to 34% of them, or approximately 6.8 million people, will develop a foot ulcer during their lifetime.[23,24] Once an ulcer has developed, the 5-year survival rate for a patient with diabetes is approximately 45%, a figure that is lower than that for both prostate and breast cancer. Despite the dangers and the risks associated with ulceration in the diabetic population, the problem has received very little press in comparison to other more politically interesting diseases.[25] For many years, foot complications have been the leading cause of hospitalization for patients with diabetes.[26] Almost 30% of diabetics aged 40 years or older have impaired sensation in the feet (ie, at least one area that lacks feeling) or approximately 8 million individuals (60–70% of people with diabetes) have mild-to-severe forms of nervous system damage affecting both sensory and motor systems.[5] The major system failure in diabetics leading to the development of an ulcer is the *loss of protective sensation* in the lower extremity. Combined with intrinsic muscle loss and extrinsic muscle imbalance, this leads to increasing biomechanical stress in areas of high pressure and eventual tissue loss. The skin breakdown is a combination of pressure ischemia, reperfusion injury, expanding sublesional microhemorrhage and micronecrosis, and shearing injury, all of which lead to an accumulation of coalescing blood and transudate within or beneath the skin. The skin eventually ruptures, opening the subcutaneous tissues to bacterial invasion from the skin surface (**FIGURES 7-11** and **7-12**).

Diabetic dyshidrosis or dry skin secondary to the loss of normal skin perspiration (a result of autonomic nervous dysfunction) is documented, and patient education about the daily use of an emollient is included in the care plan, along with consultation with a podiatric or allopathic physician to recommend an

CLINICAL CONSIDERATION

An ankle-brachial index (ABI) above 1.3 is considered unreliable for a patient with diabetes due to calcification of the arteries, in which case a toe-brachial index (TBI), or $TCPO_2$, is performed instead.

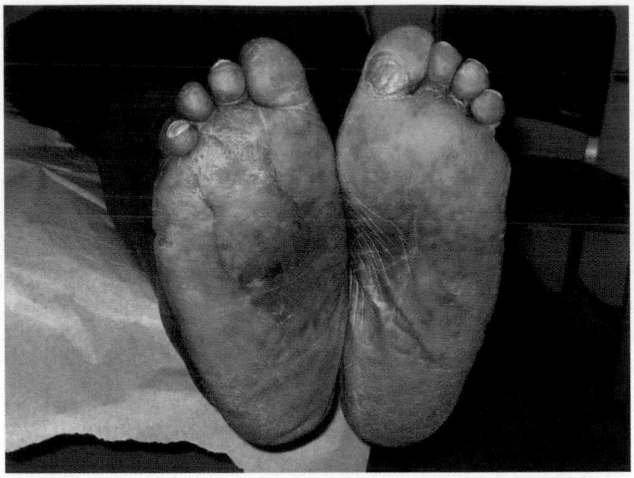

FIGURE 7-11 Charcot foot with proximal dissecting sublesional hematoma.

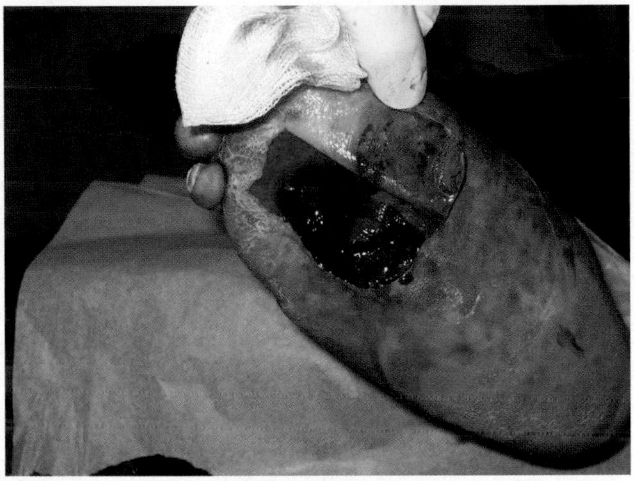

FIGURE 7-12 Deroofed hematoma with exposed full-thickness ulcer.

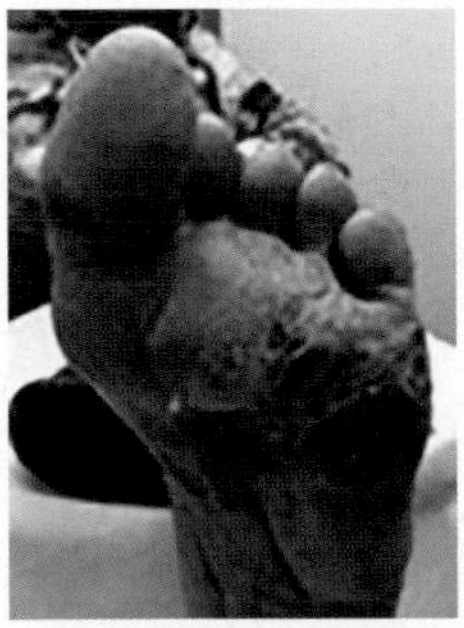

FIGURE 7-13 Severe dyshidrosis with ulceration under the fifth metatarsal.

over the counter prescription hydrating cream (**FIGURE 7-13**). Neurologic assessment includes the Semmes–Weinstein monofilament test, reflexes, biothesiometer testing, muscle strength and function, visual gait and posture analysis, and some quantification of plantar pressures (**FIGURE 7-8**).

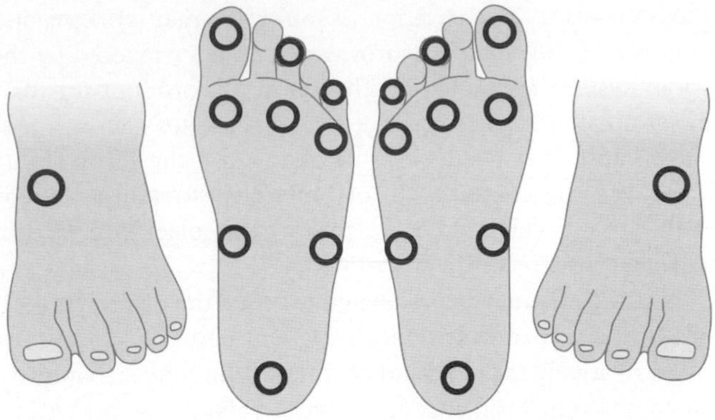

FIGURE 7-14 Diagram of sites tested with the Semmes–Weinstein monofilaments. Ten sites are tested on each foot to determine the loss of pressure sensation. This is considered one of the most reliable risk factors for diabetic foot ulceration.

FIGURE 7-14 illustrates the 10 sites that are tested with the monofilaments, and **FIGURE 7-15** illustrates an in-shoe device to measure plantar foot pressures.

The major risks for ulceration are determined by the neurologic and musculoskeletal findings, and the major risk for amputation is determined by the vascular findings. A complete vascular screening includes pulses, examination for trophic skin changes (eg, hair loss, skin thinning, nail thickening, and pigment changes), capillary refill time, and the calculation of both the ABI and the TBI. ABIs are often falsely elevated due to calcification of the arteries, leading to artificially elevated vessel occlusion pressures. The toe arteries are much less likely to become calcified, thereby providing a more accurate impression of the true distal tissue perfusion. Near-infrared spectroscopy (NIRS) is another way to measure skin perfusion. The hand-held device measures reflected light from the blood cells to determine a ratio of oxygenated to deoxygenated hemoglobin, thereby accurately measuring both the amount of blood reaching the tissue and the level of oxygenation of

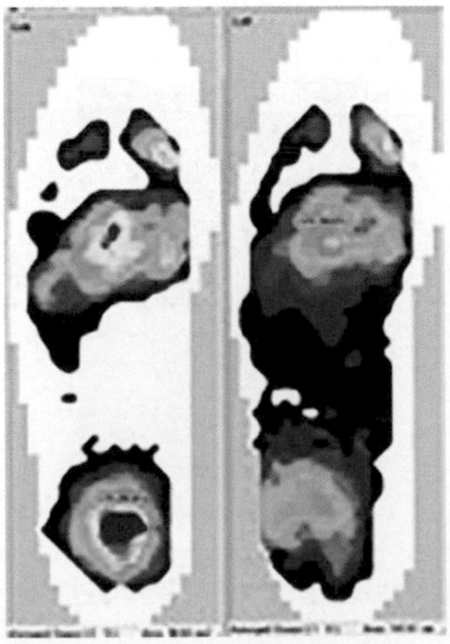

FIGURE 7-15 The in-shoe pressure assessment system is used to obtain a quantifiable estimate of dynamic plantar foot pressures. Red areas indicate high peak pressures.

TABLE 7-11 Modified Temple University Classification for Footwear Selection[a]

Degree of Deformity	Depth of Ulcer 1 Pre- or Postulcerative Lesion Fully Epithelialized	Depth of Ulcer 2 Superficial Not Involving Tendon Capsule or Bone	Depth of Ulcer 3 Deep Involving Tendon Capsule or Bone
A Mild (normal appearance to minimal deformity noted)	Standard depth footwear Simple multilaminate insoles or custom-molded foot orthoses Accommodative padding Digital orthoses	Removable cast walker Football or felted foam dressing Surgical shoe with total-contact molded orthosis PWB with ambulatory aid	TCC/iTCC Football dressing Felted foam PTB/CROW NWB with ambulatory aid
B Moderate (moderately deformed foot alignment—single focal osseous or joint deformity)	Depth footwear Modified Prefabricated Foot Orthoses, Custom orthoses Digital orthose	iTCC/TCC Removable cast walker Football dressing Felted foam PWB with ambulatory aid	TCC/iTCC Football dressing Felted foam PTB/CROW NWB with ambulatory aid Wheelchair, bedrest
C Severe (very deformed foot with multiple osseous or joint deformities)	Custom depth or molded shoes Custom orthotic inserts Custom-molded ankle Foot orthosis (TORCH/CROW/PTB Arizona/platinum orthoses)	TCC/ iTCC Football dressing or felted foam in an RCW PTB/CROW/TORCH NWB with ambulatory aid	TCC/iTCC Football dressing or felted foam in an RCW NWB with ambulatory aid Wheel chair/bedrest

Abbreviations: CROW, Charcot restraint orthotic walker; iTCC, instant total-contact cast; NWB, non-weight bearing; PTB, patellar tendon bearing; RCW, removable cast walker; TCC, total-contact cast; TORCH, total orthotic restraining custom hybrid.

[a]All shoes and fixed ankle devices have rocker soles to allow for a smooth gait and reduction of forefoot loading during ambulation.

Reproduced with permission from McGuire JB. Pressure redistribution strategies for the diabetic or at-risk foot: Part II. *Adv Skin Wound Care*. 2006;19(5):270-279.

that blood.[27] One study suggests that an oxygen flow index of less than 28% in a foot and wounded area is an indicator that the wound has poor healing potential.[28] (Refer to Chapter 4, Vascular Wounds, for more information on vascular testing.)

The musculoskeletal assessment of the foot is performed in both weight-bearing and non-weight-bearing positions. Deformities and their severity are assessed along with any motion restrictions, especially restrictions produced by the presence of equinus. A simple classification system was developed at Temple University to assess the depth of wounds and the degree of foot deformity in order to determine the type of off-loading device necessary to heal the wound (**TABLE 7-11**).

Pictorial Glossary of Transitional Off-Loading Devices

See **FIGURES 7-16** to **7-30**.

Eighty-five percent of all lower limb amputations in patients with diabetes are preceded by a foot ulcer.[23,29] Those who develop a foot ulcer have a 55 times greater risk of infection[29] and if a DFU is open for 30 days or longer the risk quadruples.[21] The cost to the healthcare system is astronomical. The annual costs of care for DFUs have been estimated to be $1.38 billion per year.[30] Using conventional care, the average cost to obtain a healed ulcer can be as high as $56,000, due in part to the relative inefficiency of what is considered good wound care.[31]

In a 1999 meta-analysis, Margolis concluded that after 12 weeks of good wound care, only 24.2% of ulcers were healed,

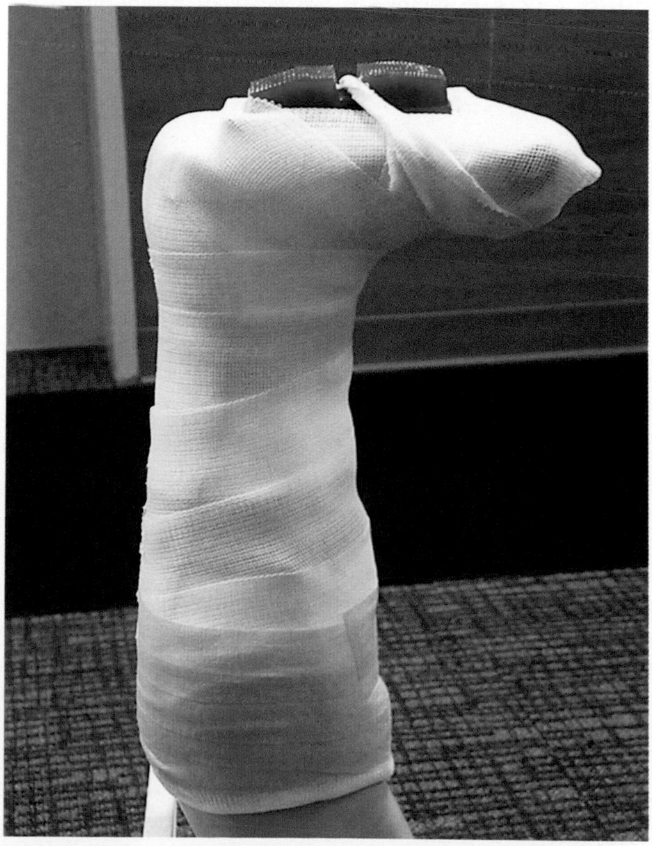

FIGURE 7-16 Total-contact cast (TCC).

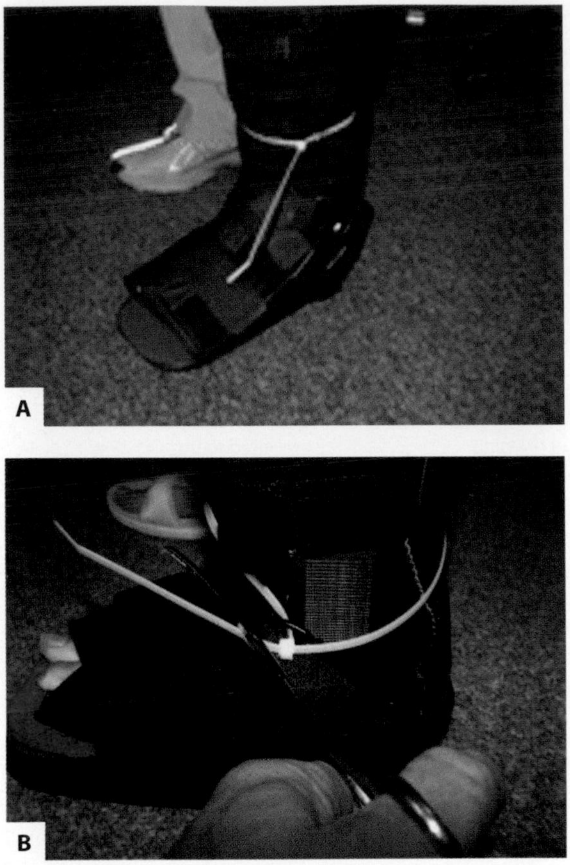

FIGURE 7-17 A, B. Removable cast walker or Instant total-contact cast (iTCC) with zip ties to ensure compliance.

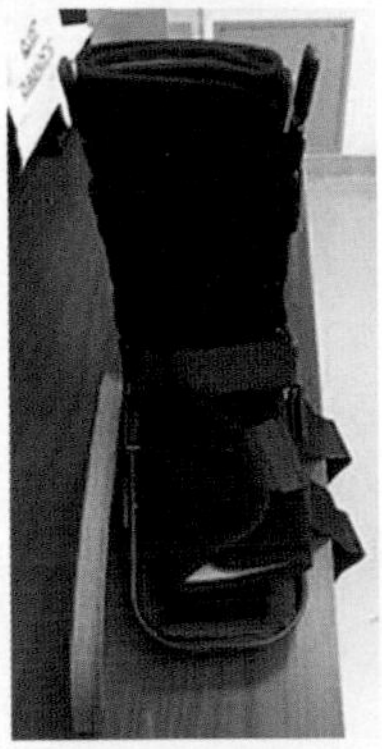

FIGURE 7-18 CAM boot with pixelated insole.

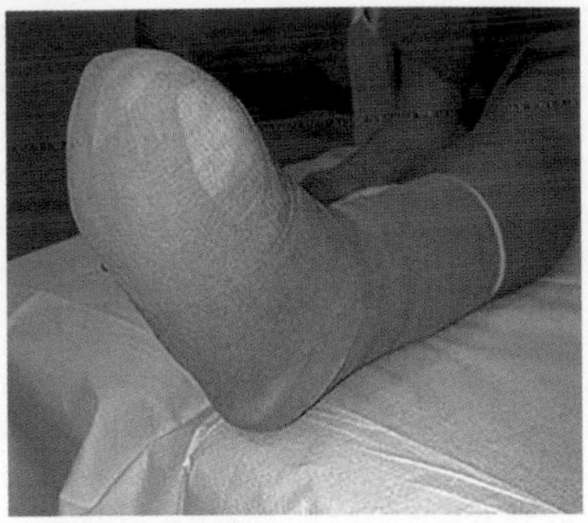

FIGURE 7-19 The Rader football dressing.

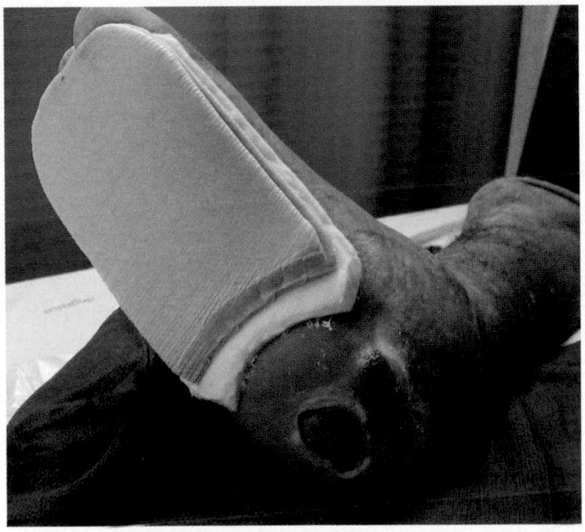

FIGURE 7-20 The felted foam dressing.

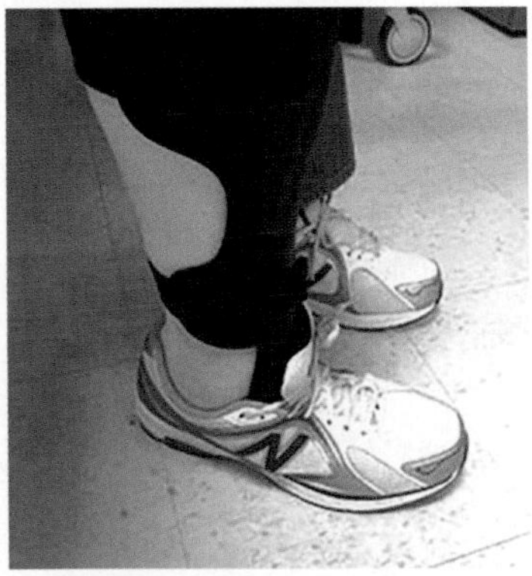

FIGURE 7-21 Carbon fiber AFO.

and after an additional 8 weeks of the same care or 20 total weeks, only 30.9% of those same wounds would have achieved complete closure.[32]

The total annual cost of diabetes treatment in 2002 (including direct and indirect costs) was estimated at $132 billion, or 1 out of every 10 healthcare dollars spent in the United States.[33,34] A patient hospitalized for a DFU can expect a 59% longer length of stay than a diabetic patient hospitalized without a foot ulcer.[35] A lower-extremity amputation (LEA) will be required by 14% to 24% of those DFU patients,[26] and unfortunately, the incidence of LEA in people with diabetes continues to rise despite deliberate efforts to prevent amputations in the last decade.[22]

Biomechanical Changes with Diabetes

Diabetes has a particularly devastating effect on the form and function of the human foot. The human foot is an intricate

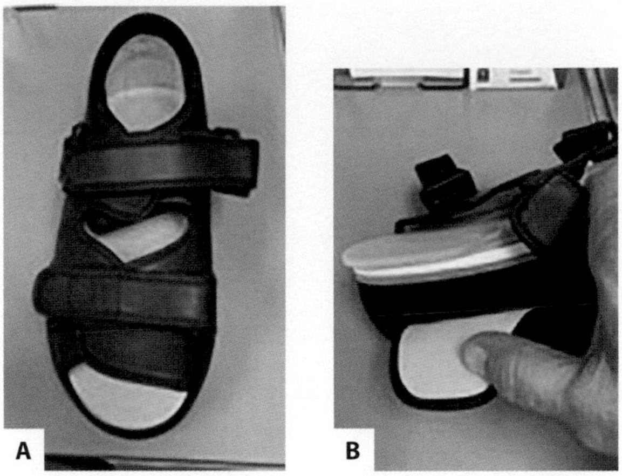

FIGURE 7-22 A. The diabetic healing shoe. The wound healing shoe consists of an open toe shoe with a rocker bottom and four layers of dense foam. Elliptical cut-outs are made in the middle two layers of foam to relieve the pressure on and around the plantar DFU. **B.** Insoles layered in the diabetic healing shoe.

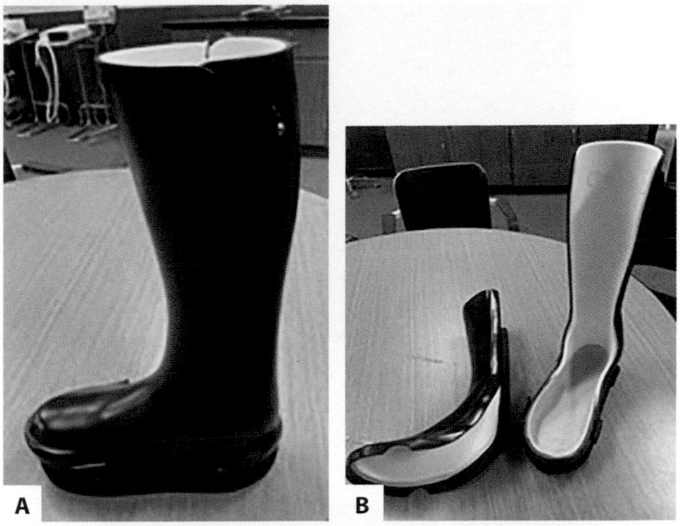

FIGURE 7-24 A. Charcot restraint orthopedic walker or CROW. B. CROW boot with custom-molded innersole.

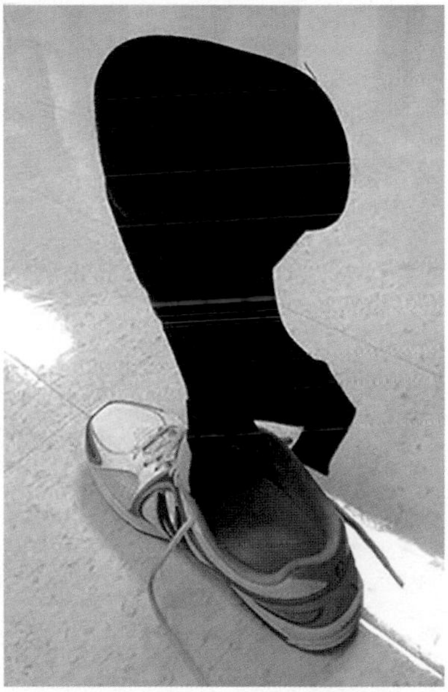

FIGURE 7-23 Carbon fiber AFO with custom-molded innersole.

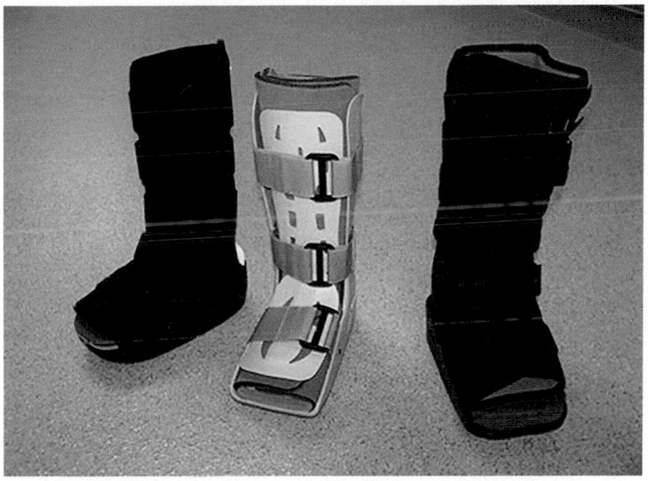

FIGURE 7-25 Removable cast walkers.

ground interface for the human body providing sensory input, balance, and stability. The 26 bones, ligaments, and muscles are organized into a highly efficient mechanical system for maintaining balance and posture, sensing ground position and surface characteristics, and converting muscular and ground reactive forces into the various movements required to stand and move. The many nerves of the plantar surface provide constant feedback to the spinal cord and brain where an elaborate system of reflex and intentional movements keep the body's center of gravity (COG) balanced between the two feet in the bipedal stance or over the weight-bearing foot in unilateral single support.

Gait is the intentional transportation of the body's COG in a forward manner. Major forces are generated in the sagittal plane with balance and control forces modulated in the frontal and transverse planes. The muscles of the lower extremity work together in an attempt to maintain the COG either between the two legs or directly over the plantigrade foot (**FIGURES 7-31** and **7-32**).

Various anatomical abnormalities or pathologies in the neuromuscular system can create imbalances in the musculoskeletal system. These imbalances necessitate an adjustment or correction in position by either reflexive or volitional muscle action in order to realign the skeletal elements and restore balance to the system. When skeletal malalignments or restrictions cannot be corrected by muscle action, the foot must accommodate to the malposition, and the body must adapt its balance mechanisms accordingly.

The individual foot adjusts position by complex muscle and postural reactions in an attempt to maintain balance around a COG or force that is located just lateral to the center

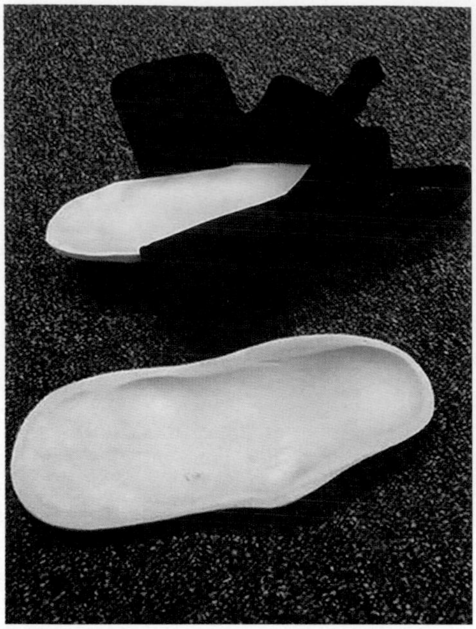

FIGURE 7-26 Modified Carville healing sandal.

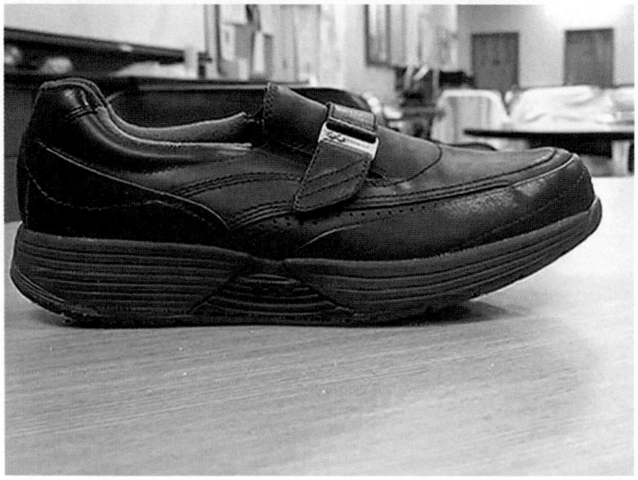

FIGURE 7-27 Rocker soled depth shoe.

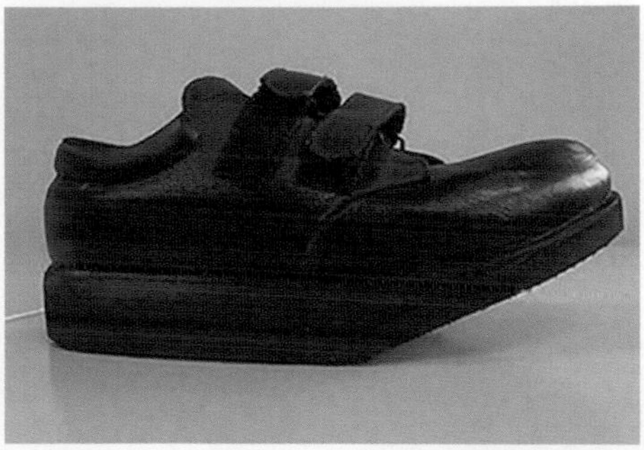

FIGURE 7-28 Depth shoe with 22-degree Carville rocker.

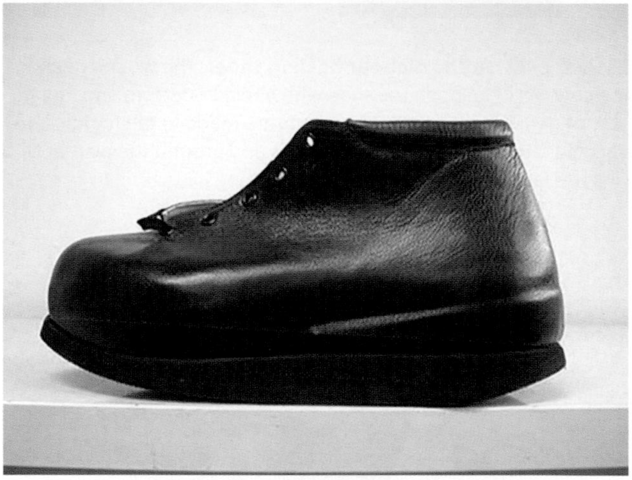

FIGURE 7-29 Chukka custom-molded shoe with heel roller and metatarsal rocker.

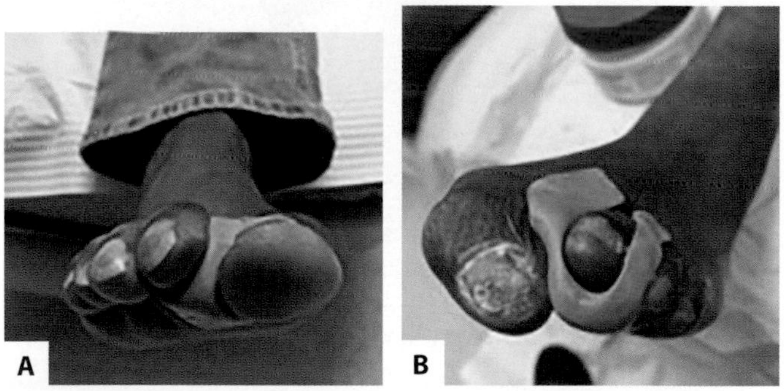

FIGURE 7-30 A, B. Silicone-molded digital orthosis.

of the second cuneiform. When functioning together, the two feet and upper body postural reactions work to maintain the COG over a point located directly between the feet. During single limb support, changes in terrain or perturbations to the body cause a shift or imbalance to this center of force in one of eight directions or vectors of imbalance (**FIGURE 7-33**).[36]

The neuromuscular system then reacts to restore balance to the system. For many years, the medical community looked at the foot using a model proposed by Merton Root.[37] In this model, the foot functioned primarily in response to various frontal plane morphologies (such as forefoot or rearfoot varus/valgus deformities or variations from an ideal normal). The subtalar joint that has a triplanar, pronatory/supinatory axis was the primary adapting articulation, and the compensations noted in each of the planes were the direct result of primary malalignments in the frontal plane. This was a useful clinical model for developing frontal plane posted foot orthoses but did not account for the planal influence of malalignments in the sagittal plane or the deforming forces that could be generated by rotational deformities in the transverse plane. Using a Rootarian approach, single or multiple ray deformities in the sagittal plane would be interpreted as frontal plane abnormalities, that is, a plantarflexed first metatarsal would be interpreted as forefoot valgus. This would lead the clinician to treat the patient with a forefoot valgus post; however, the intervention needed for proper balance was a heel elevation

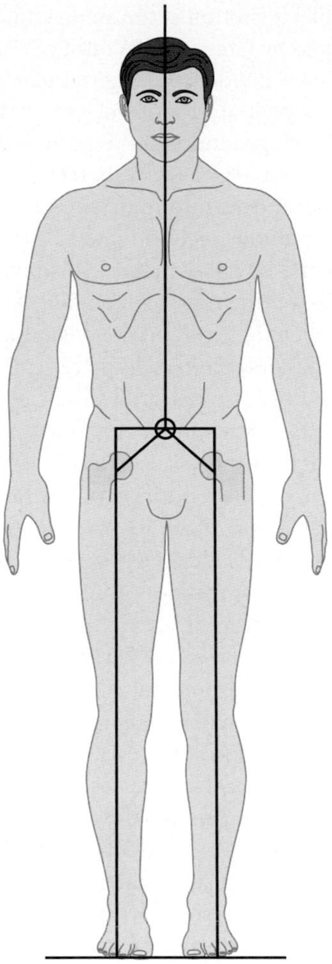

FIGURE 7-31 Center of gravity in bilateral static stance.

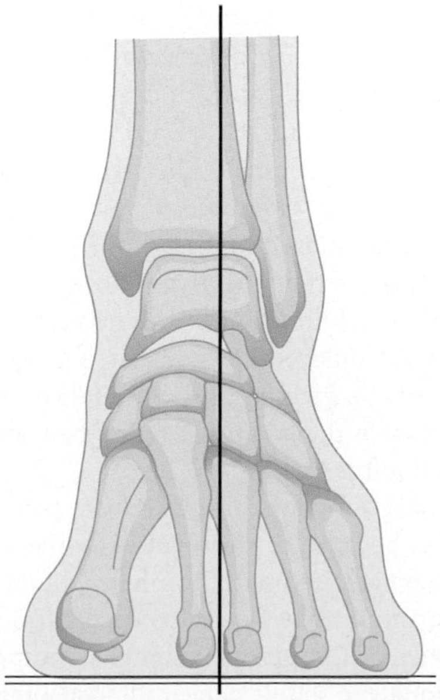

FIGURE 7-32 Center of gravity in unilateral static stance. (Courtesy of Dr. Alan Whitney.)

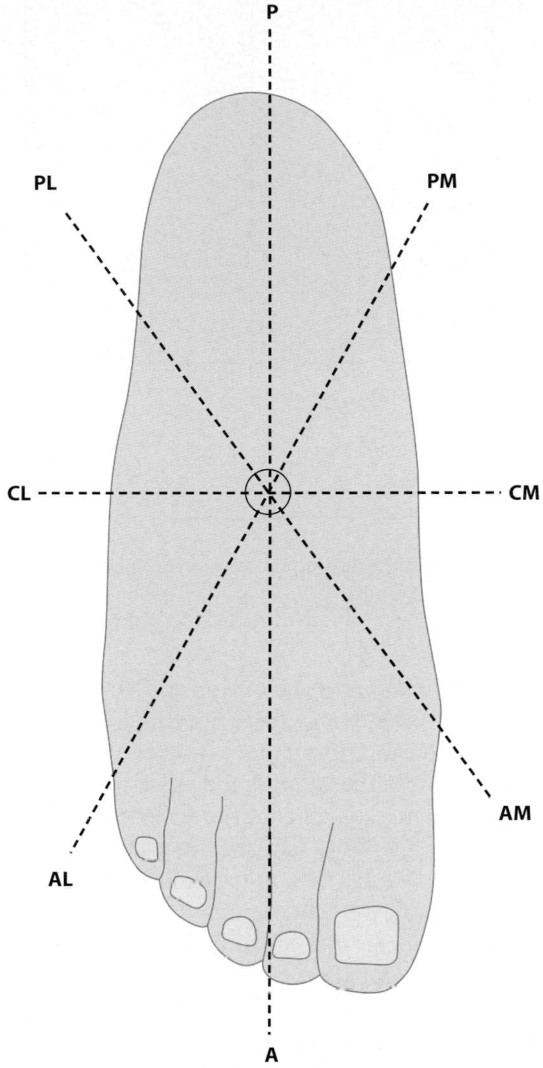

FIGURE 7-33 The eight vectors of foot imbalance. Four of these directions consist of the cardinal vectors of anterior, posterior, medial, or lateral. The remaining four vectors consist of anteromedial, anterolateral, posteromedial, and posterolateral. (Courtesy of Dr. Alan Whitney.)

and accommodation for the plantarflexed metatarsal within the orthotic shell and the forefoot extension. The weaknesses of Rootarian biomechanics led to the development of alternative foot models that attempted to account for malalignments in all three planes (triplanar). Several experts (notably those of Alan and Ken Whitney[36] and Howard Danenberg[38]) felt that the primary focus of balance lay in the sagittal plane.

The foot has a center axis of balance or "spine," which generally corresponds to the second or sometimes the second and third metatarsals with their accompanying cuneiforms. Medially, the first ray or metatarsal-cuneiform segment, and laterally, the fourth and fifth rays or metatarsal-cuboid segments function as "dynamic outriggers" by virtue of their independent supinatory/pronatory axes and their strong independent muscle attachments. If the COG deviates from the

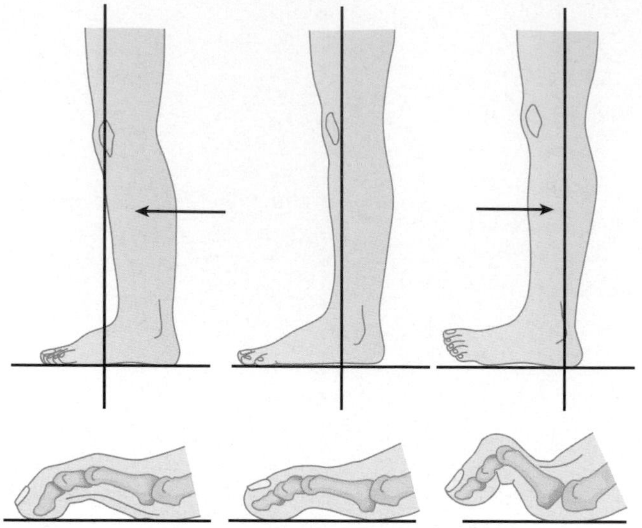

FIGURE 7-34 Digital gripping with anterior imbalance.
(Courtesy of Dr. Alan Whitney.)

center axis, the muscles of the outriggers can be activated to exert a corrective force and thereby restore central balance. Medial shifts in balance (pronation) would be resisted primarily by contractions of the anterior and posterior tibial muscles, and lateral imbalances (supination), resisted by the peroneals. Forward shifts in the COG can be corrected by contraction of ankle and digital flexors and is noted clinically as active gastrosoleus and digital flexor contractions. This action is observed as digital gripping (**FIGURE 7-34**). Posterior shifts in balance are resisted by the dorsiflexors of the ankle and toes and are noted clinically as a retraction of the digits and visible contraction of the tibialis anterior muscle.

Skeletal malalignments that produce a permanent imbalance by virtue of their axis orientation and subsequent compensations are stabilized by these same muscle groups; however, they are seen as positional deformities that are initially flexible in children but progress to fixed deformities with age. The deformities are often accompanied by degenerative arthritis due to articulation overload in one direction or another. For example, chronic anterior imbalances produced by forefoot varus or valgus or hypermobile ray segments result in relative dorsiflexion of the forefoot on the rearfoot, thereby producing a chronic digital gripping that is referred to as flexor stabilization of the toes. This alignment leads to hammertoe deformities with subsequent development of digital corns and calluses as a protective reaction to pressures caused by shoes or ground reactive forces.[39] Chronic posterior imbalances are observed with rigid plantar-flexed rays and produce sagittal plane compensations, eg, retracted digits with resultant dorsal corns and plantar calluses due to loss of digital purchase and excess pressures that are created by exposed plantar-flexed metatarsals. Any plantarflexion of the forefoot on the rearfoot must be compensated either by a segmental elevation of the affected ray(s) or by a dorsiflexion of the forefoot at the ankle. Any dorsiflexion of the ankle produces a tightening of the posterior muscle group or a reduction in available motion at the ankle joint, a term referred to as *pseudoequinus* by Green and Whitney.[40]

Jacquelin Perry divided the sagittal gait cycle into three rockers or pivots essential for normal gait.[41] At heel strike, the calcaneus strikes the ground and the body rolls over the relatively rounded plantar calcaneal tubercles, which is the first rocker. As the foot moves into midstance and comes into full contact with the ground, sagittal forward movement is transferred to the second or ankle rocker. This pivot allows the leg to move forward over the now-planted foot (**FIGURE 7-35**). The Achilles tendon then tightens and the posterior medial and lateral muscle groups contract in order to resist the rapid forward movement of the tibia over the ankle and close pack or "lock" the midtarsal joints. These muscles exert a plantarflexory force transferring motion to the third or forefoot rocker for push-off. As the body is propelled forward, the heel lifts from the ground and the ankle plantarflexes, causing the body to pivot over the metatarsal heads. Relatively small pronatory and supinatory drifts are noted as the foot progresses through a normal ideal gait cycle: pronation or anteromedial imbalance at heel strike, resupination or anterolateral imbalance during midstance, and then an anteromedial shift to the first ray in the propulsive phase. The dynamic outrigger activity of the muscle groups is generally eccentric to resist exaggerated movement in the direction of these imbalances and to act as a force couple around the virtual center axis of balance. This activity produces a stable foot and a smooth transfer of forces between each of the rockers, thereby leading to a graceful appearance to the gait.

The midfoot, and particularly the midtarsal joint, acts as both a flexible shock absorber at heel strike into midstance and a stable lever for push-off. Several mechanisms are used to accomplish this. The joint axis orientation of the subtalar, talonavicular, and calcaneocuboid joints allows for the foot to absorb pronatory forces by talar medial rotation at the subtalar joint. It also allows the forefoot to dorsiflex on the rearfoot at the midtarsal joint. Subsequently during resupination, these same joints, aided by their axis orientation, move into a position of relative stability. This positioning is also aided by derotation of the tibia as a result of forward motion of the opposite swing limb, passive tightening of the plantar fascia during heel rise utilizing the *windlass mechanism*,[42] and dynamic stabilization by concurrent contraction of the posterior tibial and peroneus longus muscles that effectively close packs or locks the midtarsal joint. The importance of dynamic stabilization has generally been downplayed in Rootarian biomechanics, favoring the more passive locking of the midtarsal joint caused by what he described as the crossing axes of the talonavicular and calcaneocuboid joints.[37]

Many people function in a relatively pronated position during push-off because of various forefoot and rearfoot planal malalignments related to their inherited foot types. Unless there is a neuromuscular weakness or control problem, the dynamic activity of the peroneus longus and posterior tibial muscles is adequate to stabilize the midtarsal joints in a number of pronated or supinated attitudes, and thus allow for efficient transfer of forces to the forefoot at the time of propulsion.[42]

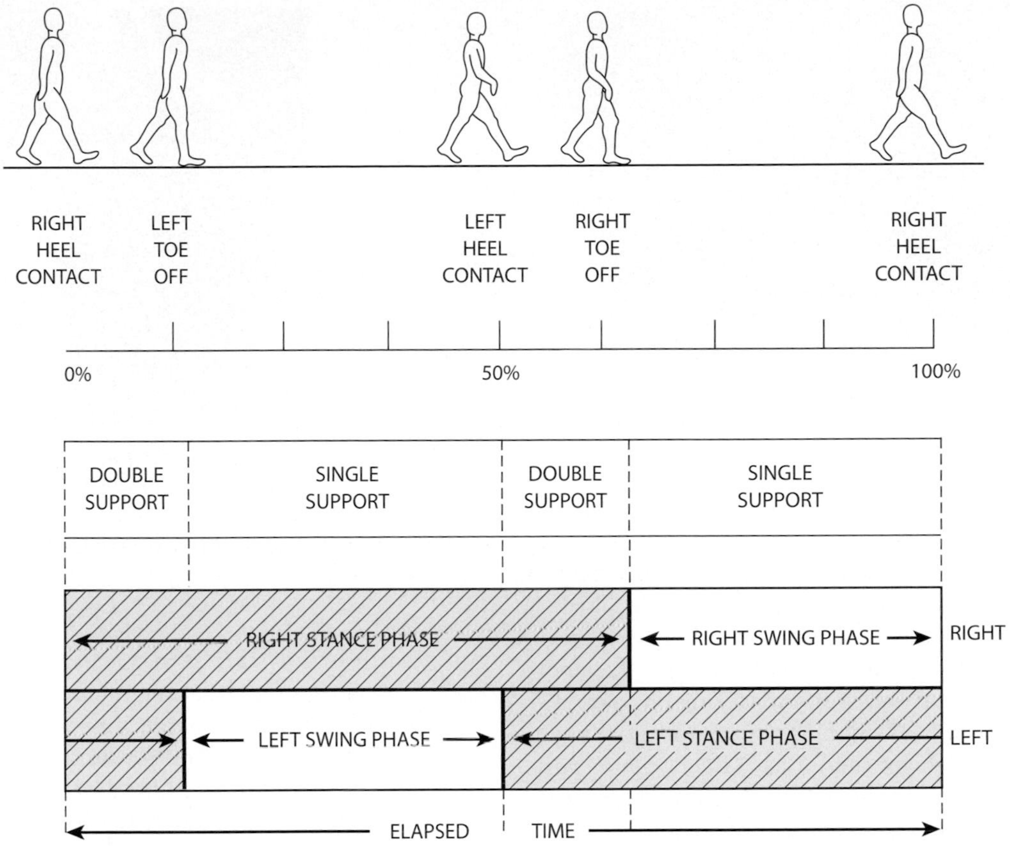

FIGURE 7-35 **Normal gait cycle.**

Inability to exert muscle force during propulsion results in a transfer of supportive responsibility from the muscles to the ligaments and passive support structures of the foot. If they are inadequate to resist the forces of weight plus momentum, the structures will either give way (tear) or attenuate over time, resulting in a midfoot collapse (**FIGURE 7-36**). Atrophy and loss of power occur over time as a result of diabetes, thereby resulting in loss of stability of the foot and a fixation of the deformities due to collagen cross-linking (see the section "Glycosylation").

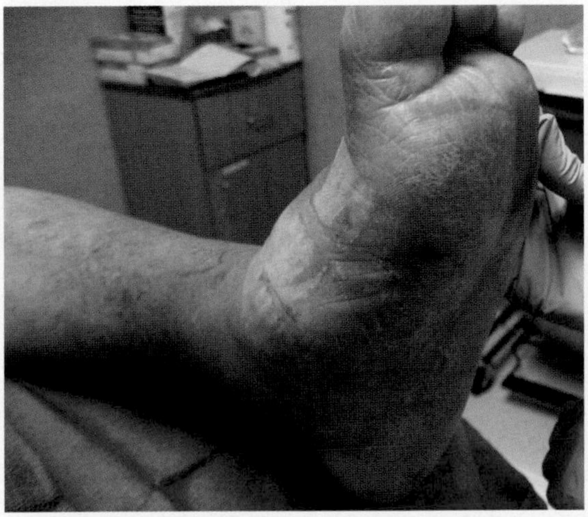

FIGURE 7-36 **Midfoot collapse.**

When these imbalances cause excessive medial or lateral translations of the center of force, and the muscles designed to correct for these translations are either at a mechanical disadvantage or compromised by weakness or paralysis, marked deformities can develop. If they are allowed to persist throughout life, they become fixed deformities.

This discussion of normal foot biomechanics is important in order to understand the diabetic foot. The diabetic foot is slowly compromised by the intersection of several component causes of ulceration.[17] These include the classic triad of neuropathy, deformity, and repetitive trauma.[43] It also includes vascular disease, footwear, lifestyle, activities, and compliance or adherence issues. These can be represented graphically by intersecting spheres (**FIGURE 7-37**). As these various factors intersect in different combinations, the demands and stresses placed on the diabetic foot can exceed its capacity to adapt and ulceration or mechanical dysfunction can ensue.

In the classic diabetic foot model, neuropathy leads to ulceration because of the inability to feel trauma and resultant ulceration at points of excess pressure and shear. Patients with diabetes have been shown to break down in areas of both high and low pressures.[44] Simple explanations are often the best to help understand complex problems, but a simple explanation

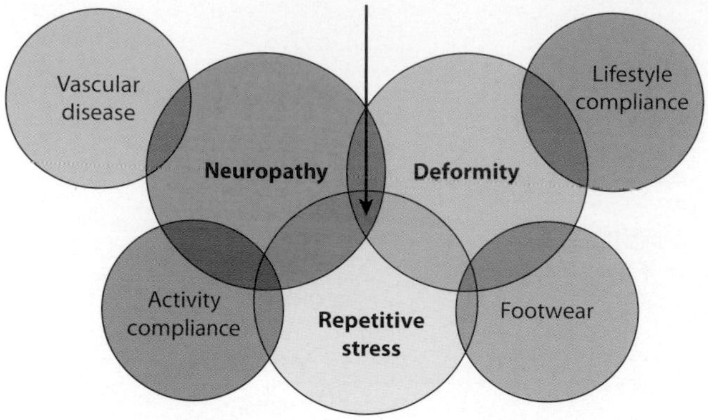

FIGURE 7-37 The intersection of component causes of the diabetic foot wound.

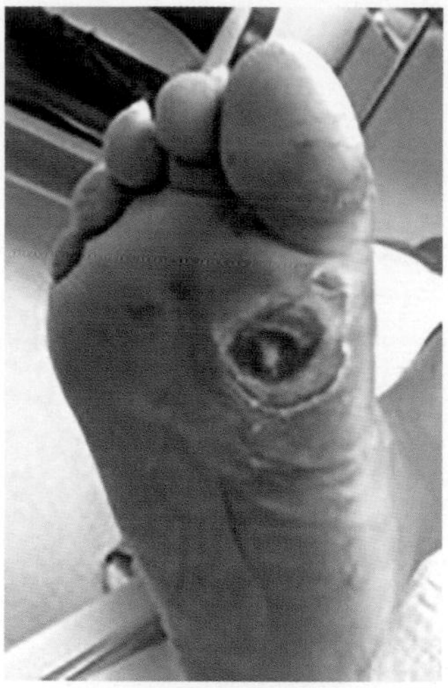

FIGURE 7-38 Large plantar shear callus with distal dissecting seroma.

for diabetic ulceration often leads providers and payers to believe that simple solutions should suffice. In reality, a much more complex and comprehensive approach is required. It cannot be assumed that only sensory neuropathy is important in diabetic foot function. Joint position sense is just as important as skin sensation, as well as more proximal balance disturbances are noted with a loss of distal proprioceptive input. When persons with diabetes cannot feel either pain or position, they are apt to compensate by using a series of destructive behaviors, including pathologic gait alterations *or* buying short or tight shoes so they can feel the shoes on their feet. They tend to lace their shoes too tight for the same reason. They develop a wider stance and a slower gait to compensate for balance losses related to muted proprioceptive input and delayed muscular balance activity. They also develop a hard heel strike and excessive digital gripping in an attempt to increase their ground perception during stance and gait. This adaptation also serves as a recruitment phenomenon when midfoot dynamic stabilization (by the peroneals and posterior tibial muscles) is delayed or inadequate to provide a rigid midfoot for propulsion. These gait alterations result in increased shear forces present on the plantar surface, exacerbating callus breakdown, and subsequent ulceration (**FIGURE 7-38**).

All aspects of the sensitive balance and control mechanism discussed above are either restricted or weakened by a progressive stiffening of the connective tissues, gradual weakening of the muscles with subsequent imbalances, and a loss of input from sensory nerves in both the skin and proprioceptors of the foot and ankle. The abnormal gait finding of late midstance pronation of the subtalar joint has been proposed as a reason for many pathologies induced by biomechanics, including plantar fasciitis, intermetatarsal neuroma, hallux limitus, hallux valgus, sesamoiditis, and low-back pain.[45]

All these entities produce pain and discomfort with resulting compensatory changes in foot position and gait in order to reduce or eliminate the discomfort. *With diabetic sensory and proprioceptive neuropathy, these pathological overloads do not produce pain and thus the patient does not initiate protective compensations.* As a result, midfoot breakdown, boney overload, and even Charcot arthropathy may ensue.

Charcot arthropathy is a particularly devastating complication of diabetes that results in multiple foot fractures and a complete loss of skeletal architecture when allowed to progress without treatment (**FIGURE 7-39**). There are three theories as to why pathological fractures develop in the neuropathic foot. The neurovascular, or French, theory suggests that increased blood flow from autonomic neuropathy leads to a "washing out" of the mineral supports of the osseous structures and a resulting osteopenia, and subsequent fracture.[46] The German theory by Virchow and Volkman proposed progressive microneurotrauma from a mechanism similar to that described above, which leads to osseous inflammation and progressive micro-fractures, resulting in macro-fractures and

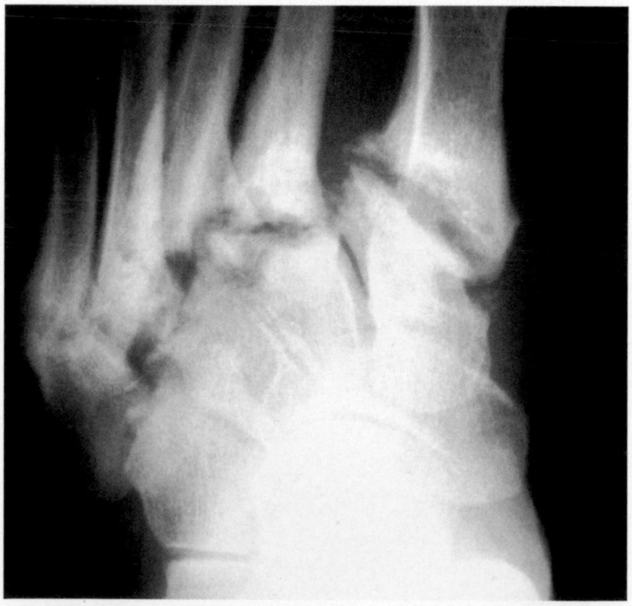

FIGURE 7-39 X-ray of severe Lisfranc's Charcot arthropathy with multiple fractures and dislocations.

eventual loss of osseous integrity.[47] The third or combined theory recognizes the contribution of both mechanisms and concludes that they contribute equally to the formation of the disorder.[48]

Glycosylation

Assessment for limited joint mobility should be part of any diabetic examination. Usually, the hands are inspected using the Prayer Sign or the Table Top Test. The Prayer Sign is performed by placing the hands together in the prayer position and observing whether the patient can get the fingers and palms together. An inability to press the palms and fingers together indicates a flexion deformity of the interphalangeal and metacarpal phalangeal joints due to limited joint mobility.[49,50] The Table Top Test is performed by asking the patient to place the hands flat on the table top and noting the ability of the hand to lie flat on the surface.[51] Although there is no similar test for the foot, the presence of equinus as measured by the Silfverskiold test and observation of the digital positions during stance perturbations can be a good substitute. According to *Wheeless' Textbook of Orthopedics*, the Silfverskiold test is performed using a goniometer to measure the degree of ankle dorsiflexion available in both the knee straight and knee bent positions (**FIGURE 7-40**).[52,53] With the knee straight the measurement is primarily looking at the gastrocnemius muscle, and should be 10 degrees or more in the normal condition.

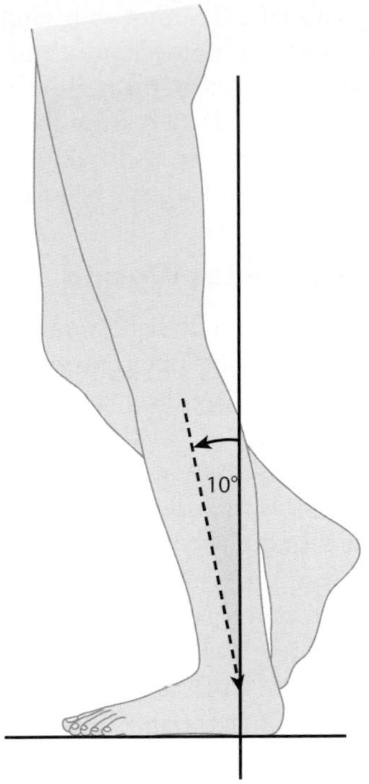

FIGURE 7-40 Measurement of ankle dorsiflexion knee bent—Silfverskiold test. With the knee straight, the measurement is primarily looking at the gastrocnemius muscle and should be 10 degrees or more in the normal condition. With the knee bent the gastrocnemius muscle, which originates above the knee joint, is placed on slack and the measurement is an approximation of the tension in the soleus muscle itself. Thus with the knee bent, there should be an additional 10 degrees of dorsiflexion or 20 degrees of total motion. If there is a restriction in dorsiflexion in both positions, then both components of the gastrosoleus complex can be assumed to be affected. (Courtesy of Dr. Alan Whitney.)

With the knee bent, the gastrocnemius muscle, which originates above the knee joint, is placed on slack and the measurement is an approximation of the tension in the soleus muscle itself. Thus, with the knee bent, there should be an additional 10 degrees of dorsiflexion or 20 degrees of total motion. If there is a restriction in dorsiflexion in both positions, then both components of the gastrosoleus complex can be assumed to be affected. Because of intrinsic muscle wasting associated with diabetic neuropathy, the toes are usually in a flexed or hammered position. When this condition exists for several years, the digital positions can become fixed or contracted, thereby making the assessment of a loss of flexibility due purely to connective tissue cross-linking difficult.

Long-standing hyperglycemia leads to a state where glucose reacts with proteins to form *advanced glycosylation end products* or AGEs. These products facilitate the formation of irreversible cross-links with collagen.[54] Along with the changes from AGEs, connective tissue changes associated with diabetic nephropathy, serum lipid peroxide, and dyslipidemia lead to a general stiffening of connective tissues in the body.[55] The result is a loss of flexibility in the foot and ankle complex with increased pressures generated across the forefoot, and gait-related changes that increase the risk for ulcer development. This risk increases the longer the person has diabetes regardless of the blood glucose levels.[56]

CLINICAL CONSIDERATION

Clinical screening for diabetic muscle wasting can be performed by observing the thenar eminence. Atrophy of the intrinsic muscles that form the thenar eminence may be a sign of diabetic motor neuropathy caused by median nerve compression.

Diabetic neuropathy not only affects the sensory nerves of the patient but the entire neuromuscular system. The annual decline in ankle strength associated with diabetic neuropathy was shown to be 3% ± 2.5%.[57] This is a progressive weakness affecting both the intrinsic and extrinsic muscles of the foot. Unlike Charcot-Marie-Tooth disease, diabetic neuropathy has a propensity for the tibial nerve over the peroneals.[58] Distal intrinsic muscles are affected first with the production of the classic "intrinsic minus foot." This deformity is seen when the intrinsic stabilizers of the metatarsophalangeal joints (MPJs) are weakened and the long flexors and extensors of the toes unopposed.[59] Loss of the function of the lumbricals and interossei of the foot leads to hammering deformity of the digits, a loss of digital stability in all planes, a loss of distal digital purchase, anterior migration of the plantar fat pad with the retracting toes, and exposure of the metatarsal heads to excessive plantar pressures.[60]

The subsequent loss of flexibility and muscle weakness due to glycosylation and diabetic myopathy produce a foot that cannot protect itself by compensatory motions and positions, skin that ulcerates because it cannot withstand the shear forces produced by the aberrant biomechanics and ulcerations that cannot heal due to the muting of the healing cascade produced by glycosylation of the cells necessary for a robust healing response. The ability to heal is also frequently compromised by some degree of peripheral arterial disease.

The Neuropathic Foot Wound

The process of developing a diabetic wound is a complicated one and is not the result of any one contributing factor. Tissues are initially compromised by the presence of neurovascular dysfunction and glycosylation of the connective tissues. The combination of lack of sensation, biomechanical imbalances, and unrelieved repetitive stress leads to soft tissue compromise, particularly in areas of high shear and pressure (**FIGURE 7-41**). Unrelieved pressure or infrequently relieved pressure produces a localized occlusion reperfusion tissue injury, which leads to cell damage and eventual cell death. Small areas of localized necrosis connect to form larger areas of necrosis, subsequently stimulating a localized inflammatory response.

This inflammatory response is detectable by skin temperature sensors (**FIGURE 7-42**). Areas where pathological inflammation is present will have an increase in temperature of ≥4°F in the area assessed when compared to the same site on the uninvolved foot. This sign is indicative of a pre-ulcerative callus or an underlying Charcot joint. Inflammation will be accompanied by the formation of pools of transudate between layers of the epidermis or between the epidermis and dermis which will be evident with callus debridement as maceration between tissue layers. These weakened tissues are unable to resist the normal shear forces produced during ambulation, thus leading to further tissue breakdown and fluid accumulation similar to that noted with a blister. Deeper tissue damage is accompanied by capillary rupture and blood in the tissues. This subcutaneous hemorrhage is evident as dark staining of the tissues beneath the surface or frank blood under the callus. If the patient continues to walk on the fluid pocket, the

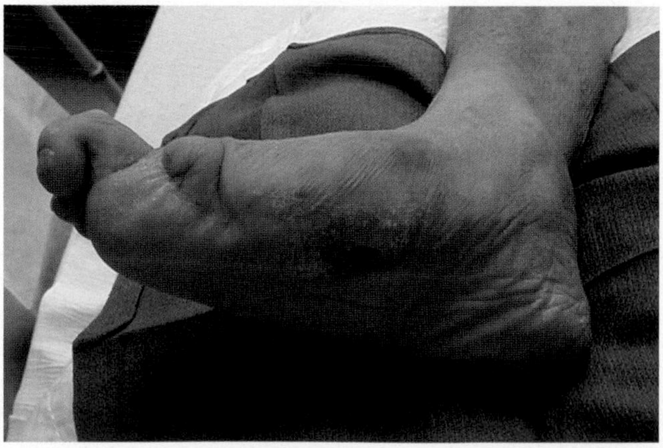

FIGURE 7-41 Neuropathic ulcer under the medial midfoot after first ray amputation. Note the severe claw toes with distal fat pad migration and exposed metatarsal heads.

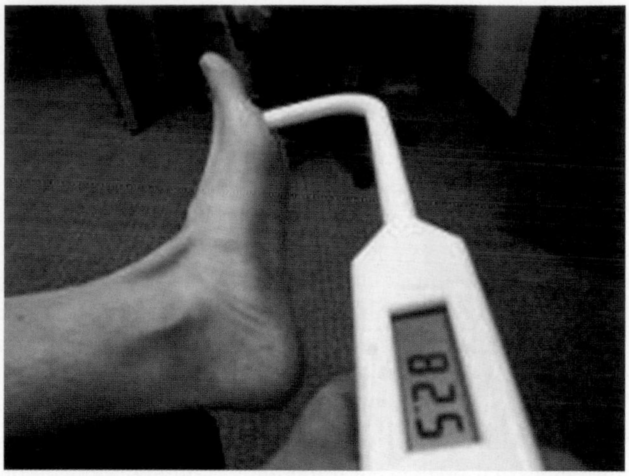

FIGURE 7-42 TempTouch temperature sensors used to detect areas of inflammation and risk for ulceration.

fluid will be pushed from side to side by shear forces and dissected into neighboring areas where there is less resistance to fluid flow (**FIGURE 7-43**). When these tissues rupture through the epidermis, the protein-rich transudate/exudate and blood are exposed to surface bacteria and easily become infected. The depth of tissue damage, the degree to which diabetes has compromised the patient, and the aggression of the microorganism determine the depth of ulceration. Continued trauma will only deepen the ulceration. Once an ulcer has formed, the patient with diabetes is at a distinct disadvantage when trying to heal the wound. The mechanisms by which the normal cellular response to wound healing is compromised are listed in **TABLE 7-12**.[61]

Off-Loading the Diabetic Foot Wound

Transitional Off-Loading The key to healing the *uninfected* diabetic foot wound is off-loading. Lack of sensation will tempt the neuropathic patient to continue to weight-bear on the wound, thus causing repetitive trauma to the delicate tissues and preventing the wound from healing. Off-loading devices shift pressure from areas of high pressure to areas of low pressure. Using a number of different mechanisms, these

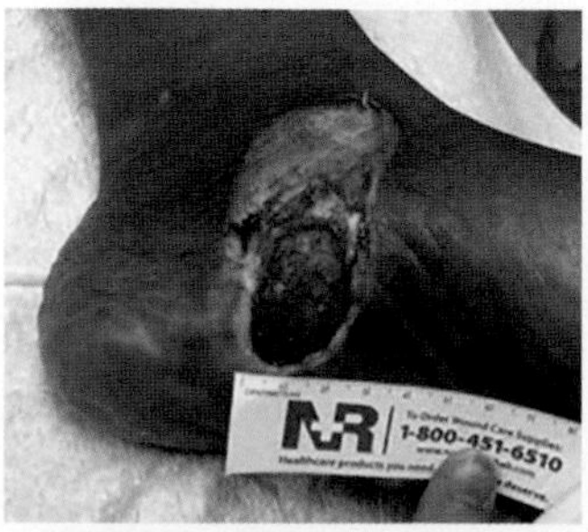

FIGURE 7-43 Dissecting sublesional midfoot hematoma after debridement.

TABLE 7-12 Impaired Cellular Function in Diabetes

- Impaired neutrophil and macrophage function
- Excessive deposition of matrix proteins (collagen and fibronectin)
- Fibroblastic growth factor receptors decreased
- Decreased endothelial cell response to angiogenic stimuli
- Interference with cell communication and need for keratinocyte migration
- Decreased keratinocyte migration
- Failure of timely and rapid wound contraction
- Impaired endothelial function (nitric oxide)

devices redistribute plantar pressures and reduce shock and shear forces that lead to tissue breakdown and delay the healing process.[62,63]

No single off-loading device is capable of reducing pressure on pedal wounds for the entire healing period. Dr. James McGuire introduced the concept of *transitional off-loading*[64] to describe the process of using different off-loading devices at different times during the phases of wound healing. In order to assess the mechanical risk for ulceration and develop a plan to treat an open ulcer, McGuire proposed a 6W assessment approach. The six Ws are based on the "who-what-when-where-why and how," or in this case, "way," of inquiry (see **TABLE 7-13**).

Normal wound healing progresses with an orderly transition from one phase to the next. The off-loading needs are different for each stage of healing. Most wound care practitioners tend to use one off-loading device throughout the healing process and then have the patient return to the pre-wound footwear, which explains the high rate of recurrence after wound healing. The component causes of ulceration unique to each patient determine the various therapies that will be utilized to manage the diabetic wound.[17] Neuropathy is the most determinant factor in wound development.[65] The most common pathway to the development of a DFU is a combination of neuropathy, deformity, secondary callus formation, and elevated peak pressure.[66] Elevated foot pressures contribute to the development of an ulceration[67]; however, it has been difficult to determine if there is a specific threshold pressure that can predict the risk of ulceration.[68] Frequently, the foot type and resultant compensatory changes are secondary to neuropathy as the primary reason for the development of ulcers in diabetic patients.[69] Biomechanical compensations such as equinus, hammer toes, and hyperpronation become fixed with prolonged glycosylation,[70] thus increasing the incidence and degree of skin irritation that results from shoe and plantar pressures and shear damage. Loss of digital purchase during ambulation leads to increased forefoot plantar pressures on the metatarsal heads compounded by the almost universal presence of equinus in the diabetic foot.[71,72]

Autonomic neuropathy produces dry skin that cracks easily and is more vulnerable to bacterial and fungal invasion.[73] Calluses form quickly, and without early detection can become limb-threatening problems. Off-loading should be designed to protect the foot from developing calluses and their subsequent ulcerations or at least slow their formation so they can be controlled by regular podiatric foot care.

As much as the clinician would like to blame the patient's choice of footwear for the problems presented by the patient with diabetes,[74] shoes are a poor predictor of wounding without an accompanying foot deformity. Therapeutic footwear, however, has been shown to reduce the incidence of foot ulceration.[75] Simply writing an off-loading prescription is not enough and the practitioner must counsel the patient regarding the amount of time they spend on the feet each day. Alterations in patient routine can have a significant effect on reducing the accumulation of pressure and shear due to

TABLE 7-13 Six-W Biomechanical Risk Assessment (Low Risk: 0–3, Moderate Risk: 4–6, High Risk: 7–12)

Six-W Biomechanical Risk Assessment	0	1	2	Total
Who	No neuropathy or deformity (0)	Neuropathy or deformity (4)	Both (7)	
What	Properly off-loaded	Adequate off-loading but not ideal	Inappropriate footwear or behavior (barefoot)	
When	Limited or no ambulation	Moderate or normal daily activity	Highly active	
Where	Indoor Limited walking on uneven surfaces	Moderate outdoor walking on some uneven surfaces	Frequent outdoor walking on multiple uneven surfaces	
Why	Compliant Highly motivated	Mostly compliant Average motivation	Noncompliant unmotivated	
Way	Short stride Slow, shuffling gait	Normal stride cadence and step length	Long stride Long step length fast, hard walker	

Who the patient is includes the intrinsic physical characteristics such as foot type, presence of deformity, severity of the diabetes, or the presence of complications such as renal disease. **What** the patient wears describes the choice of footwear and/or orthotic history. **When** the patient walks is an assessment of the amount of walking a patient does during a typical day. **Where** the patient walks describes the activities the patient engages in and the type of surfaces involved in these activities. **Why** the patient walks involves the motivation to adhere to the recommended amount of ambulation. How or the **way** the patient walks is described by the step and stride length and the aggression of ground strike. A relative risk scale was developed with each of the above variables placed on a grid and given a relative numerical weight to determine the *six-W biomechanical risk assessment* score for that patient. The higher the relative score, the greater the risk of tissue damage and the more aggressive the approach to off-loading must be.

Used with permission from McGuire J. Transitioning from open wound to final footwear: off-loading the diabetic foot. *Podiatry Today*. 2012;25(9).

unorganized activity. Walking on rough or uneven surfaces greatly increases shear forces and the risk of ulceration.

Repetitive activities such as treadmill exercise or daily walks for aerobic health need to be addressed when attempting to alter a patient's biomechanical environment. The patient's decision to cooperate with the treating clinician is the single most important factor in determining the success of wound healing (**FIGURE 7-44**). Without that, all efforts will ultimately fail no matter how expertly they are presented. To be successful, patients must understand *why* their clinician wants them to follow a certain treatment plan and *what* the consequences will be if they choose to deviate from that plan.[76] Clinicians have the tendency to expect patients to respond positively to their fact-filled presentations. This is a *provider-centered* and not a *patient-centered* approach to care.[77] It is important to treat the whole patient and not just the hole in the patient.[78]

Off-Loading Devices Off-loading the diabetic foot requires a transitional approach to the many devices available to the clinician. The total-contact cast (TCC) is considered the gold standard for off-loading a diabetic foot wound, by virtue of its ability to produce healing rates as high as 90% (see **FIGURE 7-16**).[79,80] The International Working Group on the Diabetic Foot, however, has concluded that relatively few practitioners use this modality on a routine basis despite the overwhelming research data to the contrary.[81,82] Reasons for this include established practice habits, fears of injury from the casts themselves, lack of training in its application, previous negative experiences with the device (usually by inexperienced practitioners), and reimbursement issues.[83,84] There are some instances when a patient should not be treated with a TCC. These include patients with documented PAD or an ABI of less than 0.7, fluctuating limb edema, or an active infection of the skin or the wound.[85] Other contraindications include cast claustrophobia, documented nonadherence, a sinus tract with deep extension into the foot, or inadequate training of the clinical staff in the use of the technique.

A number of alternative devices are available to off-load the DFU.[62] These include the removable cast walker (RCW) (**FIGURE 7-18**), nonremovable cast walker or instant TCC (iTCC) (**FIGURE 7-17**), D'Arco wound healing shoe (**FIGURE 7-21**) molded or double upright ankle foot orthosis (AFO) with or without a patellar tendon-bearing addition (**FIGURE 7-58**), Charcot restraint orthopedic walkers (CROWs) (see **FIGURE 7-24**), modified Carville healing sandal or shoe (see **FIGURE 7-25**), adhesive felted foam to off-load the wound in various off-loading devices (see **FIGURE 7-20**), the Rader football dressing (see **FIGURE 7-19**), and commercial off-loading shoes, such as wedge shoes (**FIGURE 7-45**), a commercial off-loading shoe with pixelated or segmented innersoles (**FIGURES 7-46** to **7-48**), or even depth or custom-molded footwear.

Devices are selected based on clinician experience, device availability, patient pressure or preference, or even insurance reimbursement with the most commonly employed device being the surgical shoe with or without internal shoe modifications.[63,86] Shoe-based devices have relatively poor evidence for healing when compared to the TCC; therefore, they are

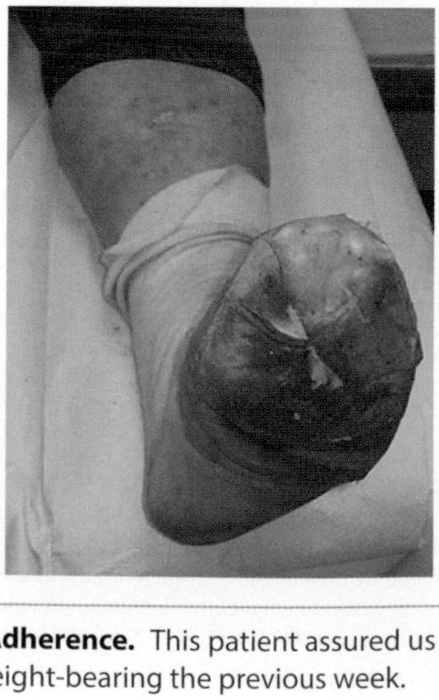

FIGURE 7-44 Adherence. This patient assured us she had remained non-weight-bearing the previous week.

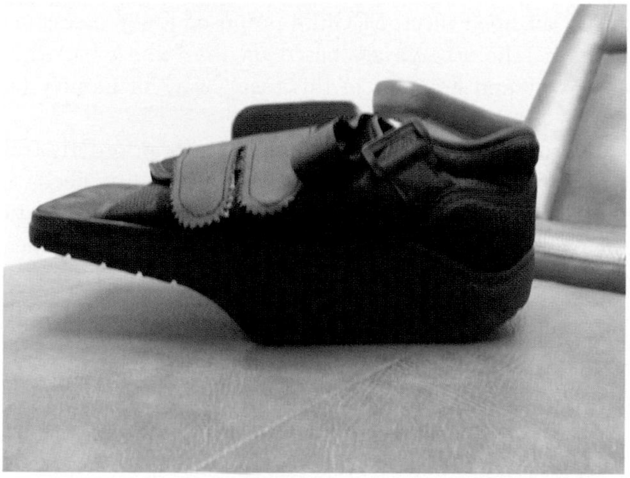

FIGURE 7-45 Orthowedge shoe.

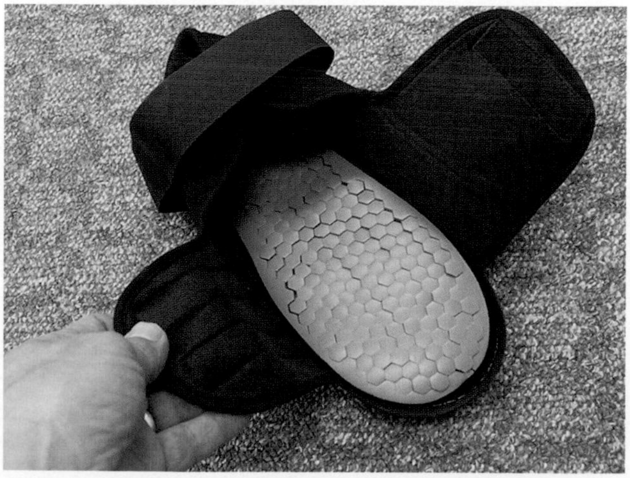

FIGURE 7-46 Diabetic healing shoe with pixelated insole.

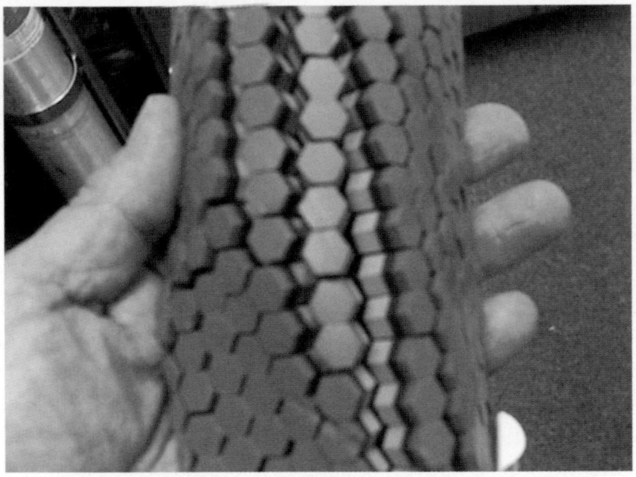

FIGURE 7-47 Hexagonal pixelated insole.

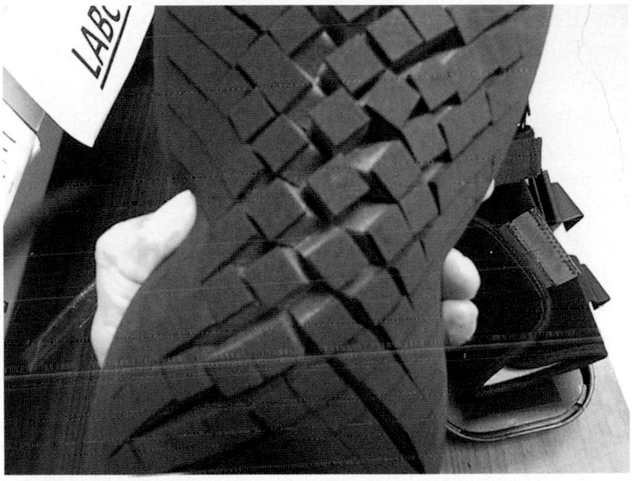

FIGURE 7-48 Diamond-shaped pixelated insole.

recommended for the transition period between the initial closure of the wound and the use of the patient's final footwear. Other than the TCC, the only other methods that have been shown to produce healing rates as high as 80% and thus considered a reasonable substitute are the iTCC, football dressings, and the felted foam technique.[87–89]

The key to healing with any of the off-loading devices is the clinician's ability to improve patient adherence by making it impossible to remove the device without the clinician's approval.[90] Knowles and Boulton found that when patients were given specialized footwear free of charge, only 20% of the patients actually wore the shoes.[91] Armstrong et al. found that when given the ability to remove the devices, RCWs were worn only 28% of the time during activities of daily living.[92] Another study found that adherence was poorest at home, and those factors that contributed to higher adherence were a low BMI, the severity of the wound, and more appealing footwear.[93]

Improving the Removable Walker Both the felted foam and football dressings can be used with RCWs, thereby increasing the effectiveness of the devices and allowing the bulky cast to be removed at night for sleeping (**FIGURE 7-23**). Removable devices allow the clinician easy access to the wound during the healing process, making it possible to apply advanced dressings to facilitate wound healing. However, any time a device can be removed by a patient there will be temptation to remove the device for comfort and thus the patient will probably walk without it.[94] A number of RCWs have been made with patellar tendon bearing (PTB) uppers or calf attachments in an effort to redistribute more weight from the foot. These devices are now available off the shelf and have only a slight edge over a standard RCW in the ability to off-load the foot. The newest type of device to be employed is the limb-load walker that uses a tight calf attachment to off-load the foot by transferring weight from the foot to the leg. These include the Torch Shoe and the Zero G brace (**FIGURE 7-49**). Once the tight upper attachment loosens because of edema reduction or weakening of the Velcro closure, the device is no better than a standard walker.

Felted Foam and the Football Dressing Felted foam dressing (FFD) utilizes a 1/4-inch adhesive felt pad with an aperture for the wound and is applied directly to the foot to reduce pressure on the ulceration (**FIGURE 7-50**). The wound is appropriately dressed, the felt applied, and a wrap of gauze or self-adherent wrap used to anchor the felt. The foot is then placed in one of several off-loading shoes or walkers to be used during ambulation. The pads are reapplied weekly or biweekly with the selected wound dressing material until the wound is healed. Birke et al. compared FFDs with a TCC and found that 93% of the ulcers treated with the FFD were healed within 12 weeks (mean time to healing of 20.9 days) compared with 92% (31.7 days) in those treated with the TCC.[89]

The football dressing can be used alone or in conjunction with the felted-foam technique. It is an excellent choice for cases where a TCC is contraindicated or a cast walker cannot

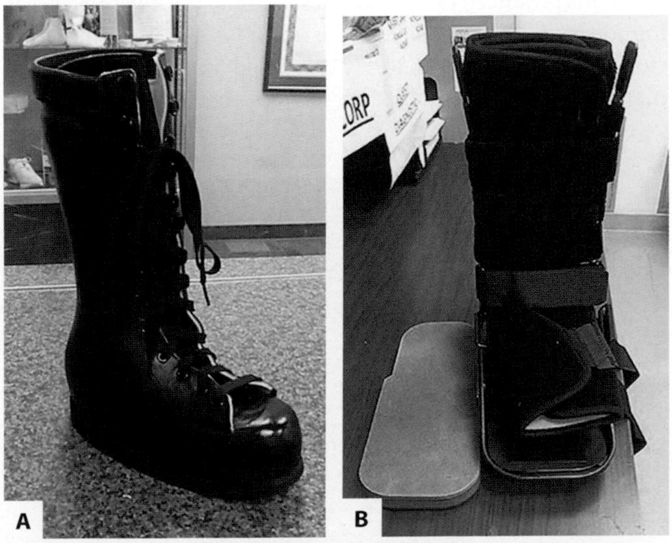

FIGURE 7-49 A. TORCH Boot. B. Zero G Brace with off-loading insole removed.

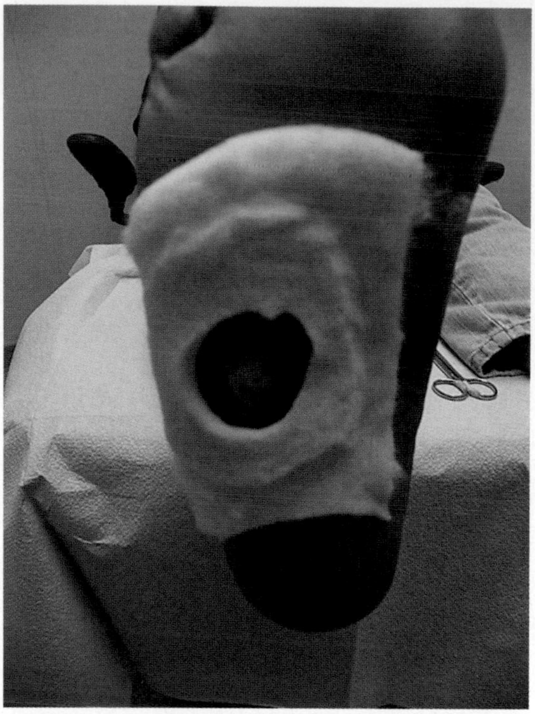

FIGURE 7-50 Felted foam dressing over a cuboid ulcer.

be obtained because of insurance limitations or other circumstances. The football dressing uses several layers of cast padding, secured with woven gauze roll bandage, overlaid by more padding, additional gauze, and finally a layer of self-adherent wrap to keep it in place (**FIGURE 7-19**). These dressings, although they are nonremovable, alleviate the feeling of claustrophobia some patients experience when they are restrained in a nonremovable device such as the TCC.

Transitional Devices Recently epithelialized scar tissue cannot withstand the stresses of normal activity or the loading problems produced by the patient's original footwear. Steed et al. found that 69% of patients broke down within 30 months after closure with a growth factor.[95,96] Pixelated innersoles or custom-made total-contact molded innersoles in footwear such as a surgical shoe with a rocker sole (**FIGURE 7-51**) or a prefabricated healing shoe (**FIGURE 7-21**) are excellent transitional devices to prepare the patient for ambulation in the final footwear.

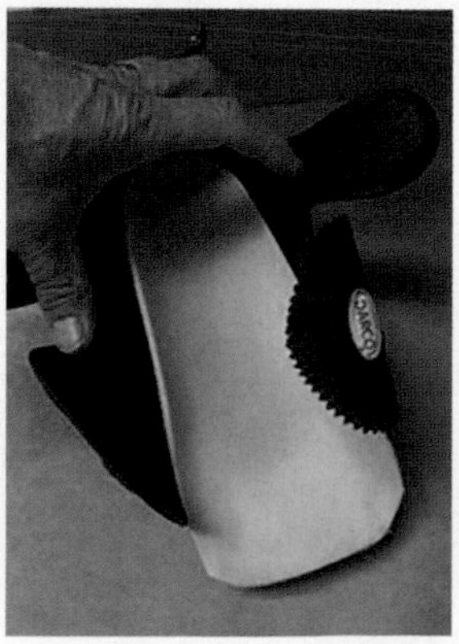

FIGURE 7-51 Surgical shoe with total-contact molded insole.

Wound Care

A comprehensive approach to wound healing begins with a thorough wound hygiene protocol such as that developed at Temple University as part of the ABCESS system for care of the diabetic foot wound (**TABLES 7-14** and **7-15**).

Conversion of the wound to a more acute stage of healing is achieved by debridement of necrotic tissues, including the periwound callus that consists of senescent cells that will inhibit wound closure. Standard wound care using the TIME principle (presented in Chapter 14, Wound Dressings) also includes the following components: treatment of infection with topical antimicrobial dressings and systemic antibiotics when indicated; moist wound dressings, beginning with absorbent dressings sufficient to manage the drainage and protect the off-loading device from moisture that will facilitate more bacterial growth; and close attention to the edges to facilitate re-epithelialization as the wound granulates. Numerous references are available to support the use of cellular and tissue products discussed in Chapter 14, Wound Dressings.[97–101]

A final note for wound care clinicians caring for patients with a history of recurrent DFUs—corrective surgery by a podiatrist or ankle/foot orthopedist experienced in caring for these patients can be beneficial in correcting bony abnormalities that underlie the soft tissue that is in a breaking down/scarring cycle. Surgeries such as metatarsal head resection, Achilles tendon lengthening, tibialis anterior lengthening, and flexor digitorum longus tenotomy are procedures that can alter foot structure and thereby influence gait mechanics in such a way that shear and pressure are relieved, sometimes more than can be done with diabetic shoes and inserts.[18]

Footwear for People with Diabetes

The choice of footwear must be a collaborative effort between the patient, the physician or physical therapist, and the pedorthist. All podiatric, and many allopathic and osteopathic physicians, receive specialized training in the skills necessary to diagnose diabetic foot disorders and prescribe interventions and footwear. Matricali et al. found that 67% of the patients developed recurrent ulcers 22 months after treatment with TCC treatments.[96]

The in-depth shoe is the basis for most footwear prescriptions. It is generally an Oxford-type or athletic shoe with an additional 1/4–1/2 inch of depth throughout the shoe, allowing the extra volume to accommodate any needed inserts or orthoses, as well as deformities commonly associated with a diabetic foot. In-depth shoes also tend to be light in weight, have shock-absorbing soles, and come in a wide range of shapes and sizes to accommodate virtually any foot. They also now come in a variety of styles to appeal to those conscious of footwear appearance.

TABLE 7-14 Temple University ABCESS Wound Protocol

All Medical Conditions: To Include a Complete History, & Physical Assessment	Wound Bed Management: Bioload/Biofilm/ Biopsy	Circulation to Include Arterial Venous and Lymphatic Circulation	Exudate Management	Skin Off-loading, Protection, and Treatment	Social, Societal, and Spiritual Factors
Control systemic disease and comorbid conditions contributing to wound healing delays.	Prevent high bacterial counts and prolonged inflammation Alter therapies based on cellular and biomarker analysis	Normalize to the extent possible with available interventions	Maintain a moist, bacteria-free wound environment	Prevent traumatic, inflammatory or iatrogenic damage	Assessment of the psychological and social environment Evaluating social support systems, spiritual strengths, and navigating societal barriers
DM, ESRD, CHF, Autoimmune Dx, KD, CVD, Nutrition, etc.	Debridement, PCR/ DNA antimicrobials, antiseptics, hydrophobics, bacterial trapping Biopsy for suspicion of malignancy CTPs Growth factors Autologous tissues	Vascular surgery Compression wraps, stockings, and segmental compression	Dressing selection or alteration, NPWT	Periwound protection, off-loading, edge effect, decrease inflammation	Establish contacts for testing. transportation. home care, educate family/ caregivers; encourage development of an emotional support network
Systemic interventions to improve local healing capacity	Low bacterial counts and controlled inflammation Restore cell migration, maceration avoided action	Maximize vascularity and healing potential	Assures a healthy environment for growing cells	Prevent unintended damage to the wound and nearby tissues	Establish a network of support to maximize the patient's ability to manage their wound

Data from McGuire J, Love E, Vlahovic TC, et al. The ABCESS system for chronic wound management: a new acronym for lower extremity wound management. *Wounds*. 2020;32(suppl 11):S1-S25.

TABLE 7-15 Temple University Hygiene Wound Protocol

- ABCESS medical history
- Observation/Measurement
- Assess biofilm/infection risk
- Culture if appropriate
- Periwound and wound bed cleansing with HOCl
- Debridement of nonviable tissue, disruption of the biofilm, reanimate wound edge
- Apply 10- minute HOCl gauze soak
- Hydrate periwound skin/limb
- Apply HOCl hydrogel and/or antimicrobial contact layer
- Choose dressing based on exudate production and biofilm history
- Off-load/Protect/Compress as needed
- Review home care instructions
- Write home care/nursing orders

According to the Medicare Therapeutic Shoe Bill, the prescribing physician is responsible for ensuring the shoes and insoles or orthoses prescribed are appropriate in both fit and function to address the needs of the patient.[102,103] The Medicare Shoe Bill is designed to provide diabetic footwear, total-contact molded inserts, and modifications for those patients or beneficiaries who meet the criteria listed in **TABLE 7-16**.

Specifics of the actual shoe prescription are best managed by a licensed podiatrist because of the specialized training in biomechanics and diabetic foot care. Diabetic footwear today is available in many styles, shapes, and sizes; the pedorthist

TABLE 7-16 Therapeutic Shoe Bill for Patients with Diabetes

This bill covers patients with diabetes and covers one pair of depth shoes and three pairs of inserts or shoe modifications per calendar year.

The following criteria must be met:

The "certifying physician" **must be** an MD or DO actively managing the patient's diabetes.

The certifying physician **must document** if the patient has one or more of the following conditions[a]:

- Peripheral neuropathy with evidence of callus formation
- Foot deformity (any type)
- A current or previous preulcerative callus (intralesional hemorrhage or maceration)
- A current or previous foot ulceration
- Amputation of all or any part of the foot
- Poor circulation

The physician must provide (**annually**) to the supplier:

- A detailed written order
- A copy of an office visit medical record indicating you are managing the patient's diabetes
- A copy of your medical office note describing one of the qualifying conditions, or an office visit note from a DPM, PA, NP, or CNS that describes one of the qualifying conditions
- The note must describe the **specific** foot deformity (bunion, hammertoe, etc.), the exact location of the foot ulcer or callus, type of amputation, and/or signs and symptoms supporting the diagnosis of peripheral neuropathy or peripheral vascular disease (venous or arterial)[92]

[a]This document **cannot be provided by** a Podiatrist (DPM), PHYSICIAN Assistant (PA), Nurse Practitioner (NP), or Clinical Nurse Specialist (CNS) but they can sign the order for the shoes and inserts themselves.

Data from http://www.medicarenhic.com.

has been trained to fill shoe prescriptions for diabetic patients and has the knowledge of the market to guide patients to make appropriate shoe choices to prevent further foot injury. The patient must be educated to make wise choices with regard to footwear and lifestyle. In order to live a long and full life, the patient must embrace the basics such as eating a proper diet, monitoring blood sugar, and purchasing and wearing protective footwear, and performing daily foot checks.

There are many shoes that on the surface appear to be an adequate substitute for the real thing, but in reality do not meet the criterion for a true extra-depth shoe as defined by the diabetic shoe bill. Regardless of education to the contrary, the majority of patients will return to their pre-ulcer shoe size and style. Patients have a strong desire to return to "normal" and convince themselves that they are different from other diabetics. Even if they have developed an ulcer, they will convince themselves that this was a fluke and that they will be able to return to their former way of life without having to make major considerations. Nothing could be further from the truth and reinforcement of the need for appropriate shoes is required from all the disciplines working with the patient.

Healthcare providers must educate the patient with diabetes and the caregiver that the time right after the first wound develops is the most critical time. For the open wound, the first 4 weeks of healing are the "golden hour" for avoiding the complications of osteomyelitis and amputation. In the same manner, the first several months after the first wound are a "momentum veritatis," or moment of truth, with regard to the patient's future health. Patients with diabetes need to understand the gravity of an open wound. When a wound is open for more than 4 weeks, its chance of healing reduces dramatically and the risk of infection increases five times. When a wound becomes infected, the patient is 155 times at greater risk for amputation secondary to overwhelming infection or osteomyelitis.[21] After a patient develops a new diabetic wound, the 5-year survival decreases drastically with mortality rates reported between 43% and 55%.[104] After a major amputation, 52% to 80% of these patients die within 5 years.[105] If patients with diabetes think they can return to their previous lifestyles, they are "dead wrong"! Healthcare providers cannot believe or trust their assurances and soft pedal their need to control the diabetes and get into the right shoe and insert combination. The very least the provider should do is provide the proper prescription or referral for shoes as well as a reputable list of pedorthotists. In addition, the patients should receive regular podiatric foot care and periodic visits with the physician who is managing the diabetes in order to continually reinforce proper maintenance of blood sugar levels, diet, and exercise routines.

Because of the digital deformities associated with the neuropathic foot, a standard shoe is *absolutely not* an option for patients. Anatomically shaped custom-molded shoes are not necessary for all patients with diabetes, and there are many styles available that provide the protection that the diabetic foot needs.

Prior to the development of an ulcer, most patients with no or low-risk factors can be managed in standard footwear. After an ulcer has developed and healed, even patients with relatively minor foot deformities and low levels of risk need to be protected from future ulceration with a total-contact molded innersole and extra-depth shoes with rocker soles.

Flexible foot imbalances that can be corrected by realignment are best treated with a corrective functional device to reduce the digital and forefoot compensations caused by the biomechanical imbalances. Rigid fixed deformities are best treated with an accommodative device with which areas of high pressure and shear specifically are addressed with relief areas in the innersole or soft inserts at the site of ulceration. Rocker soles are added to the shoes when there is a real risk of repeat ulcers in the forefoot and when the patient has enough balance to master ambulation with them. Rockers can be toe only for distal digital ulcers or metatarsal rockers to address metatarsal head lesions (**FIGURE 7-52**). Heel rollers or a cushion insert known as a SACH-style heel can be added to smooth out heel strike and prevent foot slap at heel contact, thus making it easier for the patient to adjust to the rocker platform (**FIGURES 7-53** and **7-54**). A double rocker sole can be used to provide additional pressure relief for patients who present with a rocker bottom or Charcot foot (**FIGURE 7-55**).

The concept of total-contact innersoles was first introduced by Dr Paul Brand in 1983.[106] Simple flat insoles, no matter how much cushion they provide, are not adequate to off-load the diabetic foot. Insoles that have to mold to the diabetic foot during normal ambulation, a process known

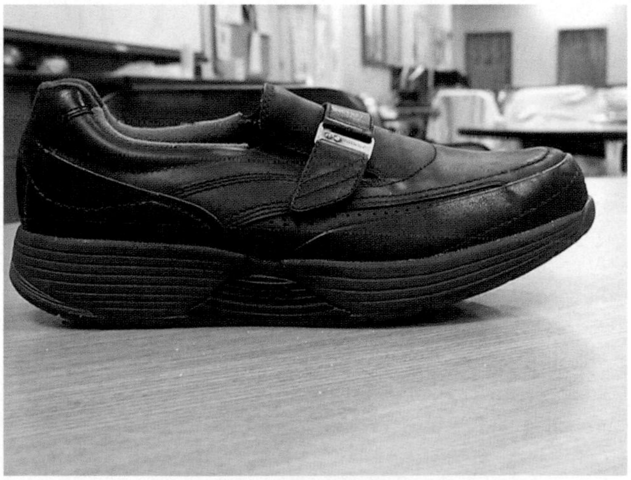

FIGURE 7-52 Commercial depth shoe with heel roller toe rocker.

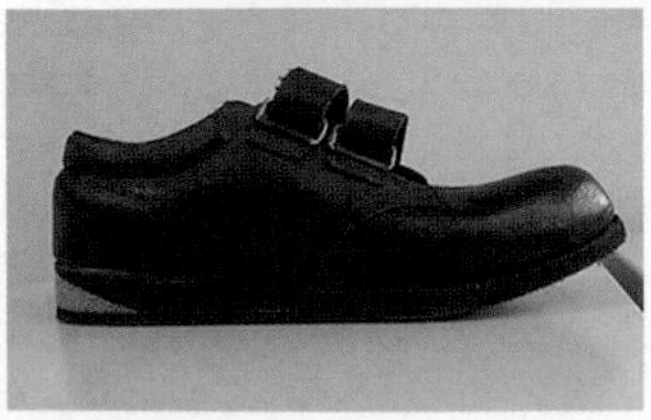

FIGURE 7-53 Customized depth shoe with metatarsal rocker and a SACH.

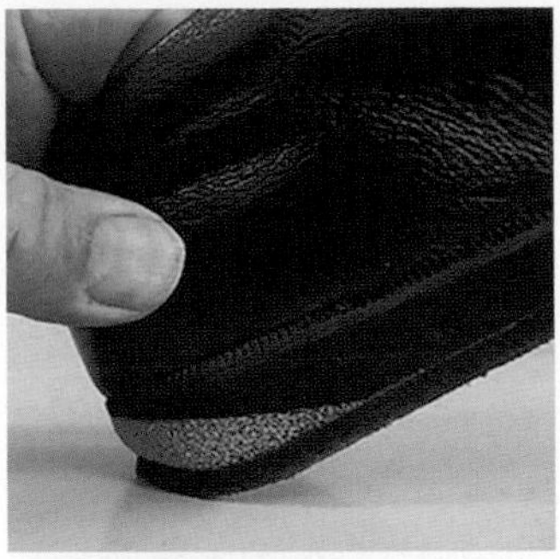

FIGURE 7-54 SACH heel insert.

as dynamic molding, are also inappropriate for off-loading a foot with demonstrated risk factors for ulceration. A contoured total-contact molded innersole is essential to distribute weight-bearing forces across the entire plantar surface and reduce anterior-posterior and medial-lateral shear forces in the shoe. Providers should not allow patients to receive unmolded innersoles to save time or money. The use of a heat gun directed into the shoe for a few seconds to warm the innersoles that come with the shoes does not provide the pressure redistribution of total-contact molding. Patients cannot use their at-risk feet to act as molding agents for insoles that are inadequate, and simple flat innersoles are inadequate to properly off-load a neuropathic foot. Molded insoles are

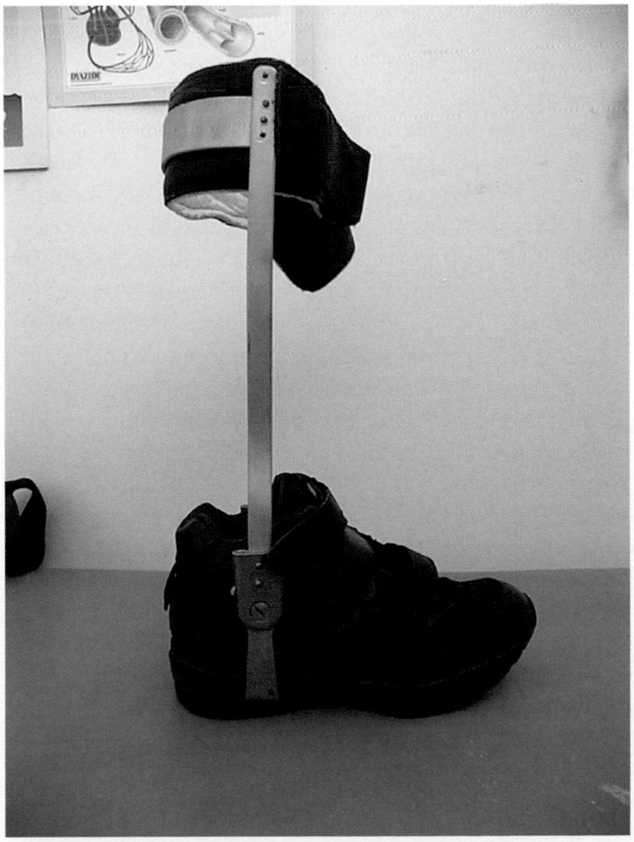

FIGURE 7-55 AFO with double rocker sole.

thick enough to fill the midfoot arches for proper pressure redistribution and to accommodate all plantar deformities. They should not, however, in any way crowd or tighten the shoe, particularly in the area of the toes (**FIGURE 7-51**). Newer orthotics and innersoles have been designed to aggressively off-load the foot in areas where ulcers are prone to form.

Penn State University has developed an innovative method for the production of a uniquely shaped therapeutic insole to alter the plantar pressure distribution of the foot. The TrueContour diabetic insoles are presently under evaluation in an active clinical trial to determine their effectiveness in the prevention of the recurrence of diabetic ulceration (**FIGURE 7-56**).[107] Rocker soles were originally proposed by Dr. Paul Brand for the prevention of ulcer recurrence after total-contact casting.[106] The original rocker design used a 22-degree metatarsal rocker with a very thick sole necessitating the use of a similar thickness insole on the opposite foot (**FIGURE 7-27**). This was very effective at off-loading the forefoot but created problems with gait and increased the fall risk for older patients. Most rocker soles today are between 12 degrees and 18 degrees and come in a number of designs based on the position and number of rockers on the sole (**FIGURE 7-55**).

Custom-molded shoes are designed to use with severe deformities that absolutely cannot be accommodated with available commercial last shoes (**FIGURES 7-28** and **FIGURES 7-57**). A version of a custom shoe with limb-loading capacity commonly used to address an unstable Charcot foot is a *Charcot restraint orthopedic walker* or *CROW* (**FIGURE 7-24**). This rigid clamshell device is custom-made to house a collapsed or collapsing foot, which needs PTB loading to reduce pressure on a delicate at-risk foot. When a patient is very heavy, additional support may be needed using a reinforced double upright AFO attached to a custom-molded shoe with a PTB upper attachment (**FIGURE 7-58**). Each of these orthoses is very expensive and should only be used when standard footwear choices have been eliminated.

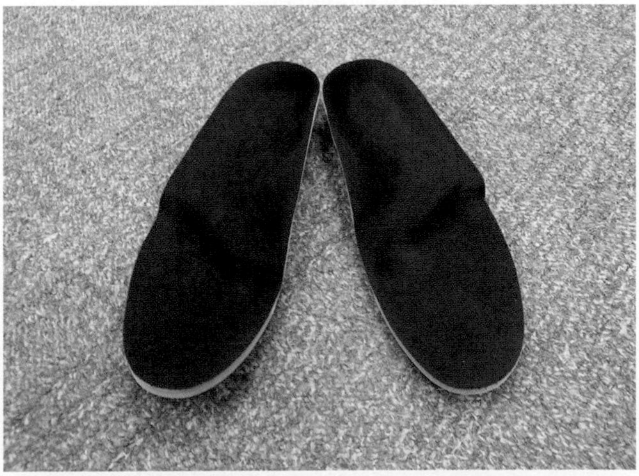

FIGURE 7-56 Diapedia insole with exaggerated metatarsal bar to off-load the metatarsal heads.

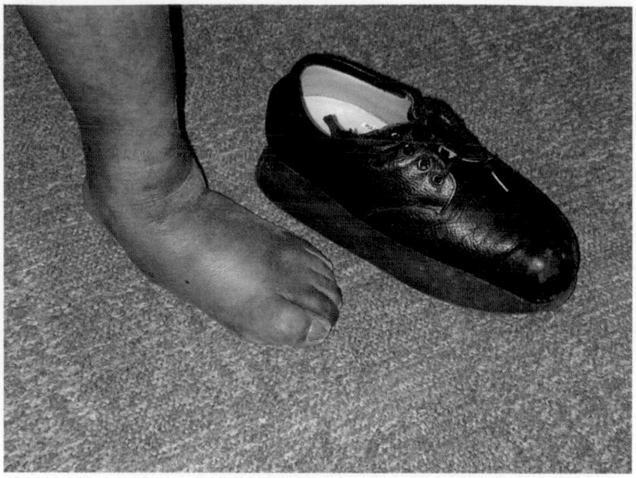

FIGURE 7-57 Custom-molded depth shoe with medial sole flare for extra control of a Charcot foot.

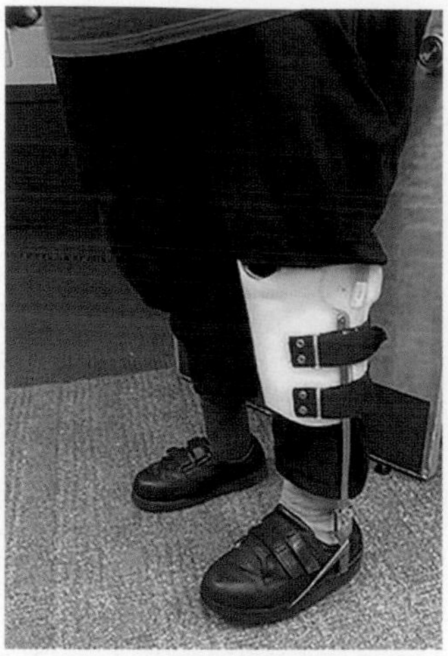

FIGURE 7-58 Reinforced double upright AFO with patellar tendon bearing upper attachment.

CASE STUDY

CONCLUSION

The vascular assessment includes trophic changes of the skin and nails, an absent pulse, and hair loss with a slightly delayed capillary filling time; these would necessitate a referral for noninvasive vascular testing that would consist of ankle-brachial indices, pulse volume recordings, and toe-brachial indices. This information would indicate whether the patient would be able to heal his wounds. An ABI of 0.7 would be required for healing in a reasonable period of time (12–16 weeks). Any limitation of blood flow to the limb would necessitate a referral to a vascular specialist to determine if revascularization surgery could improve his circulation and increase his chances of healing.

The evidence of fungal infection is typical of diabetic patients but apart from oral medications that have a slight risk of liver toxicity, there are no good topical medications available and care usually consists of regular podiatric visits for nail thinning and debridement.

The neurologic assessment indicates the presence of diabetic peripheral neuropathy, which significantly increases his risk for ulceration and complicates the healing process. Neuropathic patients are more likely to have problems with off-loading adherence because they cannot feel pain from their wound, thereby making it less likely that they will take the wound seriously.

The biomechanical assessment is the most useful part of the examination for prescribing off-loading devices, suggesting activity restrictions, and for predicting how the patient will respond to treatment. Based on our non-weight- and weight-bearing assessment, this patient ambulates on a significantly pronated foot with digital gripping making him prone to develop forefoot and digital ulcers. Equinus is a major contributing factor for elevated forefoot pressures, increased shear forces, and a transfer of forces to the midfoot, which if flexible will collapse with loading. This patient exhibits midtarsal joint hypermobility making him prone to this. Pronation also produces a shift of forces to the medial forefoot due to the abduction of the forefoot on the rearfoot and the anterior medial imbalance produced by the equinus and the inward collapse of the ankle during heel strike to midstance. Medial loading of the forefoot in this case leads to the development of a wound under the first metatarsal. This patient also has a limited range of motion of the first MPJ known as hallux limitus. As the forefoot loads and progresses from the midstance to the propulsive phase, a restriction at the first MPJ would lead to a transfer of force to the hallux interphalangeal joint or IPJ. If the force transferred is limited, a pinch callus will develop at the medial aspect of the IPJ. If these forces are excessive then an ulcer may develop at the IPJ, the most common site for a forefoot wound. This medial force transfer with pronation also leads to the development of hallux abductovalgus with a medial bunion in this patient. Assuming this patient is active and has a job that requires a lot of walking, he is much less likely to accept a restriction on activity from a wound he cannot even feel.

An open wound in this case necessitates the use of a nonremovable off-loading device, either a TCC or an iTCC. An ambulatory aid of crutches or a walker so he could remain non-weight-bearing would be best; however, at least a cane should be prescribed to slow his gait and reduce forces on the foot. If at all possible, the patient should be counseled to remain out of work for 4–6 weeks until he has demonstrated a desire to adhere to the recommendations *and* the wound has begun to heal (closed or almost fully epithelialized) sufficiently for him to transition to a removable type device. After 3 weeks in a removable walker, he could transition to a healing shoe or modified healing sandal while his final footwear is being prepared by a pedorthist. Under no circumstances should this patient return to his pre-ulcer footwear. That would be an invitation to reulcerate within a very short period of time.

SUMMARY

The person with diabetes is a challenging, often frustrating patient to treat. Each clinician must exhibit patience, persistence, and a commitment to "do the right thing."[83] It is human to fail to comply or cooperate and it is equally human to fatigue and give up in the face of difficulty. Healthcare providers cannot give up or let the fatigue of a prolonged healing course prevent them from focusing on the primary goal of a healed wound and the secondary goal of prevention of recurrence. The patient's limb and life depend on it.

STUDY QUESTIONS

1. Which of the following is one of the diagnosing criteria for diabetes?
   a. Fasting plasma glucose >140 mg/dL
   b. HbA1C of 6%
   c. 2-hour PG ≥140 mg/dL and <199 mg/dL
   d. Fasting plasma glucose ≥126 mg/dL
2. The measurement used to determine the patient's blood glucose control over a 2- to 3-month period of time is
   a. Creatinine.
   b. Fasting blood glucose levels.
   c. A1C.
   d. Oral glucose tolerance.
3. The primary goal of medical nutrition therapy in diabetes is
   a. To help the patient lose weight.
   b. To increase the amount of protein in the diet.
   c. To decrease the amount of carbohydrates and fats in the diet.
   d. To help the patient achieve optimal blood glucose levels.
4. The critical time for initiating standard care of a neuropathic wound in order to prevent infection is
   a. Within 4 weeks of the onset of the wound.
   b. After the patient first experiences pain.
   c. When the patient blood sugars are greater than 200 mg/dL.
   d. When the wound has progressed to full-thickness skin loss.
5. A patient is referred with a full-thickness wound that involves the subcutaneous tissue, but no exposed bone or tendon. Evaluation reveals severe hammer toes with fat pad migration and dropped metatarsal heads. The most appropriate off-loading device based on the Temple University classification system would be
   a. Custom orthotic inserts.
   b. Total-contact cast.
   c. Removable cast walker.
   d. Accommodative felt padding.
6. The center of axis of the foot is defined as
   a. The medial aspect of the midfoot.
   b. The midfoot from the metatarsal heads to the heel pad.
   c. The second metatarsal and the accompanying cuneiform.
   d. The line from the base of the great toe to the midfoot.
7. Which of the following mechanisms is primarily responsible for the fixation of deformities in the diabetic foot?
   a. Atrophy
   b. Loss of protective sensation
   c. Decreased muscle strength
   d. Glycosylation
8. Which of the following components is *not* considered part of the classic triad that causes a diabetic foot ulcer?
   a. Deformity
   b. Neuropathy
   c. Peripheral arterial disease
   d. Repetitive trauma

Answers: 1-d; 2-c; 3-d; 4-a; 5-b; 6-c; 7-d; 8-c

REFERENCES

1. Standards of Care in Diabetes—2023. *Diabetes Care*. 2023; 46(Supplement_1):S1-S4.
2. Garber AJ, Handelsman Y, Grunberger G, et al. Consensus statement by the American Association of Clinical Endocrinologists and American College of Endocrinology on the comprehensive type 2 diabetes management algorithm – 2020 executive summary. *Endocr Pract*. 2020;26(1):107-139.
3. *Economic Costs of Diabetes in the U.S.* https://www.cdc.gov/chronicdisease/programs-impact/pop/diabetes.htm. Accessed April 30, 2023.
4. International Diabetes Federation. *IDF Diabetes Atlas*. 10th ed. https://diabetesatlas.org/idfawp/resource-files/2021/07/IDF_Atlas_10th_Edition_2021.pdf.
5. Centers for Disease Control and Prevention. National Diabetes Statistics Report website. https://www.cdc.gov/diabetes/data/statistics-report/index.html. Accessed March 2023.
6. *The Cost of Diabetes*. https://diabetes.org/about-us/statistics/cost-diabetes. Accessed April 30, 2023.
7. Mulder G, Tenenhaus M, D'Souza GF. Reduction of diabetic foot ulcer healing times through use of advanced treatment modalities. *Int J Low Extrem Wounds*. 2014;13(4):335-346.
8. Swoboda L, Held J. Impaired wound healing in diabetes. *J Wound Care*. 2022;31(10):882-885.
9. Blakytny R, Jude E. The molecular biology of chronic wounds and delayed healing in diabetes. *Diabet Med*. 2006;23(6):594-608.
10. Burgess JL, Wyant WA, Abdo Abujamra B, Kirsner RS, Jozic I. Diabetic wound-healing science. *Medicina (Kaunas)*. 2021; 57(10):1072.
11. Rodríguez-Rodríguez N, Martínez-Jiménez I, García-Ojalvo A, et al. Wound chronicity, impaired immunity and infection in diabetic patients. *MEDICC Rev*. 2021;24(1):44-58.
12. Scarborough P. Diabetes and wound care. In: McCulloch JM, Kloth LC, eds. *Wound Healing: Evidence-Based Management*. 4th ed. Philadelphia, PA: FA Davis Company; 2010:231-247.
13. *Association of Diabetes Care and Education Specialists*. https://www.diabeteseducator.org/about-adces.
14. AADE. *AADE7™ self-care behaviors*. https://www.diabeteseducator.org/living-with-diabetes/aade7-self-care-behaviors. Accessed April 28, 2023.
15. Katsuhiro M, Teoh SH, Yamashiro H, et al. Effects on glycemic control in impaired wound healing in spontaneously diabetic torii (SDT) fatty rats. *Med Arch*. 2018;72(1):4-8.
16. Tsourdi E, Barthel A, Rietzsch H, et al. Current aspects in the pathophysiology and treatment of chronic wounds in diabetes mellitus. *Biomed Res Int*. 2013;2013:385641.
17. Pecoraro RE, Reiber GE, Burgess EM. Pathways to diabetic limb amputation: basis for prevention. *Diabetes Care*. 1990;13(5):513-521.
18. Frykberg RG, Attinger C, Smeets L, Koller A, Bal A, Kavarthapu V. Surgical strategies for prevention of amputation of the diabetic foot. *J Clin Orthop Trauma*. 2021;17:99-105.

19. Bus SA, Van Netten JJ, Hinchliffe RJ, et al. Standards for the development and methodology of the 2019 International Working Group on the diabetic foot guidelines. *Diabetes Metab Res Rev.* 2020;36(Suppl 1):e3267.
20. Sheehan P, Jones P, Caselli A, Giurini JM, Veves A. Percent change in wound area of diabetic foot ulcers over a 4-week period is a robust predictor of complete healing in a 12-week prospective trial. *Diabetes Care.* 2003;26(6):1879-1882.
21. Lavery LA, Armstrong DG, Wunderlich RP, Mohler MJ, Wendel CS, Lipsky BA. Risk factors for foot infections in individuals with diabetes. *Diabetes Care.* 2006;29(6):1288-1293.
22. Lin C, Liu J, Sun H. Risk factors for lower extremity amputation in patients with diabetic foot ulcers: a meta-analysis. *PLoS One.* 2020;15(9):e0239236.
23. Armstrong DG, Boulton AJM, Bus SA. Diabetic foot ulcers and their recurrence. *N Engl J Med.* 2017;376(24):2367-2375.
24. Reiber GE. Epidemiology of foot ulcers and amputations in the diabetic foot. In: Bowker JH, Pfeifer MA, eds. *The Diabetic Foot.* St Louis, MO: Mosby; 2001:13-32.
25. Armstrong DG, Wrobel J, Robbins JM. Guest editorial: are diabetes-related wounds and amputations worse than cancer? *Int Wound J.* 2007;4(4):286-287.
26. Frykberg RG, Banks J. Challenges in the treatment of chronic wounds. *Adv Wound Care (New Rochelle).* 2015;4(9):560-582.
27. Landsman A. Near infrared spectroscopy and predicting the likelihood of future wound healing. *Today's Wound Clinic.* 2018;12(1):12-14.
28. Leiva K, Trinidad A, Gonzalez I, et al. Development of a tissue oxygenation flow-based index towards discerning the healing status in diabetic foot ulcers. *Adv Wound Care (New Rochelle).* 2023. doi: 10.1089/wound.2022.0170. Epub ahead of print. PMID: 37060195.
29. Yates C, May K, Hale T, et al. Wound chronicity, inpatient care, and chronic kidney disease predispose to MRSA infection in diabetic foot ulcers. *Diabetes Care.* 2009;32(10):1907-1909.
30. Hicks CW, Selvarajah S, Mathioudakis N, et al. Burden of infected diabetic foot ulcers on hospital admissions and costs. *Ann Vasc Surg.* 2016;33:149-158.
31. Raghav A, Khan ZA, Labala RK, Ahmad J, Noor S, Mishra BK. Financial burden of diabetic foot ulcers to world: a progressive topic to discuss always. *Ther Adv Endocrinol Metab.* 2018;9(1):29-31.
32. Margolis DJ, Kantor J, Berlin JA. Healing of diabetic neuropathic foot ulcers receiving standard treatment. A meta-analysis. *Diabetes Care.* 1999;22(5):692-695.
33. American Diabetes Association. Economic Costs of Diabetes in the U.S. in 2017. *Diabetes Care.* 2018;41(5):917-928.
34. Ragnarson Tennvall G, Apelqvist J. Health-economic consequences of diabetic foot lesions. *Clin Infect Dis.* 2004;39(Suppl 2):S132-139.
35. Palumbo PJ, Melton LJ. Peripheral vascular disease and diabetes. In: Harris MI, Hamman RF, eds. *Diabetes in America: Data Compiled.* 1984.NIH publication No. 1-1468:1–21.
36. Whitney K. Compensatory effects of foot deformity: understanding the nature of foot deformity and imbalance. *Current Pedorthics.* 2011:14-18.
37. Root ML, Orien WP, Weed JH. *Clinical Biomechanics: Normal and Abnormal Function of the Foot.* Vol 2. Los Angeles, CA: Clinical Biomechanics Corp; 1977.
38. Danenberg HJ. Functional hallux limitus and its relationship to gait efficiency. *J Am Podiatr Med Assoc.* 1986;76(11):648-652.
39. Green DR, Ruch JA, McGlamry ED. Correction of equinus related forefoot deformities. *J Am Podiatry Assoc.* 1976;66(10):768-780.
40. Green DR, Whitney AK. Pseudoequinus. *J Am Podiatry Assoc.* 1982; 72(7):365-371.
41. Perry J. *Gait Analysis: Normal and Pathological Function.* Thorofare, NJ: SLACK; 1992.
42. Hicks JH. The mechanics of the foot. II. The plantar aponeurosis and the arch. *J Anat.* 1954;88(1):25-30.
43. Frykberg RG, Zgonis T, Armstrong DG, et al. Diabetic foot disorders. A clinical practice guideline (2006 revision). *J Foot Ankle Surg.* 2006;45(5 suppl):S1-S66.
44. Lavery L. The role of foot pressures in diabetic foot complications. *Podiatry Management.* 2002:80.
45. Kirby KA. *Foot and Lower Extremity Biomechanics: A Ten Year Collection of Precision Intricast Newsletters.* Payson, AZ: Precision Intricast; 1997.
46. Charcot J. Sur quelques arthropathies qui paraissent dependre d'une lesion du cerveau ou de la moelle epiniere. *Arch Physiol Norm Pathol.* 1868;1:161-178.
47. Armstrong DG, Lavery LA. Acute Charcot's arthropathy of the foot and ankle. *Phys Ther.* 1998;78(1):74-80.
48. Armstrong DG, Peters EJ. Charcot's arthropathy of the foot. *J Am Podiatr Med Assoc.* 2002;92(7):390-394.
49. Rosenbloom AL, Silverstein JH, Lezotte DC, et al. Limited joint mobility in childhood diabetes mellitus indicates increased risk for microvascular disease. *N Engl J Med.* 1981;305(4):191-194.
50. Shah KM, Clark BR, McGill JB, Mueller MJ. Upper extremity impairments, pain and disability in patients with diabetes mellitus. *Physiotherapy.* 2015;101(2):147-154.
51. Grgic A, Rosenbloom AL, Weber FT, et al. Joint contracture—common manifestation of childhood diabetes mellitus. *J Pediatr.* 1976;88(4 pt 1):584-588.
52. Wheeless. www.wheelessonline.com/ortho/anke_equinus_contracture_1. Accessed August 2, 2014.
53. Goss DA Jr, Long J, Carr A, Rockwell K, Cheney NA, Law TD Sr. Clinical implications of a one-hand versus two-hand technique in the silfverskiöld test for gastrocnemius equinus. *Cureus.* 2020;12(1):e6555.
54. Cooper ME. Importance of advanced glycation end products in diabetes-associated cardiovascular and renal disease. *AJH.* 2004;17:31S-38S.
55. Aoki Y, Yazaki K, Shirotori K, et al. Stiffening of connective tissue in elderly diabetic patients: relevance to diabetic nephropathy and oxidative stress. *Diabetologia.* 1993;36(1):79-83.
56. Batista F, Nery C, Pinzur M, et al. Achilles tendinopathy in diabetes mellitus. *Foot Ankle Int.* 2008;29(5):498-501.
57. Andreassen CS, Jakobsen J, Andersen H. Muscle weakness: a progressive late complication in diabetic distal symmetric polyneuropathy. *Diabetes.* 2006;55(3):806-812.
58. van Schie CH, Vermigli C, Carrington AL, Boulton A. Muscle weakness and foot deformities in diabetes: relationship to neuropathy and foot ulceration in Caucasian diabetic men. *Diabetes Care.* 2004;27(7):1668-1673.
59. Lippman HI, Perotto A, Ferrar R. The neuropathic foot of the diabetic. *Bull NY Acad Med.* 1976;52(10):1159-1178.
60. Bernstein RK. Physical signs of the intrinsic minus foot. *Diabetes Care.* 2003;26(6):1945-1946.
61. Falanga V. Wound healing and its impairment in the diabetic foot. *Lancet.* 2005;366(9498):1736-1743.
62. McGuire J. Pressure redistribution strategies for the diabetic or at-risk foot: part I. *Adv Skin Wound Care.* 2006;19(4):213-221.
63. McGuire J. Pressure redistribution strategies for the diabetic or at-risk foot: part II. *Adv Skin Wound Care.* 2006;19(5):270-277.

64. McGuire J. Transitional off-loading: an evidence-based approach to pressure redistribution in the diabetic foot. *Adv Skin Wound Care.* 2010;23(4):175-188.
65. Boulton AJ, Kirsner RS, Vileikyte L. Clinical practice. Neuropathic diabetic foot ulcers. *N Engl J Med.* 2004;351(1):4-55.
66. Lavery LA, Peters EJ, Armstrong DG. What are the most effective interventions in preventing diabetic foot ulcers? *Int Wound J.* 2008;5(3):425-433.
67. Hulshof CM, van Netten JJ, Pijnappels M, Bus SA. The role of foot-loading factors and their associations with ulcer development and ulcer healing in people with diabetes: a systematic review. *J Clin Med.* 2020;9(11):3591.
68. Armstrong DG, Peters EJ, Athanasiou KA, Lavery LA. Is there a critical level of plantar foot pressure to identify patients at risk for neuropathic foot ulceration? *J Foot Ankle Surg.* 1998;37(4):303-307.
69. Kästenbauer T, Sauseng S, Sokol G, Auinger M, Irsigler K. A prospective study of predictors for foot ulceration in type 2 diabetes. *J Am Podiatr Med Assoc.* 2001;91(7):343-350.
70. Kwon OY, Tuttle LJ, Johnson JE, Mueller MJ. Muscle imbalance and reduced ankle joint motion in people with hammer toe deformity. *Clin Biomech.* 2009;24(8):670-675.
71. Grant WP, Sullivan R, Sonenshine DE, et al. Electron microscopic investigation of the effects of diabetes mellitus on the Achilles tendon. *J Foot Ankle Surg.* 1997;36(4):272-278.
72. Orendurff MS, Rohr ES, Sangeorzan BJ, Weaver K, Czerniecki JM. An equinus deformity of the ankle accounts for only a small amount of the increased forefoot plantar pressure in patients with diabetes. *J Bone Joint Surg Br.* 2006;88(1):65-68.
73. Amin N, Doupis J. Diabetic foot disease: from the evaluation of the "foot at risk" to the novel diabetic ulcer treatment modalities. *World J Diabetes.* 2016;7(7):153-164.
74. Apelqvist J, Larsson J, Agardh CD. The influence of external precipitating factors and peripheral neuropathy on the development and outcome of diabetic foot ulcers. *J Diabetes Complications.* 1990;4(1):21-25.
75. Uccioli L, Faglia E, Monticone G, et al. Manufactured shoes in the prevention of diabetic foot ulcers. *Diabetes Care.* 1995;18(10): 1376-1378.
76. Osterberg L, Blaschke T. Adherence to medication. *N Engl J Med.* 2005;353(5):487-497.
77. Krasner DL. The interprofessional wound caring model. In: Krasner DL, Rodeheaver GT, Sibbald RG, eds. *Chronic Wound Care: A Clinical Sourcebook for Healthcare Professionals.* 4th ed. Wayne, PA: HMP Communications; 2007.
78. Sibbald RG, Williamson D, Orsted HL, et al. Preparing the wound bed-debridement, bacterial balance, and moisture balance. *Ostomy Wound Manage.* 2000;46(11):14-37.
79. Armstrong DG, Nguyen HC, Lavery LA, van Schie CH, Boulton AJ, Harkless LB. Off-loading the diabetic foot wound: a randomized clinical trial. *Diabetes Care.* 2001;24(6):1019-1022.
80. Messenger G, Masoetsa R, Hussain I. A narrative review of the benefits and risks of total contact casts in the management of diabetic foot ulcers. *J Am Coll Clin Wound Spec.* 2018;9(1-3): 19-23.
81. Apelqvist J, Bakker K, Van Houtum WH, Nabuurs-Franssen MH, Schaper NC, eds. *International Consensus on the Diabetic Foot.* Maastricht, The Netherlands: International Working Group on the Diabetic Foot; 1999.
82. Jones NJ, Harding K. 2015 International Working Group on the Diabetic Foot Guidance on the prevention and management of foot problems in diabetes. *Int Wound J.* 2015;12(4):373-374.
83. Fife CE, Carter MJ, Walker D. Why is it so hard to do the right thing in wound care? *Wound Repair Regen.* 2010;18(2):154-158.
84. Applewhite AJ. Following the evidence for total contact casting as first-line treatment of DFUs in the wound clinic. *Today's Wound Clinic.* 2016;10(10):12-16.
85. Nabuurs-Franssen MH, Sleegers R, Huijberts MS, et al. Total contact casting of the diabetic foot in daily practice: a prospective follow-up study. *Diabetes Care.* 2005;28:243-247.
86. Snyder RJ, Lanier KK. Off-loading difficult wounds and conditions in the diabetic patient. *Ostomy Wound Manage.* 2002;48(1):22-35.
87. Armstrong DG, Short B, Espensen EH, Abu-Rumman PL, Nixon BP, Boulton AJ. Technique for fabrication of an "instant total-contact cast" for treatment of neuropathic diabetic foot ulcers. *J Am Podiatr Med Assoc.* 2002;92(7):405-408.
88. Rader AJ, Barry TP. Football dressing for neuropathic forefoot ulcerations. *Wounds.* 2006;18(4):85-91.
89. Birke JA, Pavich MA, Patout CA Jr, Horswell R. Comparison of forefoot ulcer healing using alternative off-loading methods in patients with diabetes mellitus. *Adv Skin Wound Care.* 2002;15(5): 210-215.
90. Lazzarini PA, Jarl G, Gooday C, et al. Effectiveness of offloading interventions to heal foot ulcers in persons with diabetes: a systematic review. *Diabetes Metab Res Rev.* 2020;36(Suppl 1):e3275.
91. Knowles EA, Boulton AJ. Do people with diabetes wear their prescribed footwear? *Diabet Med.* 1996;13(12):1064-1068.
92. Armstrong DG, Lavery LA, Kimbriel HR, Nixon BP, Boulton AJ. Activity patterns of patients with diabetic foot ulceration: patients with active ulceration may not adhere to a standard pressure off-loading regimen. *Diabetes Care.* 2003;26(9):2595-2597.
93. Waaijman R, Keukenkamp R, de Haart M, Polomski WP, Nollet F, Bus SA. Adherence to wearing prescription custom-made footwear in patients with diabetes at high risk for plantar foot ulceration. *Diabetes Care.* 2013;36(6):1613-1618.
94. Armstrong DG, Boulton AJ. Pressure offloading and "advanced" wound healing: isn't it finally time for an arranged marriage? *Int J Low Extrem Wounds.* 2004;3(4):184-187.
95. Steed DL, Edington HD, Webster MW. Recurrence rate of diabetic neurotrophic foot ulcers healed using topical application of growth factors released from platelets. *Wound Repair Regen.* 1996;4(2):230-233.
96. Matricali GA, Deroo K, Dereymaeker G. Outcome and recurrence rate of diabetic foot ulcers treated by a total contact cast: short-term follow-up. *Foot Ankle Int.* 2003;24(9):680-684.
97. Raspovic KM, Wukick DK, Naiman DQ, et al. Effectiveness of viable cryopreserved placental membranes for management of diabetic foot ulcers in a real world setting. *Wound Repair Regen.* 2018;26(2):213-220.
98. Pacaccio DJ, Cazzell SM, Halperin GJ, et al. Human placental membrane as a wound cover for chronic diabetic foot ulcers: a prospective, postmarket, closure study. *J Wound Care.* 2018;27(suppl 7):S28–S37.
99. Guo X, Mu D, Gao F. Efficacy and safety of acellular dermal matrix in diabetic foot ulcer treatment: a systematic review and meta-analysis. *Int J Surg.* 2017;40:1-7.
100. Richmond NA, Vivas AC, Kirsner RS. Topical and biologic therapies for diabetic foot ulcers. *Med Clin N Am.* 2013;97(5):883-898.
101. Garwood CS, Steinberg JS, Kim PJ. Bioengineered alternative tissues in diabetic wound healing. *Clin Podiatr Med Surg.* 2015;32(1):121-133.
102. *Medicare Benefit Policy Manual.* Therapeutic Shoes for Individuals with Diabetes. https://www.cms.gov/search/cms?keys=Therapeutic+Shoe+Bill. Accessed May 3, 2023.

103. Stoker D. Understanding the diabetic therapeutic shoe program. *Podiatry Today*. 2005;18(10):28-32.
104. Robbins JM, Strauss G, Aron D, Long J, Kuba J, Kaplan Y. Mortality rates and diabetic foot ulcers: is it time to communicate mortality risk to patients with diabetic foot ulceration? *J Am Podiatr Med Assoc*. 2008;98:489-493.
105. Thorud JC, Plemmons B, Buckley CJ, Shibuya N, Jupiter DC. Mortality after nontraumatic major amputation among patients with diabetes and peripheral vascular disease: a systematic review. *J Foot Ankle Surg*. 2016;55(3):591-599.
106. Brand PW. The diabetic foot. In: Ellenberg M, Rifkin H, eds. *Diabetes Mellitus*. Garden City, NY: Medical Examination Publishing; 1983:829-849.
107. Cavanagh PR, Bus SA. Off-loading the diabetic foot for ulcer prevention and healing. *Plast Reconstr Surg*. 2011;127(suppl 1): 248S-2s56S.

CHAPTER EIGHT

Pediatric Wounds

Brian H. Odom, PT, PhD, CWS

CHAPTER OBJECTIVES

At the end of this chapter, the learner will be able to:

1. **Recognize the differences between pediatric and adult skin.**
2. **Identify factors affecting wound healing in neonates and the pediatric population.**
3. **Discuss common wound etiologies seen in the pediatric population.**
4. **Compare and contrast different interventions in pediatric wound care.**
5. **Apply the elements of best wound management in the pediatric population.**
6. **Utilize common skin assessment tools in evaluation of neonates and pediatric patients.**

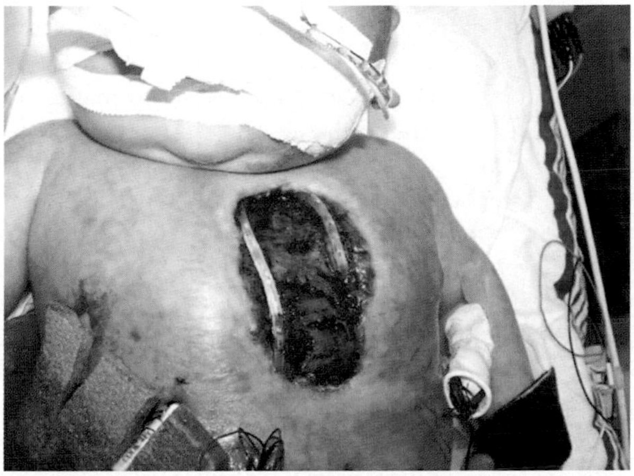

FIGURE 8-1 The complexity of treating pediatric patients is exemplified in this 3-month-old who has wounds as a result of tissue erosion from drains and pacing wires placed after a heart transplant.

INTRODUCTION

Children suffering from wounds cannot be treated as small adults. By following this flawed approach, the clinician does not fully understand the complexity and vulnerability of treating wounds in the pediatric population nor apply that knowledge to select appropriate interventions. Treatment can be daunting and clinicians may be apprehensive about treating this population due to the lack of established treatment guidelines, the paucity of available research, and an unfamiliarity with what makes pediatric skin different from adult skin. Another compounding factor is that treatment of pediatric wounds is often based on institutional preference and routine.[1] A lack of evidence-based treatment guidelines is further complicated by the fact that clinicians are apprehensive about implementing research on such a vulnerable population (**FIGURE 8-1**).

Pediatric wounds are treated successfully when the clinician conducts a thorough assessment, provides individualistic care, reviews the components of wound products, and uses a comprehensive team approach to address the child's needs. Consideration of all these factors is paramount for optimal outcomes while acknowledging that the principles of wound healing for children are comparable to adult wound healing (**FIGURE 8-2**).

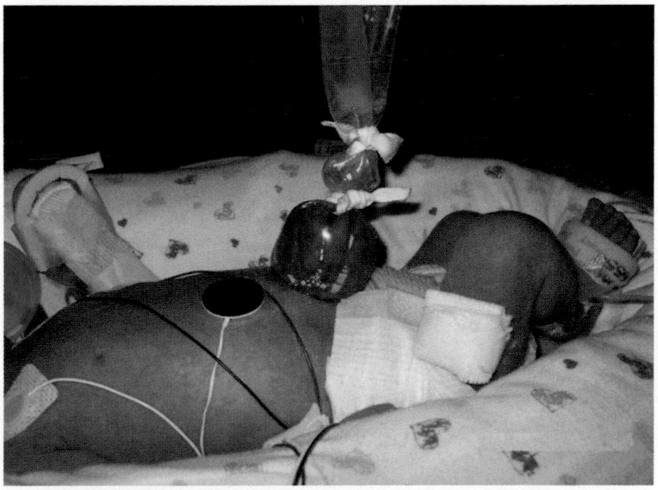

FIGURE 8-2 Gastroschisis is a rare birth defect in which a hole in the abdominal wall occurs next to the belly button allowing the intestines to herniate. A silicone pouch is used to enclose the herniated bowel which slowly returns the contents back into the abdomen. A surgeon will perform an abdominal wall repair for closure.

STAGES OF SKIN DEVELOPMENT

The developmental stages of skin are based on the age of the patient and include gestational development, neonatal and infant development, prepubescent development, and finally changes that occur during puberty (**TABLE 8-1**).

Gestational Development

The terminology used to describe the development of pediatric skin relative to age provides an important context about the developmental stage of the skin. *Infancy* refers to the first year of life.[2] During the first 28 days after birth, an infant is termed a *neonate.*[2] If born prior to 37 weeks, the infant is referred to as *preterm, premature*, or a "*premie*."[2] The development of the skin begins about week 4 of gestation with the formation of two distinct layers—the stratum basale and the stratum corneum. The first layer formed is the *basal layer* which is then covered by an outer layer called the periderm.[3] Keratinization, which is the process of skin cells differentiating and hardening to form a protective layer, begins around week 9 with stratification being apparent around the 13th week.[3] In weeks 14–20, hair follicles begin to form along with the development of sweat glands, and subsequent formation of epidermal buds in the basal layer.[3] At 24 weeks of gestation, a significant stage occurs with the formation of the *stratum corneum* and attached rete ridges.[4] Prior to the 24th week, fetal skin is characteristically able to heal without scar formation.[5] This unique characteristic remains a fervent research topic that has yet to be understood and is continually being investigated because there are currently no reliable treatments to prevent scar formation.

As development continues past the 24th week, fetal skin moves into a transitional phase and scar formation is evident; thus, the capacity for scarless wound healing is lost in the last trimester of pregnancy.[3] Starting about the 26th week and progressing through the 29th week, subcutaneous fat deposits begin to form and skin wrinkling decreases.[4] During this period, the barrier function of the skin remains poor and water loss is at a heightened risk.[4] During weeks 30–34, subcutaneous tissue becomes evident and the outer stratum corneum may contain two to three cell layers.[6]

At 33–34 weeks, epidermal maturation is considered complete.[4,7] At week 34, four layers are typically present (basal, spinous, granular, and stratum corneum) with each layer being well delineated.[8] This milestone is characterized by mature keratinocytes being present and strengthening of the dermal/epidermal junction.[4] The fetal skin progresses toward maturity but continues to be fragile and highly susceptible to damage. By week 36, which is considered full term, the skin is structurally similar to adult skin; however, it may be only 60% as thick as adult skin in the epidermal and dermal layers.[4,9] While some authors have reported that full-term neonates have a normal, well-developed thickness at the epidermal and dermal layers as compared to adults, it has also been reported that infant epidermis is thinner in relation to adult skin.[10,11]

Understanding that neonatal and infant skin is undergoing a maturing physiological process is crucial for clinicians working in neonatal practice, particularly with preterm infants or in neonatal intensive care units.

Neonatal Development

The barrier development of skin with epidermal maturation is generally accepted as occurring around the 34th week of gestation. Characteristics of the skin include mature keratinocytes which are flattened and appear to have adult-type dermoepidermal undulations.[12,13] The mature stratum corneum, which provides the barrier function of skin, typically contains between 10 and 20 layers; however, an infant's stratum

TABLE 8-1 Pediatric Skin Development

Stages	Time Frame	Key Progression
Gestational	0 to 34–36 weeks	Two distinct layers at 4th week Apparent layers at 13th week Sweat glands and hair follicles develop 14th through 20th week Scarless healing lost at 24th week Subcutaneous fat deposited at 26th week
Neonatal	34–36 weeks to birth	Vernix caseosa forming Epidermal maturity at 34th week
Infant	Birth to 3 years	Basal and corneum layers thickening Healing ability improving Melanin density increasing
Prepubescent	3 years to between 8 and 14 years (females average 11 y/o) (males average 12 y/o)	Thickening of epidermal and dermal layers Increasing collagen density
Pubescent	11–12 y/o to 19–20 y/o	Increase in hormonal influence Thickening of subcutaneous fat layer in females Thinning of epidermal and dermal layers in males Maturation of skin

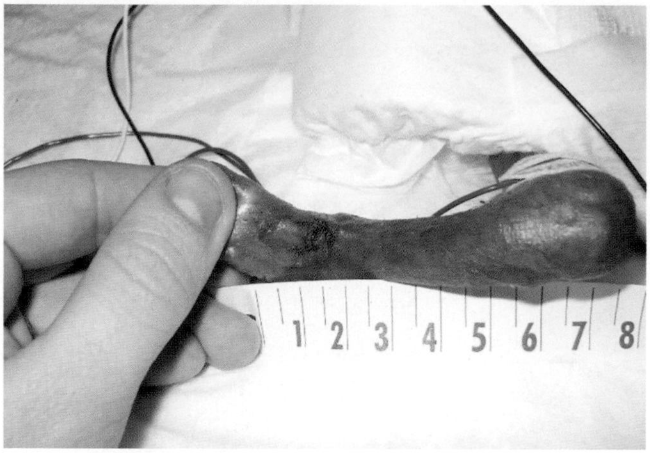

FIGURE 8-3 The fragility of neonate skin is evident in this IV infiltrate on the left dorsal ankle of a 27-week-old neonate.

corneum can be 30–40% thinner than adult skin through the first year of life (FIGURE 8-3).

During the last trimester of gestation, human fetuses form a unique skin covering called vernix caseosa (VC). This protective coat is secreted by the sebaceous glands and is composed primarily of 80% water and 20% lipids.[14] The VC also contains lysozymes, lactoferrin, linoleic acid, and other components which are anti-infective.[15,16] The VC protects the fetus from amniotic fluid maceration while in utero, contributes to epidermal cornification and stratum corneum formation, and is important for the development of a newborn's acid mantle.[15] The acid mantle is the protective layer that inhibits the growth of pathogenic microorganisms and provides immunological protection to a newborn's skin.[17] Newborn skin has a pH of about 6.0 during the first 15 days of life, then drops to more adult-like levels (pH 5.5) at 5–6 weeks of age.[18]

Infant Development

During the first 1–3 years of life, the infant's skin is competent, but lacks structural maturity, for example, the basal layer is approximately 20% thinner than adult skin.[19] The stratum corneum in infants, which contains the same number of layers as adults (10–20), is approximately 30–40% thinner than adults, contributing to an increased risk of transepidermal water loss and microbial invasion.[19,20] The development of the anchoring system and increased dermal adhesion between the epidermis and dermis also continues to mature. During development of infant skin, the number of attachments and anchoring filaments between the dermis and the basement membrane increases. This phase of skin growth is characterized by an increased ability to restore itself as a barrier as compared to adults.[14] Along with improved cohesion, the microvascular network of infant skin is developing but not yet mature. The capillary plexus is not well organized in the infant phase and has poor capacity to stretch and accept changes. This places infants at an increased risk for breakdown and loss of skin integrity. Melanin density is also increasing which protects epidermal cells from ultraviolet light damage (FIGURE 8-4).[14]

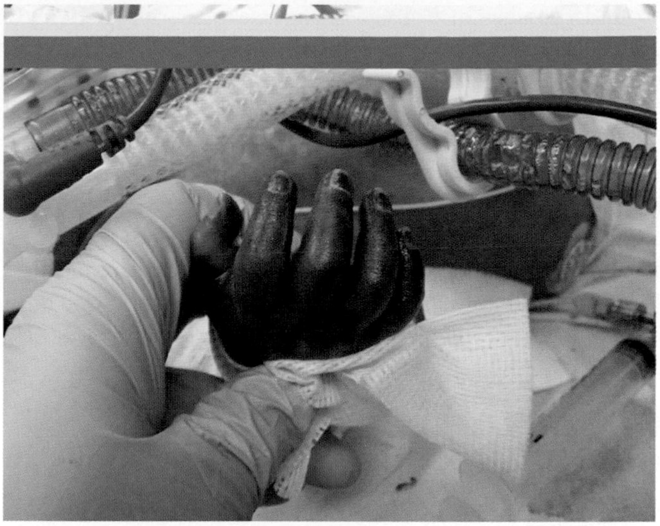

FIGURE 8-4 Microvascular damage in the fingers of a 6-month-old due to clotting that occurred after the placement of an ECMO (Extracorporeal Membrane Oxygenation) machine. Topical nitroglycerin paste and keeping the extremity warm were used to reduce ischemia and necrosis.

The development of an infant's skin after birth can be influenced by exposure to environmental microbes that occurs at or during the birthing process. The type of birth, whether it be vaginal or cesarean section, must be considered because infants delivered vaginally may have different skin characteristics or changes as compared to infants born via cesarean section. A neonate born vaginally is exposed to the mother's vaginal and intestinal microflora that results in improved resistance to commensal bacteria.[21–23] Infants born by cesarean section are only exposed to environmental microbes. Based on epidemiological data, infants born via cesarean section are prone to increased skin infections and lack healthy microbial colonization on their skin. Infants born by cesarean section may take up to 6 months to be colonized by commensal bacteria which places them at an increased risk for skin infection, microbial invasion, delayed immune development, and a host of other conditions.[19,24–29]

Prepubescent Development

During this next developmental stage, which can be described as largely uneventful, skin maturation is observed near or around the age of 3 years and continues progressing through the prepubescent years or until puberty is reached. During this period, the epidermal and dermal layers thicken and collagen density increases,[30] and males develop thicker epidermal and dermal layers as compared to females.[30]

Pubescent Development

This last phase of skin development is hallmarked by the child reaching and progressing through puberty. The phase begins around the ages of 9–13, with females generally arriving at puberty earlier than males. During this phase, hormonal influences on males and females play a key role in skin changes and alteration. In females, a thicker layer of subcutaneous fat is formed, whereas in males, this formation is not seen.[30] In males, a thinning of the epidermal and dermal layers occurs; however, in females, the epidermal and dermal layers remain a consistent thickness throughout their lives until menopause is reached.[30] After completion of puberty, skin is considered to be normal or adult-like and starts showing signs of a linear decrease in skin collagen content as ageing occurs.[30]

FACTORS AFFECTING WOUND HEALING IN CHILDREN

Children may struggle to heal a wound just as adults do; however, pediatric patients have unique challenges that can alter wound healing. While it is known that factors such as nutrition, medications, immunosuppression, and chronic disease have an impact on healing for all wound patients, pediatric patients have the following additional factors which can significantly alter healing rates: decreased skin thickness, transepidermal water loss (TEWL), altered skin pH, underdeveloped circulatory plexus, and increased physiological stress.

Decreased skin thickness is a challenge for wound healing in the premature, neonate, and infant population. The skin barrier function is disadvantaged and contributes to multiple other problems including risk for epidermal stripping, *TEWL* with resultant heat loss, and toxicity from percutaneous absorption. TEWL is water that passively evaporates through the skin leaving it dry, irritated, and at risk for further breakdown, and it is a special concern when treating the *premie* or neonate population. This passive water loss is a danger to premature infants because of the high risk of dehydration.[31–33]

An *immature circulatory skin plexus* can also affect an infant's wound-healing capacity. Because the underlying plexus is under-developed, neonates and infants are at risk for extravasation injuries due to a fragile capillary system, small caliper peripheral veins, immature skin structures, and lack of subcutaneous tissue.[34,35] Therefore, the placement and monitoring of peripheral intravenous lines is crucial (**FIGURE 8-5**).

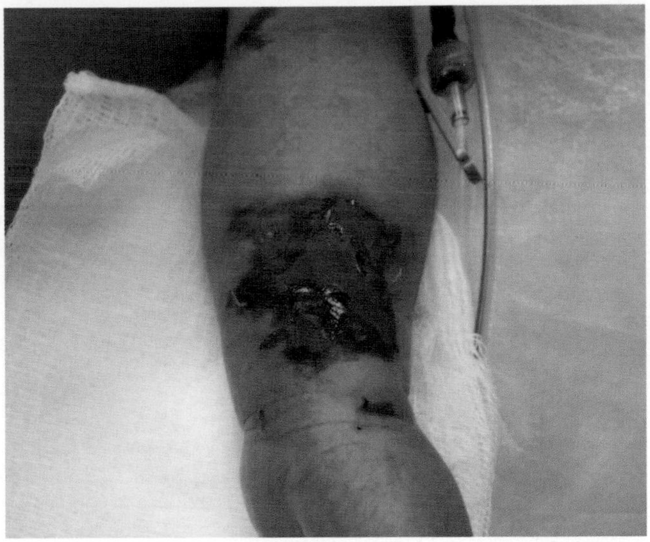

FIGURE 8-5 The wrist is a common site for extravasation injuries in infants. Severity of the injury is related to the type of drug being infused, exposure time of the vesicant fluid, and mechanical damage caused from the pressure within the tissue.

Altered skin pH is another challenge a pediatric patient may face. At birth, a newborn's skin pH is more basic with a pH of 6.0. Fully mature skin has a pH range between 4.5 and 6.0, which provides the barrier protection characteristic of an acid mantle, with ideal pH values between the range of 5.0 and 5.5.[18,36,37] Neonatal skin has a higher pH compared to older pediatric and adult patients, regardless of gestational age, sex, mode of birth delivery, or body weight.[38] This thin mantle is formed from the combination of lipids and amino acids that are secreted by oil and sweat glands and is important for assisting with retaining moisture and reducing the risk of bacterial infection. As previously mentioned, skin acidity is an important mechanism for skin defense against infection and assists with the establishment of healthy skin flora, skin barrier maturation, and normalizing skin surface lipids.[36]

Lastly, the challenge of *increased physiological stress* may alter skin function. Whether it be isolated or in combination, the stress of birthing, fighting infection, physiological instability, and/or potential pathology, in addition to all the factors previously mentioned in this section, can contribute to compromised skin function in a pediatric patient. Physiological stress of an infant, neonate, or *premie* is beyond the scope of this chapter, but should be considered when discussing pediatric skin dysfunction.

CASE STUDY

INTRODUCTION

A 10-year-old black male was referred for wound care for multiple ischemic wounds on the hands and feet with a diagnosis of polyarteritis nodosa (PAN), an autoimmune disorder of unknown etiology that causes severe inflammation of the small and medium arteries with necrosis distal to the areas of inflammation (**FIGURES 8-6 through 8-9**). The patient also had the following complaints that are common with PAN:

CASE STUDY *(Continued)*

- Severe muscle pain
- Peripheral neuropathy, worse in the feet than in the hands
- Hematuria, renal hypertension, and swollen kidneys
- Acute abdominal pain and diarrhea

The patient arrived for treatment in a wheelchair, accompanied by his mother. Ambulation was limited by the severe pain in both feet with weight-bearing, and upper extremity activities were limited by the wounds on his hands.

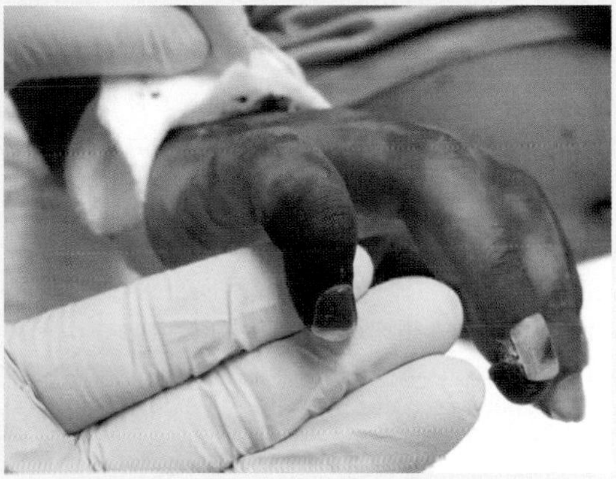

FIGURE 8-6 Right distal fifth finger.

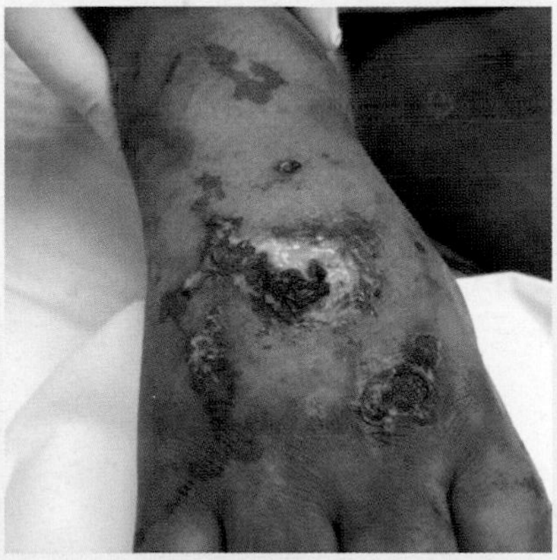

FIGURE 8-7 Right dorsal hand.

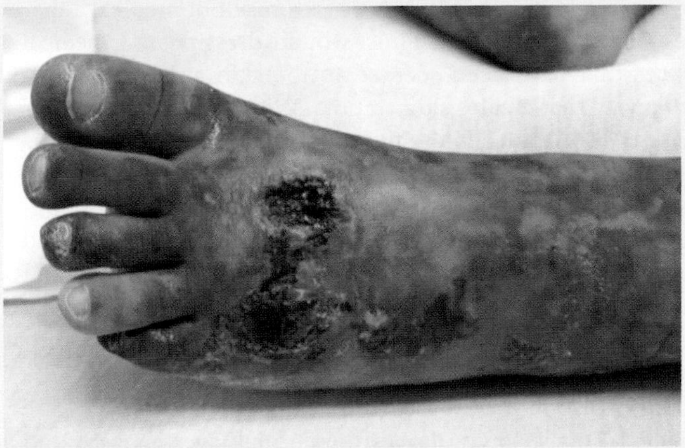

FIGURE 8-8 Left dorsal foot.

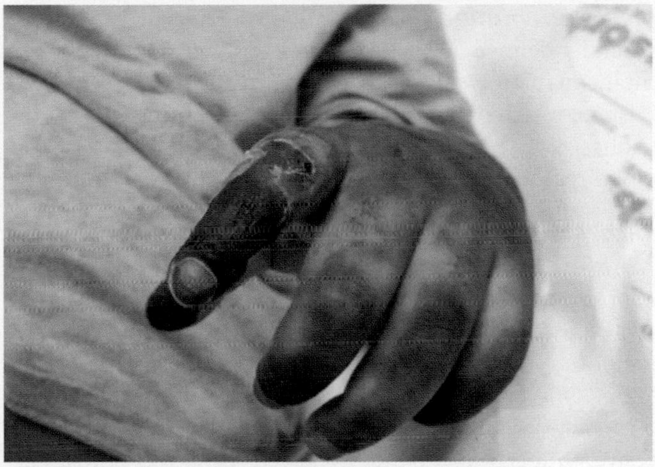

FIGURE 8-9 Left hand.

STUDY QUESTIONS

1. What are some of the special concerns when treating a pediatric patient with these wounds?
2. How can these concerns be addressed in both the development of a care plan and the treatment of the patient?
3. What other professionals might be helpful in treating this patient?

COMMON PEDIATRIC WOUND ETIOLOGIES

The common wound etiologies for pediatric patients that are discussed in this chapter include epidermal stripping, pressure injuries (PIs), extravasation injuries, surgical site wounds, thermal and chemical injuries, dermatitis associated with incontinence, and congenital defects. Along with discussion of each etiology, best practices for treatment and management, along with potential product recommendations, are provided. The most common vasculitic disorders that occur in children are included in Table 9-7.

Epidermal Stripping

Pathophysiology Epidermal stripping or medical adhesive-related skin injury (MARSI) is often a result of medical adhesives such as tapes, clear films, wound dressings, or medical devices that have been secured to the skin and removed in such a way that creates skin trauma. When adhesive products are removed, the fragile epidermis with fewer cell layers is stripped away thereby causing loss of the stratum corneum or epidermis. Trauma occurs very easily in the pediatric population because the bond between the adhesive dressing and the skin is stronger than the bond between the epidermal and dermal layers.[39] Epidermal stripping, due to adhesive and tape removal in neonates born before 27 weeks, is the most common form of skin breakdown.[4] Epidermal stripping is also the primary reason for skin breakdown in neonatal intensive care units.[40,41] This stripping leaves the dermal layer exposed and places the neonate and pediatric population at further risk for TEWL and absorption toxicity from topical substances (**FIGURE 8-10**).

Clinical Presentation Manifestation of epidermal stripping is generally defined as erythema and/or other manifestations of cutaneous abnormality which may include erosion, tearing, or blisters, which persist 30 minutes or more after removal of the adhesive.[42] The site of stripping is commonly only in the area of direct contact with the medical adhesive (**FIGURE 8-11**).

Medical Management The incidence of epidermal stripping or MARSI can be reduced by staff education and by the use of appropriate skin and wound products. Clinicians treating neonates and pediatric patients with fragile skin need to be aware of the high risk of potential injury. Adhesives and tape may not only cause stripping, but may also cause skin tears and contact dermatitis. Dressings or tape that contain strong adhesive properties are best removed with the horizontal stretch method or what is sometimes called "low and slow."[43]

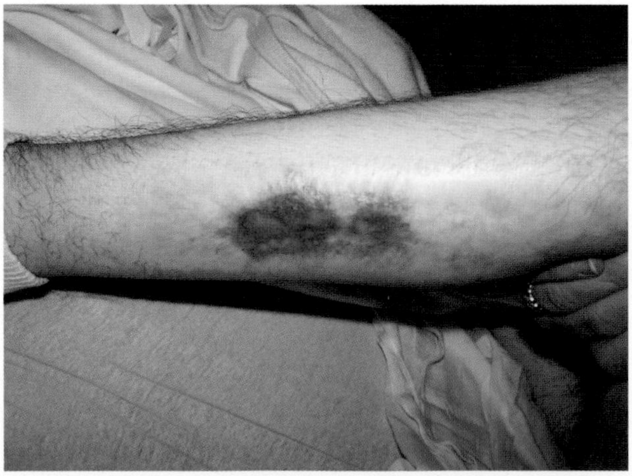

FIGURE 8-10 Epidermal stripping occurred with the improper removal of an adherent dressing in a 15-year-old male with a history of skin breakdown on the left lateral leg. Use of a skin prep may reduce damage caused by adherent dressings.

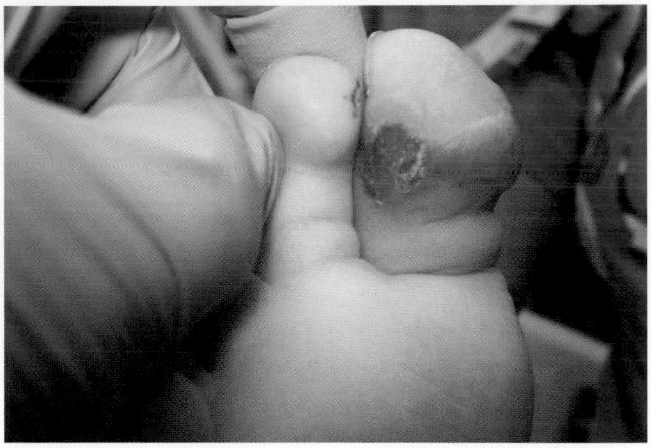

FIGURE 8-11 A MARSI (medical adhesive-related skin injury) may cause tension blisters due to improper removal of medical adhesives, tapes, or dressings.

This technique, along with stabilizing the skin, minimizes the force needed to remove a tape or dressing and reduces the incidence of a MARSI. Further incidence of skin stripping can be reduced by the use of nonalcoholic barrier sprays or liquid barrier films. However, these protective films or barrier sprays can be an irritant and the removal requires the use of a solvent which may further irritate the skin.[44] The avoidance of tape for splint securement is recommended; Velcro-padded support straps can be used instead.[45–47] If intravenous sites are secured with clear film dressings, some form of a barrier film applied to the skin is advised to reduce epidermal stripping (**FIGURES 8-12** and **8-13** illustrate the improper and safe way to remove tape).

Wound Management Recommendations for treatment of epidermal stripping or MARSI include the use of soft silicone-backed products or foam dressings which are gentle on

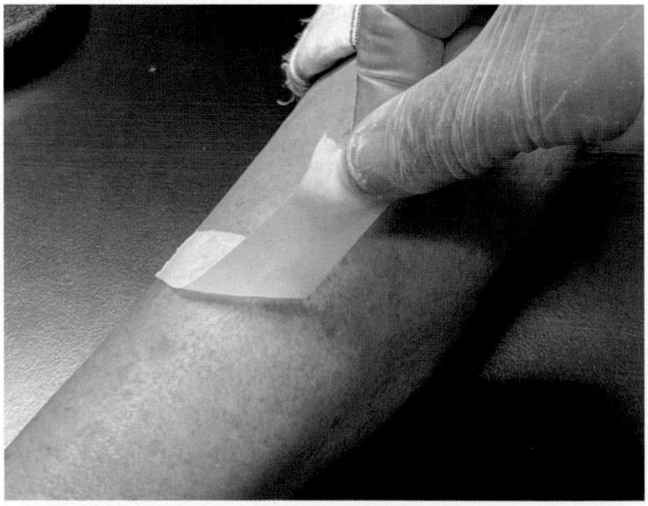

FIGURE 8-12 The improper technique of adhesive or tape removal. The clinician is pulling straight up at an angle and is not supporting the skin. This improper technique may tear or cause epidermal stripping of fragile skin.

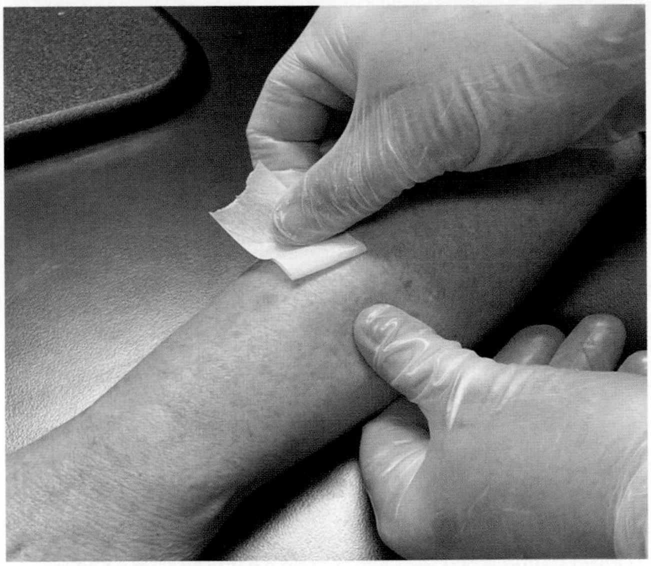

FIGURE 8-13 The "low and slow" method of adhesive or tape removal is the preferred technique for all dressing removal but is especially so for fragile or pediatric skin. The clinician supports the skin where the tape has been removed and pulls the tape slowly and back over itself in the direction of hair growth or pulls with the tape held parallel to the skin.

the skin and reduce discomfort and trauma. However, silicone dressings perform best on dry skin and their use on neonates in an incubator may present a challenge for clinicians because incubators have an environment of increased relative humidity. Hydrocolloid dressings can be used as well, but atraumatic removal of such dressings must be facilitated due to their high adhesive content. Lastly, reducing the frequency of removal and reapplication of dressings at the injured site are advised.

Pressure Injuries

Pathophysiology A PI is defined by the National Pressure Injury Advisory Panel (NPIAP) as localized damage to the skin and underlying soft tissue usually over a bony prominence or related to a medical or other device.[48] The incidence of PIs in pediatric patients in the intensive and neonatal intensive care units is as high as 27%.[49,50] Research has historically focused on adults and then extrapolated findings and subsequent care down to the pediatric population.[49,51–56] This is concerning for the following two reasons: (1) pediatric patients are more susceptible to PIs than adults because of skin development and (2) pediatric skin is immature and thus more vulnerable than adult skin.[55] The pediatric population has thinner immature skin, increased body fat allowing for increased skin deformation, and decreased muscle thickness which leads to an increase in PIs.[4,54] These characteristics, combined with medical complexity and the inability of the patient to communicate, can effectively accelerate the risk of PIs in the pediatric and neonate population (**FIGURES 8-14** through **8-16**).

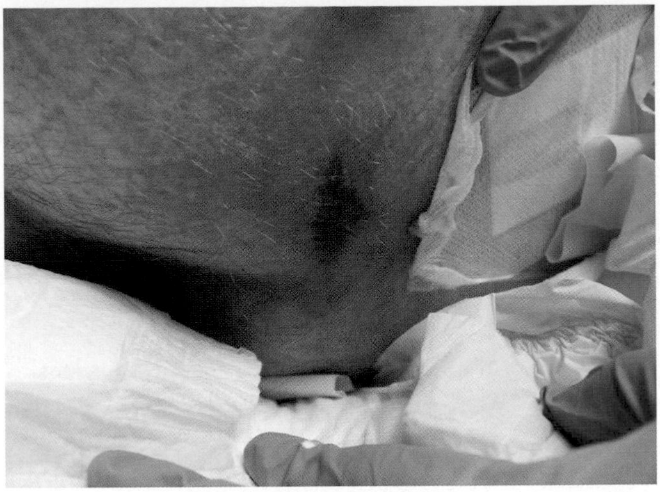

FIGURE 8-14 A deep tissue pressure injury caused by improper positioning and inadequate pressure relief. Without proper monitoring, a pressure injury can occur on the sacrum of pediatric patients who lack the ability to reposition independently.

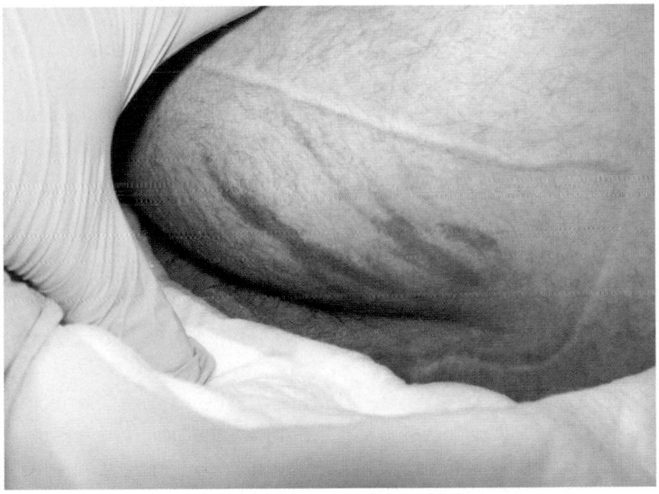

FIGURE 8-15 This pediatric patient suffered stage 1 and deep tissue injuries on the buttocks and sacrum due to sheets that were not straightened under the patient. Monitoring by caregivers and parents about sheets that are "bunching" or "rolling up" under pediatric patients is critical for prevention of these PIs.

Clinical Presentation The recommended staging of pediatric PIs was set forth by the NPIAP. (Refer to Chapter 6, Pressure Injuries and Ulcers.)

Medical Management Strategies to reduce the risk of PIs include using an age-appropriate, valid, and reliable PI assessment scale; frequent assessment; and pressure redistribution by implementing turning schedules. Pediatric and neonate patients in the intensive care units are at higher risk for developing a PI from medical devices and equipment.[50] Therefore, frequent assessment of areas beneath nasal and oxygen tubing, gastric tubing, blood pressure cuffs, tracheostomy plates,

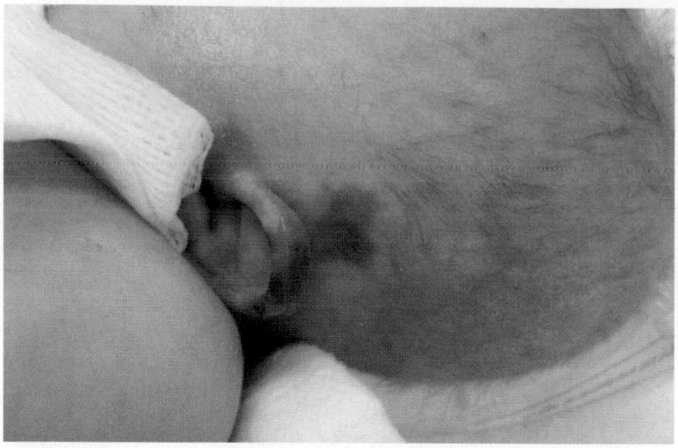

FIGURE 8-16 Pediatric patients are often at increased risk for pressure injuries on the occiput. Acute care patients need to be repositioned frequently in the pediatric intensive care.

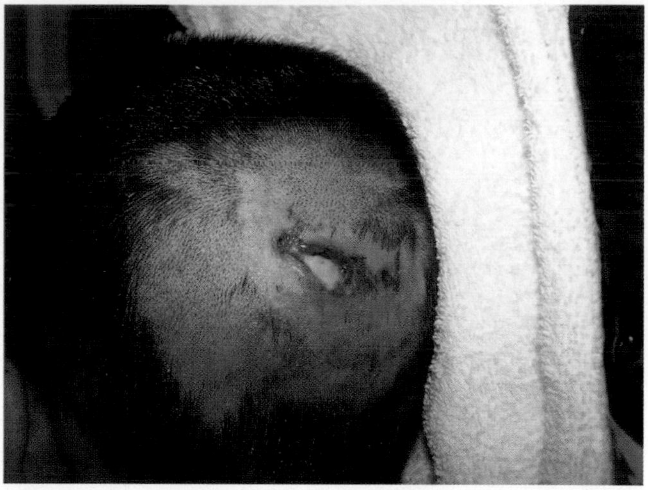

FIGURE 8-17 A stage IV full-thickness injury occurred on the occipital region while the child was on a ventilator with spine trauma. Children are often at greater risk for occiput pressure injuries due to disproportionate head size in relation to the rest of the body.

CLINICAL CONSIDERATION

In pediatric care, younger children are at greater risk for occipital PIs due to larger surface area and disproportionate weight of the head as compared to adults in whom breakdown is often seen on the heels and sacrum. Other areas of frequent breakdown in children include the nose and ears due to the lack of fat on the cartilaginous areas of the face (**FIGURES 8-17** and **8-18**).

CLINICAL CONSIDERATION

Pressure redistribution in cribs, incubators, and beds is critical; however, note that some specialty hospital beds that perform pressure redistribution often have a required minimum patient weight to be effective for turning and pressure redistribution. Extra padding or gel positioners may need to be added to incubators or cribs in the neonatal population.

IV sites, catheter straps, sites with arm boards, and respiratory devices is needed.

Wound Management Initial treatment of PIs focuses on (1) identifying the source or sources causing the PI and (2) removing or redistributing pressure. The principles of standard wound care are applied in the pediatric population, including cleansing, debridement of nonviable tissue, moist wound care, and infection management. Wound dressing recommendations include products that provide protective padding and pressure redistribution (for example foam dressings, composite foam dressings with silicone borders, hydrocolloids, or silicone sheets).

Extravasation Injuries

Pathophysiology Peripheral infiltration is defined as an inadvertent delivery of nonvesicant or nonirritating fluid into the surrounding tissue with the potential to harm or injure the skin of a pediatric patient.[57] The leakage of vesicant or irritating fluid into the tissue space is termed extravasation.[58] The vesicant fluids can be composed of, but not limited to, calcium, potassium, parenteral nutrition, and a wide variety of other substances.[59,60] Besides the substances themselves, other factors that contribute to the severity of the infiltration are the following: osmolarity of the infused agent, duration of the exposure, pH of the vesicant, chemical irritation, and the mechanical pressure caused by the fluid that has leaked into the tissue.[61] As previously noted, the pediatric population is at the greatest risk for extravasation injuries due to decreased cell-layer thickness, a fragile dermal vascular system, decreased vessel diameter, decreased adhesion between the dermis and epidermis, and highly flexible and distensible subcutaneous tissue.[62] In neonates less than 26 weeks, extravasation injuries occur more frequently due to the fragility and small caliber of the peripheral veins.[34] Reported injury rates are wide-ranging and highly variable and have been reported between 10% and 58%.[60,63] Injury rates have been reported specifically in the neonatal population ranging from 0.1% to 15% and up to reported ranges of 55–70%.[63–66]

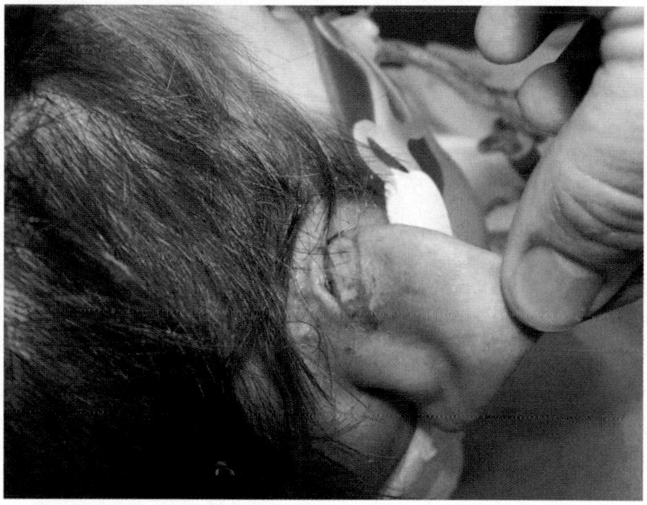

FIGURE 8-18 A device-related pressure injury on the ear caused by oxygen tubing prior to intubation.

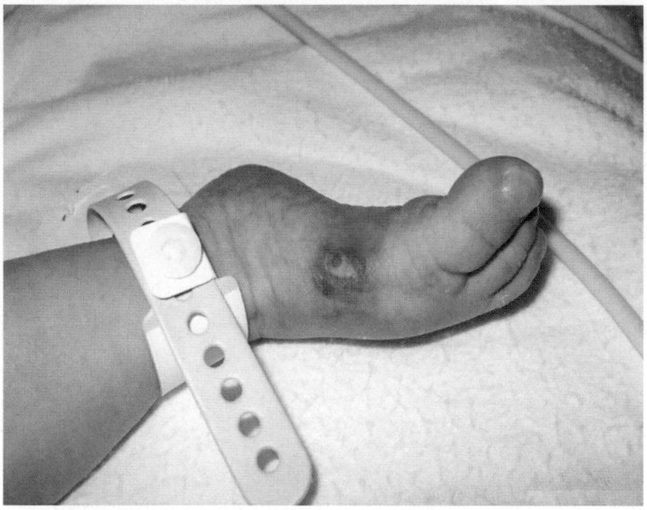

FIGURE 8-19 An extravasation injury on the foot of a 3-month-old infant. Peripheral IVs should be covered with a film dressing so the site can be monitored visually for signs of swelling and redness.

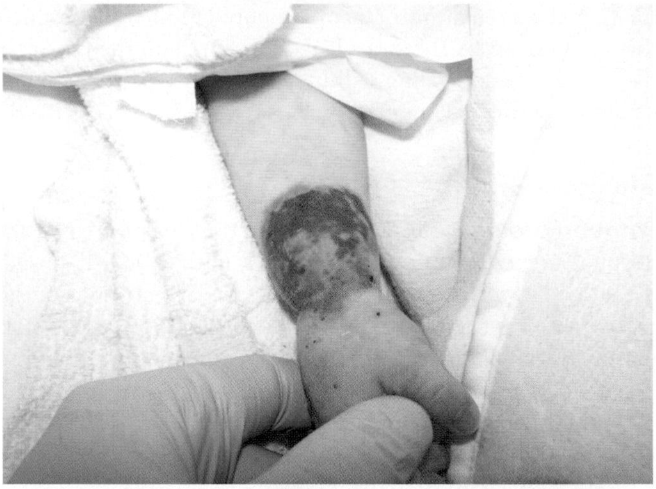

FIGURE 8-20 An extravasation injury of the right wrist of a 2-month-old. Treatment of pediatric extravasation injuries should include immediate removal of the IV and elevation of the site. Treatment protocols for pediatric extravasation injuries may vary from facility to facility.

Clinical Presentation The resulting extravasation injury may include redness, blistering of the skin, necrosis, visible pocketing of the vesicant in subcutaneous tissue, pain, infection, and in extreme cases may cause compartment syndrome (**FIGURE 8-19**).

Medical Management Evidence is lacking for appropriate treatment of extravasation injuries in neonates.[67] Treatment protocols for IV extravasation injuries should be followed based on the hospital or facility guidelines, as well as the scope of practice of the clinician treating the site. A staging scale such as the Pediatric PIV scale to evaluate the degree of damage may serve as a guideline for development of a care plan.[57] Treatment of extravasation injuries needs to be immediate in order to limit exposure to the vesicant and to reduce the possibility of necrosis. If extravasation injury causes a serious tissue defect or extensive full-thickness tissue loss injury, plastic surgery, or dermatology services are advised (**FIGURE 8-20**).

Treatment protocols include the following nonpharmacological strategies: elevation of the injury site to aid in venous return; creation of multiple puncture holes around the site using a sterile procedure in order to alleviate pressure and swelling which thus aids in removing the vesicant fluid from the site; irrigation of the site with saline through incisions made in the skin in order to drain the toxins.[68–70]

Some pharmacological interventions include the use of hyaluronidase or phentolamine. The concentrations and therapeutic dosing of these pharmacological agents may vary by facility and are largely dependent on the size, weight, and extent of injury to the pediatric patient. Hyaluronidase, a common treatment agent used to reduce inflammation and diffuse toxic fluids, is administrated subcutaneously around the peripheral borders of the injured site.[71–73] Phentolamine, also administered subcutaneously around the periphery of the injured site, is often used when the vesicant fluid is either dopamine or norepinephrine.[61] Phentolamine can also be used subcutaneously in combination with a topical application of 2% nitroglycerin ointment for injuries that occur while using vasopressors.[63] Both hyaluronidase and phentolamine are most effective when used as quickly as possible at the site of injury, and again, dosing is based up the extent of the injury, size and weight of the patient, and facility protocols.

Wound Management The principles of standard wound care for extravasation injuries in the premature, neonatal, and pediatric population include cleansing, debridement of nonviable tissue, moist wound dressings, and infection management. The multiple dressings used to treat extravasation injuries should have characteristics that manage exudate, allow adherence without tissue or wound bed damage, provide adequate bacterial protection, provide compression, and permit access for visualization. The dressings must be gentle on the skin because the neonate and infant populations are often the most at risk for suffering this type of injury. Recommended dressings include foam dressings with/without silicone borders, hydrogel dressings used with silicone component, hydrogel sheet dressings, absorbent hydrofiber dressings, or contact layers used in combination with another wound dressing to reduce adhesion. Caution is advised when applying hydrocolloid dressings to the neonate population because of its adhesive nature and the risk of skin tears with removal. Also, caution is required when

CLINICAL CONSIDERATION

Medical grade honey is effective in the treatment of extravasation injuries in neonates; however, its use may be limited due to allergic reactions in children. Although it has shown promise in facilitating healing in a variety of pediatric wounds, more controlled research is needed to determine its safety and efficacy in the neonatal and pediatric population.

treating the premature or neonate population with products that contain silver. There is a lack of research on the impact of silver and wound healing within the pediatric population and its use could be detrimental.

Surgical Sites

Pathophysiology Surgical site wounds for children in the hospital are common. Some reviews have revealed that as many as 43% of pediatric patients may have an open surgical wound or a closed incision while in the hospital.[74] Factors that may contribute to a dehiscence or infection of the surgical site include location, frequent scratching, tissue frailty, and frequent movement (**FIGURE 8-21**).

Clinical Presentation The appearance of surgical sites is based primarily on the method of closure. Surgical sites are closed one of the four ways: sutures, staples, tissue glue, or Steri strips. A post-op surgical dressing is then placed over the site to keep it clean and to reduce the potential for a surgical site infection (**FIGURE 8-22**).

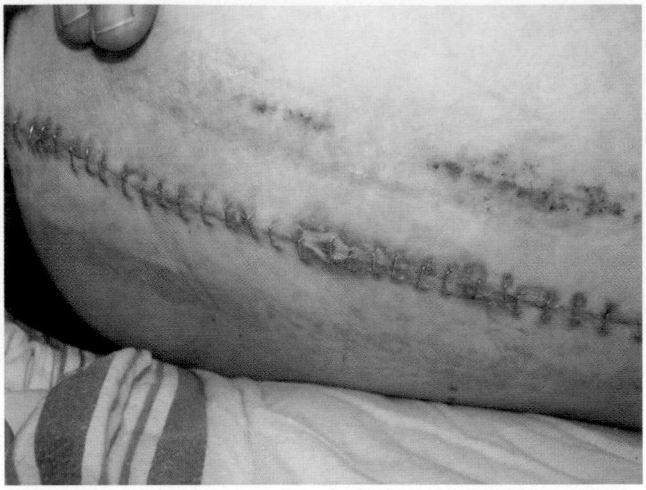

FIGURE 8-22 A surgical site incision closed with staples. Dressings to cover surgical incisions need to allow for easy visualization, as well as be absorbent and nonadherent at the incision.

Medical Management The standard of care for surgical incisions includes close monitoring for signs and symptoms of infection, visualization of the site, maintaining thermal insulation, and proper cleansing based on the type of closure used.

Wound Management Sterile technique should always be used when cleaning and changing dressings for surgical sites.[75] Antimicrobial dressings may help to reduce the rate of surgical site infections.[76,77] Dressings that can be used on open or closed surgical sites include foams, hydrogels, soft silicone dressings, and hydrofiber dressings that are placed in the open surgical wound to absorb exudate and to fill wound dead space.[45] The use of negative pressure wound therapy (NPWT) may also be appropriate for surgical sites with a larger surface area and significant amounts of exudate.[4] (See Chapter 17, Negative Pressure Wound Therapy for parameters for use on pediatric patients.) Foams with soft silicone borders that have low adherence to surgical sites are a good option and the use of contact layers over suture and staple sites reduces the possibility of adherence. Use of low adherence dressings can make dressing changes less intimidating for the pediatric patient. Precautions should be taken when using antimicrobial dressings that contain cadexomer iodine or sustained release silver. Data on these dressings lack evidence to support their use on the neonate and infant population.[45] The risk for absorption of chemicals may be greater due to an immature epidermis (**FIGURES 8-23** and **8-24**).

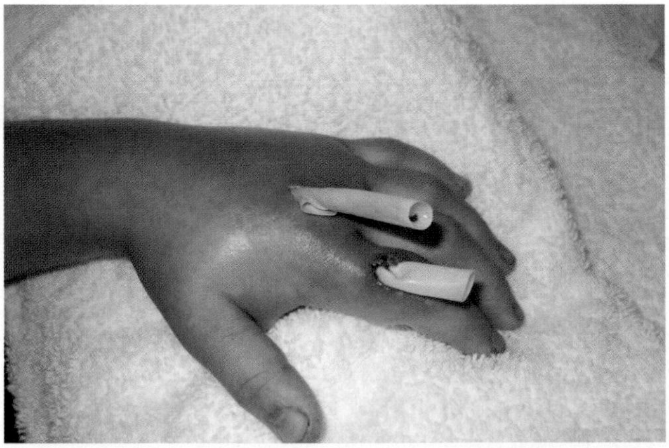

FIGURE 8-21 Surgical intervention may be required for removal of infection. A piece of sterile surgical tubing is used to assist with surgical site drainage after an animal bite occurred in this 4-year-old patient. This technique is used on any wound when there is a concern for spreading infection if the wound is surgically closed too soon.

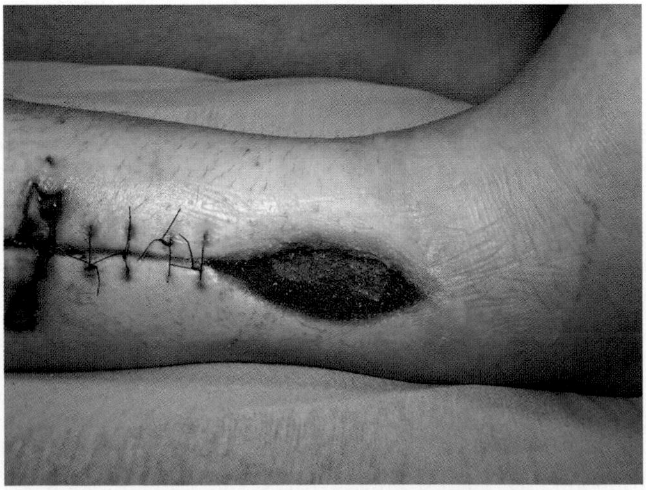

FIGURE 8-23 This surgical site dehisced on the right lateral ankle of a 15-year-old male patient. Note the beefy, red granulation tissue present after the application of negative pressure wound therapy used to assist with closure.

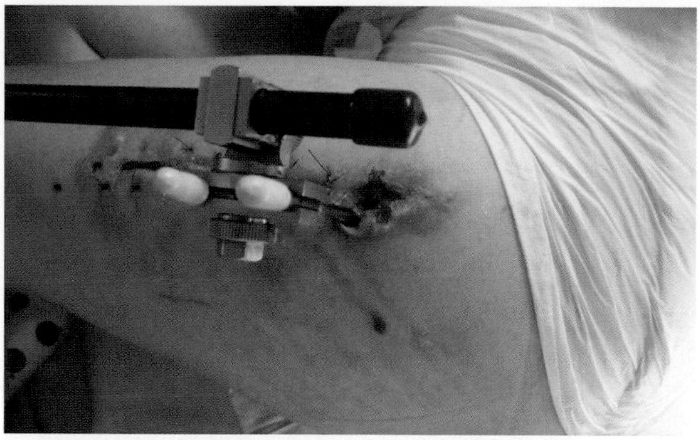

FIGURE 8-24 **After placement of external fixation, this surgical site has become infected.** There is increased redness and swelling at the pin site with seropurulent drainage. A fever higher than 100.4°F (38°C) can also indicate a sign of infection in children.

Thermal and Chemical Burns

Pathophysiology Thermal Burns Thermal burns are among the most common type of injuries in children.[77] Thermal burns occur primarily from exposure to open flames, contact with hot surface or liquid, or from some form of electrical current (this is rare).[79] Burns in children are classified the same way as they are in the adult population; however, in younger children and infants, calculating total body surface area (TBSA) is adjusted due to an infant's head being proportionally larger to overall body surface area as compared to that of the adult population. (Refer to Chapter 11, Burn Wound Management.) Neonates and infants may acquire thermal injuries in the hospital from monitoring electrodes, pulse oximetry leads, and warm ventilation tubing lying directly on the skin.

CLINICAL CONSIDERATION

NPWT is often used for wound treatment in the pediatric population. Currently, high-quality evidence providing safe guidelines and treatment parameters for the use of this biophysical modality with children and infants is scarce and often derived from case studies and expert opinion. While some clinicians consider NPWT essential to pediatric wound healing, the Food and Drug Administration (FDA) states that safety and effectiveness of NPWT have not been established for use in newborns, infants, or children. The FDA defines a child as greater than 2–12 years of age.[78]

Clinical Presentation The appearance of burns is categorized the same as adults with descriptions based on the severity of burn, such as superficial, superficial partial thickness, deep partial thickness, and full thickness (**FIGURE 8-25**).

Medical Management Immediate care includes removing the heat source and initiating a comprehensive assessment. Management of the burn wound is determined by the size and depth of the burn, duration of contact, and intensity of the heat source. Management of pain is crucial for the patient and is often insufficient in the pediatric population.[80]

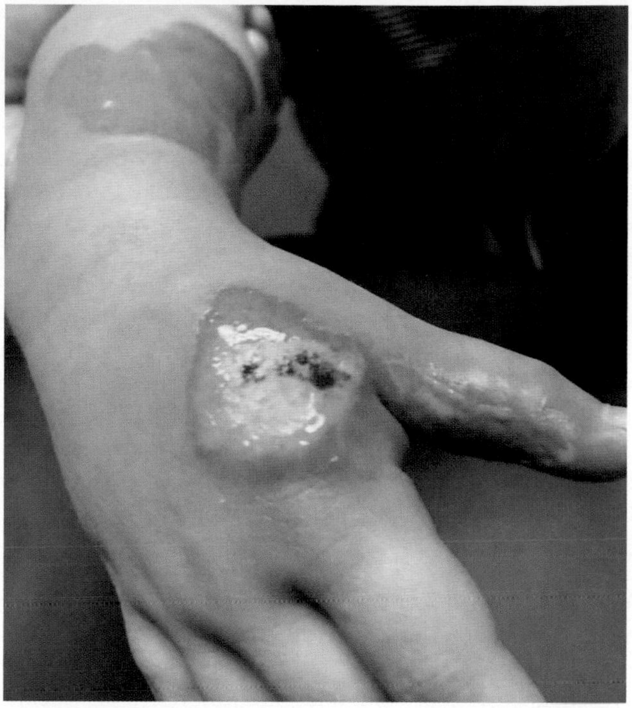

FIGURE 8-25 **Pediatric patient suffering a friction burn after falling on a moving treadmill.**

Wound Management Depending on the severity and depth of the burn, skin grafting is determined by the surgical or burn team. Management of burn wounds is similar to that of adults with focus being on debridement of the burn area, cleansing the site, and application of a proper burn dressing. Burn dressings for pediatric patients include a nonadherent component for reducing pain and a component for exudate management. The use of contact layers, soft silicone dressings, and foam dressings is appropriate for reducing pain and the number of potential dressing changes (**FIGURE 8-26**).

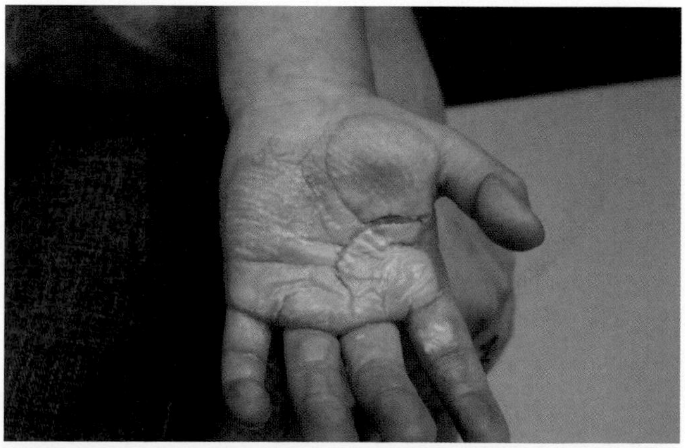

FIGURE 8-26 **This pediatric patient suffered a superficial partial-thickness burn after grabbing a hot object.** The area was debrided and treated with topical antimicrobial medication and a burn dressing. Pain control is often a challenge with pediatric patients who have this type of burn injury.

Chemical Burns

Pathophysiology Chemical Burns Chemical burns can be difficult to treat due to their progressive nature and the challenge of determining the chemical agent that contacted the child, concentration of the agent, and exposure time. Data on chemical burns in children are difficult to find, but chemical burns in children from birth to the age of 19 years have been reported to be between 1.3% and 3.0% of all reported burns in the United States.[81] Most chemical burns are the result of contact with either acids or alkalis in the home. Household products such as detergents, drain cleaner, and other common "under the sink" products are the primary sources of injury that occurs in the home. In the hospital setting, children may acquire a chemical burn related to barrier sprays, adhesive removers and solvents, betadine, cleansing agents and antiseptics, surgical bonding glue, or alcohol-based prep solutions.[82,83]

Clinical Presentation Minor chemical irritation may have the appearance of a rash or erythema at the point of contact with the chemical. More severe chemical injuries may include erythema, blistering, skin sloughing, or necrosis. Chemical burns that look mild may actually be extremely severe with progression of the chemical penetrating through multiple layers of skin and into deeper layers of tissue (**FIGURE 8-27**).

Medical Management Initial treatment for chemical burns includes neutralization of the chemical agent if the agent is known. If the chemical agent is not known, improper deactivation of the chemical may cause further toxicity and damage. In the community, if a child suffers a chemical burn, immediate medical attention or advice from Poison Control is advised. (The national, toll-free Poison Help line number is 1-800-222-1222.) In the hospital or clinical setting, if any type of chemical agent is applied to a child's skin prior to a surgical procedure, care should be taken to limit the spread of the agent, and it should be immediately removed with sterile

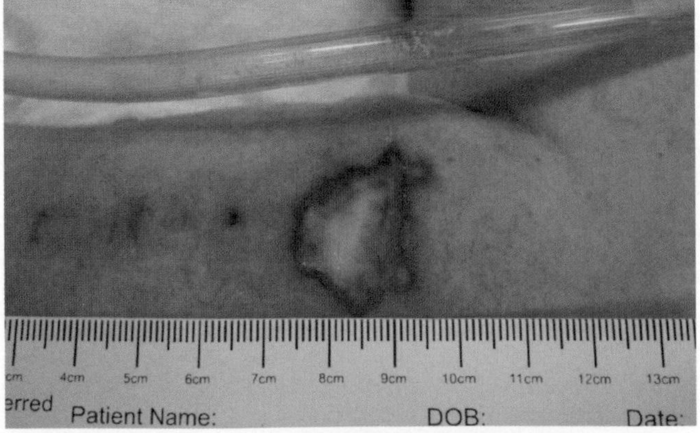

FIGURE 8-27 Upon initial examination, chemical burns may present as less severe. However, they may progress through deeper layers of the skin for multiple days after initial contact with the offending chemical.

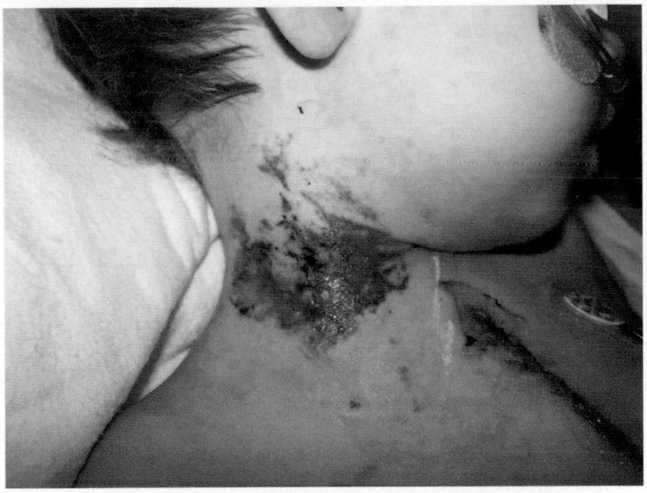

FIGURE 8-28 This patient suffered a chemical burn after reacting to an antiseptic agent used to clean an IV-line site. The area was cleaned with sterile water to remove the spread of the chemical agent and covered with a nonadherent dressing.

water after completion of the procedure in order to limit the possibility of a chemical burn. A water-based agent is recommended if possible (**FIGURE 8-28**).[83]

In the neonate population, the use of alcohol, betadine-based solutions, and skin disinfectants should be avoided; the use of chlorhexidine gluconate (CHG) as a skin disinfectant has been controversial. In 2012, the FDA required the following labeling on CHG: to "not use on premature or low birth weight infants or infants less than 2 months of age" and to "use with care in premature infants on infants under 2 months of age. These products may cause irritation or chemical burns."[67] The Centers for Disease Control and Prevention (CDC) maintains there is insufficient evidence to make recommendations about safety and efficacy of CHG products in infants younger than 2 months of age.[84] Preterm neonates may only have cell layers 3–10 layers thick; therefore, it is recommended to evaluate the risk and benefits of each product relative to efficacy, potential for percutaneous toxicity, and skin irritation.[67,85]

Wound Management As with thermal burns, the management of chemical burns is similar to that of adult care with the focus being on immediate rinsing of the site with tepid water for 15–20 minutes and covering with a clean gauze or cloth, application of a proper dressing, and debridement of nonviable tissue as needed. Dressings for pediatric patients with a chemical burn include a nonadherent component for reducing pain and exudate management. The use of contact layers, soft silicone dressings, and foam dressings is appropriate for reducing pain, and the reduction of the number of dressing changes is recommended.

CLINICAL CONSIDERATION

The progression or extent of a chemical burn may not be immediately recognized and may require several days to establish defined borders of the burn, or area and depth of damage.

TABLE 8-2 Clinical Presentation for Diaper Dermatitis

Severity	Skin Condition	Intervention
Slight to Mild	Slight dryness Erythema/redness present in small area Possible papules in a single area Skin intact	Frequent diaper changes Cleansing with diaper wipe Application of a barrier cream, barrier film, or petrolatum
Mild to Moderate	Mild dryness Redness progressing from pink to intense redness over larger area Slight scattering of papules over multiple areas Skin intact	Increased frequency of diaper changes, removal of irritant Cleansing with diaper wipe, no rubbing or "patting" dry Application of a barrier cream, barrier film, or petrolatum Application of Touchless care Zinc oxide
Moderate to Severe	Moderate dryness or scaling Severe redness in larger area Multiple areas of papules Mild edema Loss of skin integrity Slight bleeding Fungal presence	Increased frequency of diaper changes, removal of irritant Cleansing with diaper wipe, no rubbing or "patting" dry Application of a barrier film or a heavy barrier cream "like cupcake frosting" Initiation of "crusting" technique Consultation with wound care team
Severe	Scaling present Intense erythema/redness of the entire area Moderate to severe edema Erosion, ulceration, excoriated tissue Fungal presence, *Candida albicans* Numerous red papules with satellite lesions on thighs, groin, skin folds, low back	All interventions listed above Advanced care with "crusting" technique Consultation with wound care team or wound specialist Treatment for fungal infection

Incontinence-Associated Dermatitis

Pathophysiology Incontinence-associated dermatitis (IAD) or diaper dermatitis (DD) is a condition that is seen in every setting of pediatric healthcare (**TABLE 8-2**). This condition is included within a more expansive group of skin conditions termed moisture-associated skin damage (MASD) and is one of the most frequent dermatological conditions seen in the pediatric and neonatal populations.[88] Diaper dermatitis may account for up to 25% of dermatology visits seen by clinicians during the first year of life.[86–89] DD is often related to skin contacting or rubbing against wet diapers, or caused by friction between areas of wet skin that have been contaminated by feces or urine (eg, between the buttocks). This synergistic combination of fecal contact and ammonia in the urine is the primary cause of the skin irritation. Other factors that may contribute to DD include alterations of skin pH, congenital skin defects, congenital deficits, allergies, antibiotic use, or frequent loose stools. Once skin erosion or epidermal loss occurs, the site is at risk for infection by common bacteria such as *Candida albicans*, *Streptococcus*, or *Staphylococcus*.

Allergic contact dermatitis (ACD), seen less frequently, is a reaction to contact with irritants (ie, dyes, adhesives, fragrances, and preservatives in skin products) and may also occur in areas where diapers are not making direct skin contact, such as the trunk, extremities, and face (**FIGURE 8-29**).[90] A period of 1–3 weeks is needed for sensitization to occur before this type of dermatitis is observed.[91] Pediatric patients may be sensitive to the elastic, adhesives, or rubber often present in the waistline, in the elastic components, or inner contents of the disposal diaper.[89]

Clinical Presentation Diaper dermatitis is observed in diaper areas caused by direct contact between the skin and the irritant. The signs of irritation can include erythema, irritation, or chaffing. These clinical manifestations may be seen in the pubic and gluteal region with possible progression to the lower abdomen, upper thighs, and lower back. In classic cases of IAD, skin creases are often spared irritation due to the lack of contact with the diaper or irritant (**FIGURE 8-30**).

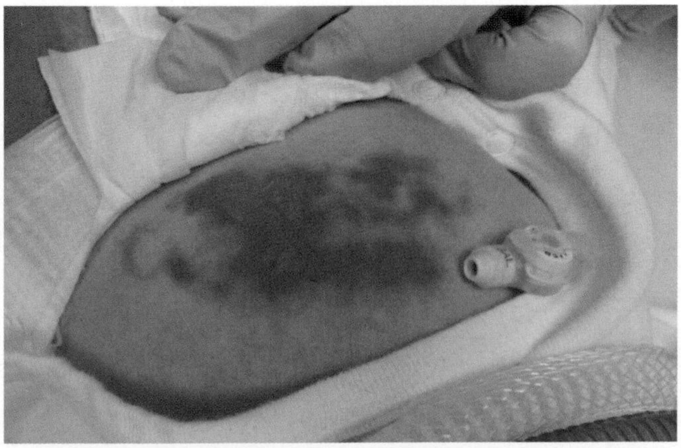

FIGURE 8-29 This patient reacted to the elastic material in a disposable diaper. Signs of irritation include erythema, edema, and blistering.

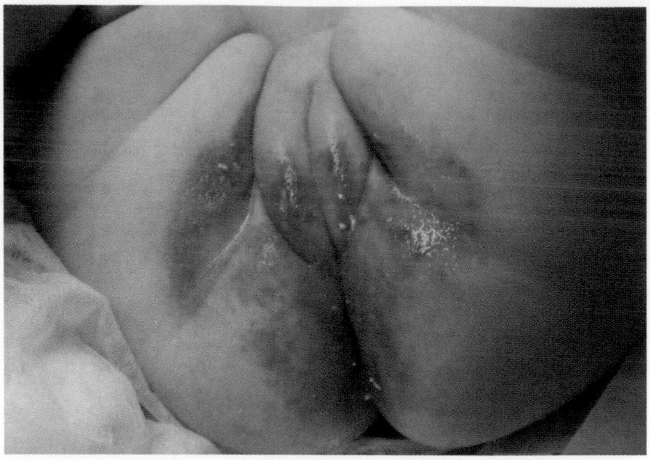

FIGURE 8-30 Classic presentation of diaper dermatitis includes redness, skin irritation, erosion, and satellite pustules. Pain control is essential when treating this skin irritation. Heavy mechanical rubbing must be avoided when providing care.

Clinical presentation of IAD varies from mild to severe symptoms. In mild cases, the epidermis remains intact, erythema is present, and scattered erythematous papules may occur. In moderate cases, there is intense redness, an increased surface area of involvement, and an increase in scattered papules. Erosion and scaling of the epidermis is present, and patients often have pain and discomfort during treatment of the area (**FIGURE 8-31**). In severe cases, there is extensive erythema, edema, and a prevalent number of painful papules/pustules. Widespread erosion of the epidermis and possible areas of inflammatory lesions may also occur. In chronic cases of IAD, *Candida albicans* will be present.

In allergic contact dermatitis, an itchy rash and pink patches or plaques often occur at the point of contact with the allergen. Extended contact with the allergen can progress to erythematous papules, small pruritic pustules, or painful swollen skin (**TABLE 8-2**).

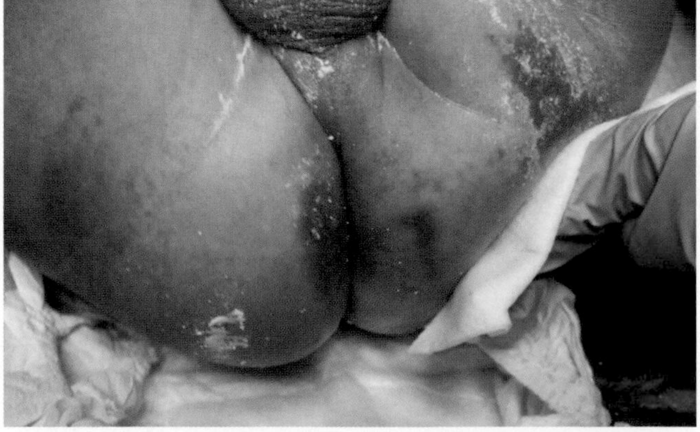

FIGURE 8-31 Healing diaper dermatitis on the buttocks. Thick barrier creams, proper care, and frequent monitoring of the area enhance healing times.

Medical Management In cases of IAD, the amount of fecal and urine exposure is critical and the frequency of diaper changes is increased in order to monitor and reduce exposure to the irritants. Medications, fluid intake, nutritionals status, and optimization of skin care should be evaluated. Urinary catheters or fecal management systems are recommended to reduce exposure to contaminants. If skin breakdown or erosion is the result of frequent acidic stools, the use of topical cholestyramine is helpful because it can bind the acid present in feces and thereby provide relief from irritation.[92] Treatment of ACD begins with identification and removal of the allergen; the skin may require 1–4 weeks to recover from the sensitizing agent. Use of emollients or topical steroid creams may reduce the symptoms of ACD.[93]

Diaper dermatitis with severe denuded skin, inflammation, and yeast, may require the use of antibiotics and antifungal therapies.

Wound Management Treatment of DD is defined in the ABC's of care (**TABLE 8-3**). Cleansing of dermatitis sites begins with the use of gentle, warm diaper wipes that contain no alcohols, fragrances, or irritants. Water-moistened cotton wipes are not recommended because they require more force to adequately clean the skin and may alter skin pH. Standard wipes are appropriately preserved, support acidic pH to protect from irritants from feces, and reduce friction.[94] The traumatized area is gently cleaned—vigorous scrubbing or abrasion of the area is discouraged. After cleansing, thick ointment-based emollients are applied. The area should be "crusted" by applying layered products,[95] for example, a combination might include applying (1) Cavilon no-sting barrier spray (3M Company, St. Paul, MN) or Cavilon Advanced Skin Protectant by 3M (3M Company, St. Paul, MN) and (2) Touchless Care Zinc Oxide protectant spray (3M Company, St. Paul, MN). The combination of zinc and protectants in the barrier spray promotes healing and provides an additional layer of protection. Some studies have shown that the use of topical barrier creams containing 2% magnesium is effective in treating diaper dermatitis.[96] Other combinations of protective layering may include applying a no-sting barrier spray, stoma powder, Vaseline, or some other form of barrier cream. The ingredients should be reviewed to determine if the product has the necessary ingredients to form a protective layer (eg, zinc oxide, silicone/dimethicone, or petroleum).

TABLE 8-3 The ABC's of Diaper Dermatitis

A Air	Expose diaper area to air, provide time when a diaper is not worn
B Barrier	Build a barrier for anyone wearing a diaper, protect area
C Clean	Clean with appropriate products, avoid abrasion or rubbing
D Diaper	Assess and change diapers frequently
E Educate	Educate healthcare workers, parents, and caregivers; teach the basics
F Follow-up	Frequent assessment and follow-up management of severe cases. Review with the wound team and caregivers

The principles of wound management for DD are (1) to avoid heavy scrubbing when cleansing the area of breakdown and (2) layer and build the "crust" or "mantle" for barrier protection. If the area is soiled with feces or urine, care should be taken to remove only the contaminated layering before reapplying the protective product. Only in the event of heavy soiling should all the layers of the protective product be removed and reapplied. Caregivers frequently remove the layers of barrier protection by wiping down to the impaired skin at every diaper change. This rubbing action only contributes to the continuation of the diaper dermatitis problem. The stigma, "my child must be absolutely clean," is common among parents because of the misconception that parental care has led to the problem of diaper dermatitis for their child.

Special consideration is required when combining multiple barrier ointments that contain antibiotics, antifungal agents, or topical steroids because some combinations are not acceptable for use on open or broken skin, and the overuse of topical steroids may cause adverse side effects including the development of Cushing's syndrome.[97,98] In cases with *Candida* infection, topical antifungal agents such as nystatin, clotrimazole, miconazole, ketoconazole, or ciclopirox can be applied with every diaper change.[99]

Prevention is the key to managing diaper dermatitis. Providing caregiver and parent education about the causative factors, as well as providing the appropriate skin care practices and treatment, will ensure a better outcome for this skin condition.

CONGENITAL CONDITIONS

Cutaneous Hemangiomas

Pathophysiology Cutaneous hemangiomas (CHs) are common vascular tumors in children and are often benign. Such tumors are present in 1.0–2.6% of neonates and in 10.5–12% of infants by 12 months of age.[100] Clinically, CHs are characterized by a typical evolution profile, consisting of rapid change or growth during the first year of life, and then starting to progressively shrink through 5–10 years of age.[101] CHs are typically asymptomatic and require no treatment, but in rare instances, they can lead to serious or even life-threatening complications.[102] The exact cause of CHs is not known, but some have theorized a familial link. Current research is focused on determining if there is a chromosomal or genetic connection.

Clinical Presentation CHs may have multiple descriptions but often present as a faint red birthmark commonly seen on the head and neck area of infants. CHs are also called port wine stains, "strawberries," or salmon patches (**FIGURE 8-32**).

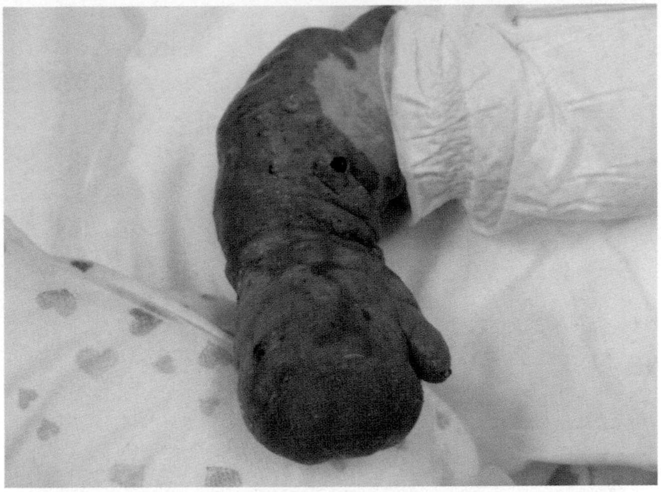

FIGURE 8-32 Presentation of a severe cutaneous hemangioma of the right lower extremity. Surgical intervention is needed to correct this malformation.

Medical Management CHs are usually non–life threatening; however, they can pose a problem based on location on the body, eg, problems with eating, vision, breathing, speaking, and diaper changes. Because CHs are often present on the face or neck and can be large and disfiguring, the psychological impact needs to be addressed for the patient and parents. Initial treatments include topical, intralesional, or systemic corticosteroids.[102] The next progression of treatment may include surgery to excise the tissue or the use of laser therapy to lighten the area. Other options for treatment include embolization, angiogenesis inhibitors therapy, radiotherapy, electrocautery, or sclerotherapy.[102] CHs need to be regularly monitored because in extreme cases, they may become malignant lesions.

Wound Management CHs are evaluated regularly to identify areas of abrasive breakdown, ulceration, and bleeding. Local wound care includes topical antibiotics to treat infectious areas and protective dressings such as foams or soft silicone products, hydrocolloid gels, and barrier creams or paste to provide protection.[103]

Epidermolysis Bullosa

Pathophysiology Epidermolysis bullosa (EB) is a heterogenous, inherited genetic group of skin disorders characterized by increased skin fragility and blister formation as a result of minor friction and trauma[104–106] (**FIGURE 8-33**). EB is caused by dysfunctional proteins that create a loss of cohesion between the anchoring fibrils of the dermal–epidermal junction which in turn results in formation of blisters and open wounds.[107] Inherited EB is grouped into the following four major types based on the depth of blister formation: EB simplex (most common), EB junctional, EB dystrophic, and Kindler syndrome.[104,106] Currently, there is no cure for EB.

Clinical Presentation On the newborn, EB presents with localized or widespread blistering at birth or within a few days after birth, often on the hands and feet.[104] The type of EB is confirmed through a series of differential diagnostic examinations and skin biopsies in the weeks following birth.[104] With EB simplex, simple forms of holding, touching, and diaper changes can elicit a blister or open wound (**FIGURE 8-34**). In more severe cases, blistering may be seen in mucosal tissue

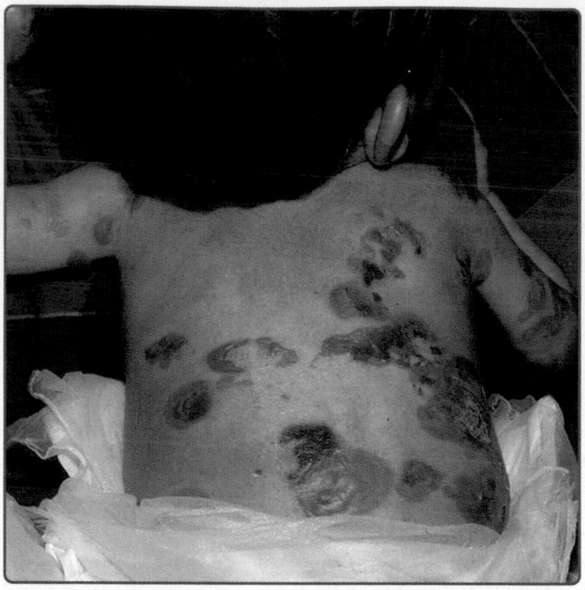

FIGURE 8-33 Widespread blistering on an infant with generalized EB simplex. (Used with permission from Kang S, Amagai M, Bruckner AL, Enk AH, Margolis DJ, McMichael AJ, Orringer JS, eds. *Fitzpatrick's Dermatology*. 9th ed. New York, McGraw Hill; 2019, Figure 60-4.)

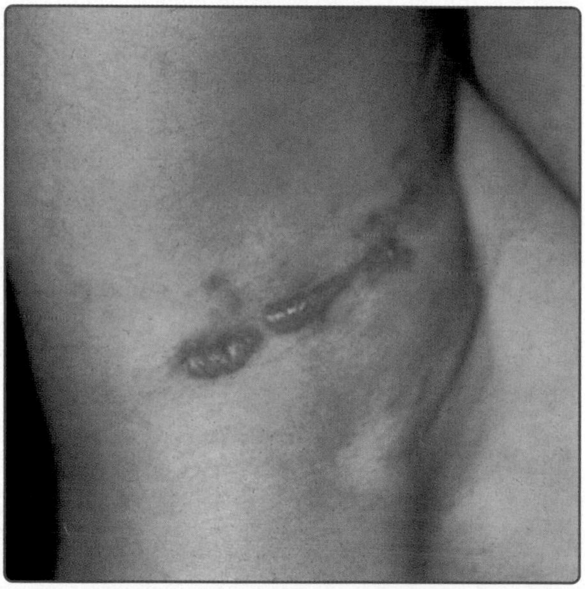

FIGURE 8-34 Trauma-induced blistering due to right clothing on a patient with localized ED simplex. (Used with permission from Kang S, Amagai M, Bruckner AL, Enk AH, Margolis DJ, McMichael AJ, Orringer JS, eds. *Fitzpatrick's Dermatology*. 9th ed. New York, McGraw Hill; 2019, Figure 60-5.)

of the mouth and throat and in the gastrointestinal tract. The routine act of swallowing or bowel movements may cause severe, painful blisters.

Medical Management Medications for pain, itching, and infection are the initial standard treatment, along with strategies to prevent new injuries and treatment complications. Surgical interventions may be needed for the following: feeding tube placement for growth and weight gain, esophageal widening due to scarring, skin grafting to increase function and appearance, and restorative surgery to allow better movement at over-scarred joints (**FIGURE 8-35**). Any monitoring devices that are attached to the skin during a hospital stay should be secured with nonadhesive products in order to prevent skin tearing with dressing changes.

Wound Management Treatment and management of EB are highly specialized and individualistic. The skin of a patient with EB should be evaluated frequently and safely, and local wound care provided for open sites and blisters. The available products used to treat this condition are limited and sometimes challenging to obtain. The use of medical gloves with latex or vinyl is discouraged because they may stick or cling to the skin and increase the risk of trauma. For newborns, the use of an incubator is discouraged because heat and humidity may further facilitate blistering. Cleansing agents need to be gentle and nonabrasive, and dressings need to be atraumatic with removal and highly absorbent (such as silicone-backed foam). Dressing management may include layering with hydrogels and contact layer dressings, applying an impregnated gauze or nonadherent bandage, and securing with a secondary retention dressing. Creams and lotions are also recommended to reduce the risk of dry skin and itching. Cloth diapers are advised as they are soft on the skin.[106] If standard disposable diapers are used, the elastic edges of the diaper need to be removed because they can cause blistering.[106] Education is critical for parents and caregivers and includes the following components: proper handling and holding of the child, pressure relief and redistribution, and types of clothing that are appropriate to reduce further blistering and trauma. Complete prevention of a blister or wound is unrealistic for a child with EB, but meticulous treatment strategies can reduce pain and trauma.

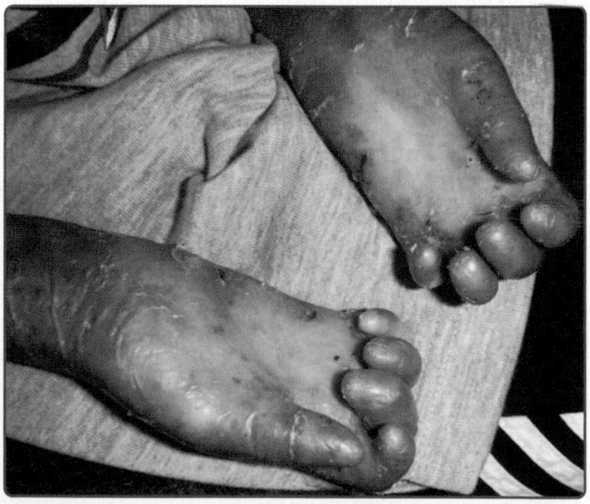

FIGURE 8-35 Scarring of the hands on a patient with recessive dystrophic EB. (Used with permission from Kang S, Amagai M, Bruckner AL, Enk AH, Margolis DJ, McMichael AJ, Orringer JS, eds. *Fitzpatrick's Dermatology*. 9th ed. New York, McGraw Hill; 2019, Figure 60-14.)

PEDIATRIC SKIN ASSESSMENT TOOLS

A routine and thorough assessment of skin is one of the foundational processes for developing an objective treatment plan for the pediatric patient; however, there are a limited number of validated and reliable skin and risk assessment tools available. This section will discuss some assessment tools and the characteristics of each, yet it is only a summary of some of the available tools and by no means exhaustive. Clinicians, interdisciplinary wound teams, and healthcare facilities need to consider the population being treated and associated risk factors for wounds before adopting an assessment tool. Risk factors that are more impactful on the neonatal and pediatric population, as compared to the adult population, include gestational age and birthweight of the neonatal or "*premie*" patient, transepidermal water loss (TEWL), medical devices or support equipment that is inserted or attached to the patient, hemodynamic and physiological instability, and the use of drug therapy.

Braden Q Pediatric Skin Risk Assessment Scale

The Braden scale, a familiar tool used to assess the risk for PIs and skin breakdown in the adult population, has been adapted and termed the Braden Q Scale. This tool is for pediatric-specific PI risk assessment in patients in the age range from 2 weeks to 8 years.[108] Seven categories of risk that are examined include the six categories of the Braden scale (sensory perception, moisture, activity, mobility, nutrition, friction, and shear), plus *tissue perfusion and oxygenation*. This tool does not consider the risk of injury associated with medical devices or immobility. The Braden Q scale should be used with caution when assessing neonates or noncritically ill pediatric patients due to limitations of clearly defined ages in neonates and limited evaluations of this tool on children who were evaluated in areas of the hospital that were considered noncritical, for example, general medical wards.[109]

Braden QD Pediatric Skin Risk Assessment Scale

The Braden QD scale appears very sensitive in predicting PI in children and useful in identifying when risk-prevention strategies need to be activated.[110] This revised Braden Q scale has removed the categories for activity or skin moisture and has been reviewed for use in patients who range in age from preterm to 21 years. This tool is different from the Braden Q by demonstrating that it reliably predicts risk for both immobility-related and medical device-related PIs across a diverse pediatric population in the hospital environment.[111] This scale is valuable in pediatric hospitals because of the risk assessment of medical devices (the "D" in QD) that are often encountered in the hospital setting (**TABLE 8-4**).[111]

Neonatal Skin Risk Assessment Scale (NSRAS)

The NSRAS is a tool designed to assess skin in neonates and has six subscales that identify risk in the areas of physical condition, mental status, mobility, activity, nutrition, and moisture.[112] The NSRAS is used worldwide and has predictive validity in the subgroups of physical condition, activity, and nutrition. The NSRAS is preferred because of its ease of use and accuracy in the prediction of skin breakdown in the neonate population.[113]

Glamorgan Pediatric Pressure Ulcer Risk Assessment Scale

The Glamorgan scale was developed in the United Kingdom for assessing PI risk in patients who range in age from 1 day to 18 years (**TABLE 8-5**). This scale measures the following variables that are associated with PI formation: difficult to position, anemia, equipment touching the skin, reduced mobility for age, prolonged surgery, and persistent fever.[114] The Glamorgan scale was found to have better predictive validity for PI risk than that of the Braden Q scale.[114]

AWHONN Neonatal Skin Condition Score Tool (NSCS)

The NSCS tool developed by the Association of Women's Health, Obstetric and Neonatal Nurses (AWHONN) evaluates the skin condition in patients ranging from low-birth-weight premature infants to healthy newborns. The tool was developed to improve clinical practice in the challenging area of the neonatal intensive care units (NICUs) by assessing the following three areas: dryness, erythema, and breakdown/excoriation.[115] The scores generated by the NSCS are then used in conjunction with evidenced-based clinical practice guidelines designed by AWHONN and National Association of Neonatal Nurses (NANN) to improve overall skin condition in infants. The use of the NSCS along with neonatal skin care research-based clinical practice guidelines have demonstrated improved skin condition outcomes in premature and full-term newborns.[115] The NSCS has also shown to be reliable and valid in assessing neonatal skin conditions.[116]

Other Skin Assessment Tools

Other tools exist for assessing skin in the pediatric population; however, some are currently being revised, lack sufficient testing to be reliable or valid, have only been evaluated in a limited population, or are under development. They include the following:

- Starkid Skin Scale[117]
- Seton Infant Skin Risk Assessment Tool (SISRA)[118]
- Neonatal/Infant Braden Q[119]
- Skin Risk Assessment and Management Tool (SRAMT)[120,121]

CASE STUDY

CONCLUSION

Conservative wound care was provided initially, allowing time for all wounds to demarcate. Medical treatment included corticosteroids to manage/decrease vessel inflammation and NSAIDs for pain. Antibiotics were prescribed as needed for local infection. Wound care was tedious due to the pain levels at all sites, and included gentle cleansing with sterile water and nonadhesive foam dressings with silver to decrease the bacterial load and manage drainage. After 3 months, the wounds appeared as shown in FIGURES 8-36 through 8-38. Upon discharge, the mother was instructed in wound care, including the use of nonstick contact layers and foam dressings, anchored with gauze rolls as a secondary dressing to avoid use of any adhesives.

Surgical intervention was required for digits that did not autoamputate (FIGURES 8-39 through 8-40).

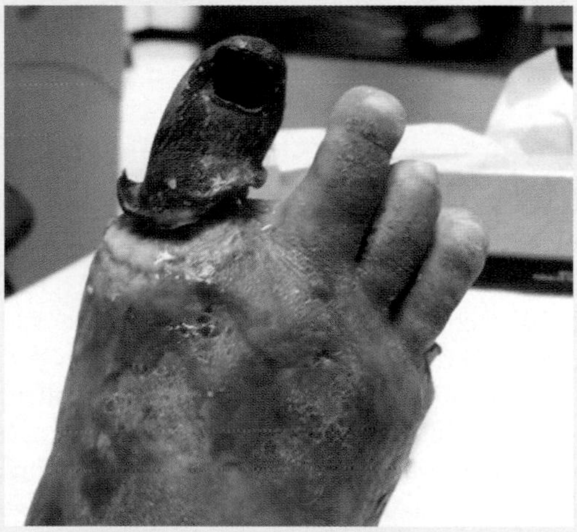

FIGURE 8-36 Three months after onset, right great toe shows signs of autoamputation.

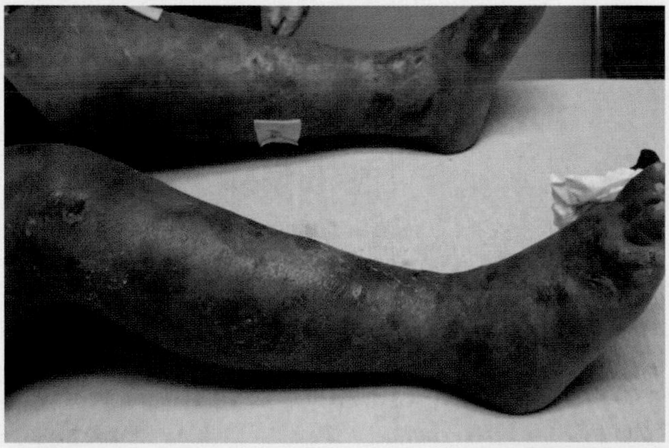

FIGURE 8-37 Three months after onset, skin integrity on both lower extremities is improving with mother's care. Right fifth toe has autoamputated, but others will need surgical removal.

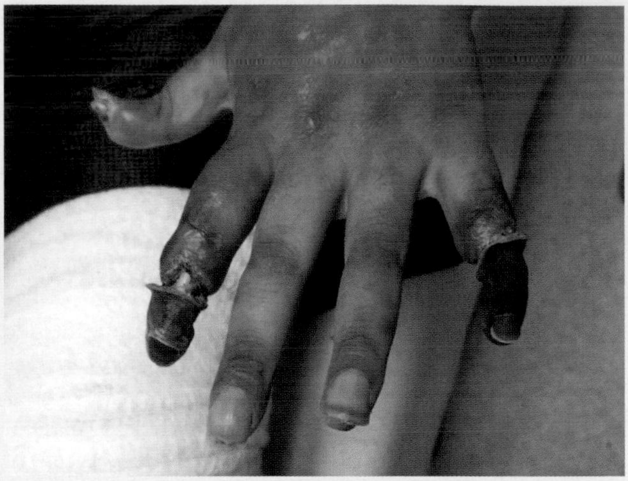

FIGURE 8-38 Three months after onset, left second and fifth digits show signs of autoamputation with exposed bone on the second finger. Note the necrosis on the end of the thumb also.

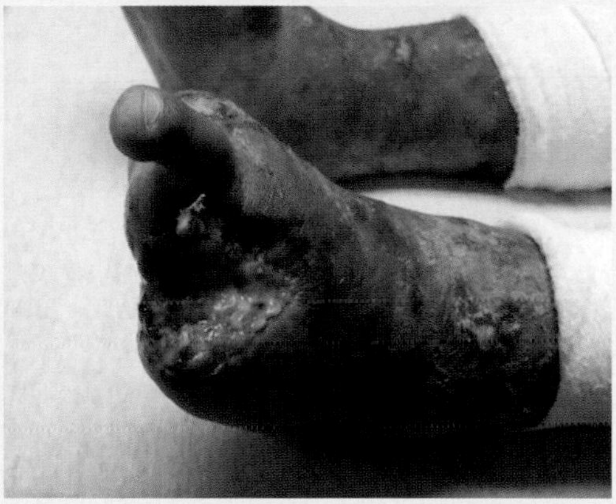

FIGURE 8-39 Five months after onset, left lateral foot required major amputation of four digits.

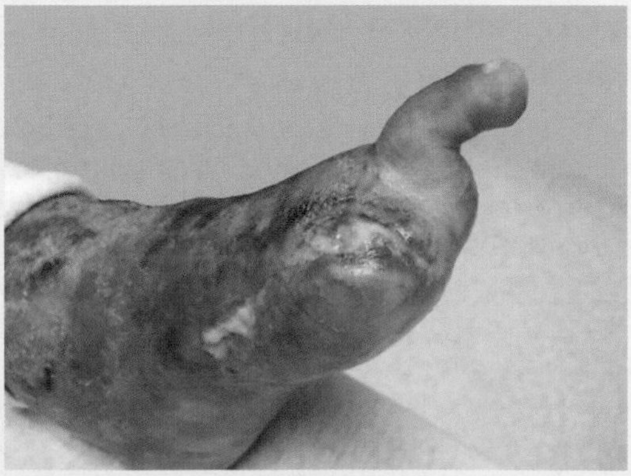

FIGURE 8-40 Five months after onset, left medial view of amputation site.

CASE STUDY *(Continued)*

DISCUSSION QUESTIONS

1. How will these impairments affect the patient's gait?
2. What type of footwear is recommended after all the wounds are healed?
3. How can the lower extremity edema be managed for a child? How is this similar to or different from how edema would be managed for an adult?

TABLE 8-4 The Braden QD Scale

Braden QD Scale				
Intensity and Duration of Pressure				**Score**
Mobility The ability to independently change and control body position	**0. No Limitation** Makes major and frequent changes in body or extremity position independently.	**1. Limited** Makes slight and infrequent changes in body or extremity position **OR** *unable* to reposition self independently (includes infants too young to roll over).	**2. Completely** Immobile Does not make even slight changes in body or extremity position independently.	
Sensory Perception The ability to respond meaningfully, in a ***developmentally*** appropriate way, to pressure-related discomfort	**0. No Impairment** Responsive and has no sensory deficits which limit the ability to feel or communicate discomfort.	**1. Limited** Cannot always communicate pressure-related discomfort **OR** has some sensory deficits that limit the ability to feel pressure-related discomfort.	**2. Completely Limited** Unresponsive due to diminished level of consciousness or sedation **OR** sensory deficits limit ability to feel the pressure-related discomfort over most of body surface.	
Tolerance of the Skin and Supporting Structure				
Friction and Shear ***Friction:*** occurs when skin moves against support surfaces ***Shear:*** occurs when skin and adjacent bony surface slide across one another	**0. No Problem** Has sufficient strength to completely lift self up during a move. Maintains good body position in bed/chair at all times. Able to completely lift patient during a position change.	**1. Potential Problem** Requires some assistance in moving. Occasionally slides down in bed/chair, requiring repositioning. During repositioning, skin often slides against surface.	**2. Problem** Requires full assistance in moving. Frequently slides down and requires repositioning. Complete lifting without skin sliding against surface is impossible **OR** spasticity, contractures, itching or agitation leads to almost constant friction.	
Nutrition *Usual* diet for age—assess pattern over the most recent 3 consecutive days	**0. Adequate** Diet for age providing **adequate** calories and protein to support metabolism and growth.	**1. Limited** Diet for age providing **inadequate** calories **OR** **inadequate** protein to support metabolism and growth **OR** receiving supplemental nutrition any part of the day.	**2. Poor** Diet for age providing **inadequate** calories **and** protein to support metabolism and growth.	
Tissue Perfusion and Oxygenation	**0. Adequate** Normotensive for age, **&** oxygen saturation ≥ 95%, **&** normal hemoglobin, **&** capillary refill ≤ 2 seconds.	**1. Potential Problem** Normotensive for age with oxygen saturation <95%, **OR** hemoglobin <10 g/dL, **OR** capillary refill > 2 seconds.	**2. Compromised** Hypotensive for age **OR** hemodynamically unstable with position changes.	
Medical Devices				
Number of Medical Devices	**Score 1 point for each medical device* up to 8 (Score 8 points maximum)** ****Any diagnostic or therapeutic device that is currently attached to or traverses the patient's skin or mucous membrane.***			
Repositionability/Skin Protection	**0. No Medical Devices**	**1. Potential Problem** All medical devices can be repositioned **OR** the skin under each device is protected.	**2. Problem** Any one or more medical device(s) can**not** be repositioned **OR** the skin under each device is not protected.	
			Total (≥13 considered at risk)	

Reproduced with permission from Martha A.Q. Curley.

TABLE 8-5 Glamorgan Pediatric Pressure Ulcer Risk Assessment Scale

Suitable for use from Birth–18 years

Admission Date............................Time..................

Consultant/GP...............................

N.B. This tool should be used to support **not replace** your clinical judgement as to whether the child is at risk of pressure ulcer development.

Risk Factor *(If data such as serum albumin or hemoglobin is not available then score 0)*	**Score**	**Date and time of assessments (reassess at least daily and every time condition changes)**						
Child cannot be moved without great difficulty or deterioration in condition/under general anesthetic >2 hours	20							
Unable to change his/her position without assistance/cannot control body movement	15							
Some mobility, but reduced for age	10							
Normal mobility for age	0							
Equipment/objects/hard surface pressing or rubbing on skin	15							
Significant anemia (Hb < 9 g/dL)# Not Known	1 0							
Persistent pyrexia (temperature > 38.0°C for more than 4 hours)	1							
Poor peripheral perfusion (cold extremities/capillary refill > 2 seconds/ cool mottled skin)	1							
Inadequate nutrition/PYMS score >2 (discuss with dietician if in doubt)	2							
Low serum albumin (< 35 g/L) Not Known	1 0							
Incontinence (inappropriate for age)	1							
Total score								
Action Taken: Yes or No If Yes complete SSKINS care plan. Refer to relevant Specialist Service, i.e. Dietetics, Tissue Viability, Orthotics								
Signature								
Designation								

Risk score	**Category**	**Suggested action**
0	Not at risk	Continue to reassess daily and every time condition changes.
10+	At risk	Inspect skin at least twice a day. Relieve pressure by helping/encouraging the child to move at least every 2 hours. Use a size- and weight-appropriate pressure redistribution surface for sitting on and/or sleeping on if necessary.
15+	High risk	Inspect skin with each repositioning. Reposition child/equipment/devices at least every 2 hours. Relieve pressure before any skin discoloration develops. Use a size- and weight-appropriate pressure redistribution surface for sitting on and/or sleeping on.
20+	Very high risk	Inspect skin at least hourly if condition allows. Move or turn if possible, before skin becomes discolored (refer to EUPAP grade 1). Ensure equipment/objects are not pressing on the skin. Consider using specialized pressure relieving equipment. Refer to local guidelines/protocol if available, if not contact/refer to TVN.

PEDIATRIC PRESSURE ULCER RECORD

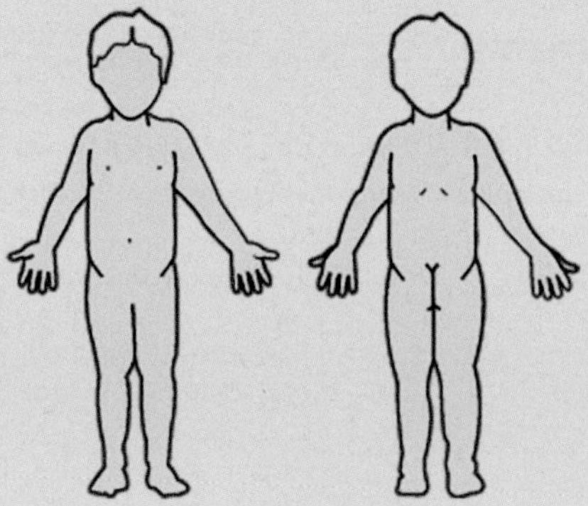

Using numbers, indicate on the diagram above any discolored areas or pressure ulcers.

TABLE 8-5 Glamorgan Pediatric Pressure Ulcer Risk Assessment Scale (*Continued*)

Use the box below. Enter the number, the date it was first observed, grade and location, and the outcome (resolved or not resolved).

Ulcer Number	Date Ulcer First Observed	Grade and Location of Ulcer(s)	Outcome (resolved/ not resolved)	Date of Reassessment	Signature

Healthcare Improvement Scotland   NATVNS SCOTLAND

GUIDANCE ON USING THE GLAMORGAN SCALE

A child's risk of developing a pressure ulcer should be assessed within 8 hours of admission and re-assessed daily and every time there are significant changes in his/her condition.

Dates & Times of assessments must be inserted in the appropriate box.

Mobility—Include the total of ALL relevant scores in this section

Child cannot be moved without great difficulty or deterioration in condition—add 20 to total score for this section.

Eg, ventilated child who desaturates with position changes, a child who becomes hypotensive in a certain position.

Children with cervical spine injuries are limited in the positions they can lie in.

Some children with contracture deformities are only comfortable in limited positions.

General anesthetic >2 hours—add 20 to total score for this section **only on the day of surgery**

Eg, a child who is on the theatre table may not have their position changed during an operation for a prolonged period and is placed on a firm surface for stability during the operation.

Unable to change his/her position without assistance—add 15 to total score for this section.

Eg, a child may be unable to move themselves, but carers can move the child and change his/her position.

Cannot control body movement—add 15 to total score for this section.

Eg, the child can make movements but these may not be purposeful (repetitive dyskinetic movements), the child is unable to consciously change his/her own position.

Some mobility but reduced for age—add 10 to total score for this section.

The child may have the ability to change their own position but this is limited/restricted. Eg, a child with developmental delay, a child in traction who can make limited movements, or a child on bed rest.

Normal mobility for age—score 0 for this section.

Mobility is appropriate for the developmental stage.

Eg, a newborn baby can move his/her limbs but is not able to roll over; a 1-year old can roll over, bottom shuffle or crawl, sit up, and pull up to standing.

Equipment/objects/hard surface pressing or rubbing on the skin—add 15 to total score.

Any object pressing or rubbing on the skin for long enough or with enough force can cause pressure damage. (These areas must be observed closely.)

Eg, pulse oximeter probes, ET tubes, masks, tubing/wires, tight clothing (antiembolic stockings), plaster casts/splints.

Significant anemia (Hb < 9 g/dL)

If the hemoglobin has been measured during this admission and is below 9 g/dL—score 1.

If the hemoglobin is 9 g/dL or above score 0.

If the hemoglobin is unknown, write NK and score 0.

Persistent pyrexia (temperature > 38.0°C for more than 4 hours)

If temperature is 38.0°C and above for more than 4 hours—score 1.

If temperature is less than 38°C and/or pyrexia lasts less than 4 hours—score 0.

Poor peripheral perfusion (cold extremities/capillary refill > 2 seconds/cool mottled skin)

If the child has any of the above symptoms whilst in a warm environment (ie, not due to low environmental temperature)—score 1.

Inadequate nutrition/PYMS score >2 (discuss with a dietician if in doubt)

If a child is identified as being malnourished (exclude pre-op fasting)—score 1.

A child who has a normal nutritional intake—score 0.

(*Continued*)

TABLE 8-5 Glamorgan Pediatric Pressure Ulcer Risk Assessment Scale (*Continued*)

Low serum albumin (<35 g/L)
If serum albumin is less than 35 g/L—score 1.
If serum albumin is 35 g/L or above—score 0.
If serum albumin has not been measured write NK and score 0.
Incontinence (inappropriate for age)
Inappropriate incontinence—score 1
Eg, A 4-year-old child who needs to wear nappies during the day and night.
Include children with special needs in this category.
Normal continence—score 0
Eg, A 5-year old who is dry during the day but may be occasionally incontinent during the night, a 12-month old who needs to wear nappies during the day and night.
Moisture lesions should not be confused with pressure ulcers.
Risk Score
Document total score; **however, scores for individual risk factors should be acted on**, ie, optimize nutrition and mobility.
If the child scores 10 or higher, he/she is at risk of developing a pressure ulcer unless action is taken to prevent it. This action may include normal nursing care, such as frequent changes of position (document how often the position is changed), encouraging mobilization, lying the child on a foam hospital mattress or on an air-filled mattress overlay, changing the position of pulse oximeter probes regularly, ensuring the child is not lying on objects in the bed such as tubing or hard toys.
Suggested action is indicated in the table; however, nurses should also use their own discretion and expertise, and if possible, seek advice from a tissue viability specialist if a high-specification pressure redistributing surface is considered necessary.
Complete SSKINS Care Plan to evidence these actions and review daily and/or if any changes to care. Adjust SSKINS Care Plan depending on patients' needs/requirements.
Pressure Ulcer Record
The diagram of the child can be used to indicate the position of any skin lesions.
If lesions are near to, or associated with any equipment such as BIPAP mask, nasogastric tube, or splint, these should also be indicated. The skin lesions indicated in the diagram should be numbered so that they can be referred to in the table below the diagram. In the table, the lesions can be described more fully, with the date they were first observed and the outcome.

Reproduced with permission from Healthcare Improvement Scotland.

SUMMARY

Healthcare clinicians may find pediatric patients with wounds challenging and sometimes intimidating to treat. Common practice tends to treat children as small adults with attempts to mitigate the risk of a more serious skin event; however, the focus of treating a pediatric patient with a wound includes the need to provide an adequate patient assessment along with wound appearance, morphology, and pathophysiology. An understanding of pediatric skin anatomy is necessary to determine the best practice for treatment. The treatment and advancement of pediatric wound care has historically been an underserved area of wound care; however, there is now the recognition for the need to increase research, establish clinical guidelines, and provide improved recommendations for treatment and product determination for the pediatric population.

STUDY QUESTIONS

1. In which developmental stage does pediatric skin lose its ability to form a scar?
   a. Gestational
   b. Neonatal
   c. Infantile
   d. Pubescent
2. Which unique factor would be specific to a pediatric patient to overcome in normal wound healing?
   a. Immunosuppression
   b. Medications
   c. Nutrition
   d. Transepidermal water loss
3. Which of the following contributes to pediatric patients' increased risk for suffering an extravasation injury?
   a. Increased vessel diameter
   b. Large caliber veins
   c. Decreased cell-layer thickness
   d. Robust vascular plexus

4. Which technique is used to form a protective barrier in children with severe diaper dermatitis?
   a. Bonding
   b. Cup caking
   c. Crusting
   d. Frosting
5. Which dressing is best used to reduce irritation and assist with binding acid that occurs in fecal material in young children?
   a. Cholestyramine
   b. Hyaluronidase
   c. Phentolamine
   d. Silver
6. What is the primary key to managing diaper dermatitis?
   a. Cleaning
   b. Barriers
   c. Education
   d. Prevention
7. Which genetic skin disorder is characterized by skin fragility and blistering in children?
   a. Cutaneous hemangiomas
   b. Diaper dermatitis
   c. Epidermal stripping
   d. Epidermolysis bullosa
8. Which is the most frequent dermatological skin condition seen in the pediatric population?
   a. Epidermal stripping
   b. Extravasation injuries
   c. Diaper dermatitis
   d. Pressure injuries

Answers: 1-a; 2-d; 3-c; 4-c; 5-a; 6-d; 7-d; 8-c

REFERENCES

1. Malloy-McDonald MB. Skin care for the high-risk neonates. *J Wound Ostomy Cont Nurs*. 1995;22:177-182.
2. Nix D, Best M, Bryant R. Skin care needs of the neonatal and pediatric patient. In: Bryant R, Nix D, eds. *Acute and Chronic Wounds: Current Management Concepts*. 5th ed. St Louis, MO: Elsevier; 2016:516-517.
3. Leung A, Balaji S, Keswani G. Biology and function of fetal and pediatric skin. *Facial Plast Surg Clin North Am*. 2013;21:1-6.
4. Baharestani M. An overview of neonatal and pediatric wound care knowledge and considerations. *Ostomy Wound Management*. 2007; 53:34-55.
5. Ulrich MMW. Fetal wound healing. In: Téot L, Mustoe TA, Middelkoop E, Gauglitz GG. eds. *Textbook on Scar Management*. Cham: Springer; 2020. https://doi.org/10.1007/978-3-030-44766-3_1
6. Eichenfield L, Hardaway C. Neonatology dermatology. *Curr Opin Pediatr*. 1999;11(5):471-474.
7. Evans NJ, Rutter N. Development of the epidermis in the newborn. *Biol Neonate*. 1989;49:74-80.
8. Visscher M, Narendran V. The ontogeny of skin. *Adv Wound Care*. 2014;3:291-303.
9. Campbell JM, Banta-Wright SA. Neonatal skin disorders: a review of selected dermatologic abnormalities. *J Perinat Neonat Nurs*. 2000; 14(1):63-83.
10. Fairley JA, Rasmussen JE. Comparison of stratum corneum thickness in children and adults. *J Am Acad Dermatol*. 1983;8:652-654.
11. Stamatas GN, Nikolovski J, Luedtke MA, et al. Infant skin microstructure assessed in vivo differs from adult skin in organization and at the cellular level. *Pediatr Dermatol*. 2010;27:125-131.
12. Nikolovski J, Stamatas GN, Kollias N, et al. Barrier function and water-holding and transport properties of infant stratum corneum are different from adult and continue to develop through the first year of life. *J Invest Dermatol*. 2008;128:1728-1736.
13. Tagami H. Location-related differences in structure and function of the stratum corneum with special emphasis on those of the facial skin. *Int J Cosmet Sci*. 2008;30:413-434.
14. Oranges T, Dini V, Romanelli M. Skin physiology of the neonate and infant: clinical implications. *Adv Wound Care*. 2015;4(10):587-595.
15. Visscher M, Utturkar R, Pickens W, et al. Neonatal skin maturation-vernix caseosa and free amino acids. *Pediatr Dermatol*. 2011;28: 122-132.
16. Walker V, Akinbi H, Meinzen-Derr J, et al. Host defense proteins on the surface of neonatal skin: implications for innate immunity. *J Pediatr*. 2008; 152:777-781.
17. Coughlin C, Taieb A. Evolving concepts of neonatal skin. *Pediatr Dermatol*. 2014;31:(suppl. 1):5-8.
18. Flurh J, Darlenski R, Lachmann N, et al. Infant epidermal skin physiology: adaptation after birth. *Br J Dermatol*. 2012;166:483-490.
19. Lawton S. Understanding skin care and skin barrier function in infants. *Nurs Child Young People*. 2013;25:28.
20. Dyer J. Newborn skin care. *Semin Perinatol*. 2013;37:3-7.
21. Hartz L, Bradshaw W, Brandon D. Potential NICU environmental influences on the Neonate's Microbiome: a systematic review. *Adv Neonatal Care*. 2015;15(5):324-335.
22. Biasucci G, Rubini M, Riboni S, et al. Mode of delivery affects the bacterial community in the newborn gut. *Early Hum Dev*. 2010; 86 (suppl):13-15.
23. Marques T, Wall R, Ross R, et al. Programming infant gut microbiota: influence of dietary and environmental factors. *Curr Opin Biotechnol*. 2010;21:149-156.
24. Faa G, Gerosa C, Fanni D, et al. Factors influencing the development of personal tailored microbiota in the neonate, with particular emphasis on antibiotic therapy. *J Matern Fetal Neonatal Med*. 2013; 26 (suppl 2):35-43.
25. Saavedra J, Dattilo A. Early development of intestinal microbiota: implications of future health. *Gastroenterol Clin North AM*. 2012;41: 717-731.
26. Collado M, Cernada M, Bauerl C, et al. Microbial ecology and host microbiota interactions during early life stages. *Gut Microbes*. 2012;3: 352-365.
27. Neu J, Rushing J. Cesarean versus vaginal delivery: long-term infant outcomes and the hygiene hypothesis. *Clin Perinatal*. 2011;38:321-331.
28. Prince A, Antony K, Ma J, Aagaard K. The microbiome and development: a mother's perspective. *Semin, Reprod Med*. 2014;32: 14-22.
29. Rigon G, Vallone C, Lucantoni V, Signore F. Maternal Factors pre- and during delivery contribute to gut microbiota shaping in newborns. *Front Cell Infect Microbiol*. 2012;2:93.
30. Tur E. Physiology of the skin-differences between women and men. *Clin Dermatol*. 1997;15:5-16.
31. Irving V. Neonatal iatrogenic skin injuries: a nursing perspective. *J Neonatal Nurs*. 1995;5:10-13.
32. Rustogi R, Mill J, Fraser J, Kimble R. The use of Acticoat in neonatal burns. *Burns*. 2005;31:878-882.

33. Lund C, Tucker J. Adhesion and newborn skin. In: Hoath SB, Maibach, HI, eds. *Neonatal Skin Structure and Function*. 2nd ed. New York, NY: Marcel Deckker, Inc; 2003. CRC Press.
34. Wilkins C, Emmerson A. Extravasation injuries on regional neonatal units. *Arch Dis Child Fetal Ed*. 2004;89:F274-F275.
35. Nix D, Best M, Bryant R. Skin care needs of the neonatal and pediatric patient. In: Bryant R, Nix D, eds. *Acute and Chronic Wounds: Current Management Concepts*. 5th ed. St Louis, MO: Elsevier; 2016:524.
36. Giusti F, Martella A, Bertoni L, et al. Skin barrier, hydration, and pH of the skin of infants under 2 years of age. *Pediatr Dermatol*. 2001;18:93-96.
37. Schmid-Wendtner M, Korting H. The pH of the skin surface and its impact on the barrier function. *Skin Pharmacol Physiol*. 2006;19: 296-302.
38. Yosipovitch G, Maayan-Metzger A, Merlob P, et al. Skin barrier properties I different body areas in neonates. *Pediatrics*. 2000; 106:105-108.
39. Kuller J. Skin care management of the low birth weight infant. In: Gunderson L, Kenner C, eds. Care of the 24-25 Week Gestational Age Infant (Small Baby Protocol). Petaluma, CA: Neonatal Network.
40. Irving V. Caring for and protecting the skin of pre-term neonates. *J Wound Care*. 2001;10:253-256.
41. Lund C, Osborne J, Kuller J, et al. Neonatal skin care: clinical outcomes of the AWHONN/NANN Evidence-Based Clinical Practice Guideline. *J Obstet Gynecol Neonatal Nurs*. 2013;30:41-51.
42. McNichol L, Lund C, Rosen T, Gray M. Medical adhesives and patient safety: state of the science: Consensus statements for the assessment, prevention, and treatment of adhesive-related skin injuries. *Orthop Nurs*. 2013;40:365-380.
43. Irving V. Wound care for preterm neonates. *Infant*. 2006;2:102-106.
44. Black P. Peristomal care: an overview of available products. *Br J Nurs*. 2007;16:1048-1056.
45. Report from an independent advisory group. Issues in neonatal wound care minimizing trauma and pain. The Tendra Academy. June 2005. Norcross., GA: Molnlycke Health Care, Inc.
46. Irving V, Bethell E, Burton F, on behalf of a Neonatal Advisory Group. Neonatal wound care: minimizing trauma and pain. *Wounds UK*. 2006;2: 33-41.
47. Irving V. Reducing the risk of epidermal stripping in the neonatal population: an evaluation of an alcohol free barrier film. *J Neonatal Nurs*. 2001;7:5-8.
48. National Pressure Injury Advisory Panel. NPIAP Pressure Injury stages. https://npiap.com/page/PressureInjuryStages. Accessed September 15, 2022.
49. Curley MA, Razmus IS, Roberts KE, Wypij D. Predicting pressure ulcer risk in pediatric patients: the Braden Q Scale. *Nurs Res*. 2003; 52:22-31.
50. Willock J, Hughes J, Tickle S, et al. Pressure sores in children: the acute hospital perspective. *Tissue Viabil Soc*. 2000;10:59-62.
51. Chapman S. Preventing and treating pressure ulcers: evidence review. *Br J Community Nurs*. 2017;22:S37-S40.
52. Wound, Ostomy and Continence Nurses Society. Guidelines for Prevention and Management of Pressure Ulcers. WOCN Clinical Practice Guidelines Series. Glenview, IL: Wound, Ostomy, and Continence Nurses Society; 2003.
53. Garvin G. Wound and skin care for the PICU. *Crit Care Nurs Q*. 1997; 20: 62-71.
54. Baharestani M, Vertichio R, Higgins MB, et al. A neonatal and pediatric evidence-linked pressure ulcer and sin care performance improvement initiative. Poster abstract presented at the Symposium on Advanced Wound and Medical Forum on Wound Repair; April 21-24, 2005; San Diego, CA.
55. Delmore BA, Ayello E. Pressure injuries caused by medical devices and other objects: a clinical update. *Am J Nurs*. 2017;117:36-45.
56. Freundlich K. Pressure injuries in medically complex children: a review. *Children (Basel)*. 2017;4:E25.
57. Odom B, Lowe L, Yates C. Peripheral infiltration and extravasation injury methodology. *J Infus Nurs*. 2018;41:247-252.
58. Gorski L, Hadaway L, Hagle M, et al. Infusion therapy standards and practice. *J Infus Nurs*. 2016;39(suppl 1):S1-S159.
59. Beall V, Hall B, Mulholland J, Gephart S. Neonatal extravasation: an overview and algorithm for evidence-based treatment. *Newborn Infant Nurs Rev*. 2013;13:189-195.
60. Gault D. Extravasation Injuries. *Br J Plast Surg*. 1993;46:91-96.
61. Thigpen J. Peripheral intravenous extravasation: nursing procedure for initial treatment. *Neonatal Netw*. 2007;26:379-384.
62. McCullen K, Pieper B. A retrospective chart review of risk factors for extravasation among neonates receiving peripheral intravascular fluids. *J Wound Ostomy Continence Nurs*. 2006;33:133-139.
63. Treadwell T. The management of intravenous injuries in infants and children. *Ostomy Wound Manage*. 2012;58:40-44.
64. Irving V. Managing extravasation injuries in preterm neonates. *Nurs Times*. 2001;97:40,43-46.
65. McLane K, Bookout K, McCord S, et al. The 2003 national pediatric pressure ulcer and skin breakdown prevalence survey: a multisite study. *J WOCN*. 2004;31:168-178.
66. Shenaq S, Abbase E, Friedman J. Soft-tissue reconstruction following extravasation of chemotherapeutic agents. *Surg Oncol Clin Am*. 1996;5: 825-845.
67. Association of Women's Health, Obstetric and Neonatal Nurses (AWHONN). *Neonatal Skin Care. Evidence-Based Clinical Practice Guideline*. Washington, DC: Association of Women's Health, Obstetric and Neonatal Nurses (AWHONN); 2018.
68. Casanova D, Bardot J, Magalon G. Emergency treatment of accidental infusion leakage in the newborn: Report of 14 cases. *Br J Plastic Surgery*. 2001;54:396-399.
69. Chandavasu O, Garrow E, Valda V, et al. A new method for the prevention of skin sloughs and necrosis secondary to intravenous infiltration. *Am J Perinatology*. 1986;3:4-5.
70. Kostogloudis N, Demiri E, Tsimponis A, et al. Severe extravasation injuries in neonates: a report of 34 cases. *Pediatr Dermatol*. 2015;32: 830-835.
71. Beaulieu M. Hyaluronidase for extravasation management. *Neonatal Netw*. 2012;31:413-418.
72. Keunsting L. Treatment of intravenous infiltration in a neonate. *J Ped Health Care*. 2010;24:184-188.
73. Sawatzky-Dicksson D, Bodnaryk L. Neonatal intravenous extravasation injuries: evaluation of a wound care protocol. *Neonatal Netw*. 2006;25: 13-19.
74. Noonan C, Quigley S, Curley M. Skin integrity in hospitalized infants and children: a prevalence survey. *J Ped Nurs*. 2006;21:445-453.
75. Brindle CT, Creehan S. Management of surgical wounds. In: Doughty D, McNichol L, eds. *Wound, Ostomy and Continence Nurses Society™ Core Curriculum: Wound Management*. Wolters Kluwer; 2016:655.
76. FDA Safety Communication (2011) UPDATE on Serious Complications Associated with Negative Pressure Wound Therapy Systems: FDA Safety Communication. http://www.fda.gov/MedicalDevices/Safety/AlertsandNotices/ucm244211.htm
77. Yin S. Chemical and common burns in children. *Clin Pediatr*. 2017; 5:8S-12S.

78. Kohler H, Schulz S, Wiebalck A. Pain management in children: assessment and documentation in burn units. *Eur J Pediatr Surg.* 2001;11:40-43.
79. American Burn Association, National Burn Repository 2019 Update. report of data from 2009-2018. https://ameriburn.org/wp-content/uploads/2017/05/2016abanbr_final_42816.pdf. Accessed September 21, 2022.
80. Lund C. Prevention and management of infant skin breakdown. *Nurs Clin N Am.* 1999;34:907-920, vii.
81. Irving V, Bethell E, Burton F, on behalf of a Neonatal Advisory Group. Neonatal wound care: minimizing trauma and pain. *Wounds UK.* 2006; 2:33-41.
82. Centers for Disease Control and Prevention (CDC). 2011 guidelines for the prevention of intravascular catheter-related infections. Retrieved from https://www.cdc.gov/hai/pdfs/bsi-guidelines-2011.pdf.
83. Noonan C, Quigley S, Curley M. Skin integrity in hospitalized infants and children: a prevalence survey. *J Ped Nurs.* 2006;21:445-453.
84. Klunk C, Domingues E, Wiss K. An update on diaper dermatitis. *Clin Dermatol.* 2014;32:477-487.
85. Ravanfar P, Wallace J, Pace N. Diaper dermatitis: a review and update. *Curr Opin Pediatr.* 2012;24:472-479.
86. Ersoy-Evans S, Akinci H, Atakan N. Diaper dermatitis: a review of 63 children. *Pediatr Dermatol.* 2016;33:332-336.
87. Coughlin C, Eichenfield L, Frieden I. Diaper dermatitis: clinical characteristics and differential diagnosis. *Pediatr Dermatol.* 2014; 31(suppl 1):19-24.
88. Di Landro A, Grevo V, Valsecchi R. "Lucky Luke" contact dermatitis from diapers with negative patch tests. *Contact Derm.* 2002;46:48-49.
89. Cohen B. Differential diagnosis of diaper dermatitis. *Clin Pediatr.* 2017;56:16S-22S.
90. White C, Gailey R, Lippe S. Cholestyramine ointment to treat buttocks rash and anal excoriation in an infant. *Ann Pharmacother.* 1996;30:954-956.
91. Alberta L, Sweeney S, Wiss K. Diaper dye dermatitis. *Pediatrics.* 2005;116: e450-e452.
92. Heimall L, Lund C. Assessment and interventions for diaper dermatitis. Retrieved from Heimall L, Storey B, Stellar J, Davis K. Beginning of the Bottom: Evidence-Based Care of Diaper Dermatitis. *Am J Maternal/Child Nurs.* 2012;37:10-16.
93. Vongsa R, Rodriguez K, Koenig D, Cunningham C. Benefits of using an appropriately formulated wipe to clean diapered skin of preterm infants. *Global Pediatr Health.* 2019;6:1-6.
94. Nourbakhsh S, Rouhi-Boroujeni H, Kheiri M, et al. Effect of topical application of the cream containing Magnesium 2% in treatment of diaper dermatitis and diaper rash in children: a clinical trial study. *J Clin Diagn Res.* 2016;10:WC04-WC06.
95. Ozdemir A, Bas VN. Iatrogenic Cushing's syndrome due to overuse of topical steroid in the diaper area. *J Tropical Pediatr.* 2014;60: 404-406.
96. Bulus AD, Andiran N, Kocak M. Cushing's syndrome: hidden risk in usage of topical corticosteroids. *J Pediatr Endocrinol Metabol.* 2014; 27:977-981.
97. Blume-Peytavi U, Kanti V. Prevention and treatment of diaper dermatitis. *Pediatr Dermatol.* 2018;35:16S-22S.
98. Jacobs AH, Cahn RL. Birthmarks. *Pediatr Ann.* 1976;5:743-758.
99. Astner S, Anderson RR. Treating vascular lesions. *Dermatol Ther.* 2005;18:267-281.
100. Musumeci M, Schlecht K, Perrotta R, et al. Management of cutaneous hemangiomas in pediatric patients. *Cutis.* 2008;81:315-22.
101. Hebert AA, Chang YC. Hemangiomas. In: Lebwohl MG, Heymann WR, Berth-Jones J, et al, eds. *Treatment of Skin Disease: Comprehensive Therapeutic Strategies.* 2nd ed. Philadelphia, PA: Mosby; 2006:264-266.
102. Gonzalez M. Evaluation and treatment of the newborn with epidermolysis bullosa. *Semin Perinatol.* 2013;37:32-39.
103. Report from an independent advisory group. Issues in paediatric wound care minimizing trauma and pain. The Tendra Academy®. June 2004. Molnlycke Health Care, Inc. Norcross., Ga.
104. Bello YM, Falabella AF, Schachner LA. Epidermolysis bullosa and its treatment. *Wounds.* 2001;13:113-118.
105. Kasperkiewicz M, Sadik C, Bieber K, et al. Epidermolysis bullosa acquisita: from pathophysiology to novel therapeutic options. *J Investig Dermatol.* 2016;136:24-33.
106. Noonan C, Quigley S, Curley MA. Using the Braden Q scale to predict pressure ulcer risk in pediatric patients. *J Pediatr Nurs.* 2010;26:566-575.
107. Liao Y, Gao G, Mo L. Predictive accuracy of the Braden Q Scale in risk assessment for paediatric pressure ulcer: a meta-analysis. *Int J Nurs Sci.* 2018;5:419-726.
108. Curley MA, Hasbani NR, Quigley SM, et al. Predicting pressure injury in pediatric patients: the Braden QD Scale. *J Pediatr.* 2018; 192:189-195.e2.
109. Chamblee T, Pasek T, Caillouette C, et al. How to predict pediatric pressure injury risk with the Braden QD scale. *Am J Nurs.* 2018;118: 34-43.
110. Huffiness B, Logsdon CM. The neonatal skin risk assessment scale for predicting skin breakdown in neonates. *Issues Comprehensive Pediatr Nurs.* 1997;20:103-114.
111. Dolack M, Huffiness B, Logsdon C, et al. Updated Neonatal Skin Risk Assessment Scale (NSRAS). University of Louisville Medical Center 530 South Jackson St., Louisville, KY 40207
112. Willock J, Baharestani M, Anthony D. The development of the Glamorgan paediatric pressure ulcer risk assessment scale. *J Wound Care.* 2009;18:17-21.
113. Lund C, Osborne J, Kuller J, et al. Neonatal skin care: clinical outcomes of the AWHONN/NANN evidence-based clinical practice guideline. *J Obstet Gynecol Neonat Nurs.* 2001;30:41-51.
114. Lund C, Osborne J. Validity and reliability of the neonatal skin condition score. *J Obstet Gynecol Neonatal Nurs.* 2004;33:320-327.
115. Suddaby E, Barnett S, Facteau L. Skin breakdown in acute care pediatrics. *Pediatr Nurs.* 2005;31:132-138, 148.
116. Vance DA, Demel S, Kirksey K, et al. A Delphi study for the development of an infant breakdown risk assessment tool. *Adv Neonatal Care.* 2015;15:150-157.
117. Wacek M, Ecklund M. Adopting Braden Q I the NICU to identify neonates at risk of developing pressure injuries. *Neonatal Netw.* 2018;37:319-323.
118. Broom MM, Burton WA, Ehrlich, et al. Developing an Australian skin risk assessment and management tool for neonates. *Wounds Pract Res.* 2017;25:15-22.
119. Broom M, Dunk AM, Mohamed ALE. Predicting neonatal skin injury: the first step to reducing skin injuries in neonates. *Health Serv Insights.* 2019;12:1-10.
120. Gaspard F, Brassard P, Alam T, et al. Impact of an antimicrobial dressing in reducing surgical site infections in cardiac surgery patients. *Wounds.* 2013;25:178-185.
121. Mueller S, Kresback L. Impact of an antimicrobial-impregnated gauze dressing on surgical site infections including methicillin-resistant Staphylococcus aureus infections. *Am J Infect Control.* 2008;36:651-655.

CHAPTER NINE

Atypical Wounds

Rose L. Hamm, PT, DPT, FACCWS and
Jayesh B. Shah, MD, MHA, CWSP, FUHM, FACHM, FACP, FACCWS

CHAPTER OBJECTIVES

At the end of this chapter, the learner will be able to:

1. **Recognize signs of an atypical wound.**
2. **Categorize an atypical wound according to a basic pathology.**
3. **Determine the appropriate medical specialist for a given wound.**
4. **Develop an evidence-based care plan for an atypical wound.**
5. **Educate the patient and family about the wound diagnosis.**

INTRODUCTION

Most wounds are diagnosed as arterial, venous, pressure, neuropathic, surgical, trauma, or burn and are treated according to the principles that have been discussed in the previous chapters. If a wound has a different appearance or does not respond to standard care, the clinician is challenged either to determine the factors that are inhibiting healing *or* to consider a different diagnosis. This chapter reviews the basic morphology of skin disease, red flags of atypical wounds, and characteristics of different diagnostic categories. The pathophysiology, clinical presentation with photographs, medical management, and wound management of each wound category are provided to assist the clinician in making sound clinical decisions.

CHARACTERISTICS OF ATYPICAL WOUNDS

The first indication that a wound is atypical is that little signal in the clinician's instinct that says, "This is just not quite what it looks to be." And usually, it behooves the clinician to follow those instincts, to at least rule out an atypical diagnosis, and to make a differential diagnosis that may change the care plan and result in wound healing. Sometimes searching for the wound diagnosis may lead to an undiagnosed underlying condition that needs to be treated in order for wound healing to occur. **TABLE 9-1** provides a list of characteristics that suggest a wound does not fall into the typical categories.[1–4]

TABLE 9-1 Characteristics of Atypical Wounds

Unusual location
Unusual age of the patient
Asymmetric lesion
Granulation extending over the wound edge
Exuberant granulation tissue or callus
Friable granulation tissue
Purple-red color around ulcer (termed *violaceous*)
Ulcer in center of pigmented lesion
History of repeated trauma
Rolled out edges
Fungating growth
History of radiation therapy
Wound secondary to burns, trauma, and diabetes
No obvious diagnosis

Diagnosis of an atypical wound frequently involves additional tests and imaging, including biopsy, blood tests, MRI, CT scan, or cultures.[3] Biopsy guidelines vary depending on the suspected diagnosis; therefore, referral to a specialist is advised. Recommended tests are discussed in the Medical Management component of each diagnosis.

MORPHOLOGY OF SKIN DISEASE

Many diseases will cause changes in the skin that are predictable and/or suggestive of a certain diagnosis. **TABLE 9-2** provides a list of terms and definitions of integumentary characteristics (based on size, texture, and color) that are used to describe abnormal skin appearance as well as atypical wound presentations.

CATEGORIES OF ATYPICAL WOUNDS

The atypical wounds discussed in this chapter can be categorized into the following groups: allergic reactions, immune-mediated tissue injury, infected wounds (bacterial, viral, and fungal), malignant wounds, and miscellaneous. Some categories will have common signs and symptoms and yet discrete but definite differences, and similar treatment strategies. The list is by no means exhaustive—that would be beyond the scope of this chapter!

TABLE 9-2 Skin Disease Morphology

Macule—A circumscribed, flat, nonpalpable lesion that is flush with the level of surrounding normal skin; smaller than 10 mm in diameter
Patch—A flat, nonpalpable lesion that is flush with the level of surrounding normal skin; greater than 10 mm in diameter
Papule—A superficial, circumscribed dome-shaped or-flat topped palpable lesion elevated above the skin surface; less than 10 mm in diameter
Plaque—A lesion that rises slightly above the surface of the skin; greater than 10 mm in diameter
Nodule—A firm lesion that is thicker or deeper than the average plaque or papule; is palpable as differentiated tissue
Vesicle—An elevated lesion that contains clear fluid; less than 10 mm in diameter
Bulla—An elevated lesion that contains clear fluid; greater than 10 mm in diameter
Pustule—An elevated lesion that contains pus
Urticarial (hives)—An allergic reaction characterized by white fluid-filled blisters (termed *wheals*) surrounded by erythema (flares)
Livedo reticularis—A mottled, lace-like purplish discoloration of the skin caused by thrombotic occlusion of the capillaries that leads to swelling of the venules
Wheals—transient and discrete areas of erythema in the epidermis and dermis; also referred to as hives

ALLERGIC REACTIONS

Allergic reactions can be either contact (the offending substance touches the skin) or systemic (the offending substance is injected or ingested). In either case, the substance is lysed by the macrophages and polymorphic neutrophilic lymphocytes (PMNs) and the resulting antigens (*anti*body *gen*erators) are presented to the host immune T cells, thereby activating the immune system. The subsequent immunological response results in the production of antibodies followed by inflammation. The reaction can cause wounds to develop, or in the case of existing wounds, prevent healing from progressing. The allergic response can vary from mild to life-threatening and will usually increase in severity with repeated exposure to the offending agent.

The first strategy for treating any allergic reaction is the identification of the offending substance and cessation of its use. Treatment of underlying comorbidities is also a critical component of successful treatment of the allergic reaction.

Contact Dermatitis

Pathophysiology Contact dermatitis can be either *allergic* or *irritant,* depending on the host immune system and the concentration of the irritant.[4] In *allergic contact dermatitis,* the offending substance or contact allergen (ie, a nonprotein chemical called *hapten*) reacts with the skin barrier to activate the innate immune response. The allergen binds to the carrier protein and creates a sensitizing antigen, the Langerhans cells carry the antigen to the T cells (specifically CD8+ T cells that are primed in lymphoid organs during sensitization and recruited in the skin upon re-exposure to the hapten),[4] and the T cells cause the release of lymphokines.[5] Subsequently, the inflammatory symptoms develop, including erythema, rash, itching, and in some cases vesicular lesions, followed by scaling and dry skin (**FIGURES 9-1** and **9-2**).[4] The allergic response can be either immediate or delayed and can involve both the skin and the subcutaneous tissue. The response usually increases in

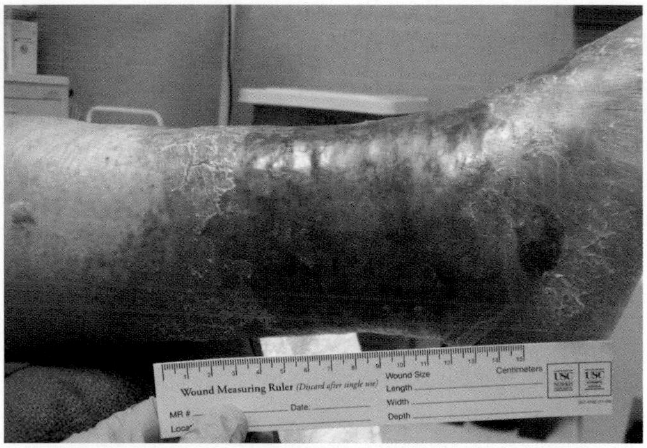

FIGURE 9-1 Contact dermatitis. Characteristics of contact dermatitis seen on the lower extremity are a well-defined border of exposure, erythema, rash (at the proximal aspect of the wound), and patient complaint of itching under the bandages. Some of the dressing components that can cause an allergic reaction are sulfa, silver, silicone, iodine, or latex. Careful subjective history about possible allergies is important to minimize the risk of reactions that may inhibit wound healing or even extend the wound.

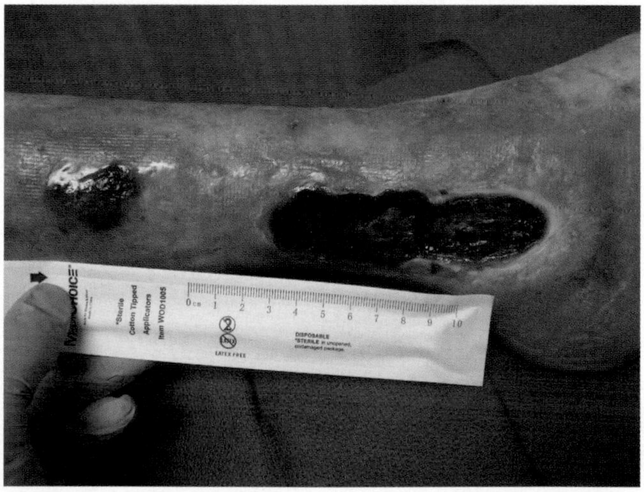

FIGURE 9-2 Contact dermatitis. This patient with a known latex allergy was being treated for a chronic venous wound using antimicrobial dressings and multilayered compression bandages. After progressing well for several months, the wound and periwound tissue began to deteriorate with numerous areas of partial thickness skin loss like the one proximal to the primary wound. Cessation of any dressings that contained silver resulted in an immediate reversal of the symptoms, confirming a suspicion that she had a silver allergy. Both infection and an allergic reaction can cause deterioration of the wound bed and are obviously treated quite differently. Confirmation of infection is by culture, and of allergy, by removing the suspected offending agent.

TABLE 9-3 Common Allergens for Contact Dermatitis

Contact allergens
Neomycin
Bacitracin
Wool
Alcohol
Formaldehyde
Parabens
Tape adhesives
Late
Perfumes
Metals (eg, nickel, silver)
Irritant allergens
Soap
Detergent
Cleaning solvents
Poison ivy or oak
Pesticides

severity after repeated exposures; sensitization upon first exposure may last 10–15 days with no clinical exposure clinical symptoms may appear within 24–72 hours.[4] **TABLE 9-3** lists the most common allergens and irritants, with nickel being the most frequent offender for both adults and children.[6]

The *irritant type of contact dermatitis* (ICD) is not an immunological response but a reaction to a caustic substance (eg, a chemical or topical liquid) and the severity of the reaction depends upon the concentration of the substance (**FIGURE 9-3**). Some antiseptics (eg, acetic acid or Dakin's solution) may cause irritant contact dermatitis if used repeatedly or in strong concentrations. ICD can also be caused by physical agents (UV radiation, X-rays, laser, ionizing radiation, and chemical warfare agents).[7] The inflammatory response is initiated by keratinocytes that produce cytokines upon exposure to the substance.[8]

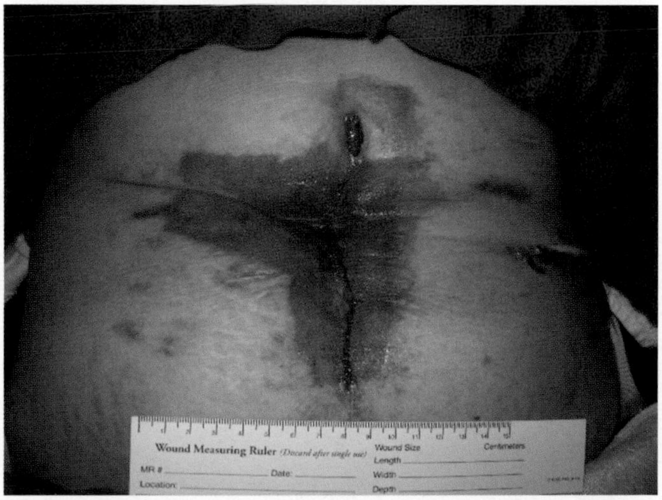

FIGURE 9-3 Irritant dermatitis. The severe erythema on the abdominal wound is a combination of contact dermatitis from the adhesive used with negative pressure therapy and irritant dermatitis from the drainage from the enterocutaneous fistula.

Patients with chronic leg wounds have an increased susceptibility to allergic contact dermatitis especially if they are being treated with compression therapy, a condition sometimes mistaken as *stasis dermatitis*. If contact dermatitis is suspected or if the patient reports a history of allergies to other substances, patch testing can be performed to confirm the diagnosis.[9]

Clinical Presentation Signs of acute allergic dermatitis include erythema, blisters, pustules, weeping, crusts, scales, and erosions, along with patient complaints of pain and itching. Chronic dermatitis is characterized by dry skin, lichenification (**FIGURE 9-4**), desquamation, and fissures. The onset of acute dermatitis is usually within 24–48 hours.[7] In severe cases, shiny skin and alopecia may develop. A visible determining factor is that the initial symptoms occur only in areas of direct contact with the irritating material, although ACD may have a tendency to spread beyond the contact border.[7]

Medical Management The most important component of treating any dermatitis is the identification and discontinuation of the medication, dressing, or other substances that might be responsible for the allergic response. In the acute phase, low-dose topical steroids and antihistamines may help decrease inflammation and discomfort; systemic steroids may be beneficial if there is an extensive area of contact dermatitis. Antibiotics are indicated only if there is evidence of secondary infection.[5]

Wound Management Patients usually require only supportive care and discontinuation of the irritating topical agent and, in the case of an existing wound, substitution of a dressing that has fewer or no allergens. Nonadherent hypoallergenic dressings are recommended for the care of open lesions. Most products that are used for wound care are available in latex-free forms, as both patients and clinicians can suffer from latex allergies. The skin will usually heal in 2–3 weeks.

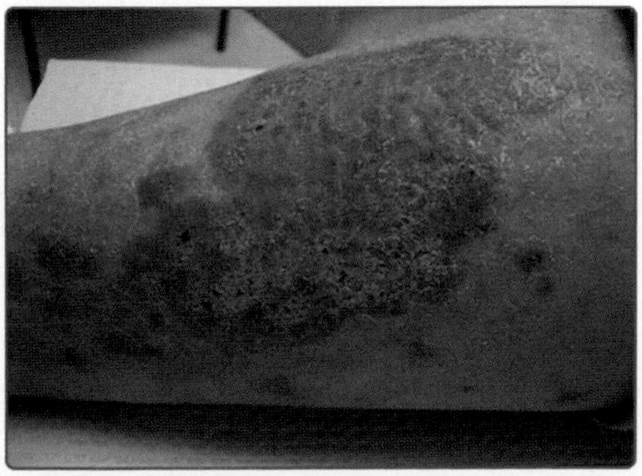

FIGURE 9-4 Lichenification. Lichenification is the thick leathery condition of the skin that can occur with chronic irritation (eg, eczema or edema from chronic venous insufficiency) especially if the patient tends to scratch the area a lot. (Used with permission from Kang S, Amagai M, Bruckner AL, et al, eds. *Fitzpatrick's Dermatology*. 9th ed. New York, NY: McGraw Hill; 2019, Figure 1-12.)

Drug-Induced Hypersensitivity Syndrome

Pathophysiology Drug-induced hypersensitivity syndrome (DIHS) is an immunologic response to a drug received either orally, by injection, or by IV. Although not fully understood, the process is similar to what occurs with skin allergies except that the immune response is activated by the causative agents and their metabolites rather than by a direct effect on the keratinocytes.[8] Recent studies show that the hypersensitivity reaction is a result of impaired function of regulatory T cells which act to suppress the immune system (termed *Tregs*) and their effect of activation of drug-specific T effector cells.[9] There are numerous DIHS syndromes based on severity, types of lesions, and underlying disease processes; however, all of them produce generalized (rather than localized) skin lesions and systemic symptoms. In the younger adult population (20–40 years), the syndrome is termed *erythema multiforme* (**TABLE 9-4**).

Adverse drug reactions have been classified as Type A: those that are predictable and dose-dependent reactions, including overdose, side effects, and drug interactions (eg, a gastrointestinal bleed following treatment with nonsteroidal anti-inflammatory drugs [NSAIDs]); and Type B, those that are unpredictable, are typically dose-independent, and may include immunologically mediated drug hypersensitivity or non-immune-mediated reactions, thus being considered allergic reactions.[10] The most commonly reported medications that cause DIHS are listed in **TABLE 9-5**.

Clinical Presentation Symptoms include generalized rash (with or without vesicles) and any of the following: local eruptions, fever, lymphedema, mucosal lesions, conjunctivitis, and epidermal sloughing (**FIGURES 9-5** to **9-7**). Onset is usually

TABLE 9-4 Drug-Induced Hypersensitivity Syndrome

Syndrome	Description
Erythema multiforme	Generalized rash with macular or popular skin eruptions; affects 20- to 40-year-olds
Drug rash with eosinophilia and systemic systems (Dress Syndrome) (**FIGURES 9-7**)	Three of the following symptoms are necessary for diagnosis: fever, exanthema, eosinophilia, atypical circulating lymphocytes, lymphadenopathy, hepatitis
Stevens–Johnson syndrome	Cutaneous lesions of papules, vesicles, or bullae covering <10% of the body surface area; mucosal lesions; conjunctivitis
Toxic epidermal necrolysis	Cutaneous lesions of papules, vesicles, or bullae covering >30% of the body surface area; mucosal lesions; conjunctivitis
Chemotherapy-induced acral erythema	Painful swelling and erythema of the palms and soles of patients on high-dose chemotherapy
Drug-induced lupus erythematosus	Lupus-type symptoms with skin signs associated with medications; resolves when medications withdrawn

Some of the more common drug-hypersensitivity syndrome nomenclature and symptoms have been reported in the literature.

Reproduced with permission from Hamm RL. Drug-induced hypersensitivity syndrome: diagnosis and treatment. *J Am Coll Clin Wound Spec.* 2012:3(4):77–81.

TABLE 9-5 Most Commonly Reported Medications That Cause Drug-Induced Hypersensitivity Reactions

Drug Class	Specific Drug	Latent Period
Angiotensin-converting enzyme inhibitors	Captopril	At any time
Xanthine oxidase Inhibitor	Allopurinol	2–6 weeks[11]
Antibiotics	Beta-lactams (pediatrics)[12]	Immediate: 1 hour Nonimmediate: ≥1 hour[13]
	Ceftriaxone	72 hours[14]
	Cyclosporine	
	Dapsone	Few days to weeks[15]
	Isoniazid	
	Levofloxacin	
	Minocycline	
	Penicillin	
	Sulfonamides	
	Trimethoprim	
Anticonvulsants	Carbamazepine	Usually 2–4 weeks; can be up to 3 months
	Lamotrigine	
	Phenobarbitone	
	Phenytoin	
	Primidone	
Antidepressants	Clomipramine (anafranil)	
Antifungals	Terbinafine	2–3 days
Antiretrovirals	Abacavir	
	Nevirapine	
Beta-blocker	Atenolol	
Biologic modifiers	Infliximab	
	Murine and humanized monoclonal antibodies	
	Recombinant interferons	
Drug-coloring agents	Blue dyes	
Calcium channel blockers	Diltiazem	2–3 days
Gold salts		
Antihypertensive	Hydralazine (apresoline)	
Immunosuppressants	Azathioprine	
Nonsteroidal anti-inflammatory drugs	Aspirin	
Antiarrhythmic	Procainamide	
Sodium channel blockers	Mexiletine	
Disease-modifying anti-rheumatic drugs	Sulfasalazine	

Reproduced with permission from Hamm, RL. Drug allergy: delayed cutaneous hypersensitivity reactions to drugs. *EMJ Allergy Immunol.* 2016;1(1):92–101. Courtesy of Dr. Rose Hamm.

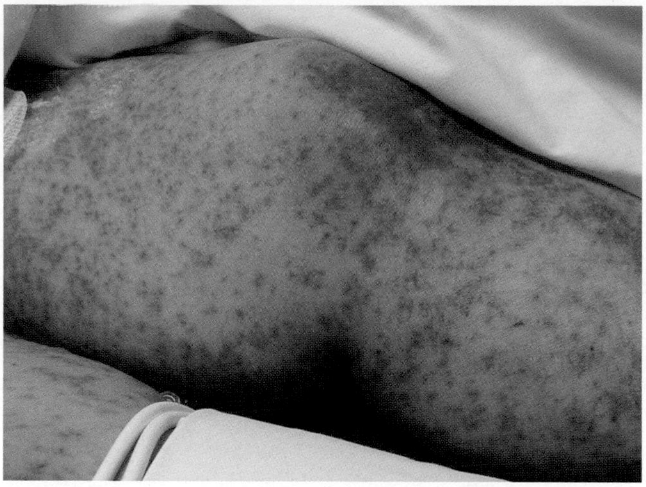

FIGURE 9-5 Drug-induced hypersensitivity syndrome. Diffuse generalized rash (with or without vesicles)—with symptoms of local eruptions, fever, lymphedema, mucosal lesions, conjunctivitis, and epidermal sloughing—can occur on any part of the body as a result of an allergic or hypersensitive reaction to ingested medications. Unlike a localized contact allergic response, DIHS involves a larger surface area without direct exposure to a specific substance.

1–3 weeks after the first exposure to the offending drug, beginning with a fever or sore throat and progressing to the cutaneous/mucosal involvement; however, in some cases, the reaction may occur up to 3 months after ingesting the drug. Other symptoms include the following:

- Epidermal blistering and sloughing with a positive Nikolsky sign, meaning lateral pressure on the edge of a blister results in dislodgement of the epidermis and extension of the blister (in toxic epidermal necrolysis and Stevens-Johnson syndrome).[16]
- Fever more than 38°C.

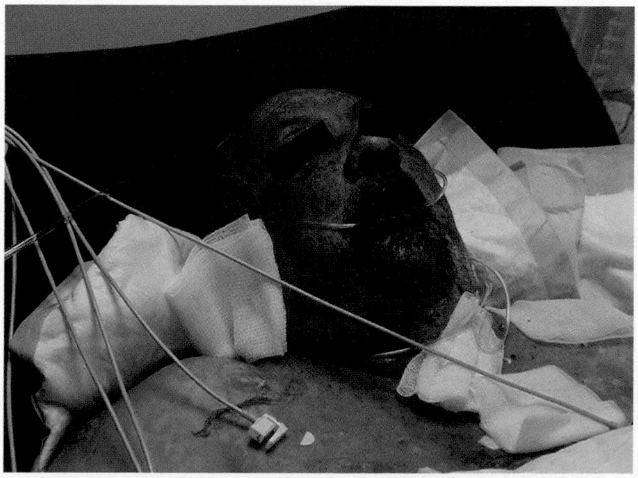

FIGURE 9-6 Mucosal lesions on a patient with toxic epidermal necrolysis.

- Symptoms that continue after discontinuation of the medication.
- Liver abnormalities (ALT > 100 U/L).
- Lymphadenopathy.
- Presence of at least one of the following leukocyte abnormalities:
  - Leukocytosis ($>11\times10^9$/L).
  - Atypical lymphocytosis (>5%).
  - Eosinophilia ($>1.5\times10^9$/L).[9]

Medical Management Medical management begins with the identification and cessation of the causative agent, which is usually the last one that the patient has initiated taking. Depending on the severity of the symptoms, corticosteroids are used to prevent progression and relieve symptoms, and supportive care is provided in an intensive care unit or a burn unit for more severe cases.

Wound Management In minor cases, cessation of the medication may be sufficient to reverse symptoms and no wound care is needed. In more severe cases with epidermal sloughing, treatment is like that of a deep superficial burn. Debate continues about debridement of the detached epidermal tissue and covering with dressings versus aspiration of blisters and leaving the epidermis intact until re-epithelialization has been achieved.[17] On any open areas, nonadherent antimicrobial dressings are recommended to help prevent infection and to avoid further skin tearing with dressing changes. Prevention of fluid loss and infection is paramount, and as the patient improves, dressings to promote re-epithelialization are advised.

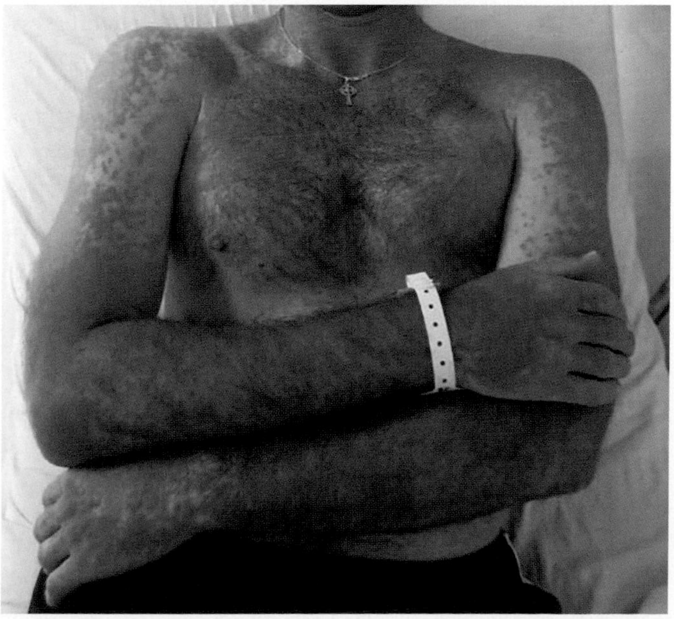

FIGURE 9-7 DRESS. (From Loscalzo J, Fauci AS, Kasper DL, et al, eds. *Harrison's Principles of Internal Medicine*. 21st ed. New York, NY: McGraw Hill; 2022, Figure 60-6. Reproduced with permission from Gildo Micheletti, MD.)

AUTOIMMUNE DISORDERS

Scleroderma

Pathophysiology Scleroderma (systemic sclerosis) is a chronic autoimmune connective tissue disorder of unknown etiology that usually affects women between the ages of 30 and 50 and results in extensive scarring and disfigurement as it progresses.[18] The skin becomes thick and hard (sclerotic) with a buildup of scar tissue, resulting in loss of skin elasticity, joint range of motion, muscle strength, mobility, and function. There is also damage to internal organs such as the heart and blood vessels, lungs, esophagus, kidneys, and other organs, which is a major factor in determining the prognosis for each individual patient.[19]

Recent studies suggest that the disease is multifactorial with immune imbalance, oxidative stress, genetics, and environmental factors contributing to its pathophysiology.[20] The most robust associations include genes for B- and T-cell activation and innate immunity; other pathways include genes involved in extracellular matrix deposition, cytokines, and autophagy (the natural, regulated mechanism of cellular activity that allows orderly degradation and recycling of cellular components).[21] The sequence of scleroderma involves the following: arteriole endothelial cells die by apoptosis and are replaced by collagen; inflammatory cells infiltrate the arteriole and cause more damage, resulting in the scarred fibrotic tissue that is the hallmark of scleroderma.[22,23]

Clinical Presentation The two main types of scleroderma are *localized* and *systemic*. Localized is further differentiated into *morphea* with discolored patches on the skin, and *linear* with streaks or bands of thick hard skin on the arms and legs. Localized scleroderma only affects the skin and not the internal organs. Systemic scleroderma can be limited (affecting only the arms, hands, and face) or diffuse (rapidly progressing, affecting large areas of the skin and one or more organs). Thirty-five percent of the patients with scleroderma develop skin ulcers that are painful, refractory, and usually over bony prominences (**FIGURE 9-8**). CREST, a limited systemic form of scleroderma, is described in **TABLE 9-6**; however, it does not reflect the internal organ involvement that may also be present. In addition, patients may experience joint pain, fatigue, depression, reduced libido, and altered body image. A third type is limited systemic sclerosis, also known as *sine scleroderma*, which includes Raynaud's phenomenon and internal involvement without sclerotic skin.[24]

TABLE 9-6 Symptoms of CREST, a Scleroderma Syndrome

Calcinosis—calcium deposits, usually in the fingers
Raynaud phenomenon—color changes in fingers and sometimes toes after exposure to cold temperatures
Esophageal dysfunction—loss of muscle control, which can cause difficulty swallowing
Sclerodactyly—tapering deformity of the bones of the fingers
Telangiectasia—small red spots on the skin of the fingers, face, or inside of the mouth

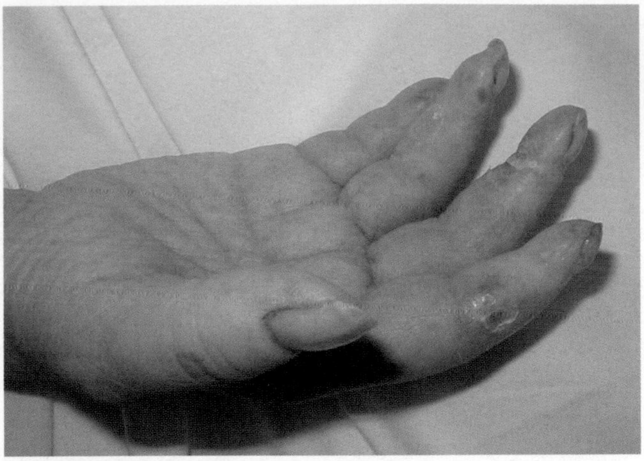

FIGURE 9-8 Scleroderma. Scleroderma causes the skin to lose its elasticity, resulting in loss of joint range of motion, strength, and function. The thick linear bands around the fingers are indicative of localized linear scleroderma.

Medical Management Because the etiology is unknown, treatment of scleroderma centers on alleviating symptoms, preserving skin integrity with protective strategies, preventing infection, and controlling inflammation to minimize severity.[25] d-penicillamine, colchicine, PUVA, relaxin, cyclosporine, and omega-oil derivatives have been used to treat the skin fibrosis. Recent studies show promise in treating sclerotic wounds with autologous adipose transplants because they are a source of stem cells and their ability to reverse skin fibrosis.[26,27] Immunosuppressive agents such as methotrexate and cyclosporine have been used to treat the systemic disease, and plasmapheresis can be used in severe cases.[1] Newer therapies for systemic scleroderma include the tyrosine kinase inhibitor Nintedanib for SSc-ILD and the IL-6 signaling inhibitor Tocilizumab.[28]

Wound Management Local wound care is tedious because of the high pain levels associated with open wounds on sclerotic skin, and wound healing is impeded by the scarring of the subcutaneous tissue and the immunosuppressive medications. Enzymatic debridement with collagenase may be helpful with painful wounds, as well as occlusive dressings to help with autolytic debridement. Nonadherent dressings are advised both to minimize pain and avoid tearing skin upon removal. Silicone-backed foam dressings are useful as secondary dressings. Patient education regarding protective measures for skin is crucial, for example, using gloves when doing housework, avoiding caustic liquids, wearing warm clothes to avoid Raynaud's phenomenon, and using moisturizers to avoid dry skin. As the disease progresses, custom shoes with molded inserts to accommodate changes in the shape of the feet can help maintain independent ambulation.

Vasculitis

Pathophysiology Vasculitis encompasses a variety of inflammatory disorders of blood vessels which can ultimately

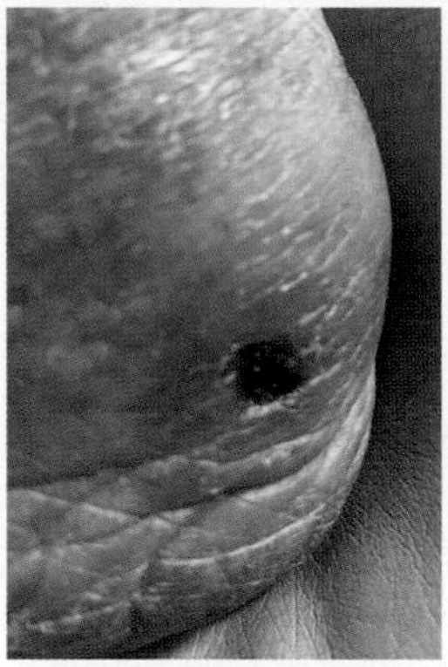

FIGURE 9-9 Wound on the heel of a patient who has been taking long-term hydroxyurea. The wound is ischemic as a result of occluded arterioles with necrotic tissue and exquisite pain.

result in organ damage, including the skin. It is classified as small, medium, or large vessel vasculitis depending on the size of the vessel involved. The etiology is often idiopathic—it is a reaction pattern that may be triggered by certain comorbidities including underlying infection, malignancy, medication (eg, hydroxyurea[29,30]) (**FIGURE 9-9**), and connective tissue diseases such as systemic lupus erythematosus (**FIGURE 9-10**). Circulating immune complexes (antibody/antigen) deposit in the blood vessel walls, causing inflammation that may be segmental or involve the entire vessel. At the site of inflammation, varying degrees of cellular inflammation and resulting necrosis or scarring occur in one or more layers of the vessel wall, and inflammation in the media of the muscular artery tends to destroy the internal elastic lamina.[31,32]

Leukocytoclastic vasculitis, a histopathologic term used to describe findings in small-vessel vasculitis, refers to the breakdown of inflammatory cells that leaves small nuclear fragments in and around the vessels. Vasculitic inflammation tends to be transmural, rarely necrotizing, and nongranulomatous. Resolution of the inflammation tends to result in fibrosis and intimal hypertrophy, which in combination with secondary clot formation can narrow the arterial lumen and account for the ischemia or necrosis of the tissue supplied by the affected vessels.[33] Clinical symptoms (ie, tissue loss) depend on the artery or arteries that are involved and the extent of lumen occlusion. Vasculitic syndromes based on the affected vessels are listed in **TABLE 9-7**.

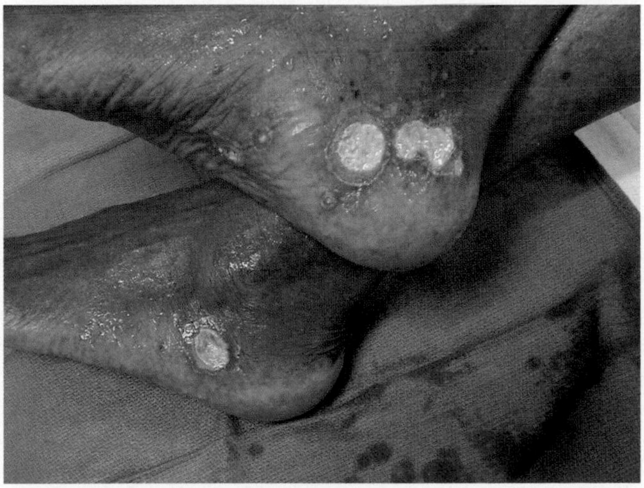

FIGURE 9-10 Vasculitis due to SLE. Vasculitis presents as dermal necrosis as a result of occluded small arterioles and is exquisitely painful, making local care very difficult. Patients with autoimmune disorders, for example, systemic lupus erythematosus (SLE), are at greater risk for vasculitis. The medications used to treat SLE further complicate and inhibit wound healing; however, the first medical priority is to suppress the inflammatory response.

Clinical Presentation Clinical presentation of cutaneous vasculitis, which varies depending on the arterial involvement, includes palpable purpura, livedo reticularis, pain, skin lesions with or without nodules, and tissue necrosis. It may present as one large necrotic lesion or several small lesions, but all are full thickness after debridement. Systemic symptoms may also be present and usually relate to kidneys, lungs, or gastrointestinal tract involvement. On some occasions, signs of vasculitis in other organs may appear before or at the same time that skin lesions appear (**FIGURES 9-11** and **9-12**). One very distinctive characteristic for differential diagnosis from chronic venous wounds is the exquisite pain that occurs with vasculitis, making the initial local treatment very tedious.

Medical Management Treatment of any vasculitis depends on the etiology, extent, and severity of the disease. Ultrasound can be used to detect abnormalities in medium- and large-vessel diseases and to determine distribution or organ involvement in small vessel vasculitides.[34] For secondary vasculitic disorders, treating the underlying comorbidity (eg, infection, drug use, cancer, or autoimmune disorder) is crucial.

Remission of life- or organ-threatening disorders is induced by using cytotoxic immune-suppressants (eg, cyclophosphamide) and high-dose corticosteroids, usually for 3–6 months, until remission occurs or until the disease activity is acceptably reduced. Adjusted treatment to maintain remission takes longer, usually 1–2 years. During this period, the goal is to eliminate corticosteroids, reduce the dosage, or use less potent immune-suppressants if needed. After tapering or eliminating corticosteroids, methotrexate or azathioprine can be substituted to maintain remission.[35]

Wound Management Initial treatment of wounds caused by vasculitis is extremely difficult because of the pain. The principles of standard wound care (debride necrotic tissue, treat inflammation and infection, apply moist wound dressings, nurture the edges, and ensure optimal oxygen supply, termed *TIMEO2*)[36] are recommended. Topical lidocaine helps reduce pain during treatments, noncontact low-frequency ultrasound helps mobilize cellular activity and interstitial fluids, and compression therapy helps manage the edema that occurs in the lower extremities because of inflammation and decreased mobility. Nonadherent dressings that promote autolysis of the necrotic tissue (eg, X-Cell, Medline, Mundelein, and IL) are excellent initially, especially in reducing pain levels with

TABLE 9-7 Vasculitic Syndromes Based on Affected Vessels

Name	Typical Vessels Involved	Symptoms
Behçet's disease	Small vessels	Recurrent painful lesions in the mouth, on the genitals, on the skin (acne-like), or in the eye (uveitis); limb claudication
Buerger's disease (thromboangiitis)	vessels to the hands and feet	Typically in smokers; thin shiny skin, thick nails, pain in hands and/or feet; cyanosis that may result in tissue necrosis
Churg–Strauss syndrome (eosinophilic granulomatosis with polyangiitis)	Small and medium vessel	Three stages: 1. Airway inflammation, asthma, allergic rhinitis 2. Hypereosinophilia 3. Vasculitis with tissue necrosis, beginning with purpura
Cryoglobulinemia	Small vessels	Often associated with hepatitis C; appears as painful purpura that progresses to full-thickness, often infected wounds, usually on these distal digits. Precipitated by exposure to cold environment that leads to presence of coagulated cryoglobulins that clog the small vessels
Giant cell arteritis	Temporal and cranial arteries	Headaches, temporal pain, visual disturbances, scalp sensitivity, dry cough with respiratory symptoms, fever, upper extremity weakness and sensory changes, unequal BP measurements or unequal/absent pulses in the limbs. May be associated with polymyalgia rheumatica
Henoch–Schönlein purpura (IgA vasculitis)	Small vessels	Purpura, arthritis, abdominal pain (usually in children)
Hypersensitivity vasculitis (allergic vasculitis, cutaneous vasculitis, or leukocytoclastic vasculitis)	Small vessels in the skin	Purpura, usually on the lower extremities or back (in bedridden patients) due to an allergic reaction to a medication
Immune complex–associated vasculitis	Small vessels to neurons	Peripheral neuropathy
Kawasaki's disease	Any of the vessels, any size	Skin erythema, enlarged lymph nodes, red mucous membranes, and in some cases heart problems; occurs in childhood
Microscopic polyangiitis	Small vessels to organs	Ischemia, hemorrhage, loss of organ function
Polyarteritis nodosa	Small and medium arteries	Subcutaneous nodules or projections of lesions; fever, chills, tachycardia, arthralgia, myositis, motor and sensory neuropathies
Primary angiitis of the CNS	Small and medium vessels in the brain and spinal cord	Brain: headache, altered mental status, focal CNS deficits; spinal cord: lower extremity weakness, bladder dysfunction
Takayasu's arteritis	Aorta, aorta branches, pulmonary arteries	Inflammatory phase with flu-like symptoms, pulseless upper extremity, claudication, renal artery disease; fatigue, night sweats, sore joints, and weight loss may occur first
Wegener's granulomatosis (granulomatosis with polyangiitis)	Small and medium vessels	Organ failure (lung and kidneys), variable including skin, depending on the vessels involved

Note: The trend is to classify the diseases by descriptive names rather than by names referring to the discovering physician.

Reproduced with permission from Hamm R. Why isn't this wound healing? In Schiffman M, ed. *Recent Clinical Techniques, Results, and Research in Wounds*. Springer; 2018.

dressing changes. Silicone-backed foam dressings are helpful in absorbing exudate as well as in reducing pain. If the patient is on steroids, local vitamin A can be used to negate the effects of steroids. As the acute inflammation recedes, pain levels decrease, and wound healing progresses to proliferation, treatment can be more aggressive with the goals of full re-epithelialization and return to the prior level of function. In the case of high-dose hydroxyurea wounds, discontinuation of the medication may result in spontaneous healing or surgical debridement may be needed to obtain full wound closure.[29,30]

Antiphospholipid Syndrome

Pathophysiology Antiphospholipid syndrome (APS) is an acquired autoimmune disorder that causes hypercoagulability which in turn results in thrombotic events (arterial, venous), pregnancy morbidity (miscarriage, late intrauterine fetal demise, severe pre-eclampsia), or catastrophic antiphospholipid syndrome (microvascular).[37] Antibodies are directed against one or more phospholipid-binding proteins (eg, anti-β2-glycoprotein I, anticardiolipin, and lupus anticoagulant) or their associated plasma proteins, resulting in hypercoagulation.[38] APS is characterized by elevated titers of different antiphospholipid antibodies.[22] The proteins normally bind to phospholipid membrane constituents and protect them from excessive coagulation activation. The autoantibodies displace the protective proteins and thus produce procoagulant endothelial cell surfaces and cause arterial or venous thrombosis.

The lupus anticoagulant is an antiphospholipid autoantibody that binds to protein-phospholipid complexes. It was initially recognized in patients with SLE; however, these patients now account for a minority of patients with autoantibodies.

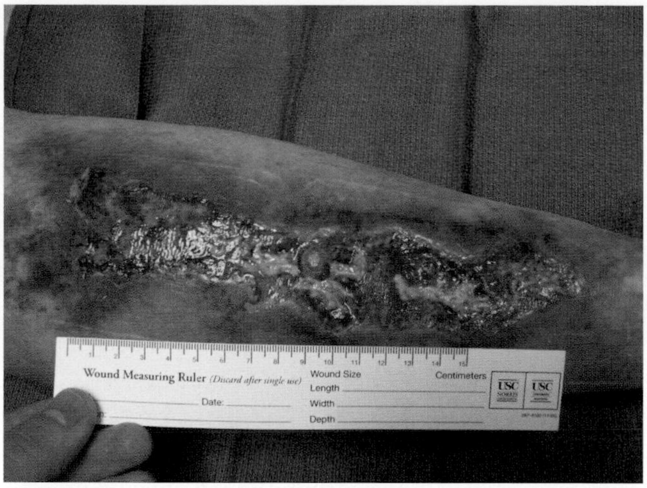

FIGURE 9-11 Vasculitis associated with other symptoms. This patient with vasculitis of the posterior calf noted the onset of pain and dermal symptoms at the same time that he experienced neurological signs associated with what was diagnosed as a CVA. Both maladies occurred after the stress of losing a family member. Note the discoloration of the proximal periwound skin, indicating that the inflammation is still evolving.

The lupus anticoagulant is suspected if the PTT is prolonged and does not correct immediately upon 1:1 mixing with normal plasma but does return to normal upon the addition of an excessive quantity of phospholipids (done by the hematology laboratory). Antiphospholipid antibodies in the patient's plasma are measured by immunoassays of IgG and IgM antibodies that bind to phospholipid-β_2-glycoprotein I complexes on microtiter plates.[22] APS can occur with or without the associated rheumatic diseases (eg, systemic lupus erythematosus).[39]

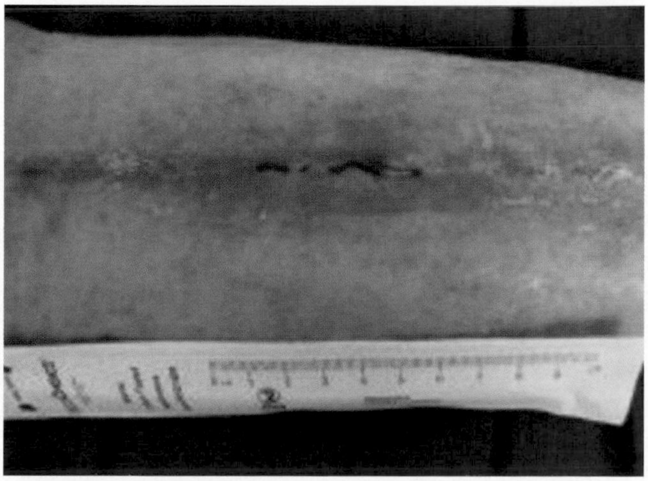

FIGURE 9-12 Vasculitis in the remodeling phase of healing. The patient in **FIGURE 9-11** was treated with low-frequency noncontact ultrasound, nonadherent dressings to facilitate autolytic debridement and compression therapy. He progressed to full closure of the wounds without surgical intervention. Topical 2% lidocaine gel was applied prior to each treatment to assist with pain management.

Clinical Presentation The arteriole thrombosis results in venous swelling, creating the typical livedo reticularis skin appearance. In addition, the lower extremities may have retiform purpura, splinter hemorrhages, Reynaud phenomenon, or superficial thrombophlebitis[40] (**FIGURE 9-13**). As the disease progresses, skin necrosis may occur, and if the disorder occurs during pregnancy, there will be fetal demise. If the thrombosis is in the venules, the result may be DVT with lower extremity edema, tachypnea due to pulmonary emboli, and ascites.[41] Other associated clinical manifestations include thrombocytopenia, hemolytic anemia, valvular heart disease, and nephropathy.[38] The catastrophic antiphospholipid syndrome may have neurologic presentations, the most common being stroke.[41]

Medical Management Asymptomatic individuals in whom blood test findings are positive do not require specific treatment. Prophylactic therapy involves the elimination of other risk factors such as oral contraceptives, smoking, hypertension, or hyperlipidemia, especially for children who test positive for the antibodies.[42] For patients with SLE, hydroxychloroquine, an anti-inflammatory that may have intrinsic antithrombotic properties, may be useful. Statins are beneficial for patients with hyperlipidemia. The standard care for the patient with thrombosis is full anticoagulation with Vitamin K antagonists (intravenous or subcutaneous heparin followed by warfarin therapy).[18,19,22,23,30,41,43] Triple therapy with anticoagulation, corticosteroids, and plasma exchange is the standard of care for patients with catastrophic antiphospholipid syndrome.[41]

Based on the most recent evidence, a reasonable target for the international normalized ratio (INR) is 2.0–3.0 for venous thrombosis and 3.0 for arterial thrombosis. Patients with recurrent thrombotic events, while well maintained on the above regimens, may require an INR of 3.0–4.0. For severe or refractory cases, a combination of warfarin and aspirin may be used. Treatment for significant thrombotic events in patients

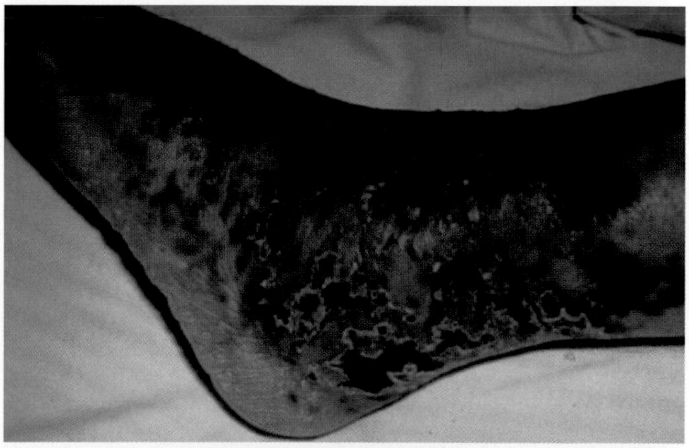

FIGURE 9-13 Antiphospholipid syndrome. Antiphospholipid syndrome is characterized in the early stages by livedo reticularis (resulting in small brown spots on the skin) and in the later stages by ischemic skin changes. (Used with permission from External Manifestations. In: Lichtman MA, Shafer MS, Felgar RE, Wang N, eds. *Lichtman's Atlas of Hematology 2016*. New York, NY: McGraw Hill; 2016, Figure XI.A.004.)

with APS is generally lifelong. Because cutaneous manifestations are the first sign of APS in up to 41% of patients, a full medical examination is advised for any patient showing clinical symptoms in order to identify and treat the underlying pathology.[44,45]

Wound Management Conservative wound care is recommended for patients with skin lesions, keeping the wound moist and following wound bed preparation principles. Healing of wounds caused by other etiologies, eg, trauma or spider bites, will be delayed in patients who have APS.

Pemphigus

Pathophysiology Pemphigus is an autoimmune blistering disease resulting from the loss of normal intercellular attachments in the skin and oral mucosal membrane. Circulating antibodies attack the cell surface adhesion molecule desmoglein at the desmosomal cell junction in the suprabasal layer of the epidermis, resulting in the destruction of the adhesion molecules (acantholysis) and initiating an inflammatory response that causes blistering. The four forms of pemphigus are the following:

- Pemphigus foliaceus (**FIGURE 9-14**) with Ig antibodies against desmoglein 1 and 3 throughout the deeper layers of the skin thus causing deeper lesions.
- Pemphigus vulgaris with Ig autoantibodies against desmoglein 1 in all layers of the epidermis with more superficial lesions.
- IgA pemphigus with antibodies that attack adhesive proteins in the epidermis; have intercellular deposition of IfA; usually occurs with an underlying autoimmune disease.[46]
- Paraneoplastic pemphigus that has Ig autoantibodies against plakins and desmogleins, always with an underlying malignant disorder, usually a lymphoproliferative disease (**FIGURE 9-15**).[47,48]

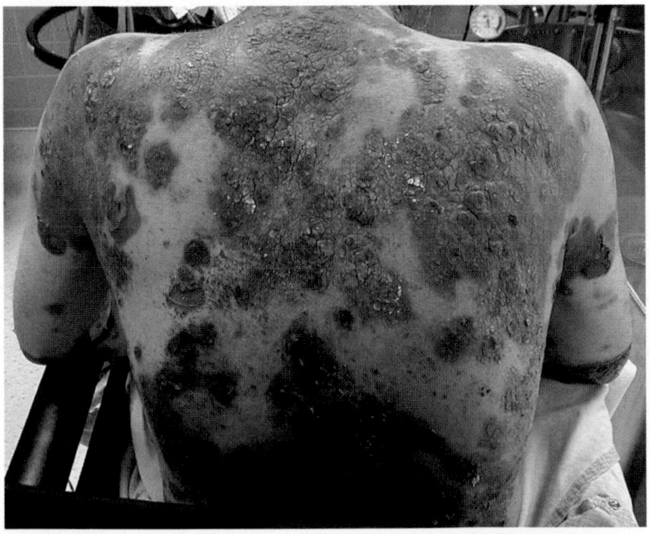

FIGURE 9-14 Pemphigus. Pemphigus foliaceous is characterized by blistering of the epidermis followed by crusting and sloughing, resulting in painful wounds and discoloration after healing. Complications include bacterial and viral infections as a result of the open wounds and immunosuppression, as well as sequelae from long-term use of corticosteroids (osteoporosis, avascular necrosis).

Desmogleins are adhesive proteins that are responsible for cell-to-cell adhesions within the epidermis. When these proteins are attacked, the cells lose their adhesion and a resulting inflammatory response causes the blistering that is characteristic of pemphigus disorders.[49]

Clinical Presentation *Pemphigus vulgaris*, the most common type, involves the mucosa and skin, especially of the scalp, face, axilla, groins, trunk, and points of pressure.

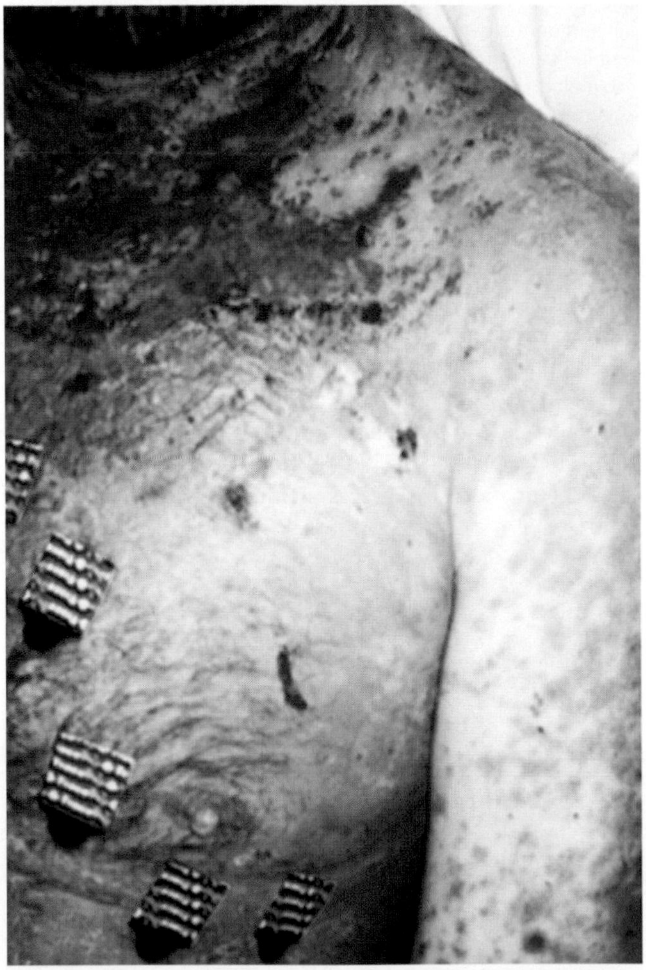

FIGURE 9-15 Paraneoplastic pemphigus. Characteristics of paraneoplastic pemphigus include extensive lesions on the lips, severe stomatitis, and erythematous macules and papules that coalesce into large cutaneous lesions. The lesions are diagnosed by biopsy that shows a mix of individual cell necrosis, interface change, and acantholysis. (Used with permission from Anhalt GJ, Mimouni D. Paraneoplastic pemphigus. In: Goldsmith LA, Katz SI, Gilchrest BA, Paller AS, Leffell DJ, Wolff K, eds. *Fitzpatrick's Dermatology in General Medicine*. 8th ed. New York, NY: McGraw Hill; 2012, Figure 55-2C.)

Patients usually present with painful oral mucosal erosions and flaccid blisters, erosions, crusts, and macular erythema in areas of skin involvement.[23,43] The primary cell adhesion loss is at the deeper suprabasal layer. *Pemphigus foliaceus* is a milder form of the disease, with the acantholysis occurring more superficially in the epidermis, usually on the face and chest. *IgA pemphigus* presents with tense bullae that transition in to clear fluid-filled blisters seen primarily in flexural areas of the proximal extremities and trunk.[49] *Paraneoplastic pemphigus*, in addition to having different autoantibodies, occurs exclusively in patients who have some type of malignancy, and because of the malignancy, mortality is high in this type of pemphigus.[50]

Diagnosis is confirmed by using immunofluorescence to demonstrate the Ig autoantibodies against the cell surface of intraepidermal keratinocytes.

Medical Management Medical treatment consists of systemic corticosteroids, immunosuppressive agents, and intravenous immune globulin with dosage depending upon the severity of the disease. For patients who have refractory pemphigus vulgaris, a combination of rituximab and intravenous immunoglobulin therapy is recommended to prevent relapse.[47,51]

Wound Management Wound management is conservative with the goal of preventing infection and promoting reepithelialization in areas where denuding occurs with the blistering. Flat antimicrobial dressings (eg, Acticoat Flex, Smith & Nephew, Largo, FL) are useful over open areas, and hydrotherapy is beneficial when the disease is widespread and in the crusty phase. Secondary dressings are required for most areas and can include surgical or fish-net garments. Silicone-backed foam dressings without adhesive borders are also recommended for easy removal of loose necrotic tissue without causing painful skin tears.

Bullous Pemphigoid

Pathophysiology Bullous pemphigoid (BP) is a subepidermal autoimmune blistering disease associated with tissue-bound and circulating autoantibodies directed against BP antigen 180 (also known as BPAG 2) and BP antigen 230 (also known as BPAG 1), both components of the basement membrane.[23,52] An immune reaction is initiated by the formation of IgG autoantibodies that target dystonin, a component of the hemidesmosomes, resulting in the infiltration of immune cells and degradation of the basement membrane. The consequence is a separation of the dermal/epidermal junction with fluid collection and blistering or bullae. The severity of the disease is IgE dose-dependent and correlates with the degree of eosinophil infiltration in the skin.[53] Diagnosis is confirmed by the presence of linear deposits of IgG and/or C3 along the dermal–epidermal junction on direct immunofluorescence and IgG class circulating autoantibodies that bind to the epidermal (roof) side of the skin basement membrane on indirect immunofluorescence.[23,54]

Triggering factors that have been associated with BP include drugs (most frequently gliptins, PD-1/PD-L1 inhibitors, loop diuretics, penicillin, and derivatives),[55] thermal or electrical burns, surgical procedures, trauma, ultraviolet irradiation, radiotherapy, chemical preparations, transplants, and infections. Predisposing factors are aging, genetics, and co-morbidities.[56]

Clinical Presentation BP occurs most commonly among the elderly, and the most common sites of involvement include inner aspects of thighs, flexor aspects of forearms, axilla, groin, and oral cavity. The extremities can also become involved. Itching is the first dominating symptom of BP, which progresses to urticarial lesions, erythematous edema, papules, eczematous lesions, and typically widespread tense bullae filled with clear fluid (**FIGURE 9-16**).[52]

Medical Management Anti inflammatory agents (corticosteroids, tetracyclines, dapsone) and immunosuppressants (azathioprine, methotrexate, mycophenolate mofetil, cyclophosphamide) are the most commonly used medications for BP, usually for 6–60 months, after which most patients will have long-term remission. Longer treatment may be required for patients who have chronic BP.[57] Omalizumab, a humanized monoclonal antibody against IgE, is used primarily for refractory cases or for cases in which aggressive immunosuppression is contraindicated; however, recent studies suggest that it may be useful as a primary treatment.[58] Identification and removal of any triggering factors may improve the prognosis.[56]

Wound Management Wound management recommendations are the same as for pemphigus, with the goal of minimizing pain, preventing infection, and promoting re-epithelialization.

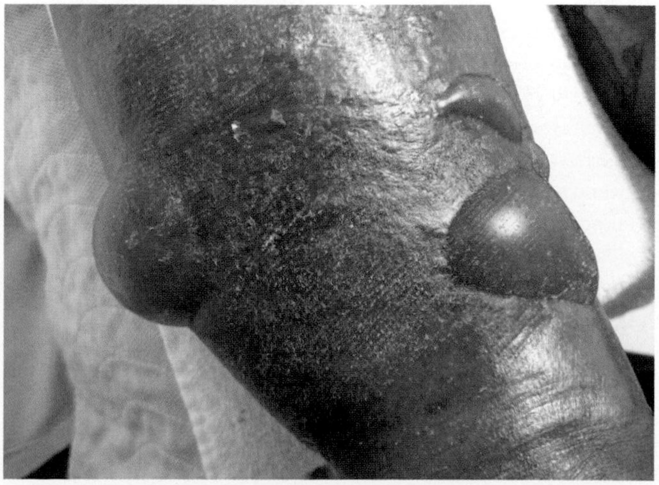

FIGURE 9-16 Bullous pemphigoid. Tense bullae filled with clear fluid (a result of the inflammatory process) are typical of bullous pemphigoid.

Cryoglobulinemia

Pathophysiology Cryoglobulins are abnormal proteins (immunoglobulins), and cryoglobulinemia is the presence of these proteins in the blood. They coagulate or become thick and gel-like in temperatures below body temperature (37°C), thereby clogging the small blood vessels and resulting in vasculitic damage that causes hypoxic skin changes, ischemic wounds, and/or other organ damage[59] (**TABLE 9-8**). The symptoms may be reversible if the environmental temperature is warmed. The disorder is grouped into three main types, depending on the type of antibody that is produced: Type I (usually with monoclonal IgM) is most often related to cancer of the blood or immune system, for example, multiple myeloma; Types II and III (polyclonal IgG), also referred to as mixed cryoglobulinemia, most often occur in people who have a chronic inflammatory condition, for example, hepatitis C, Sjögren syndrome, or systemic lupus erythematosus.[60] Type II is the most common type, and most of these patients also have hepatitis C.[1,23]

Cryofibrinogenemia is similar to cryoglobulinemia except that there are no serum cryoglobulins and the onset of skin changes is sudden and without the initial purpura that occurs with cryoglobulinemia.[61]

Clinical Presentation Symptoms vary depending on the type of cryoglobulinemia present and the organs that are affected. Systemic signs that occur with Types II and III may include difficulty breathing, fatigue, glomerulonephritis, joint pain, and muscle pain. Integumentary signs may begin with purpura and Raynaud's phenomenon (**FIGURE 9-17**). The Meltzer triad that is associated with Types II and III includes arthralgia, purpura, and weakness.[60] See **TABLE 9-8** for a list of cryoglobulinemia symptoms.

TABLE 9-8 Symptoms of Cryoglobulinemia

Local/Integumentary	General/Systemic
Type I	Type I
Lesions in head and mucosa	Retinal hemorrhage
Acrocyanosis	Arterial thrombosis
Severe Raynaud's phenomenon	Renal disease
Digital ulceration	Types II and III
Skin necrosis	Breathing difficulty
Livedo reticularis	Fatigue
Purpura	Arthralgia (PIP, MCP, knees, ankles)
Types II and III	Myalgia
Lesions in lower extremities	Immune complex deposition
Erythematous macules	Cough
Palpable purpura	Pleurisy
Raynaud phenomenon	Abdominal pain
Cutaneous vasculitis	Fever
Peripheral neuropathy	Hepatomegaly or signs of cirrhosis
Nailfold capillary abnormalities	Hypertension

Data from Edgerton CC, Diamond HS. Cryoglobulinemia clinical presentation. Available at: http://emedicine.medscape.com/article/329255. Accessed July 27, 2018.

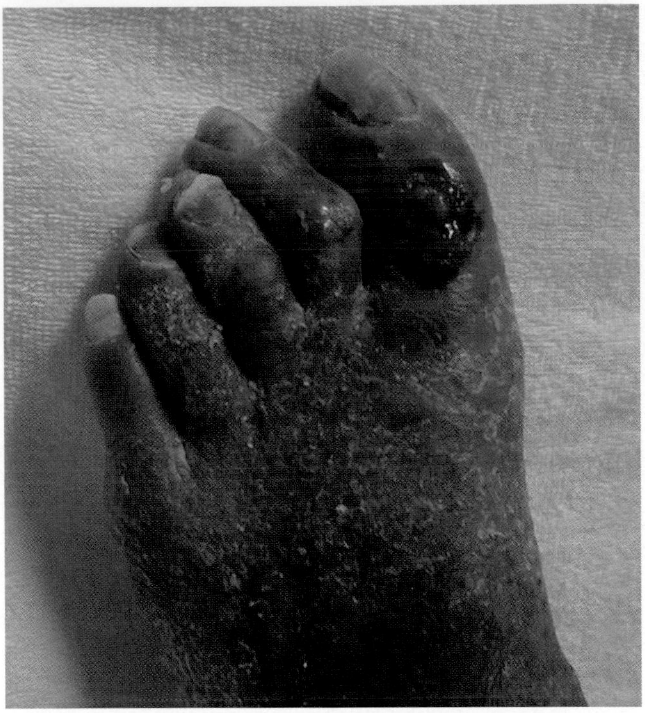

FIGURE 9-17 Cryoglobulinemia. Cryoglobulinemia on the foot of a patient with hepatitis C. Classic signs include purpura, loss of dermis due to occlusion of the small vessels to the skin, severe pain, and tendency to develop infections. This patient's wounds healed with the use of antibiotics, standard wound care, and modified compression therapy; however, when he returned to a cold climate his symptoms recurred.

Medical Management The goal of treating cryoglobulinemia is to treat the underlying cause (which will often treat or prevent cutaneous symptoms) and to limit the precipitant cryoglobulin and subsequent inflammatory effects. Simply avoiding cold temperatures can treat mild cases.[61] Standard hepatitis C treatments usually work for patients who have hepatitis C and mild or moderate cryoglobulinemia; however, the condition can return when treatment stops. NSAIDs may be used to treat mild cases that involve arthralgia and myalgia. Severe cryoglobulinemia (involving vital organs or large areas of skin) is treated with corticosteroids, immunosuppressants, interferon, or cytotoxic medications.[62] Plasmapheresis may be indicated if the complications are life-threatening.[60]

Wound Management Wound care involves the treatment of infection and pain management, especially in the early stages. Nonadherent dressings such as X-Cell (Medline, Mundelein, IL), hydrogel, Acticoat (Smith & Nephew, Largo, FL), and petrolatum gauze help minimize pain with dressing changes and promote autolytic debridement. A topical anesthetic is advised 10–15 minutes before initiating any sharp debridement; enzymatic debridement may also be beneficial but can cause stinging and burning upon application. Absorbent dressings are advised if there is wound drainage, and modified compression (eg, with short stretch bandages) helps reduce the edema that occurs with chronic inflammation, immobility, and lower extremity dependency. Compression bandages also help keep the extremities warm and facilitate vasodilation. If edema is not severe, warm hydrotherapy can help reduce the precipitation of the cryoglobulins and relieve ischemic pain. Patient education regarding avoidance of cold or wearing warm clothing such as thermal socks is a crucial component of long-term management.

Pyoderma Gangrenosum

Pathophysiology Pyoderma gangrenosum (PG) is an autoimmune disorder of unknown etiology that leads to painful skin necrosis. PG is commonly associated with other inflammatory diseases such as Crohn's disease, inflammatory bowel syndrome, arthritis, and hematologic malignancy.[63] Pathergy, the development of skin lesions around trauma or the enlargement of initially small lesions, is commonly seen with PG, especially if debridement of necrotic tissue is attempted. Neutrophilic dermatosis occurs with altered neutrophilic chemotaxis and is thought to be part of the pathology.[64]

Clinical Presentation PG ulcers usually begin as small pustules or blisters (termed *cat's paw appearance*[65] and become larger with a violaceous border and surrounding erythema. The first lesion may be at the site of minor trauma but will progress and enlarge rapidly. Often the wound edge is undermined. They are painful, necrotic, and usually recurring. Sometimes PG will appear in groups of lesions at different stages of formation or healing. They do not respond to standard care if diagnosed as another wound type and indeed may worsen if the standard TIMEO2 care, particularly aggressive debridement, is administered (**FIGURES 9-18** to **9-20**). The following variants of PG have been identified:

- Classic PG—commonly seen on the lower extremities; scars are often cribriform; patient complains of fever, malaise, arthralgia, and myalgia.
- Peristomal PG—occurs close to abdominal stomas, usually in patients with IBD, ileostomies, or colostomies for malignancy; may have bridges of epithelium that traverse the ulcer base.[66]
- Pustular PG—commonly seen on the trunk and extremity extensor surfaces of patients with IBD; stalls at the pustular stage and may persist for months.
- Bullous PG—commonly seen on upper limbs and face; associated with hematologic conditions with poor prognosis; presents as concentric bullous areas that spread rapidly.
- Vegetative PG—less aggressive and more superficial; may respond well to local treatment.[23,65,67]

Differential Diagnosis As there is no diagnostic test to confirm PG and multiple other conditions that resemble PG, a correct diagnosis relies on clinical presentation and exclusion

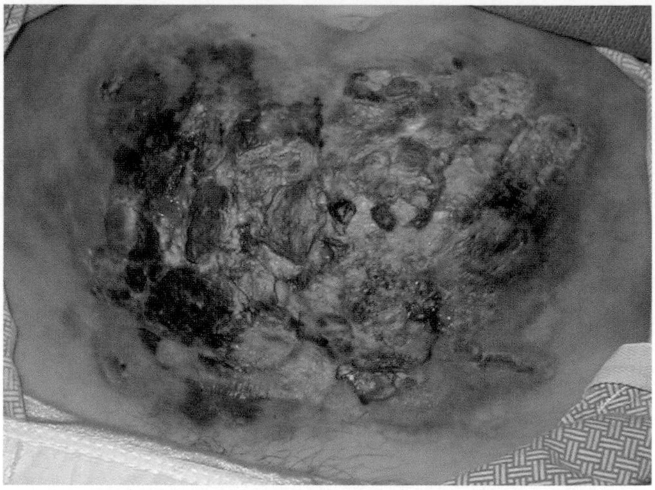

FIGURE 9-18 Pyoderma gangrenosum. Pyoderma gangrenosum on the abdomen of a female with diabetes. The PG developed after an open hysterectomy. The wounds were treated with nonadherent antimicrobial dressings (X-cell, Medline Industries, Inc., Mundelein, IL) in order to minimize pain, facilitate autolytic debridement and re-epithelialization and prevent infection. As the necrotic plaques loosened and new skin was visible beneath, they were removed with sterile forceps; however, aggressive debridement was contraindicated.

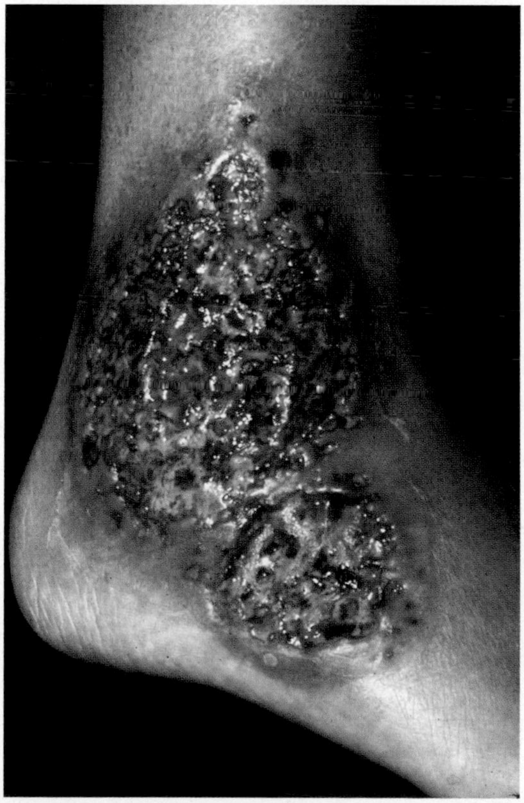

FIGURE 9-19 Pyoderma gangrenosum. Some of the characteristics of PG are seen on this lower extremity wound, including the violaceous border, purulence, and necrotic tissue. (From Usatine RP. Pyoderma Gangrenosum. In: Usatine RP, Smith MA, Chumley H, Mayeaux EJ Jr, Tysinger J, eds. *The Color Atlas of Family Medicine*. 2nd ed. New York, NY: McGraw Hill; 2013, Figure 174-5. Used with permission from Jack Resneck, Sr., MD.)

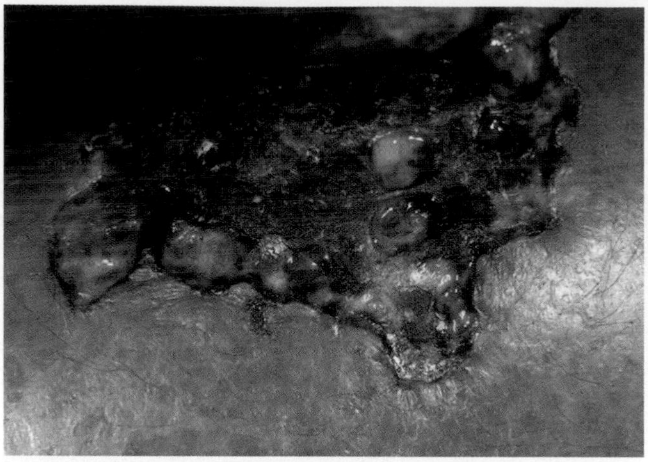

FIGURE 9-20 Pyoderma gangrenosum. The clinical appearance of PG can vary, as in this wound with both eschar and purulent subcutaneous tissue at the edges. (From Usatine RP. Pyoderma Gangrenosum. In: Usatine RP, Smith MA, Chumley HS, Mayeaux EJ Jr, eds. *The Color Atlas of Family Medicine.* 2nd ed. New York, NY: McGraw Hill; 2013, Figure 174-6. Used with permission from Jeff Meffert, MD.)

of other causes. **TABLE 9-9** lists the systemic diseases most often associated with PG. Differential diagnosis includes infections, malignancy (squamous cell or cutaneous lymphoma), vascular lesions, and antiphospholipid syndrome.

Medical Management Systemic management includes treatment of any underlying disease and long-term immunosuppression with high doses of corticosteroids or low doses of cyclosporin.[65,68] Other therapies that have been used in patients with PG include antibiotics (dapsone and minocycline), clofazimine, azathioprine, methotrexate, chlorambucil, cyclophosphamide, thalidomide, tacrolimus, mycophenolate, mofetil, IV immunoglobulin, plasmapheresis, and infliximab.[23,68]

Wound Management Topical steroids, topical tacrolimus, nicotine patches, and intralesional steroids have been used for mild or moderate diseases. *Debridement of adhered tissue is contraindicated and may cause pathergy*; however, as the necrotic tissue loosens with re-epithelialization, it may be gently removed with sterile forceps.[69] Keeping the lesions covered with a nonadherent mesh or silicone-backed wicking foam that will allow drainage to escape to a secondary dressing can help alleviate the pain associated with PD wound care. Maggot therapy has been successfully used in some cases. Split-thickness skin grafts, along with concurrent immunosuppressive therapy to reduce the risk of pathergy, have been reported. Alternative therapies include application of bioengineered skin and hyperbaric oxygen therapy.[47]

Necrobiosis Lipoidica

Pathophysiology Necrobiosis lipoidica (previously referred to as *necrobiosis lipoidica diabeticorum*) is a chronic granulomatous disorder of unknown etiology that is usually seen in morbidly obese patients with a strong family history of diabetes; however, only about one-third of the patients have diabetes, therefore the change in nomenclature.[70,71] Different pathological mechanisms have been proposed and include (1) diabetic microangiopathy as a result of glycoprotein deposition in the blood vessels, (2) abnormal collagen degeneration, (3) deposition of immunoglobulins in the blood vessel walls with enhanced platelet aggregation and coagulation, and (4) impaired neutrophil migration leading to an increased number of macrophages and subsequent granuloma formation.[72] Necrobiosis lipoidica also results in the thickening of the blood vessel walls and fat deposition, making the integumentary symptoms similar to vasculitis. The disease tends to be chronic with recurrent lesions and scarring and carries an associated risk of the development of squamous cell carcinoma.[73]

Clinical Presentation Lesions usually are bilateral but asymmetric on the tibial surface of the lower leg and begin as a rash or 1–3 mm slightly raised spots. They progress to irregular ovoid reddish- or yellow-brown plaques with shiny yellow centers and violaceous indurated borders.[74] The edges may be raised and purple, and the wound bed may have good granulation tissue but no epithelial migration. Pain and edema are also usually present. Remodeling is characterized by round patches of hyperpigmentation (**FIGURE 9-21**).[75] Direct immunofluorescence microscopy of necrobiosis lipoidica reveals IgM, IgA, C3, and fibrinogen in the blood vessels which will cause vascular thickening.[72]

Medical Management Systemic steroids or other immunotherapy can be given to patients with severe disease. Cutaneous blood enhancers such as pentoxifylline and aspirin may be helpful in facilitating cell migration to the damaged tissue and inhibiting platelet aggregation.[72] Cyclosporin,[76] mycophenolate,[77] and infliximab[78] have also been reported to successfully treat necrobiosis lipoidica. Lesions need to be monitored for transformation to malignant wounds.[74]

TABLE 9-9 Systemic Diseases Associated with Pyoderma Gangrenosum

Inflammatory Bowel Disease	Arthritis	Hematologic Abnormalities	Immunologic Abnormalities
Ulcerative colitis Regional enteritis Crohn's disease	Seronegative arthritis Rheumatoid arthritis Osteoarthritis Psoriatic arthritis	Myeloid leukemia, hairy cell leukemia, myelofibrosis, myeloid metaplasia, immunoglobulin A monoclonal gammapathy, polycythemia vera, paroxysmal nocturnal hemoglobinuria, myeloma, and lymphoma	Systemic lupus erythematous Complement deficiency Hypogammaglobulinemia Hyperimmunoglobulin E syndrome Acquired immunodeficiency syndrome

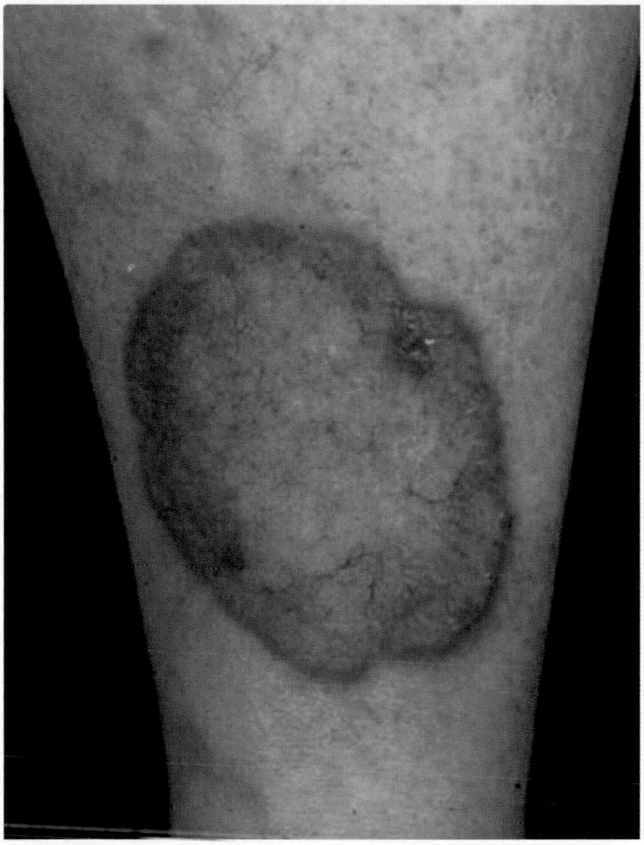

FIGURE 9-21 Necrobiosis lipoidica diabeticorum. NLD lesions are characterized by symmetrical tan pink or yellow plaques with well-demarcated, raised borders and depressed, atrophied centers. Telangiectasia is also visible throughout the wound. (Reproduced with permission from Wolff K et al. *Fitzpatrick's Color Atlas & Synopsis of Clinical Dermatology*. 5th ed. New York, NY: McGraw Hill, 2005, Figure 15-5 (Left).)

Wound Management Topical and intralesional steroids can be beneficial in treating mild to moderate cases.[70] Other reported treatments include calcineurin inhibitors,[74] 0.1% topical tacrolimus ointment,[71,75] collagen matrix dressings,[79] and phototherapy.[80] A combination of low-frequency noncontact ultrasound, topical steroid ointment, saline-impregnated cellulose dressings, and multilayer compression wraps, in conjunction with pentoxifylline, was a successful combination used by the author for a patient with chronic lesions of more than 1-year duration.

INFECTIONS (VIRAL)

Herpes Virus

Varicella is a virus that presents in three different ways: herpes simplex Type 1 (oral or cold sores), herpes simplex Type 2 (genital herpes), and herpes zoster (chicken pox and shingles).

Pathophysiology The *herpes simplex virus* (HSV) persists in an individual for a lifetime due to the presence of a latent pool of the virus in terminally differentiated neurons, usually the peripheral ganglion.[81] HSV is a DNA virus that invades the cell nucleus and replicates, thereby producing partial-thickness wounds. Herpes simplex Type 1 activation is commonly referred to as "cold sores" that occur on the mouth and lips (**FIGURE 9-22A–C**). Herpes simplex Type 2 is recognized as a sexually transmitted disease that results in lesions on the genital skin. Both can be reactivated, and in immune-compromised individuals can lead to local infection, chronic herpetic ulcers, and mucous membrane damage, as well as systemic infections in the central and peripheral nervous systems, the gastrointestinal tract, and the ocular system.[82]

Chicken pox is a childhood disorder caused by the *varicella-zoster virus* (VZV). The virus enters through the respiratory system and infects the tonsillar T cells. The infected T cells carry the virus to the reticuloendothelial system where the major replication occurs and to the skin where the rash appears (**FIGURE 9-23**).[83]

The VZV can remain latent in the dorsal sensory ganglion and reactivate in later years, usually during a period of stress or immunosuppression, as herpes varicella-zoster or "shingles" (**FIGURE 9-24A, B**).[84] Vesicles can involve the corium and dermis, with degenerative changes characterized by ballooning, multinucleated giant cells, and eosinophilic intranuclear inclusions. Infection may involve localized dermal blood vessels, resulting in necrosis and epidermal hemorrhage.[23] Individuals who are immunosuppressed (eg, patients with HIV or transplants) can have more severe cases of herpes, with the incidence of herpes zoster more than 14 times higher in adults with HIV.

Clinical Presentation Herpes simplex usually occurs initially in childhood and progresses through the stages of prodrome, erythema, papule, vesicle, ulcer, hard crust, and residual dry flaking and swelling. Lesions can become secondarily infected by *Staphylococcus* or *Streptococcus*. Individuals tend to have recurrent eruptions. Nonulcerative lesions tend to last 3 days; full-blown ulcerative lesions may last 7–10 days.

Chicken pox usually presents with prominent fever, malaise, nausea, loss of appetite, headache, and a pruritic rash that starts on the face, scalp, and trunk and spreads to the extremities. The rash is initially maculopapular and rapidly progresses to vesicles, then pustules that rupture, and then to crusts.[84]

Herpes varicella-zoster (HZV) presents as an eruption of grouped vesicles on an erythematous base limited to a single dermatome. Initial symptoms include dermatologic tingling or pain in the affected dermatome 48–72 hours before the onset of lesions, which can appear 3–5 days later. Lesions develop quickly into vesicles, then rupture, ulcerate, and dry out. They usually resolve in 10–15 days, although the pain may remain as post-herpetic neuralgia. In patients with advanced HIV, the herpetic infection may develop into chronic ulcers and fissures with a substantial degree of edema.[84]

Medical Management Chicken pox will usually heal in less than 2 weeks without medical intervention.

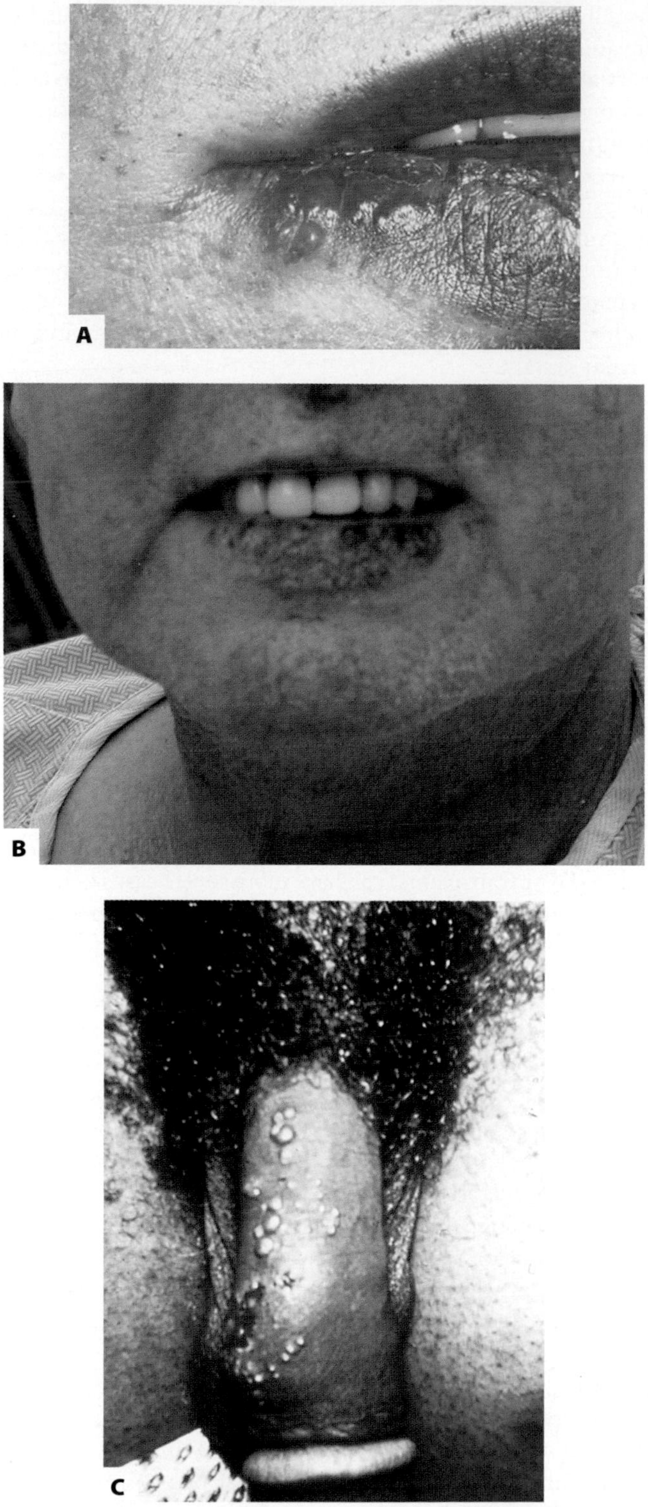

FIGURE 9-22 **Herpes simplex virus Type 1. A.** Early presentation of Herpes simplex Type 1, commonly known as a cold sore. (Used with permission from Ryan KJ, ed. *Sherris & Ryan's Medical Microbiology*. 8th ed. New York, NY: McGraw Hill; 2022, Figure 14-4.) **B.** Later progression of Herpes simplex Type 1 during the hard crust stage. **C.** Herpes simplex Type 2 that occurs on genital skin. (Used with permission from Ryan KJ, ed. *Sherris & Ryan's Medical Microbiology*. 8th ed. New York, NY: McGraw Hill; 2022, Figure 14-5.)

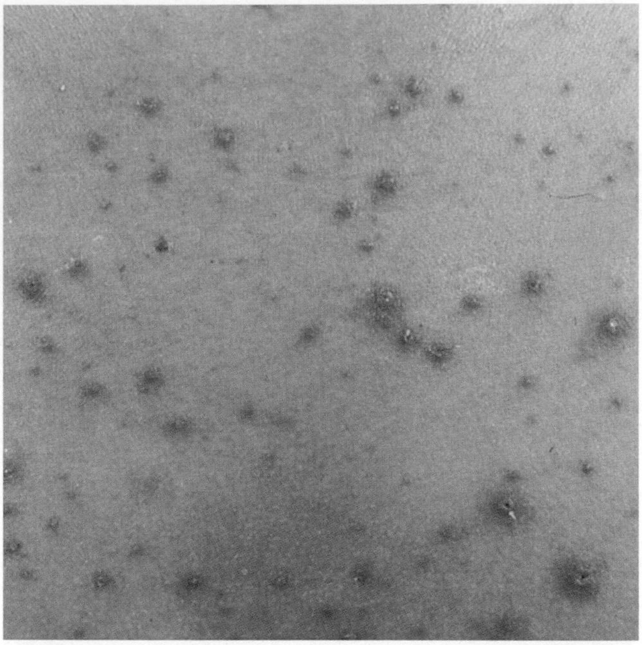

FIGURE 9-23 **Herpes zoster, chicken pox.** The dermal lesions associated with chicken pox begin as a rash and rapidly progress through the stages of papules, vesicles, pustules, and crusts. (Used with permission from Schmader KE, Oxman MN. Varicella and herpes zoster. In: Goldsmith LA, Katz SI, Gilchrest BA, Paller AS, Leffell DJ, Wolff K. eds. *Fitzpatrick's Dermatology in General Medicine*. 8th ed. New York, NY: McGraw Hill; 2012, Figure 194-3A.)

Uncomplicated HZV is treated for 7–10 days with acyclovir (Zovirax), famciclovir (Famvir), or valacyclovir (Valtrex).[85] These oral antiviral medications reduce the duration and severity of adult symptoms. Oral prednisone may decrease the risk of post-herpetic neuralgia. VariZIG injections may prevent complications in immune-compromised and pregnant patients, as well as decrease the severity of HZV symptoms.[86] As of October 2017, a new vaccine (Shingrix) is recommended to be administered twice, 2–6 months apart, and is considered 90% effective in preventing shingles and post-herpetic pain.[87] Antihistamines may help reduce the itching, and Zostrix may help reduce severe neuralgia. If the lesions have not healed in 3–4 weeks, the patient may have a drug-resistant virus that requires treatment with IV foscarnet. HSV infections are treated with antiviral medications (Acyclovir); however, long-term use of this medication in immunosuppressed patients can lead to drug resistance, requiring research for a next-generation antiviral medication.[88]

Wound Management Herpes simplex can be treated with topical acyclovir and mild corticosteroid ointment[89] or with a thin hydrocolloid dressing.[83] Moisture retentive dressings such as hydrogels, hydrocolloids, transparent films, or alginates may be helpful to facilitate autolytic debridement of necrotic tissue and healing of herpes-varicella wounds.

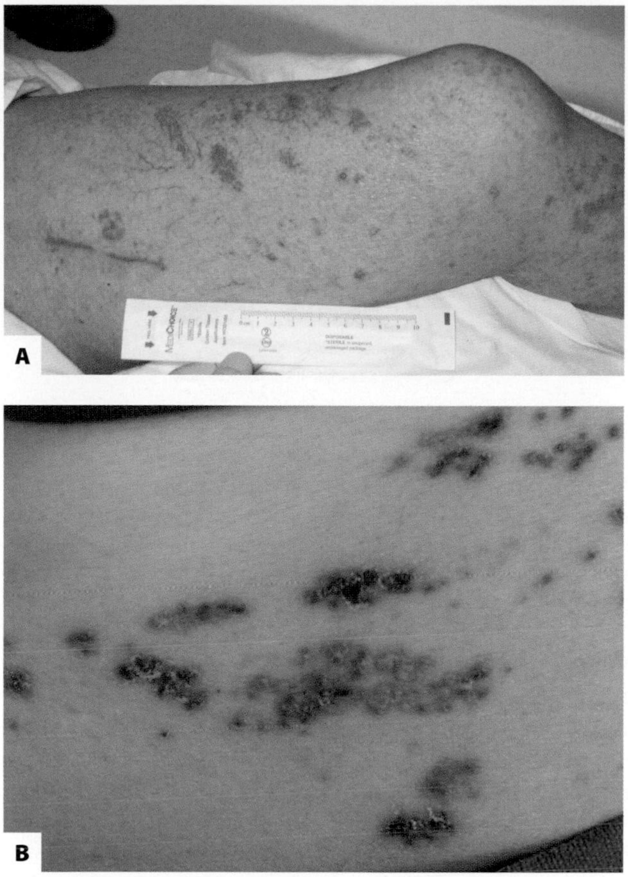

FIGURE 9-24 Herpes zoster, shingles. Herpes zoster, commonly known as shingles, begins as a rash or small vesicles and progresses to dry eruptions (**A**). The pattern follows a specific dermatome, becoming hard dry crusts (**B**), and usually resolves in 10–15 days although the post-herpetic pain may linger for months to years.

INFECTED WOUNDS (BACTERIAL)

Necrotizing Fasciitis

Pathophysiology Necrotizing fasciitis (NF) is a deep-seated infection of the subcutaneous tissue that progresses rapidly along fascial planes with severe systemic toxicity and 40% mortality. NF leads to progressive destruction of fascia, subcutaneous fat, and muscles, usually with resulting necrosis of the overlying skin.[90] Bacteria enter the skin through a cut or scratch; the most common offenders are Group A streptococcus (*Streptococcus pyogenes*), *Staphylococcus aureus*, *Clostridium perfringens*, *Bacteroides fragilis*, *Aeromonas hydrophila*, and *Klebsiella*.[90] NF has been classified into two major categories based on microbiology and location of the infection: Type 1 is polymicrobial involving at least one anaerobe with or without a facultative anaerobe (a microorganism that can live and grow with or without molecular oxygen) and is localized on the trunk, abdomen, or perineum; Type 2 is monomicrobial, usually caused by group A beta-hemolytic streptococci and/or other streptococci or staphylococci and occurs on the extremities.[91] The bacteria release toxins that produce an exotoxin that in turn activates T cells. This process produces increased cytokines that lead to severe systemic symptoms known as toxic shock syndrome, which can be fatal if the initial necrosis and infection are not immediately controlled.[1,23]

Risk factors for NF include IV drug use, diabetes, renal failure, pulmonary diseases, liver cirrhosis, peripheral vascular disease, obesity, malnutrition, and drug abuse.[90] A 50% mortality rate is associated with any combination of three or more risk factors.

Clinical Presentation NF is frequently preceded by a minor skin trauma that serves as a portal for the causative bacteria (**FIGURE 9-25**). This is followed by a sequence of the following clinical manifestations:

- Low-grade fever
- Pain, usually out of proportion to the initial clinical findings
- Swelling with massive, "sausage-like" edema
- Erythema with bullous skin changes
- Gray or "dishwater" colored drainage from the wounds (**FIGURE 9-26**)

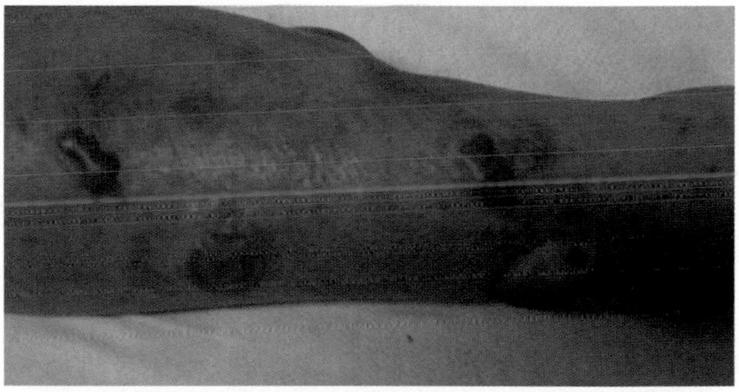

FIGURE 9-25 Necrotizing fasciitis. Necrotizing fasciitis begins with edema and erythema with bullae as a result of the underlying, fast-spreading infection. Any patient suspected of having necrotizing fasciitis requires emergent surgical debridement in order to prevent systemic complications. (Used with permission of Dr. Jayesh Shah.)

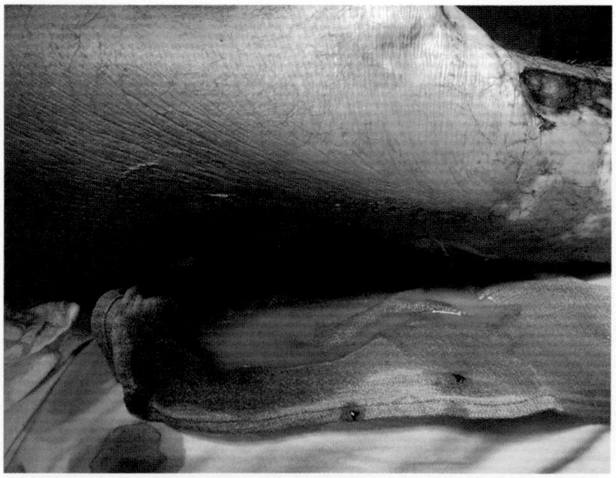

FIGURE 9-26 Dishwater drainage from incision and drainage of necrotizing fasciitis.

- Lack of adenopathy (bacteria miss immune recognition)
- Skin necrosis with hypoesthesia or anesthesia
- Striking indifference to one's clinical state
- Toxic-shock appearance with a rapid demise

Basic antigen testing may identify *Streptococcus* but does not establish a diagnosis. A basic rapid strep test is helpful, and polymerase chain reaction testing can help identify streptococcal pyrogenic exotoxin genes (SPE=B). Low serum procalcitonin (<0.87 ng/mL) has been associated with a high probability of NF.[92] The Laboratory Risk Indicator for Necrotizing Fasciitis (LRINEC) has been validated as an emergency department tool for rapid diagnosis.[90,93,94] (See **TABLE 9-10**.) Imaging with radiography, CT scan, or MRI can identify pockets of soft tissue gas (**FIGURE 9-27**).

Medical Management Medical management includes appropriate antibiotics, aggressive surgical debridement of all infected subcutaneous and dermal tissue (the saying is that the patient goes straight from the ER to the OR), medical stabilization as needed, and adjunctive hyperbaric oxygen therapy.[95] Initial empiric therapy includes broad-spectrum coverage of polymicrobial infections including an MRSA-active agent such as vancomycin, daptomycin, linezolid, or ceftaroline, as well as an agent against gram-negative pathogens such as piperacillin-tazobactam, ampicillin-sulbactam, ticarcilin-clavulanate, extended-spectrum cephalosporins or carbapenems.[96] Intravenous immunoglobulin therapy has been suggested for patients with toxic shock syndrome.[96]

TABLE 9-10 The LRINEC (Laboratory Risk Indicator for Necrotizing Fasciitis) Score to Differentiate Necrotizing Fasciitis from Other Soft Tissue Infections

C Reactive Protein (mg/L)	<150	0
	≥150	4
White Blood Cells (cells/mm³)	<15	0
	15–25	1
	>25	2
Hemoglobin (g/dL)	>13.5	0
	11.1–13.5	1
	<11	2
Sodium (mmol/L)	>135	0
	<135	2
Creatinine (mg/dL)	<1.6	0
	>1.6	2
Glucose (mg/dL)	<180	0
	>180	1

Interpretation: 0–5, less than 50% probability for developing NF; 6–7, 50–75% risk of having NF; >8, more than 75% risk of having NF. The score has high specificity but low sensitivity.

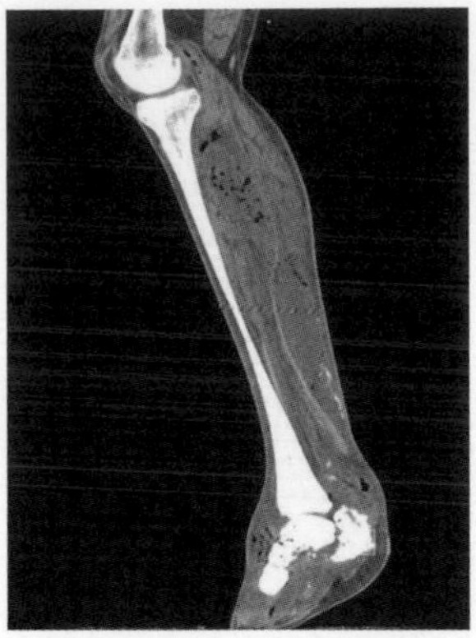

FIGURE 9-27 Lower extremity CT scan shows extensive soft tissue gas confirming a diagnosis of necrotizing fasciitis.
(From Knoop KJ, Stack LB, Storrow AB, Thurman RJ, eds. *The Atlas of Emergency Medicine*. 5th ed. New York, NY: McGraw Hill; 2021, Figure 12.15. Reproduced with permission from photo contributor: Lawrence B. Stack, MD.)

Wound Management Wound management depends on the amount of debridement performed surgically, as well as the amount and quality of the residual soft tissue. Negative pressure wound therapy with antibiotic instillation has become standard care post debridement to treat residual infection, facilitate wound contraction and angiogenesis, and prepare the wound for skin grafts or flaps.[96] Pain management during wound care is essential, and if the wounds are extensive, rehabilitation services and/or psychological care may be needed.[97]

Fournier's Gangrene

Fournier's gangrene is an aggressive form of necrotizing infection of the perineum that may extend to the anterior abdominal wall, gluteal muscles, and in males, to the penis and scrotum. The causative organisms are a mixed collection of aerobic gram-negative bacteria, enterococci, and anaerobes, including Bacteroides and peptostreptococci.[98] Penetrating trauma, recent surgery, and immunosuppression (eg, diabetes and neutropenia) are risk factors associated and predictors of poorer outcomes.[99] Medical and wound management include strategies for any necrotizing fasciitis.

Myonecrosis (Gas Gangrene)

Pathophysiology Myonecrosis, also known as gas gangrene, occurs after a deep penetrating injury compromises the blood supply, thus creating the anaerobic conditions ideal for infection. The majority of the infections in this situation are caused by *Clostridium perfringens,* although other species of *Clostridium* have been implicated, eg, *Clostridium septicum* has been associated with malignancy.[100,101] *C. perfringens* produce multiple toxins (including bacterial proteases, phospholipases, and cytotoxins) that cause aggressive necrosis of the skin and muscles.[102] The same bacteria can cause clostridial cellulitis, which also occurs after trauma or surgery. Known risk factors for developing myonecrosis are essentially the same as for any necrotizing soft-tissue infection, especially immunosuppression, diabetes, cancer, and vascular disease.[72,103–105] Patients with myonecrosis have a higher mortality rate than those with NF due to early septic shock caused by clostridial toxins.[106]

Clinical Presentation The patient presents with severe pain and skin color changes from pale to bronze to purplish-red with bullae formation. Gas in the tissue is evident from physical examination as crepitus upon palpation or by radiography. **TABLE 9-11** presents a detailed list of integumentary signs and symptoms associated with gas gangrene (**FIGURE 9-28**). In addition, renal failure may occur as a result of hemoglobinuria and myoglobinuria, as well as bacteremia and hemolysis. The patient may rapidly progress to shock and multiorgan failure with toxic psychosis.

Medical Management Medical management of gas gangrene is predicated on the debridement of all devitalized and infected tissue, appropriate IV antibiotics, and systemic support treatment.[107] Adjunctive hyperbaric oxygen therapy is recommended to control infection and decrease further extension of necrosis.[108] Strict blood glucose control is essential in patients with diabetes.[105]

Wound Management Wound care consists of negative pressure wound therapy (with the instillation of an antibiotic solution if needed), followed by skin grafts or flaps.[106]

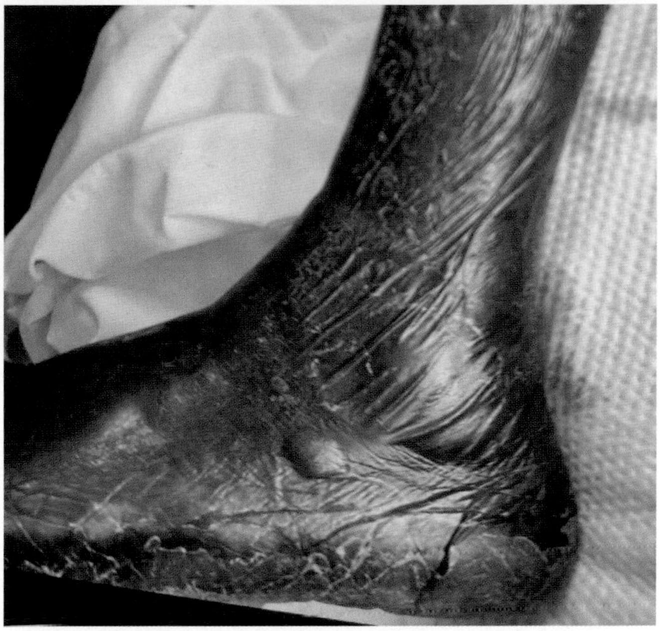

FIGURE 9-28 Myonecrosis (gas gangrene). Myonecrosis of the foot after trauma with subsequent clostridial infection. The collection of gas causes the bullous on the dorsum of the foot. Pockets of myonecrosis that form in deep tissue will expel an odor of gas when opened during debridement. (Used with permission from Dr. Jay Shah.)

Actinomycosis

Pathophysiology Actinomycosis is caused by a gram-positive, non-spore-forming anaerobic bacilli, the most common being *Actinomycosis israelii* which is normally found in the nose, throat, gastrointestinal tract, or genitourinary tract.[109,110] The most common locations for infections are cervicofacial, abdominal, or thoracic; however, actinomycosis on the foot has also been reported.[111,112] Cervicofacial actinomycosis can also be associated with local tissue damage caused by neoplastic conditions and irradiation. The infection is usually accompanied by the presence of some other bacteria that facilitates its invasion of tissue.[113]

Clinical Presentation The clinical presentation of actinomycosis, which is usually chronic and difficult to eliminate, varies with the location. Cervicofacial actinomycosis develops slowly; the area becomes markedly indurated and the overlying skin becomes reddish or cyanotic. In addition, the wound may produce particles (similar to, and frequently called, sulfur particles because of their yellow color)[109] that carry the bacteria, frequently into adjacent soft tissue and bone (**FIGURE 9-29A** and **B**). Pulmonary actinomycosis occurs in individuals with poor oral hygiene, preexisting dental disease, alcoholism, and chronic lung disease; it begins with fever, cough, and sputum production.[109] Other signs include night

TABLE 9-11 Integumentary Signs and Symptoms of Gas Gangrene

Early Signs and Symptoms	Skin Changes	Late Signs and Symptoms	Other Findings
Incubation period of about 48 hours	Shiny and tense skin	Myonecrosis	Ischemia and inoculation
Fever	Tense, bronzed, and tender skin	Hemolytic anemia	Bacterial proliferation
Pain out of proportion to the injury	Blue-black bullae	Hematuria	Exotoxin production
Tachycardia	Gas and crepitation	Myoglobinuria	Tissue destruction
Diaphoresis	Odor	Acute renal failure	Edema and necrosis
Gray Pallor		Metabolic acidosis	Decreased redox potential
Anoxemia		Consumptive coagulopathy	Gangrene
Apprehension		Seizures and death	Hemorrhagic bullae
Disorientation			Gas in muscles
Obtundation			Limited joint range of motion

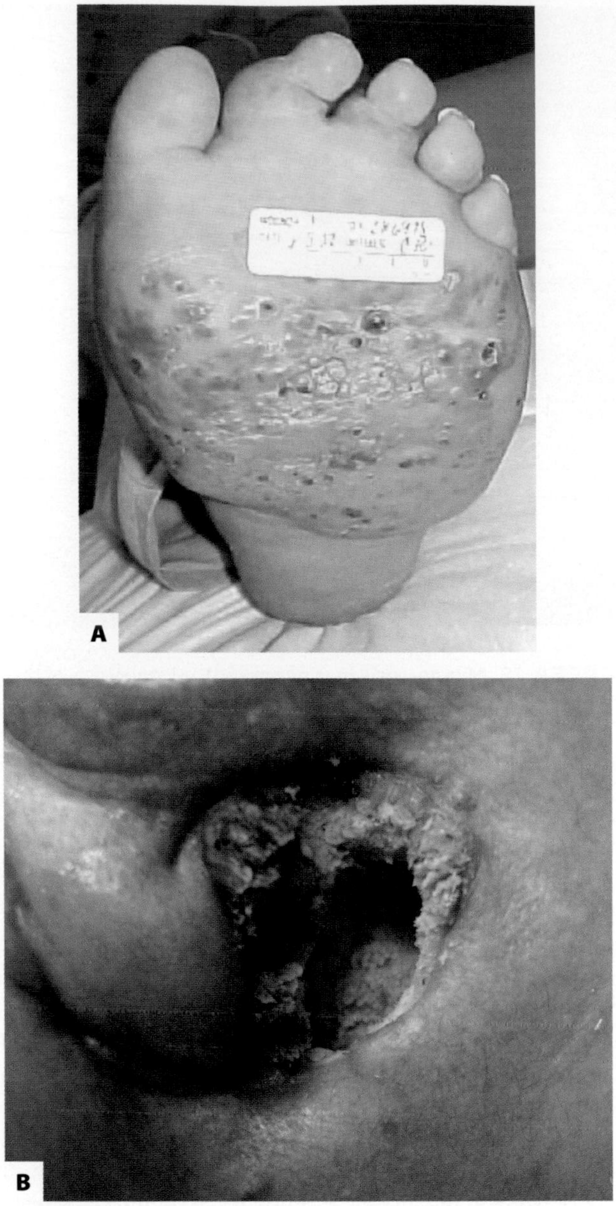

FIGURE 9-29 Actinomycosis. A. Clinical signs of actinomycosis include the white particles that accumulate on the wound surface and induration and edema of the periwound tissue, resulting in deformity of the structure. **B.** Advanced actinomycosis on a patient who had a history of two surgeries to remove a tumor from the suborbital area and ultimately had surgical removal of the infected tissue with plastic reconstruction.

sweats, weight loss, and pleuritic pain. Abdominal actinomycosis usually causes pain in the ileocecal region, spiking fever and chills, vomiting, and weight loss[114] This type may be confused with Crohn's disease.

Medical Management Surgical excision is usually required for actinomycosis, and IV or oral antibiotics (beta-lactams such as ampicillin, penicillin, or amoxicillin) are recommended for 6 months to 1 year.[115] Doxycycline and sulfonamides may also be used; however, medical treatment is slow.[114]

Wound Management Actinomycosis is treated locally with antibiotic solutions or with local antibiotic cream or anti-infective agents. Open surgical incisions are treated with moist wound therapy.

Mycobacteria

Pathophysiology Mycobacteria can be typical or atypical, and the bacteria are neither gram-positive nor gram-negative. Atypical strains were not reported as human pathogens until the 1950s. Mycobacterial cutaneous infections usually result from exogenous inoculations, and predisposing factors include a history of preceding trauma, surgery (especially cosmetic procedures), indwelling medical devices (eg, prosthetic implants), immunosuppression, or chronic disease (especially diabetes). Human pathogenic mycobacteria are divided into the following groups: *mycobacterium tuberculosis* complex; nontuberculosis mycobacteria (further divided into slow-growing and rapid-growing); and *mycobacterium leprae* and *mycobacterium lepromatosis* (or leprosy).[116,117]

Clinical Presentation The cutaneous lesions vary depending on the causative pathogen and may present as granulomas, small superficial ulcers, sinus tracts, abscesses, or large ulcerated lesions localized in exposed areas (**FIGURE 9-30A–D**). Tissue cultures are required to make an accurate diagnosis of any mycobacterial infection.

Medical Management The primary medical treatment of mycobacterial infections is pathogen-specific antimycobacterial therapy, sometimes in conjunction with steroids. Some first-line medications are Isoniazid, Rifampicin, dapsone, pyrazinamide, ethambutol, and streptomycin.[117–119] Drug resistance is a global problem and numerous second-line defense medications have been presented in the literature.

Wound Management Wound management is based on the use of antimicrobial dressings, the management of exudate, and the use of an aseptic technique to prevent further infection. Larger lesions may require surgical excision and skin grafts. The use of airborne precautions by all caregivers is required if the strain is tuberculin.

Osteomyelitis

Pathophysiology Osteomyelitis, or infection of the bone, derives its name from *osteo* (meaning bone) and *myelo* (relating to myeloid tissue in the bone marrow). Osteomyelitis can be acute (diagnosed within 2 weeks of the onset of signs and symptoms) or chronic (reoccurs in a patient with a history of osteomyelitis).[120] It can be further classified as hematogenous (caused by pathogens carried in the blood stream from sites of infection in other parts of the body) or exogenous (caused by pathogens that enter from outside the body, eg, from open fractures, surgical sites, and penetrating wounds).[121] Acute hematogenous osteomyelitis occurs most frequently in children, especially those with sickle cell disease, and affects the long bones (femur, tibia,

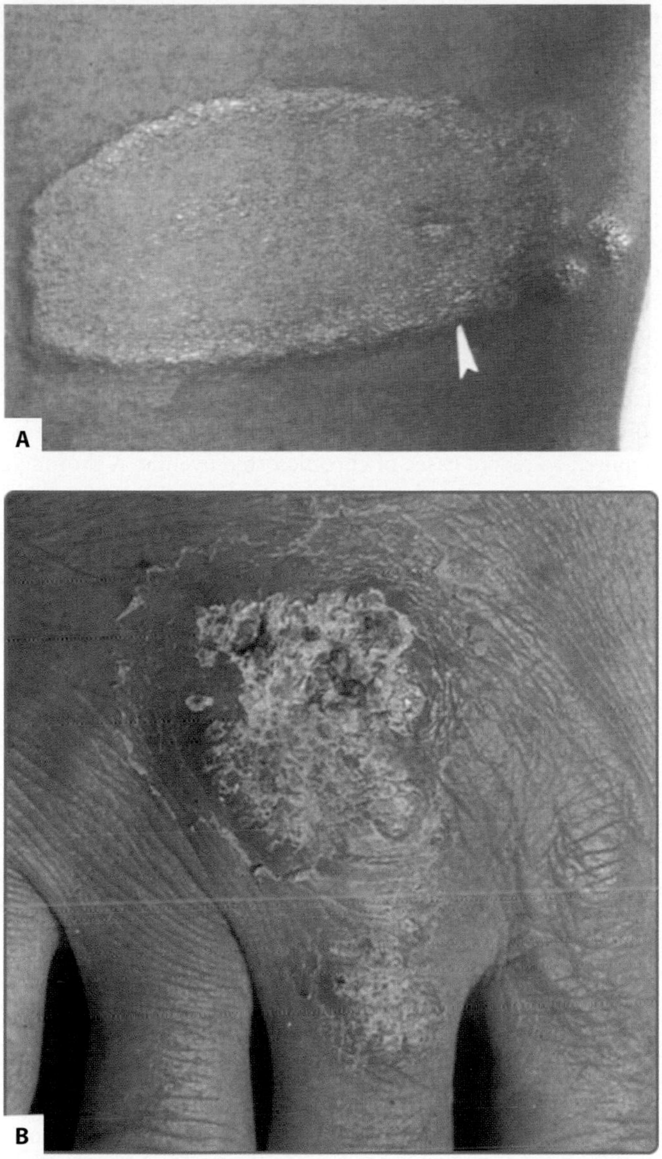

FIGURE 9-30 Mycobacterial wounds. A. Tuberculoid leprosy. Tuberculoid leprosy typically has a single, flat, hypopigmented lesion with absent sensation. (Used with permission from Longo DL, Fauci AS, Kasper DL, et al, eds. *Harrison's Principles of Internal Medicine*. 18th ed. New York, NY: McGraw Hill; 2012, Figure 166-2.) **B.** Tuberculosis verrucosa cutis. Tuberculosis verrucosa cutis on the hand. (Used with permission from Kang S, Amagai M, Bruckner AL, et al, eds. *Fitzpatrick's Dermatology*. 9th ed. New York, NY: McGraw Hill; 2019, Figure 157-4.)

humerus, pelvis). *Chronic osteomyelitis* occurs most frequently in adults, especially those with diabetes, open fractures, implanted hardware, and vascular insufficiency. In the diabetic population with vascular insufficiency, the bones most affected are the small bones in the foot.[120]

The sequence of osteomyelitis involves the following stages: Stage 1—the pathogen, usually *Staphylococcus aureus*,[122] invades the medullary canal of the bone and becomes a nidus of infection; Stage 2, the acute phase—the infection results in pus from the inflammatory process and spreads to the vascular channels in the bone; and Stage 3, the chronic phase—the inflammatory process obliterates the vascular channels with subsequent ischemia and bone necrosis.[120] The pieces of necrotic bone may separate from the healthy bone (termed *sequestrum*) and can occur on any infected bone (**FIGURE 9-31**).

Clinical Presentation Acute hematogenous osteomyelitis usually presents with focal tenderness, swelling, or difficulty with weight-bearing activities, especially in the lower extremities. The clinical diagnosis is supported by acute inflammatory serum studies (including white blood cell count, ESR, C-reactive protein) along with radiologic studies.[120] MRI studies and technetium 99 m bone scans are very sensitive, and a definitive diagnosis is made with biopsies. Although X-rays may not be definitive until 10–14 days after the onset of symptoms, they will show edema in the adjacent soft tissue and areas of sclerosis.

Osteomyelitis in adult patients usually occurs with surgical reduction and internal fixation of fractures, prosthetic devices, open fractures, and soft tissue infections. The symptoms will usually occur about 1 month after the introduction of the pathogen and include low-grade fever, drainage, pain, and loss of bone stability. The overlying soft tissue may be edematous, erythematous, or necrotic. Exposed bone in the wound bed, a positive "probe-to-bone" test, or a wound more than 2 cm^2 on the foot of a patient with diabetes is very suspicious of underlying osteomyelitis (**FIGURE 9-32**).[123] Digit edema that causes the toe to have a "sausage" appearance is

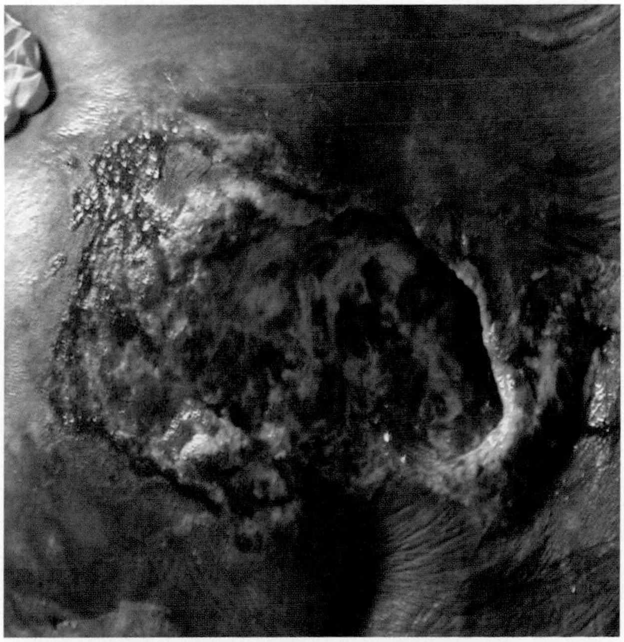

FIGURE 9-31 Osteomyelitis of the sacrum. The exposed bone in this sacral pressure ulcer has chronic osteomyelitis with necrosis and sequestrum of the cortical layer of the bone.

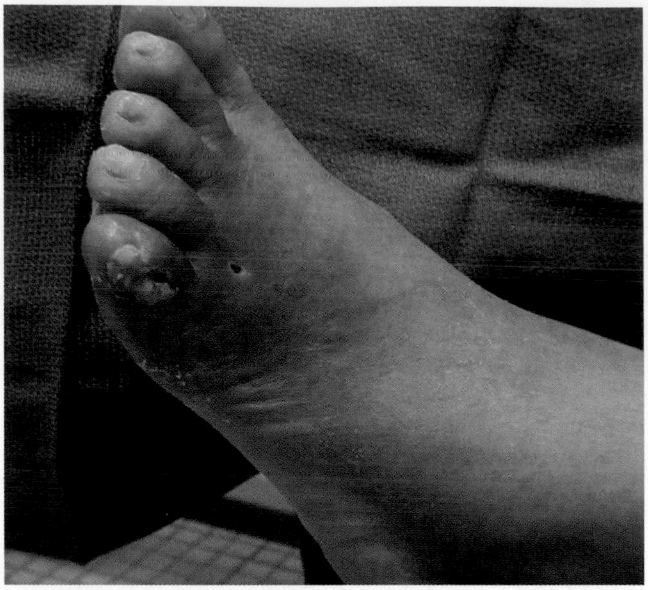

FIGURE 9-32 Chronic osteomyelitis in a diabetic foot. Signs of osteomyelitis in the foot of a patient with diabetes includes open tunneling wounds, positive probe-to-bone test, edema, erythema, "sausage" appearance of the fifth toe, and patient complaints of pain with weight-bearing. Note the discoloration of the skin which is an indication of the extent of subcutaneous soft tissue damage.

another indication of possible osteomyelitis (**FIGURE 9-33**). Bone biopsy confirms osteomyelitis and identifies the specific pathogen; however, increased leukocyte count, ESR greater than 70 mm/h, and plain films provide 89% sensitivity and 88% specificity.[124]

Medical Management The mainstay of treatment for all cases of osteomyelitis is identification of the pathogen, through biopsy or surgical debridement, and pathogen-specific antibiotics. Surgical debridement is advised for a wound that includes tissue invasion, abscess, open purulence, fistulae, or acute osteomyelitis, all of which could lead to sepsis; however, this may lead to dead spaces in the bone structure that require allograft or autograft to promote bone healing.[125] Antibiotic therapy can consist of 6–12 weeks of systemic antibiotics; however, more recent approaches are local targeted delivery of the antibiotic via poly-methyl methacrylate (PMMA) beads, biodegradable bone scaffolds, polyurethane scaffolds, or polymer microspheres.[125] Newer antibiotics that have been developed due to the resistance to traditional drugs for osteomyelitis (eg, vancomycin) include the following: dalbavancin, oritavancin, tedizolid, ceftaroline, and Debio-1450.[125] Amputation, foot reconstruction, osteotomies, or musculocutaneous flaps may be required in severe cases of chronic osteomyelitis. A thorough vascular assessment is vital for any patient with a history of peripheral vascular disease (see Chapter 4, Vascular Wounds).

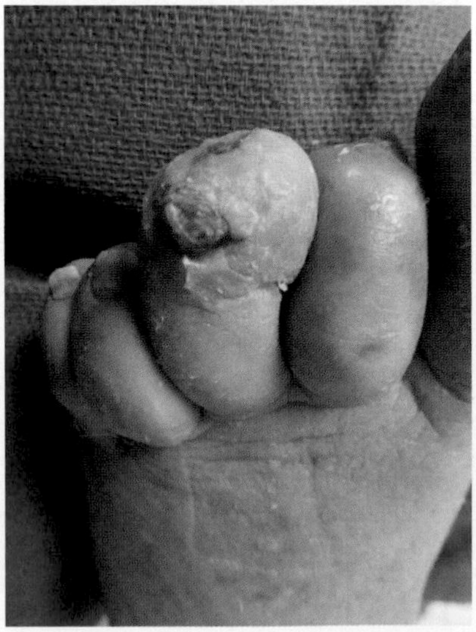

FIGURE 9-33 Osteomyelitis of the third toe with an open wound and the "sausage" appearance.

Wound Management Wounds are treated with standard moist wound care both before and after surgical debridement, which may include topical antimicrobial dressings, absorbent dressings until drainage abates, and off-loading strategies for any plantar foot wound. Negative pressure wound therapy may be used for post-surgical open wounds with adequate vascular supply, and hyperbaric oxygen therapy may be helpful for patients with diabetes and marginal blood supply (see Chapter 20, Hyperbaric and Topical Oxygen Therapy).

INFECTED WOUNDS (FUNGAL)

Sporotrichosis

Pathophysiology Sporotrichosis is a subacute or chronic fungal infection caused by one of the 53 species of the fungus *Sporothrix,* with *sporothrix schenckii* being the most common.[126] The infection occurs because of the traumatic implantation of the fungus into a break in the skin. This condition is also called rose-gardener's disease because it is usually seen in nursery workers, florists, and gardeners who have exposure to soil, sphagnum moss, or decaying wood.[127] Cats can be infected with sporotrichosis and thus become a carrier.

Clinical Presentation The patient usually presents with non-tender, red maculopapular granulomas, usually 2–4 mm in diameter, at the site of the injury (**FIGURE 9-34**). The primary lesion is typically painless and may be surrounded by raised erythema.[128] The infection can spread proximally via the lymphatics over a course of 1–4 weeks; thus, it is often associated with lymphangitis. Inhalation of the fungus can lead to pulmonary infection and subsequently spread to the bones, eyes, central nervous system, and viscera; however, this complication is uncommon.[126]

Medical Management Treatment for sporotrichosis depends upon the clinical form of the disease, the immune status of the host, and the *Sporothrix* species involved and usually includes antifungal systemic medications (itraconazole, fluconazole, terbinafine, and amphotericin B for severe life-threatening cases).[126]

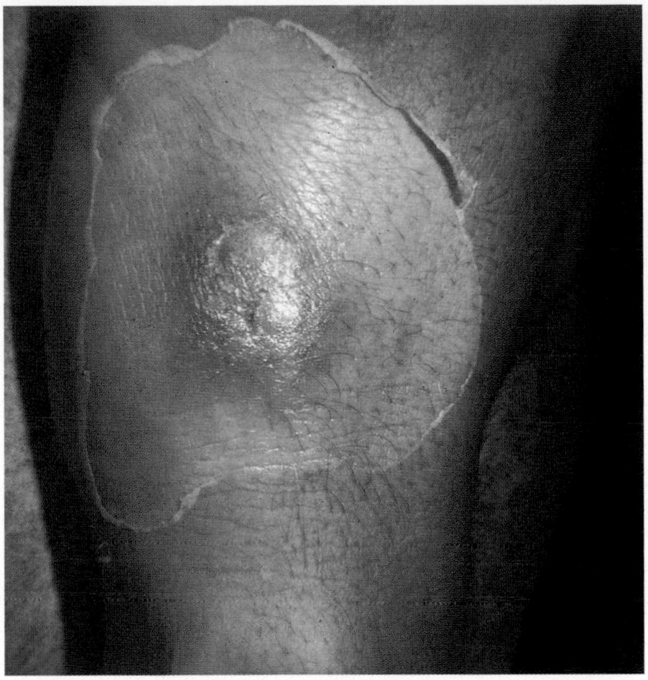

FIGURE 9-34 Sporotrichosis. Cutaneous lesions of sporotrichosis are characterized by erythema around the primary wound. The sloughing of the epidermis is a result of the inflammatory response in the periwound skin. (From Knoop KJ, Stack LB, Storrow AB, Thurman RJ, eds. *The Atlas of Emergency Medicine*. 4th ed. New York, NY: McGraw Hill; 2016, Figure 16.131. Reproduced with permission from photo contributor: Edward J. Otten, MD.)

Wound Management Local wound management includes topical antifungal agents, topical application of a saturated solution of potassium iodide, and topical application of heat (the sporotrichosis organism grows at low temperatures). Other nonpharmaceutical interventions include phototherapy, cryosurgery, and thermotherapy.

Tinea Infections

Pathophysiology Tinea infections are specific fungal infections caused by dermatophytes that obtain their nutrition exclusively from keratin (eg, stratum corneum, hair, and nails).[129] The most common tinea infections are caused by epidermophyton, trichophyton, or microsporum.[130] Histological features of tinea infections include neutrophils in the stratum corneum, often with parakeratosis and a variable inflammatory response in the dermis. The organisms are best visualized by histological biopsy with periodic acid-Schiff (PAS) staining, and potassium hydroxide (KOH) prep may show branching septate hyphae.[23]

Clinical Presentation Clinical signs of fungal infections are scaly skin, erythematous plaques, and annular plaques. A definitive fungal odor may sometimes be present. Rarely are the lesions vesicular or pustular. The specific disorder is named according to the body part infected and is described in

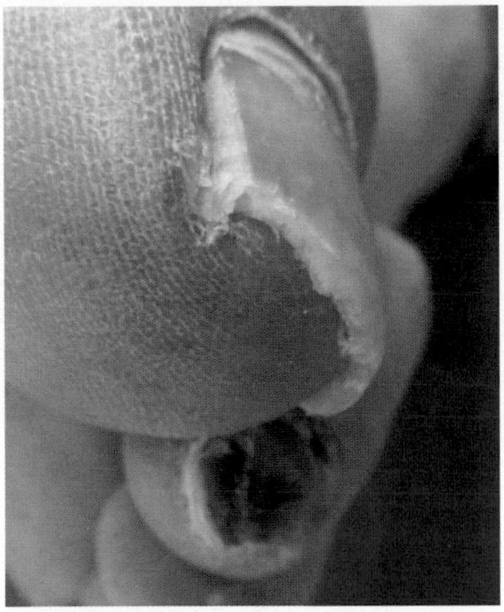

FIGURE 9-35 Onychomycosis with the "cottage cheese" appearance under the nail.

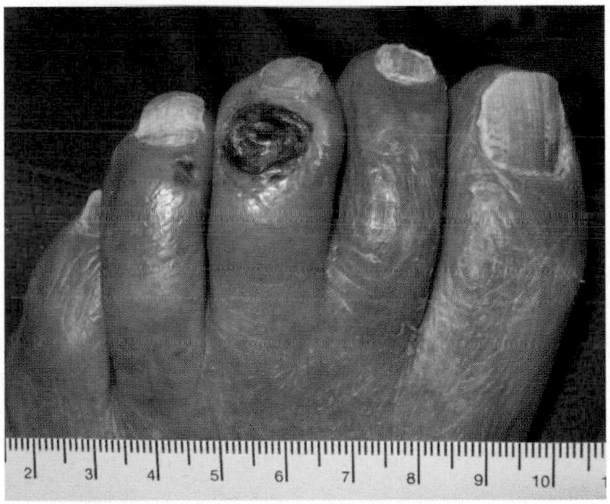

FIGURE 9-36 Onychomycosis characterized by thickened, discolored nails and banding of the great toe nail. The debris under the nail causes it to lift off the nail bed and frequently the nail will detach itself.

TABLE 9-12 (**FIGURES 9-35** to **9-41A, B**). Tinea corporis may occur under compression bandages if the skin tends to be moist, and candidiasis (a yeast-like fungus caused by *Candida albicans*) can affect the mucous membranes, the gastrointestinal tract, and the vagina (frequently seen on the skin of patients with urinary infections).[144]

Medical Management Systemic treatment with antifungal agents is indicated if the lesion is extensive, deep, recurrent, chronic, or unresponsive to topical antifungal treatment; if the patient is immunodeficient; or if there are multiple site lesions.[145] Itraconazole, fluconazole, and terbinafine are recommended for tinea corporis[146]; itraconazole and terbinafine, for onychomycosis and tinea capitis.[147]

TABLE 9-12 Name, Location, Clinical Signs, and Treatment of Tinea Infections

Name	Location	Signs and Symptoms	Treatment
Onychomycosis (also called tinea unguium)	Nail plates, especially in individuals who are elderly, immunocompromised, or have diabetes or PAD.	▪ Nail dystrophy ▪ Nail discoloration ▪ Separation of nail from underlying skin ▪ With or without odor ▪ Possible tendency to affect adjacent skin ▪ Possible infection[131]	▪ Oral antifungal agents ▪ Terbinafine ▪ Itraconazole (pulse regimen)[132] ▪ Topical fungal agents ▪ Efinaconazole ▪ Tavaborole[133] ▪ CO2 laser therapy[134,135] ▪ Urea (in conjunction with topical or oral antifungal treatment)[136]
Tinea capitis	Scalp, usually in pre-puberty children, males more than females Termed *tinea barbae* when in the beard	▪ Itching scalp ▪ Patches of hair loss with "black dots" where the hair breaks off ▪ Perifollicular scales and pustules ▪ Trichoscopic findings: Comma or corkscrew hair, Morse code-like hairs, zigzag or bent hairs[131] ▪ May develop kerions, or painful spongy masses with pustules and crusts	▪ Oral antifungal agents ▪ Itraconazole ▪ Terbinafine ▪ Griseofulvin[131,137]
Tinea corporis (ringworm)	Skin, usually the arms and legs, especially glabrous skin If on the hands, termed *tinea manuum* May occur under compression bandages if the skin tends to be moist	▪ Enlarged raised red rings with clear centers ▪ Itching ▪ Scales ▪ Hair loss	▪ Topical azoles ▪ Topical steroid and antifungal combination ▪ Terbinafine ▪ Naftifine[138]
Tinea cruris (jock itch)	Groin, inner thighs, genitals, buttocks	▪ Itching ▪ small erythematous, scaling patches ▪ vesicles with well-defined borders	▪ Topical azoles ▪ Topical steroid and antifungal combination ▪ Terbinafine ▪ Naftifine[134]
Tinea nigra	Palms or soles, primarily in tropical and subtropical regions	▪ Well-circumscribed brown-black macules	▪ Potassium hydroxide test to confirm diagnosis and rule out acral lentiginous melanoma ▪ Topical 2% ketoconazole cream twice daily for 2 weeks[139]
Tinea pedis	Feet, especially in athletes whose feet become sweaty; can spread to the hands	▪ Usually begins between the toes ▪ Begins as a scaly rash ▪ May cause maceration, peeling, and fissuring of toe interspaces ▪ Causes itching, burning, stinging ▪ Is contagious[140]	▪ Instruction in good pedal hygiene ▪ Topical antifungal sprays or ointments ▪ Oral antifungal medications for severe cases
Tinea versicolor (pityriasis versicolor)	Upper arms, trunk, and neck where the concentration of sebaceous glands is great; occurs mostly in humid weather[141]	▪ Well-defined round or egg-shaped macules ▪ White, erythematous, or brown pigment[141]	▪ Fluconazole ▪ Itraconazole ▪ Pramiconazole[142] ▪ Ketoconazole 2% shampoo[143]

From Hamm R, Carey JN. *Essential Elements of Wound Diagnosis*. New York, McGraw Hill; 2021, Table 8-5.

Wound Management The mainstay of treatment for fungal infections is topical antifungal creams, for example, imidazoles, triazoles, and allylamines. They are applied twice daily, extending the application 2 cm beyond the lesion edge, for 2–4 weeks.[146] Application needs to continue for a week or more after symptoms have resolved. Topical treatment of onychomycosis may take several months before visible changes in the nail can be observed.

MALIGNANT WOUNDS

Basal Cell Carcinoma

Pathophysiology Basal cell carcinoma is the most common type of skin cancer affecting one in every six Americans. The neoplasm arises from damaged undifferentiated basal cells usually as a result of prolonged exposure to ultraviolet (sun) light. UV exposure leads to the formation of thymine dimers,

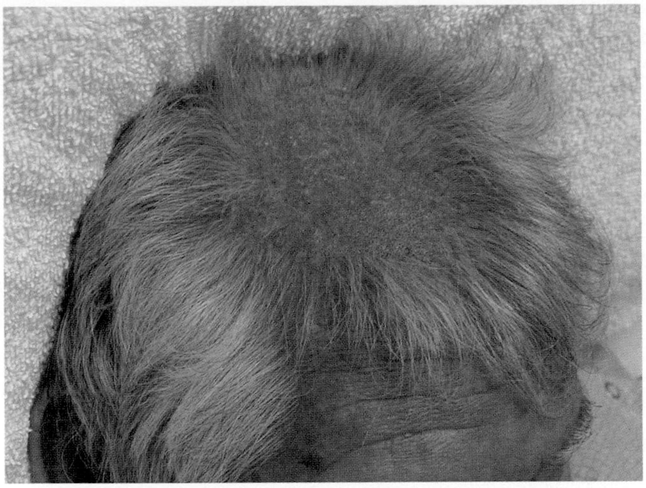

FIGURE 9-37 Tinea capitis. Symptoms of tinea capitis include patches of hair loss, "black dot" pattern within the patches, broken-off hairs, scaling, and itching.

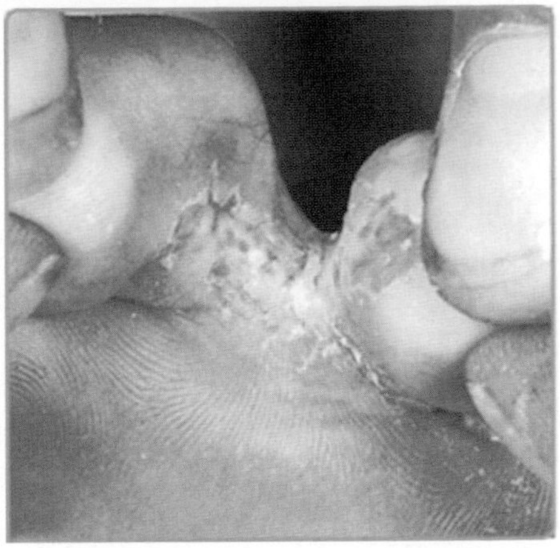

FIGURE 9-40 Tinea pedis with maceration between the toes, often referred to as athlete's foot. It is frequently accompanied by a distinctive odor and usually has to be treated with oral medications. (Used with permission from Kang S, Amagai M, Bruckner AL, et al, eds. *Fitzpatrick's Dermatology*. 9th ed. New York, NY: McGraw Hill; 2019, Figure 160-14A.)

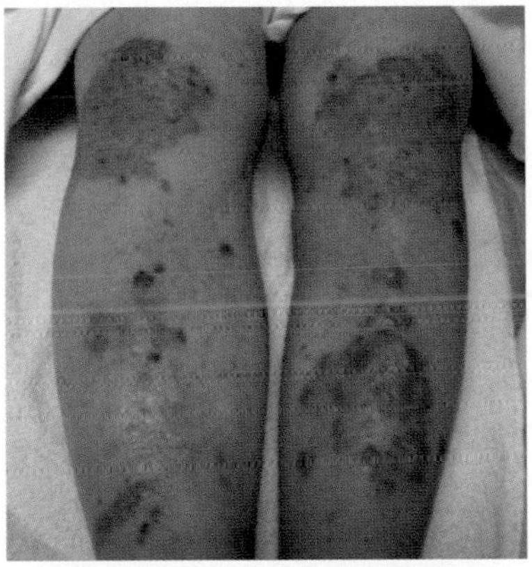

FIGURE 9-38 Tinea corporis that occurred under compression wraps.

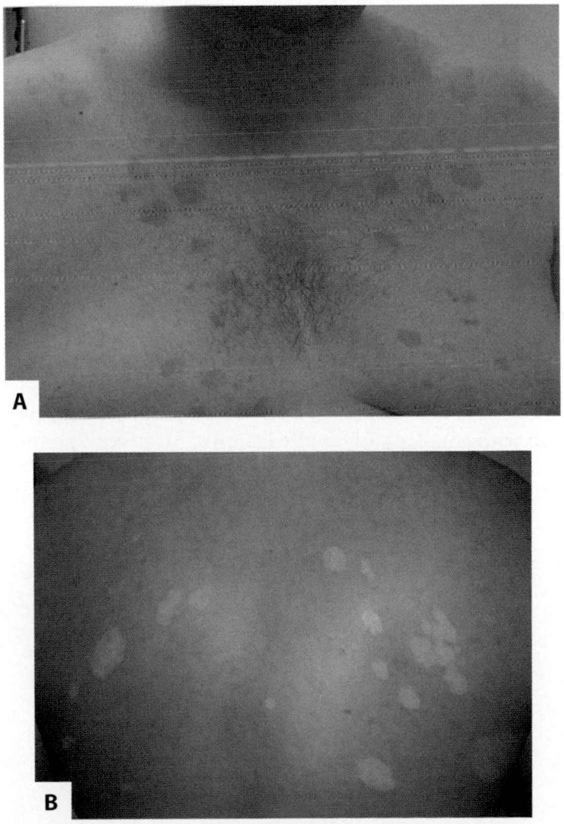

FIGURE 9-41 Tinea versicolor appearing as hyperpigmentation in lighter skin (A) and as hypopigmentation in darker skin (B). (From Usatine RP, Smith MA, Mayeaux EJ Jr, Chumley HS, eds. *The Color Atlas and Synopsis of Family Medicine*. 3rd ed. New York, NY: McGraw Hill; 2019, Figures 147-3 and 147-2, respectively. Reproduced with permission from Richard P. Usatine, MD.)

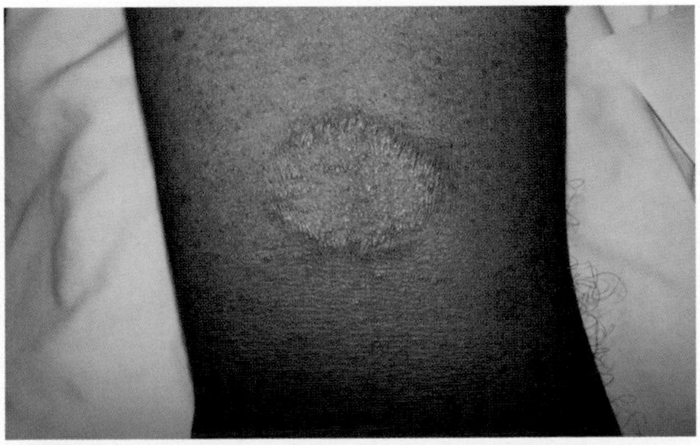

FIGURE 9-39 Tinea corporis, sometimes referred to as ring worm because of its round shape, appears lighter on skin of color, as compared with darker on lighter skin.

a form of DNA damage. BCC occurs when the DNA damage is greater than what the cells can naturally repair.[148] Abnormal activation of the intracellular signaling pathway that controls cell proliferation has also been discovered, which results is tumor development.[149]

Genetic factors predisposing an individual to BCC include light skin (Fitzpatrick I and II), light eye color, freckles, and red hair.[149] Exposure to UV light is the number one environmental factor; others include childhood sunburns, family history, photosensitizing medicines, ionizing radiation, use of tanning beds, chronic immunosuppression, and exposure to carcinogenic substances.[149]

Clinical Presentation BCC presents as a small pearly-white, scaly wound that outgrows its blood supply, eventually erodes, and subsequently ulcerates. Other characteristics include prominent telangiectatic surface vessels, rolled edges, or a slightly raised or dome-shape, as well as being painless and slow growing.[150] BCC usually occurs on the head, neck, back, or chest where there has been sun exposure. Multiple variants include superficial, infiltrative, and nodular basal cell carcinoma (with papules present) (**FIGURES 9-42** to **9-44**).

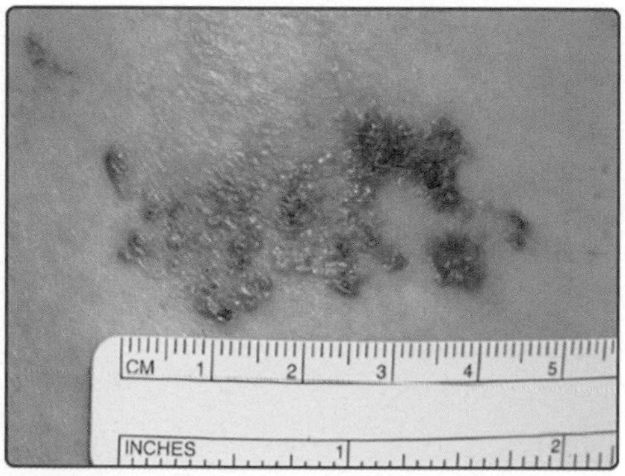

FIGURE 9-42 Basal cell carcinoma can begin as what appears to be a rash with small, pearly-white lesions. (Used with permission from Kang S, Amagai M, Bruckner AL, et al, eds. *Fitzpatrick's Dermatology*. 9th ed. New York, NY: McGraw Hill; 2019, Figure 111-4.)

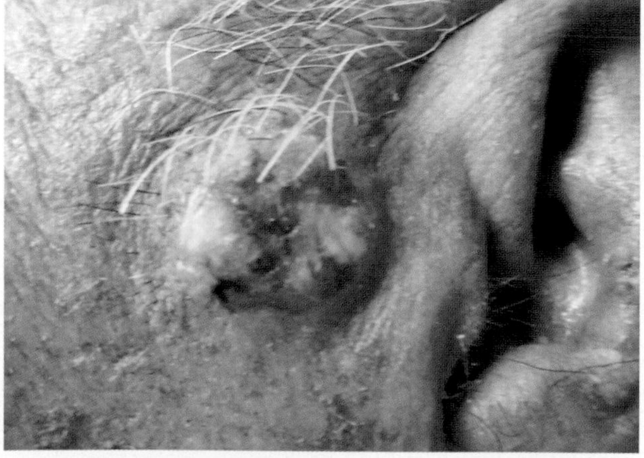

FIGURE 9-43 Basal cell carcinoma. Basal cell carcinoma is the least dangerous of the skin cancers but can become large ulcerated lesions if not removed early.

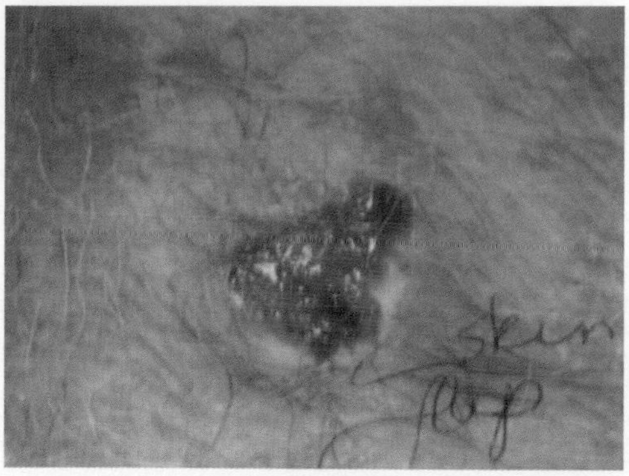

FIGURE 9-44 Basal cell carcinoma that developed 7 years after an IV insertion in the forearm.

Medical Management Treatment consists of biopsy to confirm the diagnosis and excision of the lesion with curettage, electrodessication, or Mohs micrographic surgery.[151] Close follow-up with full-body skin inspection by a dermatologist or other medical specialist is advised for early detection of additional lesions that may occur. Superficial, primary BCC can be treated noninvasively with 5% imiquimod cream.[152]

Wound Management Wound management is not usually indicated unless an excision becomes infected or for some other reason fails to heal. In such a case, moist wound healing is recommended. Cleansing with hydrogen peroxide is contraindicated as it is cytotoxic, has no antibacterial properties, and can instead prevent wound closure (**FIGURE 9-45**).

Patient education regarding avoidance of sun exposure and the use of sunscreens is necessary for the prevention of further lesions.

Squamous Cell Carcinoma

Pathophysiology Squamous cell carcinoma (SCC), the second most common form of skin cancer, is a malignant neoplasm of the keratinizing epidermal cells.[153] Tumor development is a gradual process with several histological and pathological defined stages along its malignant evolution from actinic keratosis to full dermal invasion (superficial SCC) or

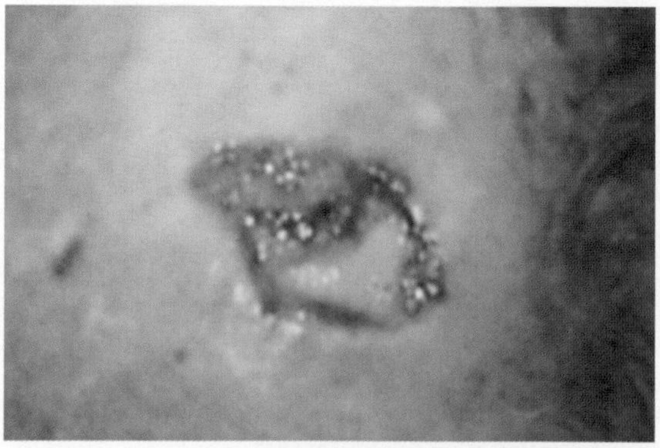

FIGURE 9-45 Excision of a basal cell carcinoma that failed to heal after 6 weeks due to the application of hydrogen peroxide twice daily.

invasion to the dermis or deeper tissue (invasive SCC).[154] The development of SCC has been reported in chronic wounds secondary to burns, trauma, hidradenitis suppurativa, radiotherapy, diabetes, and draining sinus tracts of chronic osteomyelitis. Nodal metastasis occurs in 4–6% of patients, and metastasis to other tissues is termed *advanced SCC*.[153] Risk factors for SCC include the following: exposure to ultraviolet A and B light, fair skin and blue eyes, radiation therapy, and antirejection medications after organ transplant.[155] A recent study by Lipper confirmed that the antihypertensive drug hydrochlorothiazide (HCTZ) is a potent photosensitizer and increases the risk of SCC, especially on the lip, and recommends that patients with other risk factors for SCC be placed on alternative antihypertensive agents.[156]

If the SCC occurs in a previous wound, for example, a burn, venous ulcer, or traumatic wound, years after the initial wounding, it is termed *a Marjolin ulcer*. This type of SCC is usually very aggressive and requires excision plus radiation therapy.[153,157,158]

Clinical Presentation SCC usually presents as a firm smooth red papule, nodule, or plaque; however, there are numerous presentations (**FIGURES 9-46** to **9-51**). The edges are usually poorly defined, the surrounding skin is scaly, and the center may be tender to pressure. Superficial SCC is commonly hyperkeratotic and invasive SCC is ulcerated and may metastasize and grow rapidly.[150]

Medical Management Smaller, low-risk SCCs are treated with surgical excision, electrodessication and curettage, or cryotherapy; larger, high-risk lesions are best treated with Mohs micrographic surgery with the excision going 4–9 mm beyond the lesion edge.[150,153] For advanced SCC, immunotherapy is recognized as the first line of treatment, as well as the excision of nodules and any regional lymph nodes that are involved.[153]

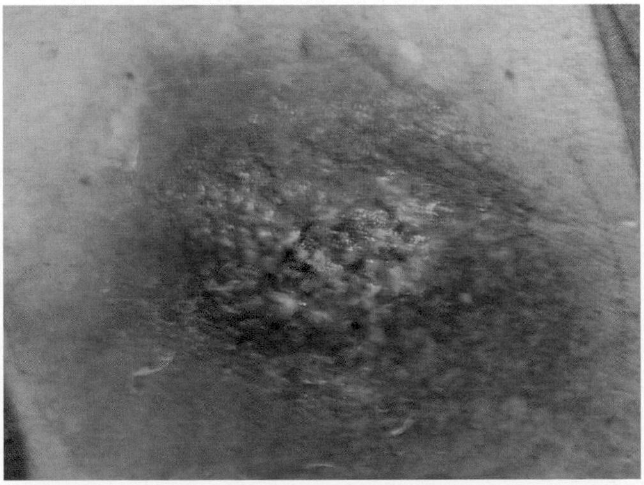

FIGURE 9-46 Squamous cell carcinoma, early-stage. Squamous cell carcinoma begins as a hyperkeratotic patch that can ulcerate and metastasize rapidly. This SCC was on a patient who had a double lung transplant with subsequent antirejection medication.

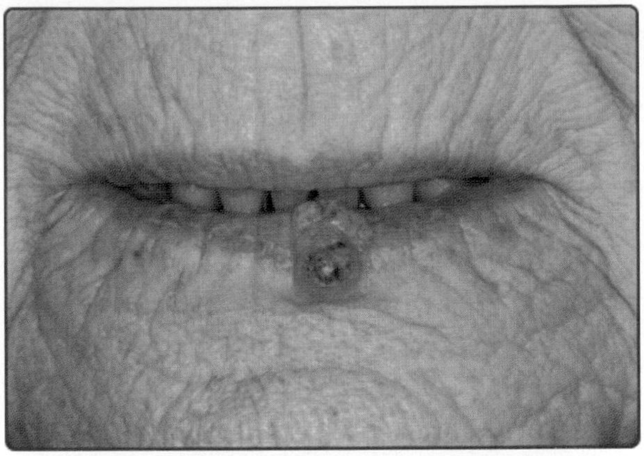

FIGURE 9-47 Squamous cell carcinoma on the lip. (Used with permission from Kang S, Amagai M, Bruckner AL, et al, eds. *Fitzpatrick's Dermatology*. 9th ed. New York, NY: McGraw Hill; 2019, Figure 112-4.)

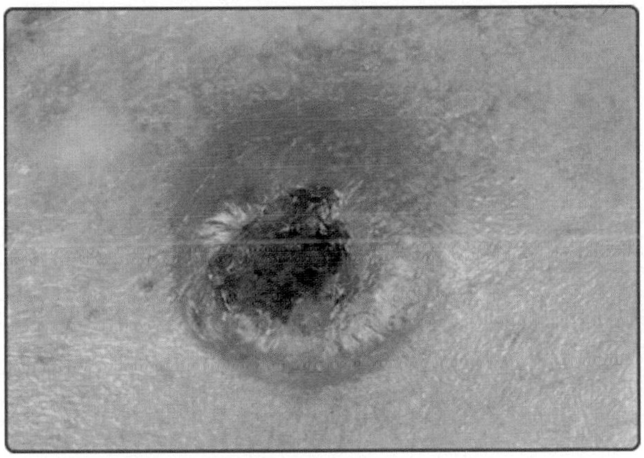

FIGURE 9-48 Squamous cell carcinoma with raised periwound border. (Used with permission from Kang S, Amagai M, Bruckner AL, et al, eds. *Fitzpatrick's Dermatology*. 9th ed. New York, NY: McGraw Hill; 2019, Figure 112-5.)

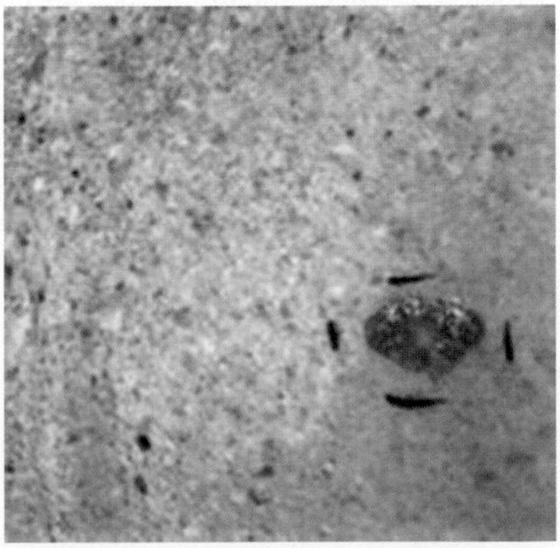

FIGURE 9-49 Invasive squamous cell carcinoma.

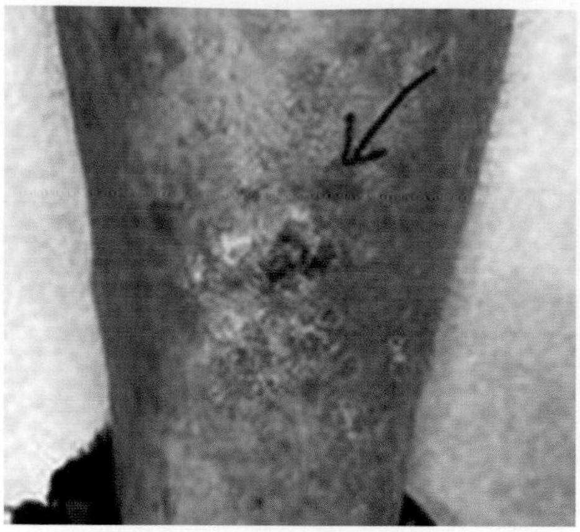

FIGURE 9-50 Squamous cell carcinoma with scaly crust in the center as well as periwound scaliness.

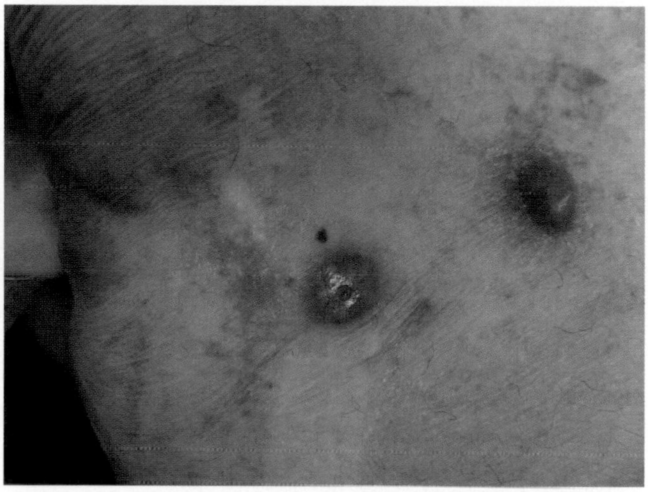

FIGURE 9-51 Squamous cell carcinoma, late-stage. Recurrent squamous cell carcinoma can occur at any place on the body; primary lesions that occur on inner tissue such as the vocal cords, larynx, or esophagus are treated with surgery and radiation. Dermal lesions such as the ones shown here are usually a sign of late-stage metastasis.

Wound Management Because of the chemotherapy and radiation of affected tissue, wounds are not uncommon after the excision of SCC. Supportive wound care is required, including infection control, pain management, lymphedema management, and frequent inspection for new lesions. Absorbent antimicrobial dressings are useful in preventing secondary infections, in managing drainage, in preventing further skin maceration at the wound site, and for facilitating wound closure. There is also evidence showing that biologic dressings are helpful in wound healing after Moh's surgery.[159,160] If the wound is on the lower extremity, compression to manage edema may be indicated to facilitate healing.

Melanoma

Pathophysiology Cutaneous melanoma, the most lethal form of skin cancer, is a tumor of the melanocytes of the epidermis. **TABLE 9-13** lists the different types of melanomas based on location[161,162] and **TABLE 9-14** presents the Breslow depth scale, which is used as a prognostic indicator. The scale indicates how deeply the tumor cells have invaded the epidermis/dermis in micrometers.[163] The cause of cutaneous melanoma is exposure to ultraviolet light in the sun and from tanning beds which results in DNA mutations. The exact mutation varies among the different types of melanoma.[161] Other risk factors include fair skin, the presence of naevi, genetic susceptibility, and a family history of melanoma.[164]

TABLE 9-13 Types of Melanoma Based on Location

Cutaneous—skin exposed to UV light
In situ—epidermis
Invasive—dermis
Superficial spreading melanoma
Nodular melanoma
Lentigo maligna melanoma
Acral—palms, soles, and nail beds
Mucosal—internal mucous membranes
Uval—eyes

Clinical Presentation Melanomas are best described by the ABCDE presentation (**FIGURES 9-52** and **9-53**).

- **A**symmetry of the discolored area
- **B**orders that are uneven and distinct
- **C**olor that is dark brown or black
- **D**iameter more than 1 cm
- **E**volution to a larger, darker lesion

Medical Management The first line of treatment is a surgical or shave biopsy to at least the dermal layer, which is essential to determine the entire area of concern. Treatment begins with wide local excision, sentinel node biopsy, chemotherapy, and radiation if needed. Treatment of metastatic melanoma is driven by genomic sequencing and consists of patient-specific combinations of targeted chemotherapy and immunotherapy.[164]

TABLE 9-14 Breslow Depth Scale for Melanoma

Stage	Depth	Depth of Tissue Involvement
Stage I	≤0.75 mm	Confined to the epidermis (*in situ*)
Stage II	0.75–1.5 mm	Invasion into the papillary dermis
Stage III	1.51–2.25 mm	Fills papillary dermis and compresses the reticular dermis
Stage IV	2.25–3.0 mm	Invasion of the reticular dermis (localized)
Stage V	>3.0 mm[1]	Invasion of subcutaneous tissue (regionalized by direct extension)

The Breslow depth scale is a prognostic indicator for melanoma based on the depth of penetration of the tumor cells into the tissue and correlates with the Clark scale of description of tissue involvement.[1]

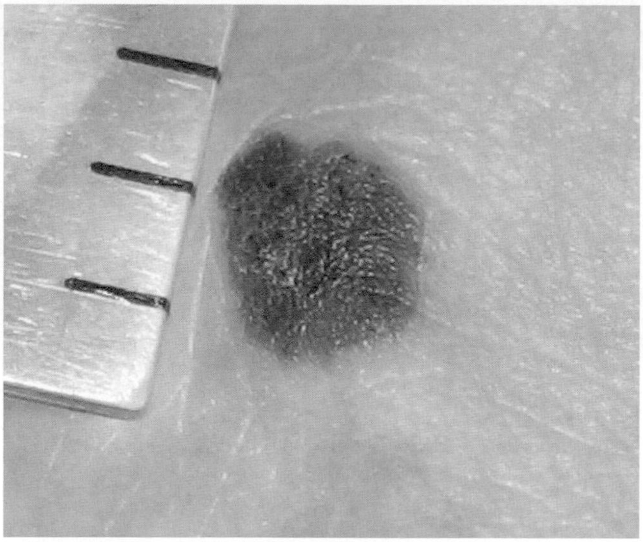

FIGURE 9-52 Melanoma. Melanoma is diagnosed by asymmetry, uneven borders, dark brown or black color, diameter greater than 1 cm, and visible changes in appearance. Early excision is necessary to prevent metastasis.

Wound Management Wound care is not indicated unless there is failure of the incisional wound to heal, in which case principles of moist wound healing are applied.

Kaposi Sarcoma

Pathophysiology Kaposi sarcoma (KS) is a malignant tumor of the lymphocytic and endothelial cells linked to the herpetic viruses and HIV. The pathogenesis of KS has now been identified as the human herpes virus type 8.[165] Four clinical variants have been identified:

- Localized, slowly progressing form in older men (classic KS)
- Endemic African KS
- Immunosuppressive KS, usually associated with organ transplant recipients
- Rapidly progressive form associated with HIV or AIDS[166]

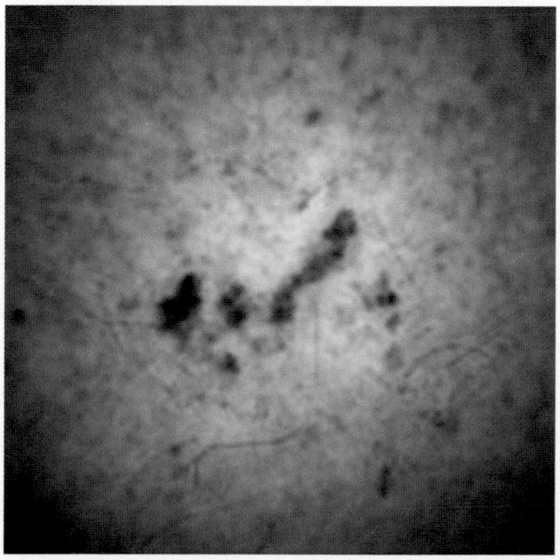

FIGURE 9-53 Melanoma with more than one lesion, all with asymmetric borders.

Clinical Presentation KS lesions can appear anywhere on the body, including the mucous membranes. The lesions are slightly raised, elongated with poorly demarcated edges, and may have rust or purple-red maculae or patches. They progress slowly into firm necrotic plaques with underlying nodules.[166] Marked edema may develop when the tumors involve the lymphatic vessels, leading to diffuse edema and subsequent skin breakdown (**FIGURES 9-54** and **9-55**).

Medical Management KS associated with AIDS is treated with herpes viral DNA polymerase inhibitors. Surgical excision, local radiation therapy, chemotherapy, and cryotherapy are used for isolated cutaneous lesions.[167] For immunosuppressed patients, rapamycin or reduction of immunosuppressive therapy is recommended.[166]

Wound Management Immediate treatment of KS may include topical application of 9-*cis*-retinoic acid (alitretinoin gel), which has been proven superior to previously used vehicle gel.[165,168]

Because of the radiation, lymphatic involvement, and edema, chronic wounds may develop (especially if the lesion

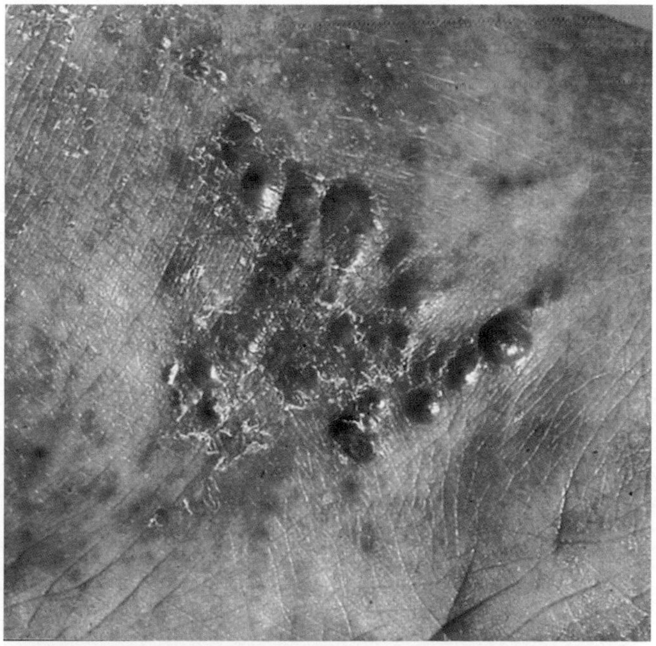

FIGURE 9-54 Kaposi sarcoma. Kaposi sarcoma is most frequently associated with HIV/AIDS, although it can occur in other immunosuppressed individuals. It is slow growing and treatable with excision and radiation. (Used with permission from Tschachler E. Kaposi's sarcoma and angiosarcoma. In: Goldsmith LA, Katz SI, Gilchrest BA, Paller AS, Leffell DJ, Wolff K. eds. *Fitzpatrick's Dermatology in General Medicine.* 8th ed. New York, NY: McGraw Hill; 2012, Figure 128-1.)

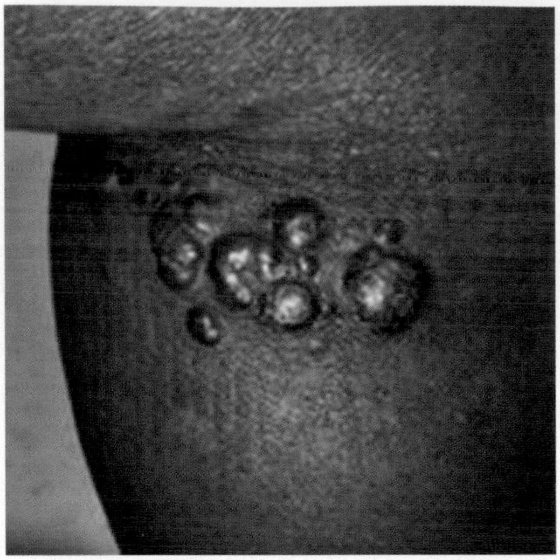

FIGURE 9-55 **Kaposi sarcoma on dark skin.**

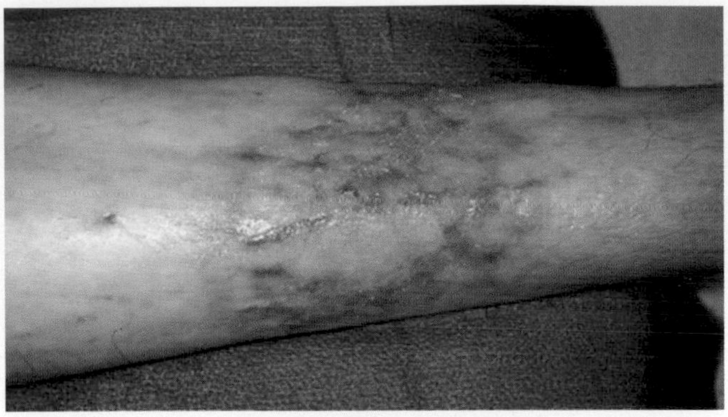

FIGURE 9-57 **Healed traumatic wound after treatment with biological matrix product, electrical stimulation, and hair follicle transplants.**

is on the lower extremity) even years after the tumor has been eliminated. Standard wound care using the TIMEO2 principles and compression therapy are recommended, and adjunctive therapies such as HBOT and electrical stimulation may be beneficial *if* there are no signs of malignant cells, eg, on wounds occurring years after radiation therapy (FIGURES 9-56 and 9-57).

Merkel Cell Carcinoma

Pathophysiology Merkel cell carcinoma (MCC) involves the Merkel cells in the basal layer of the epidermis and progresses to the dermis and subcutaneous tissue. It is a skin cancer associated with UV exposure that tends to occur in older individuals who are also immunosuppressed and have Merkel cell polyomavirus (MCPyV) infection. MCC advances to subclinical node metastasis in 30–50% of the patients.[169] Because it can advance rapidly and has a poor prognosis with metastasis, early diagnosis and intervention are critical.

Clinical Presentation Initial MCC presentation is much like a cyst, often resulting in misdiagnosis (FIGURES 9-58 and 9-59). MCC can be identified using the acronym AEIOU as defined in TABLE 9-15 and if three of the five characteristics are present, there is a high probability of MCC and a biopsy is recommended.[170]

Medical Management Medical management is based on staging and begins with surgical excision to healthy tissue with clean margins if there are no signs of metastasis, preferably with the Mohs technique. Radiation and chemotherapy are required for metastatic disease (especially for palliative care of advanced disease or for patients who cannot undergo surgery).[170] Avelumab is an FDA-approved immunotherapy drug also used for metastatic disease.[169]

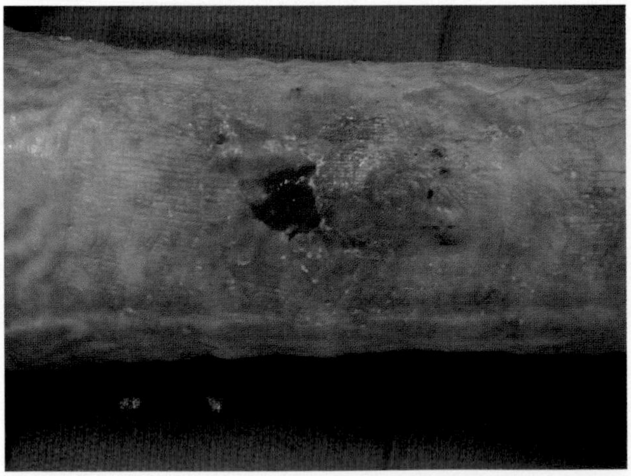

FIGURE 9-56 **Nonhealing traumatic wound on a lower extremity site that was treated with radiation for Kaposi sarcoma about 20 years prior to the first wound assessment.**

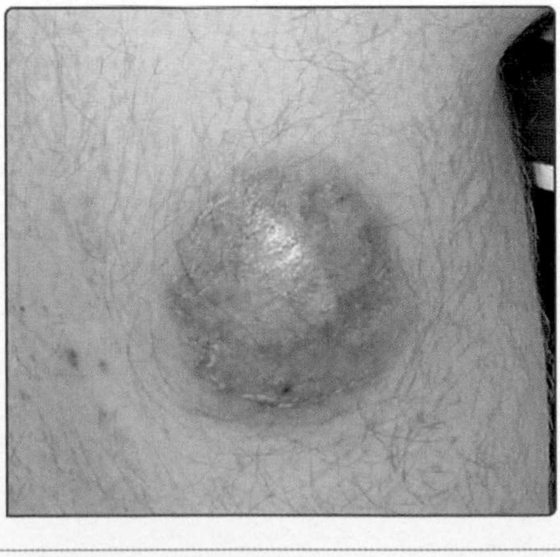

FIGURE 9-58 **Merkel cell carcinoma.** Initially a Merkel cell carcinoma may have the appearance of a cyst or small nodule. (Used with permission from Kang S, Amagai M, Bruckner AL, et al, eds. *Fitzpatrick's Dermatology*. 9th ed. New York, NY: McGraw Hill; 2019, Figure 113-1A.)

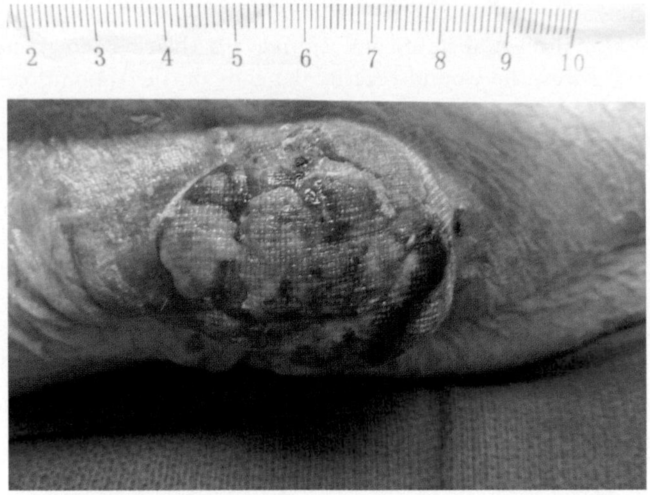

FIGURE 9-59 Merkel cell carcinoma. Advanced Merkel cell carcinoma on the elbow of an 85-year-old lady. She had four of the five characteristics of MCC and was treated with surgical excision.

Wound Management Prior to surgery, exudate can be managed with absorbent dressings. After surgery, any excision wounds are managed with standard wound care.

Cutaneous Lymphoma

Pathophysiology Although lymphomas generally originate in the lymph nodes or in collections of lymphatic tissue in organs, such as the stomach or intestines, the skin may also be affected. Cutaneous lymphomas represent the clonal proliferation of neoplastic B cells or T cells that migrate to the skin and cause progressive lesions.[171] **TABLE 9-16** presents a list of primary cutaneous lymphomas, the most common being mycosis fungoides (**FIGURE 9-60**).[172]

Clinical Presentation Cutaneous lymphoma (CT) may present as various types of skin lesions, but rarely as an open wound (**FIGURE 9-61**). Mycosis fungoides begin as patches of scaly erythema and progress to plaques of sharply demarcated, scaly, elevated lesions that are dusky red to violet. The next, most severe stage is nodular in which the malignant cells cause the formation of reddish-brown or purplish-red

TABLE 9-15 Signs and Symptoms of Merkel Cell Carcinoma

Asymptomatic (nontender, firm, red, purple, or skin-colored papule or nodule; ulceration is rare)
Expanding rapidly (significant growth noted within 1–3 months of diagnosis, but most lesions are <2 cm at the time of diagnosis)
Immune suppression (eg, HIV/AIDS, chronic lymphocytic leukemia, solid organ transplant)
Older than 50 years
Ultraviolet-exposed site on a person with fair skin (most likely presentation, but can also occur in sun-protected areas)

A lesion with three or more of these signs should be biopsied to rule out Merkel cell carcinoma.

TABLE 9-16 Classification of Primary Cutaneous Lymphoma (WHO-EROTC)

Cutaneous T-Cell and NK-Cell Lymphomas
▪ Mycosis fungoides
▪ Mycosis fungoides variants and subtypes • Folliculotropic mycosis fungoides • Pagetoid reticulosis • Granulomatous slack skin
▪ Sézary syndrome
▪ Adult T-cell leukemia/lymphoma
▪ Primary cutaneous CD30-positive lymphoproliferative disorders • Primary cutaneous anaplastic large-cell lymphoma • Lymphomatoid papulosis
▪ Subcutaneous panniculitis-like T-cell lymphoma
▪ Extranodal NK/T-cell lymphoma, nasal type
▪ Primary cutaneous peripheral T-cell lymphoma, unspecified • Primary cutaneous aggressive epidermotropic $CD8^+$ T-cell lymphoma (provisional) • Cutaneous γ/δ T-cell lymphoma (provisional) • Primary cutaneous $CD4^+$ small- or medium-sized pleomorphic T-cell lymphoma (provisional)
▪ Cutaneous B-cell lymphomas • Primary cutaneous marginal zone B-cell lymphoma • Primary cutaneous follicle center lymphoma • Primary cutaneous diffuse large B-cell lymphoma, leg type • Primary cutaneous diffuse large B-cell lymphoma, other • Intravascular large B-cell lymphoma (provisional) • Precursor hematologic neoplasm • $CD4^+/CD56^+$ hematodermic neoplasm (blastic NK cell lymphoma)

Reproduced with permission from Beyer M, Sterry W. Cutaneous lymphoma. In: Goldsmith LA, Katz SI, Gilchrest BA, Paller AS, Leffell DJ, Wolff K, eds. *Fitzpatrick's Dermatology in General Medicine*. 8th ed. New York, NY: McGraw-Hill; 2012.

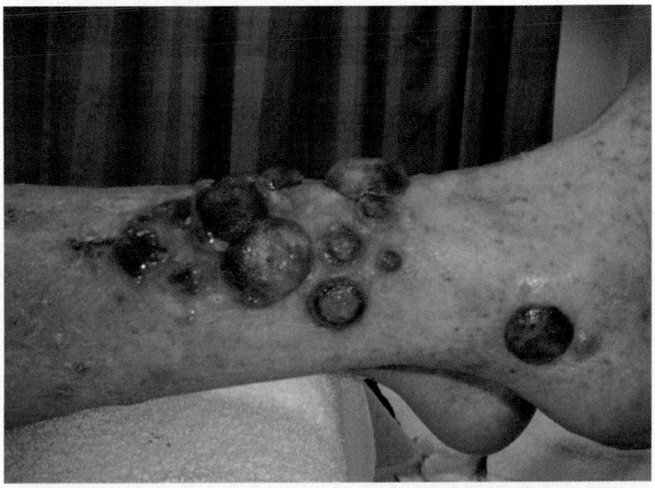

FIGURE 9-60 Cutaneous lymphoma. Mycosis fungoides have three stages: patches, plaques, and nodules as seen in the lower extremity of this patient with systemic metastasis as well as diffuse ulcerated lesions. Patients who have progressed to this stage have a poor prognosis.

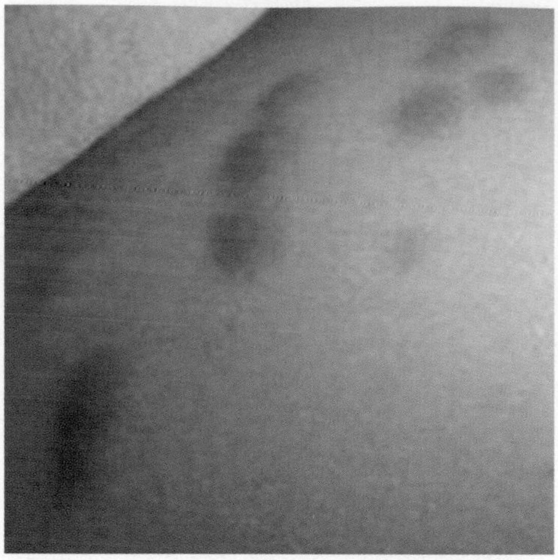

FIGURE 9-61 Early presentation of cutaneous lymphoma.

and smooth-surfaced nodules, which often ulcerate and often become secondarily infected.[172] Cutaneous B-cell lymphomas present as solitary or multiple erythematous to violaceous domed papules, plaques, nodules, or tumors (usually on the arms, face, or trunk).[173] Ulcerative cutaneous lymphomas are associated with poor prognosis; they are increasingly observed in severely immune-compromised patients. A punch biopsy of at least 6 mm is preferred for histopathological confirmation of the diagnosis.[173]

Medical Management Treatment ranges from minimal intervention with skin-directed therapy to aggressive systemic therapies that include multiagent chemotherapy with consideration for hematopoietic stem cell transplants, depending upon the type of CT and the severity of the disease.[174] Spot radiotherapy is used to treat isolated cutaneous lesions; topical chemotherapy can be useful for patches and plaques. Chemotherapy in conjunction with immunotherapy is used for progressive, diffuse lesions or systemic disease. Psoralen+UVA (PUVA) phototherapy is used for long-term maintenance therapy of patches and plaques.[175] A combination of interferon-alpha 2b and low doses of methotrexate was shown to have a good survival rate and minimal toxicity in a study done on patients with relapsed cutaneous T-cell lymphoma by Aviles et al.[176]

Wound Management Supportive wound care is indicated for any nonhealing ulcerated lesions. Because the lesions are oxygen-deprived as a result of the lymphoma, they tend to be exquisitely painful. Nonadherent absorbent dressings and mild compression on the lower extremities are effective in managing drainage and minimizing pain with dressing changes.

MISCELLANEOUS

Spider Bites

Pathophysiology More than 50 spider species in the United States have been implicated in causing significant medical conditions; however, there are two main species that are most known for causing skin necrosis and open wounds: *Loxosceles reclusa* (brown recluse) and *Latrodectus* (black widow). In both cases, the wound severity depends on the venom load and the host's immune response. The venom responsible for skin necrosis is a water-soluble substance that contains eight enzymes (including sphingomyelinase D, hyaluronidase, esterase, and alkaline phosphatase) that destroy the tissue they invade, a process termed *loxoscelism*. Approximately 10% of spider bites progress to necrosis.[177] The brown recluse is so named because it tends to reside in dark, secluded places such as closets, attics, and woodpiles and is not aggressive. It bites only when it is disturbed and requires counter pressure to inject the venom.[178]

Clinical Presentation Because most spiders are not seen at the time of the bite (80%), making a definitive diagnosis can be difficult. Only about 12% of the victims can bring the spider to the medical facility after the bite. The initial response is minor stinging or burning, followed by the development of an erythematous macule surrounding a central papule.[177] If there is sufficient venom or the host is immunosuppressed, the bite may progress to severe inflammation with a "bull's-eye" appearance, followed by a red, white, and blue discoloration as the lesion enlarges (**FIGURES 9-62** and **9-63**). If the tissue becomes anoxic, necrosis with an eschar will develop, usually after 72 hours, with underlying fatty necrosis. Viscerocutaneous loxoscelism or systemic signs may include rash, fever, chills, nausea, vomiting, malaise, arthralgia, and myalgia. In severe rare cases, renal failure may occur with hemolysis, hemoglobinuria, leukocytosis, leukopenia, or thrombocytopenia.[179–181]

Diagnosis is made by positive identification of the spider, complete blood count if there are systemic effects, urinalysis if there is renal failure, and ELISA (enzyme-linked immunosorbent assay), which can check for the specific antigen.[182]

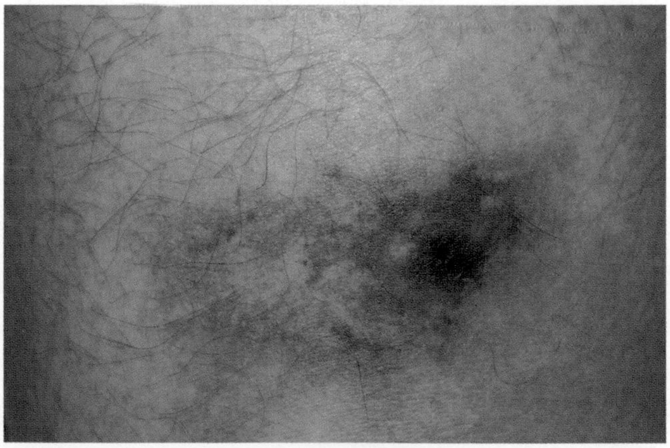

FIGURE 9-62 Bull's eye sign of spider bite. Within hours after a brown recluse spider bite, there will be a distinctively visible spot where the venom was injected, termed the "bull's eye." (From Knoop KJ, Stack LB, Storrow AB, Thurman R, eds. *The Atlas of Emergency Medicine*. 4th ed. New York, NY: McGraw Hill; 2016, Figure 16.62. Reproduced with permission from photo contributor: Lawrence B. Stack, MD.)

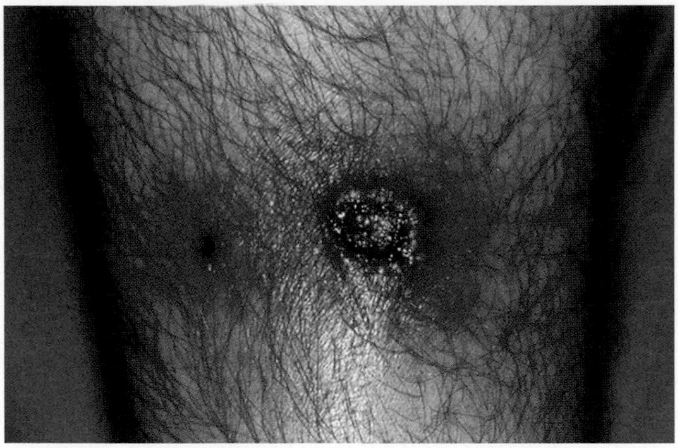

FIGURE 9-63 Recluse necrosis. Within about 2–5 weeks, significant brown recluse envenomations may produce a deep, poorly healing ulcer with necrosis. At this point, the patient may require excision of the necrotic tissue with wound healing by secondary intention. (From Knoop KJ, Stack LB, Storrow AB, Thurman RJ, eds. *The Atlas of Emergency Medicine*. 4th ed. New York, NY: McGraw Hill; 2016, Figure 16.64. Reproduced with permission from photo contributor: Kevin J. Knoop, MD.)

Medical Management Treatment of spider bites may begin with excision of the bite location. Dapsone administered within 24 hours may inhibit neutrophil migration (except in the case of G6PD deficiency), and systemic steroids may prevent enlargement of the necrotic area. Other medical interventions include oral antihistamines, glucocorticoids, and antivenom. Diethyl azelate, a plasma membrane fluidizer with a broad range of immunomodulatory activities, has also shown promise as a potential treatment for the brown recluse spider bite.[183] Prophylactic antibiotics are indicated for immunosuppressed victims.

Wound Management Initial first aide includes cooling the bite site to prevent the spreading of the venom. If tissue necrosis occurs, debridement and moist wound principles are indicated. Hyperbaric oxygen therapy may also be useful, especially if the patient has a marginal oxygen supply due to peripheral arterial disease.[177]

Calciphylaxis

Pathophysiology Calciphylaxis, also known as calcific uremic arteriolopathy, is a potentially fatal condition characterized clinically by progressive cutaneous necrosis as a result of calcification and thrombosis of the dermal arterioles.[184] Calciphylaxis is seen in 1% of patients with chronic renal failure and in 4.1% of patients receiving hemodialysis. In addition, it usually occurs in patients with Type 2 diabetes and end-stage renal disease who have been on hemodialysis for more than 10 years.[185] Other risk factors for calciphylaxis include female sex, obesity, recurrent hypotension, hypo- or hyperparathyroidism, hypercalcemia, Vitamin K deficiency, elevated time-averaged serum phosphorous levels, reduced time-averaged serum albumin levels, and warfarin therapy.[186,187] More than 50% of the patients die within 1 year of diagnosis, usually from sepsis.[184]

The pathogenesis of calciphylaxis is still poorly understood. Patients who are on long-term dialysis usually develop abnormal calcium-phosphorus products, which in turn lead to tertiary hyperparathyroidism. This results in elevated calcium-phosphate products and the development of microvascular calcification that in turn leads to tissue necrosis.[184] Diagnosis is confirmed with a skin biopsy which shows calcification of the intima and media of small and medium vessels in the dermis and subcutaneous tissue.[187–189]

Clinical Presentation The cutaneous manifestations of calciphylaxis begin as sudden-appearing red or violaceous mottled plaques in a livedo reticularis pattern. The early ischemic lesions often progress to gangrenous, poorly defined, black plaques and/or nodules. With time, the plaques ulcerate and become exquisitely tender. Ulcers are usually on the lower extremities, bilateral, asymmetric, and may extend deep into muscle (**FIGURES 9-64** and **9-65**).

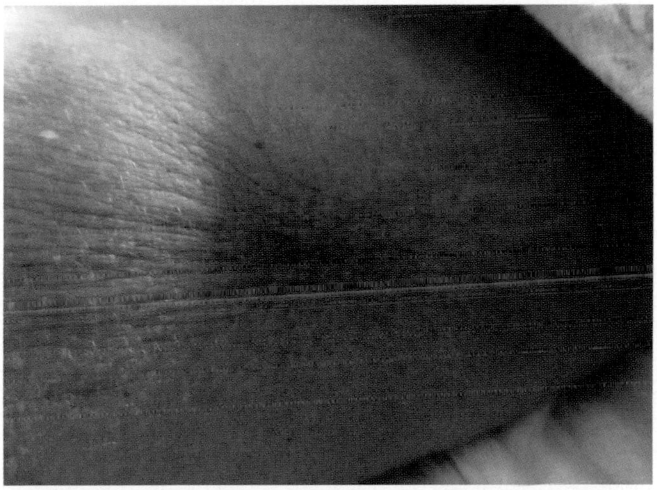

FIGURE 9-64 Calciphylaxis, early onset. Early onset of calciphylaxis appears as erythema and ischemia with severe anoxic pain.

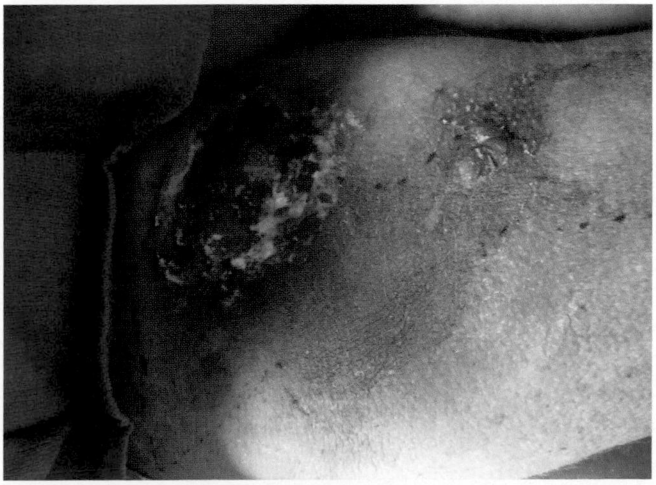

FIGURE 9-65 Calciphylaxis, progression of skin lesion. As the disease progresses, the skin necrosis becomes more extensive and more painful; the patient is at higher risk for mortality.

Medical Management Multiple approaches to the medical management of calciphylaxis are recommended to prevent infection, manage pain, and optimize outcomes by chelating arterial calcium. Reported treatment strategies include the following:

- Systemic antibiotics if there is evidence of infection
- Opioid pain medication (morphine can cause hypotension and slow blood flow in the arterioles, as well as diminished appetite that can lead to malnutrition and impaired wound healing)
- Phosphate binders such as sevelamer
- Sodium thiosulfate as a chelating agent for calcium deposits in the tissue
- Bisphosphonate therapy to help remove arterial calcification
- Low calcium hemodialysis for patients who are on hemodialysis
- Cinacalcet to lower parathyroid levels and improve calcium-phosphorus homeostasis
- Hyperbaric oxygen therapy to increase local tissue oxygen perfusion
- Low calcium diet to optimize nutrition and provide adequate calorie and protein intake for wound healing[184,190]

In the past, parathyroidectomy was performed in an effort to increase calcium uptake; however, this procedure has not been shown to be significantly effective and is reserved for patients with known hyperparathyroidism.[191] Also, systemic corticosteroids and blood transfusions are not recommended as they may exacerbate arteriolar calcification.[191]

Wound Management Debridement of necrotic tissue and calcified vessels is needed for the reversal of the inflammatory response to calciphylaxis; however, this is difficult to perform bedside if the necrosis is extensive because of the intense pain levels associated with the disease. Surgical debridement followed by negative pressure wound therapy is the most expeditious approach if the patient is medically stable for surgery. This is complemented by skin grafting with either autologous or cellular, acellular, or matrix products (CAMPs).[192] Intralesional sodium thiosulfate (250 mg/mL) injected or instilled into areas of clinically active disease has been shown to reduce pain and resolve the purpura of calciphylaxis lesions, and pentoxifylline can facilitate vasodilation.[193] Electrical stimulation and hyperbaric oxygen therapy may be beneficial adjunct therapies. In addition to the meticulous wound care (using aseptic technique to prevent infection), nutritional supplements and monitoring are advised because patients may have difficulty eating sufficient calories for wound healing given the amount of pain medicine required to manage the anoxic pain.

Warfarin-Induced Skin Necrosis

Pathophysiology Warfarin-induced skin necrosis is a rare complication of anticoagulation therapy in individuals who have a thrombophilic history or after administration of a large dose of warfarin, particularly without the simultaneous initial use of heparin.[194] Although the exact pathogenesis is unknown, it is understood that protein C deficiency, protein S deficiency, Factor V Leiden, hyperhomocysteinemia, antiphospholipid antibodies, and antithrombin III deficiency are common underlying factors. Other risk factors include female gender, obesity, perimenopausal age, viral infections, hepatic disease, large doses of warfarin, and drug interactions.[195] Dermatopathologic findings include diffuse dermal microthrombi with endothelial cell damage and red cell extravasation that progresses to full-thickness coagulative necrosis.[196] Symptoms usually begin between the 3rd and 10th days after starting anticoagulation therapy.[194]

Clinical Presentation Skin changes usually appear on the breasts, buttocks, abdomen, thighs, and calves, probably due to the reduced blood supply to adipose tissue.[192] Initial symptoms include patient complaints of paresthesias, sensations of pressure, and exquisite pain, followed by presentation of erythematous flush that becomes edema with *peau d'orange* appearance. Within 24–48 hours, petechiae and purpura appear and become hemorrhagic bullae that progress to hemorrhagic necrosis (**FIGURE 9-66**).[195,197]

Medical Management The most important aspect of treatment is discontinuation of the anticoagulant, along with pain management and infection prevention. IV heparin or low-molecular-weight heparin may be substituted for warfarin,[192] and fresh frozen plasma and subcutaneous vitamin K are used to reverse the warfarin effect quickly.[195,197]

Wound Management Wound management includes debridement (surgical, sharp, or autolytic, depending on the depth and amount of necrotic tissue), moist wound therapy, skin grafts, and/or bioengineered skin. If surgical debridement involves loss of subcutaneous tissue, negative pressure wound therapy may assist in wound bed preparation for surgical closure.

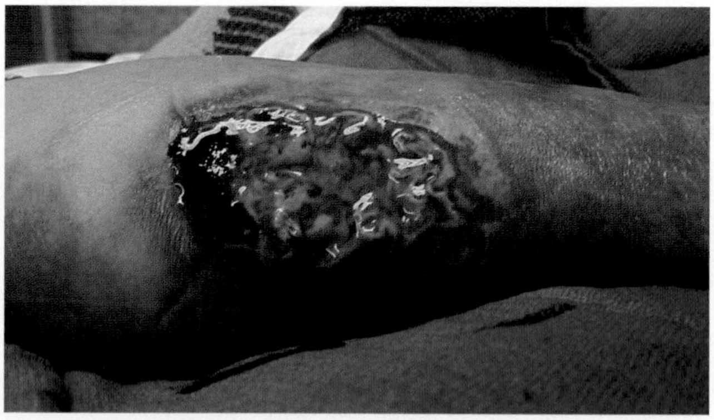

FIGURE 9-66 Coumadin-induced skin necrosis. Coumadin-induced skin necrosis usually develops days after beginning the medication. Treatment involves first stopping the medication, debridement of the necrotic tissue, and moist wound care.

Sickle Cell Wounds

Pathophysiology Sickle cell ulcers are a complication of sickle cell anemia, an inherited genetic disorder in which the red blood cells have a sickle shape, rendering them incapable of binding hemoglobin. This leads to hypoxia that can cause severe pain crises and can also deprive injured tissue of the oxygen necessary for healing. The patient with the homozygous form of sickle cell disease is most likely to develop a sickle cell ulcer. Studies have shown that males are more likely than females to develop leg ulcers due to sickle cell disease.[198]

In sickle cell disease, the abnormal hemoglobin molecule in the red blood cell causes a change in the shape of the RBC. In addition, when cells are in sickled shape, they tend to increase blood viscosity. This causes slowing of the blood flow in small vessels, which also contributes to ischemia of tissue and organs. Over time, the patient suffers repeated episodes of pain, tissue damage, and eventually, organ failure. Although the exact cause of sickle cell ulcers is not clear, they have been associated with trauma, infection, severe anemia, warm temperatures, and venous insufficiency.[199,200]

Clinical Presentation Sickle cell ulcers are found on the lower third of the leg, usually over the medial and/or lateral malleoli of the ankle (**FIGURE 9-67**). They are exquisitely painful and can have a thick layer of fibrinous tissue, slough, or biofilm. The edges tend to be even like an arterial wound, and the wound bed is slow to granulate. Because of the chronic inflammatory state and reduced ankle function due to pain, lower extremity edema may be present and thus complicate the healing process.

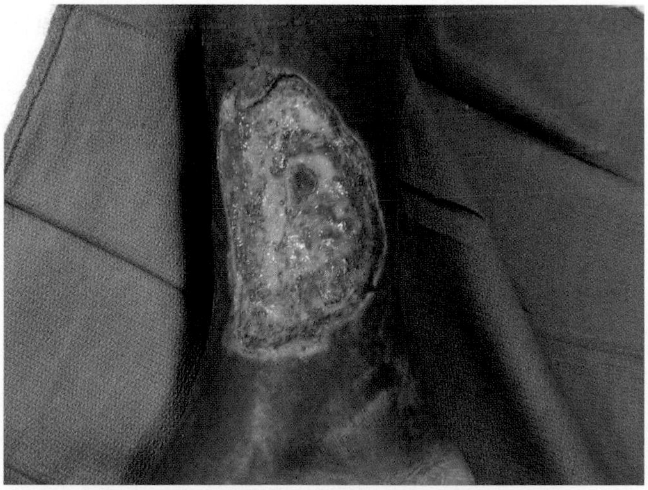

FIGURE 9-67 Sickle cell wound. The patient with sickle cell disease may develop a spontaneous ulcer or may have difficulty healing a wound that has another etiology. This patient had a chemical burn on the lower leg that became chronic and was debilitating because of the pain, drainage, and resultant loss of ankle function. He was treated medically with transfusions and deferasirox to chelate the iron; locally, with nonadherent antimicrobial dressings, compression therapy, exercise to increase the ankle range of motion and strength of the venous pump, and gait training. He healed fully and was able to return to work.

Medical Management Treating patients who have wounds and sickle cell anemia requires a combination of therapies in order to optimize healing. Stem cell transplantation has become more prevalent as a treatment for SCD in children.[201] Medical management of the sickle cell disorder includes oral zinc sulfate (200 mg three times per day)[130] and a combination of l-methylfolate calcium, pyridoxal-5 phosphate, and methylcobalamin (Metanx). Hydroxyurea and oral glutamine have also been recently approved by the FDA for treating SCD.[201] The goal is to decrease endothelial cell homocysteine levels and raise nitric oxide levels, resulting in improved wound healing. It also helps reduce pain associated with sickle cell ulcers and increase blood flow in the microcirculation at the wound margin.[202,203]

Transfusion therapy is advised with the goal of keeping the hematocrit level between 30 and 35 and the level of normal hemoglobin (hemoglobin A) greater than 70% of the total. The transfusions are continued until the ulcers heal or for 6 months at which time they are discontinued.[204] In conjunction with transfusions, deferasirox is administered to chelate the excess iron that accumulates with transfusions.[204]

IV arginine butyrate can also help change the concentration of abnormal hemoglobin, thus facilitating wound healing.[203] Pentoxifylline (Trental) is a vasodilator used to treat peripheral arterial disease that may also help increase peripheral tissue perfusion.

Wound Management Basics of good wound care include debridement of devitalized tissue, control of infection, assurance of adequate circulation, and maintenance of a moist wound environment.[204] Specific strategies that have been included in the literature include the following[205–207]:

- Negative pressure wound therapy
- Antibiotics
- Biofilm removal
- Compression therapy
- Topical growth factor (granulocyte-macrophage colony-stimulating factor)
- Honey-based dressing
- Bioengineered skin
- Split-thickness skin graft
- Hyperbaric oxygen therapy
- Electrical stimulation or electromagnetic therapy

COVID Skin

Pathophysiology Cutaneous changes have been reported with COVID-19 with the following suggested pathologies:

- Viral particles in the cutaneous blood vessels lead to a lymphocytic vasculitis similar to that seen in thrombophilic arteritis, a disorder in which blood immune complexes activate cytokines.[208]

- An immune response to the infection leads to Langerhans cells activation, resulting in vasodilation and spongiosis.[208]
- Accumulation of microvascular thromboses that originate in other organs as a result of a systemic procoagulant state, and thus reduce the blood flow to the cutaneous microvascular system.[208,209]
- Low-grade disseminated intravascular coagulation and hypoxia-related accumulation of deoxygenated blood leads to hypoperfusion in the extremities.[209]

The onset of the skin lesions ranges from 3 days prior to COVID-19 diagnosis to 13 days after diagnosis,[208] and can occur in critically ill patients, the pediatric population,[210] and recently vaccinated individuals.[211,212] COVID toes associated with vaccination tend to occur 4–9 days after vaccination, and histology shows inflammatory infiltrates suggesting that there may be an inflammatory response rather than infection causing the changes (**FIGURE 9-68**).[213] Thus, it would appear to be a hypersensitivity reaction to the vaccine.[209]

Clinical Presentation A study by Genovese[214] identified the following six main clinical patterns of skin changes associated with COVID-19 (**FIGURE 9-69**):

- Urticarial rash
- Confluent erythematous/maculopapular/morbilliform rash
- Papulovesicular exanthema
- Chilblain-like acral pattern
- Livedo reticularis/racemosa-like pattern
- Purpuric "vasculitic" pattern

COVID toes are pernio-like purple, painful, ill-defined acral purpuric lesions with acrocyanosis (**FIGURE 9-70A, B**). As with any inflammatory disorder, changes in skin are different and sometimes more difficult to discern in skin of color. Rashes will have the same color as unaffected skin, maculopapular and morbilliform rashes may increase the skin temperature more than cause a change in color, lichenification will occur more frequently in darker skin than in lighter skin, and scaliness may be more easily detected than pigment changes in skin of color.[215]

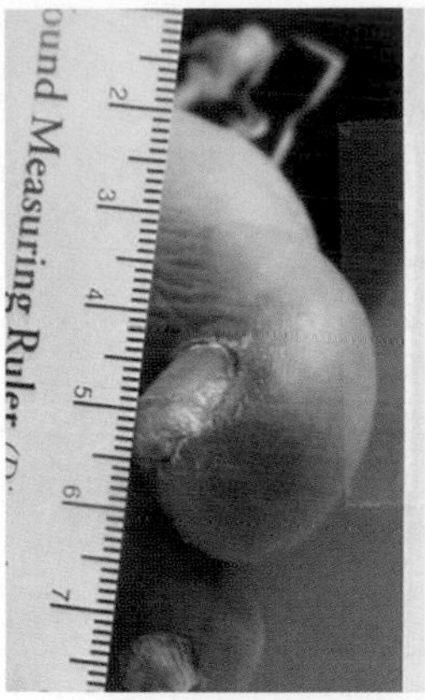

FIGURE 9-69 Hypoxia gives an ischemic appearance to the toe of a patient with COVID.

Medical Management Medical management of any skin changes is predicated on the treatment of the coronavirus and the severity of each patient's acute respiratory syndrome.[215] In cases when the patient has been treated with medications, it is necessary to determine if the skin changes are a result of the virus or a drug-induced hypersensitivity reaction.[216]

Wound Management Ischemic tissue requires protection from trauma (shear, pressure, friction) during critical care;

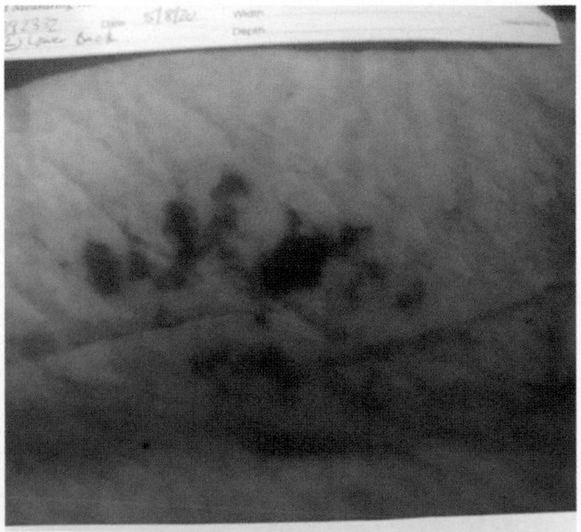

FIGURE 9-68 Rash associated with COVID skin.

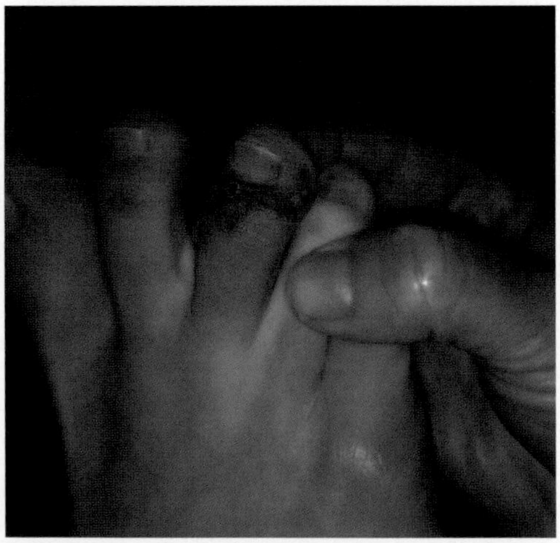

FIGURE 9-70 COVID toe on a 16-year-old vaccinated for the virus approximately 5 days prior.

any open lesions require moist wound management. Severe cases of urticarial rash can be treated with antihistamines and steroids for symptom relief. The chilblain-like acral pattern in toes has been treated with heating, NSAIDs, topical steroids, and vasodilators; however, this reported treatment was not COVID-related.[216] COVID toes after vaccination resolve spontaneously after about 6 weeks and require only protection from trauma during that time.[217]

Polymorphous Light Eruption

Pathophysiology Polymorphous light eruption (PMLE) is the most common form of photodermatosis which usually occurs in spring or early summer upon first intense exposure to the sun. Although the pathology is not fully understood, PMLE appears to involve immunologic mechanisms with ultraviolet radiation-induced immunosuppression and a subsequent delayed-type hypersensitivity response to a photoantigen.[218,219] The UVA-induced oxidative stress elicits a cellular stress response affecting keratinocyte gene expression and skin immune function.[219]

Clinical Presentation PMLE is characterized by pruritic skin lesions on areas not previously exposed to the sun. The lesions begin as papules, rash, or eczema hours to days after exposure to sunlight and may progress to plaques, vesicles, or nodules.[220] The lesions usually resolve spontaneously within 2 weeks of onset without any scarring (**FIGURES 9-71** and **9-72**).

Medical Management No medical care is indicated unless there are rare systemic symptoms. Vitamin D replacement may be needed if a susceptible individual elects to avoid sun exposure.

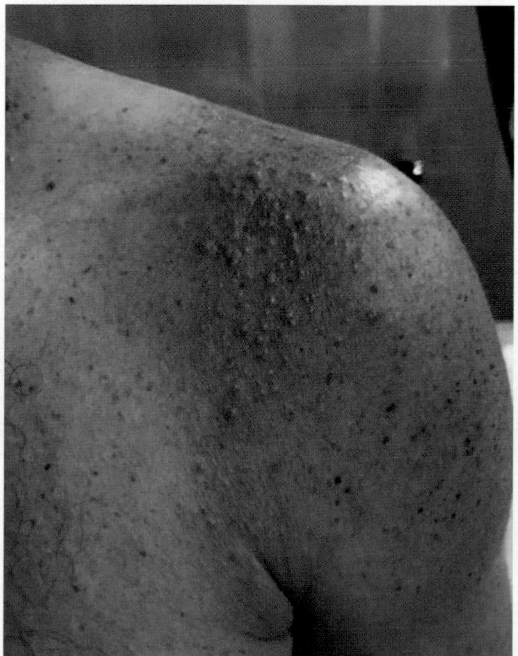

FIGURE 9-71 Polymorphous light eruption after the first exposure to intense sunlight.

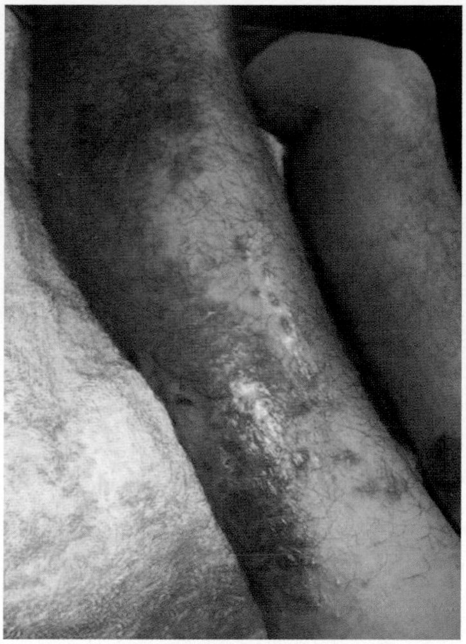

FIGURE 9-72 Polymorphous light eruption on the lower extremity.

Wound Management Prevention of PMLE involves the application of a broad-spectrum, water-resistant semi-opaque SPF 50+ sunscreen before sun exposure and every 2 hours thereafter or covering with densely woven material. Photohardening with suberythemal dosages of NB-UVB administered two to three times per week for 4–6 weeks, at a starting dose of 0.2 J/cm^2 and in dose increments of 0.05–0.1 J/cm^2 per treatment, as tolerated, has been shown to decrease incidence for patients with a history of PMLE.[221]

Topical corticosteroids may be used to mitigate symptoms.[222]

Factitious Wounds

Pathophysiology Patients with factitious disorder (FD) use false symptoms or self-injury in order to appear sick and/or to gain access to medical care. More than 62% of the patients are female and the mean age is 34.2 years. FD is similar to somatic symptom disorder, another mental disorder that involves the presence of skin lesions that are not due to actual physical illnesses. Rather the wounds are deliberately and consciously self-inflicted and not allowed to heal because of patient interference with care.[223]

Clinical Presentation Factitious wounds usually have geometric edges and healthy granulation tissue and are located on areas of the body that are easily accessible with the hands (eg, face, arms, torso, legs, but rarely on the back) (**FIGURE 9-73**). Of most importance is the patient denial of any responsibility for the wound and lying about compliance with care.[224]

Medical Management Once the clinician is suspicious that a nonhealing wound is the result of self-inflicted behavior,

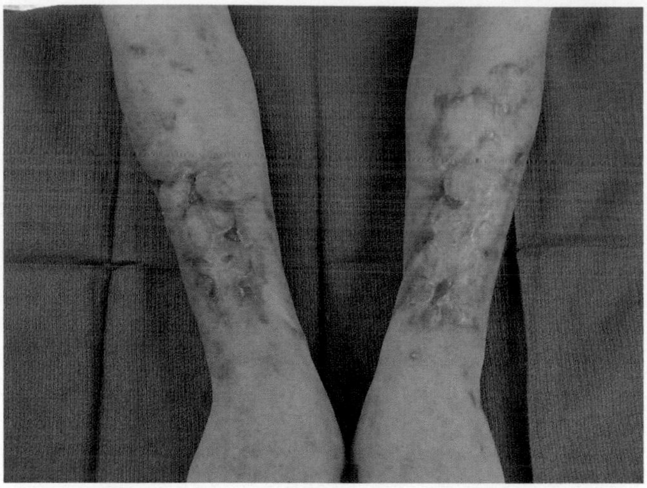

FIGURE 9-73 Factitious wounds. When wounds that should heal with standard care fail to do so, factitious behavior is a consideration. Suspicious signs are failure to retain dressings between treatments, evidence of "picking" at the wound, or waxing and waning of wound progression. This patient who had extensive wounds on the upper extremities from skin-popping drugs exhibited factitious behavior after being released from the hospital. She was inconsistent in keeping appointments, arrived without dressings, and had the typical granulated wound base with geometric edges.

differential diagnosis of factitious wounds is dependent on the diagnosis of an underlying psychological or psychiatric disorder (eg, delusional disorder, depression, anxiety, emotional deprivation, personality disorder with borderline features, schizophrenia).

Medical management must include treatment of the underlying psychiatric disorder, as well as treatment of any comorbidities and other complications that may arise from the induced illness.[224]

Wound Management Standard wound care with occlusive dressings, avoidance of invasive procedures, supportive emotional care, thorough documentation, and close observation are required for the clinician caring for a patient with factitious wounds.[224] Adherence to treatment strategies will need continuous reinforcement for both the patient and family/care givers.

Subcutaneous Injections (Skin Popping)

Pathophysiology Illicit drug use is usually done intravenously; however, after prolonged use the veins may become inaccessible and the user resorts to injecting the drugs subcutaneously (termed *skin popping*). In some cases, the medication is administered intramuscular[225] (FIGURE 9-74). The injection sites are susceptible to skin and soft tissue infection which can spread subcutaneously, resulting in very difficult–to-treat wounds. The most common bacteria causing skin infections is *Staphylococcus aureus* either alone or in combination with anaerobic bacteria.[226]

Clinical Presentation Initial signs of skin popping include round, fibrotic, depressed, hyperpigmented lesions on the affected area. Soft tissue infections present as abscesses and/or cellulitis (FIGURE 9-75). In some cases, the contaminants can create cutaneous granulomas.

Medical Management Appropriate systemic antibiotics and in some cases surgical debridement are the initial treatments, along with intense patient education about the risks of skin popping, dirty needles, and poor hygiene.

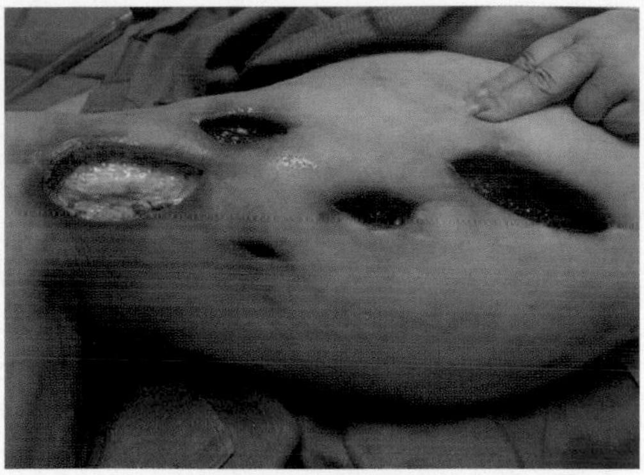

FIGURE 9-74 Open wounds on the lower extremity of a patient who was receiving intramuscular morphine injections for pain secondary to malignancy. Necrotic, infected subcutaneous tissue was surgically debrided.

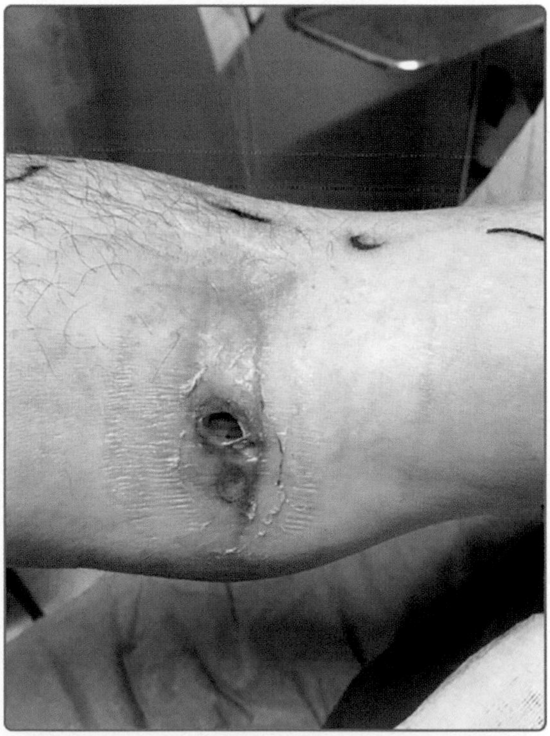

FIGURE 9-75 Soft tissue infection with an open wound from skin popping; changes in the periwound skin texture and color indication the extent of subcutaneous infection. (Used with permission from Kang S, Amagai M, Bruckner AL, et al, eds. *Fitzpatrick's Dermatology*. 9th ed. New York, NY: McGraw Hill; 2019, Figure 101-3.)

Wound Management Wound management is tedious because of the subcutaneous extension of the infected and necrotic tissue. Pain management can also be difficult for the patient addicted to opioids. Debridement, antimicrobial dressings, and compression therapy for the lower extremities are the mainstay of wound care. Patients who have a history of vein injections may develop chronic venous insufficiency due to the vein injury, making compression therapy even more critical.[227] There are numerous articles related to the prevalence, history, and clinical signs of skin popping; however, guidelines for wound care were not reported.

SUMMARY

When wounds have an unusual appearance or fail to respond to standard care, further evaluation is required to determine the diagnosis of what is termed *atypical wounds*. Signs of atypical wounds include unusual location, unusual age, poor or friable granulation tissue, overgrowth, red or purple periwound skin, or a history of diseases that suggest other wound diagnoses. Atypical wounds can be generally categorized into allergic reactions, infections (viral, bacterial, or fungal), autoimmune disorders, malignancies, or factitious behavior. Successful treatment of the wound is predicated on making the correct diagnosis of underlying diseases as well as the wound or integumentary disorder. Referral to the appropriate medical specialist is also an integral part of caring for a patient with an atypical wound.

STUDY QUESTIONS

1. Which of the following symptoms is not an indication that the patient has an atypical wound?
   a. Fungating growth of abnormal tissue
   b. Mild-to-moderate pain
   c. Unusual location for the apparent wound diagnosis
   d. Failure to respond to standard care for the apparent diagnosis
2. A patient with diabetes presents with systemic signs of fever, malaise, and weakness with erythema of the lower extremity after getting a scratch while doing yard work. The erythema is quickly spreading and small blisters are forming in the area. The recommended initial treatment for a wound of this type is
   a. Anti-inflammatory medications.
   b. Local wound care and compression.
   c. Hospital admission, antibiotics, surgical debridement
   d. Antiviral medications.
3. Irritant contact dermatitis is caused by
   a. Allergic reaction to oral medication.
   b. Contact with a caustic substance such as cleaning fluids or poison ivy.
   c. Allergic reaction to a specific substance such as latex or perfume.
   d. Psychological response to a stressful event.
4. An elevated lesion less than 10 mm in diameter that contains clear fluid is termed a
   a. Vesicle.
   b. Bulla.
   c. Pustule.
   d. Macule.
5. The first and most important treatment of toxic epidermal necrolysis is
   a. Determining and giving the correct antibiotic.
   b. Identifying and halting the causative medication.
   c. Isolation of the patient to prevent the spread of the disease.
   d. Topical steroids to treat epidermal inflammation.
6. Which of the following vasculitic disorders is most likely to have cutaneous lesions?
   a. Giant cell arteritis
   b. Microscopic polyangiitis
   c. Polyarteritis nodosa
   d. Takayasu arteritis
7. For which of the following diseases is sharp or selective debridement contraindicated?
   a. Cryoglobulinemia
   b. Necrotizing fasciitis
   c. Pyoderma gangrenosum
   d. Wegener granulosum
8. Squamous cell carcinoma, Merkel cell carcinoma, and basal cell carcinoma are found in patients who
   a. Have a history of other types of cancers.
   b. Are less than 50 years old.
   c. Have a history of drug abuse.
   d. Have had prolonged exposure to ultraviolet light.

Answers: 1-b; 2-c; 3-b; 4-a; 5-b; 6-c; 7-c; 8-d

REFERENCES

1. Shah JB. Approach to commonly misdiagnosed wounds and unusual leg ulcers. In: Sheffield PJ, Smith APS, Fife CE, eds. *Wound Care Practice*. 2nd ed. Flagstaff, AZ: Best Publishing; 2007:579-602.
2. Issoherranen K, O'Brien JJ, Barker J, et al. Atypical wounds: best clinical practices and challenges. *J Wound Care*. 2019;28(S6):S1-S92.
3. Ansert E, Tickner A, Cohen D, Murry W, Gorelik S. Understanding the zebras of wound care: an overview of atypical wounds. *Wounds*. 2022;34(5):124-134.
4. Vocanson M, Hennino A, Rozières A, Poyet G, Nicolas JF. Effector and regulatory mechanisms in allergic contact dermatitis. *Allergy*. 2009;64(12):1699-714.
5. Al-Otaibi ST, Alqahtani HAM. Management of contact dermatitis. *J Dermatol Surg*. 2015;19(2):86-91.
6. Riedel F, Aparicio-Soto M, Curato C, Thierse HJ, Siewert K, Luch A. Immunological mechanisms of metal allergies and the nickel-specific TCR-pMHC interface. *Int J Environ Res Public Health*. 2021;18(20):10867.
7. Novak-Bilić G, Vučić M, Japundžić I, Meštrović-Štefekov J, Stanić-Duktaj S, Lugović-Mihić L. Irritant and allergic contact dermatitis – skin lesion characteristics. *Acta Clin Croat*. 2018;57(4):713-720.

8. Frempah B, Luckett-Chastain LR, Calhoun KN, Gallucci RM. Keratinocyte-specific deletion of the IL-6RA exacerbates the inflammatory response during irritant contact dermatitis. *Toxicology.* 2019;423:123-131.
9. Shiohara T, Mizukawa Y. Drug-induced hypersensitivity syndrome (DIHS)/drug reaction with eosinophilia and systemic systems (DRESS): an update in 2019. *Allergol Int.* 2019;68:301-308.
10. Wheatley LM, Plaut M, Schwaninger JM, et al. Report from the National Institute of Allergy and Infectious Diseases workshop on drug allergy. *J Allergy Clin Immunol.* 2015;136(2):262-271.e2.
11. Allopurinol Drug report. Available at: http://livertox.nih.gov/Allopurinol.htm. Last update December 26, 2020. Accessed April 3, 2023.
12. Ponvert C, Perrin Y, Bados-Albiero A, et al. Allergy to betalactam antibiotics in children: results of a 20-year study based on clinical history, skin and challenge tests. *Pediatr Allergy Immunol.* 2011;22(4):411-418.
13. Blanca M, Romano A, Torres MJ, et al. Update on the evaluation of hypersensitivity reactions to betalactams. *Allergy.* 2009;64:183-193.
14. Kumar AA, Siddrama R, Baig MJ, Reddy GA. A case report on ceftriaxone induced hypersensitivity reactions (uticaria). *Int J All Med Sci Clin Res.* 2015;3(2):82-84.
15. Dapsone drug report. Available at: http://livertox.nih.gov/Dapsone.htm. Last update, December 6, 2017. Accessed April 3, 2023.
16. Maity S, Banerjee I, Sinha R, Jha H, Ghosh P, Mustafi S. Nikolsky's sign: a pathognomic boon. *J Family Med Prim Care.* 2020;9(2):526-530.
17. Frantz R, Huang S, Are A, Motaparthi K. Stevens-Johnson syndrome and toxic epidermal necrolysis: a review of diagnosis and management. *Medicina (Kaunas).* 2021;57(9):895.
18. Hafner J, Schneider E, Gunter B, Paolo C. Management of leg ulcers in patients with rheumatoid arthritis or systemic sclerosis: the importance of concomitant arterial and venous disease. *J Vasc Surg.* 2000;32(2):322-329.
19. Gabrielli A, Avvedimento EV, Krieg T. Scleroderma. *N Engl J Med.* 2009;360:1989-2003.
20. Singh D, Parihar AKS, Patel S, et al. Scleroderma: an insight into causes, pathogenesis and treatment strategies. *Pathophysiology.* 2019;26(2):103-114.
21. Tsou PS, Sawalha AH. Unfolding the pathogenesis of scleroderma through genomics and epigenomics. *J Autoimmun.* 2017;83:73-94.
22. Alarcon–Segovia D, Deleze M, Oria CV, et al. Antiphospholipid antibodies and the antiphospholipid syndromein systemic lupus erythematosus. A prospective analysis of 500 consecutive cases. *Medicine.* 1989;68(6):353-365.
23. Falanga V, Phillips T, Harding K, Moy R, Peerson L. *Text Atlas of Wound Management.* London, UK: Martin Dunitz; 2000:61-97, 189-227.
24. Furst EA. Scleroderma: a fascinating, troubling disease. *Topics Adv Pract Nursing eJournal.* 2004;4(2). Available at: http://www.medscape.com/viewarticle/473349. Accessed August 2, 2018.
25. Li SC. Scleroderma in children and adolescents. *Pediatr Clin N Am.* 2018;65:757-781.
26. Giuggioli D, Spinella A, Cocchiara E, et al. Autologous fat grafting in the treatment of a scleroderma stump-skin ulcer: a case report. *Case Reports Plast Surg Hand Surg.* 2021;8(1):18-22.
27. Wang J, Cai J, Zhang Q, Wen J, Liao Y, Lu F. Fat transplantation induces dermal adipose regeneration and reverses skin fibrosis through dedifferentiation and redifferentiation of adipocytes. *Stem Cell Res Ther.* 2022;13(1):499.
28. Rosendahl AH, Schönborn K, Krieg T. Pathophysiology of systemic sclerosis (scleroderma). *Kaohsiung J Med Sci.* 2022;38(3):187-195.
29. Michalak J, Simman R, Oostra D. A case of thrombotic vasculopathy in the setting of high-dose hydroxyurea use. *Wounds.* 2021;33(12):E79-E84.
30. Sirieix ME, Debure C, Baudot N, et al. Leg ulcers and hydroxyurea: forty-one cases. *Arch Dermatol.* 1999 Jul;135(7):818-20.
31. Weinstein D. Atypical wounds. In: Baronski S, Ayelo E, eds. *Wound Care Essentials: Practice Principles.* Philadelphia, PA: Lippincott Williams & Wilkins; 2012;491-511.
32. Lawley TJ, Kubota Y. Vasculitis. *Dermatol Clin.* 1990;8(4):681-687.
33. Fauci A, Braunwald E, Isselbacher KT, et al. *Harrison's Principles of Internal Medicine.* New York, NY: McGraw Hill; 1998:989–991, 1004-1019.
34. Schmidt W. Role of ultrasound in the understanding and management of vasculitis. *Ther Adv Musculoskelet Dis.* 2014;6(2):39-47.
35. Ntatsake E, Carruthers D, Chakravarty K, et al. BSR and BHPR guideline for the management of adults with ANCA-associated vasculitis. *Rheumatology.* 2014;53(12):2306-2309.
36. Shah JB, Isselbacher KJ. Correction of hypoxia, a critical element for wound bed preparation guidelines: TIMEO2 principles of wound bed preparation. *J Am Coll Certif Wound Spec.* 2011;3(2):26–32.
37. Petri M. Antiphospholipid syndrome. *Transl Res.* 2020;225:70-81.
38. Sammaritano LR. Antiphospholipid syndrome. *Best Pract Res Clin Rheumatol.* 2020;34(1):101463.
39. Movva S. Antiphospholipid syndrome. Medscape/Drugs & Diseases/Rheumatology. Available at: http://www.emedicine.medscape.com/article/333221. Updated July 21, 2022. Accessed April 3, 2023.
40. Zhang Y, Riddle ND, Seminario-Vidal L. Post-partum cutaneous manifestation of antiphospholipid syndrome. *Human Pathology: Case Reports. 2019.* Available at: https://doi.org/10.1016/j.ehpc.2019.200334. Accessed March 22, 2023.
41. Mustafa R. Neurologic manifestations of catastrophic antiphospholipid syndrome. *Curr Neurol Neurosci Rep.* 2022;22(10):589-600.
42. Islabão AG, Trindade VC, da Mota LMH, Andrade DCO, Silva CA. Managing antiphospholipid syndrome in children and adolescents: current and future prospects. *Paediatr Drugs.* 2022;24(1):13-27.
43. Falanga V. *Cutaneous Wound Healing.* London: Martin Dunitz; 2001:247-263.
44. Silverberg JI, Votava HJ, Smith BL. Antiphospholipid antibody syndrome secondary to trimethoprim/sulfamethoxazole. *J Drugs Dermatol.* 2012;11(9):1117-1118.
45. Thronsberry LA, LoSicco KI, English JC III. The skin and hypercoagulable states. *J Am Acad Dermatol.* 2013;69(3):450-462.
46. Kridin K, Patel PM, Jones VA, Cordova A, Amber KT. IgA pemphigus: a systematic review. *J Am Acad Dermatol.* 2020;82(6):1386-1392.
47. Ahmed AR, Spigelman Z, Cavacini LA, Posner MR. Treatment of pemphigus vulgaris with Rituximab and intravenous immune globulin. *N Engl J Med.* 2006;355:1772-1779.
48. Warren SJP, Argeaga LA, Diaz LA, et al. The role of subclass switching in the pathogen of endemic pemphigus foliaceous. *J Invest Dermatol.* 2003;120(1):1-5.
49. Malik AM, Tupchong S, Huang S, Are A, Hsu S, Motaparthi K. An updated review of pemphigus diseases. *Medicina (Kaunas).* 2021;57(10):1080.
50. Anhalt GJ, Mimouni D. Paraneoplastic Pemphigus. In: Kang S, Amagai M, Bruckner AL, et al, eds. *Fitzpatrick's Dermatology.* 9th ed. New York, NY: McGraw Hill; 2019. Available at: https://accessmedicine.mhmedical.com/content.aspx?bookid=2570&sectionid=210425528. Accessed April 4, 2023.

51. Grando SA, Rigas M, Chernyavsky A. Rationale for including intravenous immunoglobulin in the multidrug protocol of curative treatment of pemphigus vulgaris and development of an assay predicting disease relapse. *Int Immunopharmacol.* 2020;82:106385.
52. Kulczycka-Siennicka L, Cynkier A, Waszczykowska E, Wazniacka A, Zebrowska A. The role of interleukin-31 in pathogenesis of itch and its intensity in a course of bullous pemphigoid and dermatitis herpetiformis. *Biomed Res Int.* 2017;2017:5965492.
53. Lin L, Hwang BJ, Culton DA, et al. Eosinophils mediate tissue injury in the autoimmune skin disease bullous pemphigoid. *J Invest Dermatol.* 2018;138(5):1032-1043.
54. Wieland CN, Comfere NI, Gibson LE, Weaver AL, Krause PK, Murray JA. Anti-bullous pemphigoid 180 and 230 antibodies in a sample of unaffected subjects. *Arch Dermatol.* 2010;146(1):21-25.
55. Verheyden MJ, Bilgic A, Murrell DF. A systematic review of drug-induced pemphigoid. *Acta Derm Venereol.* 2020;100(15):adv00224.
56. Moro F, Fania L, Sinagra JLM, Salemme A, Di Zenzo G. Bullous pemphigoid: trigger and predisposing factors. *Biomolecules.* 2020;10(10):1432.
57. Chan LS. Bullous pemphigoid. Updated October 14, 2020. Available at: https://emedicine.medscape.com/article/1062391-overview. Accessed April 4, 2023.
58. Lonowski S, Sachsman S, Patel N, et al. Increasing evidence for omalizumab in the treatment of bullous pemphigoid. *JAAD Case Reports.* 2020;6(3)228-233.
59. Retamozo S, Quartuccio L, Ramos-Casals M. Cryoglobulinemia. *Med Clin (Barc).* 2022;158(10):478-487.
60. Edgerton CC. Cryoglobulinemia treatment and management. Available at: https://emedicine.medscape.com/article/329255-treatment. Updated May 25, 2021. Accessed April 4, 2023.
61. Panuncialman J, Felanga V. Unusual causes of cutaneous ulceration. *Surg Clin North Am.* 2021;90(6):1161-1180
62. Silva F, Pinto C, Barbosa A, Borges T, Dias C, Almeida J. New insights in cryoglobulinemic vasculitis. *J Autoimmun.* 2019;105:102313.
63. Montagnon CM, Fracica EA, Patel AA, et al. Pyoderma gangrenosum in hematologic malignancies: a systematic review. *J Am Acad Dermatol.* 2020;82(6):1346-1359.
64. Powell FC, Su PW, Perry HO. Pyoderma gangrenosum: classification and management. *J Am Acad Dermatol.* 1996;34(3):395-409.
65. Brooklyn T, Dunnill G, Probert C. Diagnosis and treatment of pyoderma gangrenosum. *Br Med J.* 2006;333(7560):181-184.
66. Afifi L, Sanchez IM, Wallace MM, Braswell SF, Ortega-Loayza AG, Shinkai K. Diagnosis and management of peristomal pyoderma gangrenosum: a systematic review. *J Am Acad Dermatol.* 2018;78(6):1195-1204.e1.
67. Wines N, Wines M, Ryman W. Understanding pyoderma gangrenosum: a review. *Med Gen Med.* 2001;3(3):6.
68. Wollina U. Clinical management of pyoderma gangrenosum. *Am J Clin Dermatol.* 2002;3(3):149-158.
69. Barbe M, Batra A, Golding S, et al. Pyoderma gangrenosum: a literature review. *Clin Podiatr Med Surg.* 2021;38(4):577-588.
70. Hashemi DA, Nelson CA, Elenitsas R, Rosenbach M. An atypical case of papular necrobiosis lipoidica masquerading as sarcoidosis. *JAAD Case Rep.* 2018;4(8):802-804.
71. Ginocchio L, Draghi L, Darvishian F, Ross FL. Refractory ulcerated necrobiosis lipoidica: closure of a difficult wound with topical tacrolimus. *Adv Skin Wound Care.* 2017;30(10):469-472.
72. Kota SK, Jammula S, Kota SK, Meher LK, Modi KD. Necrobiosis lipoidica diabeticorum: a case-based review of literature. *Indian J Endocrinol Metab.* 2012;16(4):614-620.
73. Lim C, Tschuchnigg M, Lim J. Squamous cell carcinoma arising in an area of long-standing necrobiosis lipoidica. *J Cutan Pathol.* 2006;33:581-583.
74. Sibbald C, Reid S, Alavi A. Necrobiosis lipoidica. *Dermatol Clin.* 2015;33(3):343-60.
75. Clayton TH, Harrison PV. Successful treatment of chronic ulcerated necrobiosis lipoidica with 0.1% topical tacrolimus ointment. *Br J Dermatol.* 2005;152(3):581-582.
76. Stanway A, Rademaker M, Newman P. Healing of severe ulcerative necrobiosis lipoidica with cyclosporin. *Australas J Dermatol.* 2004; 45:119-122.
77. Reinhard G, Lohmann F, Uerlich M, Bauer R, Bieber T. Successful treatment of ulcerated necrobiosis lipoidica with mycophenolate mofetil. *Acta Derm Venereol.* 2000;80:312-313.
78. Kolde G, Muche JM, Schulze P, Fischer P, Lichey J. Infliximab: a promising new treatment option for ulcerated necrobiosis lipoiidica. *Dermatology.* 2003;206:180-181.
79. Spenceri EA, Nahass GT. Topically applied bovine collagen in the treatment of necrobiosis lipoidica diabeticorum. *Arch Dermatol.* 1997;133(7):817-818.
80. Heidebheim M, Jemec GB. Successful treatment of necrobiosis lipoidica diabeticorum with photodynamic therapy. *Arch Dermatol.* 2006;142(12):1548-1550.
81. Suzich JB, Cliffe AR. Strength in diversity: understanding the pathways to herpes simplex virus reactivation. *Virology.* 2018;522: 81-91.
82. Staikov IN, Neykov NV, Kazandjieva JS, Tsankov NK. Is herpes simplex a systemic disease? *Clin Dermatol.* 2015;33(5):551-555.
83. Karlsmark T, Goodman JJ, Drouault Y, Lufrano L, Pledger GW, Cold Sore Study Group. Randomized clinical study comparing cold sore patch to acyclovir cream 5% in the treatment of herpes simplex labialis. *J Eur Acad Dermatol Venereol.* 2008;22(10):1184-1192.
84. Freer G, Pistello M. Varicella zoster virus infection: natural history, clinical manifestations, immunity and current and future vaccination strategies. *New Microbiol.* 2018;41(2):95-105.
85. Junior HP, de Oliveira MB, Gambero S, Amazonas RB. Randomized clinical trial of famciclovir or acyclovir for the treatment of herpes zoster in adults. *Int J Infect Dis.* 2018;72:11-15.
86. Updated recommendations for the use of VariZIG—United States 2013. Available at: https://www.cdc.gov/mmwr/preview/mmwrhtml/mm6228a4.htm. Accessed July 30, 2018.
87. What everyone should know about shingles vaccine (Shingrix). Available at: https://www.cdc.gov/vaccines/vpd/shingles/public/shingrix/index.html. Accessed July 30, 2018.
88. Zinser E, Krawczyk A, Muhl-Zurbes P, et al. A new promising candidate to overcome drug resistance herpes simplex virus infections. *Antiviral Res.* 2018;149:202-210.
89. Harmenberg J, Oberg B, Spruance S. Prevention of ulcerative lesions by episodic treatment of recurrent herpes labialis: a literature review. *Acta Derm Venereol.* 2010;90(2):122-130.
90. Ali SS, Lateef F. Laboratory risk indicators for acute necrotizing fasciitis in the emergency setting. *Journal of Acute Disease.* 2016; 5(2):114-116.
91. Lancerotto L, Tocco I, Salmaso R, Vindigni V, Bassetto F. Necrotizing fasciitis: classification, diagnosis, and management. *J Trauma Acute Care Surg.* 2021;72(3):560-566.
92. Novoa-Parra CD, Wakhwani J, Puig-Conco MA, et al. Usefulness of a risk scale based on procalcitonin for early discrimination between necrotizing fasciitis and cellulitis of the extremities. *Med Clin (English Edition).* 2019;153(9):347-350.

93. Bechar J, Sepehripour S, Hardwicke J, Filobbos G. Laboratory risk indicator for necrotising fasciitis (LRINEC) score for the assessment of early necrotising fasciitis: a systematic review of the literature. *Ann R Coll Surg Engl*. 2017;99(5):341-346.
94. Wong CH, Khin LW, Heng KS, Tan KC, Low CO. The LRINEC (Laboratory Risk Indicator for Necrotizing Fasciitis) score: a tool for distinguishing necrotizing fasciitis from other soft tissue infections. *Crit Care Med*. 2004;32(7):1535-41.
95. Mindrup SR, Kealey GP, Fallon B. Hyperbaric oxygen for the treatment of Fournier's gangrene. *J Urol*. 2005;173(6):1975-1977.
96. Bonne SL, Kadri SS. Evaluation and management of necrotizing soft tissue infections. *Infect Dis Clin North Am*. 2017;31(3):497-511.
97. Balbierz JM, Ellis K. Streptococcal infection and necrotizing fasciitis—implications for rehabilitation: a report of 5 cases and review of the literature. *Arch Phys Med Rehabil*. 2004;85(7):1205-1209.
98. Czymek R, Schmidt A, Eckman C, et al. Fournier's gangrene: vacuum-assisted closure versus conventional dressings. *Am J Surg*. 2009;197(2):168-176.
99. Joury A, Mahendra A, Alshehri M, Downing A. Extensive necrotizing fasciitis from Fournier's gangrene. *Urol Case Rep*. 2019;26:100943.
100. Chipp E, Phillips C, Rubin P. Successful management of spontaneous Clostridium septicum myonecrosis. *J Plast Reconstr Aesthet Surg*. 2009;62(10):e391-e393.
101. Wright WF. Clostridium septicum myonecrosis presenting as an acute painful foot. *Am J Emerg Med*. 2012;30(1):253.e3-5.
102. Bryant AE, Stevens DL. Gas gangrene and other clostridial infections. In: Longo DL, Fauci AS, Kasper DL, Hauser SL, Jameson JL, Loscalzo J, eds. *Harrison's Principles of Internal Medicine*. 18th ed. New York, NY: McGraw Hill; 2012:chap 142. Available at: http://www.accessmedicine.com/content.aspx?aID=9120982. Accessed August 2, 2018.
103. Griffin AS, Crawford MD, Gupta RT. Massive gas gangrene secondary to occult colon carcinoma. *Radiol Case Rep*. 2016;11:67-69.
104. Thompson KM, Kruse BT, Hedges MAS. Atraumatic clostridial myonecrosis in an immunocompromised host. *J Emerg Med*. 2018;54(6):e121-e123.
105. Gupta S, Goyal P, Sharma P, et al. Recurrent diabetic myonecrosis – an under-diagnosed cause of acute painful swollen limb in long standing diabetics. *Ann Med Surg (Lond)*. 2018;35:141-145.
106. Leiblein M, Wagner N, Adam EH, Frank J, Marzi I, Nau C. Clostridial gas gangrene - A rare but deadly infection: case series and comparison to other necrotizing soft tissue infections. *Orthop Surg*. 2020;12(6):1733-1747.
107. Yang Z, Hu J, Qu Y, Sun F, Leng X, Li H, Zhan S. Interventions for treating gas gangrene. *Cochrane Database Syst Rev*. 2015;2015(12):CD010577.
108. Korhonen K. Hyperbaric oxygen therapy in acute necrotizing infection with a special reference to the effects on tissue gas tensions. *Ann Chir Gynaecol Suppl*. 2000;214:7-36.
109. Valour F, Senechal A, Dupieux C, et al. Actinomycosis: etiology, clinical features, diagnosis, treatment, and management. *Infect Drug Resist*. 2014;7:183-197.
110. Gandhi K, van der Woerd BD, Graham ME, Barton M, Strychowsky JE. Cervicofacial actinomycosis in the pediatric population: presentation and management. *Ann Otol Rhinol Laryngol*. 2022;131(3):312-321.
111. Creighton RE. Actinomycosis: a rare pedal infection. *J Am Podiatr Med Assoc*. 1993;83(11):637-640.
112. Mahgoub ES, Yacoub AA. Primary actinomycosis of the foot and leg: report of a case. *J Trop Med Hyg*. 1968;71(10):256-258.
113. Bettesworth J, Gill K, Shah J. Primary actinomycosis of the foot: a case report and literature review. *J Am Coll Clin Wound Spec*. 2009;1(3):95-100.
114. Russo TA. Actinomycosis. In: Loscalzo J, Fauci A, Kasper D, Hauser S, Longo D, Jameson J, eds. *Harrison's Principles of Internal Medicine*. 21st ed. New York, NY: McGraw Hill; 2022. Available at: https://accessmedicine.mhmedical.com/content.aspx?bookid=3095&sectionid=263964355. Accessed April 5, 2023.
115. Sheikh MA, Alenzi S, Ahmadi AA, Mashragi A, Alsayid H, Abdullah A. Actinomycosis of the middle ear and mastoid. *Med Arch*. 2018; 72(4):295-296.
116. Dodiuk-Gad R, Dyachenko P, Ziv M, et al. Nontuberculous mycobacterial infections of the skin: a retrospective study of 25 cases. *J Am Acad Dermatol*. 2007;57(3):413-420.
117. Franco-Paredes C, Marcos LA, Henao-Martínez AF, et al. Cutaneous mycobacterial infections. *Clin Microbiol Rev*. 2018;32(1):e00069-18.
118. Nienhuis WA, Stienstra Y, Thompson WA, et al. Antimicrobial treatment for early, limited mycobacterium ulcerans infection: a randomised controlled trial. *Lancet*. 2010;375(9715):664-672.
119. Mycobacteria. In: Riedel S, Hobden JA, Miller S, et al, eds. *Jawetz, Melnick, & Adelberg's Medical Microbiology*. 28th ed. New York, NY: McGraw Hill; 2019. Available at: https://accessmedicine.mhmedical.com/content.aspx?bookid=2629&sectionid=217771812. Accessed April 5, 2023.
120. Groll ME, Woods T, Salcido R. Osteomyelitis: a context for wound management. *Adv Skin Wound Care*. 2018;31(6):253-262.
121. Mourad LA, McCance KL. Alterations of musculoskeletal function. In: Huether SE, McCance KL, eds. *Understanding Pathophysiology*. St. Louis, MO: Mosby; 2008;1036-1070.
122. Wassif RK, Elkayal M, Shamma RN, Elkheshen SA. Recent advances in the local antibiotics delivery systems for management of osteomyelitis. *Drug Deliv*. 2021;28(1):2392-2414.
123. Lavery LA, Armstrong DG, Peters EJ, Lipsky BA. Probe-to-bone test for diagnosing diabetic foot osteomyelitis: reliable or relic? *Diabetes Care*. 2007;30(2):270-274.
124. Goldman RJ, Deleaon JM, Popescu A, Salcido R. Chronic wounds. In: Cifu DX, ed. *Braddom's Physical Medicine and Rehabilitation*. 5th ed. New York, NY: Elsevier Health Sciences; 2015.
125. Ford CA, Cassat JE. Advances in the local and targeted delivery of anti-infective agents for management of osteomyelitis. *Expert Rev Anti Infect Ther*. 2017;15(9):851-860.
126. Rodrigues AM, Gonçalves SS, de Carvalho JA, Borba-Santos LP, Rozental S, Camargo ZP. Current progress on epidemiology, diagnosis, and treatment of sporotrichosis and their future trends. *J Fungi (Basel)*. 2022;8(8):776.
127. Ramos-e-Silva M, Vasconcelos C, Carneriro S, et al. Sporotrichosis. *Clin Dermatol*. 2007;25(2):181-187.
128. Zafren K, Thurman R, Jones ID. Sporotrichosis. In: Knoop KJ, Stack LB, Storrow AB, Thurman R, eds. *The Atlas of Emergency Medicine*. 5th ed. New York, NY: McGraw Hill; 2021. Available at: https://accessmedicine.mhmedical.com/content.aspx?bookid=2969&sectionid=250461219. Accessed April 05, 2023.
129. Lupi O, Tyring SK, McGinnis MR. Tropical dermatology: fungal tropical diseases. *J Am Acad Dermatol*. 2005;53(6):931-951.
130. Raffanti SP, Person AK. Dermatophyte (Tinea) infections. In: Knoop KJ, Stack LB, Storrow AB, Thurman R, eds. *The Atlas of Emergency Medicine*. 5th ed. New York, NY: McGraw Hill; 2021. Available at: https://accessmedicine.mhmedical.com/content.aspx?bookid=2969&sectionid=250462555. Accessed April 5, 2023.

131. Waskiel-Burnat A, Rakowska A, Sikora M, Ciechanowicz P, Olszewska M, Rudnicka L. Trichoscopy of tinea capitis: a systematic review. *Dermatol Ther (Heidelb)*. 2020;10(1):43-52.
132. Kreijkamp-Kaspers S, Hawke K, Guo L, et al. Oral antifungal medication for toenail onychomycosis. *Cochrane Database Syst Rev*. 2017;7:CD010031.
133. Thomas J, Peterson GM, Christenson JK, Kosari S, Baby KE. Antifungal drug use for onychomycosis. *Am J Ther*. 2019;26(3): e388-e396.
134. Ma W, Si C, Kasyanju LM, et al. Laser treatment for onychomycosis: a systematic review and meta-analysis. *Medicine (Baltimore)*.2019;98(48):e17948.
135. Yeung K, Ortner VK, Martinussen T, Paasch U, Haedersdal M. Efficacy of laser treatment for onychomycotic nails: a systematic review and meta-analysis of prospective clinical trials. *Lasers Med Sci*. 2019;34(8):1513-1525.
136. Dars S, Banwell HA, Matricciani L. The use of urea for the treatment of onychomycosis: a systematic review. *J Foot Ankle Res*. 2019; 12:22. Available at https://doi:10.1186/s13047-019-0332-3. eCollection 2019. Accessed April 18, 2020.
137. Gupta AD, Mays RR, Versteeg SG, et al. Tinea capitis in children: a systematic review of management. *J Eur Acad Dermatol Venereol*. 2018;32(12):2264-2274.
138. El-Gohary M, vanZuuren EJ, Fedorowicz Z, et al. Topical antifungal treatments for tinea cruris and tinea corporis. *Cochrane Database Syst Rev*. 2014; (8):CD009992.
139. Eksomtramage T, Aiempanakit K. Tinea nigra mimicking acral melanocytic nevi. *IDCases*. 2019;18:e00654. Available at https://doi.org/10.1016/j.dcr.2019.e00654. Accessed April 18, 2020.
140. Thapa RK, Choi JY, Han SD, et al. Therapeutic effects of a novel DA5505 formulation on a guinea pig model of tinea pedis. *Dermatolog Sinica*. 2017;35:59-65.
141. El Housiny S, Eldeen M, El-Attar YA, et al. Fluconazole-loaded solid lipid nanoparticles topical gel for treatment of pityriasis versicolor: formulation and clinical study. *Drug Deliv*. 2018;25(1):78-90.
142. Gupta AK, Lane D, Paquet M. Systematic review of systemic treatments for tinea versicolor and evidence-based dosing regimen recommendation. *J Cutan Med Surg*. 2014;18(2):79-90.
143. Lange D, Richards HM, Guarnieri J, et al. Ketoconazole 2% shampoo in the treatment of tinea versicolor: A multicenter, randomized, double-blind, placebo-controlled trial. *J Am Acad Dermat*. 1998;39(6):944-950.
144. Hahnel E, Lichterfeld A, Blume-Peytavi U, Kottner J. The epidemiology of skin conditions in the aged: a systematic review. *J Tissue Viability*. 2017;26(1):20-28.
145. Rajagopalan M, Inamadar A, Mittal A, et al. Expert consensus on the management of dermatophytosis in India (ECTODERM India). *BMC Dermatol*. 2018;18(1):6.
146. Leung AK, Lam JM, Leong KF, Hon KL. Tinea corporis: an updated review. *Drugs Context*. 2020;9:2020-5-6.
147. Ringworm information for healthcare professionals. Available at: https://www.cdc.gov/fungal/diseases/ringworm. Accessed April 4, 2023
148. Kyrgidis A, Tzellos TG, Vahtsevanos K, Triadidis S. New concepts for basal cell carcinoma. Demographic, clinical, histological risk factors, and biomarkers. A systematic review of evidence regarding risk for tumor development, susceptibility for second primary and recurrence. *J Surg Res*. 2010;159(1):545-556.
149. Naik PP, Desai MB. Basal cell carcinoma: a narrative review on contemporary diagnosis and management. *Oncol Ther*. 2022; 10(2):317-335.
150. Firnhaber JM. Diagnosis and treatment of basal cell and squamous cell carcinoma. *Am Fam Physician*. 2012;86(2):161-168.
151. Macfarlane L, Waters A, Evans A, Affleck A, Fleming C. Seven years' experience of Mohs micrographic surgery in a UK center, and development of a UK minimum dataset and audit standards. *Clin Exp Dermatol*. 2013;38(3):262-269.
152. Jansen MHE, Mosterd K, Arits AHMM, et al. Five-year results of a randomized controlled trial comparing effectiveness of photodynamic therapy, topical imiquimod, and topical 5-fluorouracil in patients with superficial basal cell carcinoma. *J Invest Dermatol*. 2018;138(3):527-533.
153. Rabinowits G, Migden MR, Schlesinger TE, et al. Evidence-based consensus recommendations for the evolving treatment of patients with high-risk and advanced cutaneous squamous cell carcinoma. *JID Innov*. 2021;1(4):100045.
154. Fania L, Didona D, Di Pietro FR, et al. Cutaneous squamous cell carcinoma: from pathophysiology to novel therapeutic approaches. *Biomedicines*. 2021;9(2):171.
155. Green AC, McBride P. Squamous cell carcinoma of the skin (non-metastatic). *BMJ Clin Evid*. 2014. Available at: https://www.ncbi.nlm.nih.gov/pmc/articles/PMC4144167/. Accessed July 31, 2018.
156. Lipper GM. Hydrochlorothiazide and skin cancer: raise the red flag. Available at: https://medscape.com/viewarticle/895942?nlid=122267_1521&src. Accessed August 2, 2018.
157. Franco R. Basal and squamous cell carcinoma associated with chronic venous leg ulcer. *Int J Dermatol*. 2001;40:539-544.
158. Kirsner RS, Spencer J, Falanga V, Garland LE, Kerdel FA. Squamous cell carcinoma arising in osteomyelitis and chronic wounds. Treatment with Mohs microsurgery versus amputation. *Dermatol Surg*. 1996;22(12):1015-1028.
159. Lyons AB, Chipps LK, Moy RL, Herrmann JL. Dehydrated human amnion/chorion membrane allograft as an aid for wound healing in patients with full-thickness scalp defects after Mohs micrographic surgery. *JAAD Case Rep*. 2018;4(7):688-691.
160. Loh CY, Loh M, Mashhadi SA. Integra as a temporary method of wound cover post Mohs surgery. *Int Wound J*. 2016;13(1):143.
161. Newell F, Johansson PA, Wilmott JS, et al. Comparative genomics provides etiologic and biological insight into melanoma subtypes. *Cancer Discov*. 2022;12(12):2856-2879.
162. Weiss JM, Hunter MV, Cruz NM, et al. Anatomic position determines oncogenic specificity in melanoma. *Nature*. 2022;604(7905):354-361.
163. Markovic SN, Erickson LA, Rao RD, et al. Malignant melanoma in the 21st century, Part 2: Staging, prognosis, and treatment. *Mayo Clin Proc*. 2007;82(4):490-513.
164. Scatena C, Murtas D, Tomei S. Cutaneous melanoma classification: the importance of high-throughput genomic technologies. *Front Oncol*. 2021;11:635488.
165. Gill K, Shah JB. Kaposi sarcoma in patients with diabetes and wounds. *Adv Skin Wound Care*. 2006:19(4):196-201.
166. Chumley HS, Baraki A. Aids and Kaposi Sarcoma. In: Usatine RP, Smith MA, Mayeaux EJJr, Chumley HS. eds. *The Color Atlas and Synopsis of Family Medicine*. 3rd ed. New York, NY: McGraw Hill; 2019. Available at: https://accessmedicine.mhmedical.com/content.aspx?bookid=2547&sectionid=206782025. Accessed April 5, 2023.
167. Naimo E, Zischke J, Schulz TF. Recent advances in developing treatments of Kaposi's sarcoma herpesvirus-related diseases. *Viruses*. 2021;13(9):1797.
168. Walmsley S, Northfelt DW, Melosky B, Conant M, Friedman-Kien AE, Wagner B. Treatment of AIDS-related cutaneous Kaposi's sarcoma with topical alitretinoin (9-cis-retinoic acid) gel. *J Acqir Immune Defic Syndr*. 1999;22(3):235-246.

169. Stachyra K, Dudzisz-Śledź M, Bylina E, et al. Merkel cell carcinoma from molecular pathology to novel therapies. *Int J Mol Sci*. 2021; 22(12):6305.
170. Tegeder A, Afanasiev O, Nghiem P. Chap. 120: Merkel cell carcinoma. In: Wolff K, ed. *Fitzpatrick's Dermatology in General Medicine*. 8th ed. New York, NY: McGraw Hill; 2012: Available at: http://www.accessmedicine.com/content.aspx?aID=56061397. Accessed August 2, 2018.
171. Pulitzer M. Cutaneous T-cell lymphoma. *Clin Lab Med*. 2017;37(3): 527-546.
172. Beyer M, Sterry W. Chap. 145: Cutaneous lymphoma. In: Goldsmith LA, Katz SI, Gilchrest BA, Paller AS, Leffell DJ, Wolff K, eds. *Fitzpatrick's Dermatology in General Medicine*. 8th ed. New York, NY: McGraw Hill; 2012. Available at: http://accessmedicine.mhmedical.com/content.aspx?bookid=392&sectionid=41138867. Accessed August 1, 2018.
173. Goyal N, O'Leary D, Carter JB, et al. Practical review of the presentation, diagnosis, and management of cutaneous B-cell lymphoma. *Dermatol Clin*. 2023;41(1):187-208.
174. Oh Y, Stoll JR, Moskowitz A, et al. Primary cutaneous T-cell lymphomas other than mycosis fungoides and Sézary syndrome. Part II: Prognosis and management. *J Am Acad Dermatol*. 2021; 85(5):1093-1106.
175. Non-hodgkin lymphoma types. Available at: https://www.cancercenter.com/non-hodgkin-lymphoma/type. Accessed August 1, 2018.
176. Aviles A, Neri N, Fernandez-Diez J, Silva L, Nmbo MJ. Interferon and low doses of methotrexate versus interferon and retinoids in the treatment of refractory/relapsed cutaneous T-cell lymphoma. *Hematology*. 2015;20(9):538-542.
177. Haddany A, Fishlev G, Bechor Y, Meir O, Efrati S. Nonhealing wounds caused by brown sider bites: application of hyperbaric oxygen therapy. *Adv Skin Wound Care*. 2016;29(12):560-566.
178. Hogan CJ, Barbaro KC, Winkel K. Loxoscelism: old obstacles, new directions. *Ann Emerg Med*. 2004;44(60):608-624.
179. Isbister GK, White J. Clinical consequences of spider bites: recent advances in our understanding. *Toxicon*. 2004;43(5):477-492.
180. Suchard JR. "Spider bite" lesions are usually diagnosed as skin and soft-tissue infection. *J Emerg Med*. 2011;41(5):473-481.
181. Talib U, Abdelfattah AH, Talib M, et al. Brown recluse spider bite resulting in coombs negative hemolytic anemia in a young male requiring blood transfusion. *Cureus*. 2022;14(7):e26574.
182. Thompson AL. Laboratory testing in monitoring the effects of brown recluse spider bites. *Lab Med*. 2013;44(4): 300-303.
183. Streeper RT, Izbicka E. Diethyl azelate for the treatment of brown recluse spider bite, a neglected orphan indication. *In Vivo*. 2022; 36(1):86-93.
184. Bhambri A, Del Rosso JQ. Calciphylaxis: a review. *J Clin Aesthet Dermatol*. 2008;1(2):38-41.
185. Weening RH, Sewell D, Davis MD, et al. Calciphylaxis: natural history, risk factor analysis, and outcome. *J Am Acad Dermatol*. 2007;56(4):569-579.
186. Zhang Y, Corapi K, Luongo M, Thadhani R, Nigwekar S. Calciphylaxis in peritoneal dialysis patients: a single center cohort study. *Int J Nephrol Renovasc Dis*. 2016;2019(9):235-241.
187. Kodumudi V, Jeha GM, Mydlo N, Kaye AD. Management of cutaneous calciphylaxis. *Adv Ther*. 2020;37(12):4797-4807.
188. Dauden E, Onate MJ. Calciphylaxis. *Dermatol Clin*. 2008;26(4): 557-568.
189. Weening RH. Pathogenesis of calciphylaxis: Hans Selye to nuclear factor kappa-B. *J Am Acad Dermatol*. 2008;58(3):458-471.
190. Nigwekar S, Brunelli SM, Meade D, Wang W, Hymes J, Lacson E. Sodium thiosulfate therapy for calcific uremic arteriolopathy. *Clin J Am Soc Nephrol*. 2013;8(7):1162-1170.
191. Strand N, Maloney J, Wu S, et al. Perioperative management of calciphylaxis: literature review and treatment recommendations. *Orthop Rev (Pavia)*. 2022;14(3):37573.
192. Solanky D, Hwang SM, Stone G, Gillenwater J, Carey JN. Successful surgical treatment of severe calciphylaxis using a bilayer dermal replacement matrix. *Wounds*. 2015;27(11):302-307.
193. Strazzula L, Nigwekar SU, Steele D, et al. Intralesional sodium thiosulfate for the treatment of calciphylaxis. *JAMA Dermatol*. 2013;149(8):946-949.
194. Despoina DK, Papanas N, Karadimas E, Polychronidis A. Warfarin-induced skin necrosis. *Ann Dermatol*. 2014;26(1):96-98.
195. Wali M, Latif MT, Lockwood M, Saeyeldin A, Borz-Baba C. Warfarin-induced skin necrosis despite enoxaparin bridging therapy. *Cureus*. 2022;14(1):e20883.
196. Nazarian RM, Van Cott E, Zembosicz A, Duncan LM. Warfarin-induced skin necrosis. *J Am Acad Dermatol*. 2009;61(2):325-332.
197. Cheng A, Scheinfeld NS, Mcdowell B, et al. Warfarin skin necrosis in postpartum woman with protein S deficiency. *Obstet Gynecol*. 1997;90(4 pt 2):671-672.
198. Treadwell T. Sickle cell ulcers. In: Baronski S, Ayelo E, eds. *Wound Care Essentials, Practice Principles*. Philadelphia, PA: Lippincott Williams & Wilkins; 2012:447-460.
199. Powars DR, Chan LS, Hiti A, Ramicone E, Johnson C. Outcome of sickle cell anemia: a 4-decade observational study of 1056 patients. *Medicine*. 2005;84(6):363-376.
200. Tessema FA, Lapping-Carr G, Affini MI, et al. Sickle cell trait and multisystem trauma: an unaddressed urgent knowledge gap. *Trauma Surg Acute Care Open*. 2022;7(1):e000955.
201. Bernaudin F. Why, Who, When, and How? Rationale for considering allogeneic stem cell transplantation in children with sickle cell disease. *J Clin Med*. 2019;8(10):1523.
202. The Sickle Cell Information Center. *Evidence-based Management of Sickle Cell Disease*. 4th ed. Available at: http://scinfo.org/index.php?option+com_contents&view=category& id=15:the-management-ofcell-disease-4th-ed&Itemid=27&layout=default. Accessed April 5, 2023.
203. Morris C, Kuypers FA, Larkin S, et al. Arginine therapy: a novel strategy to induce nitric oxide production in sickle cell disease. *Br J Haematol*. 2000;111(2):498-500.
204. Hamm RL, Weitz I, Rodrigues J. Pathophysiology and multi-disciplinary management of leg wounds in sickle cell disease: a case discussion and literature review. *Wounds*. 2006;18(10):277-285.
205. Schultz GS, Sibbald RG, Falanga V, et al. Wound bed preparation: a systemic approach to wound management. *Wound Repair Regen*. 2003:11(suppl 1):S1-S28.
206. Mery L, Girot R, Aractingi S. Topical effectiveness of molgramostim (GM-CSF) in sickle cell leg ulcers. *Dermatology*. 2004;208(2):135-137.
207. Gordon S, Bui A. Human skin equivalent in the treatment of chronic leg ulcers in sickle cell disease patients. *J Am Podiatr Med Assoc*. 2003;93(3):240-241.
208. Sachdeva M, Gianott R, Shah M, Lucia B, Tosi D, Veraldi S, et al. Cutaneous manifestation of COVID-19: report of three cases and a review of the literature. *J Dermatol Sci*. 2020;98:75-81.
209. Magro C, Nuovo G, Mulvey JJ, Laurence J, Harp J, Crowson AN. The skin as a critical window in unveiling the pathophysiologic principles of COVID-19. *Clin Dermatol*. 2021;39(6):934-965.

210. Andina D, Belloni-Fortina A, Bodemer C, et al. Skin manifestations of COVID-19 in children: Part 1. *Clin Exp Dermatol.* 2021;46(3): 444-450.
211. Hodge B, Daniel CR, Elewski BE. Vaccine toes are the new COVID toes. *Skin Appendage Disord.* 2022;37(4):1-4.
212. Davido B, Mascitti H, Fortier-Beaulieu M, Jaffal K, de Truchis P. 'Blue toes' following vaccination with the BNT162b2 mRNA COVID-19 vaccine. *J Travel Med.* 2021;28(4):taab024.
213. Cavazos A, Deb A, Sharma U, Nugent K. COVID toes following vaccination. *Proc (Bayl Univ Med Cent).* 2022;35(4):476-479.
214. Genovese G, Moltrasio C, Berti E, Marzano AV. Skin manifestations associated with COVID-19: current knowledge and future perspectives. *Dermatology.* 2021;237(1):1-12.
215. Akuffo-Addo E, Nicholas MN, Joseph M. COVID-19 skin manifestations in skin of colour. *J Cutan Med Surg.* 2022;26(2):189-197.
216. Singh H, Kaur H, Singh K, Sen CK. Cutaneous manifestations of COVID-19: a systematic review. *Adv Wound Care (New Rochelle).* 2021;10(2):51-80.
217. Kelso JM, Coda AB, Keating RM, Vaccari DM. "COVID Toes" after mRNA COVID-19 vaccines. *J Allergy Clin Immunol Pract.* 2021; 9(8):3196-3197.
218. Gruber-Wackernagel A, Byrne SN, Wolf P. Polymorphous light eruption: clinic aspects and pathogenesis. *Dermatol Clinic.* 2014;32: 315-334.
219. Duteil L, Queille-Roussel C, Aladren S, et al. Prevention of polymorphic light eruption afforded by a very high broad-spectrum protection sunscreen containing ectoin. *Dermatol Ther (Heidelb).* 2022;12(7):1603-1613.
220. Chen Y, Lee J. Clinicopathologic study of solar dermatitis, a pinpoint popular variant of polymorphous light eruption. *J Formos Med Assoc.* 2013;112:125-130.
221. Gruber-Wackernagel A, Hofer A, Legat F, Wolf P. Frequency of occurrence of polymorphic light eruption in patients treated with photohardening and patients treated with phototherapy for other diseases. *Photodermatol Photoimmunol Photomed.* 2019;35(2): 100-105.
222. Lembo S, Raimondo A. Polymorphic light eruption: what's new in pathogenesis and management. *Front Med (Lausanne).* 2018; 5:252.
223. Montero EC, Sanchez-Albisua B, Guisado S, Martin-Diaz MA, Balbin-Carrero E, Dobao P. Factitious ulcer misdiagnosed as pyoderma gangrenosum. *Wounds.* 2016;28(2):63-67.
224. Amr A, Schmitt C, Kuipers T, Schoeller T, Eckhardt-Henn A, Werdin F. Identifying and managing patients with factitious wounds. *Adv Skin Wound Care.* 2017;30(12):1-7.
225. Freibott CE, Phillips KT, Anderson BJ, Stewart C, Liebschutz JM, Stein MD. Under the skin: the relationship between subcutaneous injection and skin infections among people who inject drugs. *J Addict Med.* 2022;16(2):164-168.
226. Saporito RC, Lopez Pineiro MA, Migden MR, Silapunt S. Recognizing skin popping scars: a complication of illicit drug use. *Cureus.* 2018;10(6):e2726.
227. Smith ME, Robinowitz N, Chaulk P, Johnson KE. High rates of abscesses and chronic wounds in community-recruited injection drug users and associated risk factors. *J Addict Med.* 2015;9(2): 87-93.

CHAPTER TEN

Skin Grafts and Flaps

Cynthia Sung, MD; Haig Manoukian, BS; Nicholas D. Hamelin, MD, DMV, MBA, FRCSC; and Alex K. Wong, MD, FACS

CHAPTER OBJECTIVES

After studying this chapter, the learner will be able to:

1. **Define the types of skin grafts.**
2. **Recognize skin anatomy relevant to flaps.**
3. **Integrate skin graft healing physiology into a plan of care.**
4. **Recognize signs of graft failure.**
5. **Explain relevant elements of donor site selection.**
6. **Describe a pedicle and a free flap.**
7. **Assess and determine an appropriate classification for a specific flap.**
8. **Distinguish the vascular anatomy of the skin, muscle, fascia, and perforator flaps.**
9. **Integrate the concepts and effects of angiosomes and venosomes on flap design.**
10. **Discuss flap physiology, including delay phenomenon and tissue expansion.**
11. **Assess and monitor a flap for tissue viability.**
12. **Recognize common flap complications.**

INTRODUCTION

Primary closure of a surgical wound is the simplest and fastest way of approximating wound margins; however, in many instances, it is neither feasible nor desirable to close a wound with this method. Using principles of moist wound healing results in a wound being left open to heal by secondary intention. Primary closure results in minimal scarring and re-epithelialization; wounds healing by secondary intention may have more extensive scarring with subsequent contraction and deformity.

When there is a relative or absolute soft tissue deficit appropriate for coverage, a skin graft or flap can be used to fill the defect. The extent of the deficit and its location, among other factors, dictate the type of coverage needed. The first section of this chapter discusses the principles and applications of skin grafting. The second section illustrates different types of flaps, followed by a succinct description of flap monitoring and common complications.

While this chapter is not an exhaustive reference on the subject, it is intended to be comprehensive for wound care providers, focusing on essential concepts related to grafts and flaps that will help the clinician understand the indications and postoperative care. For those readers who require more detailed information on the topics presented in this chapter, a thorough reference list is provided for further study.

SKIN GRAFTS

Definition

A skin graft is composed of epidermis as well as a variable amount of dermis (**FIGURE 10-1**). Human skin thickness varies greatly within the body, ranging from 0.5 to 4.0 mm.[1] Eyelid skin is among the thinnest of the body; back and scalp skin are the thickest. It is, therefore, the quantity of dermis that is variable in a skin graft. By definition, a graft *is tissue that is removed from the body, is completely devascularized, and is replaced in another location.*[2] A skin graft can be defined as epidermis and a proportion of dermis completely separated from its donor site that is transferred to a distant recipient bed.

Classifications

By Thickness The principal approach to classify a skin graft is by thickness. A graft that comprises the entire dermis and epidermis is termed a *full-thickness skin graft* (FTSG). If only a fraction of the dermis is harvested with the epidermis, the graft is termed a *split-thickness skin graft* (STSG). Within the STSG spectrum, a graft may be thin, medium, or thick. The instrument used to harvest a skin graft is called a *dermatome* and can be handheld or power assisted. Mechanical instruments are calibrated to harvest a specific skin thickness, measured in one thousandth of an inch (1/1000 inch) or in millimeters (mm) (**TABLE 10-1**).

By Origin Skin grafts may also be classified by their origin. Grafts can be harvested from humans or animals. If the donor and the recipient of the graft are the same individual, it is termed an *autograft*. If a graft is exchanged between two identical twins, it is termed an *isograft*. When the donor and the recipient are two different individuals but from the same species, it is termed *allograft*. If a graft is exchanged between two different species (eg, pig to human), it is termed *xenograft*.[3]

Autografts are routinely performed as part of plastic surgery procedures. For example, a free latissimus dorsi muscle flap may be covered by an STSG taken from the same patient (**FIGURE 10-2**).

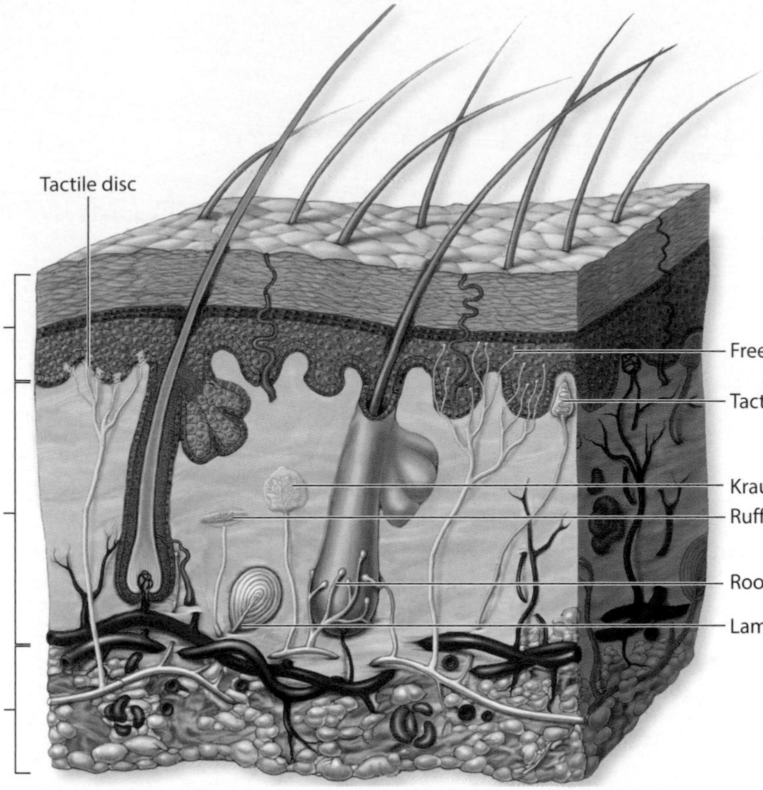

FIGURE 10-1 Skin anatomy. Skin grafts can be split-thickness (using the epidermis and part of the dermis) or full-thickness (using all of the epidermis and dermis).

TABLE 10-1 STSG Thickness

Thickness	/1000 inch	mm
Thin	8–10	0.020–0.025
Medium	12–14	0.030–0.036
Thick	18–22	0.046–0.056

The use of allografts is more restricted due to the high cost and limited indications. Allografts are harvested from cadavers and distributed for temporary skin coverage (**FIGURE 10-3**). Most allografts are used on burn patients to bridge the period between debridement and final coverage with autografts. If left in place for an extended period of time, a rejection reaction may occur and the skin allograft will be lost.

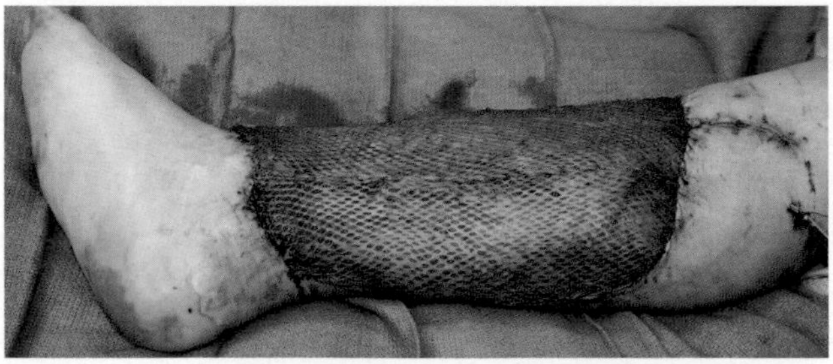

FIGURE 10-2 Free latissimus dorsi muscle flap covered with STSG. The split-thickness skin graft on the lower extremity is composed of the epidermis and part of the dermis, thus the red presentation from the presence of skin capillaries. In this patient, both the flap and the skin graft are examples of autografts, meaning the grafted tissue is taken from the patient's own body.

Because of the morbidity of harvesting skin autograft and its paucity in patients with extensive burns, animals have been considered as a skin source, with the hope of developing a reliable and nonhuman source of skin coverage. Unfortunately, xenografts were found to be expensive and immunogenic; therefore, they may be used as biologic dressings but not for durable long-term skin coverage. Xenograft tissue transplantation is an active area of research. Recently, there has been growing interest in using decellularized animal tissues such as porcine dermis, pericardium, and bladder for wound care indications. However, long-term outcome studies are limited.

Skin Anatomy

Human skin is the largest organ of the human body and represents 8% of the body, covering 1.2–2.2 m^2.[4] Skin is composed of epidermis and dermis, with an underlying subcutaneous fat layer (which is not per se part of the skin). The dermis contains a rich vascular supply, innervation, lymphatic drainage, glands, and hair follicles.

Epidermis and Dermis The outermost layer of skin is the epidermis and is defined as a keratinized stratified squamous layer that continuously renews itself. It is composed of five different

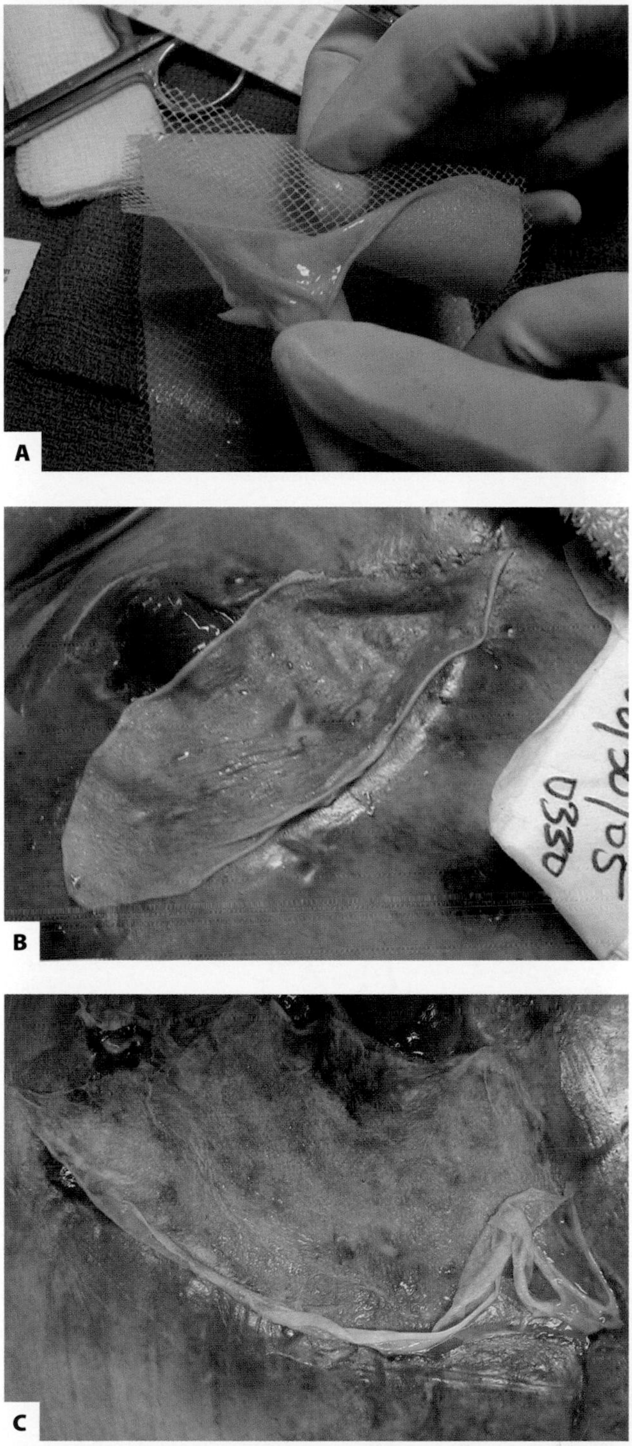

FIGURE 10-3 Allografts for temporary wound coverage. A. Allograft prior to application. **B.** Allograft applied to an abdominal wound with an enterocutaneous fistula. The goal was to facilitate wound healing prior to resection of the fistula. **C.** Four days after application, part of the allograft is being sloughed off (lower edges); in the center, granulation tissue is visible under the allograft that is still adhered to the underlying wound.

histologic sublayers, with a total thickness of 0.075–0.15 mm (**FIGURE 10-4**).[4] Epidermis is the host of four cell populations including keratinocytes, melanocytes, Langerhans cells, and Merkel cells. Keratinocytes, which are responsible for maintaining a physical barrier against external pathogens, represent at least 80% of epidermal cells.[4]

The layer between the epidermis and the underlying subcutaneous fat is termed the dermis. It is significantly thicker than the epidermis, ranging from less than 1 mm for the eyelid to over 4 mm for skin on the back.[4] The dermis contains vascular and nervous structures as well as glands and hair follicles (**FIGURE 10-5**). Fibroblasts are the principal cell population of the dermis, along with macrophages and adipocytes.

Dermal cells are contained in the extracellular matrix (ECM), which acts as a support for cells within the dermis. ECM is composed of collagen and gel-like substances, including glycosaminoglycans, proteoglycans, and glycoproteins. The non-collagenous component of ECM is referred to as the ground substance. Fibroblasts are responsible for the production of collagen fibrils as well as components of the ground substance. Approximately 75% of the dry weight of skin is collagen. There are many types of collagen but type I is the most abundant in the dermis.[4] Collagen is responsible for the tensile strength and elasticity of the skin, along with elastin (another protein synthetized by fibroblasts). Elastin allows the skin to stretch and return to its resting position without deformation. The dermis is divided into a superficial layer termed papillary dermis and a deeper layer termed reticular dermis.

Blood Supply Skin is vascularized by networks of blood vessels termed plexuses. The arterioles and venules within the dermis form two horizontal plexuses: an upper horizontal network in the papillary dermis and a lower horizontal plexus at the dermis–subcutaneous tissue junction.

Skin Appendages The various glands and hair follicles located in the dermis are termed *skin appendages.* The pilosebaceous units, comprising hair follicles and sebaceous glands, are located in the vast majority of the skin, with the exception of mucous membranes, palms, and soles. Eccrine sweat glands are ubiquitous on skin except for mucous membranes. Apocrine sweat glands are localized in specific locations, namely the axilla, perineum, areolae, eyelid, and external auditory canal.[4]

The relevance of skin anatomy in skin graft harvesting is important; for example, an STSG of 12/1000 inch (0.03 mm) from the back includes epidermis and part of the papillary dermis; however, hair follicles and sweat glands are not harvested with the split-thickness skin graft. The consequence is that the grafted site will not have hair nor glandular structure, and after healing, the donor site will regrow hair and keep its glandular potential. An FTSG from the abdomen that is transferred to the axilla carries all of the skin appendages to the newly grafted site. Thus, if hair were present on the abdomen, then hair would grow in the axilla, assuming an uneventful healing of the skin graft. Also, after STSG harvest, numerous small foci of bleeding are present representing the tangential cut of the upper horizontal plexus.

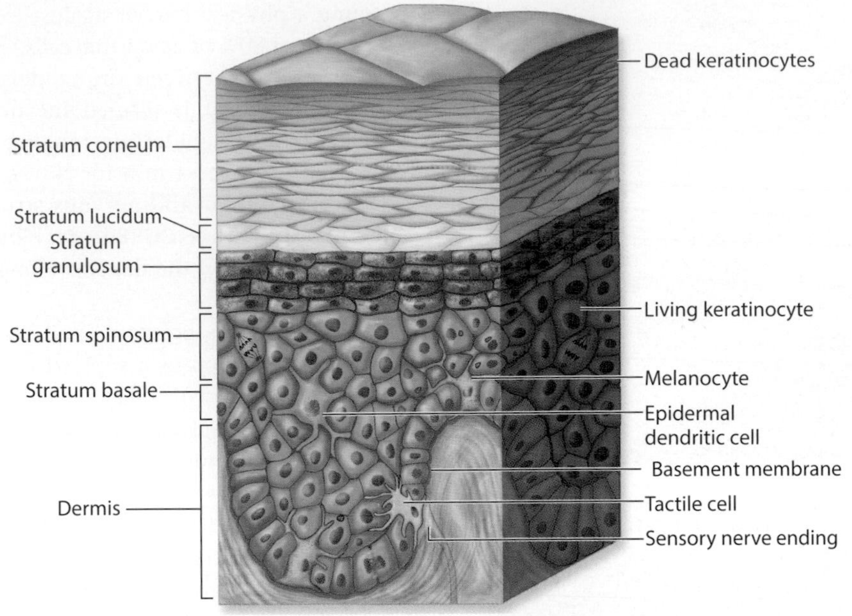

FIGURE 10-4 Layers of the epidermis.

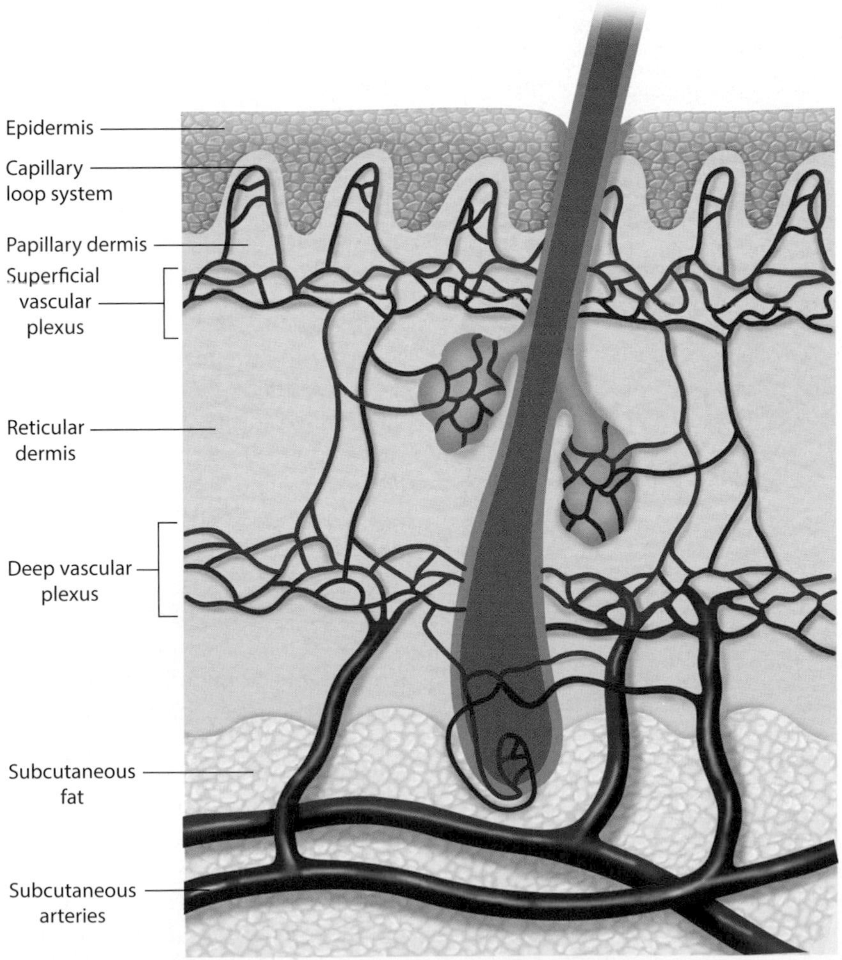

FIGURE 10-5 Vascular anatomy of dermis. The dermis contains networks of capillaries, termed plexuses. The upper horizontal network is in the papillary dermis, and the lower horizontal plexus is at the dermis–subcutaneous tissue junction. Random skin flaps that are not supplied by named axial blood vessels are viable secondary to perfusion from both dermal plexuses.

Physiology

Understanding the skin graft survival physiology is of paramount importance since it allows the surgeon to carefully prepare the recipient graft site and adequately immobilize the graft after placement. The first step before harvesting any skin graft is to prepare the recipient site. Since a skin graft does not have any intrinsic vascular supply when transferred, it relies solely on the resource of the recipient bed for survival during the postoperative period. An adequate recipient site must, therefore, be well vascularized, devoid of necrotic material, and free from pathogenic agents. Failure to achieve a proper recipient site will result in "non-take" of the skin graft, resulting in failure for the patient and the surgeon (**FIGURE 10-6**). Following are examples of patients who would not be good candidates due to high risk of failure:

- *Patient with lower extremity trauma with exposed tibia stripped of its periosteum*. The periosteum is essential to deliver nutrients to the graft and bone devoid of periosteum cannot be an adequate recipient bed.
- *Patient with burn wounds that are colonized with Staphylococcus aureus*. The wound may appear ready for skin graft after debridement; however, chances of failure are high because the graft may be inhibited by bacterial-derived collagenases.
- *Patient who is taking high doses of steroids or anti-inflammatory medications*. The same medications that inhibit wound healing will cause a graft to have a high risk of failure.
- *STSG on a plantar ulcer for a patient with diabetes and severe peripheral vascular disease*. The graft will not receive enough nutrients to survive and may be subjected to both friction and shear forces if the graft is not adequately off-loaded.

Normal Skin Graft Healing

The normal healing of a skin graft goes through three steps: serum imbibition, inosculation, and revascularization.

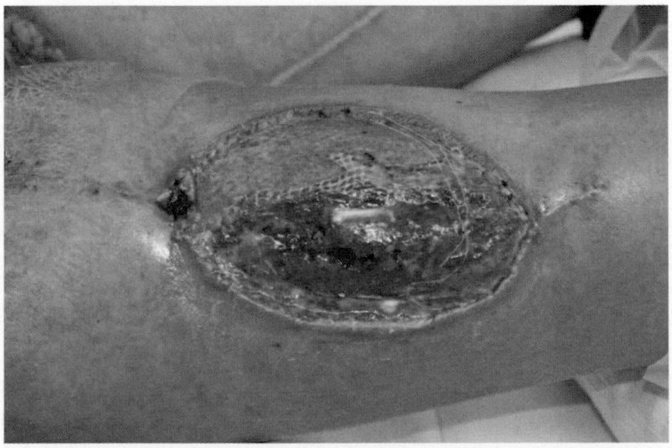

FIGURE 10-6 Skin graft with areas of both normal "take" and "non-take."

Serum Imbibition At the time it is harvested, a skin graft loses its vascular supply and in order to survive, it needs to receive nutrients from the recipient bed. Vascular connections cannot be reestablished instantaneously; therefore, during the first 48 hours, oxygen and nutrients diffuse passively from the recipient bed to the skin, a period termed the *serum imbibition* phase. Fibrin fixes the skin graft to the wound bed as fibrinogen is transformed into fibrin. During this phase, skin grafts gain up to 40% in weight compared with their initial weight in the first 24 hours; however, this gain is only 5% 1-week postgrafting.[5,6] Thickness of the graft is important, as thicker grafts need more diffusion of nutrients to survive. A poor recipient bed may have difficulty feeding a skin graft, for example, the plantar ulcer in a patient with vascular disease.

Accumulation of fluid in the interface between the bed and the graft, termed a *seroma*, affects survival of the graft because nutrients have to pass through the seroma to reach the graft. Clinically, a localized area with a seroma within a skin graft translates into a graft failure in the localized area. In addition, during this phase, skin grafts need to be protected from external trauma because any shearing of the graft may compromise its outcome.

Inosculation The second phase of skin graft healing, *inosculation,* takes place between 48 hours and 5 days postsurgery. Inosculation originates from Latin, *in* and *osculare*; it can be translated as "to unite by a small opening." It was originally thought that capillaries in the basal membrane would realign and connect with the skin graft; however, the process is in fact quite complex, involving anastomosis, neovascularization, and endothelial cell proliferation.[6] This phase marks the beginning of the process to achieve "normal" circulation by creating the foundation for a more definitive vascular support of the graft. Clinically, the graft appears congested and swollen. During this phase, the graft is still fragile and must be protected by a dressing. Any trauma, especially shearing of the graft, would disrupt the tiny capillary network developing to revascularize the graft.

Revascularization The final phase of skin graft healing is revascularization during which vascular channels form afferent and efferent vessels, as well as lymphatic drainage. The swollen appearance disappears and is replaced by a more natural texture and color. This is also a maturation phase during which contraction and remodeling of the surrounding tissues take place. Skin grafts take at least 1 year to complete maturation, and can take even longer in burned victims and children.[7] Long-term contraction of the graft varies according to its thickness. Skin graft contraction is divided into two types: the immediate contraction after harvest (termed *primary contraction*) and the long-term contraction after maturation (termed *secondary contraction*). Immediately after harvest, the thinner the graft, the lesser the amount of contraction; a full-thickness skin graft (FTSG) contracts the most. However, during the maturation phase, thinner grafts contract the most while FTSGs contract the least (**FIGURE 10-7**).

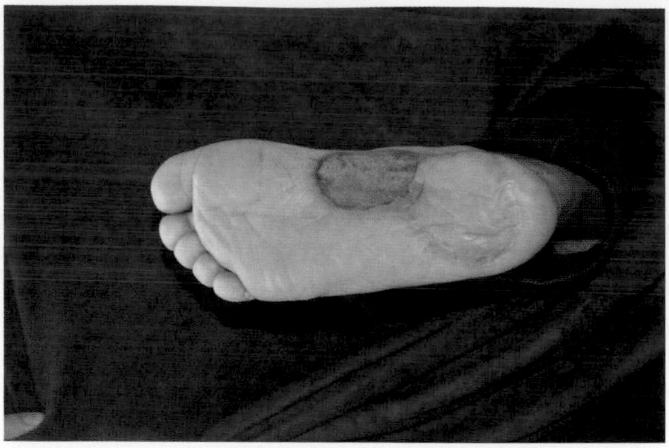

FIGURE 10-7 Healed STSG and FTSG. The plantar surface of the foot illustrates both a split-thickness and a full-thickness skin graft in the maturation or remodeling phase of wound healing.

Graft Immobilization

As mentioned earlier, skin grafts need to be protected from external distress to increase graft survival. Since contact of the graft with the wound bed is important, especially for the serum imbibition phase, a typical skin graft dressing includes a degree of pressure on the graft. If the wound bed is not a flat surface and is irregular, the graft has to be secured to the wound bed with stitches or staples in order to maintain close contact and prevent seroma or hematoma accumulation. Lack of appropriate contact between the graft and the recipient bed predictably results in graft failure.

Bolster Dressing The classic skin graft dressing, termed a bolster dressing, is simply a method to maintain close contact of the graft to the recipient bed and to protect it against trauma, primarily shearing forces (**FIGURE 10-8**). An example of a bolster dressing consists of a non-adherent dressing on the skin graft such as an Adaptic (Johnson & Johnson, New Brunswick, NJ). This layer maintains a moist environment and prevents tearing or ripping of the graft during dressing removal. The dressing is then padded by a cotton ball layer to perfectly "mold" the contour of the skin graft. The last step is to use sutures to ensure no movement of the dressing.

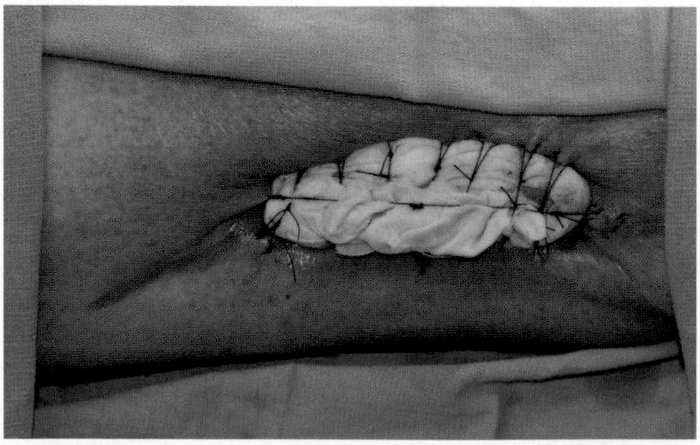

FIGURE 10-8 Example of a bolster dressing. A bolster dressing is used to maintain good contact of the graft with the recipient wound bed and to protect it against trauma. In this case, the graft is covered with several layers of nonadherent Xeroform gauze and sutured in place to ensure no movement of the dressing.

Negative Pressure Therapy Negative pressure therapy dressings are also used to protect skin grafts. This dressing maintains adequate graft-bed contact, protects the graft from trauma, and removes excess fluid by the negative pressure therapy. A negative pressure of 75 mmHg is normally sufficient to allow graft survival. NPWT may be difficult to apply in some areas of the body where a vacuum may be hard to achieve, for example, a cheek skin graft. (Refer to Chapter 17, Negative Pressure Wound Therapy, for more information on negative pressure wound therapy.)

Skin graft survival can be achieved without any dressing depending on the location and functional activities of the involved body part. For example, an STSG on a latissimus dorsi-free flap typically is not covered by bolster or negative pressure therapy dressing; pressure on the graft may compromise flap survival (**FIGURE 10-9**). As long as the skin graft is protected from trauma, is kept moist, and has no seroma or hematoma accumulation, it can survive if the recipient bed is appropriate. In the free latissimus dorsi example, grafts are often expanded (see the section "Graft Expansion") to prevent fluid accumulation and minimize the amount of skin needed. Muscle is an excellent recipient bed; in fact, STSG on a well-vascularized muscle adheres in only a few minutes due to fibrin exudation. In addition, fibrin glue may be used to create better contact between the graft and the recipient bed and is sprayed on the wound bed before apposing the skin graft.

The length of time required for a skin graft postoperative dressing to stay in place arises from an understanding of graft healing. The first 5 days are critical for graft survival as discussed earlier; thus, dressings are normally removed after 5 days. The graft still needs to be protected after initial dressing removal because it may be damaged if subjected to trauma, especially shear or friction forces. The maturation process is variable among individuals and clinical evaluation is warranted to assess adequate healing. Of note, some clinicians do not wait 5 days; they prefer to remove dressings earlier and evaluate the graft for fluid accumulation, position, or any other problem. If accumulated, fluid is drained or graft repositioned early, graft survival can still be achieved.

Graft Failure

Unfortunately, skin graft survival may be partial, leaving an area where the graft does not take to its underlying bed. These areas can be regrafted or left to heal by secondary intention. Skin grafting demands meticulous harvesting, in-setting, and dressing technique. Any failure along the chain of events from harvesting to dressing will lead to skin graft failure (**FIGURE 10-10**).

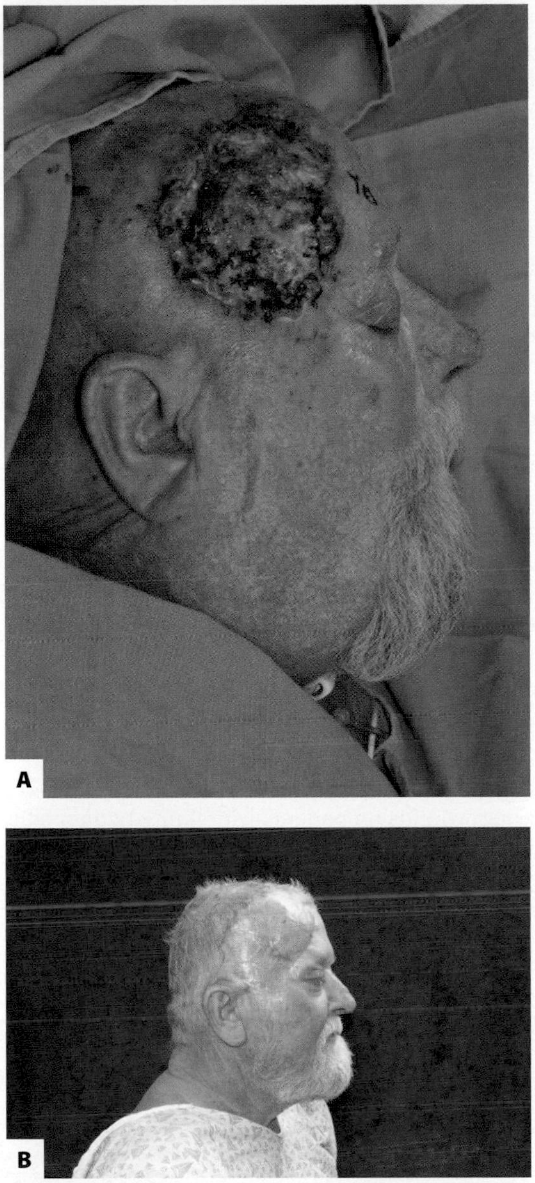

FIGURE 10-9 STSG on a free latissimus dorsi muscle flap. **A.** Basal cell carcinoma of the scalp. **B.** Postoperative result after wide excision of tumor and reconstruction with free latissimus dorsi flap and STSG.

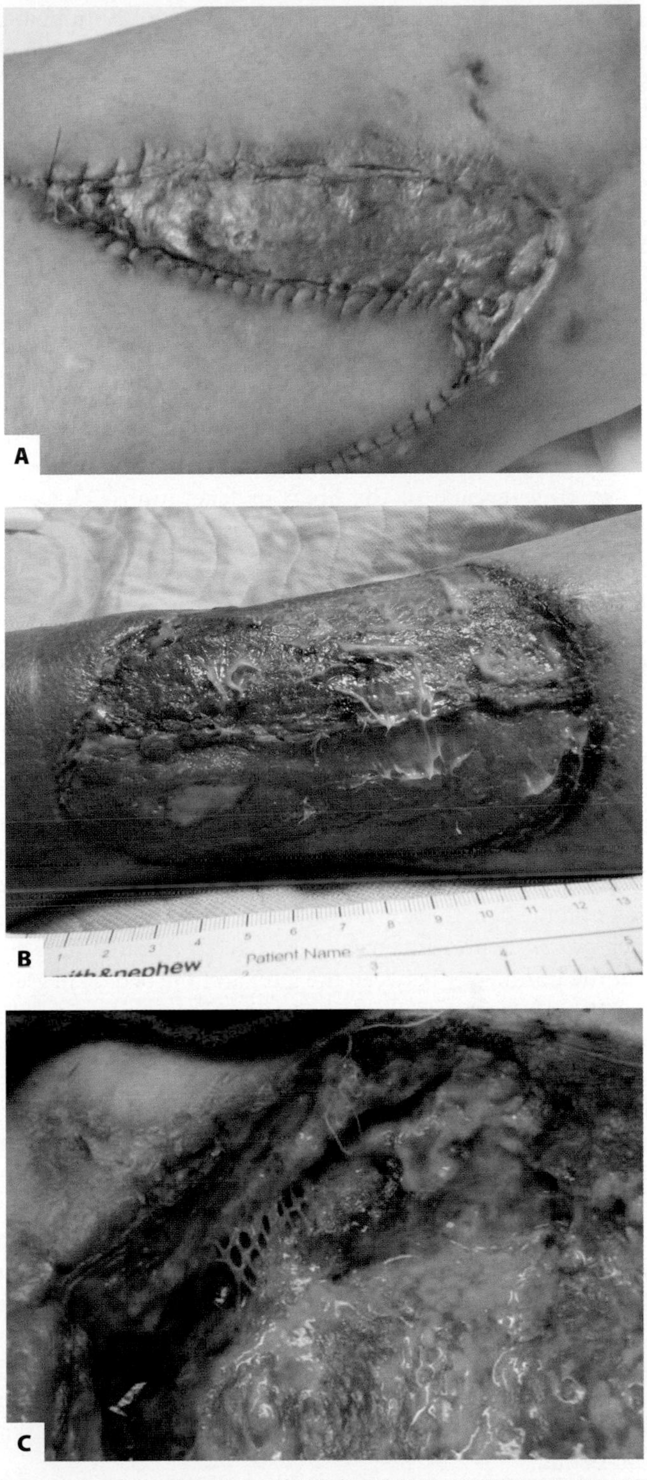

FIGURE 10-10 Examples of skin graft failure. Impending skin graft failure may be detected by changes in skin color, eg, dark red indicates hematoma formation beneath the skin; white, infection; black, necrosis; yellow slough, autolysis of nonviable tissue. **A.** The dark edges, loss of graft at the left edge, and dusky color of the skin around the lower incision are signs that part of the graft did not take. **B.** The white nonviable tissue in the graft site indicates possible infection. **C.** Remnants of meshed graft, along with large amounts of slough and necrotic tissue, are observed in this dehisced surgical incision after a hernia repair.

Factors of Skin Failure Skin graft failures have multiple origins, and the first cause is a technical error, eg, harvesting the skin graft too thick; placing the epidermal side of the skin to the recipient bed (rather than the dermal side); not placing the graft properly in the recipient bed, thus allowing movement or not creating close contact with the bed; and applying a dressing inadequately so that the graft is not properly protected from friction or shear. Again, a meticulous technique is mandatory to achieve skin graft survival.

A second cause of skin graft failure relates to fluid accumulation between the recipient bed and the skin graft. Fluid accumulating in the interface disrupts the serum imbibition process and causes skin graft failure. Seromas (clear fluid) or hematomas (blood) originate from the recipient bed; it is therefore essential to have a properly prepared bed. Adequate hemostasis prevents hematoma; drainage holes in the skin graft prevent seromas.

Drainage holes in a skin graft are performed in various ways. Skin expansion (see the next section), with its meshed network, allows easy drainage of any fluid. But drainage pits can also be performed by creating holes or lacerations in the skin graft. This process is termed *pie crusting* and is performed using a scalpel or fine scissors. The number of holes or incisions is dictated by the size and location of the skin graft. Ultimately, openings in the skin graft will heal by secondary intention, causing small areas of scarring in each of the holes or lacerations. However, for cosmetic reasons, a skin graft can be applied without any drainage openings. For example, an FTSG on the face generally does not have pie crusting; attention must then be focused on a recipient bed with proper hemostasis and a good bolster dressing with close contact between the graft and the bed.

Infection, either bacterial or fungal, is another potential cause of skin graft failure. Typically, a count of more than 10^5 organisms per gram of tissue leads to graft failure. The exception is *Streptococcus* infection, where less than 10^5 organisms per gram of tissue are needed to cause graft failure. When infection occurs, purulence may accumulate between the graft and the bed, thereby preventing revascularization. When *Streptococcus* is present, enzymes secreted by the microbes disrupt the fibrin layer between the graft and the bed. Skin grafting without proper antimicrobial treatment will lead to skin failure.

Finally, a poor recipient bed with inadequate vascular supply that is insufficient to nourish the graft will fail. Venous congestion, arterial insufficiency, and lymphedema are examples of vascular factors that may be responsible for a poor recipient bed.

Skin graft failure can be observed months after grafting. Contraction of the skin graft can be detrimental and may turn what appears to be a healthy graft into a functional failure. Clinicians in burn units, with especially challenging patients, can observe this phenomenon. For example, an axillary region can be grafted with an STSG only to realize, after months of healing, that arm movement restrictions are present due to skin contraction.

Graft Expansion

Skin is a scarce resource, especially for severely burned patients. For cosmetic reasons, several techniques can be used to conserve skin and minimize scarring of the harvest site. An elegant way to expand the surface of skin grafts is to create multiple windows and stretch the graft to increase the total surface area. This process is termed *graft expansion* and is accomplished with a *skin graft mesher* that uses blades with built-in cutting ratios. For example, a blade with a skin ratio of 1.5:1 expands harvested skin 1.5 times the initial surface area. Blades with ratios up to 9:1 are available. A blade with a higher ratio allows for more expansion but also leaves larger open areas in the graft.

Healing of the meshed skin graft occurs in two different ways. The expanded skin heals as previously described with open areas healing by second intention. Keratinocytes from the margin of the expanded skin colonize and fill open areas. Aesthetically, a meshed skin graft may have an unequal and rough appearance with multiple asperities (**FIGURE 10-11**). If hypergranulation is present, the result can be quite displeasing. The anatomic location of the skin graft recipient site often guides the type of meshing. For example, a face skin graft will not be meshed while a skin graft over a muscle-free flap for a lower extremity trauma may be meshed (**FIGURE 10-12**).

As mentioned earlier, the meshed area permits evacuation of fluid that may cause loss of contact between the graft and the recipient bed. A compromise between a better aesthetic result and a functioning drainage system is to mesh the graft without expanding it. Since the open areas heal by second intention and create an unpleasing appearance, an unexpanded mesh graft prevents fluid accumulation while at the same time minimizing scarring.

Larger wounds on patients with limited donor skin available for autologous skin grafting may be covered temporarily with allografts or xenografts until either more skin is available or until re-epithelialization occurs beneath the biomaterial

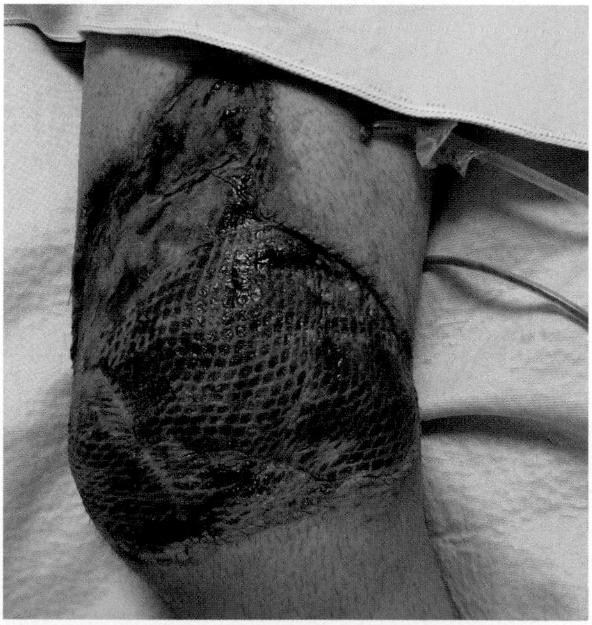

FIGURE 10-11 A meshed skin graft. A meshed skin graft immediately after placement over a lower extremity traumatic wound. The meshed texture of the skin graft allows the harvested skin to be stretched to cover a larger area than the donor site, thereby minimizing the size of the donor wound.

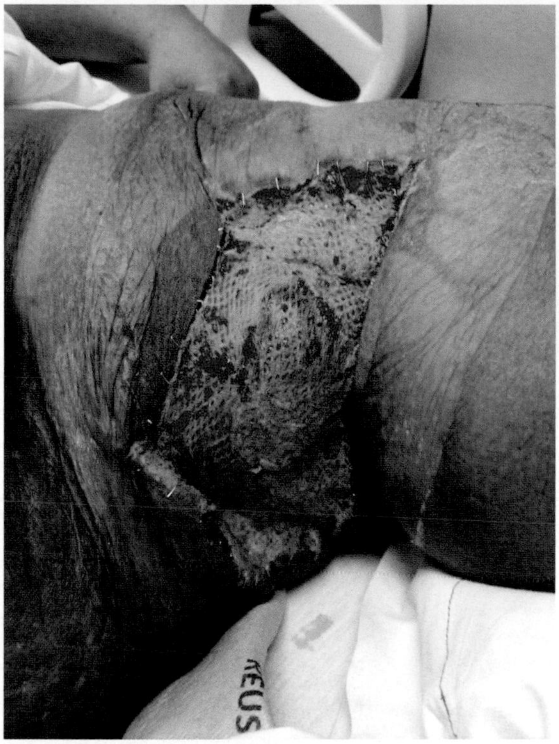

FIGURE 10-12 Expanded mesh skin graft on the lower extremity. A meshed graft that allows drainage to escape is especially important on the lower extremity where the wound may interfere with lymphatic flow and result in edema below the graft site. Modified compression with short-stretch bandages may help manage edema, improve the graft take, and result in a better outcome.

covering (see Chapter 14, Wound Dressings, for more information on biomaterials or cellular/tissue products).

Donor Site Selection and Morbidity

An autologous skin graft is usually harvested from a body site that is distant from the recipient defect. The consequence is termed *donor site morbidity*. Selecting an appropriate donor site is not trivial and demands careful consideration. Ideally, a skin graft would exactly match the skin it replaces; it would have the same color, texture, thickness, and appendages; however, this is rarely achieved.

The main consideration in donor site selection is the area that it will cover. Certain areas dictate an FTSG while others can be accommodated with an STSG. The face generally needs an FTSG for aesthetic concerns. In this example, color is a major factor in selecting a donor site. A distinctly different color in an area of the face attracts the eye and is cosmetically displeasing. Skin from the pre- or postauricular region or the supraclavicular region is often selected as a donor site for a facial skin graft.

However, a skin graft to cover a lower extremity trauma may not carry as many aesthetic considerations; also the same leg can often be selected as a donor site. For example, a skin graft needed to cover a calf defect may be taken from the thigh region of the same leg.

FTSG donor sites are usually closed primarily. Since all of the dermis is taken with the graft, leaving the donor site open would lead to secondary intention healing, thus creating a scar. For example, an FTSG can be harvested from the groin region to fill an axilla skin defect. The skin deficit in the groin region is then undermined to allow primary closure. For an STSG, part of the dermis is left on the donor site and is key to healing, which occurs in 7–21 days[8] by a process called *re-epithelialization*. The source of precursor cells comes from the periphery of the donor site and from the hair follicle stem cells. Once healed, an STSG generally leaves a distinctive texture that is different from the surrounding skin so that it is noticeable; it tends to have a shiny or polished appearance and is less pliable. Pigmentation is often affected, ranging from hypo- to hyperpigmented (**FIGURE 10-13**). If appendages have been incorporated into the graft, they are not replaced. Ultimately, the overall thickness of the graft compared to the total dermis thickness is a significant factor in the final look and feel of the donor site.

Donor site healing can be affected by common complications affecting any type of surgery (**FIGURE 10-14**). For example, a donor site can bleed excessively, be infected, or develop a hypertrophic scar/keloid. Meticulous wound care with occlusive dressings, with or without antimicrobial agents, is helpful in preventing donor site complications and in minimizing pain with dressing changes and functional activities. An informed discussion with patients about all of the aforementioned potential complications is essential to achieve a successful result.

The ultimate outcome for any skin graft is to have an aesthetically acceptable appearance and to recover full function of the affected part (**FIGURE 10-15**).

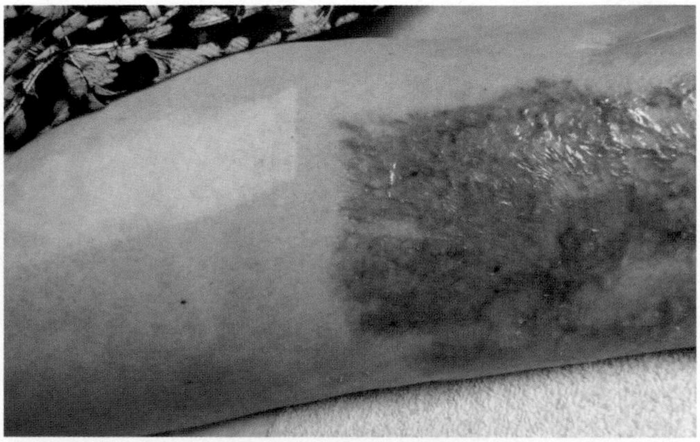

FIGURE 10-13 Hypopigmented or reddish healed donor site. Two donor sites on the thigh illustrate the color changes that occur. On the left, the hypopigmented area is from an older donor site that is completely healed, and on the right, the signs of neoangiogenesis give the donor site a reddish vascular appearance. As the re-epithelialized tissue remodels, the red scar tissue will diminish and the site will probably become hypopigmented.

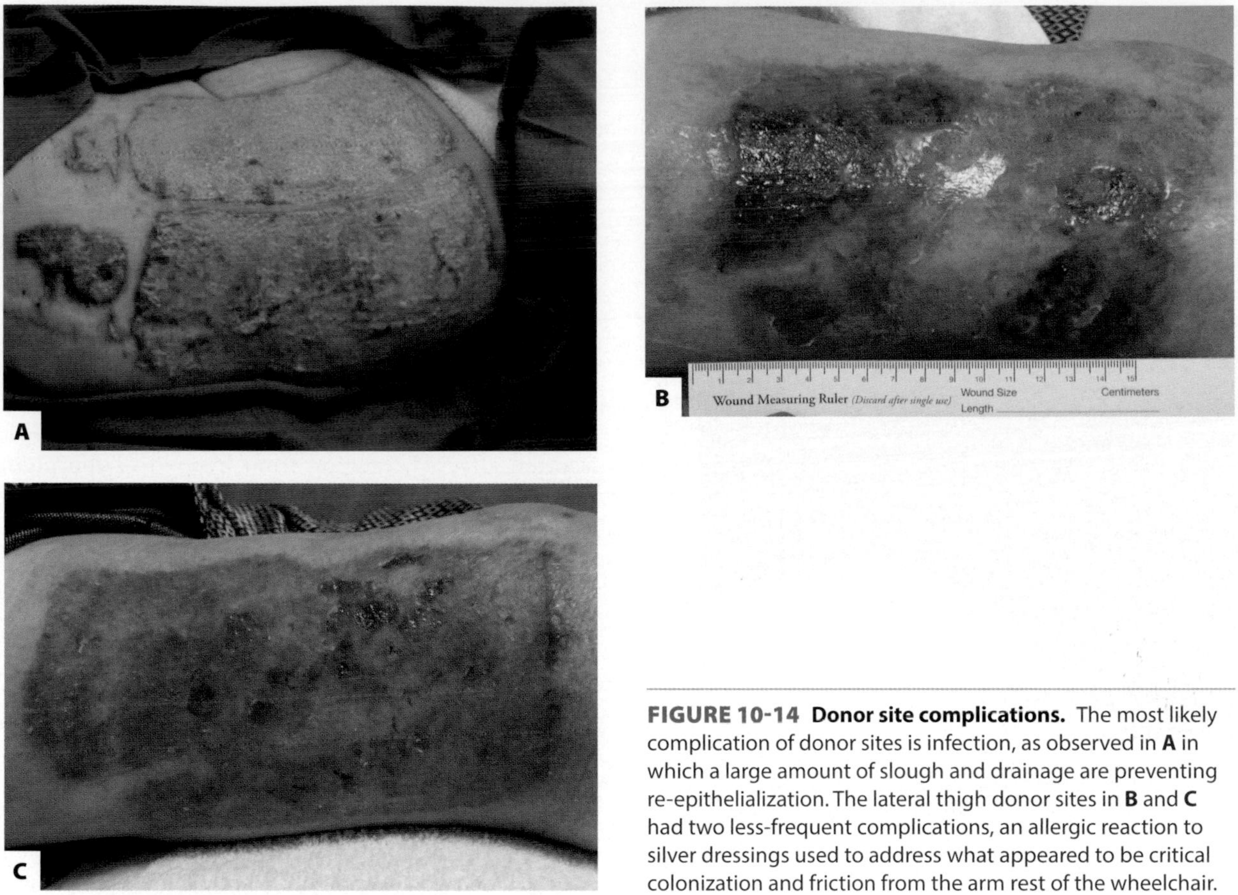

FIGURE 10-14 Donor site complications. The most likely complication of donor sites is infection, as observed in **A** in which a large amount of slough and drainage are preventing re-epithelialization. The lateral thigh donor sites in **B** and **C** had two less-frequent complications, an allergic reaction to silver dressings used to address what appeared to be critical colonization and friction from the arm rest of the wheelchair.

CASE STUDY

STSG

A healthy 30-year-old male sustained burn injuries to his hands and forearms while trying to start a campfire with gasoline. Because of the location of his injuries, he was transferred to a burn center. Evaluation of his injuries revealed a combination of superficial and deep partial-thickness burns. The initial treatment was debridement and moist dressings. He had no other injuries.

Superficial burns heal by re-epithelialization leaving no scar, but deep partial-thickness burns heal by second intention, creating scars if not treated.

DISCUSSION QUESTIONS

1. What is the most important treatment for a burn injury?
2. Why is skin grafting important in the overall medical management of this patient?
3. List pros and cons of an STSG versus FTSG treatment for this patient.

The key point of the reconstruction for this patient is to remove all nonviable tissue (debridement) and prevent limiting and disfiguring scarring. The best way to achieve this result is by skin grafting the lesion, and STSG is preferred over FTSG. STSG can be taken from any normal skin area of the body and the donor site will re-epithelialize. Thin skin grafts have a better "take" than thicker skin grafts due to the initial diffusion process involved in the first days postgrafting. FTSG donor sites have to be closed primarily, thus limiting the overall surface area that can be collected. FTSG is not an option for this patient.

The location from which the STSG is taken is determined after consulting the patient. For a patient with dark skin, hypo- or hyperpigmentation post-STSG is possible and has to be discussed with the patient. In this case, STSG would be harvested from the thigh.

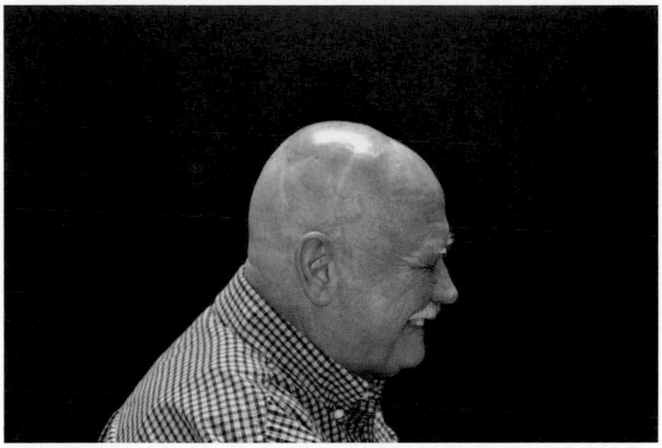

FIGURE 10-15 Long-term outcomes for an STSG. The goal of every STSG is to have an aesthetically acceptable outcome for the patient. The skin graft on this patient's scalp is barely visible; however, the full healing process from onset through maturation can take up to 2 years.

FLAPS

Definition

A flap is a unit of vascularized tissue that is transferred from one part of the body to another.[9] More simply defined, it is specific tissue that is mobilized on the basis of its vascular anatomy.[1] A flap may contain a single tissue (eg, skin, muscle, fascia, fat, bone, tendon, nerve) or a combination of tissues. A flap may also be comprised of enteric components such as jejunum, colon, stomach, or omentum. The critical concept about flaps is the relationship to its blood supply, which is necessary for the flap to survive. Because of the thickness and/or composite nature of flaps, the tissue being transferred cannot initially survive by diffusion from the recipient bed like a skin graft; it must have its own inflow and outflow of blood. A flap is termed *pedicled* if it maintains its blood vessel continuity at all times and is raised and/or transposed on the pedicle; it is termed a *free* flap if the vein and artery of the pedicle are cut and reanastomosed to other blood vessels. The term *free tissue transfer* may also be used to describe a *free flap*.

Classification

The dichotomy between a pedicle and a free flap is easy to understand but fails to classify flaps in a useful way. Over the years, different classifications have been used to categorize flaps according to various predominant factors, including vascular supply, tissue composition, transfer method, and vascular orientation.

Vascular Supply Classification by vascular supply is based on the type of vascularization of the flap and is used to describe cutaneous flaps, whether alone or combined with another tissue.

Random Flap Random cutaneous flaps apply only to skin and are based on random non-dominant contributions from the dermal and subdermal plexus.[9] Rather than having a definite blood vessel system to supply its surface, a random flap relies on the interconnection between specific vascular territories and the vascular skin plexus.[9] The critical concept in a random flap is its width-to-length ratio. A length twice as long as its base (ratio 2:1) is generally considered the limit for most tissue; however, it may be greater in the face and scalp but smaller in the lower extremity.[10] Exceeding a 2:1 length-to-width (base) ratio predictably results in distal flap necrosis. A classic example of a random flap is a transposition flap as illustrated in **FIGURE 10-16**.

Axial Flap An axial flap is based on longitudinal vessels along the pathway of the flap. The significant advantage of an axial flap over a random flap is the capability to extend the design outside the 2:1 ratio. In fact, an axial flap can be as long as the length of the blood vessel included in the flap. In an axial flap, the main axial artery with its *venae comitantes* gives rise to multiple branches that feed and drain the cutaneous portion adjacent to the flap. A classic example is the groin flap, based on the superficial circumflex iliac artery.

Musculocutaneous A musculocutaneous flap involves a combination of skin and muscle. The vascular pedicle supplies a muscle, which at the same time provides perforator branches to the skin. An example of a musculocutaneous flap is the transverse rectus abdominis flap (TRAM) used frequently in breast reconstruction.

Fasciocutaneous In a fasciocutaneous flap, the fascia is the recipient of a named vessel. Once the artery reaches the fascia, it gives perforator branches to the skin. An example of a fasciocutaneous flap is the anterolateral thigh flap (ALT) with the lateral circumflex femoral artery (LCFA) as a pedicle. The artery reaches the vastus lateralis and its fascia before giving perforator branches to the skin.

Septocutaneous When perforator branches do not have to go through a muscle or a fascial layer, they travel between

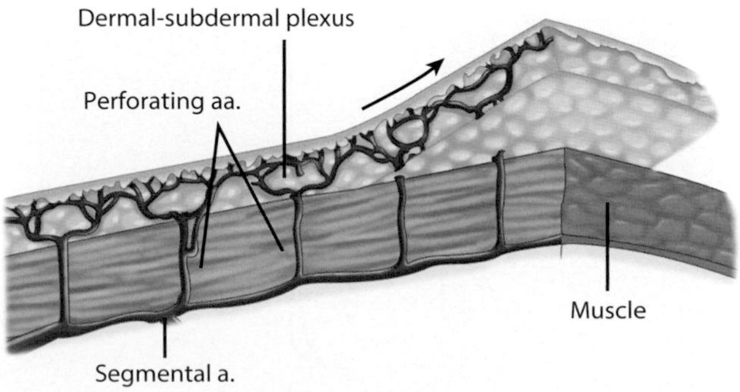

FIGURE 10-16 Random flap. Illustration of a random pattern flap in a transposition rectangular flap (2:1 ratio). (Reproduced with permission of Losee JE, Gimbel M, Rubin J, Wallace CG, Wei F. Plastic and reconstructive surgery. In: Brunicardi F, Andersen DK, Billiar TR, et al, eds. *Schwartz's Principles of Surgery.* 10th ed. New York, NY: McGraw-Hill; 2015.)

structures. The space where these vessels travel is termed a *septum*; therefore, the term septocutaneous flap. The ALT flap, with the same pedicle (LCFA), may have perforator branches traveling in the septum between the vastus lateralis and the rectus femoris muscles, reaching the skin without crossing through the vastus lateralis or its fascia. In this case, the flap is labeled a septocutaneous flap.

Tissue Composition The tissue composition classification is based on the actual tissue type involved in the flap, which can be a single tissue or a composite of tissues. The vascular supply is indirectly implied as being included in the flap and, therefore, is not named.

Single Tissue A single tissue flap is referred to by its main tissue. For example, a flap containing only the rectus abdominis muscle is a muscle flap; a flap composed of the temporoparietal fascia is a fascial flap. A flap can also contain skin, bone, omentum, or colon. (This list is not exhaustive.)

Composition of Tissues When more than one tissue is combined into a flap, it is labeled using the main tissues involved. Examples include a musculocutaneous flap or an osteofasciocutaneous flap. Many potential combinations are possible.

Transfer Method Classification by transfer method refers to the spatial displacement of a flap from a fixed point or a base. Consequently, it applies only to local pedicle flaps.

Advancement Flap Advancement flap describes the procedure when a flap is advanced directly forward into a defect without any rotation or lateral movement (**FIGURE 10-17**).[11]

Rotational Flap A rotational flap describes the procedure in which a semicircular flap is rotated about a pivot point into the defect to be closed (**FIGURE 10-18**).[12]

Transposition Flap A transposition flap is a combination of rotation and advancement of a single flap to close a defect (**FIGURE 10-19**).

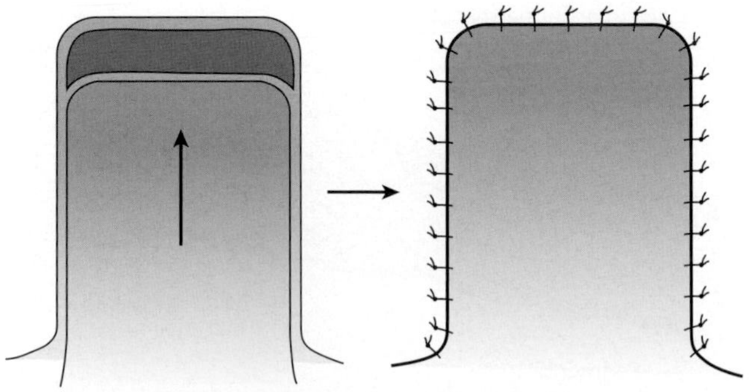

FIGURE 10-17 Example of advancement flap. Advancement flap describes the procedure when a flap is advanced directly forward into a defect without any rotation or lateral movement. (Reproduced with permission from Thorne CH. Techniques and principles in plastic surgery. In: Thorne CH, Beasley RW, Aston SJ, et al. eds. *Grabb and Smith's Plastic Surgery.* 6th ed. Philadelphia, PA: LWW; 2007.)

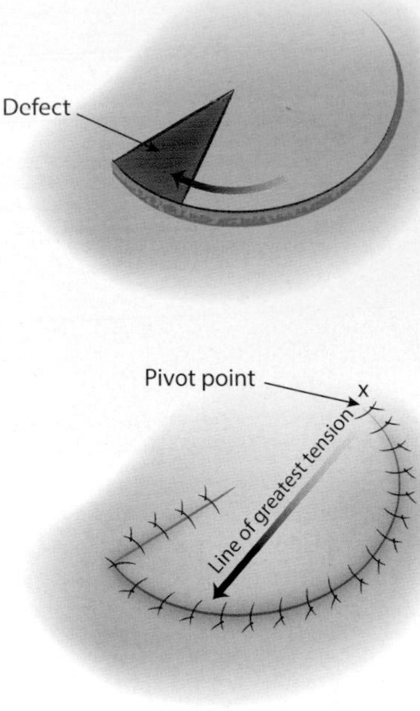

FIGURE 10-18 Example of rotational flap. A rotational flap is a semicircular flap that is rotated about a pivot point into the defect to be closed. (Reproduced with permission from Mathes SJ, Levine J. Muscle flaps and their blood supply. In: Thorne CH, Beasley RW, Aston SJ, et al. eds. *Grabb and Smith's Plastic Surgery.* 6th ed. Philadelphia, PA: LWW; 2007.)

Interpolation Flap An interpolation flap is a two-stage tissue flap in which the base of the flap is not immediately adjacent to the recipient site.[13] For this type of flap, normal tissue is interposed between the base of the flap and its insertion. The forehead flap is a classic example (**FIGURE 10-20**).

Vascular Orientation A flap can be named according to the direction of its blood flow. This classification is not specific to tissue, rather to a specific pattern of vascularization.

Anterograde Flow Flap An anterograde flow flap maintains the normal pattern of the arterial flow. For example, a pedicle radial forearm flap based proximally has an anterograde arterial flow in the radial artery.

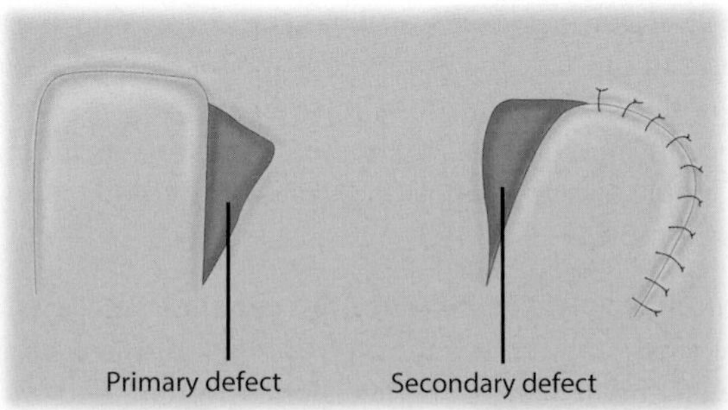

FIGURE 10-19 Example of transposition flap. A transposition flap is a combination of rotation and advancement of a single flap to close a defect.

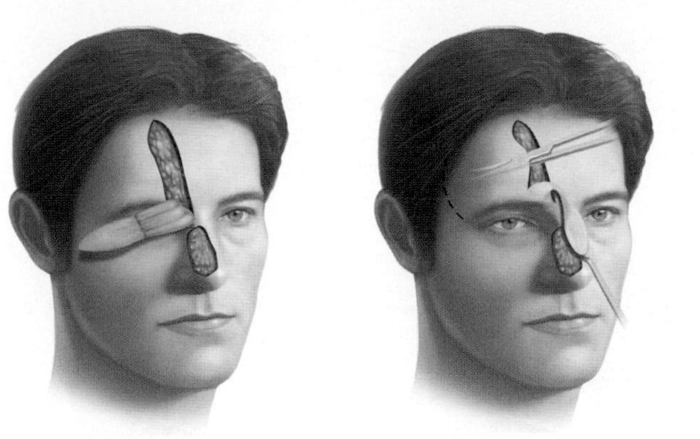

FIGURE 10-20 Example of interpolation flap. An interpolation flap is a two-stage tissue flap in which the base of the flap is not immediately adjacent to the recipient site.[6] In this type of flap, normal tissue is interposed between the base of the flap and its insertion. The forehead flap is a classic example, as shown here as a paramedian forehead flap.

Retrograde Flow Flap In a retrograde flow flap, the arterial blood flow does not travel through the usual pattern but instead has its flow reversed due to transection of the antero-grade dominant blood flow. An example is a reverse posterior interosseous flap in which the arterial flow in the posterior interosseous artery (PIA) originates normally from the ulnar artery and the common interosseous artery. In this flap, when the PIA is transected proximally, blood is flowing reversely from an anastomotic branch of the anterior interosseous artery located in the distal forearm.

Flow-Through Flap A flow-through flap can be used to bridge an interrupted arterial flow by anastomosing the proximal and distal pedicle, thereby restoring flow distally. The first flow-through flap is used to connect the external carotid to the facial artery with a radial forearm flap. In this case, the radial artery is used to reestablish arterial circulation.

Venous Flap A venous flap has no arterial pedicle, only a venous pedicle(s). The physiology of these flaps is more complex and only small flaps can survive on venous inflow only.[14]

Vascular Anatomy Flaps are based on an absolute understanding of their vascular supply. A thorough appreciation of the delicate and complex vascular anatomy of each specific tissue is necessary for a flap to be harvested in a safe and efficient way. Most flaps are composite flaps with each component having its own vascular territory. For the sake of clarity, in this text, a *perforator artery* is defined as an artery that supplies the skin; a *branch artery* is defined as an artery that supplies a muscle or fascia.

Vascular Supply of the Skin The skin can be nourished via direct connections from an artery; otherwise, the artery has to penetrate through various tissues, the most important being muscle and fascia. Once the artery reaches the skin, its vascular supply forms five different plexuses.[1,12] A vascular plexus can be simply described as a network of anastomoses between blood vessels (**FIGURE 10-21**).

The skin microcirculation can be described using another model. The arterioles and venules within the dermis form

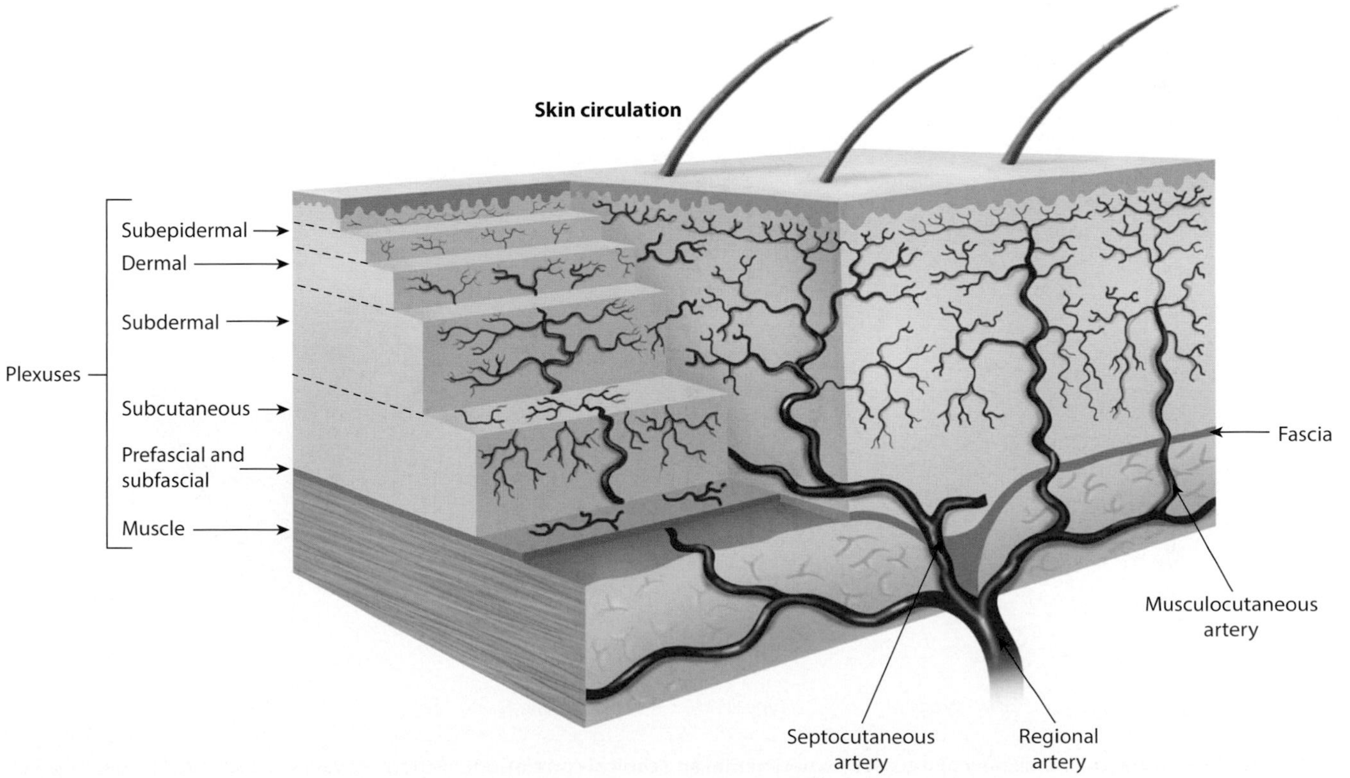

FIGURE 10-21 Skin circulation. Once the artery reaches the skin, it forms multiple different plexuses through which blood is supplied to the layers of the skin.

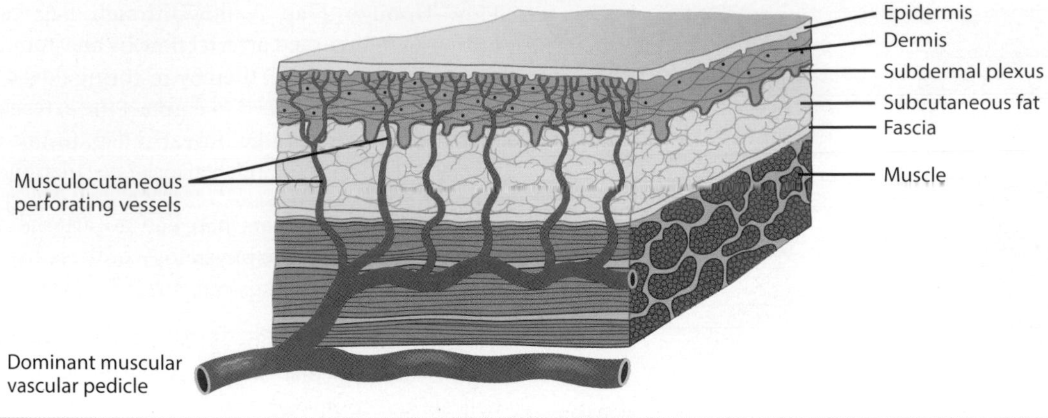

FIGURE 10-22 Perforator arteries to the skin. The artery in the muscle provides smaller branches that perforate the fascia to provide the blood supply to the skin layers.

two horizontal plexuses: an upper horizontal network in the papillary dermis and a lower horizontal plexus at the dermis-subcutaneous tissue junction. Muscle and fat tissues host the perforating vessels, which ultimately create the lower plexus. The newly formed arterioles and venules connect to the upper horizontal plexus, irrigating epidermal appendages at the same time (**FIGURE 10-22**).[1,13]

Muscle Flaps Muscle flaps are, in their simplest form, individual muscles harvested with the vascular pedicle. However, muscles are not vascularized uniformly and the understanding of the vascularization pattern is of paramount importance when harvesting a muscle flap. In a landmark article published in 1981, Mathes and Nahai described five patterns of muscle vascular anatomy (**FIGURE 10-23** and **TABLE 10-2**).[15]

Type I: *One vascular pedicle.* In this type of flap, the entire muscle is dependent on its main blood supply, meaning that the entire muscle can survive on a single artery and vein. The disadvantage of a type I muscle flap is that if the vascular pedicle is severed, the muscle will not survive. The *tensor fascia lata* or the *gastrocnemius* are muscles that can be used for type I flaps.[16]

Type II: *One or more vascular pedicle(s) and minor pedicle(s).* Muscles in this group have a dominant pedicle that can sustain the whole muscle and a minor blood supply that is incapable of solely maintaining muscle viability. In this case, a muscle flap can be harvested on a dominant pedicle and minor pedicles can be ligated without affecting the subsistence of the flap. Examples include the *gracilis* or *rectus femoris* muscles.

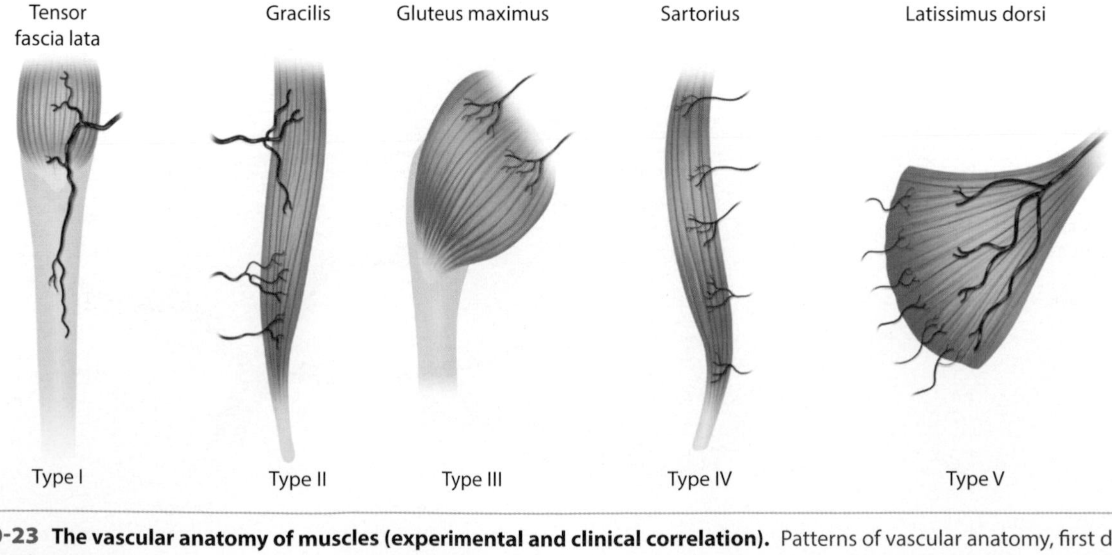

FIGURE 10-23 The vascular anatomy of muscles (experimental and clinical correlation). Patterns of vascular anatomy, first described by Mathes and Nahai in 1981, are also described in Table 10-2. (Reproduced with permission from Mathes SJ, Nahai F. Classification of the vascular anatomy of muscles: experimental and clinical correlation. *Plast Reconstr Surg.* 1981;67(2):177-187.)

TABLE 10-2 Patterns of Muscle Vascular Anatomy

Classification	Vascular Supply	Example
Type I	One vascular pedicle	Gastrocnemius Tensor fascia lata
Type II	Dominant and minor pedicles (the flap cannot survive based only on the minor pedicles)	Gracilis Rectus femoris
Type III	Two dominant pedicles	Rectus abdominis Pectoralis minor
Type IV	Segmental pedicles	Sartorius External obliques
Type V	One dominant pedicle with secondary segmental pedicles (the flap can survive based only on the secondary pedicles)	Pectoralis major Latissimus dorsi

Type III: *Two dominant pedicles.* These muscles have two dominant pedicles that can each maintain adequate blood flow if harvested individually. As long as one of the two pedicles is intact, the flap will remain viable. A classic example is the *rectus abdominis* in the TRAM flap with two main vascular trunks. A pedicled TRAM uses the superior epigastric artery and veins while a free TRAM utilizes the inferior epigastric system. Another example is the *pectoralis minor* muscle, which can be harvested using the thoracoacromial artery or the lateral thoracic artery.

Type IV: *Segmental vascular pedicles.* These muscles are vascularized by multiple branches that are each responsible for the survival of a segment of the muscle. The origin and insertion of the muscle are considered pedicles. The primary limitation of a type IV muscle becomes obvious during flap harvest. Since each segment is not well connected to the other vascular segment, only a limited number of branches can be safely ligated and still maintain survival of the entire muscle flap. If too many branches are severed, segmental flap necrosis will occur. Examples include the *sartorius* or the *external oblique* muscles. These muscles cannot be used as a free tissue transfer but are useful as a rotational pedicle flap. Sartorius flaps, raised by ligation of two to three branches, can be used to cover an exposed femoral artery and vein.

Type V: *One dominant and secondary segmental pedicles.* In these muscles, the multiple segmental pedicles are capable of adequately vascularizing the flap as well as the single dominant pedicle. The flap can then be based on either of the pedicles for a pedicle flap. If free tissue transfer is performed, then the flap must be based on the dominant pedicle. Examples include the *latissimus dorsi* or the *pectoralis major*. A latissimus dorsi flap can be distally based on its lumbar branches or it can be used as a free tissue based on the thoracodorsal vascular trunk.

A muscle flap can be combined with other tissues to create a composite flap, the most common being the musculocutaneous flaps. Muscles give rise to multiple arterial branches, termed perforator arteries, which travel through the fascia to supply the skin. In order to achieve better vascularization of the skin, the connections between the muscle and skin are maximized during flap surgery. Every muscle that has skin in continuity can include a portion of skin when it is used for a flap. This attached section of skin is termed a skin paddle. A rectus abdominis or a latissimus dorsi muscle can easily be combined with a skin paddle. A pectoralis minor flap, however, does not have direct connection to any skin and, therefore, cannot include a skin paddle.

Fasciocutaneous Flaps A fasciocutaneous flap is composed of skin, subcutaneous fat, and fascia. Its main vascular supply irrigates deep fascia that permits vascularization to a more or less well-defined skin territory. The first fasciocutaneous flap was described by Pontén in 1981[17] and a more formal classification was developed by Cormack and Lamberty in 1984. Four types of vascular patterns were originally identified.[18]

Type A: *Multiple fasciocutaneous vessels.* These flaps have multiple perforators oriented in the long axis of the flap in the predominant direction of the arterial plexus and at the level of the deep fascia. An example is a rotational flap in a lower extremity.[18] As in segmental muscle flap (type IV), survival of the flap is directly related to the number of segmental vessels included in the flap.

Type B: *Single fasciocutaneous vessel.* These flaps have a single vessel responsible for vascularizing the entire flap. According to the authors, the essential characteristic of the flap is a T-junction on the single vessel feeding the fascial plexus.[18] An example is the medial arm flap based on the superior ulnar collateral artery.

Type C: *Multiple small fasciocutaneous vessels in a septum.* These flaps have branches originating from an axis vessel; however, they travel between muscles in a septum. A classic example is the radial forearm flap where the numerous perforators to the skin and fascia originate from the radial artery and travel in between the brachioradialis (BR) and the flexor carpi radialis (FCR). The main difference between type A and type C is the fact that the main vessel is included in the flap in type C. Therefore, type C can be converted into a free tissue transfer but type A cannot.

Type D: *Osteomyofasciocutaneous flap.* This flap is an extension of type C and as such is often included in this category. In this flap, the fascial septum is included as well as the adjacent muscle and bone along with their blood supply. An example is the radial forearm osteofasciocutaneous flap including the radius bone with a cuff of muscle including fascia and skin.

Fascial flaps do not need a skin paddle and therefore are often harvested as a pure fascial flap without a skin paddle. Examples include a temporoparietal fascia flap or a radial forearm fascia flap.

TABLE 10-3 Nahai–Mathes Classification of Fasciocutaneous Flaps

Classification	Vascular Supply	Example
Type A	Direct cutaneous vessel that penetrates the fascia	Temporoparietal fascial flap
Type B	Septocutaneous vessel that penetrates the fascia	Radial artery for earm flap
Type C	Musculocutaneous vessel that penetrates the fascia	Transverse rectus abdominis myocutaneous flap

Reproduced with permission of Losee JE, Gimbel M, Rubin J, Wallace CG, Wei F. Plastic and reconstructive surgery. In: Brunicardi F, Andersen DK, Billiar TR, Dunn DL, Hunter JG, Matthews JB, Pollock RE, eds. *Schwartz's Principles of Surgery.* 10th ed. New York, NY: McGraw-Hill; 2015.

For fasciocutaneous flaps, another classification by Mathes and Nahai deserves mentioning because of its simplicity and frequency of use. This classification is based on the pathway of the perforator to the skin and includes three types (**TABLE 10-3**).[1,10,12]

Type A: *Direct cutaneous perforator*. In these flaps, a perforator artery originates from an axial vessel and travels directly to the skin without having to travel through a muscle or a septum. Examples include the groin flap, based on perforators from the superficial circumflex femoral artery or the temporoparietal fascia based on branches from the superficial temporal artery.

Type B: *Septocutaneous perforator*. In these flaps, perforators travel from the originating vessel to the skin between muscles via a septum. The primary advantage of these perforators is that during harvesting of the flap, the vessel course is easily identifiable in a septum and because of the absence of side branches, dissection is rapid and straightforward.

Type C: *Musculocutaneous perforators*. Perforators that travel through a muscle to access the skin are termed musculocutaneous perforators. Unlike type B perforators, vessels in muscle are more difficult to dissect if the muscle is not included in the flap. Close proximity of muscle fibers to blood vessels and numerous small branches makes dissection of perforators more tedious.

Perforator Flaps The concept of perforator flaps emerged from the postulate that a single perforator artery could vascularize a definite skin territory and its subcutaneous component without having to include the adjacent muscular tissue. The first reported perforator flap was described by Koshima in 1989 in which an abdominal skin paddle was harvested without the rectus abdominis muscle, including only the skin and adipose tissue, and was vascularized by a single perforator of the deep inferior epigastric artery.[19] This flap is now known as the *deep inferior epigastric perforator* (DIEP) flap.

Numerous perforator flaps have since been described. When an artery is dissected from its arborization into the skin to its proximal origin, it is termed a perforator flap. Perforator flaps differ from conventional musculocutaneous or fasciocutaneous flaps by way of their anatomic origin. Skin and subcutaneous tissues are supplied by the following five vascular plexuses: subepidermal, subdermal, dermal, subcutaneous, and fascial (sub- and suprafascial). Conventional flaps originate from vessels beneath muscle layers or within the fascia. In contrast, perforator flaps are supplied by the more distal subcutaneous or subdermal vessels, which allows for elevation of just the skin paddle without the requirement of other tissues.[20]

In an attempt to define and classify perforator flaps, Blondeel et al. defined a perforator flap as the following: "A perforating vessel, or, in short, a perforator, is a vessel that has its origin in one of the axial vessels of the body and that passes through certain structural elements of the body, besides interstitial connective tissue and fat, before reaching the subcutaneous fat layer."[21] Some authors make a distinction between a direct (only goes through fascia before reaching skin) and an indirect perforator (goes through other tissues before reaching skin).[22] In 2003, the Gent consensus was published proposing a classification and a nomenclature scheme (**TABLE 10-4** and **FIGURE 10-24**).[21]

This classification was simplified in 2003 with only three types of flaps included (**TABLE 10-5** and **FIGURE 10-25**).[23] Despite these efforts, controversy still exists among the definition of perforator flaps, and there have been calls to refine the terminology.[1,24]

To standardize nomenclature of perforator flaps, the Gent consensus proposed that "A perforator flap should be named

TABLE 10-4 Gent Classification of Perforator Flaps

Type 1: Direct perforators perforate the deep fascia only. The perforator artery runs from its main vessel directly to the deep fascia.
Type 2: Indirect muscle perforators predominantly supply the subcutaneous tissues. A perforator travels through a muscle but mainly vascularizes a skin territory; few branches are going into the muscle.
Type 3: Indirect muscle perforators predominantly supply the muscle but have secondary branches to the subcutaneous tissues.
Type 4: Indirect perimysial perforators travel within the perimysium between muscle fibers before piercing the deep fascia.
Type 5: Indirect septal perforators travel through the intermuscular septum before piercing the deep fascia.

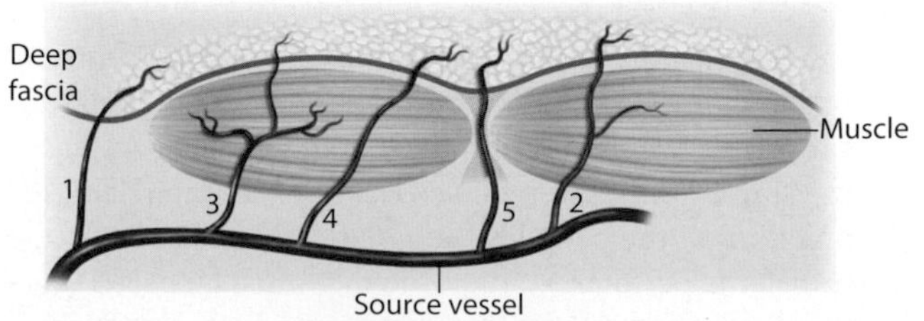

FIGURE 10-24 The Gent classification illustrated. (Reproduced with permission from Blondeel PN, Van Landuyt KH, Monstrey SJ, et al. The "Gent" consensus on perforator flap terminology: preliminary definitions. *Plast Reconstr Surg.* 2003;112(5):1378-1387.)

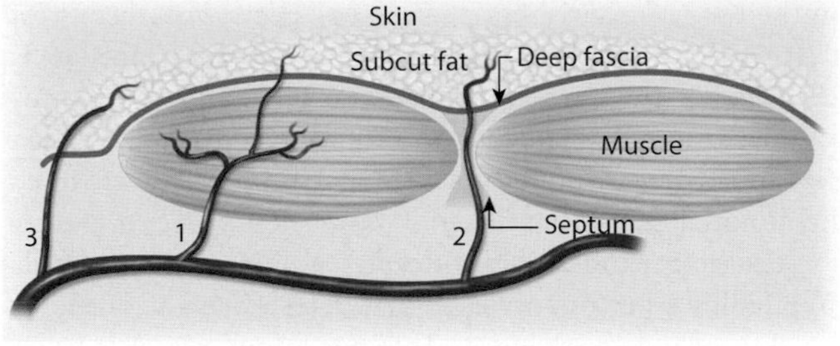

FIGURE 10-25 Illustration of the three types of perforator flaps.

TABLE 10-5 Simplified Classification of Perforator Flaps

Type 1: Indirect "muscle" or myocutaneous perforators traverse through muscle to pierce the outer layer of the deep fascia to supply skin.
Type 2: Indirect "septal" or septocutaneous perforators traverse only through a septum to reach the deep fascia and the skin.
Type 3: "Direct" perforators perforate the deep fascia only. (From Blondeel PN, Van Landuyt K, Hamdi M, Monstrey SJ. Perforator flap terminology: update 2002. *Clin Plast Surg*. 2003;30(3):343–346.)

after the nutrient artery or vessels and not after the underlying muscle. If there is a potential to harvest multiple perforator flaps from one vessel, the name of each flap should be based on its anatomical region or muscle."[21] For example, a perforator flap based on the thoracodorsal vessels, the main vessel for the latissimus dorsi, should be labeled a *thoracodorsal artery perforator flap* (TAP flap).

Since their discovery, over 350 perforators have been identified. Perforator flaps can be elevated as pedicled or free flaps.[25] In 2009, Saint-Cyr et al. introduced the term "perforasome" to describe the cutaneous territories supplied by various perforator vessels (**FIGURE 10-26**).[26] The authors mapped and compiled the perforators and their associated tissues via injection and imaging. This concept is similar to the term angiosome which describes the vascular territory supplied by each artery (more information on angiosomes is given in the following section).

Perforator flaps have become a mainstay of reconstruction. The DIEP flap is now the preferred technique in breast reconstruction as it offers excellent aesthetic outcomes and decreased donor site morbidity compared to previous techniques such as the transverse rectus abdominis myocutaneous (TRAM) flaps.[27] Other techniques such as profunda artery perforator (PAP), thoracodorsal artery perforator (TDAP), and superior gluteal artery perforator (SGAP) flaps have been described and are now commonly used for a variety of reconstructive purposes, including but not limited to head and neck reconstruction, abdominal wall reconstruction, and extremity reconstruction.[28,29]

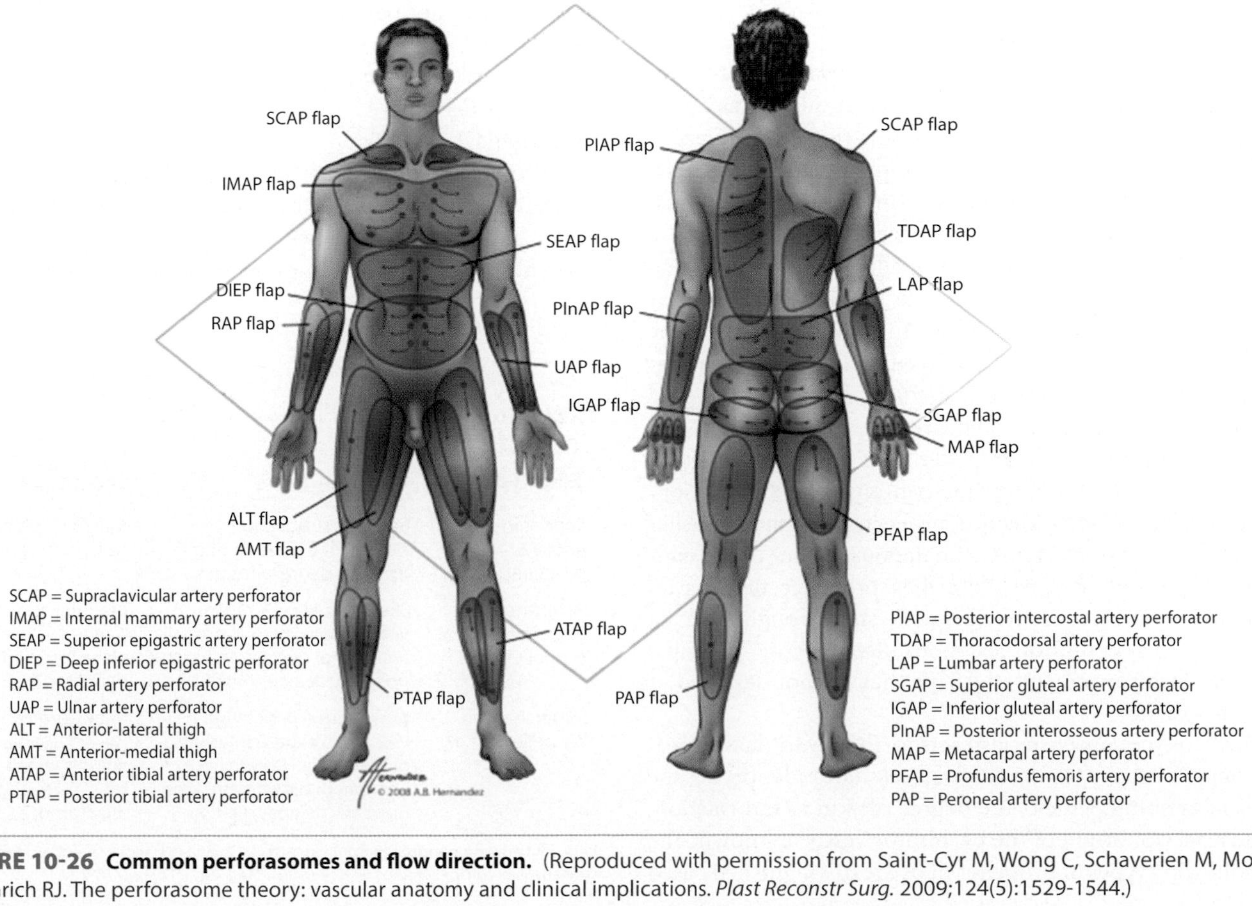

FIGURE 10-26 Common perforasomes and flow direction. (Reproduced with permission from Saint-Cyr M, Wong C, Schaverien M, Mojallal A, Rohrich RJ. The perforasome theory: vascular anatomy and clinical implications. *Plast Reconstr Surg*. 2009;124(5):1529-1544.)

The perforator flap offers many advantages over the conventional myocutaneous flap. The wealth of perforators provides an abundance of donor sites. Perforator flaps do not require elevation of the underlying muscle; therefore, the muscle can be spared and donor site function is preserved, as opposed to myocutaneous or myofascial flaps. Unlike conventional flaps, perforator flaps can be oriented in any direction on the perforator, which allows for optimal defect coverage. Perforator flaps can be much more versatile than conventional flaps because they can be readily thinned and shaped to conform to the defect, they can be oriented freely based on the pedicle, and they have a longer pedicle.[30] These properties may stem from the observed phenomenon that pedicled flaps are hyperperfused compared to normal circulation.[31] However, these benefits also pose disadvantages. Perforator flaps often require tedious, time-consuming dissection, which can prolong operative time. In addition, the distribution of perforator vessels is less consistent than larger vessels, necessitating more preoperative studies and intraoperative effort.[32]

Perforator flaps are a powerful tool in the reconstructive surgeon's armamentarium. The increase in popularity of these flaps has been supported by improved understanding, which has enabled perforator flaps to supplant many conventional flaps. The mantra of "flap of choice" is slowly fading away as the versatility of perforator flaps continues to evolve and expand.[33] Continued study is needed to better characterize and define the vascular distribution, and future investigation will refine the use of these flaps as well as potentially discover their new applications.

Propeller Flaps Since its inception in 1991, the propeller flap has undergone a series of transformations to maximize tissue coverage and improve its use in soft-tissue defect reconstruction throughout the body. The original flap described by Hyakusoku et al. was adipocutaneous in nature and consisted of a skin island with two "propeller blades" at each end of a vascular pedicle.[34] Much like a propeller, the flap was then rotated 90 degrees around its pedicle for the release of scar contractures at the axilla and elbow. A modified version of the original propeller flap was later described by Hallock and included two major changes: as skeletonized perforating vessel and a flap rotation angle of 180 degrees.[35]

The different types of propeller flaps commonly used in current practice are described in a consensus by the Advisory Panel of the First Tokyo Meeting on Perforator and Propeller Flaps.[36] The "Tokyo" consensus, analogous to the "Gent" consensus on perforator flaps, describes propeller flaps as an "island flap that reaches the recipient site through an axial rotation."[37] This definition excludes flaps whose principal movement is advancement and flaps that are not designed as a complete island.

The "Tokyo" consensus also sets forth how to classify propeller flaps.[36] Proper terminology necessitates identifying the type of nourishing pedicle, the degree of skin island rotation, and the artery of origin of the perforator vessel, if known. The three following types of propeller flaps are distinguished based on the type of nourishing pedicle: (1) The *subcutaneous pedicled propeller flap* is analogous to the original propeller flap described in 1991, where a subcutaneous pedicle of unknown vascular origin is rotated 90 degrees without the need to visualize or isolate perforator vessels, followed by direct closure of the donor site. (2) The *perforator pedicled propeller flap* incorporates the perforator flap concept, leading to a propeller flap supplied by a perforator vessel that determines the borders of the skin island overlying it. This perforator vessel is visualized, dissected, and skeletonized, allowing for a rotation up to 180 degrees as opposed to the original subcutaneous propeller flap. Freeing the vessel from fascial adhesions minimizes the risk of vessel buckling during flap rotation. The greater range of rotation inherent in the pedicled propeller flap design makes it the most commonly used type of propeller flap. (3) The *supercharged propeller flap* is a modified version of the pedicled propeller flap that allows for greater tissue coverage. Its design involves the dissection and anastomosis of an extra vascular pedicle to enhance arterial inflow, venous outflow, or both. As such, it is used if extra flap length is needed that would not be sufficiently supplied by a single perforator vessel, or for salvage procedures (**FIGURE 10-27** and **TABLE 10-6**).

An updated "Tokyo" consensus was proposed by Toia et al. in 2017, whereby a new type of propeller flap is described that does not fit into the established classification. The newly proposed *axial pedicled propeller flap* is by definition a propeller flap since it involves an island of tissue that reaches its recipient site through axial rotation; however, its pedicle is neither subcutaneous nor perforator, but rather comes out of the bone to enter the flap perpendicularly.[38] Two such types of flaps have been reported in the literature: the supratrochlear artery axial propeller (STAAP) flap and the deep lingual artery axial propeller (DLAAP) flap.[38]

Propeller flaps are an attractive reconstructive option due to their versatility. Reconstruction can be performed in the upper and lower extremities, the head and neck, the trunk, abdomen, and buttocks. In order to be successful, the defect

TABLE 10-6 Propeller Flap Types and Their Characteristics

Flap Type	Characteristics	Technique
Subcutaneous pedicled propeller	Random subcutaneous pedicle of uncertain origin, up to 90 degrees rotation	Macroscopic (vessel not visualized)
Perforator pedicled propeller	Skeletonized perforating vessel, origin known from anatomy or directly visualized, up to 180 degrees rotation	Magnification needed (vessel visualized and dissected)
Supercharged propeller	Skeletonized perforating vessel plus extra vein, artery, or both, origin known from anatomy or directly visualized, up to 180 degrees rotation	Microsurgical (vessel visualized and dissected, plus microsurgical anastomosis)

Reproduced with permission from Pignatti M, Ogawa R, Hallock GG, et al. The "Tokyo" consensus on propeller flaps. *Plast Reconstr Surg.* 2011;127(2):716-722..

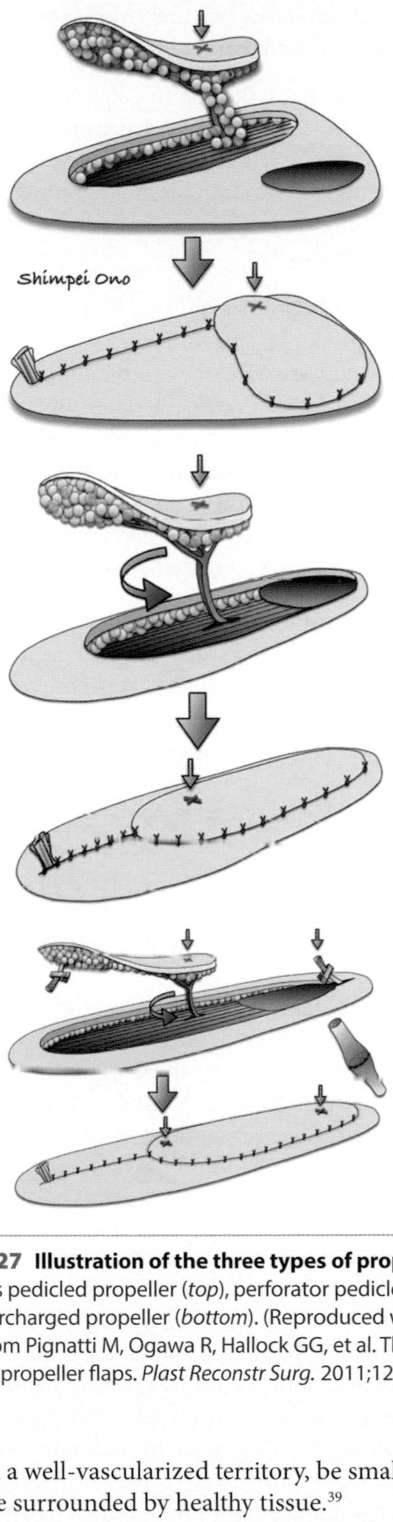

FIGURE 10-27 Illustration of the three types of propeller flaps. Subcutaneous pedicled propeller (*top*), perforator pedicled propeller (*middle*), supercharged propeller (*bottom*). (Reproduced with permission from Pignatti M, Ogawa R, Hallock GG, et al. The "Tokyo" consensus on propeller flaps. *Plast Reconstr Surg.* 2011;127(2):716-722.)

should be in a well-vascularized territory, be small to medium sized, and be surrounded by healthy tissue.[39]

There are many advantages to using propeller flaps, which set it apart from other techniques. The most obvious benefit is the great mobility, which can reach 180 degrees of rotation, allowing for maximum utilization of the flap. The design of the flap allows for partial coverage of the secondary defect (often by primary closure) and scar manipulation, which is especially beneficial in cosmetically sensitive areas. Another advantage of propeller flaps is their ability to exceed the traditional 3:1 length-to-width ratio; in fact, successful flaps with a ratio of greater than 6:1 have been reported.[40] This may be due in part to the ability of perforator vessels to adequately perfuse beyond their angiosome/perforasome territory into those of their neighbors.[41] In all, these flaps offer robust coverage with skin that offers similar quality and type, which can be used in a variety of applications.[20]

No flap is perfect, and propeller flaps have disadvantages that must be carefully considered when they are used. The complication rate can be as high as 31% in lower extremity reconstruction due to the lack of well-vascularized recipient tissue. Certain demographics such as infants and the elderly have higher rates of complications as well.[39] As stated, these flaps cannot cover as great of an area as can others, due to being elevated on a single pedicle. Rotation of the flap can cause undue tension on the pedicle and the donor site, which must be carefully monitored. Finally, as with other flap modalities, the dissection can be arduous, as perforator anatomy can be varied.[39]

Propeller flaps, when properly utilized, can be an excellent reconstructive option that may become more prevalent as they are continually studied. Although propeller flaps have lower complications than conventional pedicled flaps, there are currently few studies analyzing risk variables and propeller flap complications, such as venous congestion, superficial necrosis, and flap failure.[42,43] Consistent risk variable documentation by providers and future multicenter studies will help identify what patient factors and flap characteristics are more likely to result in success or complications.

The Angiosome Concept and the Choke Vessels In 1987, Taylor and Palmer defined the concept of an *angiosome*. They described the skin perfusion as a 3D jigsaw puzzle where each artery originating from a source vessel perfuses a skin territory with its underlying structure.[44] For example, the deep inferior epigastric system vascularizes a skin territory labeled the deep inferior epigastric angiosome. Each defined artery supplying the skin has its own angiosome.

Angiosomes are not isolated entities and are related to each other by connecting vessels called *choke vessels*. These vessels are at the margin of adjacent angiosomes and can be more or less open to allow perfusion from one territory to another. This concept will be later explained in the delay phenomenon section.

Veins and Venosomes The venous system is composed of a deep and a superficial system, connected by perforator veins. An artery may have one or two veins with a similar anatomical pathway. Such a vein is labeled *vena comitans* or *venae comitantes* in the plural form (*comitans* comes from Latin and means to accompany). For example, a radial forearm flap may have the cephalic vein as a superficial venous drainage system as well as two *venae comitantes* along the radial artery. These two systems ultimately join near the elbow via a communicating vein. Of note, some arteries do not have *vena comitans*. For example, the carotid artery does not have any accompanying vessels per se.

Using the same concept as angiosomes, Taylor et al. described a comparable venosome concept. A close relationship was found between the arterial and venous territories of each muscle.[44] Instead of having choke vessels on the periphery of their territories, venosomes have *oscillating veins* that have the unique characteristic of no valves. In contrast, venae comitantes have valves to direct blood flow toward the source artery.[45]

Physiology

Vascular Sequence Following Flap Harvest The elevation of a flap has a major impact on local blood flow. The angiosome concept explains the interconnection between different vascular territories. During a flap harvest, blood inflow and outflow are often restricted to a single pedicle; the numerous small connections between the flap and its surrounding tissues are severed. Microcirculation undergoes a reorganization to allow adequate blood inflow and outflow; this process lasts up to 4 weeks. The sequence for pedicle flaps can be described as follows[46]:

0–24 hours: The immediate response of the microcirculation is vasospasm attributed to a local axon reflex phenomenon and hyperemia caused by hypoxia and loss of sympathetic control. The overall effect is a decrease in blood flow. There is a decrease in circulation during the initial 6 hours, reaching a plateau at 6–12 hours postharvest, followed by a progressive increase at 12 hours postharvest. Congestion and edema are frequently observed during this postsurgical period.

1–3 days: An improvement in pulse amplitude is noted when spontaneous vascular tone returns around the third day. There is an increase in the number and caliber of longitudinal anastomoses as well as the number of small vessels in the pedicle. *It is imperative for flap survival to avoid shear and congestion during this period.*

3–7 days: Circulation increases progressively with a plateau on day 7. Anastomoses noted earlier become significantly functional at 5–7 days, and there is an increase in both vessel size and number.

1 week: Blood circulation is well established between pedicle and recipient bed. Pulse amplitude approaches preoperative levels.

7–14 days: No further significant increase in vascularization occurs and maximum inflow is achieved. Circulation efficiency is superior to preoperative levels during the period of 10–21 days.

2 weeks: There is a progressive regression of the vascular system. Maturation of the new anastomoses between flap and recipient bed takes place.

3 weeks: The vascular pattern is similar to preoperative levels. Vascular connections between the pedicle flap and the recipient bed are fully developed.

4 weeks: There is a decrease in diameter of all vessels, including preexisting vessels. Circulation efficiency is normal and skin color becomes more normal without the increased vascularity.

The sequence that follows a free flap harvest and anastomosis is similar but retains a major distinction. When blood vessels are sectioned, they lose direct nervous regulation by sympathetic and parasympathetic fibers. However, the reestablishment of circulation between the flap and its recipient bed shares similitudes.

Microcirculation Regulation Local blood flow in the microcirculation is regulated by multiple factors, each one ultimately causing vasoconstriction or vasodilation. The summation of these opposing forces eventually determines the final local blood flow. In the case of a flap in which microvascular rearrangements are multiple secondary to flap dissection, these factors are of paramount importance. They must be carefully evaluated and controlled to allow flap survival. These factors can be classified as being regulated systemically or locally.

Systemic Regulation Systemic regulation has two components: neural regulation and humoral regulation. *Neural regulation* is the dominant effect of systemic regulation and is mostly via sympathetic adrenergic fibers. Vasoconstriction is induced by α-adrenergic receptors while vasodilation is the result of β-adrenergic receptors. Other fibers have also been implicated in the overall vascular tone. Serotoninergic fibers induce vasoconstriction while parasympathetic cholinergic fibers, via muscarinic receptors, cause vasodilation. The combination of all these forces ultimately determines the neural basal tone of vascular smooth muscle fibers in blood vessel.[47]

Humoral regulation is controlled by circulating hormones. The most important are epinephrine and norepinephrine acting on α-adrenergic receptors, thereby causing vasoconstriction. Serotonin, thromboxane A_2, and prostaglandin $F_{2\alpha}$ also cause vasoconstriction. Substances causing vasodilation are prostaglandin E_1, prostaglandin I_2, histamine, bradykinin, and leukotrienes C_4 and D_4.[47]

Local Regulation Local regulation is also known as autoregulation and is divided into two separate components. The first local control is exercised through metabolic factors; for example, hypercapnia, hypoxia, and acidosis cause vasodilation. The second component relates to physical factors. Increased tissue perfusion pressure can initiate a myogenic reflex that causes vasoconstriction in order to maintain constant capillary blood flow. Hypothermia causes vasoconstriction via stimulation of vascular smooth muscles. Hyperthermia causes vasodilation by the opposite effect. Finally, it has been speculated that blood rheology, defined as the study of blood flow, can affect perfusion. High blood viscosity can diminish flap perfusion and viability.[47]

Delay Phenomenon The final design of a flap is limited by the previously described vascular territories; however, the flap dimension can be extended using a delay procedure (**FIGURE 10-28**). In physiological conditions, each angiosome has a peripheral area connecting to other angiosomes through choke vessels. These vessels are not aligned in a specific direction and are of small caliber.

In a delay procedure, only a portion of a flap is elevated and then sutured back in place for 2–3 weeks. The goal is to "induce a level of ischemia in the distal portion of the flap that does not cause necrosis yet conditions the tissue so that the flap will survive after later elevation."[48] The vascular sequence following flap harvest was previously described and indicates that the blood flow is near normal or normal after 2–3 weeks. For this reason, final flap harvest is usually performed between 2 and 3 weeks after the initial procedure.

The results of a delay procedure are multiple. (1) There is an opening of choke vessels that are normally closed. (2) There is a reorientation of the flap vessels in a more longitudinal pattern. (3) There is a sprouting of new vessels within the flap via angiogenesis. (4) The physiologic stress of the delay procedure increases the vessel caliber.[9]

As an example, the deltopectoral fasciocutaneous flap, initially described by Bakamjan, is frequently used for head and neck reconstruction and can be extended using a delay procedure. The original design, based on internal mammary artery perforators, can only extend up to the medial border of the deltoid muscle. This anatomic consideration significantly limits the reach of the flap. Using a delay procedure, the skin paddle can be extended to the lateral aspect of the deltoid muscle. During the initial procedure, the distal skin paddle covering the deltoid is elevated but sutured back in place; however, the base of the flap is not elevated. Three weeks later, the entire skin paddle is elevated.

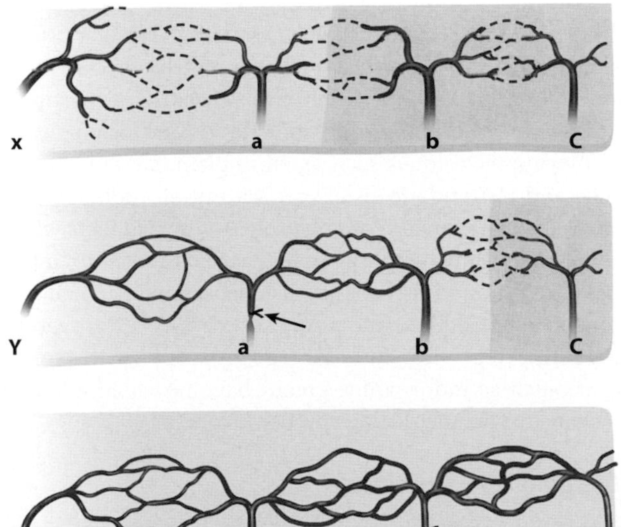

FIGURE 10-28 The delay phenomenon for a flap procedure. Surgical delay of a flap induces vasodilation of choke vessels, leading to increased perfusion and venous drainage of the distal portion of a flap. The shaded area in flap "X" represents distal necrosis. After surgical delay or vascular bundle "a" in flap "Y," there is increased distal flap perfusion secondary to changes in choke vessels between "a" and "b" but necrosis in the distal tip because vessel "b" was not delayed. In flap "Z" both vascular bundles "a" and "b" have been delayed, thus leading to increased perfusion via choke vessels between both a/b and b/c segments. Maximal surgical delay in flap "Z" leads to the most distal flap survival.

Tissue Expansion Tissue expansion may be used for skin deficits where a specific color match or texture of skin is desired for reconstruction (**FIGURE 10-29**). For example, in a burned patient, scalp skin expansion may be employed to reconstruct deficits of hair bearing skin. In tissue expansion, an expander device is inserted subcutaneously and after a week to 10 days of acclimation is gradually inflated (eg, once a week for 6 weeks) so that a force stretches the targeted tissue over weeks

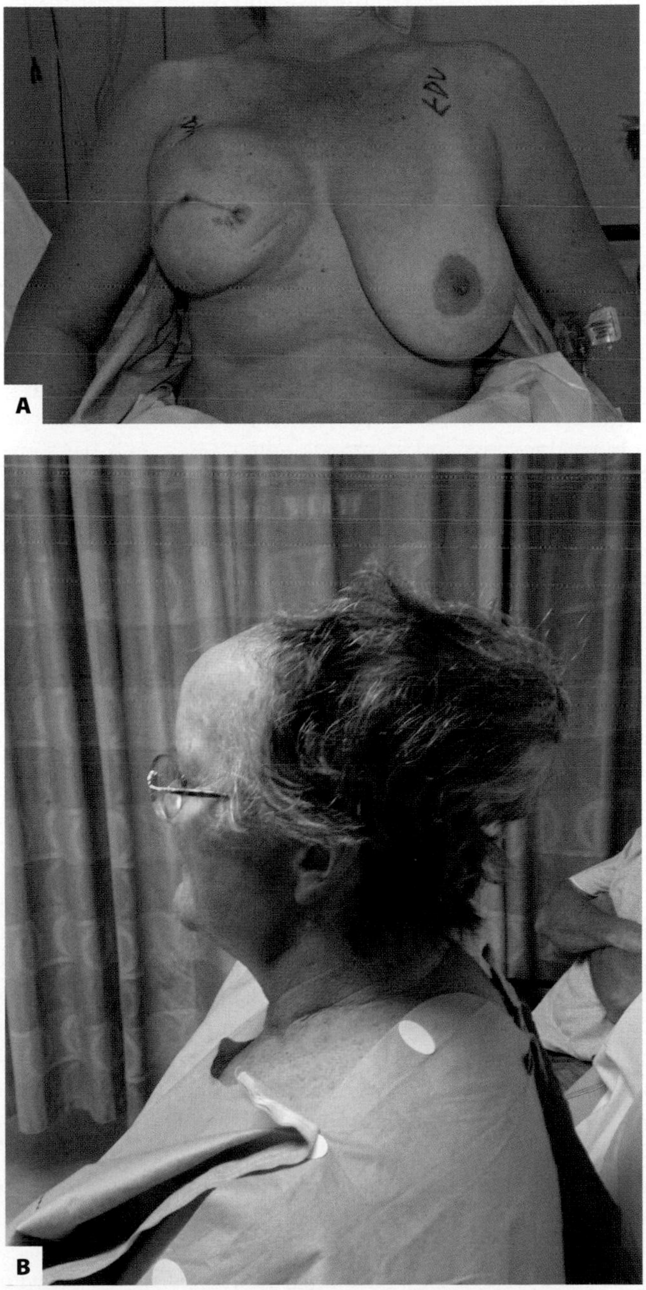

FIGURE 10-29 Examples of tissue expansion. A. Breast expansion with tissue expanders placed under the pectoralis muscle. **B.** Scalp expansion with tissue expanders placed under the scalp.

to months prior to transfer. Tissue expanders are used for a variety of applications, the most common of which are breast reconstruction and repair of scalp defects.

The tissue to be expanded initially undergoes mechanical creep, which is comprised of realignment of collagen fibers and displacement of water from the ground substance. Chronic distension initiates stretch responses (collectively termed biological creep) that include increased rates of mitosis, upregulated angiogenesis, and new tissue production.[49] The final result is a mixture of tissue stretching and growth.

The device, generally a silicone envelope that is progressively inflated with saline, creates a capsule around itself and causes specific changes to the skin and the underlying tissues. The capsule is composed of dense fibrous fibers and becomes less cellular over time, reaching maximal thickness after 2 months of expansion. Fibroproliferation and capsular contracture are potential complications that are associated with radiation therapy.[50]

During expansion of the skin, the epidermis initially increases in thickness while the dermis and the subcutaneous adipose tissue are significantly thinner after expansion.[51] Skin appendages are not histologically affected but develop decreased density and the muscle atrophies.[52] An expander compressing a bone causes a decrease in bone thickness and volume but does not affect bone density, for example, during a scalp expansion. At the periphery of the expander, an increase in bone thickness and volume is noted.[53] Research has shown that many of these changes are reversible. The capsule resolves after expander removal and little histological evidence persists after 2 years following the removal of the device. Similarly, dermis and subcutaneous tissue regain thickness after expander removal.[52]

Tissue expanders come in three varieties: round, rectangular, and crescentic (crescent-shaped). van Rappard et al. calculated that rectangular devices provide the largest increase in surface area, 38% expansion compared to 32% of cresenteric and 25% of round.[54] Various claims have been reported regarding the required width of the expander relative to the defect, but most authors claim a requirement of 2.5–3 times the diameter of the defect.[55]

Expanded flaps provide several advantages over unmodified ones, the most obvious being increased coverage of defects with the same donor footprint. Coverage can be achieved via advancement or transposition.[56] Tissue expansion provides matching skin tone, texture, and hair patterns, which are especially valuable in aesthetically sensitive areas. Expanded tissue can be closed primarily, which can help minimize donor site morbidity. Since the entire sequence of tissue expansion is planned, scar placement and size can be manipulated to be minimally disruptive. Finally, tissue expansion is a reliable and well-understood technique that can be utilized with known results.

As with any surgical technique, tissue expansion is not without disadvantages. At least two operations are required for tissue expansion, one to implant and one to remove the expander. Reconstruction must be delayed for the duration of the expansion process, which, especially in aesthetically sensitive areas such as the head and neck, can be very disruptive to a patient's quality of life. The implant creates a dramatic and instantly noticeable deformity that the patient must be prepared to face.

Complications of tissue expander use can delay or prevent reconstruction. Minor complications include hematoma or seroma formation, exposure of the valve, or insufficient expansion; major complications include infection, exposure of the implant, implant deflation, or flap necrosis. Lower extremity expansion confers the highest risk, which may be secondary to anatomic limitations and decreased vascularity of the tissue, as compared to the head, neck, or trunk.[55]

Monitoring

The ultimate success of any flap transfer is not measured immediately after surgery but only after adequate *healing and remodeling* of the flap have occurred. As noted earlier, it takes several days to reestablish satisfactory blood supply and, therefore, ensure flap survival. The first 5–7 days are critical because the entire flap relies on its vascular pedicle for blood supply. At 1-week postsurgery, additional blood supply has been reestablished, consequently decreasing the overall dependency from the main pedicle. However, flaps have been lost later than 7 days postoperatively, illustrating the variability of flap healing. Since flap salvage procedures are available and can be successful, appropriate monitoring is essential to detect early signs of flap insufficiency.

The monitoring of a flap can be performed in various ways. The most common include clinical parameters such as color, temperature, and turgor. These metrics are very sensitive for flap danger to the point that some authors question the need for any other monitoring modality.[57] That stated, invasive monitoring techniques such as an implantable Doppler flow probe and transcutaneous oxygen saturation probe are available to the clinician and can be useful for buried flaps without skin paddles. Implantable Doppler has been shown to improve postoperative monitoring of at-risk flaps, which can allow for more prompt response and salvage of the flap.[58] More recently, modalities (eg, near-infrared spectroscopy with contrast agents such as indocyanine green) have provided additional mechanisms for measuring flap perfusion.[59,60]

Physiological Parameters

Vital Signs As with the evaluation of any specific medical condition, vital signs are of critical importance when monitoring a patient with a flap. Normal circulation is influenced by temperature, blood pressure (BP), heart rate (HR), and/or respiratory rate (RR). For a flap where the only vascular supply is limited to a single artery and one or two veins, slight variations of these parameters can have a significant influence on both arterial and venous blood flow.

As discussed earlier, hypothermia can lead to vasoconstriction and is a cause of significant blood redistribution in the body. For example, a flap on a lower extremity may suffer from vasoconstriction if the body needs to conserve heat and maintain normal core body temperature. As a consequence, vasoconstriction in a flap can lead to transient ischemia and induce a cascade of events that leads to flap failure.

The importance of maintaining adequate systemic blood pressure for flap perfusion is straightforward and because flaps have relatively small conduits for arterial inflow and venous outflow, periods of systemic hypotension are poorly tolerated. Respiratory rate can also influence flap survival by its influence on blood pH. Hypercapnia, hypoxia, and acidosis cause vasodilation and have a direct effect on flap tissue perfusion.

Capillary Refill Time (CRT) Normal skin perfusion fills the capillaries in the dermal layer of the skin. By simple digital pressure, these capillaries can be emptied and will again refill. The time needed to refill capillaries is directly related to the local arterial and venous pressures; normal CRT is less than 2 seconds.[61,62] When monitoring a flap, a CRT between 1 and 3 seconds is considered normal. If CRT is 1 second or less, it is an indicator of *venous congestion*.[23] This phenomenon may be explained by the following: since perfusion pressure on the arterial capillary side is two times the pressure of the venous capillary,[63] digital pressure on the skin forces blood to the venous side of the capillaries. If venous drainage is impaired, venous capillary blood pressure will increase and blood emptying will be limited by the increased venous blood pressure. Thus, CRT is then faster than expected in venous congested flaps. However, a CRT of more than 3 seconds is a sign of arterial insufficiency. A prolonged CRT can be explained by the fact that when arterial capillary pressure is lower than normal, the time to refill capillaries is longer (**FIGURE 10-30**).

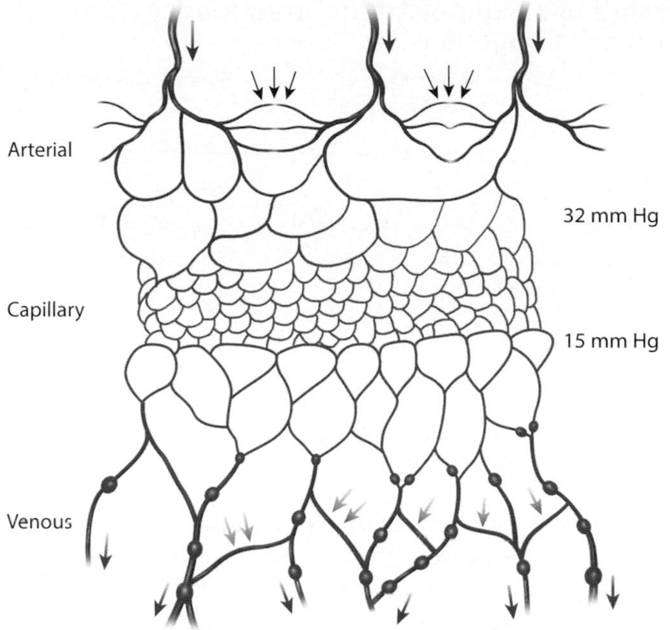

FIGURE 10-30 Capillary bed pressures. The capillary bed has a pressure of 32 mmHg on the arterial side and 15 mmHg on the venous side. If there is venous congestion in a flap, pressure on the skin does not force fluid into the venules; therefore, the capillary refill time is less than normal. In contrast, if the arterial flow is impaired, refill time will be longer than the normally expected 2–3 seconds. This screening test can be used to monitor vascularization following flap surgery and to detect early perfusion impairments. (Reproduced with permission from Moris SF, Taylor GI. Vascular territories. In: Neligan PC, ed. *Plastic Surgery*. 3rd ed. Philadelphia, PA: Elsevier; 2013:480.)

Color Skin color of a flap can be readily monitored for viability (**FIGURE 10-31**). Depending on the patient's skin complexion, pale or dusky skin can be assessed in a few seconds. Pallor is associated with under-perfusion while pink, bluish, or dusky skin is associated with venous congestion. Skin transferred from one region of the body to another may not have the same basal color. For example, a TRAM flap for breast reconstruction can have a much lighter skin paddle than the chest wall skin. A baseline assessment of skin color by digital photography is recommended as a reference for postoperative monitoring.

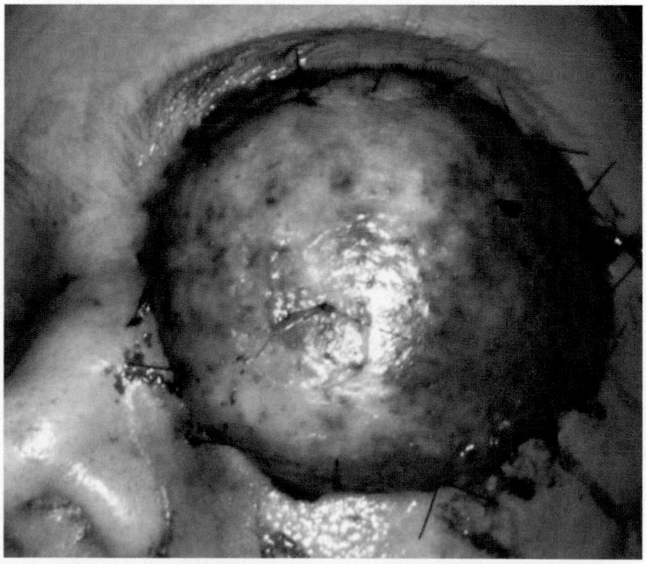

FIGURE 10-31 Color monitoring for flap viability. Congested purple skin in a free radial forearm flap for ocular exenteration. The purple color is indicative of venous congestion. This situation warrants surgical re-exploration but in some cases is treated with leech therapy to relieve the congestion temporarily until capillary ingrowth is reestablished.

Flap Temperature Any flap, including a skin flap, can be evaluated for temperature. An abnormal temperature is a symptom of inadequate perfusion. This examination is performed subjectively with the dorsum of the hand or objectively with an infrared skin thermometer, comparing the temperature of the flap with its surrounding environment. A cool flap compared to its adjacent tissue is a sign of hypoperfusion. Flap hyperthermia is less of a concern and hard to evaluate clinically as flaps are often externally warmed in the immediate postop period to reduce vasoconstriction.

Needle Prick A simple method to assess perfusion is by creating a small puncture wound on the flap using a 21-gauge needle. Whereas a healthy flap would exude bright red blood,

TABLE 10-7 Signs of Arterial Insufficiency and Venous Congestion

	Arterial Insufficiency	Venous Congestion
Color	Pale, white, mottled	Purple, dusky
Temperature	Cool	Warm
Turgor	Decreased, prune-like	Increased, swollen, tense
Needle prick	Scant, serous	Rapid, dark cyanotic
Capillary refill	Sluggish	Brisk

the absence of blood can be interpreted as arterial insufficiency while dark cyanotic blood would be a sign of venous congestion (**TABLE 10-7**).

Ancillary Monitoring Methods In situations where clinical parameters are not available (eg, buried flap) or not reliable (eg, on a darker skin patient), more objective measurement tools are utilized to better assess flap viability.

Doppler Blood flow in the vascular pedicle can be evaluated by ultrasonography using a pencil-type Doppler probe, which measures the velocity of the blood flow in the artery and vein (**FIGURE 10-32**). Arterial flow is classically triphasic while venous flow is monophasic. Although a Doppler signal is not always available because of flap configuration and the signal quality can vary, the Doppler study is reliable when it is audible. The loss of a previously good signal is correlated with flap failure, although the rate of false-positive loss of a signal may be important.[64] Evaluation of the appropriate artery may be difficult, for example, in a patient with a partially missing cranial vault after a cranioplasty where a latissimus dorsi flap is used to cover the deficit. The recipient vessels chosen are often the superficial temporal artery and veins. Without the bony structure covering the brain, a positive Doppler signal from the cerebral circulation can be mistakenly assessed as a positive flap pedicle signal. For this reason, more sophisticated methods have been developed, including an implantable Doppler probe directly around the vessels.

Transcutaneous Oximetry Another method of evaluating flap perfusion is through pulse oximetry. Pulse oximetry, which is based on absorption of a specific wavelength of light by the patient's hemoglobin, is a reliable indicator of arterial perfusion. In the case of a replanted finger, a simple pulse oximetry sensor can be placed around the tip of the finger to get constant saturation measurement. For flaps with skin, transcutaneous probes, which can be affixed with adhesive tape, have been developed to measure flap saturation. As with the Doppler signal, a sudden change in saturation, as opposed to the absolute value of the saturation, is an indicator of potential flap failure.

Contrast Agents for Assessment of Tissue Perfusion Indocyanine green (ICG) dye has been utilized to directly visualize flap perfusion (**FIGURE 10-33**). When injected into the bloodstream, it tightly binds to plasma proteins and is, therefore, confined to the vascular system. A laser is used to detect the dye, which has a peak spectral absorption at 800 nm. Since ICG dye has a short half-life of 3–4 minutes, it quickly enters vascularized tissue flaps but then also rapidly washes out prior to being metabolized by the liver. For example, after a mastectomy, random skin flaps that have questionable perfusion can be assessed by ICG angiography intraoperatively when perfusion is not always clinically obvious. Real-time data can be used to guide excision of marginally perfused tissue.[65,66]

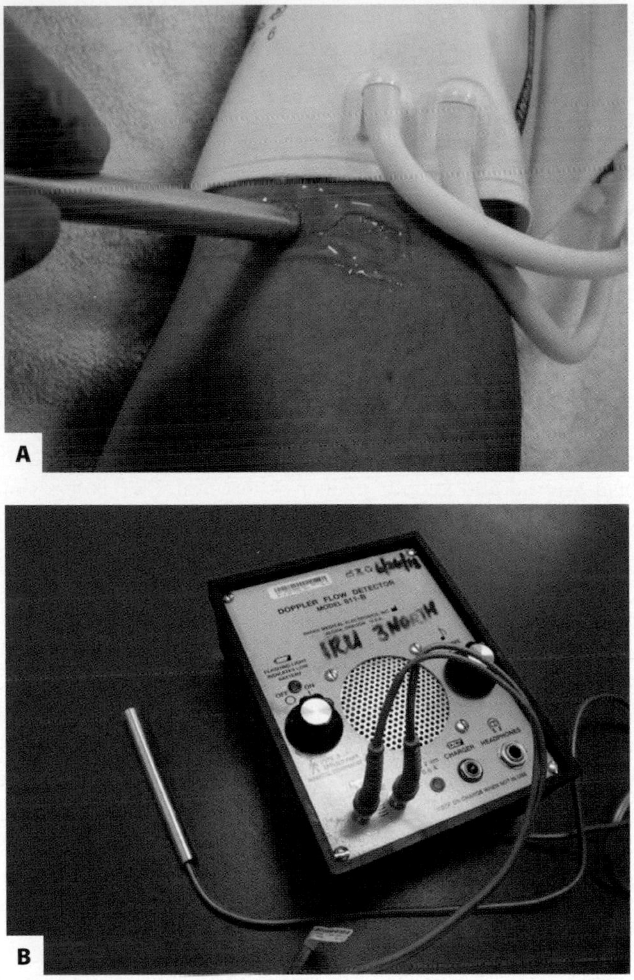

FIGURE 10-32 A handheld Doppler. The pencil-style handheld Doppler is used to monitor blood flow in the pedicle artery and to detect any decrease in flow that may compromise flap perfusion.

Complications

Besides the usual complications associated with a surgical procedure under general anesthesia, unique difficulties are specific to flap procedures. Complications can be to the flap itself or they can be associated with its donor site. Morbidity from the donor site may be quite significant, such as a ventral hernia following a TRAM flap or a persistent seroma following a latissimus dorsi harvest. Complications involving flaps can be arbitrarily divided into two categories: extrinsic and intrinsic.

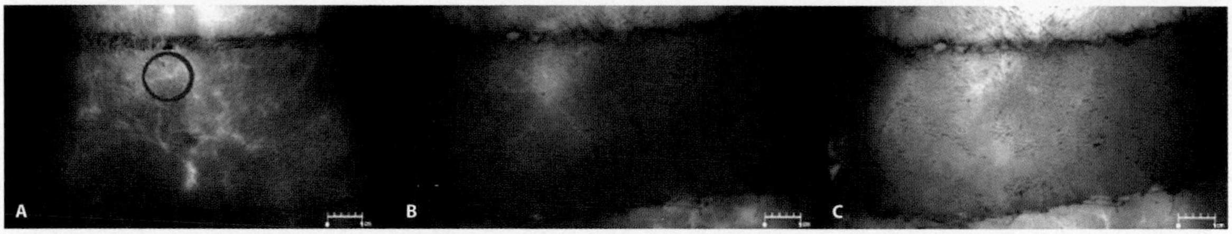

FIGURE 10-33 Indocyanine green staining of a breast flap. Indocyanine green angiography is used to monitor flap perfusion in an animal study involving abdominal perforator flaps. **A.** A preoperative view of the target perforator. **B.** Early injection showing localization of the perforator. **C.** Late injection phase with hyperlucent and hyperopaque zones. (Used with permission from Monahan J, Hwang BH, Kennedy JM, Chen W, Nguyen GK, Schooler WG, Wong AK. Determination of a perfusion threshold in experimental flap surgery using indocyanine green angiography. *Ann Plast Surg*. 2014;73(5):602–604. https://journals.lww.com/annalsplasticsurgery/Abstract/2014/11000/Determination_of_a_Perfusion_Threshold_in.26.aspx.)

Extrinsic Factors

Local Factors Extrinsic factors are not related to the flap per se and can be a result of either local and/or systemic factors. Local factors are generally any impediment to the circulation of the flap, including tight dressings or strangulating stitches that cause circulation impairment. Another example is a hematoma or seroma that compresses the flap pedicle.

Systemic Factors Systemic factors have an overall effect on the body as well as on the flap itself. Hypovolemia can lead to flap hypoperfusion; hypothermia can lead to vasoconstriction. Systemic diseases can also affect flap survival; for example, arteriosclerosis can significantly affect the quality of recipient vessels, therefore decreasing blood supply to a flap especially in the lower extremity. Refer to Chapter 12, Factors That Impede Wound Healing, for other factors that may inhibit wound healing, including the postsurgical healing of a flap.

CLINICAL CONSIDERATION

Rehabilitation of a patient with a flap begins when the surgeon deems it safe for the patient to perform bed mobility and transfers. Patients with sacral flaps are usually in a fluidized air bed and require longer periods of bed rest than those with extremity flaps. A primary principle of any mobility is to avoid shear, which can disrupt capillary growth and lead to flap failure, undermining, and sinus formation.

CLINICAL CONSIDERATION

Elevation of the extremity with a flap is a basic principle to help avoid venous congestion. This is especially important for any patient with a known history of chronic venous insufficiency. Transfers and positioning are performed with techniques to maintain elevation (eg, the foot is higher than the knee and the knee is higher than the hip) and using equipment that provides support without direct pressure on the flap.

Intrinsic Factors Intrinsic factors that complicate healing are those related to the flap itself. Aside from an improper flap design or flawed harvest technique, failure is related to poor arterial inflow or venous outflow.

Arterial Insufficiency Arterial insufficiency can have its origin anywhere along the vascular pathway of the flap, from the beginning of the pedicle to the end of a perforator. For example, vasoconstriction at the base of the pedicle secondary to sympathetic stimulation can cause arterial insufficiency. However, a flap isolated on a single small perforator can be insufficient to vascularize a large flap. No matter where the occlusion is located, the consequence is the same—inadequate blood supply leads to arterial insufficiency and flap compromise, which is usually followed by partial or complete necrosis (**FIGURE 10-34**).

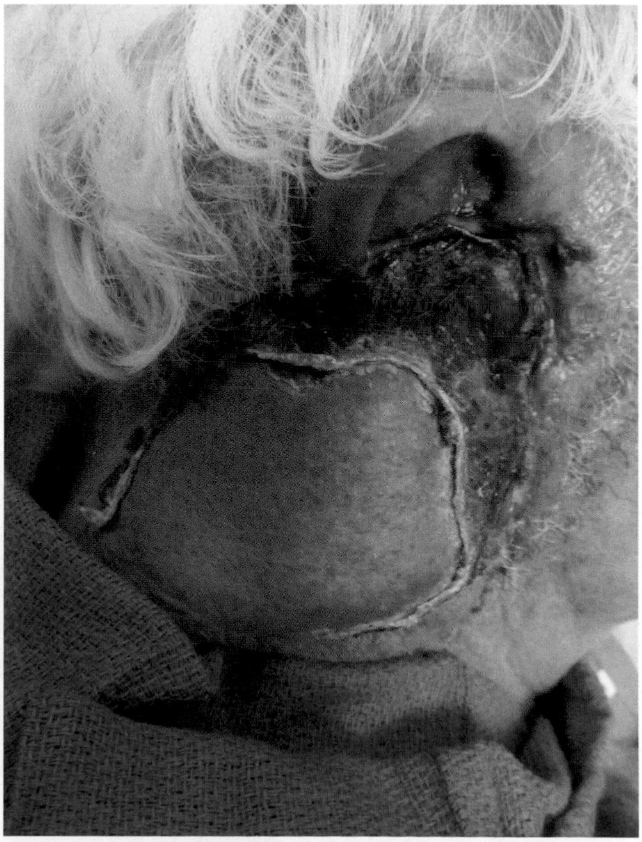

FIGURE 10-34 Example of arterial insufficiency. Changes in skin tone to a more pale skin flap and a long capillary refill time (>3 seconds) are indications of arterial insufficiency. The result can be a heavy eschar with necrosis of the subcutaneous tissue. Other clinical symptoms include drainage, loosening of the flap edges, and odor.

Venous Insufficiency Venous insufficiency can be caused by a deficit anywhere from the capillaries to the pedicle vein(s). Contrary to arterial inflow, venous drainage is often divided into a deep and a superficial system. The proportion of drainage between the two systems is variable among patients and is not always predictable. Since these two systems are not located contiguously to each other, both drainage systems cannot always be harvested at the same time due to flap design constraint. For example, a radial forearm flap can be harvested with two *venae comitantes* (deep venous system) of the radial artery as well as with the cephalic vein (superficial system) without affecting flap design significantly. However, an abdominal flap is harvested with the deep inferior epigastric artery and veins for a DIEP flap or it can be harvested with the superficial inferior epigastric artery and veins for a superficial inferior epigastric artery (SIEA) perforator flap. Because of different anatomic locations, a flap is based on one of the two systems.

The consequence of inadequate venous drainage is venous congestion (also referred to as secondary or venous ischemia). Clinically, congested flaps appear blue or purple, dusky, and edematous with elevated intravascular pressure in the venous system of the flap. Physically, congested blood occupies volume in the flap, thus increasing intraflap pressure. This elevation can be enough to compress remaining venous outflow (therefore worsening the situation), as well as the arterial inflow, leading ultimately to flap failure. For example, a venous thrombosis has the following sequence of events: (1) venous thrombosis leads to flap congestion, (2) venous congestion leads to compression of arterial inflow, (3) compressed arterial flow causes an arrest in tissue perfusion, and (4) ischemia causes flap failure (**FIGURE 10-35A, B**). Since arterial pressure is significantly higher than venous pressure, blood continues to flow into the flap long after complete venous thrombosis has occurred, resulting in even greater intraflap pressure and leading the flap into a *no-reflow* condition with poor outcomes for both the patient and the surgeon. In selected cases, leeches can be applied to the flap to drain congested blood and decrease the overall flap pressure (**FIGURE 10-35C**). However, the appropriate treatment for venous congestion remains exploration in the operating room when possible.

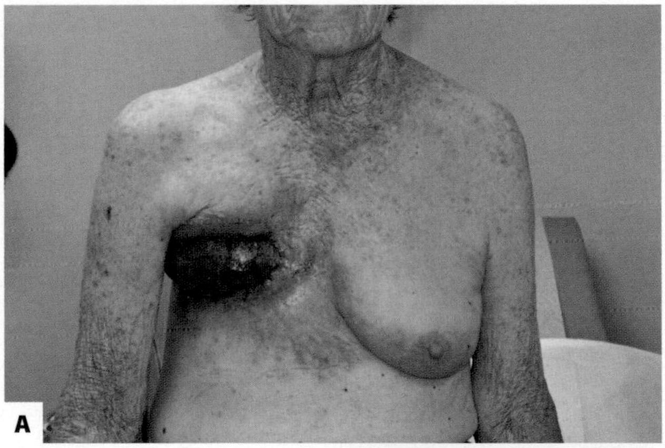

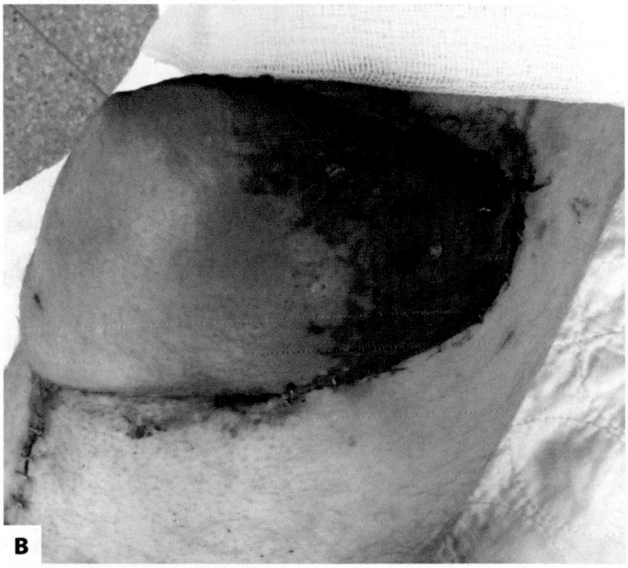

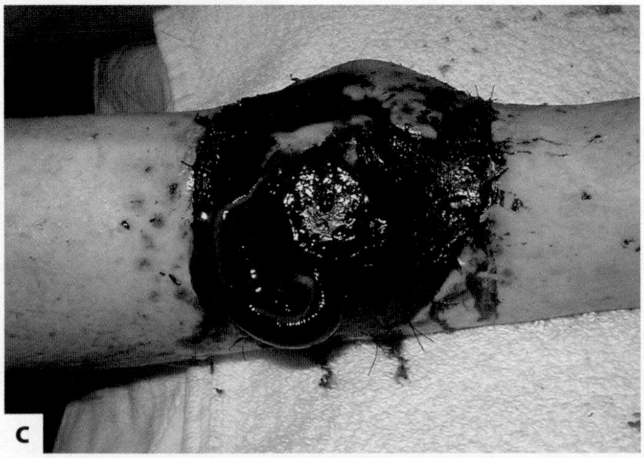

FIGURE 10-35 Example of flap with venous congestion. A. Total failure of a breast flap due to venous outflow obstruction/congestion. **B.** Partial flap necrosis can occur in a flap with venous congestion, as seen on the medial part of the flap. **C.** Venous congestion is sometimes treated with leeches that attach to the flap and suction out the excess venous blood.

CASE STUDY

FLAPS

A 57-year-old woman sustained a necrotizing soft tissue infection of her left lower leg and ankle. One week postinjury, the plastic surgery team was consulted for management of exposed bone, tendons, and joint surfaces. After serial debridement in the operating room, the patient had a 15 × 15 cm soft tissue defect. The patient had no significant medical comorbidities, tissue cultures were negative, and nutritional markers for protein were normal (**FIGURES 10-36** and **10-37**).

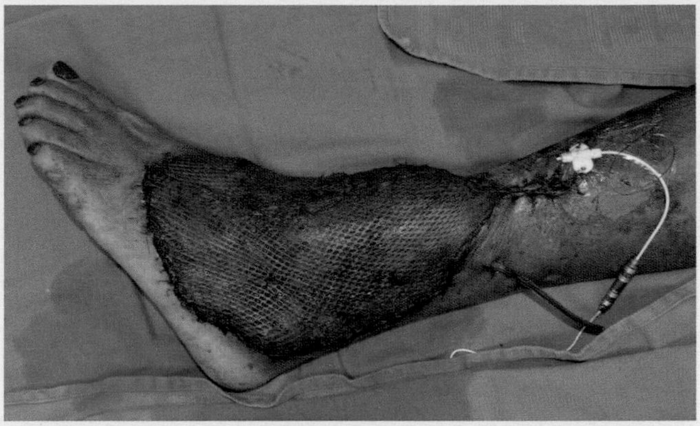

FIGURE 10-36 A lower extremity soft tissue defect posttrauma covered with a latissimus dorsi muscle free flap and a split-thickness skin graft.

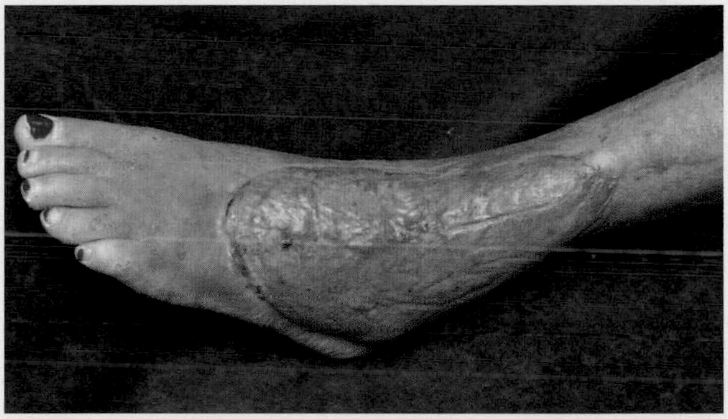

FIGURE 10-37 The same flap during the remodeling phase of healing during which the edema noted in the flap can be treated with mild compression to help reshape the ankle and foot.

DISCUSSION QUESTIONS

1. What is the main goal of the surgery?
2. What kind of coverage is needed for this patient?
3. List specific concerns or important factors in the selection of a durable coverage for this patient.

The key point of this reconstruction is to ensure that all infection has been controlled with surgical debridement and IV antibiotics. The next goal is to provide stable vascularized soft tissue coverage over the exposed bone, tendon, and ankle joint capsule. If it is not reconstructed properly, the patient is at risk for persistent infection and resultant amputation. A skin graft would be insufficient in this case because of the exposed bone and tendon. Biological dressings (cellular/tissue products) would be inadequate for a defect of this complexity because of the inability of bone and tendon to support granulation tissue needed for re-epithelialization. Therefore, a flap is needed to cover the defect. Because of the location of the injury on the distal third of the leg, a pedicled flap is not an option because it has limited arc of rotation. A free flap is the best option to achieve full coverage of this complex wound.

The choice of flap takes into consideration the size and anatomic location of the defect, thickness of the flap, length and orientation of the pedicle, possibility of subsequent surgeries, long-term aesthetic result, donor site morbidity, and functional aspects of the reconstruction. Of course, patient preference is also important. In this case, a free latissimus dorsi muscle flap covered with an STSG or an anterolateral thigh fasciocutaneous flap would be the first-line option. For this patient, a latissimus dorsi muscle-free flap was performed.

SUMMARY

Skin grafts are classified as full or partial thickness. The normal process of skin graft healing includes serum imbibition, inosculation, and revascularization. Factors affecting graft survival include proper immobilization after surgery, meticulous technique, prevention of infection, and adequate vascularization.

Free flaps are defined as units of tissue that may be transferred from donor to recipient sites while maintaining their blood supply. Flaps can be defined by their vascular supply, tissue composition, methods of transfer, or vascular orientation. Free flaps can be defined by the relevant vascular anatomy, including muscle flaps, fasciocutaneous flaps, and perforator flaps. The concept of angiosomes and venosomes further defines the vascular anatomy and circulation required for flap survival. Basic physiology concepts specific to the intrinsic nature of free tissue transfers include local and systemic effects after a free flap harvest. Flap monitoring techniques, including physiological parameters and ancillary methods (Doppler, oximetry, and tissue staining), are used to monitor flaps after surgery. Extrinsic and intrinsic factors can lead to flap failure.

STUDY QUESTIONS

1. Which of the following *best* describes a split-thickness skin graft (STSG)?
   a. A graft composed of epidermis and some dermis
   b. A graft composed of only epidermis
   c. A graft composed of only dermis
   d. A graft that leaves a donor site to be closed primarily
   e. A graft that will never contract after being harvested
2. Which of the following is *not* a factor to consider in order to prevent skin graft failure?
   a. A well-vascularized wound bed
   b. The skin pigmentation
   c. A sterile environment
   d. A bolster dressing creating close contact between the graft and the wound bed
   e. A flawless technique during harvest and application of the graft
3. Among the following, which one *best* describes the environment needed for a free tissue transfer (a free flap) to survive?
   a. A well-vascularized wound bed
   b. An adequate arterial inflow and venous outflow
   c. A sterile environment
   d. An adequate arterial inflow without venous outflow
   e. A maximum ratio length to width of 2:1
4. The Mathes and Nahai classification of muscle flaps describes a type III muscle flap as
   a. Composed of only one dominant pedicle.
   b. Composed of one or more vascular pedicle(s) and minor pedicle(s).
   c. Composed of two dominant pedicles.
   d. Composed of segmental vascular pedicles.
   e. Composed of one dominant and secondary segmental pedicles.
5. Which of the following *best* describes a delay phenomenon in a flap?
   a. A transposition of a 3 × 3 cm skin paddle with a 45 degrees angle
   b. A free latissimus dorsi flap for a scalp defect
   c. Insertion of an expander implant under the pectoralis major muscle during breast reconstruction
   d. A pedicle TRAM flap after ligation of both deep inferior epigastric arteries 2 weeks earlier
   e. A deltopectoral flap performed immediately after a neck mass removal
6. Which of the following is an indicator of venous congestion?
   a. A capillary refill time of 3 seconds
   b. A hypothermic flap
   c. A hypoperfused flap
   d. A pale or light pink flap
   e. A swollen bluish flap

Answers: 1-a; 2-b; 3-b; 4-c; 5-d; 6-e

REFERENCES

1. Mathes SJ, Hansen SL. Flap classification and applications. In: Mathes SJ, ed. *Plastic Surgery*. 2nd ed. Philadelphia, PA: Saunders; 2005:367.
2. Nguyen GK, Hwang BH, Zhang Y, et al. Novel biomarkers of arterial and venous. Ischemia in microvascular flaps. *PLoS One*. 2013;8(8):e71628.
3. Thorne CH. Techniques and principles in plastic surgery. In: Thorne CH, Beasley RW, Aston SJ, Bartlett SP, Gurtner GC, Spear SL, eds. *Grabb and Smith's Plastic Surgery*. 6th ed. Philadelphia, PA: LWW; 2007:7.
4. Scherer-Pietramaggiori SS, Pietramaggiori G, Orgill DP. Skin graft. In: Neligan PC, ed. *Plastic Surgery*. 3rd ed. Philadelphia, PA: Elsevier; 2013:319.
5. Bichakjian CK, Johnson TM. Anatomy of the skin. In: Baker SR, ed. *Local Flaps in Facial Reconstruction*. 2nd ed. Philadelphia, PA: Mosby; 2007:4.
6. Converse JM, Uhlschmid GK, Ballantyne DL. "Plasmatic circulation" in skin grafts. The phase of serum imbibition. *Plast Reconstr Surg*. 1969;43(5):495-499.
7. Scherer-Pietramaggiori SS, Pietramaggiori G, Orgill DP. Skin graft. In: Neligan PC, ed. *Plastic Surgery*. 3rd ed. Philadelphia, PA: Elsevier; 2013:323.
8. Scherer-Pietramaggiori SS, Pietramaggiori G, Orgill DP. Skin graft. In: Neligan PC, ed. *Plastic Surgery*. 3rd ed. Philadelphia, PA: Elsevier; 2013:333.
9. Mathes SJ, Levine J. Muscle flaps and their blood supply. In: Thorne CH, Beasley RW, Aston SJ, Bartlett SP, Gurtner GC, Spear SL, eds. *Grabb and Smith's Plastic Surgery*. 6th ed. Philadelphia, PA: LWW; 2007:42-52.
10. Mathes SJ, Nahai F. *Reconstructive Surgery: Principles, Anatomy, & Techniques*. Philadelphia, PA: Churchill Livingston; 1997:16.
11. Thorne CH. Techniques and principles in plastic surgery. In: Thorne CH, Beasley RW, Aston SJ, et al. eds. *Grabb and Smith's Plastic Surgery*. 6th ed. Philadelphia, PA: LWW; 2007:12.
12. Mathes SJ, Levine J. Muscle flaps and their blood supply. In: Thorne CH, Beasley RW, Aston SJ, et al. eds. *Grabb and Smith's Plastic Surgery*. 6th ed. Philadelphia, PA: LWW; 2007:10.
13. Ramsey ML. Pedicle/interpolation flaps. Available at: http://emedicine.medscape.com/article/1128874-overview. Updated October 8. 2021. Accessed March 15, 2023.
14. Thatte MR, Thatte RL. Venous flaps. *Plast Reconstr Surg*. 1993; 91(4):747-751.
15. Mathes SJ, Nahai F. Classification of the vascular anatomy of muscles: experimental and clinical correlation. *Plast Reconstr Surg*. 1981;67(2):177-187.
16. Wong AK, Pu LLQ, Sherman R. Gastrocnemius flap. In: Pu LLQ, Levine JP, Wei FC, eds. *Reconstructive Surgery of the Lower Extremity*. St. Louis, MO: QMP Press; 2013:591-608.
17. Pontén B. The fasciocutaneous flap: its use in soft tissue defects of the lower leg. *Br J Plast Surg*. 1981;34(2):215-220.
18. Cormack GC, Lamberty BG. A classification of fascio-cutaneous flaps according to their patterns of vascularisation. *Br J Plast Surg*. 1984;37(1):80-87.
19. Koshima I, Soeda S. Inferior epigastric artery skin flaps without rectus abdominis muscle. *Br J Plast Surg*. 1989;42(6):645-648.
20. Saint-Cyr M, Schaverien MV, Rohrich RJ. Perforator flaps: history, controversies, physiology, anatomy, and use in reconstruction. *Plast Reconstr Surg*. 2009;123:132e-145e.

21. Blondeel PN, Van Landuyt KHI, Monstrey SJM, et al. The "Gent" consensus on perforator flap terminology: preliminary definitions. *Plast Reconstr Surg*. 2003;112(5):1378-1383.
22. Hallock GG. Direct and indirect perforator flaps: the history and the controversy. *Plast Reconstr Surg*. 2003;111(2):855-865.
23. Blondeel PN, Van Landuyt K, Hamdi M, Monstrey SJ. Perforator flap terminology: update 2002. *Clin Plast Surg*. 2003;30(3):343-346.
24. Sinna R, Boloorchi A, Mahajan AL, Qassemyar Q, Robbe M. What should define a "perforator flap"? *Plast Reconstr Surg*. 2010;126:2258-2263.
25. Koh K, Goh TLH, Song CT, et al. Free versus pedicled perforator flaps for lower extremity reconstruction: a multicenter comparison of institutional practices and outcomes. *J Reconstr Microsurg*. 2018; 34(8):572-580.
26. Saint-Cyr M, Wong C, Schaverien M, Mojallal A, Rohrich RJ. The perforasome theory: vascular anatomy and clinical implications. *Plast Reconstr Surg*. 2009;124:1529-1544.
27. Ireton JE, Lakhiani C, Saint-Cyr M. Vascular anatomy of the deep inferior epigastric artery perforator flap: a systematic review. *Plast Reconstr Surg*. 2014;134:810e-821e.
28. Neligan PC, Lipa JE. Perforator flaps in head and neck reconstruction. *Semin Plast Surg*. 2006;24(3):237-254.
29. Hamdi M, Craggs B, Stoel A-M, Hendrickx B, Zeltzer A. Superior epigastric artery perforator flap: anatomy, clinical applications, and review of literature. *J Reconstr Microsurg*. 2014;30:475-482.
30. Prasetyono TO, Bangun K, Buchari FB, Rezkini P. Practical considerations for perforator flap thinning procedures revisited. *Arch Plast Surg*. 2014;41:693-701.
31. Rubino C, Coscia V, Cavazzuti AM, Canu V. Haemodynamic enhancement in perforator flaps: The inversion phenomenon and its clinical significance. A study of the relation of blood velocity and flow between pedicle and perforator vessels in perforator flaps. *J Plast Reconstr Aesthet Surg*. 2006;59(6):636-643.
32. Karunanithy N, Rose V, Lim AKP, Mitchell A. CT angiography of inferior epigastric and gluteal perforating arteries before free flap breast reconstruction. *Radiographics*. 2011;31:1307-1319.
33. Kim JT, Kim SW. Perforator flap versus conventional flap. *J Korean Med Sci*. 2015;30:514-522.
34. Hyakusoku H, Yamamoto T, Fumiiri M. The propeller flap method. *Br J Plast Surg*. 1991;44:53-54.
35. Hallock GG. The propeller flap version of the adductor muscle perforator flap for coverage of ischial or trochanteric pressure sores. *Ann Plast Surg*. 2006;56:540-542.
36. Pignatti M, Ogawa R, Hallock GG, et al. The "Tokyo" consensus on propeller flaps. *Plast. Reconstr Surg*. 2011;127(2):716-22.
37. Blondeel PN, Van Landuyt K, Monstrey SJ, et al. The "Gent" consensus on perforator flap terminology: preliminary definitions. *Plast Reconstr Surg*. 2003;112:1378-1382.
38. Toia F, D'Arpa S, Pignatti M, et al. Axial propeller flaps: a proposal for update of the "Tokyo consensus on propeller flaps." *J Plast Reconstr Aesthet Surg*. 2017;70(6):857-860.
39. Sisti A, D'Aniello C, Fortezza L, et al. Propeller flaps: literature review. *In Vivo*. 2016;30:351-373.
40. Teo TC. The propeller flap concept. *Clin Plast Surg*. 2010;37: 615-626, vi.
41. Callegari PR, Taylor GI, Caddy CM, Minabe T. An anatomic review of the delay phenomenon: I. Experimental studies. *Plast Reconstr Surg*. 1992;89:397-407; discussion 417.
42. Innocenti M, Menichini G, Baldrighi C, et al. Are there risk factors for complications of perforator-based propeller flaps for lower extremity reconstruction? *Clin Orthop Relat Res*. 2014;472: 2276-2286.
43. Tajsic N, Winkel R, Husum H. Distally based perforator flaps for reconstruction of post-traumatic defects of the lower leg and foot. A review of the anatomy and clinical outcomes. *Injury*. 2014;45: 469-477.
44. Taylor GI, Palmer JH. The vascular territories (angiosomes) of the body: experimental study and clinical applications. *Br J Plast Surg*. 1987;40(2):113-141.
45. Watterson PA, Taylor GI, Crock JG. The venous territories of muscles: anatomical study and clinical implications. *Br J Plast Surg*. 1988;41(6):569-585.
46. Hoopes JE. Pedicle flaps—an overview. In: Krizek TJ, Hoopes JE, eds. *Symposium on Basic Science in Plastic Surgery*. St. Louis, MO: Mosby; 1976:241-259.
47. Vedder NB. Flap physiology. In: Mathes SJ, ed. *Plastic Surgery*. 2nd ed. Philadelphia, PA: Saunders; 2005:484.
48. Vedder NB. Flap physiology. In: Mathes SJ, ed. *Plastic Surgery*. 2nd ed. Philadelphia, PA: Saunders; 2005:494.
49. De Filippo RE, Atala A. Stretch and growth: the molecular and physiologic influences of tissue expansion. *Plast Reconstr Surg*. 2002;109:2450-2462.
50. Marks MW, Argenta LC. Principles and applications of tissue expansion. In: Neligan PC, ed. *Plastic Surgery*. 3rd ed. Philadelphia, PA: Elsevier; 2013:623.
51. Pasyk KA, Argenta LC, Hassett C. Quantitative analysis of the thickness of human skin and subcutaneous tissue following controlled expansion with a silicone implant. *Plast Reconstr Surg*. 1988;81(4):516-523.
52. Pasyk KA, Argenta LC, Austad ED. Histopathology of human expanded tissue. *Clin Plast Surg*. 1987;14(3):435-445.
53. Argenta LC, Marks MW. Principle of tissue expansion. In: Mathes SJ, ed. *Plastic Surgery*. 2nd ed. Philadelphia, PA: Saunders, 2005:541.
54. van Rappard JH, Sonneveld GJ, Borghouts JM. Geometric planning and the shape of the expander. *Facial Plast Surg*. 1988;5:287-290.
55. Wagh MS, Dixit V. Tissue expansion: concepts, techniques and unfavourable results. *Indian J Plast Surg*. 2013;46:333-348.
56. Bauer BS, Margulis A. The expanded transposition flap: shifting paradigms based on experience gained from two decades of pediatric tissue expansion. *Plast Reconstr Surg*. 2004;114:98-106.
57. Cervenka B, Bewley AF. Free flap monitoring: a review of the recent literature. *Curr Opin Otolaryngol Head Neck Surg*. 2015;23:393-398.
58. Hosein RC, Cornejo A, Wang HT. Postoperative monitoring of free flap reconstruction: a comparison of external Doppler ultrasonography and the implantable Doppler probe. *Plast Surg (Oakv)*. 2016;24:11-19.
59. Yano A, Orihashi I, Yoshida Y, Kuriyama M. Near-infrared spectroscopy for monitoring free jejunal flap. *J Plast Reconstr Aesthet Surg*. 2021;74(1):108-115.
60. Bai W, Guo H, Ouyang W, et al. Intramuscular near-infrared spectroscopy for muscle flap monitoring in a porcine model. *J Reconstr Microsurg*. 2022;38(4):321-327.
61. Braverman IM. The cutaneous microcirculation. *J Investig Dermatol Symp Proc*. 2000;5(1):3-9.
62. Champion HR, Sacco WJ, Hannan DS, et al. Assessment of injury severity: the triage index. *Crit Care Med*. 1980;8(4):201-208.
63. Hall JE. The microcirculation and lymphatic system: capillary fluid exchange, interstitial fluid, and lymph flow. In: Hall JE, ed. *Guyton and Hall Textbook of Medical Physiology*. 12th ed. Philadelphia, PA: Saunders; 2011:182.

64. Rosenberg JJ, Fornage BD, Chevray PM. Monitoring buried free flaps: limitations of the implantable Doppler and use of color duplex sonography as a confirmatory test. *Plast Reconstr Surg.* 2006;118(1):109-113.
65. Phillips BT, Lanier ST, Conkling N, et al. Intraoperative perfusion techniques can accurately predict mastectomy skin flap necrosis in breast reconstruction: results of a prospective trial. *Plast Reconstr Surg.* 2012;129(5):778e-788e.
66. Liu DZ, Mathes DW, Zenn MR, Neligan PC. The application of indocanine green fluorescence angiography in plastic surgery. *J Reconstr Microsurg.* 2011;27(6):355-364.

Burn Wound Management

Zachary J. Collier, MD, MS; Joseph N. Carey, MD, FACS; and T. Justin Gillenwater, MD

CHAPTER OBJECTIVES

At the end of this chapter, the learner will be able to:

1. **Classify burn wounds according to the depth of tissue injury using the American Burn Association terminology.**
2. **Estimate the percentage of total body surface area of a burn using the three main techniques—Lund & Browder Chart, Wallace Rule-of-Nines, and Palmar Surface Area.**
3. **Appreciate the different mechanisms of burn injuries.**
4. **Recognize the critical aspects of the initial evaluation and assessment of a burn injury.**
5. **Estimate the fluid and caloric requirements of a burn patient.**
6. **Understand the different nonsurgical and surgical treatment modalities for burns and identify when surgical treatment is required.**
7. **Distinguish the discrete complications that can occur after a burn injury and discuss how they are managed.**
8. **Address the major physical and psychological objectives of rehabilitation in a burn patient.**

INTRODUCTION

Epidemiology

The World Health Organization estimates that more than 10 million people are burned worldwide annually, accounting for more than 180,000 deaths and 8 million adjusted-life years of disability due to nonfatal burn injuries.[1] The global burden of burn disease is further impacted by the high incidence of women and children who are disproportionately burned, particularly in lower-income countries. Each year in the United States, over 486,000 individuals receive medical care for burns, 40,000 patients require hospitalization, and 30,000 are treated at hospital burn centers.[2] Thus, burns create a significant burden for the health care system due to the complex inpatient and outpatient care of burned patients needed to facilitate optimal recovery. It is important to note that over 90% of burn injuries are deemed preventable occurrences, which means that ongoing burn prevention efforts are critical to further reduce burn morbidity and mortality.

Mortality has significantly decreased with the development of regional burn units, the establishment of multidisciplinary treatment teams, as well as improved critical care strategies focused on optimizing resuscitation, early surgical interventions, infection control, and nutrition. The American Burn Association reports the current survival rates are greater than 96% for patients having survived burns involving as much as 95% of the body.[2] With the increasing survival of this patient population, especially those with severely disabling burn injuries that were previously fatal, greater emphasis has been placed on long-term rehabilitation geared at the restoration of function and activities of daily living, correction of aesthetic deformities, and improvement of psychosocial well-being. With this paradigm shift in burn care toward optimizing post-burn quality of life, newer interventions are being rapidly developed and applied during both the acute and reconstructive phases of burn care to facilitate such improvements for burn survivors.

Pathophysiology

The term *burn injury* is often employed as an umbrella term that encompasses a vast array of unique mechanistic etiologies, all of which eventually result in injury to the skin and underlying structures. These mechanisms can be separated into five main categories: thermal, chemical, radiation, electrical, and friction. Thermal etiologies include flame, contact, scald, and frostbite. Thermal injury to the skin is the result of the direct energy transfer to or from the tissue and severity is dependent upon temperature and contact or exposure time. Temperature is a derivative of the average kinetic energy of the molecules within a system, or in the case of burn injury, a substance (i.e., boiling water or hot iron), such that the temperature of any substance represents a potentially transferable molecular kinetic energy ($KE_{avg} = 3/2\ \kappa T$; κ = Boltzmann's constant, T = Kelvin) to some other substance (i.e., skin). Transfer of this stored kinetic energy to cellular structures of the skin results in the denaturation of proteins, vaporization of water, and thrombosis of cutaneous blood vessels, thus resulting in tissue and cell death. The rapid coagulation of protein occurs in the setting of irreversible thermal cross-linking that may limit depth progression when compared to other burn mechanisms such as chemical and radiation exposure. Frostbite is the inverse direction transfer of energy in which the "heat" (aka kinetic energy of the skin) is transferred to the surrounding environment or material causing rapid cooling of the skin and underlying structures.

This process of tissue injury may be immediate in the case of very high or low temperatures and/or prolonged contact time but may also be potentiated by the patient's premorbid condition(s), injury status, and local inflammatory factors. The delineation between hot and cold thermal mechanisms (i.e., flame, contact, scald) strictly translates to the interface through which the stored kinetic energy is transferred and has implications with respect to the contact time required to facilitate such a transfer. For example, contact burns occur when a solid substance (i.e., hot iron) contacts skin; a burn injury of a specific depth will occur at a much shorter exposure interval than that of a liquid or gas of the same temperature. This is because the solid substance has a significantly greater molecular energy density, which allows it to transfer a greater magnitude of energy across the contact interface in a short period of time in comparison to less energetically dense liquid and gas. This means that in order for liquid and gas to achieve the same depth burn as that of a contact mechanism, a higher temperature or longer contact time is required.

This nuance is important when comparing the burn mechanism to the pattern of a burn injury. For example, a mixed mechanism such as hot noodles (boiling liquid and hot solid) will often result in variable burn depths—deeper where the solid makes contact relative to the depth in the liquid contact areas—despite both components of the substance having the same "temperature." This delineation also plays an important role when examining burn patterns and comparing observations to the reported mechanism for investigations related to burn abuse and neglect. Other mechanisms of burn injury related to chemicals, electricity, radiation, and friction will be discussed in further detail later in the chapter as tissue damage in these instances is not always a direct result of kinetic energy but rather more complex biochemical and electrophysical interactions.

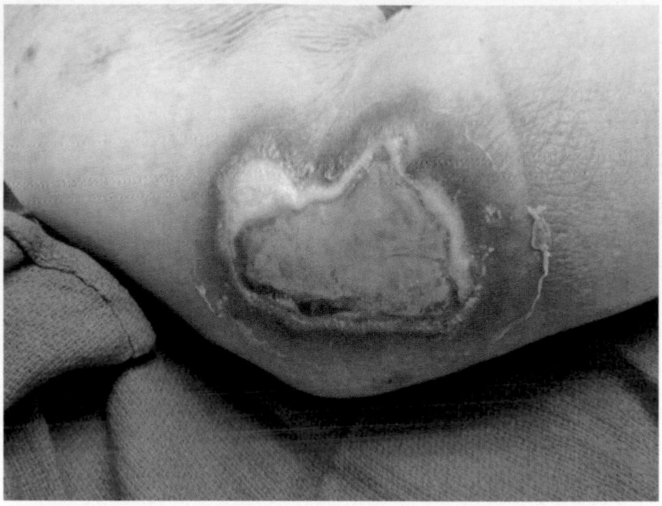

FIGURE 11-1 Jackson's concentric zones of burn tissue. Jackson's burn theory classifies three concentric zones in relation to the potential viability of the tissue. These regions from the center of the wound to the periphery were labeled as the zone of coagulation, the zone of stasis, and the zone of hyperemia. The center zone of coagulation is the area of maximum contact with the thermal source. Tissues in this area undergo a coagulation necrosis as proteins of the extracellular matrix are denatured and vascularity is impaired. Cells will not recover and emphasis is placed on early debridement and prevention of infection. The intermediate zone of stasis is characterized by hypoperfusion and hypometabolism as the numbers of viable cells are substantially reduced. Phenotypically this area appears as blanching erythema when pressure is applied. There is a risk of tissue progression to necrosis if proper care is not taken to preserve tissue perfusion by adequate fluid resuscitation, avoidance of vasoconstrictors, and prevention of infection. Patients with significant comorbidities that impair blood flow such as diabetes, peripheral vascular disease, and tobacco use are at increased risk for irreversible injury. The outer zone of hyperemia also appears as erythema as the result of local vasodilatation. Cells in this zone are completely viable and will recover if protected from further trauma and/or infection.

Zones of Injury

In 1953, Douglas M. Jackson published a classic article in the *British Journal of Surgery* describing three histological zones of thermal burn injury. These "zones of injury" have been adapted by burn literature and are still applicable to this day (**FIGURE 11-1**).[3] *Zone 1* is considered the *Zone of Coagulation* and refers to the area of burned tissue that is irreversibly damaged or "coagulated" and is no longer viable. Depending on burn size and depth, this area may be addressed with immediate mechanical or subsequent operative debridement. *Zone 2* is also known as the *Zone of Stasis* due to the diminished or "static" perfusion to this area of burned tissue. The tissue injury in this zone is potentially reversible if appropriate and expedient post-burn interventions are administered to restore or improve perfusion to the area. Adequate intravascular resuscitation, infection prevention, early removal of necrotic or nonviable tissues, nutrition optimization, and restoration of physiologic core body temperature are all components of the treatment algorithm that can minimize the conversion of *Zone 2* to irreversible *Zone 1* injury. *Zone 3* is the *Zone of Hyperemia*, which is the area of "unburned" tissue surrounding *Zone 2* that is exposed to the nearby release of inflammatory cytokines (e.g., interleukins, prostaglandins, bradykinin, substance P, histamine) and subsequently develops vasodilation and increased capillary permeability leading to flushing or "hyperemia." As there is no direct tissue injury, *Zone 3* is completely reversible unless uncontrolled infection or expanding necrosis of adjacent *Zone 2* burn results in the involvement of the *Zone 3* tissue.

BURN WOUND CLASSIFICATION

Depth of Injury

Burn severity and the subsequent treatments are largely determined by the depth of injury and the percent of the surface area of injured skin in relationship to the total body surface area (% TBSA) of the patient. The previous designations of *first-*, *second-*, and *third-degree* burns have been replaced by newer terminology—*superficial thickness*, *superficial* or *deep partial thickness*, and *full thickness*—because of an improved understanding of burn physiology. This system redirects the focus to anatomic descriptors of injury which help guide treatment. While researchers and clinicians have transitioned to the aforementioned depth descriptors, medical coding still utilizes the degree system, so it is important for practitioners treating burn wounds to understand both systems and the translation between the two.

Superficial thickness injuries are burns limited to the epidermis without disruption of underlying dermal integrity (**FIGURE 11-2**). This injury was previously designated as a *first-degree burn* and is characterized by erythema of the skin secondary to vasodilatation of local capillaries and may be very painful due to the intact yet inflamed cutaneous nerve endings within the dermis. Sunburns are examples of superficial burns and after 3–4 days, the damaged epithelium desquamates and is replaced by regenerating keratinocytes.[4] Importantly, *superficial* or *first-degree* burns are not included in TBSA calculations as this injury does not violate the dermis and therefore the physiologic derangements from such burns are inconsequential during the treatment of deeper burns. Referring providers will often incorrectly include *superficial* or *first-degree* burns in TBSA calculations, which leads to burn size overestimation, excessive or unnecessary treatments and interventions, and inappropriate initiation of Parkland fluid resuscitation.

Partial-thickness, previously *second-degree*, burns are heterogeneous in nature due to regional variability in dermal thickness and therefore encompass a spectrum of injury patterns and pathophysiology related to the involvement of superficial and deep dermal tissues and structures. The defining characteristic of a *partial-thickness* burn compared to *full-thickness* is that dermal structures are still intact, so spontaneous healing may occur through the migration of epithelial progenitor cells from remaining dermal appendages. However, the healing potential of a *superficial partial-thickness* burn is much better than a *deep partial-thickness* burn because of the density of dermal appendages, adnexal structures, and progenitor cells that remain viable within the preserved reticular dermis. This variability in healing potential based on the depth of injury within the dermal layer has resulted in the further designation of *partial-thickness* burns into two subgroups—*superficial and deep*—which subsequently have different treatment requirements and expected outcomes.

Superficial partial-thickness burns are dermal injuries that extend into the papillary dermis while sparing most, if not all, of the deeper reticular dermis (**FIGURE 11-3**). These wounds are sensate to nociceptive, proprioceptive, and light touch stimuli, blanch with pressure, and typically result in blistering

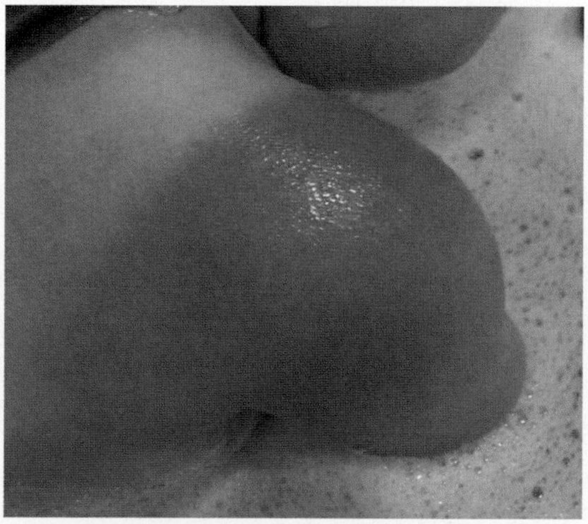

FIGURE 11-2 Superficial burn. Superficial burns involve only the epidermis and will heal in 3–4 days without scarring or medical intervention. Sunburn on the shoulder of this toddler is an example of a superficial burn.

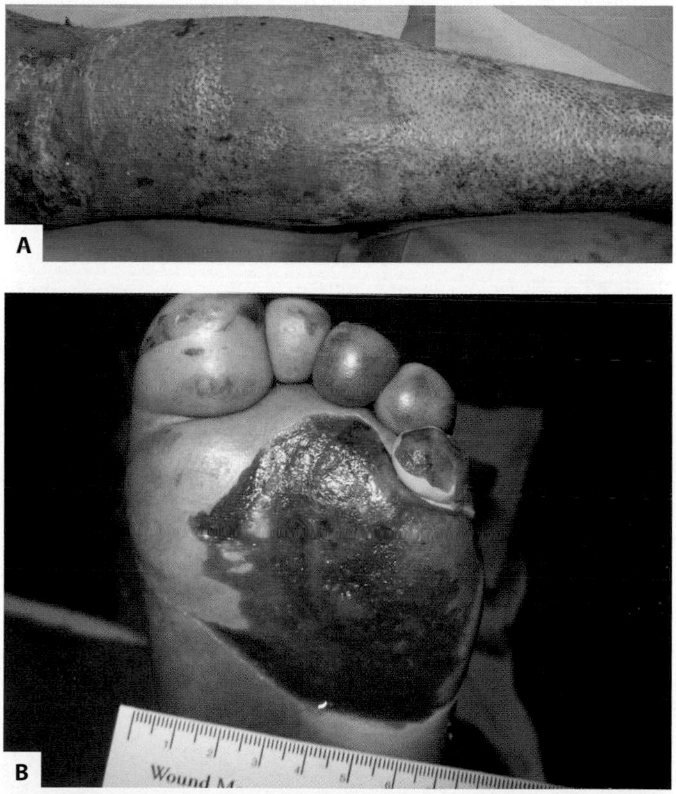

FIGURE 11-3 A. Superficial *partial-thickness* burns. Superficial *partial-thickness* burns involve the epidermis and the superficial dermis. They are characterized by intense pain, blanching with pressure, and blistering as a result of the local inflammatory process between the dermis and epidermis. These wounds heal within 2–3 weeks by epithelization and rarely form hypertrophic scarring and/or wound contracture. A scald burn on the lower extremity with sloughing of the epidermis is an example of a superficial *partial-thickness* burn; the areas that are mottled and nonblanching are deep *partial-thickness* burns. **B.** Superficial *partial-thickness* burn re-epithelializing. The thermal burn on the plantar foot is superficial partial thickness, and islands of new epithelium can be observed in the middle of the wound. The blistered tissue was debrided, but the wound healed without grafting.

as a result of the local inflammatory process between the dermis and the remaining epidermis. In particular, blistering in *superficial partial-thickness* burns is the result of an exudative accumulation of interstitial fluids at the site of the damaged epidermal–dermal interface and these blisters are often intact at the time of initial presentation. The blistering can be serious in nature; thus, a hemorrhagic appearance often correlates with *deeper partial-thickness* burns where the reticular vascular plexus has been damaged. Superficial partial thickness wounds usually heal within 2–3 weeks by re-epithelialization from retained dermal appendages (i.e., bulge stem cells from the base of hair follicles), so they rarely form hypertrophic scars and/or wound contractures. Due to their healing potential and ability to re-epithelialize within 3 weeks, they frequently do not require excision and grafting.

Deep partial-thickness burns extend into the reticular dermis and are often nociceptively insensate or diminished, have a mottled white or "fixed pink" appearance, and do not blanch with pressure as the result of impaired vascularity and capillary refill along with irreversibly denatured dermal proteins that give the fixed white or pink coloring (**FIGURE 11-4**). Because the free nerve endings responsible for nociception are more superficial within the dermis compared to the other somatosensory nerve receptors contained within skin, *deep partial-thickness* burns remain sensate to light touch (i.e., Merkel's cells, Meissner's corpuscles), vibration and rapid pressure (i.e., Pacinian corpuscle), and stretch and sustained pressure (i.e., Ruffini's corpuscles) even when no longer sensitive to pain. This delineation of the type of sensation that is lost within a burn wound helps further clarify the depth of the burn when a mixed clinical examination is present. Furthermore, *deep partial-thickness* burns may also be pink rather than white due to the different ways in which the proteins are denatured. The characteristic that helps to differentiate this pink appearance from that of more superficial burns is the blanching which will be diminished compared to other more superficial areas. There is often a transition point rather than a clear demarcation between these areas of different depths and the physical examination can help identify the transition zones. The reticular dermis contains skin appendages, so injury in this area can cause permanent damage to hair follicles and sebaceous glands, two critical sources of epidermal stem cells required for re-epithelialization and skin healing. The reticular dermis also possesses a distinct lineage of fibroblasts compared to those of the papillary dermis that are specifically responsible for the deposition of new extracellular matrix proteins and wound closure. *Deep partial-thickness* burns damage this fibroblast population that is crucial for wound healing. As a result of damage to stem cell-containing hair follicles and sebaceous glands as well as loss of reticular fibroblasts, *deep partial-thickness* burns heal in 3–9 weeks by a mix of contraction and epithelialization, which results in extended periods of inflammation and subsequently significant hypertrophic scarring and wound contracture. Because of the sequelae of delayed healing in *deep partial-thickness* burns that are allowed to heal by contraction—causing hypertrophic scarring and contractures with significant cosmetic and functional impairments—they are best treated by debridement of necrotic or nonviable tissue followed by an appropriate method of defect coverage, including autologous skin grafting, local tissue rearrangement, or local and free flaps.

Full-thickness, previously third-degree, burns are cutaneous injuries extending through the entire dermis and into or across the subdermal plexus, causing complete loss of the skin's barrier function (**FIGURE 11-5**). This designation also implies that there is no possibility of healing from the wound base since all dermal regenerative cells have been obliterated.

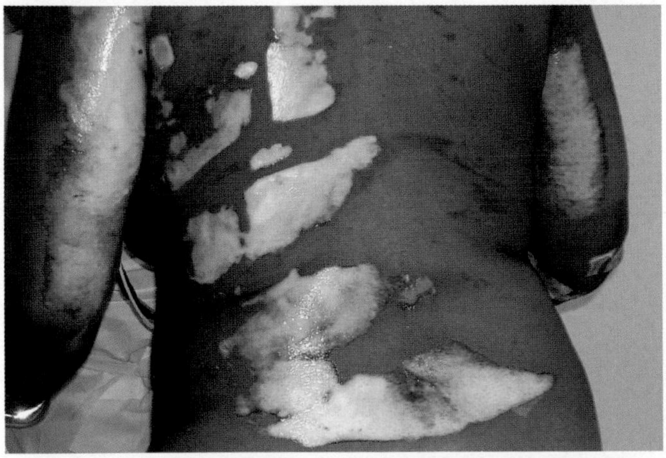

FIGURE 11-4 Deep *partial-thickness* burn. Deep *partial-thickness* injuries extend into the reticular dermis and are insensate, have a mottled white appearance, and do not blanch with pressure as the result of impaired vascularity and capillary refill. Deep *partial-thickness* burns heal in 3–9 weeks, sometimes with significant hypertrophic scarring and wound contracture; therefore, they are best treated by debridement of necrotic tissue and skin grafts.

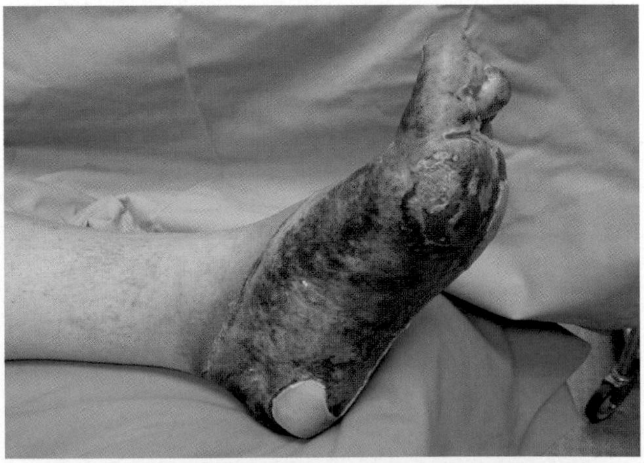

FIGURE 11-5 *Full-thickness* burn. *Full-thickness* burns extend through the entire dermis and into the subcutaneous tissue. The appearance is leathery brown or black eschar with no capillary refill. The wounds are insensate and treatment is focused on early excision and grafting to prevent infection, hypertrophic scarring, and wound contracture. This foot with extensive eschar and exposed subcutaneous tissue is an example of a *full-thickness* burn.

The physical appearance is often leathery brown or a black eschar with no blanching or capillary refill, although pink and white pigmentation may be present due to protein fixation. The key delineation is that no blanching is present due to coagulation of the subdermal plexus. Furthermore, *full-thickness* burn tissue is nonviable and shrinks or contracts as opposed to *partial-thickness* tissue, which is damaged but viable, and therefore swells from the release of inflammatory cytokines from injured cells. The saying "dead tissue shrinks, damaged tissue swells" is helpful to remember when assessing burn depth. The wounds are insensate with respect to all forms of somatosensation because of the loss of all dermal and subdermal nerve endings. Treatment is focused on early excision of necrotic tissues to prevent infection, hypertrophic scarring, and wound contracture. Depending on size and location, most *full-thickness* injuries are treated with excision and grafting procedures, although excision and delayed primary closure or more complex reconstructive options such as local or free vascularized tissue transfer or coverage with cellular/acellular matrix products may be employed when the wound is small, critical structures are exposed, or ideal graft-receptive wound beds are not available.

The full extent of burn depth may not be readily apparent at the time of initial evaluation because the burn eschar often impairs the delineation of true depth in *deep partial* and *full-thickness* burns. Although many tools have been used as predictive indicators of the depth of injury (e.g., wound biopsy, ultrasound, infrared, or perfusion techniques), none have proven to be as reliable as a physical examination at 48–72 hours postinjury.[5,6] The initial nonsurgical debridement of burn wounds with mechanical methods such as rigorous scrubbing to remove blisters, exudate, coagulum, and eschar is crucial to the accurate assessment of the burn depth.

Size of Burn Injury

An estimate of the burn wound surface area in proportion (%) to the total body surface area (TBSA) is used to estimate the initial total fluid and caloric requirements while also guiding other interventions and serving as a predictor of morbidity and mortality. Since the concept of estimating burn size with TBSA was created, many different techniques have been utilized from photography to molds to ruler measurements to apps and now even AI. While a myriad of options exists for TBSA estimation, there are a few well-validated and readily applicable methods that may be effectively employed. These include the *Lund & Browder Chart*, the *Rule of Nines*, the *Rule of Sevens*, and the *Palmar Surface Area*. For an adult patient with larger burns that involve significant portions of a body region, the burn area is often generalized utilizing the "Rule of Nines" for rapidity and ease of assessment (**FIGURE 11-6**). When assessing burn size for patients with BMIs greater than 35, the adaptation of the Rule of Nines to the Rule of Sevens [**FIGURE 11-7**] is indicated to reduce inaccuracies that occur when generalizing the Rule of Nines to obese patients. In particular, the anterior and posterior torsos represent 28% TBSA, respectively, whereas the lower extremities are 14% and the upper extremities are 7%. While the Rule of Nines and Sevens are useful for larger, contiguous burns, the Palmar Surface Area (PSA) technique (**FIGURE 11-8**) equates the patient's own palm and fingers to a specific percent TBSA; it is best used for smaller and scattered patterns. It is important to note that age, gender, and BMI all impact PSA relative to TBSA, and can result in twofold errors in estimation when not accounted for by the practitioner. The most common PSA adjustments are shown in **FIGURE 11-8**. For pediatric patients, their PSA represents 1% TBSA whereas adults' PSA is 0.8% TBSA if BMI < 40 and PSA is 0.6% if BMI > 40.[7] More complex charts such as the Lund–Browder chart are available for more accurately estimating the body surface in relationship to age and may be more useful particularly in the pediatric population (**TABLE 11-1**). The Lund–Browder chart, although more accurate, is also more time-consuming in application, so it is

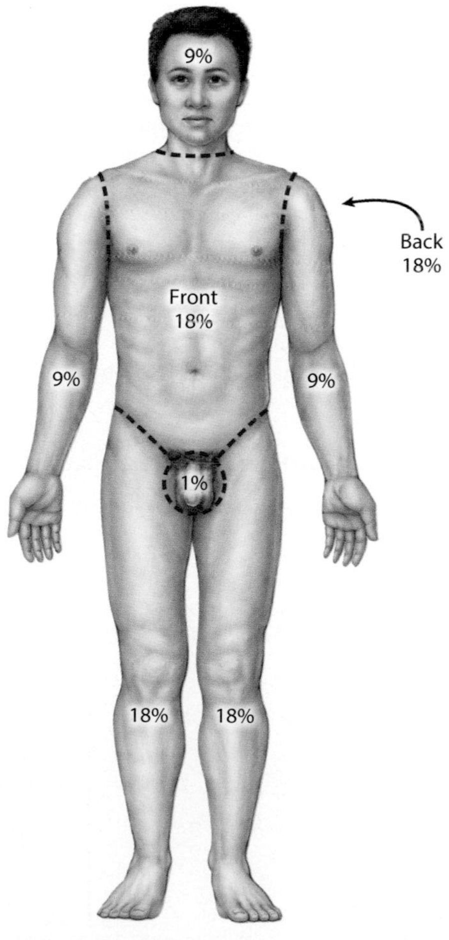

FIGURE 11-6 Rule of Nines. The Rule of Nines is used to determine the total body surface area that is burned and estimates that each upper extremity accounts for 9% of the total burn surface area or TBSA, and each lower extremity, 18%. In addition, the anterior and posterior trunk is predicted to be 18%, the head and neck 18%, and the perineum 1%. For burns spanning anatomical regions, the volar surface area of the hand may be considered 1% of the TBSA.

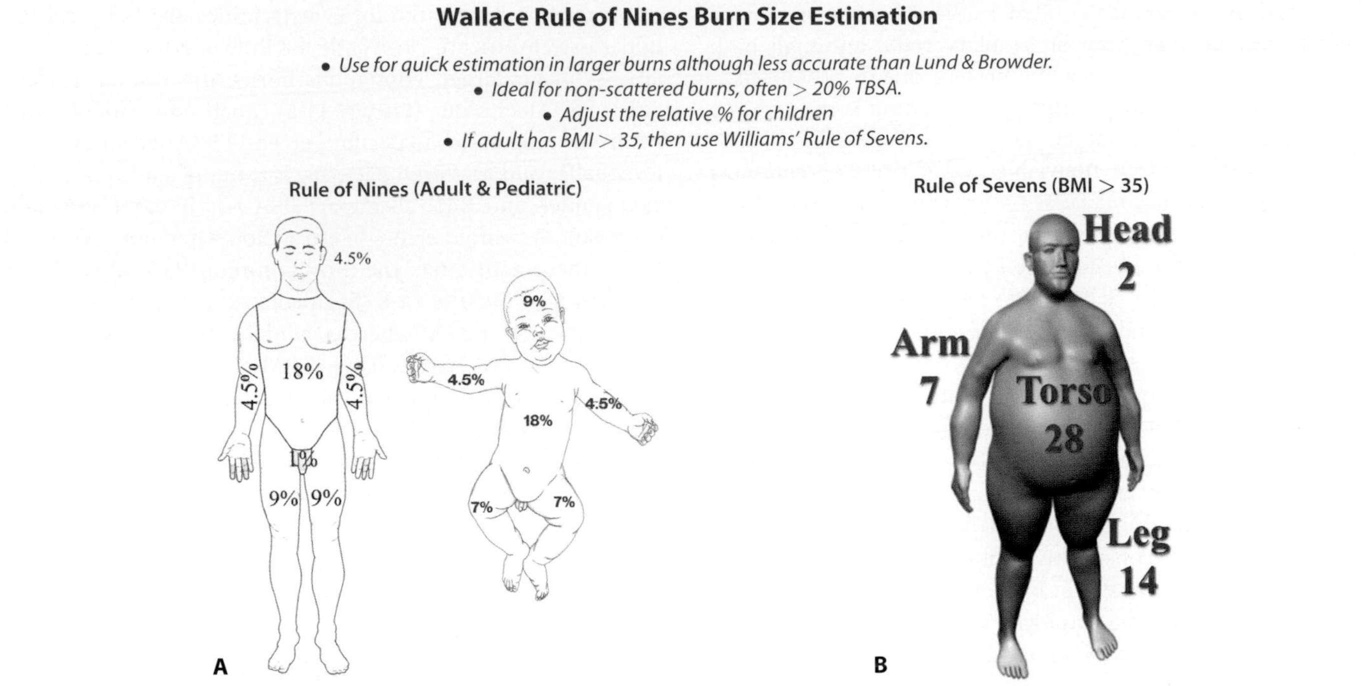

FIGURE 11-7 A. The Rule of Nines used to determine total body surface area (TBSA) of both adult and pediatric patients with burns (Reproduced with permission from American Burn Association. Advanced Burn Life Support Providers Manual, American Burn Association 2005.) **B.** The Rule of Sevens is used to determine TBSA for obese adults with a BMI > 35. (Data from Williams RY, Wohlgemuth SD. Does the "rule of nines" apply to morbidly obese burn victims? *J Burn Care Res.* 2013;34(4):447-452.)

often not employed by nonburn and prehospital providers. In order to reduce the significant errors or variability that often occur in TBSA estimation, even among experienced practitioners, computer- and mobile app–based methods such as Burn Case 3D (RISC Software GmbH), BurnMed (Johns Hopkins University), and uBurn Medic (JAMB Innovations, LLC) have been developed.[7] Validation continues to progress with these and many other digital techniques with the ultimate goal of overcoming the current limitations that exist with manual estimation methods. The depth of the injury and the burn TBSA are major determinants by the American Burn Association for referral to a regional burn center for a higher level of care, so ensuring that both aspects of the diagnosis are accurate is critical to ensuring patients receive proper care (**TABLE 11-2**).

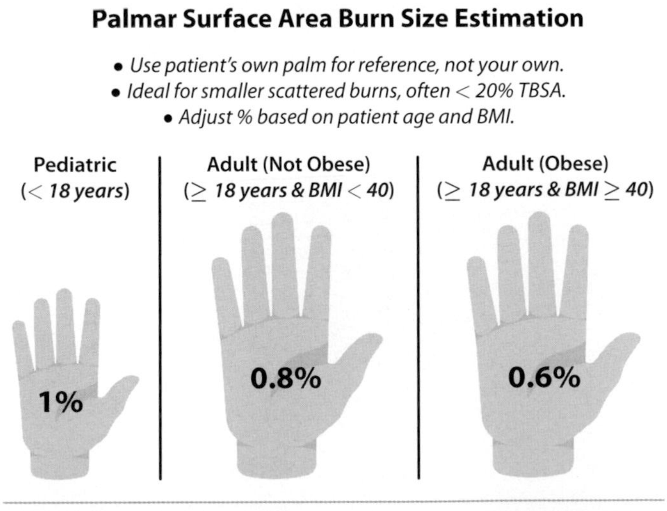

FIGURE 11-8 Palmar surface area. The palmar surface area is used for smaller wounds and those with scattered patterns. The size of the wound is equated to the patient's palm and fingers to determine a specific TBSA. (Palmar TBSA estimates for adults adapted from Butz DR, Collier Z, O'Connor A, Magdziak M, Gottlieb LJ. Is palmar surface area a reliable tool to estimate burn surface areas in obese patients? *J Burn Care Res.* 2015;36(1):87-91.)

PROGNOSIS

When a patient first enters a burn center and the initial evaluation is completed, prognostication is performed to facilitate a better understanding of injury severity as well as discussions with the patient and family members regarding the overall prognosis. Initially, when the Parisian surgeon Serge Baux first devised his mortality scoring system in 1961, this calculated score (i.e., Baux Score = patient age + % TBSA) translated directly to the patient's mortality rate. In other words, a 60-year-old patient with a 40% TBSA burn had a Baux Score of 100 (60 + 40) and therefore had a 100% mortality rate. However, due to significant advances in burn critical care, infection prevention and control, and surgical management, this score is now used as a marker of injury severity but not as a direct measure of mortality risk. Recently, to account for the influence of inhalation injury on mortality in burn injury, the Revised Baux Score (rBaux) was formulated by Osler et al. in 2010.[8–10] This method calculates a score by summating a patient's age,

TABLE 11-1 Estimating Total Surface Burn Area with Lund & Browder Chart

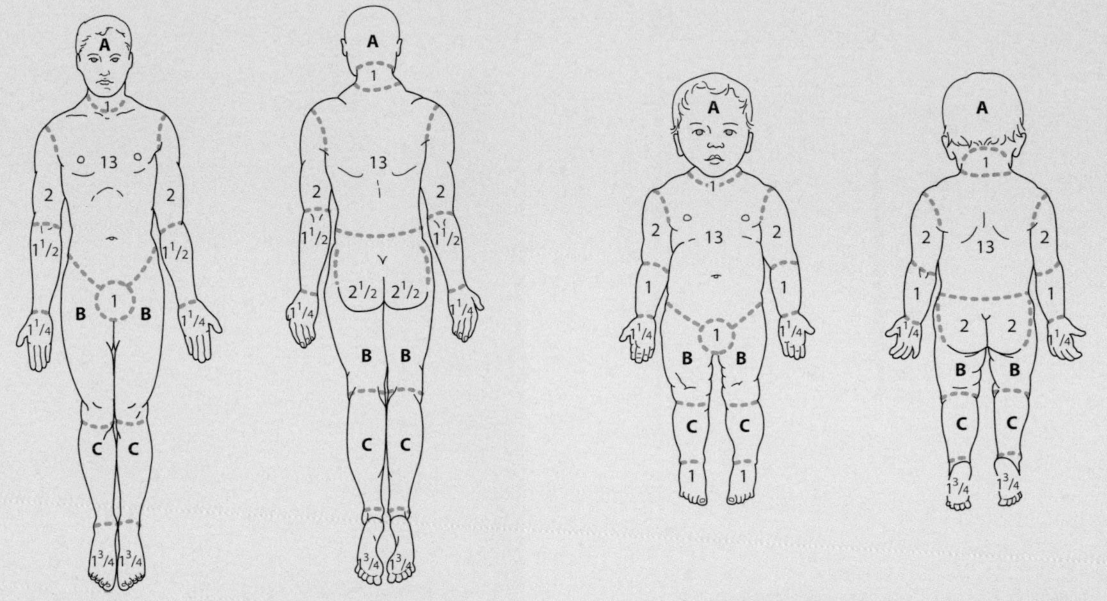

Relative Percentages of Areas Affected by Growth

Area	Age 10	Age 15	Age Adult
A = half of head	5 1/2	4 1/2	3 1/2
B = half of one thigh	4 1/4	4 1/2	4 3/4
C = half of one leg	3	3 1/4	3 1/2

Relative Percentages of Areas Affected by Growth

Area	Age 0	Age 1	Age 5
A = half of head	9 1/2	8 1/2	6 1/2
B = half of one thigh	2 3/4	3 1/4	4
C = half of one leg	2 1/2	2 1/2	2 3/4

TABLE 11-2 Criteria for Referral to a Regional Burn Center

American Burn Association Criteria for Referral to Regional Burn Unit
▪ Partial-thickness burns that encompass greater than 10% TBSA
▪ Burns that involve the face, hands, feet, hands, feet, genitalia, perineum, or major joints
▪ Full-thickness burns in any age group
▪ Electrical burns, including lightning injury
▪ Chemical burns
▪ Inhalation injury
▪ Burn injury in patients with preexisting medical conditions that can complicate management, prolong recovery, or affect mortality
▪ Any patients with burns and concomitant trauma, in which burn injury poses the greatest risk of morbidity and mortality
▪ Burn children in hospitals without qualified personnel or equipment for the care for children
▪ Burn injury in patients who will require special social, emotional, or rehabilitative intervention

Data from www.ameriburn.org. Accessed April 12, 2023.

% TBSA, and adding an additional 17 points in the presence of any inhalation injury. For example, a 50-year-old patient with a 30% TBSA burn and inhalation injury would have a total Revised Baux Score of 97 (50 + 30 + 17). With the rBaux, a conversion nomogram may be used to determine predicted mortality, and for the example above, the predicted mortality from the rBaux nomogram would be 21% as opposed to only 7% if inhalation injury was not considered (**FIGURE 11-9**).

While the rBaux provides a relatively accurate estimate of predicted mortality after severe burn injury, it does not account for other clinical indicators of prognosis such as comorbidities or concomitant trauma. As a result, the entirety of the patient must be considered while placing their burn injuries into the context of the greater picture—baseline health, premorbid conditions, new postinjury comorbidities, and concomitant injuries.

MECHANISMS OF BURN INJURIES

Scald

Scald burns are the result of contact with hot liquids and are the most common burn etiology in most countries. The extent of injury is primarily dependent on the temperature and viscosity of the liquid as well as the duration of exposure; however, patient factors and anatomical location also play a role. Exposure to hot water above 60°C for 3 seconds can result in *deep partial-thickness* or *full-thickness* injury. These injuries typically appear less severe in exposed areas of the body. Clothed areas typically have more extensive injuries because clothing absorbs the heated liquid, prevents evaporative heat dissipation, and maintains contact with the skin for a longer duration of time. In the pediatric population, immersion scald

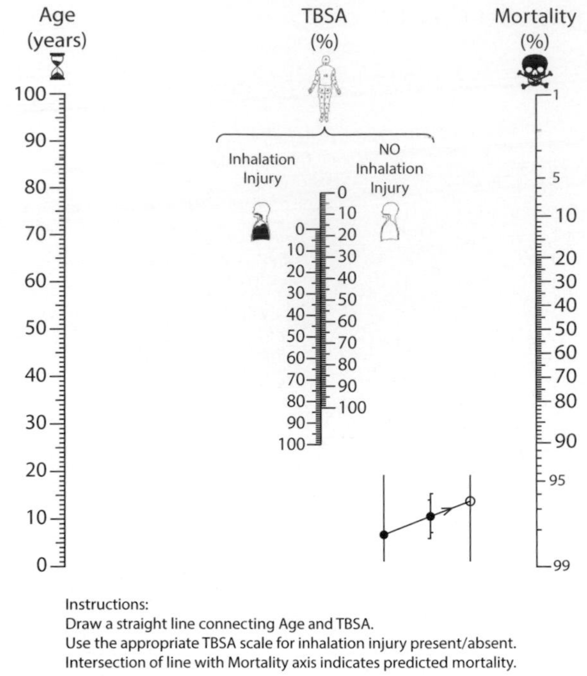

FIGURE 11-9 Revised Baux Nomogram for burn mortality. (Reproduced with permission from Williams DJ, Walker JD. A nomogram for calculation of the Revised Baux Score. *Burns.* 2015;41(1):85-90.)

burns with a symmetric distribution and linear demarcations of the upper extremity or lower extremity and/or crease-sparing of the perineum and buttocks warrant suspicion of abuse, and health care professionals are required to notify appropriate child protective agencies (**FIGURE 11-10**). While not within the scope of this chapter, a detailed discussion on the evaluation and management of suspected abuse and negligent burns may be found in "Negligent and Inflicted Burns in Children" by Collier *et al.* in the July 2017 issue of *Clinics in Plastic Surgery*.[11] A provider taking care of patients with burns needs to know what signs to look for when evaluating for negligent and/or inflicted burn injuries. Recognizing the signs can help save the patient from future injuries and also identify families who may benefit from additional resources at home.

Scald burns from grease may result in more severe injuries because grease is more viscous than water, therefore resulting in a longer duration of contact due to the decreased evaporative losses and increased difficulty removing the offending agent. Although grease can reach higher temperatures (usually around 200°C) compared to water, water has a significantly higher heat capacitance and therefore contains more stored thermal energy for a given temperature. As a result, water can transfer greater energy in a given period of time and cause greater damage per second of exposure. The combination of boiling water and oil results in the greatest degree of damage compared to either in isolation because the oil prevents evaporation of water which then facilitates prolonged delivery of stored thermal energy in water to the contacted tissues. These burns therefore frequently result in *deep partial-thickness* to *full-thickness* injuries.

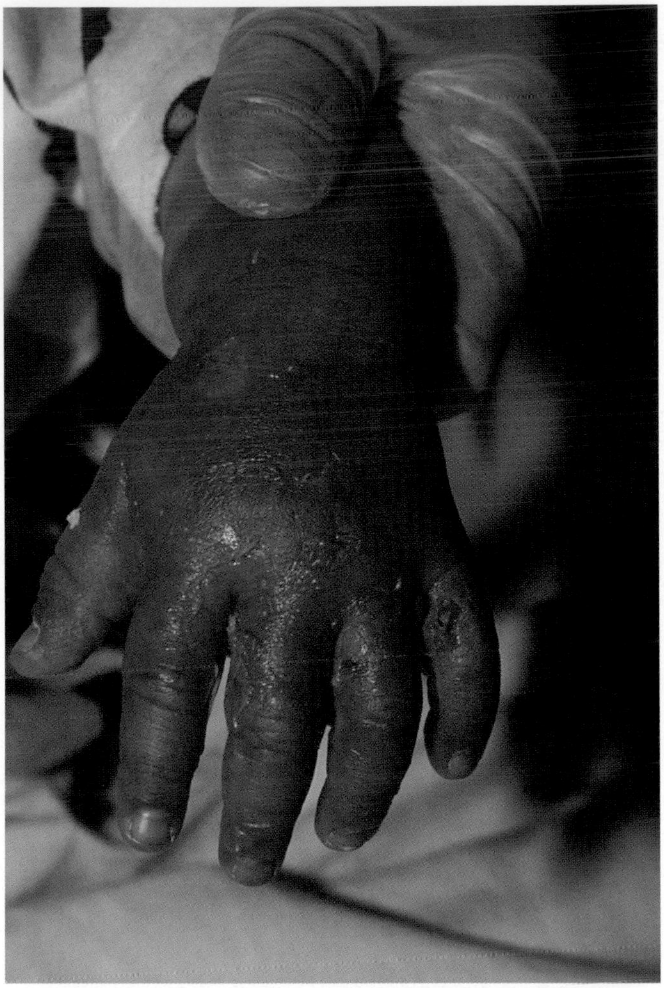

FIGURE 11-10 Scalding burn. This toddler's hand is an example of a superficial *partial-thickness* burn due to scalding water. The depth of tissue injury depends on the liquid temperature and time of exposure. Any suspicion of child abuse with this type of burn should be reported to the Children's Protective Services.

Tar is a unique type of scald burn that requires specialized management because it becomes adherent to the skin as it cools and creates a secondary alkaline chemical injury. Treatment is initially focused on rapidly cooling the tar with ice packs to reduce continued thermal injury followed by the slow removal of the tar with petroleum-based ointment such as Neosporin (Johnson & Johnson, New Brunswick, NJ) and Medi-sol (Medi-sol, Oklahoma City, OK) or simple mineral oil. The ointment or oil may need to be applied multiple times in order to totally dissolve the tar. Rapid intervention is warranted even after cooling measures have stopped thermal-based injury because the alkaline composition of tar can continue to cause underlying liquefactive necrosis. Once dissolved, an appropriate assessment can be made regarding the depth of penetration and extent of injury.

Flame

Flame injuries are the second most common mechanism of burns and the most common mechanism requiring hospitalization. Flame injuries account for 44% of burn admissions in the United States annually.[2] The incidence of flame burns has significantly decreased with the implementation of prevention programs and improved detection methods such as smoke detectors and fire alarms. The major determinant of morbidity and mortality in this patient population is the presence of concomitant inhalation injury.[12] Inhalation injury is suspected if the burn occurred within an enclosed space; the patient was found unconscious or after prolonged extraction from a fire; or if physical examination reveals singed nasal hair, voice changes (e.g., coarse or hoarseness), inspiratory stridor, and/or carbonaceous sputum.

Electrical

Electrical burns have been described as the most devastating burn injuries because they not only involve the skin, but also underlying organ systems (e.g., the cardiovascular, musculoskeletal, and nervous systems). Electrical burn pathophysiology, like that of chemical injury, has a mixed contribution from direct and indirect mechanisms to create tissue injury to both cutaneous and deeper structures. Electrical current is directly damaging to cell membranes as the flow of electrons will generate heat as they flow through the relative "high resistance" of these cellular structures. This mechanism creates entry and exit wounds often seen in electrical injury. As electrical energy travels through the body, it is converted to heat, and the severity of the injury is dependent on voltage, type of current (alternating vs. direct), the pathway traveled through the person's body, and the electrical resistance of tissues through which the electricity passes (least-to-most resistance: blood vessels, nerves, muscle, skin [wet < dry], tendon, fat, and bone). Bone has the highest resistance compared to other tissues, so it heats up the most with the conduction of electrical current. As a result, thermal injury to adjacent muscles can be severe, leading to occult compartment syndrome. Because of the hidden nature of this injury, often occurring underneath "normal" appearing skin, it is hard to recognize and can be fatal if missed. As a result, it is important to keep a high suspicion when triaging these patients.

Electrical injuries may be classified as either low voltage (<1000 V) or high voltage (≥1000 V). Low voltage typically damages tissues immediately surrounding the point of initial contact, while high voltage usually results in penetration to deeper organ systems. High-voltage injuries, especially from alternating current sources, create significant tetany of muscles throughout the body that may result in skeletal fracture, even of the spine, and sustained high-intensity contractions can lead to myocyte necrosis. This muscle damage causes myoglobinuria that can result in renal failure and hyperkalemia, which in turn may lead to life-threatening arrhythmias. Alternating current causes tetanic contractions that can prevent the victim from releasing the source, called the *no-let-go-phenomenon*, thereby resulting in prolonged contact with the electricity and thus more devastating injuries. Smaller body parts such as the hands, fingers, and feet tend to heat up to a greater extent because their heat dissipation capacity is less than larger body regions. In many cases, injuries to these structures will therefore result in greater tissue necrosis and subsequent morbidity (**FIGURE 11-11**).

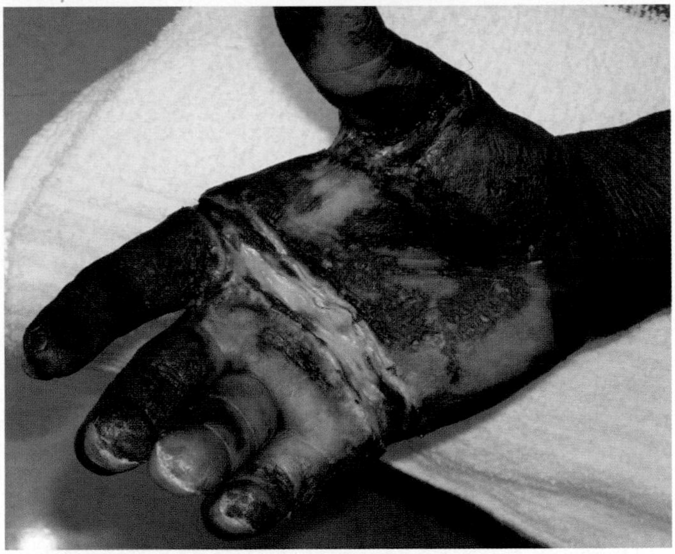

FIGURE 11-11 Electrical burn. Electrical burns on smaller body parts such as the hand frequently result in *full-thickness* tissue loss with necrosis. The patient with this type of wound should be referred to a regional burn center.

An electrical burn typically has three injury components that need to be evaluated: a true electrical energy injury from current flow, an arc or flash flame injury by a current arcing at a temperature around 7200°F from the source to the ground, and a flame injury via ignition of clothing. The extent of injury can be easily underestimated because the cutaneous phenotypic appearance may be limited, while underlying muscle necrosis may be extensive. Complications of electrical injuries include rhabdomyolysis leading to hyperkalemia, cardiac injury and arrhythmias, metabolic acidosis, myoglobinemia, and renal failure.

Treatment of electrical burns is focused on robust fluid hydration, correction of electrolyte abnormalities, and ensuring perfusion of damaged tissues. Muscle edema may also lead to compartment syndrome and should be suspected if the patient complains of progressive pain on passive extension and/or paresthesias. While compartment syndrome is often associated with the "5 Ps"—pale, paresthesias, poikilothermia, pain out of proportion on passive ranging, and pulselessness—it is important to recognize compartment syndrome early before pulselessness develops because the tissue damage is already extensive and irreversible by the time the extremity has lost pulses. Pain out of proportion to visible exam findings, particularly with passive ranging is often one of the earliest findings and should not be ignored. Once compartment syndrome is diagnosed, an emergent fasciotomy of all involved compartments is required to prevent progressive tissue hypoperfusion and necrosis. Cardiac arrest, ventricular fibrillation, and other arrhythmias are common within the first 48 hours

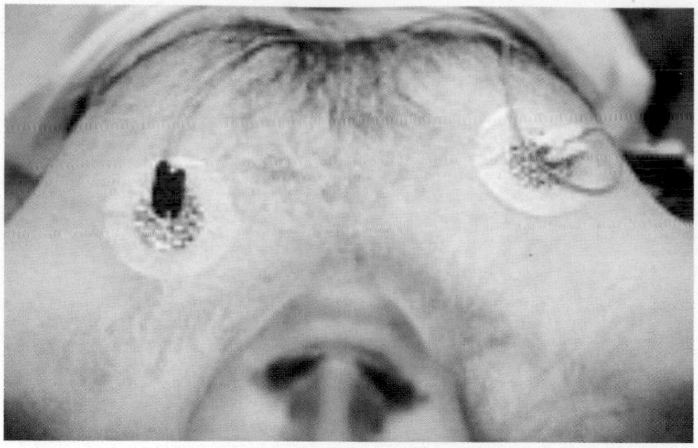

FIGURE 11-12 Lichtenberg figures with lacy ferning pattern seen on the upper chest. (Used with permission from Zafren K, Thurman R, Jones ID. Environmental conditions. In: Knoop KJ, Stack LB, Storrow AB, Thurman R, eds. *The Atlas of Emergency Medicine*. 3rd ed. New York, NY: McGraw-Hill; 2010: Chap. 16.)

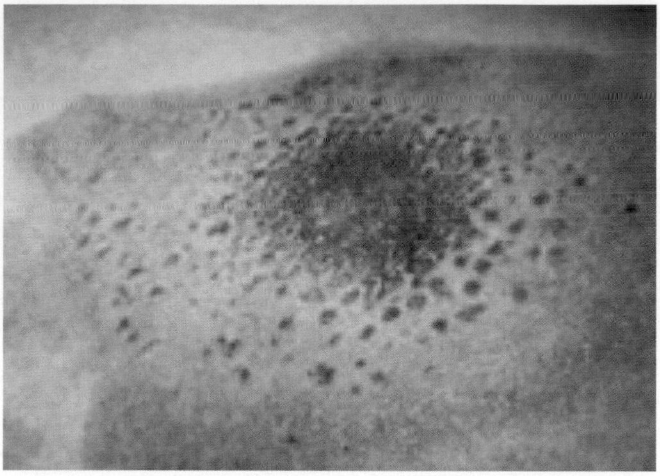

FIGURE 11-13 Punctate lightning burn. (Used with permission from Zafren K, Thurman R, Jones ID. Environmental conditions. In: Knoop KJ, Stack LB, Storrow AB, Thurman R, eds. *The Atlas of Emergency Medicine*. 3rd ed. New York, NY: McGraw-Hill; 2010: Chap. 16.)

and can be life-threatening. Indications for cardiac monitoring include documented ECG abnormalities, observed arrhythmias, postinjury electrolyte disturbances (e.g., hyper/hypokalemia, hyper/hypocalcemia), high voltage (≥1000 V) mechanism, large TBSA burn (>20%), and/or advanced age (>50 years). In addition, transient and permanent nerve injuries, including peripheral neuropathy, delayed transverse myelitis, and anterior spinal syndrome have been reported.

Lightning strikes are a rare type of electrical injury resulting from a direct current that can generate heat as high as 50,000°F. Due to the short duration of action, usually of 1–2 milliseconds, frank skin necrosis is uncommon. Patients typically demonstrate superficial skin manifestations of a fernlike pattern, termed *Lichtenberg figures*, which are related to the flow of electrons over the body surface (**FIGURE 11-12**). These lesions are transient, lasting only for 24 hours, and death is usually the result of cardiac arrest and apnea from direct effects of the current on the central nervous system. Lightning can also cause punctate wounds as seen in **FIGURE 11-13**.

Chemical

Chemical burns occur secondary to contact of the skin with strong acids or bases. The concentration of the agent, quantity, duration of contact, and the mechanism of action in a biological system are factors that determine the severity of the chemical burn injury. Acidic burns tend to be less severe since contact results in coagulation necrosis of the tissue that creates a denatured protein eschar which then acts as a physical barrier that impairs further penetration of the acid. In contrast, basic agents result in liquefactive tissue necrosis, which causes a deeper extension of injury due to protein hydrolysis and fat saponification, thereby creating a liquefied area of tissue that allows the base to penetrate underlying structures. Hydrofluoric acid (HF) is unique among acidic substances in that it also causes liquefactive necrosis, so the lack of a physical barrier from coagulative necrosis allows it to penetrate much deeper than other types of acid.

Initial management of chemical burns is focused on the removal of the agent from the skin by copious cool water irrigation for extended periods of time, often beyond 30 minutes. The use of warm water should be avoided because it can increase cutaneous porosity and chemical absorption. It is imperative that the irrigation be carried out in the form of lavage instead of submerging the patient in a contained space such as a tub, which will prolong skin contact with the caustic source. In addition, neutralization of the acid or base must never be performed as such a chemical reaction is exothermic in nature and would cause a concomitant thermal injury.

Although neutralization products are usually discouraged, there may be a known specific antidote when the chemical exposure is the result of a single agent. For example, a common acid used in industrial jobs is hydrofluoric (HF) acid. The fluoride ions chelate with positively charged ions in the body such as calcium and magnesium, causing an efflux of intracellular calcium that inhibits biological reactions which require these cations and/or specific transmembrane charge gradients. Fluoride ions will continue to react until neutralized by bivalent cations, thus, calcium gluconate gel or calcium gluconate injections may be used for the treatment of these wounds. For severe systemic disturbances of calcium from HF, intravenous calcium gluconate may be given to prevent life-threatening arrhythmias and atony (i.e., life-threatening, complete loss of muscle tone). For most chemical agents, antidotal information is available on the material safety data sheets (MSDS)—often found in labs, containers, or online—and should be reviewed to identify potential systemic toxicities as well as recommended treatment protocols. In addition, regional poison control agencies can be contacted for information on the toxicities of common household products.

In many cases, the exact chemical substance is unknown, so the MSDS or antidote cannot be determined; this is why aggressive water irrigation is recommended. However, newer neutralizing agents like Diphoterine have been developed to work against both acidic and basic substances. Diphoterine has multiple binding sites, allowing it to be effective with multiple chemicals, while not inducing a significant exothermic reaction.[13] It is both amphoteric (chelates both acids and bases) as well as hypertonic (prevents the penetration of the chemical into the tissue by drawing the fluid out of the cell) which makes it more effective for a broad range of caustic agents. For pH normalization, up to 17 times less volume of Diphoterine is required compared to water alone, and when compared with using distilled water or normal saline, it is known to remove the offending chemical up to four times faster. This reagent along with others is becoming increasingly available in Emergency Departments, so it is helpful to ask hospitals and clinics what is available in order to be prepared if a patient with an acute chemical burn requires care.

Radiation

With the increasing use of ionizing radiation as treatment for disease, particularly in oncology, more research has focused on understanding the effects of radiation on biological systems. The manifestations of radiation injury are dependent on the type of energy source, total dose and time administered, and the location and size of the exposed field (**TABLE 11-3**). Radiation is most effective on rapidly proliferating cells, making it efficacious for cancer therapy. However, it can also cause "bystander" effects to other normal rapidly proliferating cells in structures such as the skin, gastrointestinal tract, and hematopoietic system.

Radiation-induced skin injury can result in acute and chronic changes to tissues. Acute effects manifest within 6 weeks of radiation exposure as the radiation reacts with water molecules within the cell, causing free radical formation, double-stranded DNA breaks, cell cycle arrest, and apoptosis. In addition to damage to the epithelial and parenchymal cells, radiation induces blood vessel dilation, increased capillary permeability, activation of coagulation, and further necrosis of endothelial cells. Phenotypic changes associated with acute injury include erythema which appears similar to a superficial burn, and higher doses can result in *partial-thickness* injuries characterized as wet and dry desquamation (**FIGURE 11-14**). *Full-thickness* ulceration and frank necrosis can result from doses higher than 25 Gy (**FIGURE 11-15**). Acute effects are usually transient and are amenable to recovery through DNA repair mechanisms. After initial exposure to radiation, it takes up to 6 weeks for reversibly damaged epithelial and endothelial cells to recover. Chronic effects, however, can manifest months to years after radiation exposure and are progressive and permanent. The exact mechanism of chronic skin injury is not completely understood; however, there is persistent upregulation of many inflammatory cytokines. One of the most studied pathways in chronic radiation injury is TGF-β and downstream mediator SMAD3 that can signal fibroblasts to produce collagen and lead to extensive dermal fibrosis.[14,15]

TABLE 11-3 Skin Changes Associated with Radiation Dose

Dose	Skin Change
≥2 Gy	Erythema
12–20 Gy	Dry desquamation
>20 Gy	Moist desquamation
≥35 Gy	Necrosis

One Gy is the international system of units equivalent of 100 rads, which is equal to an absorbed dose of 1 J/kg of tissue.

Adapted from Kawamura M, Yoshimura M, Asada H, et al. A scoring system predicting acute radiation dermatitis in patients with head and neck cancer treated with intensity-modulated radiotherapy. *Radiat Oncol.* 2019;14(1):14.

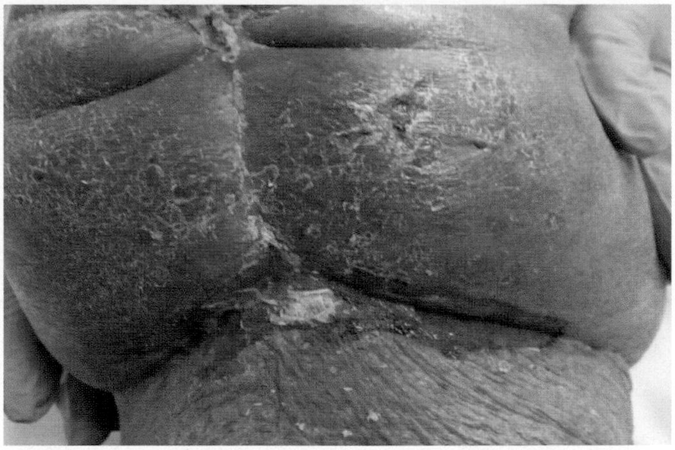

FIGURE 11-14 Acute radiation burn. Changes associated with acute radiation injury include erythema, which appears similar to a superficial burn. Higher doses can result in *partial-thickness* injuries characterized as wet and dry desquamation, as seen in this patient's face and neck radiation burns.

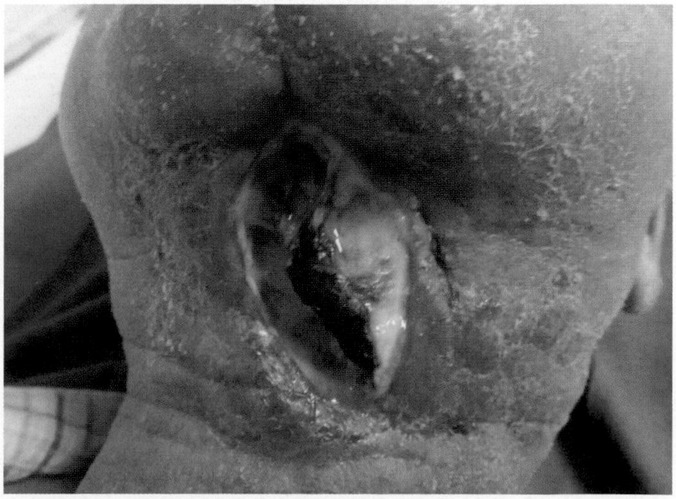

FIGURE 11-15 Chronic radiation burn. The necrosis, slough, and periwound skin changes including dry desquamation are a result of higher doses of radiation.

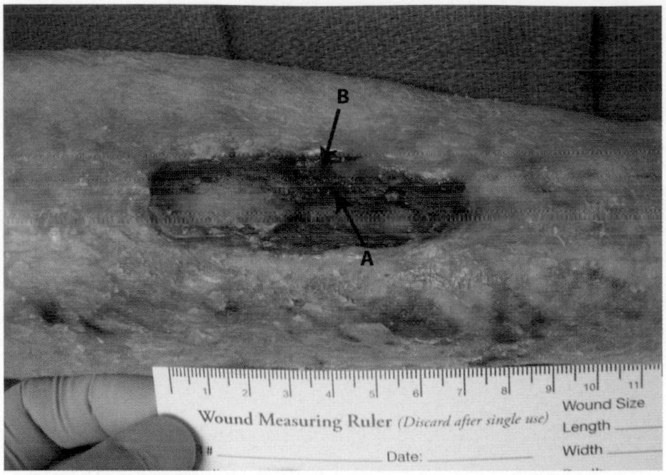

FIGURE 11-16 Chronic radiation wound. Chronic radiation wounds rarely heal without surgical intervention. Visible signs of radiation damage include necrotic bone, periwound skin changes with increased vascularity and sloughing, and loss of hair. Note (**A**) the granulation buds that are coming from the trabecular bone under the necrotic cortical layer (in the center) and (**B**) the recurrence of tumor tissue at the edge of the wound.

This is thought to be partly due to sclerosis of small arteries and arterioles, which results in local tissue ischemia and the subsequent release of inflammatory cytokines that promote T-lymphocyte recruitment and further activation of fibroblasts within the injured tissue—a process that creates fibrosis.

Other phenotypic characteristics of chronic radiation injury are alopecia, pigmentation changes, telangiectasia, impaired vascularity, the development of nonhealing wounds, secondary malignancies, and delayed wound healing after trauma or surgical procedures (**FIGURE 11-16**). There are limited treatment options for these patients and most wounds have low rates of complete resolution (**FIGURE 11-17**). Many patients require local debridement beyond the radiated tissue margins and autologous tissue coverage with local or free flaps.

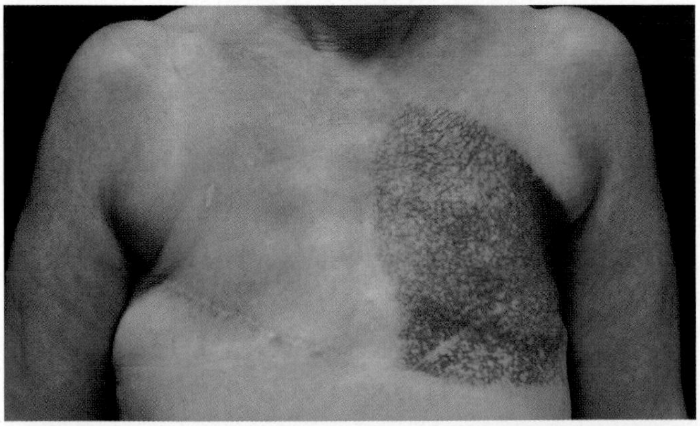

FIGURE 11-17 Chronic skin changes after radiation. Chronic skin changes after radiation can include pigmentation changes, telangiectasia, and impaired vascularity as seen in this patient who had radiation and reconstructive surgery for breast cancer.

Of recent interest in the literature is the use of lipoaspirated fat or adipose-derived stem cells for the treatment of radiation-induced chronic wounds. Studies have demonstrated that the application of autologous fat can lead to improvement and even complete resolution of chronic lesions induced by radiation.[16] Additional research needs to be conducted on the safety and efficacy of its potential therapeutic use, the long-term survival of the adipose tissue, and the potential malignant transformation of these multipotent stem cells.

Friction

A more recently recognized type of burn injury results from friction mechanisms and is often referred to as road rash (**FIGURE 11-18**). Friction burns create complex treatment challenges for burn providers because they consist of both the friction/tissue avulsion mechanism as well as the thermal component from the heat generated by the friction force. This dual mechanism usually creates an extensively contaminated wound bed that contains deeply imbedded environmental bacteria and foreign debris. The peripheral thermal injury along with the high levels of contamination increases patients' risk for soft tissue infections, significant scarring (e.g., hypertrophic or keloid), wound healing delays, and

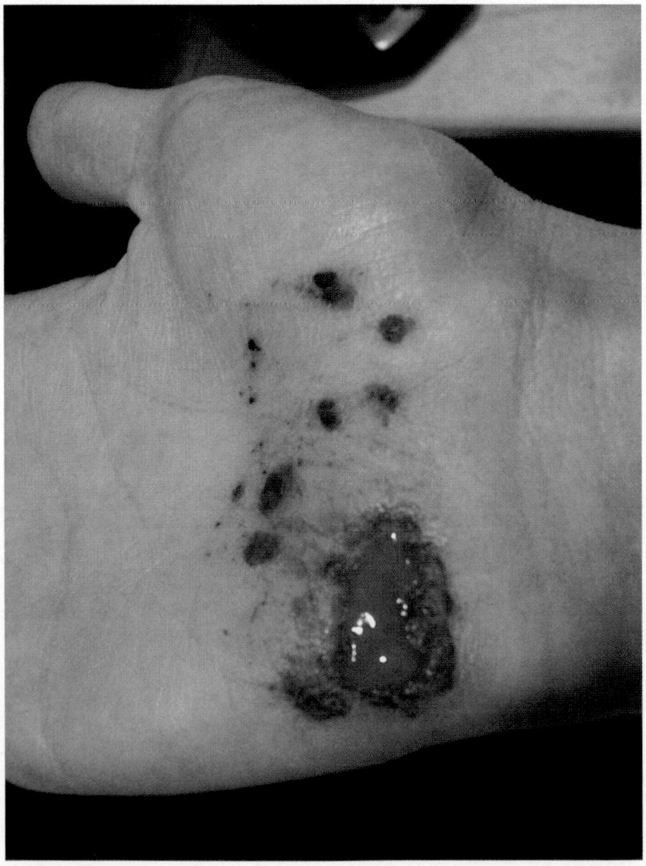

FIGURE 11-18 Friction wound. Friction wounds usually happen with moving vehicle accidents and are thus referred to as road rash. This patient's road rash on the hand was the result of a bicycle accident.

traumatic tattooing. Friction burns often occur due to high-force mechanisms such as motorcycle and car accidents that cause sheering and avulsing of tissues which can create Morel-Lavallee lesions as well as injury to underlying neurovascular and musculoskeletal structures. Because of this, practitioners should evaluate patients for injuries to the nerve, blood vessels, tendon, and bone on extremities that have friction burns.

Contact

Contact burns are the result of direct skin contact with hot or cold objects including metals, plastic, glass, or coal. The depth of penetration is related to the duration of contact and the temperature of the object. Although these burns are usually small in size, they may have deeper penetration that can result in extensive myonecrosis. One common area for contact burns is the hand, which can result in a significant functional impairment due to nerve and tendon necrosis. The severity of tissue injury often leads to wound contracture if the burn is allowed to heal without any surgical intervention. Treatment is therefore focused on expedient debridement of necrotic tissue and early grafting of areas with *deep partial-thickness* or *full-thickness* injuries in order to prevent functional impairments from the development of contracted hypertrophic scars. Evaluation of contact burns in susceptible populations such as children and the elderly must assess for inflicted or nonaccidental etiologies when clear lines of demarcation and multiple sites are observed, often with stories that do not match the burn pattern. Suspicion for nonaccidental injuries should be especially high in pediatric contact burns that have small circular patterns such as those arising from cigarettes.

Cold

Thermal injuries from temperatures at the cold end of the spectrum are often overlooked when addressing burn injuries because their geographical dependence often limits presentation to specific regional burn centers. Cold injuries have a slightly different categorization than other thermal injuries and are designated as frostnip (reversible, analogous to *first-degree* or *superficial* burns), superficial frostbite (irreversible; *partial-thickness* injury), and deep frostbite (irreversible; *full-thickness* injury). Cold injuries most commonly occur at temperatures below 28.4°F (−2°C) due to the slow freezing of tissues and subsequent intra- and extra-cellular crystal formation. The cellular damage is further exacerbated in the setting of repeated freeze-thaw cycles. Unlike high-temperature thermal injuries that tend to spread out from a central heat source, low-temperature etiologies result in injury that progresses along extremities from distal to proximal and involves other exposed structures such as the ears and nose. Because the insulating medium is mostly cold air, the injuries are circumferential in nature and rarely spare skin folds or creases, the opposite of what is seen in scald and contact mechanisms.

The factors that influence the extent of local tissue cold injury are the nadir tissue temperature, duration of exposure, rate of cooling, ischemia time, number of freeze-thaw cycles, and rewarming conditions. From a pathophysiological perspective, low temperatures result in vasoconstriction of peripheral vascular beds (i.e., extremities, nose, ears) to redirect blood from counter-exchange systems that would result in heat loss in order to preserve core temperature. This further exacerbates the cooling of the peripheral tissue, and additional counterproductive vasoconstriction occurs. At 15°C, maximal vasoconstriction is reached (local blood flow = 20–50 mL/min). To counteract this deleterious cycle, once skin temperatures drop below 15°C, the body undergoes a process called the *hunting response*—defined as cycles of vasodilation and vasoconstriction transiently every 5–10 minutes to facilitate rewarming of extremities and to minimize cold-induced tissue damage. The drawback of the *hunting response* is that it results in the delivery of cold blood to the central circulation, cooling the core, and eventually, the body must blunt the *hunting response* to maintain core temperatures. Once skin temperature reaches 10°C, neuropraxia occurs; and, below 0°C, cutaneous circulation is nearly absent, skin temperature drops 0.5°C/min, and true freezing occurs. Smaller vessels and the venous system are the first to freeze as the increased blood viscosity more easily occludes smaller diameters and lower flow rate vessels.

While rapid freezing—often seen with liquid nitrogen and other industrial accidents—causes intracellular ice crystal formation, the more common slow cooling from environmental exposure starts with extracellular crystal formation. The extracellular crystals create an osmotic pressure gradient that dehydrates cells, creates electrolyte shifts, and induces acid–base disturbances. The ice crystals may further cause direct harm to adjacent cell membranes. Endothelial cells are also injured, which, when combined with the increased blood viscosity and activation of clotting cascade from adjacent tissue damage, results in thrombosis of the microvasculature and further tissue ischemia. Studies show that the greatest degree of tissue injury is actually caused by the thawing or rewarming of the tissue due to the initiation of reperfusion injury. In particular, restoration of perfusion to the ischemic tissues results in the generation of free oxygen radicals, prostaglandin-induced vasoconstriction, leukocyte diapedesis, and clot formation through platelet aggregation.

Superficial frostbite often presents with hyperemia, numbness, and clear or serous blisters (**FIGURE 11-19**). These injuries often are painful on rewarming and sensation is a positive prognostic factor. Deep frostbite results in hemorrhagic blisters due to the propagation of tissue injury into the reticular dermis and the underlying subdermal vascular plexus that can further involve muscle and bone (**FIGURE 11-20**). Poor prognostic findings include hemorrhagic blebs proximally distributed on the affected limb in the setting of cold distal tissue that appears ischemic and insensate. Deep frostbite has a firm, woody feel with a blue-gray appearance as opposed to the supple hyperemic character of superficial frostbite. Furthermore, unlike superficial injuries, deeper injuries remain insensate after thawing.

Although the evaluation and treatment of thermal injuries are addressed in the following section, the unique nature of

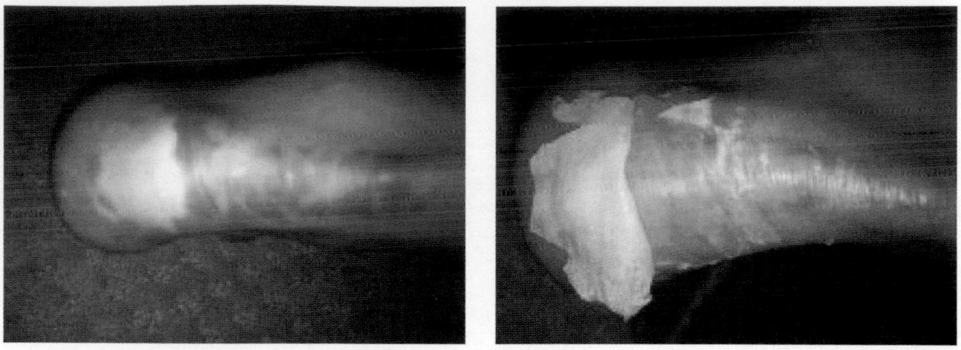

FIGURE 11-19 Superficial frostbite. **A.** Superficial frostbite on the Achilles of an individual who placed a commercial cold pack directly onto the skin with no protective interface material. **B.** The thick blister peeling off with new epithelium beneath. The wound healed with no intervention except time and protection.

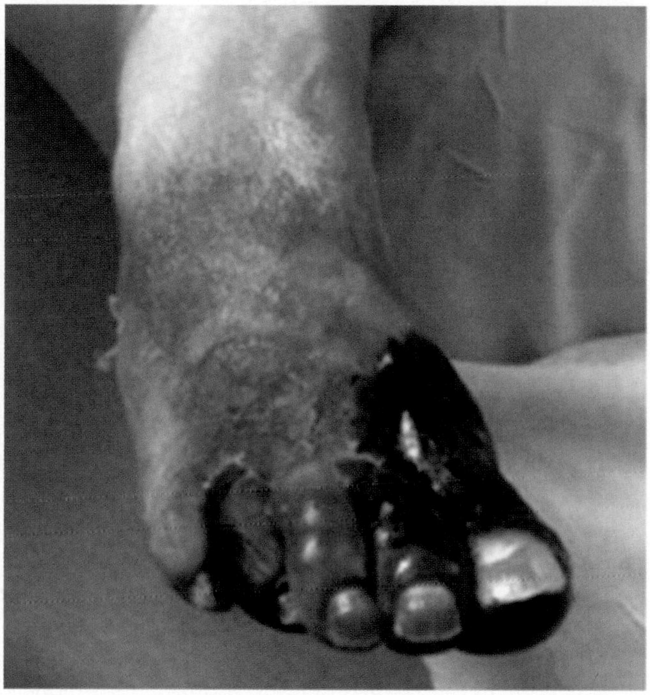

FIGURE 11-20 Deep frostbite. Deep frostbite shows signs of deep tissue injury, edema, erythema, and necrosis. (Used with permission from Dean SM, Satiani B, Abraham WT. *Color Atlas and Synopsis of Vascular Diseases*. New York: McGraw-Hill; 2014, Figure 86-2.)

frostbite treatment is discussed in this section. The first step in the management of frostbite injuries is to rapidly rewarm the affected extremity for 15–20 minutes with water heated to 38–42°C. Conversion of the frostbitten area to a pliable, soft, and red or purple color indicates the end of rewarming. Numerous studies have looked at the value of different interventions for improving post-rewarming outcomes with varied results. Some studies have shown that amputation rates are decreased with tissue plasminogen activator (tPA) administration within 24 hours of rewarming. The practice of blister deroofing in frostbite is controversial but numerous burn specialists have advocated for aspirating or debriding clear and yellow blisters which classically contain prostaglandin F_{2a} and thromboxane A_2, both of which damage underlying tissue through platelet aggregation and thrombosis. Hemorrhagic blisters are often left intact as these injuries are deeper and often do not benefit from deroofing like the clear or yellow blisters. The exposed wound beds from denuded blisters may be dressed with topical antimicrobials in a similar fashion to other burn injuries. Some data exist to specifically support the use of aloe vera, a topical thromboxane inhibitor, on frostbite injuries. Surgical interventions in frostbite injury are often deferred at least 10–14 days to allow the irreversible cell injury to fully declare itself and the wound to demarcate. Acute surgery is rarely performed but may be done in the case of compartment syndrome associated with severe frostbite injury. Multiple authors including D. Shenaq and L. Gottlieb have emphasized the value of triple-phase bone scans in identifying delineations between viable and nonviable bone by their ability to track bone perfusion over the course of the first few days, thereby providing a high predictive value for final amputation level.[17,18]

INITIAL EVALUATION AND MANAGEMENT OF A BURN WOUND

Healing a burn injury depends on appropriate decision-making, which begins at the time of initial assessment. The history and exact mechanism of injury, plus a comprehensive physical examination and extent of the burn, are critical to providing an optimal outcome. The evaluation of the entire patient includes a thorough medical and surgical history, systemic premorbid conditions such as diabetes and cardiovascular disease, current medications, prior trauma to the affected area, and any preinjury functional deficits. This is critical to planning the treatment of a patient with a burn injury. Burns can be relatively small and self-limiting or can be massively devastating and lead to multisystem derangements. Accurate initial evaluation determines the path to success.

Initial Assessment

Initial evaluation of the burned patient should be focused on determining whether the patient would be best treated in an outpatient or inpatient setting, and if treatment at an ABA-certified center and critical care in an intensive care unit are required. This may be rapidly accomplished by applying the ABCs of trauma evaluation and ABA Burn Center Transfer Criteria. Concern for airway stability is evaluated by history and physical examination. Burns that include flame injury or explosions are suspicious for inhalation injury, especially those that occurred in a burning structure or enclosed space. Facial burns, singed facial hair, coughing, hoarseness, voice changes, and stridor may indicate the presence of inhalation injury. Physical examination of breathing and ventilatory capacity should be rapidly evaluated with lung auscultation and observation of a patient's breathing mechanics. Progressively worsening tachypnea, labored breathing, accessory muscle use, and other signs of pending respiratory failure need to be identified rapidly and treated immediately with endotracheal intubation and mechanical ventilation. Even small surface burns can have severe inhalation injury, so patients who present with these findings should be quickly triaged to critical care pathways. Following intubation, formal bronchoscopy should be performed to assess whether or not inhalation injury is present and to what extent (e.g., how far down the bronchial tree, degree of mucosal sloughing, amount of carbonaceous debris) in order to help guide ventilation management, respiratory and systemic treatments, and fluid resuscitation. In addition to the impact of inhalation injury on respiratory status, circumferential burn wounds located around the torso can form leathery eschar that compresses and compromises chest expansion, perfusion, and ventilation. Noncircumferential torso injuries that are *full-thickness* can create a noncompliant eschar that impairs chest excursion and thereby prevent adequate ventilation. As such, it is important to closely examine diaphragmatic dynamics and chest wall mechanics during respiration in the setting of any circumferential or *full-thickness* injury to the torso.

Similarly, circumferential burns around the extremities can constrict perfusion to the more distal tissues through a tourniquet effect, resulting in ischemia and compartment syndrome. Frequent examination of peripheral pulses and neuromuscular exams are critical in identifying patients who may require escharotomies. In these cases, prompt escharotomy (defined as a sharp or electrocautery incision through the entirety of the eschar into adjacent unburned tissue) is warranted to separate the constricting band of eschar and relieve compression (**FIGURE 11-21**). Other areas where burn eschar may create restrictive complications in the setting of progressive burn wound edema are around the neck and orbit. Circumferential neck burns require frequent reassessment of airway patency and evaluation for any signs of neurological decline. Severe facial burns with periorbital eschar can result in orbital compartment syndrome, in which case frequent intraocular pressure assessments are required to identify patients who may require decompressive lateral canthotomies. When assessing burn depth, the single most important maneuver on the physical exam is palpation of the burn wound. A single maneuver such as dragging a finger across the wound bed with moderate pressure will facilitate the assessment of blanching, moisture, and sensation within seconds. Very rapidly, details for determining burn depth may be acquired.

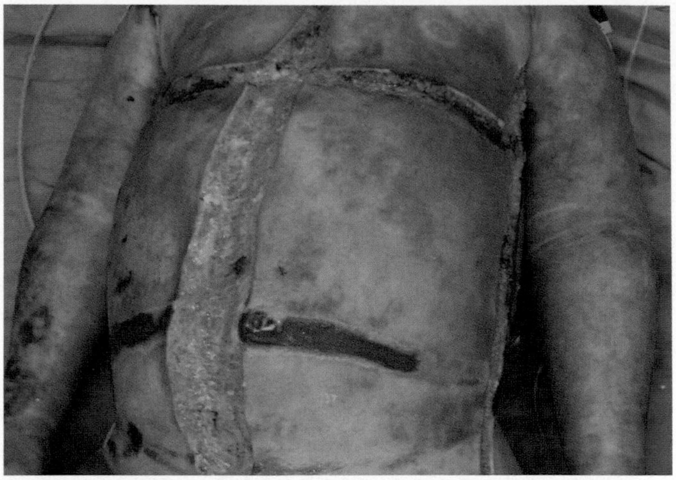

FIGURE 11-21 Escharotomy of a circumferential burn. Circumferential burn wounds located around the torso can form leathery eschar that compresses and compromises chest expansion, perfusion, and ventilation. Similarly, circumferential burns around the extremities can constrict perfusion to the extremities, resulting in compartment syndromes. In these cases, prompt escharotomy is warranted to separate the constricting band of eschar to relieve compression.

Fluid Requirements

Patients who sustain over 20% TBSA burns are at risk of circulatory abnormalities (a.k.a., burn shock) that compromise tissue perfusion and can lead to end-organ failure as well as progression of the burn wound to a deeper depth. The goal of fluid resuscitation, therefore, is to maintain adequate end-organ perfusion in the setting of burn shock. The pathophysiology of burn shock is not completely understood; however, significant fluid shifts caused by the leakage of fluid and protein from the intravascular space into the interstitial space due to increased capillary permeability create hypovolemia. In addition, the release of inflammatory mediators from the burn area creates a hyperdynamic response in extreme cases and can lead to excessive systemic inflammatory responses with coagulopathy, excessive vasodilation, hemodynamic instability, and organ failure. Patients with critical-sized burns—often greater than 20% TBSA—require large amounts of fluid resuscitation to prevent organ damage. The Parkland formula is often used to estimate the initial fluid requirement in relation to the body surface area of burn and the patient's weight. The current formula is:

$$4\text{ cc} \times \text{weight (kilograms)} \times \%\text{TBSA burn} = \text{24-hour intravenous fluid (IVF) requirement}$$

An alternative, the Brooke Formula uses 2 cc instead of 4 cc in the calculation and is favored by many burn units due to

CASE STUDY

INTRODUCTION

A 30-year-old female presents to the emergency department with a scald injury to her abdomen and left thigh sustained when a pot of boiling water accidentally spilled on her while she was cooking She has no significant past medical history, allergies, or social issues and her BMI is 25 (**FIGURES 11-22** and **11-23**).

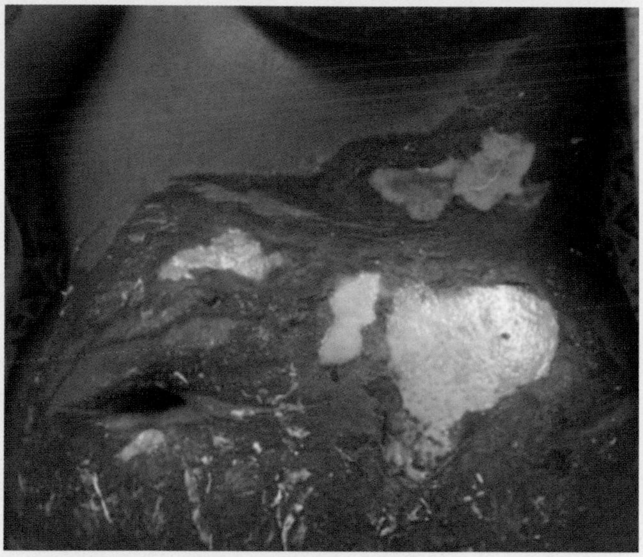

FIGURE 11-22 Abdominal burn wound.

DISCUSSION QUESTIONS

1. How is the patient's burn classified?
2. What would be the total burn surface area using the Rule of Nines? How about Palmar Surface Area?

Evaluation reveals extensive blistering of the skin that is painful, consistent with *superficial partial-thickness* injury. There are also areas of pale, nonblanching, and dry dermis with diminished sensation, consistent with either *deep partial-thickness* or *full-thickness* injury. The TBSA is

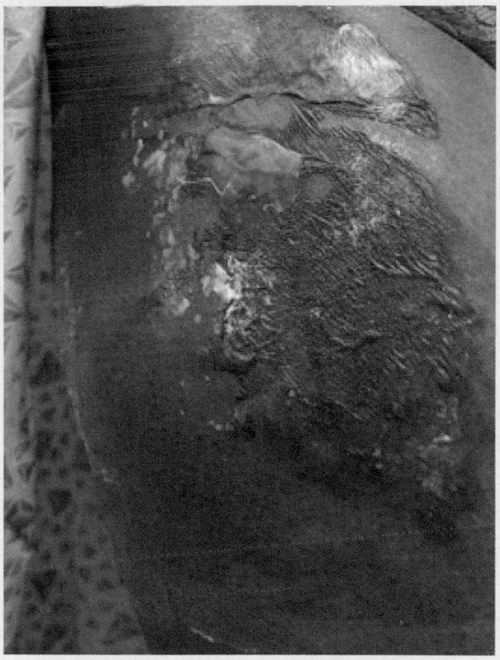

FIGURE 11-23 Burn wound on the left thigh.

determined to be 8% (5% for the abdomen and 3% for the left thigh). The patient is determined to be hemodynamically stable with no substantial fluid loss. She remains alert and oriented ×4, but complains of 8–10/10 pain using the analog scale.

DISCUSSION QUESTIONS

1. What would be the immediate plan of action seconds after sustaining the burn?
2. What would be the best plan of care based on evaluation in the emergency room?
3. What are the major concerns for a patient with scalding wounds during the first 48 hours of treatment?
4. Should this patient be admitted to the intensive care or burn unit?

multiple studies showing over-resuscitation with the 4 cc estimation. Whether 2 or 4 cc is used in the equation, the standard implementation of the calculated number is to give one-half of the estimated fluid requirement over the first 8 hours and the remaining half over the following 16 hours. It is important to note that the *target time intervals for resuscitation start from the initial time of burn injury*, not the time that intravenous fluids are started. In other words, if a patient is extricated from a car fire and arrives in an emergency room 3 hours after the initial injury, the first half of calculated fluids should be delivered over the next 5 hours as opposed to 8 hours. This formula provides only a rough estimate to guide the initial hourly infusion rate and theoretical 24-hour requirement with subsequent adjustments based on clinical response. Proper fluid resuscitation must be assessed by closely monitoring the patient's hourly urine output, which should be maintained at 0.5–1.0 cc/kg/h, through the insertion of an indwelling Foley catheter. Resuscitation infusion rates are then titrated to achieve the desired urine output (UOP) goals and to maintain mean arterial pressures greater than 60-65 mmHg. Vigilant titration of fluids to the target parameters is important to avoid under- and over-resuscitation, both of which can have significant clinical sequelae. Under-resuscitation can lead to burn wound conversion and/or global end-organ damage due to hypoperfusion, whereas over-resuscitation can cause excessive local and systemic interstitial edema that may result in extremity and abdominal compartment syndromes as well as impaired wound healing. After the first 8 hours of resuscitation, increasing IVF requirements to maintain UOP goals may indicate a phenomenon known as "*fluid creep*" (defined as increased third spacing of IVFs). The initiation of colloid resuscitation helps preserve intravascular volume while reducing overall IVF requirements due to third space losses. If a patient has a large enough burn—often above 20% TBSA—to require fluid resuscitation, intubation, or ICU care, direct management should be provided by a physician trained in burn critical care. The details of managing burns to this extent are beyond the scope of this chapter, but it is important to appreciate their complexity so that patients can be appropriately transferred to specialized care when indicated.

Nutritional Requirements

Large burn injuries result in a hypermetabolic state that begins soon after injury and can persist for weeks to months, even after complete coverage of the wound. Burns greater than 30% TBSA in adults and 20% in children may increase basal metabolic rates by up to twofold, necessitating intensive nutritional supplementation protocols. Even in smaller TBSA burns, the increased caloric requirements are significant, and failure to achieve those needs results in burn wound conversion and delayed healing. Two equations commonly used to predict the caloric requirements are the *Curreri* formula and the *Harris–Benedict* formula (**TABLE 11-4**). The *Curreri* equation has been reported to overestimate and the *Harris–Benedict* formula to underestimate the exact requirements; thus, an average of the two equations is commonly used. A significant amount of protein is required to prevent protein catabolism and muscle wasting. An estimated requirement of 2 g/kg/day is used by some groups, while others take into consideration the TBSA using the equation of 1 g/kg/day + (3 g × % TBSA). Nitrogen balance studies are recommended on a regular basis in order to ensure that sufficient protein intake is maintained. The goal is to start enteral feeding within the first 48 hours to preserve mucosal integrity throughout the gastrointestinal tract and prevent bacterial translocation through the compromised mucosal lining. Insertion of nasogastric tubes (e.g., Dobhoff tube) facilitates early initiation of enteral feeding. Previously, post-pyloric positioning was preferred over gastric placement as studies showed decreased rates of feeding intolerance and potentially aspiration events. Furthermore, studies in general surgery and burn populations showed continuous perioperative feeding with post-pyloric placement did not increase aspiration rates and ensured continued caloric supplementation. However, gastric feeding has benefits, such as gastroprotective effects against Curling's Ulcers, the ability for bolus feeding, and a more physiologic activation of the digestive cascade. Parenteral feeding may also be used in patients who have contraindications to enteral feeding such as bowel obstruction, ileus, intestinal discontinuity, abdominal compartment syndrome, or some other malabsorptive pathology; but it has been associated with increased infection and mortality rates, so it is frequently avoided unless absolutely indicated.

TABLE 11-4 Formulas for Nutritional Requirements of a Burn Patient

Curreri Formula
25 kcal × Weight (kg) + 40 kcal × %TBSA burn
Harris–Benedict Equation
$\frac{\text{Men}}{66.4730} + (13.7516 \times \text{Weight (kg)}) + (5.0033 \times \text{Height (cm)}) - (6.7550 \times \text{Age (years)})$
$\frac{\text{Women}}{655.0955} + (9.5634 \times \text{Weight (kg)} + (1.8496 \times \text{Height (cm)}) - (4.6756 \times \text{Age (years)})$

Note: The Curreri formula and Harris–Benedict equation can both be used to calculate the calorie requirements for a patient recovering from burns. The hypermetabolic state, especially in cases of large total burn surface area, requires greater calorie and protein intake in order for the body to synthesize new tissue.

Pain Control

Patients with burns may experience significant pain that is both challenging to control and may persist for a very long time. Current recommendations focus on the management of three aspects of pain: breakthrough, background, and procedural. The goals of pain management are to provide a sufficient amount of pain relief without oversedation in order to allow the burn patient to comfortably engage in dressing changes and participate in rehabilitation exercises.[19] Treatment strategies should be individualized and multimodal in nature, including the use of analgesics, sedatives, and anxiolytics. Utilization of multiple analgesics that alter pain signaling through different pathways (e.g., mu-opioid, arachidonic, Cox-2, GABA, local or regional blocks) or at different sites within the pain pathway is ideal to maximize the total anesthetic effect.[20] Conscious sedation with agents such as fentanyl, ketamine, and propofol is becoming increasingly popular for procedural interventions and dressing changes to provide analgesic and anxiolytic benefits with a potential reduction in treatment-related trauma.[21,22] Other well-validated strategies for pain management in burned patients include cognitive behavior therapy,[23] music,[24,25] virtual reality,[26] and computer tablet distraction (studied in the pediatric population[27]). Adequate pain control is assessed by monitoring the patient's vital signs, administration of pain scales, and patient reporting using one of the pain scales discussed in Chapter 3, Examination and Evaluation of the Patient with a Wound. Appropriate pain management is crucial as the literature indicates that uncontrolled pain acts as a major physiologic stress that can negatively impact wound healing and patient recovery while also contributing to post-burn depression, anxiety, and posttraumatic stress disorder.[28] The psychological sequelae of inadequate pain control has been shown to be even more severe in pediatric populations due to numerous contributing factors, but, because of this increased propensity, it is important to be aware of children's pain and adequately treat it when identified.

TREATMENT

Once the initial patient evaluation is completed and life-threatening injuries are assessed and managed, care is directed toward assessing the extent of burn injury and wound treatment. Evaluation of the burn wound is directed at identifying the location, extent, and depth of the burn injury. These characteristics of the burn can then be used to assess the healing potential of the wound and determine which interventions will be necessary.

Superficial Burns

Once a *superficial* burn is diagnosed according to the specifications noted above, treatment is generally supportive. Initial treatment with cool, not cold, compresses can provide relief. Ice packs, while they may provide pain relief, can actually cause burn wounds to convert to deeper injuries due to excessive vasoconstriction and subsequent hypoperfusion of the already injured tissue. These burns can be quite painful, so appropriate analgesia with nonsteroidal anti-inflammatory drugs or codeine may be used as needed. The dermal barrier is not violated, but epidermal desquamation or "peeling" occurs; this can be treated effectively with topical moisturizing lotions. In addition, aloe vera provides both cooling and analgesic effects in *superficial* burns. Because the barrier function of the skin is intact in a *superficial* burn, topical antimicrobial treatment is not required. Ultimately, long-term contraction and scarring are not encountered, although occasionally transient skin color changes may be noted, especially in patients of *Fitzpatrick Type III* and above.

Superficial Partial-Thickness Burns

Burns that completely disrupt the epidermal barrier are more serious and must be promptly evaluated and diagnosed. *Superficial partial-thickness* burns often have large fluid-containing blisters that should be drained and the skin debrided so that the true depth of the wound can be evaluated. These burns, as a result of this epidermal disruption, are at risk for infection and should be treated with some form of antimicrobial dressing. Prophylactic systemic antibiotics have consistently been shown to be unnecessary while also predisposing patients to colonization by multidrug-resistant organisms. Because of this, systemic antibiotics are not given prophylactically regardless of burn size.

Topical Antibiotic Dressings

Silver sulfadiazine (Silvadene) has been the most widely used ointment in the burn population. Silvadene has broad-spectrum antibiotic coverage; however, the silver ion carrier has limited potential for penetrating the burn eschar, making it useful for *superficial* and *deep partial-thickness* injuries. Side effects of Silvadene include thrombocytopenia and neutropenia, which may be monitored through labs but is often unnecessary as the neutropenia that develops is not functionally significant and has no impact on infection rates. In addition, this medication should be avoided in patients with sulfonamide allergies, pregnant or nursing women, and infants younger than 2 months.[29] Another downside of Silvadene is the tendency for it to form a pseudoeschar on deeper *partial-thickness* burns. This pseudoeschar develops when old Silvadene is not completely removed prior to the application of new cream, and it creates a thickened, yellowish eschar that complicates burn wound assessment, may be mistaken for pus or infection, and can impair wound healing. As a result, its use in an outpatient setting should be avoided in patients where pain control or compliance with daily dressing changes may be a concern.

Mafenide acetate (Sulfamylon) is another topical antimicrobial agent that has broad-spectrum coverage; however, unlike Silvadene, it has good penetration of burn eschar and cartilage. One side effect of Sulfamylon is that systemic absorption can cause metabolic acidosis through inhibition of carbonic anhydrase, although it is reversible when application is stopped. Also, Sulfamylon can cause burning pain during application that may limit its use in certain patient populations like children and those with larger TBSA burns. As a result, Sulfamylon is often reserved for wounds infected with *Pseudomonas aeruginosa*, deep burns over cartilaginous structures (e.g., ears, nose), and burns with thick eschars.

Silver nitrate is another topical antimicrobial agent with broad coverage and, in contrast to Sulfamylon, does not induce pain upon application. Side effects include hyponatremia, hypochloremia, and on rare occasions methemoglobinemia. Silver nitrate is no longer used as frequently as in the past given its suboptimal coverage spectrum, especially in the setting of newer topical antimicrobials and silver-based non-daily dressings.

Of the commonly used silver delivery dressings, nanocrystalline silver has been shown to be the most potent silver delivery system as compared to hydrofiber and foam dressings that are impregnated with silver and thus more effective in preventing infection, facilitating healing, and shortening the length of stay.[30]

Sodium Hypochlorite and Hypochlorous Acid

Classically, Dakin's solution was used as a topical antimicrobial solution deriving its effect from sodium hypochlorite (NaOCl). In order to avoid severe cytotoxicity, it has been progressively diluted down to 0.5% and has consequently lost more than 95% of its antimicrobial effects. Newer products composed of 0.03% hypochlorous acid (H^+OCl^-) have antimicrobial and antifungal effects without the cytotoxicity seen with clinically effective doses of Dakin's solution. As a result, the use of 0.03% hypochlorous acid as an irrigating agent for skin grafts, debrided wounds, and with other topical enzymatic debriding agents has become an increasingly useful option in the burn wound management arsenal.

Silver-Impregnated Dressings

The use of silver-impregnated dressings has gained favor since they are changed less frequently than other antimicrobial dressings (i.e., every 3-7 days as opposed to daily) and can provide adequate antimicrobial coverage of the burn wound due to the silver. These dressings come from a variety of manufacturers and can be used with or without sterile water, allowing for both the moist wound environment and the elution of the active silver ions to prevent infection. These dressings are less ideal in dynamic *deep partial-thickness* wounds where the nondaily nature of the dressing change may result in delayed identification of wound progression and missed opportunity to intervene.

Enzymatic Debridement

For over two decades, various organic extracts from citrus fruits and bacteria have been used as enzymatic debriding agents. Enzymatic debriding agents derived from pineapple (i.e., bromelain) contain proteolytic and hydrolytic capabilities that result in the decomposition of collagen and other necrotic tissue components in *partial-thickness* burn wounds. Other enzymatic debriding agents such as collagenase, which are derived from fermenting *Clostridium histolyticum*, provide a slower yet effective chemical debridement of *partial-thickness* burn wounds in comparison to the faster-acting yet more painful citrus-derived enzymes. Enzymatic debridement is optimally used in mixed *partial-thickness* burns to facilitate the removal of pseudoeschar, coagulum, and other debris over the course of hours to days to allow for a more accurate burn depth assessment. After 1–3 days of enzymatic debridement, it is often easier to delineate between *superficial* and *deep partial-thickness* burns to determine which will require surgery for debridement and grafting. Studies have shown that enzymatic topical ointments decrease the rate of surgical interventions such as tangential debridement and grafting for mixed *partial-thickness* burns due to their ability to eliminate inflammatory necrotic tissues from the wound while also preventing infection.[31]

Deep Partial-Thickness and *Full-Thickness*

Partial-thickness injuries are divided into *superficial* and *deep* designations, primarily to define those wounds which need surgical intervention. *Superficial partial-thickness* injuries will likely heal within 2–3 weeks if appropriate antibiotic dressings are applied due to the preservation of the stem cell and fibroblast populations within the reticular dermis. As discussed above, the use of enzymatic debridement may decrease the number of *superficial* and mixed *partial-thickness* burns that would otherwise require surgical debridement. *Deep partial-thickness* and *full-thickness* injuries will often take longer than 3 weeks to heal due to their lack of necessary skin appendages and cell populations; therefore, the delayed healing of these burns leads to more scarring and tissue distortion. The prolonged inflammatory response present in wound beds with protracted closure times stimulates increased fibroblast activity that results in more collagen deposition and matrix metallopeptidase activity which in turn impairs collagen reorganization and stabilization of the extracellular matrix. These are two of the main reasons that burn wounds that take longer than 3 weeks to heal have a significantly higher risk (56% vs. 8%)[32] for developing hypertrophic scarring and their associated sequelae. For this reason, early identification of *deep partial-thickness* and *full-thickness* burns facilitates timely debridement and wound coverage to avoid or ameliorate these scar contracture issues.

Surgical Treatment

Surgical management is required for *full-thickness* injuries as well as many *deep partial-thickness* injuries that do not show signs of timely re-epithelialization. The goal of surgical management is the removal of nonviable tissue, restoration of the physioimmunologic barrier, and recreation of ideal aesthetics in sensitive areas (e.g., face, hands, genitalia, breasts, and feet). Tangential excision is employed to remove necrotic and nonviable tissues in consecutive layers until healthy viable tissue is encountered. Surgical debridement can be challenging because of the large amount of blood loss that is associated with this procedure. Careful excisional procedures that employ intralesional epinephrine injections (frequently at dilutions of 1:1,000,000 in normal saline) and application of epinephrine-soaked telfa nonadherent gauze (1:100,000 dilution for topical application) can decrease blood loss and increase the amount of surface area that can be safely covered in a single surgery. Excision procedures are performed with the goal of sparing viable tissue while removing nonviable tissue in preparation for coverage with skin grafts or flaps from an unburned part of the body. This level of debridement is also a critical step toward the application of cellular/acellular matrix products that are frequently used in burn care.[33,34]

Autologous tissue, most often in the form of skin grafts, is the gold standard for permanent wound coverage in most *deep partial* and *full-thickness* burn wounds. Skin grafts can be split-thickness (STSG), which involves the epidermis and part of the dermis, or *full-thickness* (FTSG), which involves the entirety of the epidermis and dermis. STSGs can be meshed—frequently 1:1.5, 1:2, and 1:3 but up to 1:8—to expand for maximal coverage relative to the donor site size. In addition, meshing may promote better graft survival because the graft is less prone to retaining fluid collections (e.g., hematoma, seroma) beneath the skin (**FIGURE 11-24**). FTSGs are thought to be more aesthetically pleasing since color match and texture may better match the reconstructed area while having lower contracture and scarring rates in comparison to burns covered with STSG. However, there is limited donor site availability for FTSGs, the harvesting process is more labor-intensive, the risk of graft

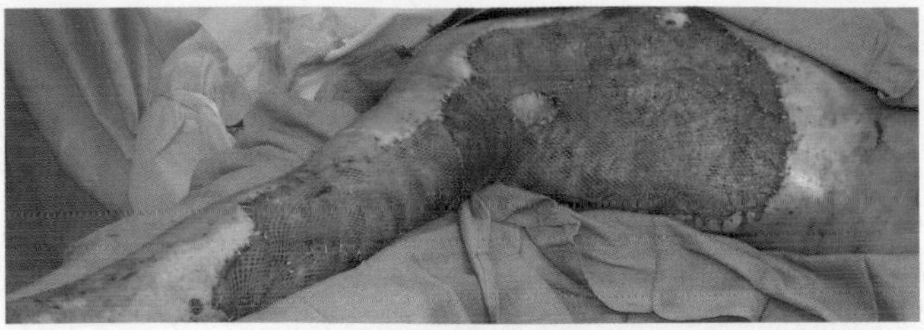

FIGURE 11-24 Meshed split-thickness skin graft. Meshing the donor skin of a STSG enables the skin to cover a larger area and prevents the pooling of fluid under the graft.

loss is higher due to greater metabolic demands of the tissue, and they are subject to greater failure from hematoma and seroma formation under the grafts. Along with the aesthetic benefits of FTSGs, they develop less secondary contracture (graft contracture during the course of the healing process) than STSGs because they have the entire dermal extracellular matrix that better resists contractile fibroblast forces. As a result, they are better suited to covering joints and other highly mobile regions where the consequences of graft contracture are more severe and disabling. Due to their limited donor site availability, FTSGs are generally reserved for use in secondary reconstruction of the face, hands, and genitalia (**FIGURE 11-25**) where contracture may lead to debilitating functional and aesthetic deficits. Skin can be harvested from unburned parts of the patient's body in a manner that minimizes further disfigurement by hiding the donor sites within "short" and "shirt" clothing boundaries. Patients who sustain large surface area burns may have limited donor site availability and therefore any available donor site must be used to achieve coverage. These patients benefit from staged coverage procedures that allow the donor sites to re-epithelialize for later repeat harvest—a process that often takes two or more weeks depending on a patient's healing potential and nutrition optimization.

Biologic dressings (also referred to as cellular/acellular matrix products or CAMPs) can be used as a temporizing method of wound coverage to prevent further fluid evaporation and heat loss while also lowering the rates of wound infection.

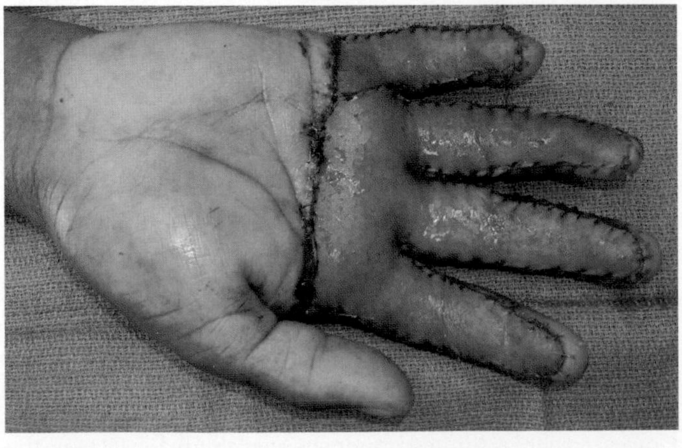

FIGURE 11-25 ***Full-thickness* skin graft on a hand.**

The most commonly used biologic dressing is *allograft* (i.e., human cadaveric skin). When placed on a healthy wound bed, it promotes revascularization and prevents desiccation, but it will undergo rejection within 1–2 weeks as the newly formed capillary beds facilitate delivery of immune cells to the allograft's dermis and immune-mediated rejection occurs. A potential disadvantage is the transmission of communicable diseases from the donor to the patient, in particular, there is a risk of cytomegalovirus. *Xenografts* (i.e., skin from another species, commonly porcine) are another option for temporary coverage. Xenografts have suboptimal adherence, higher incidence of infections, and poor revascularization which decreases their desirability.

Integra (Integra LifeSciences, Plainsboro, NJ) is a dermal matrix composed of bovine collagen cross-linked with shark chondroitin 6-sulfate glycosaminoglycan and an outer silicone dual-layer membrane. It serves as a scaffold for the ingrowth of fibroblasts and blood vessels, and the silicone membrane acts as a temporary barrier to retain heat and water while reducing infection risk compared to open burn wounds (**FIGURE 11-26**). Another newer option with similar application is NovoSorb Biodegradable Temporizing Matrix (BTM) (PolyNovo Biomaterials Pty Ltd, Victoria, Australia) which consists of a synthetic 2-mm bioabsorbable polymer matrix covered by a

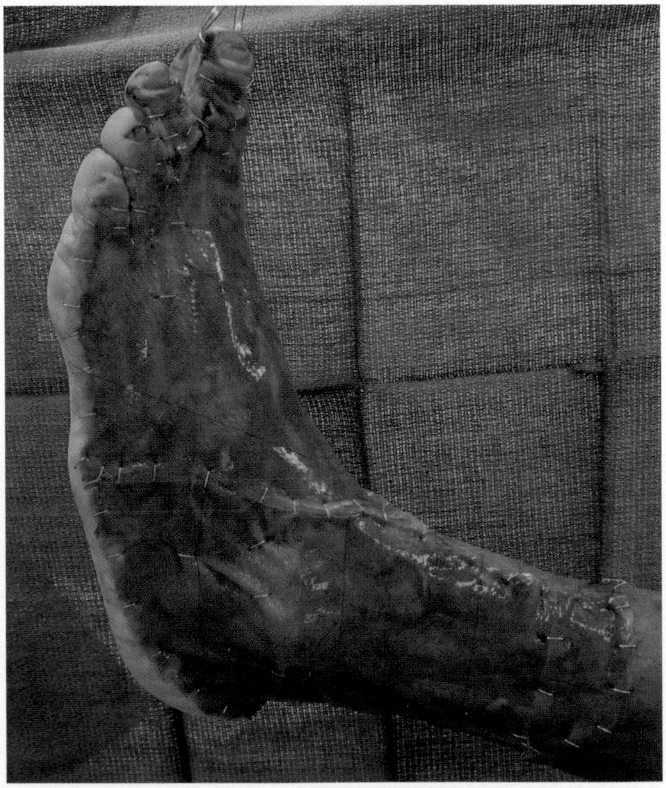

FIGURE 11-26 Biological skin equivalent dressings. Integra is a dermal matrix composed of bovine collagen cross-linked with glycosaminoglycan and an outer silicone membrane. It serves as a scaffold for the in-growth of fibroblasts and blood vessels and the silicone membrane acts as a temporary barrier. These biological dressings are termed *living skin equivalents*.

dual-layered silicone membrane. The polymer is broken down over the course of 18 months as neovascularization and collagen formation occurs.[35] Whether using Integra or BTM, vascularization of the matrix is usually complete in 14–21 days, at which time the outer silicone membrane is removed to reveal the "neodermis," and is covered by an autologous skin graft. Integra and BTM are valuable reconstructive options when poorly vascularized structures such as bone without periosteum, tendon without peritenon, and neurovascular bundles are in the base of the wound bed and direct application of a skin graft would result in either graft failure or undesired adherence to underlying critical structures. No comparative studies of Integra and BTM exist, but practitioners have used both for similar clinical indications with success, which is often dependent upon clinician experience with the product. The use of negative pressure therapy over these products has been shown to increase success rates due to improved vascularization of the matrices and decreased infection rates.[36,37]

Other cellular and tissue biologic dressings that have been reported as beneficial in treating burns include Apligraf (Organogenesis, Canton, MA), dehydrated Human Amnion/Chorion Membrane (dHACM) allografts (EpiFix, AmnioFix, EpiBurn; MiMedx Group Inc., Marietta, GA[38]), and MatriStem burn matrix (ACell, Columbia, MD). A newer product, ReCell Spray-On Skin system, uses a skin biopsy sample to immediately create a cell suspension for spraying onto an exposed area either from a burn, in the mesh graft interstices, or on the STSG donor site. Typically, a 4 cm^2 biopsy is converted into a spray containing a suspension of keratinocytes, melanocytes, Langerhans cells, and fibroblasts that can be used to cover an area of 320 cm^2.[39]

The function of these cellular/tissue biologics is to promote wound closure through increased cellular migration, stem cell proliferation and differentiation, and/or synthesis of extracellular matrix.

COMPLICATIONS

Hypertrophic scarring is the result of wounds that heal with an excessive amount of collagen formation. Unlike keloids, they do not extend beyond the area of the initial wound, and thus appear as a raised scar within defined boundaries (**FIGURE 11-27**). Ethnic populations with *Fitzpatrick* types 4 and above (more melanated skin) are at increased risk of both hypertrophic scarring and keloid formation. Hypertrophic scars most commonly develop when *deep partial-thickness* or *full-thickness* injuries are allowed to heal by contraction, not re-epithelialization, and in functional areas, these can lead to contractures and joint mobility impairment (**FIGURES 11-28** and **11-29**). Treatment of hypertrophic scars includes pressure therapy with custom-made compression garments, corticosteroid and 5-FU injections, silicone gel dressings, therapeutic scar massage, and laser therapy, all with varying degrees of scar improvement depending on the timing of intervention and frequency. In the event of wound contracture causing functional impairment, surgical release, local tissue rearrangement, skin

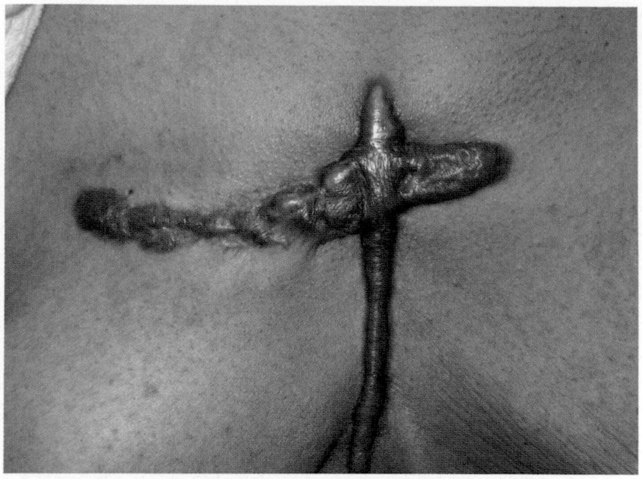

FIGURE 11-27 Keloid scarring. (Used with permission from Keloids. In: Usatine RP, Smith MA, Chumley HS, Mayeaux EJ Jr, eds. *The Color Atlas of Family Medicine.* 2nd ed. New York, NY: McGraw-Hill; 2013, Figure 204-1.)

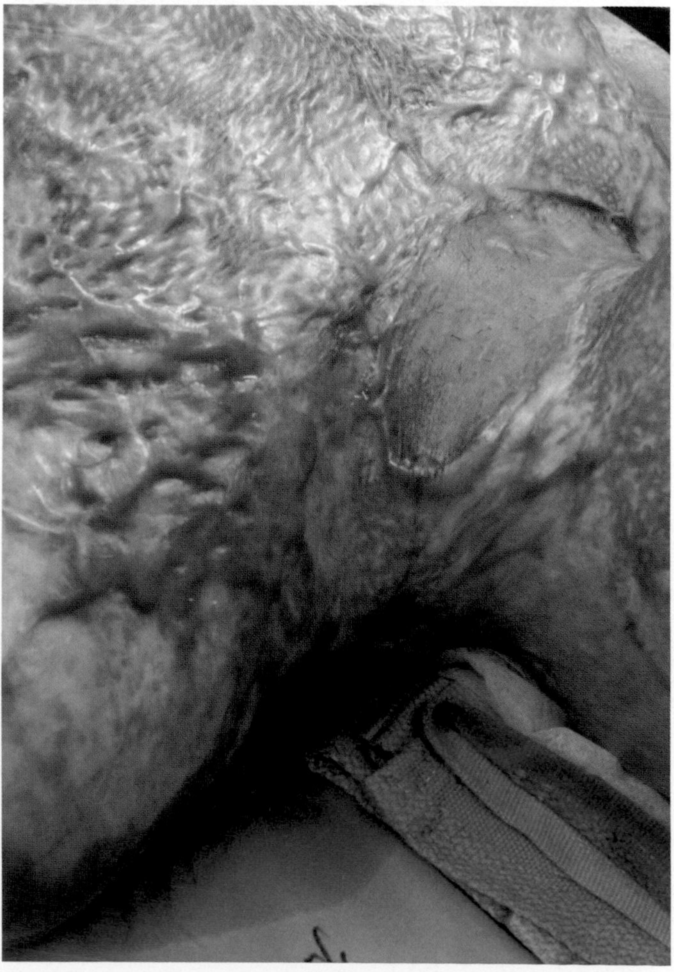

FIGURE 11-28 Hypertrophic scarring.

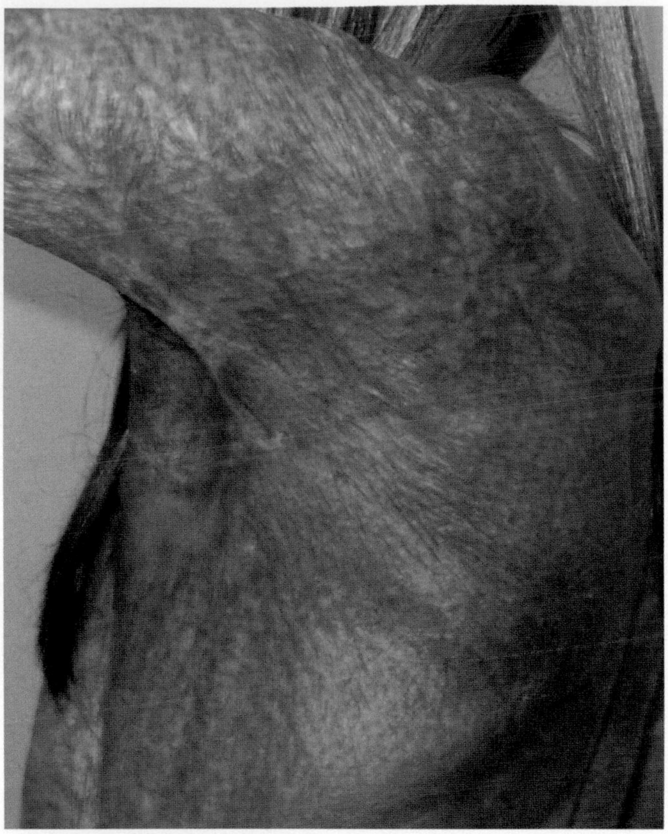

FIGURE 11-29 Hypertrophic scarring with joint impairment at the shoulder.

grafting, and/or free vascularized tissue transfer may be warranted (**FIGURES 11-30** and **11-31**).

Burn wound infections, cellulitis, and burn sepsis are currently the greatest contributors to burn morbidity and mortality in patients admitted for burn treatment. Infectious sequelae following burn injury account for over 75% of in-hospital

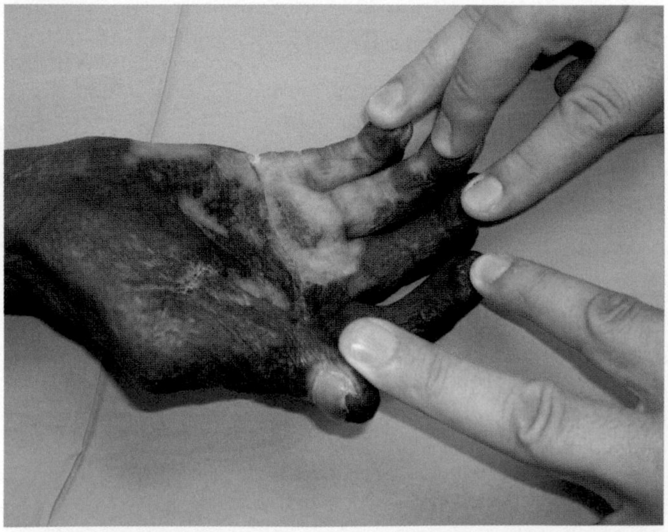

FIGURE 11-30 Hypertrophic scarring with severe contractures and functional impairments of the hand.

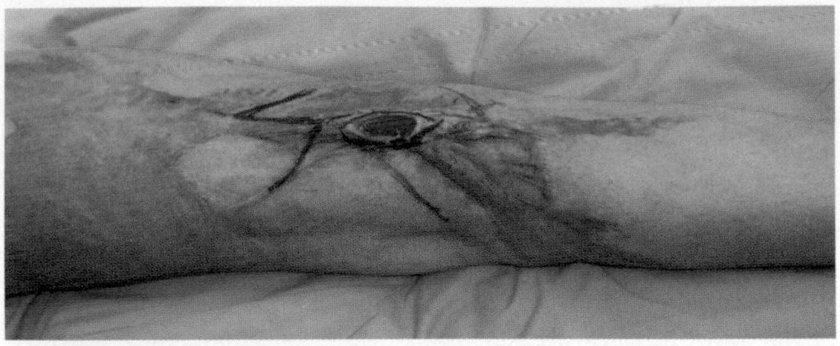

FIGURE 11-31 Surgical excision of hypertrophic scarring may be required for both function and aesthetics.

post-burn complications.[40] Burn infection is diagnosed by assimilation of clinical examination, laboratory tests, and quantitative tissue biopsy to identify the causative organism(s) for directing antimicrobial and surgical interventions. These complications are addressed aggressively as wound-derived sepsis is the primary cause of mortality in patients with large burn injuries.

Curling Ulcers can occur in the gastric or duodenal mucosa of the gastrointestinal tract of severely burned patients as a result of reduced plasma volume, decreased tissue perfusion, and subsequent gastric mucosal ischemia and necrosis. If allowed to progress, these ulcers can result in hemorrhage and perforation. The incidence of Curling Ulcers has significantly decreased with the initiation of prophylactic treatment with H_2 blockers, proton pump inhibitors, and early enteral gastric feeding. These ulcers previously contributed to significant morbidity and even mortality in burn patients, which is why prophylactic treatment should be initiated as early as possible if gastric enteral feeding is not initiated early on in treatment.

Burn wounds can result in chronic inflammation that predisposes the area to malignant transformation termed *Marjolin Ulcers* (MU), which are aggressive ulcerating squamous cell carcinomas. MUs are suspected if there is a chronic, slow-growing lesion in the area of an old burn wound that classically progresses beyond the boundaries of the initial burn wound. Diagnosis is made by wedge resection; however, these cancers tend to be aggressive and are associated with a poor prognosis. Wide local excision with at least 1 cm margins is required to provide some survival benefit in this population. Burns account for about 64% of all MUs, although any chronic wound can develop them.[41] The average time between initial injury and onset of MU (latency period) is 29 ± 11 years with a recurrence rate of 23% that is greatest in the head, neck, and upper extremities.[41]

Heterotrophic ossification (HO) is a rare complication related to *full-thickness* burns near joints due to elevated TGF-β cross-reactivity with bone morphogenic protein (BMP) pathways present in the nearby periosteum. HO usually occurs 1–3 months postinjury and has a higher incidence in the upper extremities, especially at the elbows. Calcium is deposited in soft tissues surrounding the involved joint, thus leading to impaired movement as heterotrophic bone is formed within the soft tissue. Plain films

CASE STUDY

CONCLUSION

The patient arrived at the emergency room with clothes still intact, so they were carefully removed to avoid further skin damage. Because of the pain levels, intravenous narcotic medication was administered to initially control pain. The burns were irrigated and debrided of devitalized tissue once adequate pain control was established. Because the wounds were *partial-thickness*, a topical antibiotic dressing was applied, and no systemic antibiotics were indicated since the patient had no other comorbidities or risk factors. Classic choices include topical silver dressings, such as silver sulfadiazine, which are inexpensive but laborious, requiring daily dressing changes. In addition, at each dressing change the old silver sulfadiazine must be completely removed to prevent buildup of residue. If a thick residue or pseudoeschar develops, removing it can be painful and failure to do so can inhibit evaluation of the burn. Other options include silver-impregnated gauze that can be placed after initial debridement and left for up to 7 days. These dressings are cost-effective and prevent the pain associated with daily dressing changes while effectively preventing infection. Also, because it was too early to determine if the wounds were *superficial* or *deep partial-thickness*, the patient was admitted for daily wound care until it could be determined if further surgical debridement of any devitalized tissue would be needed. If the injuries only result in *superficial partial-thickness* injuries, re-epithelialization should occur with normal wound healing without any additional intervention provided there is no infection. However, if the patient has *deep partial-thickness* injuries, early surgical debridement and grafting are warranted to prevent future hypertrophic scarring and wound contracture which causes pain, impairs activities of daily living, and has significant psychological sequelae.

demonstrating calcification of the soft tissue and muscle (myositis ossificans) around the involved joint can be used to confirm the diagnosis. Treatment in many cases involves excision of the deposits to restore the range of motion. Unfortunately, rates of recurrence may be as high as 35% even after surgical resection and early initiation of postoperative therapy.

REHABILITATION

Early rehabilitation of the burn patient focuses on the range of motion exercises, positioning, and splinting to prevent wound contracture and functional limitations. In many burn centers, rehabilitation starts from the very first day of the injury and continues well beyond discharge from the hospital or clinic. Long-term rehabilitation places greater emphasis on the restoration of activities of daily living, correction of cosmetic deformities, and physiological adaptation. Occupational and physical therapists play an integral role in the treatment plan even in the initial stages of burn treatment. Many of these injuries are life-changing experiences, leading to dramatic physical adjustments that cause severe psychological stress. Newer strategies of burn rehabilitation integrate psychological assessment to identify and treat early signs of posttraumatic stress disorders and/or depression. The incorporation of virtual reality paradigms to simulate important daily tasks as well as to motivate pediatric patients has become an area of increasing interest and success. This integral approach of physical and occupational therapy involvement from initial hospital admission through long-term outpatient follow-up aims to address all levels of recovery with the ultimate goal of returning the patient to the previous level of function.

STUDY QUESTIONS

1. A 20-year-old 70-kg female presents to the emergency room after sustaining a 48% TBSA burn. Estimate the initial fluid requirements and nutritional requirements for this patient.
2. A 32-year-old male was brought in by paramedics after being extricated from a house fire. He is alert, talking, and responding appropriately to commands. Describe the initial assessments and critical aspects of evaluation taking into consideration the mechanism of the burn injury.
3. A 10-year-old male sustains a 3% TBSA to the perineum. Does he require a referral to a regional burn unit? Explain why or why not.
4. A 45-year-old male sustains an electrical burn to his right hand 6 hours prior to presentation to the emergency room. On evaluation, the right hand is swollen and red. Passive flexion-extension of the fingers elicits severe pain. What is the concern of this physical examination finding? What would be the management of this condition?
5. A 4-year-old girl sustains greater than 60% TBSA circumferential flame burns to the chest, back, abdomen, and legs in a house fire. She was intubated in the field due to respiratory distress. After being hospitalized for 24 hours in the intensive care unit, she develops increasing peak pressures on the ventilator. What concerns would you have at this point in time?
6. A 33-year-old male presents to his physician for evaluation of the right arm for limited movement at the

elbow. Three months prior he sustained a deep *partial-thickness* scald burn to the right antecubital area while cooking and managed the injury at home with over-the-counter antibacterial ointment. What concerns would you have regarding the physical examination finding? How would you manage this condition?

Answer 1: The Parkland formula would be utilized to estimate the initial fluid requirements of an adult burn patient. Therefore, 4 cc × 70 kg × 48% TBSA = 13,440 cc of fluid, in which one-half (6720 cc) should be given over the first 8 hours, and the remaining half given over the following 16 hours. However, the Parkland formula only gives an estimate of the total fluid requirements, and fluid should be adjusted appropriately to ensure urine output of 0.5–1 cc/kg/hr. There are many formulas available to estimate the caloric requirements of a burn patient; however, nitrogen balance should be assessed to ensure the patient maintains an anabolic state.

Answer 2: The initial assessment should start off with the standard ABCs of a trauma evaluation assessing the airway, breathing, and circulation status. Since this patient was found in an enclosed space, he is at risk for inhalation injury. The evaluator should note if there is any hoarseness or stridor on the initial evaluation. Even if the patient is able to vocalize initially, as airway edema progresses, he could rapidly go into respiratory distress and intubation could potentially be difficult. Most institutions advocate early intubation if there are any signs of inhalation injury in order to avoid this scenario.

Answer 3: This patient would require referral to a regional burn unit because of the sensitive area that is involved. In addition, burns in a pediatric population could indicate abuse, and time should be taken to obtain a thorough history. If abuse is suspected, notification to the proper child protective agency is warranted.

Answer 4: This physical examination finding is concerning for compartment syndrome. This patient is at high-risk because he sustained an electrical injury to his hand. With electrical injuries, even if there are little superficial manifestations of injury, the underlying injury could be extensive due to the path of the current. Hands are particularly at risk for more severe injuries because they dissipate less heat. Treatment for compartment syndrome is an emergent fasciotomy.

Answer 5: The patient sustained a circumferential wound to the chest, and, therefore, eschar could be limiting ventilation. This would be managed by an escharotomy in which the devitalized tissue is removed.

Answer 6: This patient sustained a *deep partial-thickness* burn across a joint which he treated with local antibiotic ointment. This would make him at risk for hypertrophic scarring and wound contracture due to its location across a joint. Treatment for wound contracture is the surgical release of constricting bands of scar tissue. Depending on the extent of a defect after release, the patient may need subsequent skin graft coverage.

REFERENCES

1. Burns. World Health Organization. Available at: https://www.who.int/news-room/fact-sheets/detail/burns#. Accessed April 12, 2023.
2. National Burn Repository Report. American Burn Association. Available at: https://ameriburn.org/who-we-are/media/burn-incidence-fact-sheet/. Accessed April 12, 2023.
3. Jackson DM. The diagnosis of the depth of burning. *Br J Surg.* 1953;40(164):588-596.
4. Pham TN, Gibran NS, Heimbach DM. Evaluation of the burn wound: management decisions. In: Herndon DN, ed. *Total Burn Care.* 3rd ed. Philadelphia, PA: Saunders Elsevier; 2007:119.
5. Devgan L, Bhat S, Aylward S, Spence RJ. Modalities for the assessment of burn wound depth. *J Burns Wounds.* 2006;5:7-15.
6. Huang S, Dang J, Sheckter CC, Yenikomshian HA, Gillenwater J. A systematic review of machine learning and automation in burn wound evaluation: a promising but developing frontier. *Burns.* 2021;47(8):1691-1704.
7. Butz DR, Collier Z, O'Connor A, Magdziak M, Gottlieb LJ. Is palmar surface area a reliable tool to estimate burn surface areas in obese patients? *J Burn Care Res.* 2015;36(1):87-91.
8. Parvizi D, Giretzlehner M, Wurzer P, et al. BurnCase 3D software validation study: burn size measurement accuracy and inter-rater reliability. *Burns.* 2016;42(2):329-335.
9. Osler T, Glance LG, Hosmer DW. Simplified estimates of the probability of death after burn injuries: extending and updating the baux score. *J Trauma.* 2010;68(3): 690-697.
10. Williams DJ, Walker JD. A nomogram for calculation of the revised Baux score. *Burns.* 2015;41(1):85-90.
11. Collier ZJ, Roughton MC, Gottlieb LJ. Negligent and inflicted burns in children. *Clin Plast Surg.* 2017;44(3):467-477.
12. Hassan G, Wong JK, Bush J, Bayat A, Dunn KW. Assessing the severity of inhalation injuries in adults. *Burns.* 2010;36(2):212-216.
13 Alexander KS, Wasiak J, Cleland H. Chemical burns: diphoterine untangled. *Burns.* 2018;44(4):752-766.
14. Martin M, Lefaix J, Delanian S. TGF beta1 and radiation fibrosis: a master switch and a specific therapeutic target? *Int J Radiat Oncol Biol Phys.* 2000;47(2):277-290.
15. Flanders KC, Major CD, Arabshahi A, et al. Interference with transforming growth factor-beta/Smad3 signaling results in accelerated healing of wound in previously irradiated rats. *Am J Pathol.* 2003;163(6):2247-2257.
16. Rigotti G, Marchi A, Galie M, et al. Clinical treatment of radiotherapy tissue damage by lipoaspirate transplant: a healing process medicated by adipose-derived adult stem cells. *Plast Reconstr Surg.* 2007;119(5):1409-1422.
17. Greenwald D, Cooper B, Gottlieb BL. An algorithm for early aggressive treatment of frostbite with limb salvage directed by triple phase bone scanning. *Plast Reconstr Surg.* 1998;102:1069-1074.
18. Shenaq DS, Gottlieb LJ. Cold injuries. *Hand Clin.* 2017;33(2): 257-267.
19. Faucher L, Furukawa K. Practice guidelines for the management of pain. *J Burn Care Res.* 2006;27(5):659-668.
20. Meyer WJ, Martyn JAJ, Wiechman S, Thomas CR, Woodson L. Management of pain and other discomforts in burned patients. In Herndon DN (ed.). *Total Burn Care.* 5th ed. Amsterdam, the Netherlands: Elsevier; 2018:679-699.
21. Pardesi O, Fuzaylov G. Pain management in pediatric burn patients: review of recent literature and future directions. *J Burn Care Res.* 2017;38(6):335-347.

22. Griggs C, Goverman J, Bittner E, Levi B. Sedation and pain management in burn patients. *Clin Plast Surg.* 2017;44(3):535-540.
23. James DL, Jowza M. Principles of burn pain management. *Clin Plast Surg.* 2017;44(4):737-747.
24. Ghezeljeh TN, Ardebili FM, Rafii F, Haghani H. The effects of patient-preferred music on anticipatory anxiety, post-procedural burn pain and relaxation level. *Eur J Integr Med.* 2017;9(1):141-147.
25. Hsu K, Chen LF, Hsiep PH. Effect of music intervention on burn patients' pain and anxiety during dressing changes. *Burns.* 2016;42(8):1789-1796.
26. Small C, Stone R, Pilsbury J, Bowden M, Bion J. Virtual restorative environment therapy as an adjunct to pain control during burn dressing changes: study protocol for a randomised controlled trial. *Trials.* 2015;16:329.
27. Burns-Nader S, Joe L, Pinion K. Computer tablet distraction reduces pain and anxiety in pediatric burn patients undergoing hydrotherapy: a randomized trial. *Burns.* 2017;43(6):1203-1211.
28. Young DM. Burn and electrical injury. In: Mathes SJ, Hentz VR, eds, *Mathes Plastic Surgery.* 2nd ed. Philadelphia, PA: Saunders Elsevier; 2006:811-833.
29. Moss LS. Treatment of the burn patient in primary care. *Adv Skin Wound Care.* 2010;23(11):517-524.
30. Nherera L, Trueman P, Roberts C, Berg L. Silver delivery approaches in the management of partial thickness burns: a systematic review and indirect treatment comparison. *Wound Repair Regen.* 2017;25(4):707-721.
31. Loo YL, Goh BKL, Jeffery S. An overview of the use of bromelain-based enzymatic debridement (Nexobrid®) in deep partial & full thickness burns: appraising the evidence. *J Burn Care Res.* 2018;39(6):932-938.
32. Chipp E, Charles L, Thomas C, Whiting K, Moiemen N, Wilson Y. A prospective study of time to healing and hypertrophic scarring in paediatric burns: every day counts. *Burns Trauma.* 2017;5:3.
33. Palackic A, Duggan RP, Campbell MS, et al. The role of skin substitutes in acute burn and reconstructive burn surgery: an updated comprehensive review. *Semin Plast Surg.* 2022;36(1):33-42.
34. Jeschke MG, van Baar ME, Choudhry MA, Chung KK, Gibran NS, Logsetty S. Burn injury. *Nat Rev Dis Primers.* 2020;6(1):11.
35. Lo CH, Brown JN, Dantzer EJG, et al. Wound healing and dermal regeneration in severe burn patients treated with NovoSorb® Biodegradable temporising matrix: a prospective clinical study. *Burns.* 2022;48(3):529-538.
36. Austin CL, Draper B, Larson KW, Thompson SJ. Biodegradable temporising matrix: use of negative pressure wound therapy shows a significantly higher success rate. *J Wound Care.* 2023;32(3):159-166.
37. Diehm YF, Fischer S, Gazyakan E, et al. Negative pressure wound therapy as an accelerator and stabilizer for incorporation of artificial dermal skin substitutes – A retrospective, non-blinded, and non-randomized comparative study. *J Plast Reconstr Aesthet Surg.* 2021;74(2):357-363.
38. Peirce SC, Carolan-Rees G. ReCell® Spray-on skin system for treating skin loss, scarring and depigmentation after burn injury: a NICE medical technology guidance. *Appl Health Econ Health Policy.* 2019;17(2):131-141.
39. Glat PM. The evolution of burn injury management: using dehydrated human amnion/chorion membrane (dHACM) allografts in clinical practice. *Ann Plast Surg.* 2017;78(suppl 1):S1-S26.
40. American Burn Association. 2015 National Report of Data from 2005 to 2018. Available at: http://www.ameriburn.org/NBR.php. Accessed December 12, 2018.
41. Cheng KY, Yu J, Liu EW, Hu KC, Lee JJ. Prognostic factors of Marjolin ulcers: a meta-analysis and systematic review assisted by machine learning techniques. *Plast Reconstr Surg.* 2023;151(4):875-884.

Factors That Impede Wound Healing

Rose L. Hamm, PT, DPT, FACCWS

CHAPTER OBJECTIVES

At the end of this chapter, the learner will be able to:

1. **Identify wounds that are not healing due to the influence of impeding factors.**
2. **Identify the impeding factors based on subjective and objective evaluations.**
3. **Select the tests necessary to confirm suspected impeding factors.**
4. **Adapt a plan of care to minimize the effect of impeding factors on the wound healing process.**
5. **Educate patients and caregivers on strategies to mitigate or eliminate the effects of impeding factors.**

INTRODUCTION

Chapter 3, Examination and Evaluation of the Patient with a Wound, presented the two questions that need to be answered in order to successfully treat a patient with a wound: (1) Why does the patient have a wound? and (2) Why is the wound not healing? Once a wound diagnosis has been determined and standard care has been initiated, the wound should progress through the stages of wound healing discussed in Chapter 2, Healing Response in Acute and Chronic Wounds. When progress is not observed, the second question—Why is the wound not healing?—becomes even more imperative to answer. Sometimes the wound will respond initially and make measurable progress, then stall again for no apparent reason. This chapter focuses on those factors that are known to impede wound healing, some more obvious than others, and provides suggestions on how to identify and minimize the effect on the healing process. The factors are categorized into infection, medications, nutritional deficits, comorbidities, and extrinsic/psychosocial behaviors.

TABLE 12-1 provides laboratory values, always a good starting place for solving the conundrum, with normal values, trends that are typical when a patient does not have the normal healing response, and clinical presentations that may accompany abnormal lab values.

CASE STUDY

INTRODUCTION

A 45-year-old male is evaluated for a 3+ year history of a nonhealing wound on the right anterior leg (**FIGURE 12-1**). The patient states that the initial wound was the result of trauma while working outside. His medical history includes the following:

- History of HIV for more than 15 years
- History of Kaposi sarcoma on the right anterior leg at the site of the current wound, treated with radiation and chemotherapy (doxol or doxorubicin) about 20 years prior to the wound occurring
- History of recurrent lower extremity cellulitis, treated with both IV vancomycin and oral Xyvox

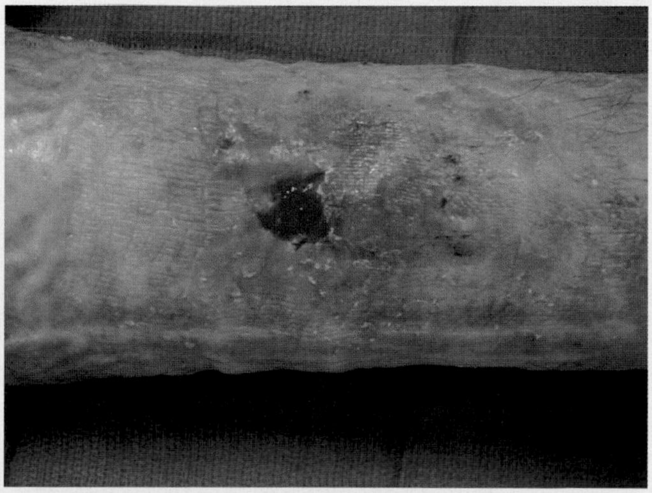

FIGURE 12-1 Case study at the time of initial evaluation. Nonhealing wound on the lower extremity of a patient with multiple factors that impede wound healing.

DISCUSSION QUESTIONS

1. What subjective information is needed to determine the factors that have prevented this wound from healing?
2. What questions would be helpful in obtaining this information?
3. What tests and measures are indicated in order to establish a plan of care?

TABLE 12-1 Laboratory Values with Implications for Wound Healing

Laboratory Test	Normal Range	Values Affecting Wound Healing	Clinical Presentation
CBC			
WBC	4.5–11 × 10^3/mm^3	Increased Decreased	Signs of infection, inflammation, necrosis, trauma, or stress Failure to initiate an immune response against bacteria
RBC	M 4.5–5.5 × 10^6/mm^3 F 4.1–4.9 × 10^6/mm^3	Decreased	Pale or anemic granulation or failure to progress
Hemoglobin	M 13.5–18 g/dL F 12–15 g/dL	Decreased Increased	Pale or anemic granulation or failure to progress Failure to progress (patient may show signs of congestive heart failure or COPD)
Hematocrit	M 37–50% F 36–46%	Decreased Increased	Pale or anemic granulation or failure to progress Signs of thrombi or emboli
Platelet count	150–400 × 10^3/mm^3	Decreased Increased	Bleeds easily, fatigue Signs of infection or inflammation
AUTOMATED DIFFERENTIAL			
Neutrophil rel	57–67% of leukocyte count	Increased	Bacterial infection Chronic inflammation
Lymphocyte rel	25–33% of leukocyte count	Increased Decreased	Signs of bacterial infection Opportunistic infections
Monocyte rel	3–7% of leukocyte count	Increased	Tissue injury Early healing response
Eosinophil rel	1–4% of leukocyte count	Increased Decreased (with corticosteroid use)	Allergic reaction Parasitic infection Delayed inflammatory response
Basophil rel	0–0.75% of leukocyte count	Increased	Allergic reaction
Neutrophil abs	4300–10,000 cells/mm^3	Increased	Signs of infection
Lymphocyte abs	2500–3300 cells/mm^3 2000–2500/μL	Increased Decreased	Signs of bacterial infection Opportunistic infections
Monocyte abs			
Eosinophil abs			
Basophil abs	0–1000 cells/mm^3	Increased	Allergic reaction
COAGULATION STUDIES			
PT (prothrombin time)	12.3–14.2 seconds	Increased (>2.5 × reference range)	Bleeds easily
PTT (partial thromboplastin time)	25–34 seconds		
INR	Normal 0.9–1.1 Therapeutic range 2–3 Mechanical heart valves 2.5–3.5	Elevated	Bleeds easily Skin bruising
ROUTINE CHEMISTRY			
Sodium	135–145 mEq/L		
Potassium	3.5–5.3 mEq/L		
Chloride	95–105 mEq/L		
CO_2	22–29 mEq/L 35–45 mmHg (arterial)		
Glucose	70–115 mg/dL	Decreased (<70) Increased (>200)	Headache, dizziness, altered mental status, malaise Arrested healing processed Signs of infection Increased risk of abscess formation
Calcium	8.8–10.5 mg/dL		

(Continued)

TABLE 12-1 Laboratory Values with Implications for Wound Healing (*Continued*)

Laboratory Test	Normal Range	Values Affecting Wound Healing	Clinical Presentation
Phosphate	2.5–5.0 mg/dL		
BUN	7–18 mg/dL	Increased (renal failure, dehydration) Decreased (liver failure)	Edema Poor healing Jaundiced skin Yellow fluids
Creatinine	0.1–1.2 mg/dL	Increased (renal failure) Decreased	Edema Decreased lean body mass
Albumin	3.5–5.5 g/dL	Decreased Increased	Lack of granulation tissue Bilateral edema Muscle wasting Signs of dehydration
Prealbumin level	15–36 mg/dL	Decreased	Poor wound healing Lack of granulation formation
Globulin	2.5–3.5 g/dL		
Fibrinogen	200–400 mg/dL		
A/G ratio	1.5:1–2.5:1	Decreased (liver damage) Increased (iron deficiency)	
Bilirubin total	0.1–1.0 mg/dL	Increased	Yellow wound fluids Jaundiced skin
Alkaline phosphate	30–85 U/L		
OTHERS			
Hemoglobin A1C	4–6%	Increased	Delayed healing
C-reactive protein (CRP)	0–1.0 mg/dL or <10 mg/L	Increased	Inflammation Infection
Erythrocyte Sedimentation Rate (ESR)	Male <15 mm/h Female ≤20 mm/h Child ≤10 mm/h Newborn 0–2 mm/h	Increased	Infection Inflammation Tissue damage
Retinal binding protein	10 mg/L 0.002 g/kg body wt	Increased	Delayed healing due to protein deficits
Magnesium	1.5–2.5 mEq/L		
Phosphorus	2.5–4.5 mg/dL		
Iron		Decreased Increased	Lack of granulation Hemochromatosis
Ferritin		Decreased Increased	Anemic granulation Lack of granulation Hemosiderosis
Transferrin	204–360 µg/dL <0.1 g/kg body wt	Decreased Increased	Delayed wound healing due to protein deficits Iron deficiency
Zinc	>60 µg/dL	Decreased	Delayed wound healing Lack of epithelialization Bullous—pustular dermatitis Intercurrent infections Weight loss
MICROBIOLOGY			
Wound culture	Negative	Positive	Poor wound healing Wound degradation
Blood culture	Negative	Positive	Systemic signs of infection

Data from Goodman CC, Fuller KS, Boissonnault WG. *Pathology: Implications for the Physical Therapist*. 2nd ed. Philadelphia, PA: Saunders; 2003 and Huether SE, McCance KL. *Understanding Pathophysiology*. 4th ed. St Louis, MO: Mosby; 2008.

INFECTIONS

Definition of Terms

Pathogens, defined as any microorganism that can cause disease in its host, can either damage or infect any wound tissue, or they can adhere to and colonize the wound surface. One distinguishing feature of pathogenic (vs. nonpathogenic) microorganisms is their ability to evade the host's innate and adaptive immune defenses. Pathogens have developed a variety of strategies to avoid immediate destruction by the host, including covering themselves in a thick polysaccharide capsule termed *biofilm*,[1,2] or in the case of mycobacterium (eg, *Mycobacterium leprae*, *Mycobacterium tuberculosis*), growing inside the macrophage phagosomes while inhibiting the phagosomal acidification and subsequent fusion with lysosomes.[3] Bactericidal agents (eg, toxic oxygen-derived products, nitric oxide, AMPs, and enzymes) are released by the phagocytic cells and are intended to render the invader harmless; however, these agents have consequences—they damage the surrounding host tissue and may potentiate the chronic proinflammatory state observed in chronic wounds (see **FIGURES 12-2** and **12-3**).

Just as the skin is known to have certain flora residing on the surface, so the wound bed has a variable amount of microbial presence that is defined as contaminated, colonized, locally infected, or deep infected (see **TABLE 12-2**).[4] The effect of the microbes on the wound bed is dependent on the type of bacteria, the number of colony-forming units (CFUs) per gram of tissue, and the host immune system. Colonization and local infection may respond to topical antimicrobials (see Chapter 14, Wound Dressings); deep infection and sepsis require that the patient receive systemic antibiotics specific to the invading microbe.[4]

Bacterial Infection

The innate immune response is initiated with the engagement of primary host cells and conserved bacterial components, defined as the repetitive arrays of carbohydrates, lipids, and proteins that are contained in the bacteria cell walls. These repetitive arrays are termed pathogen-associated molecular patterns (PAMPs) and the receptors that recognize them are termed pattern recognition receptors (PRRs). Host cells (eg, macrophages) constitutively express PRRs that recognize essential and highly conserved microbial components. The PRRs recognize the microbe by contact with its living extracellular components or its phagocytosed components after it has been ingested. Although the PRRs have a limited degree of specificity, they are specific enough to engage the host's innate immune system.

Gram-positive bacteria carry a number of proinflammatory cell wall components including peptidoglycan (PGN), teichoic acid, lipoteichoic acid, and other surface proteins. Gram-negative organisms express an extremely potent proinflammatory lipopolysaccharide (LPS). As a result, the evolution of the host innate immune system includes separate and

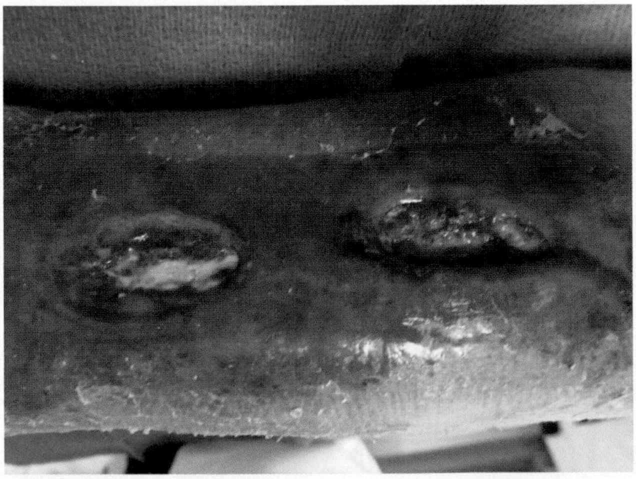

FIGURE 12-2 Infected wound. Wound infected with *Staphylococcus aureus*. The bacteria are not visible; however, the signs of persistent periwound erythema, drainage, epidermal sloughing, and failure to heal are signs of infection. Pain and warmth are other signs of infection that may be present.

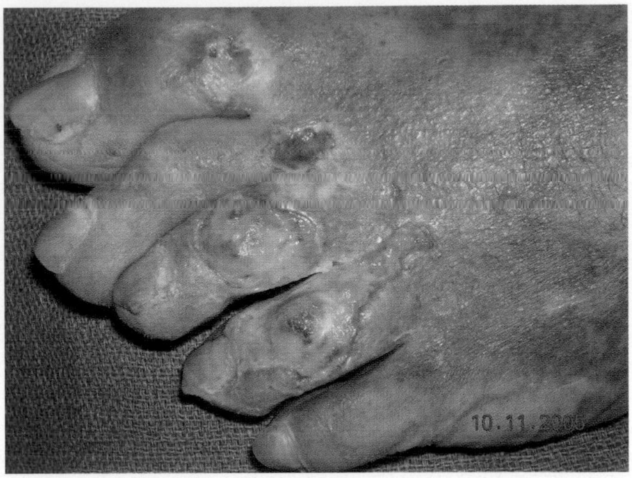

FIGURE 12-3 Infected wound. Biofilm, the polysaccharide covering produced on the surface of a wound by bacteria, may not be visible; however, the thick film on the surface of the toe wounds is an indication of possible infection. In this case, the wound culture was positive for MRSA.

TABLE 12-2 Terms Defining the Presence of Bacteria on a Wound

Contaminated
▪ **Contamination**—presence of nonreplicating bacteria on the wound surface without any effect upon the wound healing process
▪ **Colonization**—presence of replicating bacteria attached to the wound surface with no harm to the host and no effect on the wound healing process
▪ **Local infection**—presence of replicating bacteria on the wound surface with sufficient numbers to visibly affect the wound healing process
▪ **Deep infection**—presence of replicating bacteria that have invaded the surrounding tissue with visible effects in the wound healing process and in the periwound tissues. Clinical infection for most bacteria is defined as 10^5 CFUs/g of tissue
▪ **Sepsis**—presence of replicating bacteria that produces a whole-body inflammatory state termed systemic inflammatory response syndrome (SIRS)

TABLE 12-3 Microorganisms Most Commonly Present in Chronic Wounds

Aerobes (need oxygen to survive)
Acinetobacter baumannii
Coliforms*
Corynebacterium spp
Enterococcus faecalis
Methicillin-resistant *Staphylococcus aureus*
*Pseudomonas aeruginosa**
*Staphylococcus aureus**
Staphylococcus epidermidis
Streptococcus pyogenes
Anaerobes (do not need oxygen to survive)
Bacteroides spp
Fusobacterium spp
Peptostreptococcus spp
Porphyromonas spp
Prevotella spp
*Proteus mirabilis**
Veillonella spp

The microbes starred were identified by Bessa et al. as those found most frequently in infected wounds.[6]

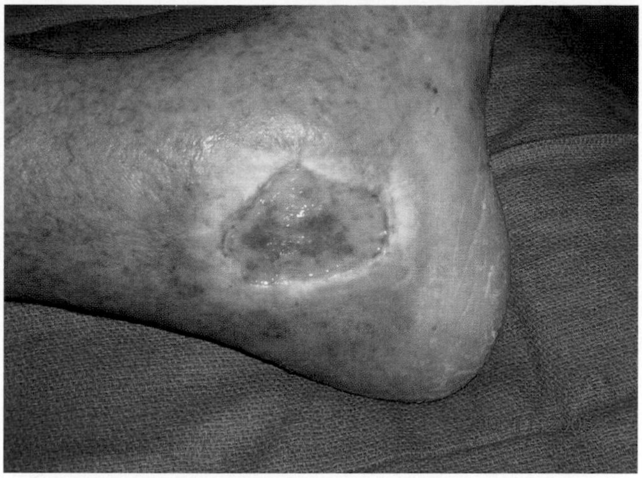

FIGURE 12-4 Biofilm on the wound surface. Biofilm can appear as a thin, adhered yellow layer on the wound that is difficult to penetrate with antimicrobial dressings. Usually sharp debridement, in combination with contact low-frequency ultrasound or an iodine-based topical dressing, is required to remove the film and attached bacteria.

distinct, although sometimes overlapping, sets of sensors to detect the components of both gram-positive and gram-negative organisms. The detection of the organism then sets into motion a cascading proinflammatory response from resident macrophages and leukocytes.[1] Bacteria are further characterized as aerobic (needing oxygen to survive) and anaerobic (able to survive without oxygen) and can coexist in chronic wounds, especially if there is necrotic tissue present.[5] **TABLE 12-3** provides a list of bacteria most commonly found in chronic wounds.[6]

Biofilms

Colonizing pathogens establish an attachment to the host epithelium or wound surface that is composed of an exopolymeric matrix of polysaccharides, proteins, and DNA synthesized by the bacteria.[5] The substance is adherent to the wound bed, providing an environment for the bacteria to live and replicate, and thus it is not easily removed by mechanical force or competing bacteria. Studies indicate that the first microorganism to establish host attachment has an advantage over subsequent colonizers even though competition of bacteria often occurs at the level of attachment to host receptors.[7] The biofilm can sometimes resemble a layer of slough on the wound surface or it can be invisible (**FIGURE 12-4**). In order for the wound to progress from chronic to healing, the biofilm must be removed, preferably with sharp debridement as most antimicrobial dressings will not penetrate the biofilm to kill the bacteria although they can suppress biofilm formation.[2]

Fungus Infections

Recent studies indicate that the fungal response to phagocytosis actively modulates the host immune cell function. Fungal pathogens avoid detection by masking PAMPs (such as cell wall carbohydrates) and by down-regulating the complement cascade. Once detected, various species of fungi actually interfere with phagocytosis and can repress the production of antimicrobial substances like NO. Some fungi successfully replicate while inside the host macrophage. It is becoming readily apparent that fungi manipulate the host–pathogen interaction to their advantage (**FIGURE 12-5**).[8]

In the wound care clinic, fungal infections are sometimes observed in conjunction with compression therapy, especially if using dressings and compression systems that stay in place up to 7 days. The moisture of both wound drainage and perspiration creates an environment where fungi thrive. The infection can usually be managed with a topical antifungal medication, adequate absorbent dressings to manage the wound fluid, and more frequent dressing changes.

Identification of an infected wound is not always easy for even the most astute clinician. The most common signs are persistent periwound erythema, drainage, epidermal sloughing, odor, and failure to respond to standard care. Friable granulation tissue in a previously progressing wound bed is another sign of infection. Specific to the diabetic foot ulcer, erythema that extends more than 2 cm from the edge of the wound is highly correlated with infection; and if the wound can be probed to bone, there is a possibility of osteomyelitis.[9] Accurate identification of any bacteria or fungi that are impeding wound healing is necessary for effective treatment, and effective treatment is necessary for wound healing to progress. A recent study found that swabs and biopsies yield the same culture results when taken from the same location, suggesting that biopsies are indicated only when needed for a pathological diagnosis, not for bacteria identification.[10,11] Fluorescence imaging provides immediate information on the presence, location, and load of wound bacteria at the

CASE STUDY

CONTINUED

The following subjective information was obtained at the time of the evaluation:

- Works as a landscape artist
- Spends a lot of time standing and walking
- Is compliant with all medications, takes vitamins
- Works out at the gym 3–4 days a week
- Eats a healthy diet
- Has no history of smoking; occasional alcohol
- Has no history of drug abuse

The following objective information was obtained:

- Wound size: 2 × 2 cm
- Friable granulation tissue that bled very easily
- Periwound erythema
- Moderate serous drainage
- Moderate pitting edema with severe venous reflux
- 2–3/10 pain with touch or prolonged standing
- 3+ dorsalis pedis and posterior tibialis pulses
- No hair growth on the periwound skin

DISCUSSION QUESTIONS

1. What red flags indicate that local or deep infection may be present?
2. What risk factors does the patient have that make him susceptible to infection?
3. Are referrals to a medical specialist indicated? Which ones?

point of care, thus facilitating prompt removal of bacterial burden to reduce wound infection and facilitate healing.[12]

MEDICATIONS

Steroids

Anti-inflammatory steroids, including glucocorticosteroids, are known to significantly affect many aspects of wound healing. When steroids have been part of the patient's medication regime

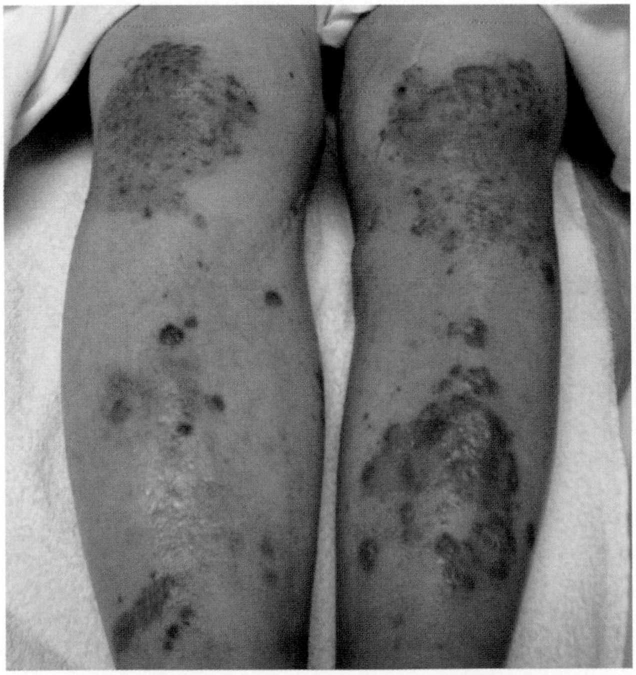

FIGURE 12-5 Fungal infection. Fungal infections can occur under compression wraps if the skin becomes a supportive moist environment. Note the circular presentation of the infections, which has given some fungal infections the laymen's nomenclature of ringworm.

prior to wounding, the elevated corticosteroid levels delay the appearance of inflammatory cells and fibroblasts; decrease the deposition of ground substances and collagen; and inhibit angiogenesis, wound contraction, and epithelial migration (**FIGURE 12-6A, B**).[13,14] The effect of steroid-mediated, delayed healing has been demonstrated to occur largely through the down-regulation of TGF-β and ILGF-1 and is apparent in all phases of wound healing. The effects of TGF-β on ECM formation are more profound than any other growth factor, and in the absence of TGF-β, matrix deposition, and angiogenesis are impaired.[15] Specifically TGF-β is mitogenic for fibroblasts and stimulates the production of fibronectin and collagen. Insulin-like growth factor (ILGF-1) is a major regulator of wound healing. Wounds deprived of 90% of their IGFs demonstrate impairment in cell replication and deposition of collagen and a constitutive decrease in wound macrophage numbers. ILGF-1 also directly engages fibroblasts, endothelial and epithelial cells.[16,17]

The wound healing trajectory is affected in several ways in patients who have been or are currently taking steroids. Decreased leukocyte infiltration, delayed insufficient inflammatory response to injury, and reduced autolysis of necrotic tissue are characteristics of a dampened response early in the healing process. The healing process and clearance of the debris and/or pathogen are inhibited secondary to decreased macrophage recruitment and proliferation. In the proliferative phase of healing the effects of steroids can be observed in the formation of less ground substance, decreased angiogenesis, and diminished fibroblast function, which directly decrease the amount of collagen synthesis.[18] Fibroblasts do not differentiate into myofibroblasts, thus decreasing wound contraction and overall tensile strength. The effects of steroids on each phase of wound healing may lead to vulnerability for ulcer recurrence.[19]

Numerous studies have looked at the results of orthopedic surgery on patients (specifically with rheumatoid arthritis) who are on anti-inflammatory medications, either steroidal or disease-modifying antirheumatic drugs (DMARDs) such as

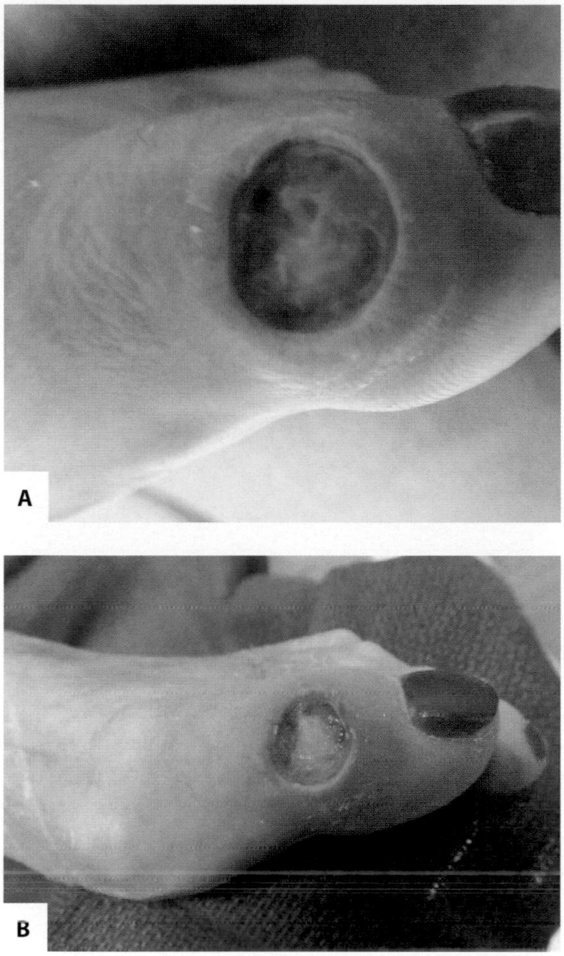

FIGURE 12-6 A. Wound on the patient taking steroids. The wound on the great toe of a patient who takes steroids for severe rheumatoid arthritis has impaired healing. **B. The wound after 10 days of treatment.** Debridement of necrotic tissue, low-frequency noncontact ultrasound, and antimicrobial dressings have decreased the periwound inflammation; however, the ability to move from inflammation to proliferation is slow.

methotrexate. A study on adverse events with craniovertebral junction fusion concluded that prednisone dosages <7.5 mg and/or methotrexate were safe with no effect on outcomes, whereas daily prednisone dosages >7.5 mg may impact clinical outcomes, as measured by the Nurick score.[20] Three studies on postoperative complications (surgical site infections and delayed wound healing) in patients taking DMARDs found no statistically significant difference in wound healing in those patients taking the medications.[21–23] In their review of perioperative use of DMARDs on patients undergoing plastic surgery, Tsai and Borah[24] suggest that in younger patients who have been placed on the medications recently, "it is reasonable to withhold therapy based on 3–5 half-lives of the specific agent," whereas in older patients with more advanced disease, discontinuing therapy must be carefully considered by the patient and the rheumatologist. However, a conflicting case study reported the failure of a skin graft on a patient taking methotrexate.[25]

Two specific guidelines were issued by the British Society for Rheumatology: (1) methotrexate is unlikely to increase the risk of surgical complications if continued,[26] and (2) anti-TNFα drugs (infliximab, etanercept, adalimumab) "should be withheld for 2–4 weeks prior to major surgical procedures" and resumed when wound healing is satisfactory.[27] The decisions regarding steroid management for patients with chronic wounds demand careful consideration and observation from all the medical providers involved in their care.

Another potential side effect of long-term corticosteroid use that may affect wound healing is the development of drug-induced diabetes.[28] This condition may not be diagnosed initially; therefore, if a patient receiving corticosteroid therapy has poor wound healing, monitoring blood glucose levels is advised.[29] In addition, patients on steroids develop thin fragile skin that is at risk for skin tears (**FIGURE 12-7**).

Nonsteroidal Anti-Inflammatory Drugs

Nonsteroidal anti-inflammatory drugs (NSAIDs) are used to treat both autoimmune diseases and acute injuries because of their ability to decrease inflammation, prevent disease progression, and mitigate pain. (See **TABLE 12-4** for a list of commonly used NSAIDs.) These medications work by inhibiting both COX-1 and COX-2 enzymes, thereby decreasing the production of prostaglandins and leukotrienes.[30] The positive therapeutic effects of decreased production of prostaglandins are well known; however, the negative effects on wound healing are especially evident when given long-term and in higher doses.[31,32] The mechanisms through which wound healing may be impeded include the following:

- Decreased production of thromboxane A_2, which decreases platelet aggregation and increases the propensity for bleeding and hematoma formation, especially postoperatively[33]

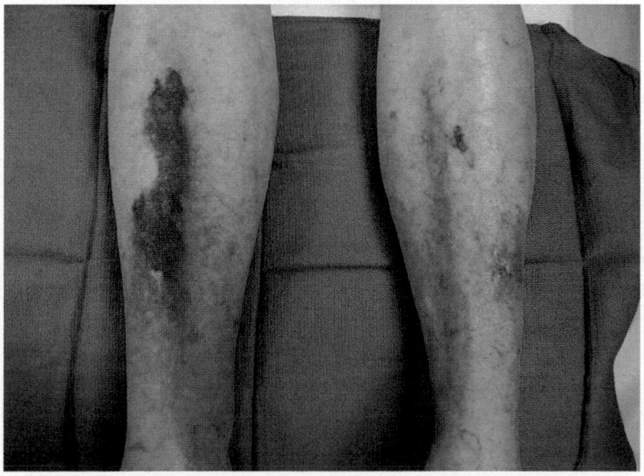

FIGURE 12-7 Skin on the patient taking steroids. Patients on long-term steroid therapy have thin, fragile skin and tend to bruise easily, thus creating frequent superficial trauma wounds that are difficult to heal. Protection of the extremities with foam sleeves is beneficial, and meticulous wound care is required to prevent infection.

TABLE 12-4 Commonly Used NSAIDs That May Affect Wound Healing

Nonselective NSAIDs	Cyclooxygenase (COX)-2 Inhibitors	Disease-Modifying Antirheumatic Drugs (DMARDs)
Aspirin Diclofenac (Voltaren) Fenoprofen (Nalfon) Ibuprofen (Motrin, Rufen) Indomethacin (Indocin) Ketoprofen (Orudis) Meclofenamate (Meclofen, Meclomen) Naproxen (Anaprox, Naprosyn) Piroxicam (Feldene) Sulindac (Clinoril) Tolmetin (Tolectin)	Celecoxib Parecoxib Rofecoxib Valdecoxib	Azathioprine Penicillamine Methotrexate

- Inhibition of hyaluronic acid production with less granulation formation during the proliferative phase of healing
- Decreased neutrophil migration to the wound site with increased risk of infection
- Decreased collagen synthesis with a decreased tensile strength of new tissue

In addition, there is evidence that NSAIDs and COX-2 inhibitors inhibit PGE2 production which in turn might exacerbate excessive scar formation. Both overproduction of TGF-β and suppression of PGE2 are found in excessive scarring as compared with normal wound healing. This effect seems to be more prevalent in the later proliferative phase of healing; therefore, the use of these medications has to be balanced between the effects on healing and the cytokines needed to suppress inflammation.[34]

The results of several studies have led to the recommendation that NSAIDs be discontinued 1–4 weeks before surgery, depending on the half-life of the drug being taken by the patient, and some suggest that they should be withheld after surgery until the incision has healed.[19,35,36] Many of the studies are based on animal models and results are sometimes inconsistent, so the decision to discontinue their use before surgery needs to be weighed against the effects on the patient's pain and disease progression.[30]

Some of the clinical signs that may be observed if the NSAIDs are affecting wound healing include failure to progress through inflammation to the proliferative phase, tissue that bleeds easily, poor-quality granulation tissue that will not support re-epithelialization, tendency to develop infections, and vulnerability to break down during the remodeling phase (FIGURE 12-8). Patients who are taking NSAIDs for pain relief and not for anti-inflammatory effects may have better healing by substituting acetaminophen, especially if the NSAID dosage is high. If patients are on high doses of any anti-inflammatory medications, it is advised that they be tapered off in order to avoid the side effects of sudden withdrawal.

Anticoagulants

Anticoagulants (eg, warfarin, apixaban, rivaroxaban, and dabigatran) inhibit the coagulation cascade and thereby may prevent fibrin deposition and delay the healing process.[31,37] Two patient populations that were found to have significantly higher rates of postoperative wound and bleeding complications were women who received anticoagulation during pregnancy and required Cesarean delivery[38] and patients who were female and/or received oral anticoagulation and had lower extremity bypass surgery for critical limb ischemia. This does not undermine the importance of continuing anticoagulation therapy for those patients who require it for cardiac or thrombosis reasons. For any patient undergoing surgery and on anticoagulation therapy, the decision to continue medication

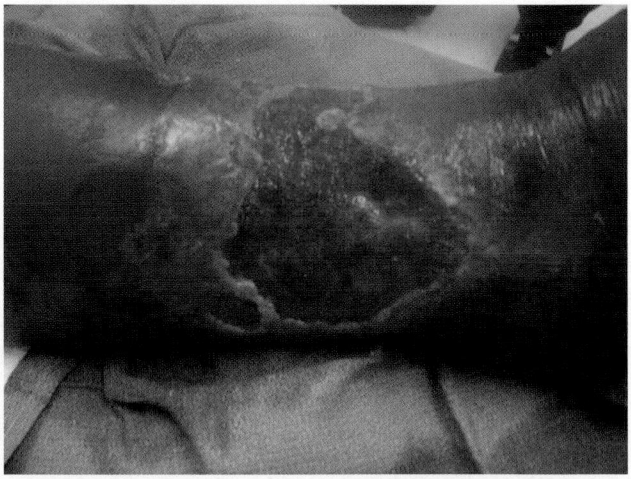

FIGURE 12-8 Stalled wound on a patient who is taking NSAIDs. The venous wound is clean and granulating; however, it has stalled and is not epithelializing. The patient, who had initially reported only medication for hypertension, told the therapist she was taking 800 mg of ibuprofen each day. Medications were discussed with her primary care physician; she was started pentoxifylline (vasodilator), discontinued ibuprofen, and changed hypertension medications. Within a week the wound had signs of epithelial migration at the edges.

during the perioperative period requires careful consultation between the surgeon and the prescribing physician to consider benefits and potential complications.

Cutaneous reactions to anticoagulation that have been reported are heparin-induced bullous hemorrhagic dermatosis, hematomas, ecchymoses, erythematous plaques, nodules, contact dermatitis, and urticarial,[39] as well as warfarin-induced skin necrosis (**FIGURE 12-9**). Although these conditions are rare, they are differential diagnoses to be ruled out in patients who develop skin necrosis, especially within 2 weeks of initiating therapy.[40]

Antirejection Medications

The hallmark of successful organ transplantation is suppressing the immune system so that the host does not activate the immune cells to a level sufficient to reject the allograft. **TABLE 12-5** provides a list of commonly used antirejection medications; most of which act by interfering with "discrete sites in the T- and B-cell cascades."[41] Specifically, the actions include inhibition of cytokine transcription, inhibition of nucleotide synthesis, inhibition of growth factor signal transduction, inhibition of the stimulation of T-cell interleukin (IL)-2 receptor sites, and diminished chemotaxis.[41,42] In addition, the effects of the corticosteroids include decreased counts of lymphocytes, monocytes (thus decreased macrophages), and basophils while increasing the number of senescent cells.[43] These altered cellular functions are known to impede wound healing, resulting in frequent dehiscence of the transplant surgical incision (**FIGURE 12-10**).

Acute adverse effects of the antirejection medications may include increased risk of infection; nausea, vomiting, and diarrhea; and loss of appetite, all of which result in a diminished nutritional state with subsequent insufficient calories, proteins, and vitamins needed for incisional healing (**FIGURE 12-11**).

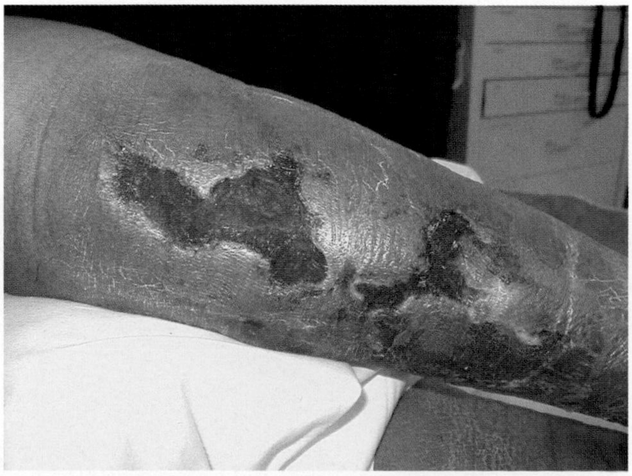

FIGURE 12-9 Coumadin-induced skin necrosis. Patient with warfarin- or Coumadin-induced skin necrosis on the posterior lower leg. Treatment included discontinuing warfarin, sharp debridement, and moist wound healing.

TABLE 12-5 Antirejection Medications Used for Organ Transplantation

Azathioprine (AZA, *Imuran*)
Corticosteroids
Primary endogenous glucocorticoid
Cortisol
Prednisone
Methylprednisolone
Cyclosporine (CsA)
Tacrolimus (Prograf)
Mycophenolate mofetil (Cellcept)
Sirolimus (SRL, *Rapamune*)
Polyclonal antibodies
Thymoglobulin
Atgam
Monoclonal antibodies (OKT3)
Daclizumab (Xanapax)
Basiliximab (Simulect)
Calcineurin inhibitor (CI)
CsA (Sandimmune, Neoral, and SangCya)
Mycophenolate mofetil (MMF)

Data from Lake DF, Briggs AD, Akporiaye ET. Immunopharmacology. In: Katzung BG, Masters SB, Trevor AJ, eds. *Basic & Clinical Pharmacology*. 12th ed. New York, NY: McGraw Hill; 2012: Chap 55.

Because antirejection medications are required for the life of the recipient, the effects on wound healing are long-term and may result in hard-to-heal wounds unrelated to the transplant surgery.[44] This is especially a problem if the patient develops drug-induced diabetes. Another long-term effect of the medications is a significantly higher rate of aggressive squamous cell carcinoma (SCC), a malignant skin cancer linked to the increased number of senescent cells,[43] and an oxidative environment.[45,46] Careful skin inspections are advised in order to detect SCC in the early stages and to increase survival rates.

CLINICAL CONSIDERATION

Even though they are acting as a foreign body, the blue sutures in a transplant incision cannot be removed because they are anchoring the deep fascial layers. Discussion with the surgeon will give the clinician direction on when and if sutures can be removed.

COMORBIDITIES

Diabetes

Diabetes has multiple inhibitory effects on wound healing, including neuropathic, macrovascular, and microvascular changes, as well as altering cytokine and growth factor signaling.[47] Regardless of the etiology of the wound (surgical, neuropathic, pressure, venous, arterial, acute, or chronic) the patient with diabetes or routinely uncontrolled blood glucose levels is at risk for delayed healing. At the cellular level, diabetes is associated with decreased PDGF receptor expression[48] on epithelial and endothelial cells, thereby altering the wound healing process at the initial phase of hemostasis. In addition,

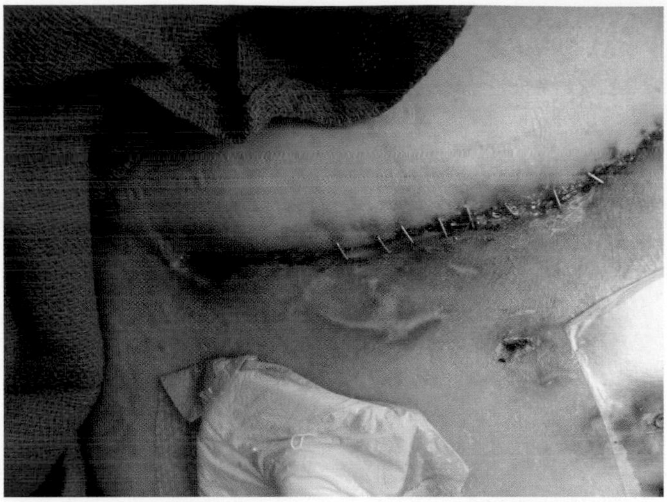

FIGURE 12-10 Surgical incision on a transplant patient. The patient on antirejection medications (Prednisone and Cellcept) after a liver transplant. Note the poor epithelial bridging of the approximated edges and the opening at the right side of the incision, indicating poor healing of the subcutaneous tissue with tunneling under the incision. The wound may require surgical I&D and negative pressure therapy to promote healing and prevent infection.

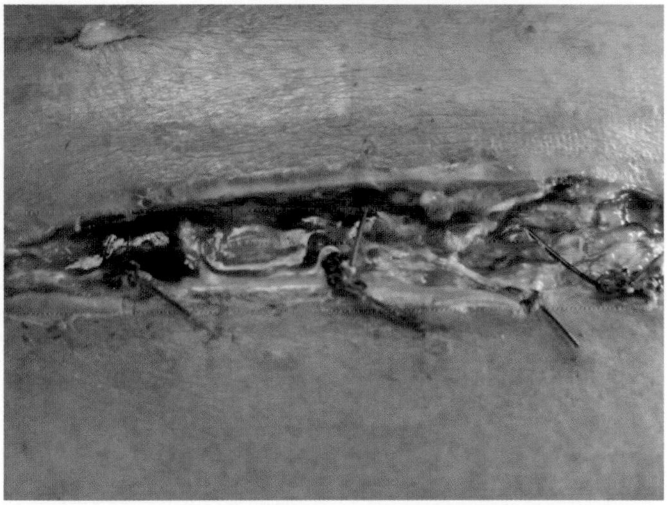

FIGURE 12-11 Close view of surgical wound. Evidence of protein deficiency is visible in the poor quality of the tissue in this surgical incision, including lack of granulation tissue, slough, rolled edges, and extrusion of the deep sutures, which are acting as a foreign body.

patients with diabetes exhibit a prolonged inflammatory phase attributed to the following:

1. A disproportionate expression of vascular cell adhesion molecules by endothelial cells, which increases extravasation and inflammatory cell accumulation at the wound site.
2. The presence and increased infiltration of wound-activated macrophages (WAMs), which contribute to an increased and prolonged expression of inflammatory cytokines.[49,50]
3. Higher levels of neutrophil-formed extracellular traps (termed NETs[51]).

In the proliferative phase, diabetic wounds exhibit the following characteristics:

1. Increased accumulation of fibrotic ECM at wound edges results in stalled keratinocyte migration (**FIGURE 12-12**).[52]
2. Impaired fibroblast signaling further contributing to poor granulation tissue formation.[53,54]
3. Glycation of the ECM, which causes ECM instability and disrupts matrix assembly and interactions between collagen and proteoglycans.[55,56] The ECM instability is compounded by the fact that high glucose levels stimulate MMP production by fibroblasts, macrophages, and endothelial cells.[57]
4. Poor ECM maturation secondary to elevated MMPs and reactive oxygen species (ROS) from inflammatory cells.[56] Early cell senescence diminishes the effectiveness of newly arriving progenitor cells and biases the local cellular environment toward one of oxidation and proinflammation.[43] The triad of early cell senescence, diminished cell proliferation, and impaired cellular migration escalates the challenge of wound healing in the patient with diabetes.[58]
5. An imbalance of free radical and antioxidants results in the overproduction of ROS and oxidative stress which lead to delayed wound healing.[56]

Finally, there is an altered sensitivity to VEGF[59] resulting in decreased endothelial progenitor cell numbers and recruitment in response to injured tissue, thereby leading to poor revascularization. The impact of these cell signaling defects in the wound healing phase is illustrated in **FIGURE 12-13**.

The American Diabetes Association (ADA) and the American College of Endocrinology (ACE) have established guidelines for blood glucose and hemoglobin A1C levels for patients with diabetes in order to minimize complications (**TABLE 12-6**).

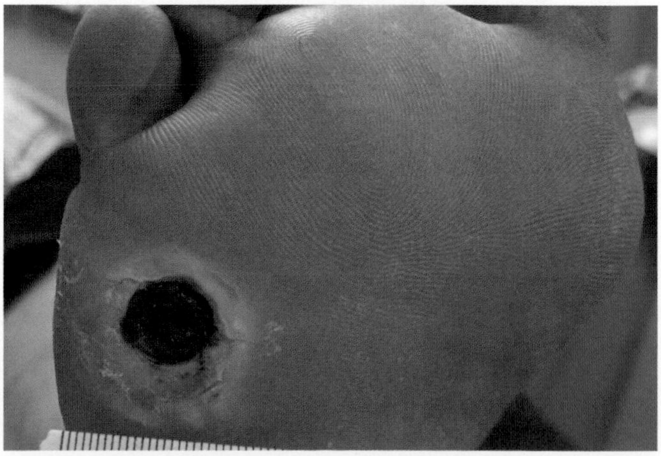

FIGURE 12-12 Diabetic foot ulcer. The heavy callus at the edge of a diabetic foot wound is a result of stalled keratinocyte migration and a probable lack of total off-loading of the injured tissue.

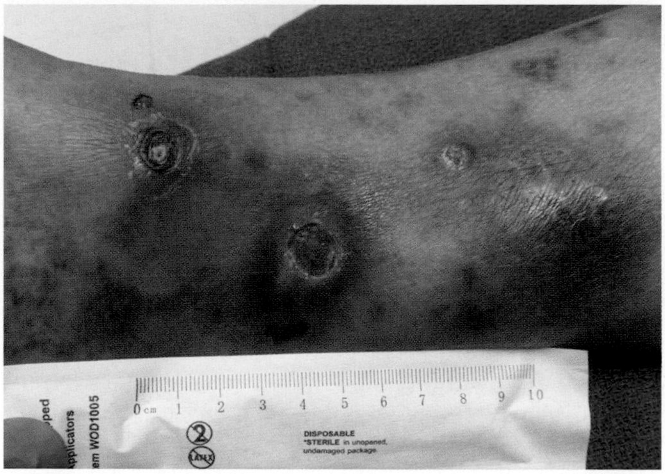

FIGURE 12-13 Skin on the lower extremity of a patient with diabetes. The brawny skin with multiple wounds is characteristic of poorly controlled diabetes, especially if the patient has renal failure. The punctuate appearance is a result of poor vascularization of the injured tissue.

The ACE recommends that postoperative blood glucose levels be maintained at less than 180 mg/dL and further states that patients with hyperglycemia have higher infection rates.[61] Clinically, patients with diabetic foot ulcers who have A1C levels less than 7.1% have shorter healing times than those who have higher levels, and patients with higher A1C levels had more frequent ulcer recurrence.[62] Another review recommended that presurgical glucose levels be maintained in the 100–180 mg/dL range in order to prevent infection, decrease the risk of hypoglycemia, and prevent dehydration as a result of osmotic diuresis.[63,64] Studies also suggest that the medications used for treating diabetes actually facilitate wound healing by controlling ROS levels.[56]

CASE STUDY

CONTINUED

As treatment continued on the patient's lower extremity wound, it was noted that the wound was granulated but not epithelializing. The patient had not reported diabetes at the time of evaluation and did not have the bodybuild or diet to indicate he was high risk for diabetes. However, in exploring every possible cause of poor healing, in addition to the radiated tissue, the patient reported that his grandmother had diabetes with lower extremity complications that led to amputation. He agreed to have his fasting blood glucose levels tested and did indeed have type 2 diabetes. He initially tried to control his blood glucose levels with diet and exercise; however, when he developed other medical issues including a gastrointestinal bleed, he required oral medication.

DISCUSSION QUESTIONS

1. What are the mechanisms by which diabetes impedes wound healing?
2. What are the visible signs that would indicate a wound is not healing because of diabetes?
3. What risk factors does this patient have for diabetes?

TABLE 12-6 Recommendations for Glycemic Control for Patients with Diabetes

	Hemoglobin A1C	Fasting Plasma Glucose	Postprandial Plasma Glucose
ADA	<7%	90–130 mg/dL 5–7.2 mmol/L	<180 mg/dL <10 mmol/L
ACE[60]	6.5%	<110 mg/dL 4.4–7.2 mmol/L	<180 mg/dL <10 mmol/L

Data from ADA—American Diabetes Association. Management of Hyperglycemia in Type 2 Diabetes: A Patient-Centered Approach. Available at: http://care.diabetesjournals.org/content/35/6/1364.full.pdf+html. Accessed August 29, 2018 and Garber AJ, Handelsman Y, Grunberger G, et al. Consensus statement by the American Association of Clinical Endocrinologists and American College of Endocrinology on the comprehensive type 2 diabetes management algorithm—2020 executive summary. *Endocr Pract*. 2020;26(1):107-139.

An extensive review of diabetes and diabetic foot wounds is found in Chapter 7, Diabetes and the Diabetic Foot. However, the effect of diabetes, sometimes undiagnosed, on poor wound healing regardless of the wound etiology is a factor that always needs to be considered, especially if the patient has a known or suspected risk for diabetes or has a family history of diabetes.

Obesity

The health consequences of obesity (defined as BMI greater than 30[65]) include a range of negative outcomes, including cardiovascular disease,[66] diabetes,[67,68] physical limitations,[60] and decreased mobility.[69] Excess body weight influences the onset and progression of chronic illness through multiple pathways.[63] Adipose tissue is active, releasing nonesterified fatty acids, hormones (including leptin, glycerol, proinflammatory cytokines, eg, tumor necrosis factor-α), interleukin-6, and chemokines (including monocyte chemotactic protein-1), as well as other bioactive mediators.[70,71] In overweight or obese individuals, the increased number of adipocytes results in higher levels of all of these factors, thereby changing the regulation of basic physiologic processes at a systemic level,[70] and supposedly at the local level of the wound environment as well.[72]

There is now evidence that obesity also contributes to delayed wound healing by creating an aberrant low-level inflammatory state[73] as well as disturbed macrophage differentiation. In addition,[74] studies have shown that obese patients have higher risks for surgical site infections, wound dehiscence, and delayed wound healing.[75–78] This may be in part due to the decreased vascularity of adipose tissue with relatively decreased oxygen tension, resulting in decreased collagen synthesis, decreased immunity to infection, overall decreased ability to support the processes of wound healing, and increased tissue necrosis (**FIGURE 12-14**).[79] The decreased vascularity may be inherent (with chronic low-grade inflammation and increased glucocorticoids that suppress angiogenesis) or acquired (as a result of surgical and trauma tissue injury that disrupts the adipose tissue); however, either mechanism can disrupt the normal healing process.[79] The heightened inflammatory state can also result in part from chronic venous insufficiency and thereby affect wound healing, especially in the lower extremities.[80] The specific mechanisms involved in the chronic low-grade inflammatory process have been studied primarily in obese mice studies and have consistently shown increased proinflammatory cytokine production resulting from the activation of invariant natural killer T cells by the excess lipid.[79] Other inflammatory mediators that have been shown to increase with obesity include angiotensinogen, tumor necrosis factor-alpha, leptin, interleukin 6, and transforming growth factor-beta.[73,81] In addition, decreased adiponectin concentration (which occurs with obesity even though it is produced by adipocytes) impairs adequate profusion and wound epithelialization.[79] Other factors that may cause wounds or impede wound healing in the obese population are the prevalent comorbidities, nonadherence to treatment plans, poor nutrition, increased risk of friction/shear with resulting pressure ulcers, and confirmed infection.[82,83] Most strategies to address poor wound healing in the obese have concentrated on maintaining blood glucose levels, proper nutrition for optimal healing, preventing infections, and meticulous wound care. However, one animal study using obese mice suggests that physical exercise may help improve cutaneous healing in obese individuals.[73] Research on both cellular causes and interventions and holistic treatments such as exercise is still investigational but much needed, given the increased prevalence of obesity in our society.

Protein Energy Malnutrition

Healing a wound without protein is like building a house without bricks and lumber—amino acids are the building blocks needed for the growth of new tissue, as was so exquisitely detailed in Chapter 2. Ingested proteins are metabolized into amino acids and peptides that serve as enzymes, hormones, cytokines, growth factors, and components of antibodies, all of which play a very important role in tissue maintenance and wound healing. Patient populations who are known to be at risk for protein energy malnutrition (PEM), defined as inadequate energy and protein intake to meet bodily demands, including the elderly,[84] HIV-positive patients,[85] and liver/cirrhosis patients (**FIGURE 12-15**).[86] **TABLE 12-7** lists the protein requirements for wound healing, and when these proteins are not available from daily nutrition, they are taken from the skeletal muscle stores.

The normal body is 75% lean body mass (protein and water) and 25% fat (the calorie reservoir). If there is a loss of lean body mass, the host takes precedent over the wound and healing will not occur (**FIGURE 12-16**).[87] In addition, the individual will exhibit attenuated physical and mental function with poorer clinical outcomes, including wound healing. **TABLE 12-8**[88] provides the relationship between loss of lean body mass and wound formation and/or healing. Laboratory values used to detect or measure PEM are given in **TABLE 12-1**, and include albumin, prealbumin, transferrin, and retinal binding protein. Albumin is commonly measured especially as an indicator for chronic malnutrition; however, it has the disadvantage of having a long half-life (20 days) and may not accurately reflect the protein substrates available for healing if the patient is acutely ill, dehydrated, or in hepatic or renal failure.[89] Advantages of prealbumin include the following: has a short half-life (48–72 hours), is not affected by dehydration

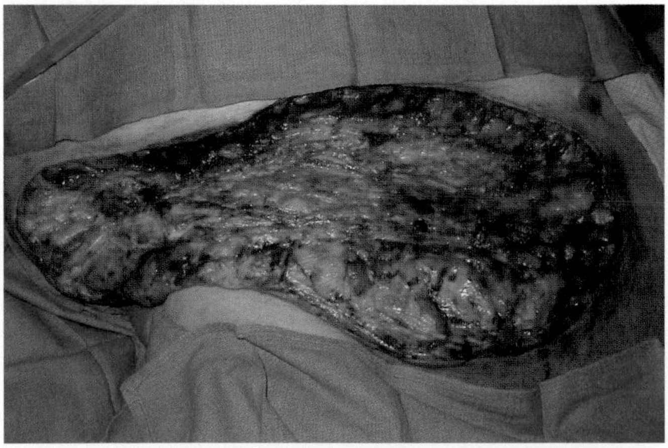

FIGURE 12-14 Abdominal wound on postsurgical patient. Obese patients are prone to poor healing of abdominal surgical wounds because of poor nutrition, prevalence of diabetes, poor vascularity of adipose tissue, and high risk of infection. These wounds frequently require surgical debridement, prolonged negative pressure wound therapy, and continued serial debridement and pulsed lavage with suction.

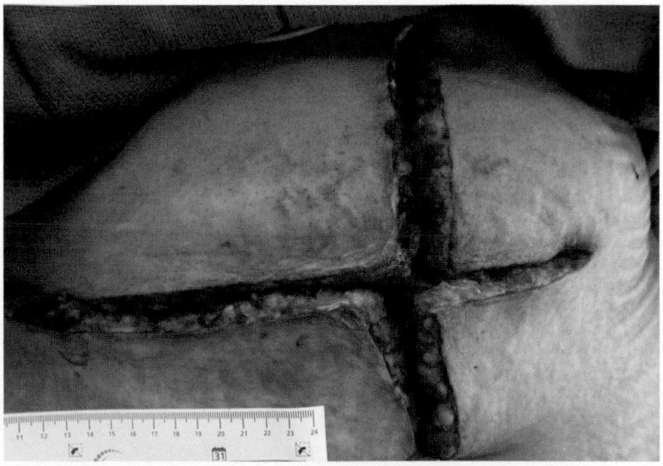

FIGURE 12-15 Dehisced incision on a patient with liver transplant. Patients who have liver cirrhosis are at risk for protein energy malnutrition, which impedes wound healing, as seen in this dehisced incision after a liver transplant. Healing is further compromised by the antirejection medications, which the patient has to take. Note the yellow jaundiced color of the skin, typical of patients with elevated bilirubin levels due to liver failure.

TABLE 12-7 Nutritional Requirements for Wound Healing

	Calories[a]	Protein[b]
Normal (at rest)	20–25 kcal/kg/day (age dependent)	0.8 g/kg/day 60–70 g
Postoperative/ill/injured	30–50% above normal	1.2–2 g/kg/day
Large open wounds, burns	30–35 kcal/kg/day (normal weight) 40 kcal/kg/day (underweight)	1.5–2 g/kg (adults) 2.5–2 g/kg/day (children)[c]
Malnourished	50% above normal	1.5 g/kg/day plus anabolic agent[a]

[a]Data from Demling RH, Nutrition, anabolism, and the wound healing process: an overview. *ePlasty.* 2009;9:65-94.

[b]Data from Huckleberry Y. Nutritional support and the surgical patient. *Am J Health Syst Pharm.* 2004;61(7):671-682.

[c]Data from Clark A, Imran J, Madni T, Wolf SE. Nutrition and metabolism in burn patients. *Burns Trauma.* 2017;5:11.

or renal failure, does not increase with stress, decreases with sepsis and stress, and is easily monitored. Therefore, it is considered a more accurate reflection of a patient's nutritional status.[87] Transferrin is a glycoprotein that binds and transports iron, and its level decreases with inflammation and malnutrition. However, it is less reliable (may increase with iron deficiency) and more expensive, thus not used as frequently as the other measures.[90,91] Retinal binding protein levels have been shown to decrease with protein malnutrition and vitamin A deficiency, and it is especially sensitive in patients with acute stress, inflammation, and infection, as well as in women and children.[92]

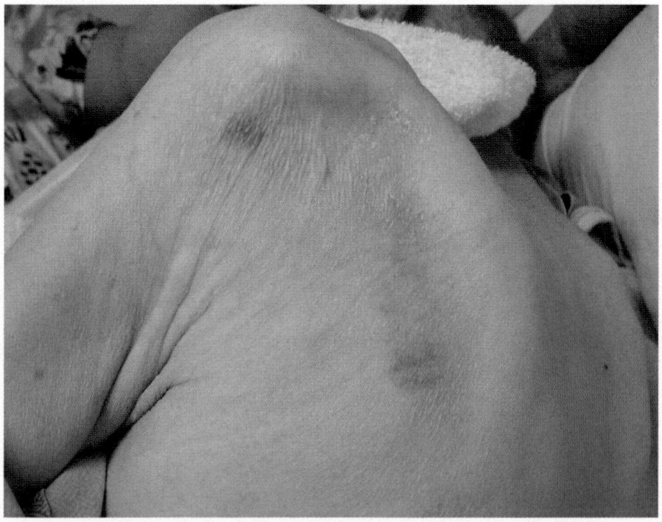

FIGURE 12-16 Patient with loss of lean body mass. Patients who have a 30% loss of lean body mass are at high risk for developing pressure ulcers. Note the severe muscle atrophy and lack of soft tissue to protect the bony prominences, with resulting Stage I pressure ulcers on the scapula. Whether or not pressure ulcers in these patients are preventable remains controversial.

TABLE 12-8 Loss of Lean Body Mass Relative to Wound Healing

% Loss of Total Lean Body Mass	Implication for Wound Healing
10%	Impaired immune response, increased risk of infection
20%	Impaired or delayed wound healing, increased risk of infection, thin skin
30%	No wound healing, increased incidence of pressure ulcers
40%	Death, usually from pneumonia

Used with permission from Demling RH. Nutrition, anabolism, and the wound healing process: an overview. *ePlasty.* 2009;9:65-94.

Recent literature discusses the limitations in using these values to determine malnutrition because the inflammatory process can affect these levels in almost all chronic conditions, terming the values "negative acute-phase reactants" and, thus, no longer valid to use alone as a basis for providing nutritional interventions.[93,94] A decline in serum albumin and prealbumin are therefore inflammatory markers associated with nutrition risk which is defined as "the risk of developing malnutrition and/or poor clinical outcomes if nutrition support is not provided." In 2012[95] the Academy of Nutrition and Dietetics (Academy) and the American Society for Parenteral and Enteral Nutrition (ASPEN) released a joint consensus statement that proposes a three-pronged etiology-based definition of malnutrition (**TABLE 12-9**), as well as the following six characteristics for the diagnosis:

- Insufficient energy intake
- Weight loss
- Loss of muscle mass
- Loss of subcutaneous fat
- Localized or generalized fluid accumulation that may sometimes mask weight loss
- Diminished functional status as measured by hand-grip strength.[94]

Guidelines state that the presence of two or more of these criteria constitutes a diagnosis of malnutrition.[94] Thus, one of the most important aspects of diagnosing malnutrition is the subjective patient history (including recent food intake,

TABLE 12-9 Etiology-Based Definitions of Malnutrition

1. Malnutrition in the context of social or environmental circumstances (starvation-related malnutrition). May be pure starvation due to financial or social reasons or caused by anorexia nervosa.
2. Malnutrition in the context of acute illness or injury, such as organ failure, pancreatic cancer, rheumatoid arthritis, or sarcopenic obesity.
3. Malnutrition in the context of chronic illness, such as major infections, burns, trauma, or closed head injury.

CLINICAL CONSIDERATION

For very active patients, for example, runners, who are having difficulty with wound healing, assessing the caloric intake along with the energy expenditures during exercise may be helpful, in which case limiting the exercise until wound healing is completed may be the solution.

unintentional loss of body weight, and medications), physical examination, and functional assessment.

Laboratory values for inflammation (C-reactive protein, white blood count, and blood glucose levels) can help determine if the malnutrition is due to starvation, chronic disease, or acute disease/injury.[94] Two other screening tools that have been published are the Canadian Nutrition Screening Tool and the MEAL Scale. The Canadian Tool asks the patient the following two questions:

1. Have you lost weight in the past 6 months without trying to lose this weight? (If the patient reports a weight loss but gained it back, consider it as no weight loss.)
2. Have you been eating less than usual for more than a week?

Two "yes" answers indicate malnutrition risk, and this was shown to be valid with or without considering the patient's body mass index. Validity testing of the Canadian Tool was performed on 1015 patients admitted to 18 Canadian hospitals for more than 2 days.[96] Fulton et al.[97] looked at 18 factors thought to be associated with malnutrition and found only 4 to be statistically significant: the presence of multiple wounds, eating less than usual, eating less than 3 meals per day, and a low activity level. Using this information, they developed the MEAL scale (**TABLE 21-10**) for nutrition screening in the wound patient population.

The Mini Nutritional Assessment (MNA) was developed by the Nestle Research Center and Toulouse University, France, for the older population but is also useful in other patient groups. The MNA consists of 18 easily measurable items classified into the following 4 categories:

1. Anthropometric measurements (four questions on weight, height, and weight loss)
2. Dietary questionnaire (six questions related to number of meals, food and fluid intake, autonomy of feeding)
3. Global assessment (six questions related to lifestyle, medication, and mobility)
4. Subjective assessment (two questions on self-perception of health and nutrition)

Validation studies demonstrated the strong capacity of the MNA to evaluate the nutritional status of older adults and had a strong correlation with biochemical parameters, especially albumin. The full tool with explanations for administering is available at: https://www.swrwoundcareprogram.ca/UPLOADS/CONTENTDOCUMENTS/HCPR%20-%20MNA%20GUIDE.PDF[98] or on their website https://www.mna-elderly.com/forms/mini/mna_mini_english.pdf.[99]

Imaging tools such as dual-energy X-ray absorptiometry, bioelectrical impedance, ultrasound, and computed tomography scan are being used for muscle mass assessment and have the potential to be a "biomarker" for standardized objective nutrition assessment in the future.[100] Hand dynometry and sit to stand are two functional tests that have been related to nutrition status.[101]

TABLE 12-10 The MEAL Scale for Nutrition Screening in the Wound Patient Population

Multiple wounds	Do you have >1 open wound?	
	0	No
	1	Yes
Eats <3 meals	How many meals, not including snacks, do you eat in a typical day?	
	0	≥3 meals
	1	≤3 meals
Appetite loss	Thinking about your normal food intake, would you say you are eating about the same, more, or less than usual?	
	0	About the same or more than usual
	1	Less than usual
Level of activity	Thinking about your normal level of activity, how would you consider your activity level over the past month?	
	0	Normal
	0	Not quite normal, but able to do most things
	1	Not feeling up to most things, in bed or chair less than half the day
	1	Able to do little activity and spend most of the day in bed or chair
	2	Pretty much bedridden, rarely out of bed

Total points: 0–1, not at risk; 2–4, at risk.

Reproduced with permission from Way LW, ed. *Current Surgical Diagnosis and Treatment*. 11th ed. New York, NY: McGraw-Hill; 2003.

The macronutrients needed for wound healing include carbohydrates which stimulate insulin production and help in the anabolic process of wound healing, fats which supply additional calories, proteins which are needed for collagen synthesis and granulation formation, and fluids (particularly water) which maintain skin turgor and promotes tissue perfusion and oxygenation.[93] The micronutrients (including amino acids, vitamins, and minerals) are also vital to wound healing; however, the need for supplementation is less definitive.[65] **TABLE 12-11** contains a list of micronutrients important for cellular function, survival, and thus for wound healing. These nutrients tend to be deficient during severe stress and with PEM and thus amplify stress, metabolic derangements, and catabolism.[86]

Arginine is an amino acid used in the biosynthesis of protein, a necessary process for wound healing to occur. Benefits of arginine supplementation include increased collagen deposition, increased lymphocyte mitogenesis, increased production of growth hormone, and increased activation of T cells.[102] A study by Leigh et al.[103] of patients with pressure ulcers found

TABLE 12-11 Micronutrients Needed for Wound Healing

Vitamin A	Stimulant for the onset of wound healing, epithelialization, and fibroblast deposition of collagen; is anti-inflammatory by increasing the number of monocytes and macrophages at early wound onset; facilitates epithelial cell differentiation; counteracts effects of steroids
Vitamin C	Cofactor for collagen synthesis, immunity, fatty acid metabolism
Vitamin D	Regulates structural integrity of its receptor signaling; induces cathelicidin, an antimicrobial peptide that promotes wound healing
Copper	Cofactor for connective tissue production, collagen cross-linking, and cytochrome oxidase for energy production
Iron	Cofactor in collagen synthesis; deficiency results in impaired T cell and phagocyte function
Manganese	Cofactor for collagen and ground substance synthesis
Selenium	Antioxidant, role in wound healing under investigation
Zinc	Cofactor for DNA, RNA, and polymerase for collagen and ground substance synthesis; increases immunity

Data from Demling RH. Nutrition, anabolism, and the wound healing process: an overview. *ePlasty.* 2009;9:65-94. Department of Surgery, Brigham and Women's Hospital, Boston, MA, and Burn and Wound Program, Health South Braintree Rehabilitation Hospital, Braintree, MA and Quain AM, Khardori NM. Nutrition in wound care management: a comprehensive overview. *Wounds.* 2015;27(12):327-335.

that 4.5 g/day supplementation of arginine was sufficient to facilitate wound healing but must be given with adequate protein intake to be effective. Vitamins A, C, and D all play a role in the wound healing process, and deficits have been shown to impede the progression of the healing cascade.[104–106] The most common use of Vitamin A supplementation is to offset the effects of steroids on wound healing.[105] Supplementation of other vitamins is recommended only if there are measured deficits with the following recommendations for amounts:

1. Vitamin A—10,000–15,000 IU/day administered in a short course of 10–14 days to prevent toxicity
2. Vitamin C—500–1000 mg in divided doses for wound healing and 1–2 g/day for severe wounds, eg, extensive burns
3. Vitamin D—deficient in patients with venous ulcers and pressure ulcers; dosages not given[93]

The minerals which have been suggested as critical in wound healing, specifically in enzyme and metalloenzyme structure, include zinc, selenium, and iron. Zinc deficiency affects all phases of wound healing; however, supplementation is recommended only in the case of deficiency.[104] Recommended supplementation in the zinc-deficient patient range varies from 40 mg/day to 220 mg twice a day for 10–14 days and must be carefully monitored because excessive zinc supplementation can interfere with the absorption of iron and copper.[93] Negative pressure wound therapy, particularly for open abdominal wounds, has been shown to significantly reduce the amounts of micronutrients; therefore, these patients need to be nutritionally monitored and supplements provided as needed.[107]

One of the most helpful questions to use in the subjective examination is "What did you have for breakfast this morning?" and "What did you have for dinner last night?" The answers can give useful insight into the patient's eating habits such as protein intake, caloric intake, and consumption of high-glycemic index foods (especially important for patients with pre- or diagnosed diabetes). Concerns that are raised as a result of the answers can be followed up with additional tests and measurements. Nutritional supplements are an integral part of treating patients who have PEM, and oral or enteral nutrition is preferred over parenteral nutrition.

In summary, all patients with nonhealing wounds need to be screened for nutritional deficiencies. Any patient found at risk by a screening tool or who has other red flags that indicate inadequate nutrition may be a factor in poor healing capacity is advised to have further testing for specific deficits, counseling by a registered dietician, and supplements when deemed appropriate.[108]

Arterial Insufficiency

A nonhealing wound may be the first visible sign of undiagnosed peripheral arterial disease (PAD). Arterial ulcers typically result from PAD, either macro- or microvascular disease, which can be a result of arteriosclerosis or atherosclerosis. Progressive narrowing of the vessels manifests as poor circulation, decreasing the delivery of oxygen and nutrients to tissues while simultaneously preventing the removal of metabolic waste products, both of which contribute to delayed healing.[109] Ischemic pain, a major problem with severe PAD and possibly with an arterial ulcer, further debilitates the individual. See Chapter 4, Vascular Wounds, for a detailed discussion of the diagnosis and treatment of PAD.

Other less common diseases that also cause arterial insufficiency with decreased oxygen perfusion of distal injured tissue, include but are not limited to the following: large and medium vessel disease as a result of arteriosclerosis obliterans, thromboangitis obliterans, arteriovenous malformation, Raynaud's phenomenon (microthrombotic disease), antiphospholipid syndrome, cholesterol emboli, Takayasu arteritis, sickle cell anemia and polycythemia vera, and acute trauma or previous lower extremity fracture.[110] The reduction in arterial blood supply results in tissue hypoxia and ischemic damage.[111] (Refer to Chapter 4.)

Risk factors for the development of atherosclerosis, a common cause of arterial insufficiency, include increasing age, smoking, hypertension, dyslipidemia, family history, diabetes, sedentary lifestyle, and obesity. Obesity, although associated with atherosclerosis, has not been directly correlated to arterial ulcers or insufficiency.[85] Further complicating the clinical picture is the fact that arterial insufficiency may be present in concert with other pathological conditions, which must be ruled out or addressed in tandem. Unlike venous ulcers that can be successfully treated with therapeutic compression, chronic wounds caused by arterial insufficiency require the restoration of arterial function via revascularization.[112]

Chronic Edema

Patients with chronic venous insufficiency suffer from ambulatory venous hypertension, meaning that the venous pressure remains elevated during ambulation.[113,114] The mechanism by which the sustained ambulatory venous hypertension causes ulcers remains unclear. Proposed theories include pericapillary fibrin cuff deposition, abnormalities of the fibrinolytic system, trapping of growth factors by macromolecules in the dermis,[115] an increase in the percentage of local senescent cells,[43] and leukocyte plugging in lower extremity vessels.[116] Ineffective pumping of the calf muscle combined with venous valve dysfunction or incompetence contributes to pooling of the blood in the dependent venous circulatory system. This triggers capillary damage and activates the inflammatory process implicated in the theory of leukocyte-mediated endothelial damage and cuffing.[117] The accumulation of fibrin itself has direct negative effects on wound healing by down-regulating the synthesis of collagen.[118] In addition, the presence of fibrin cuffing creates a barrier to normal vessel function and traps blood-derived growth factors.[119,120]

Chronic venous insufficiency is discussed in Chapter 4 and lymphedema in Chapter 5. In addition to wounds developing specifically as a result of these pathologies, wounds of other etiologies will have slower or halted healing rates if edema is present. Frequently, if there is ankle hypomobility with resulting lower leg muscle atrophy, edema is undetected based on apparent girth (FIGURE 12-17). Performing the pitting test (pressing on the tissue with the forefinger for 5 seconds and watching for poor tissue rebounding) will detect edema. Even if the wound is not related to the edema (eg, trauma or pressure), management of the edema is a necessary component of the care plan in order to optimize healing.[121,122] When cellular debris and necrotic cells are trapped in the interstitial spaces and healing tissue is further from the arterial supply, delayed wound healing affects the return to optimal function.

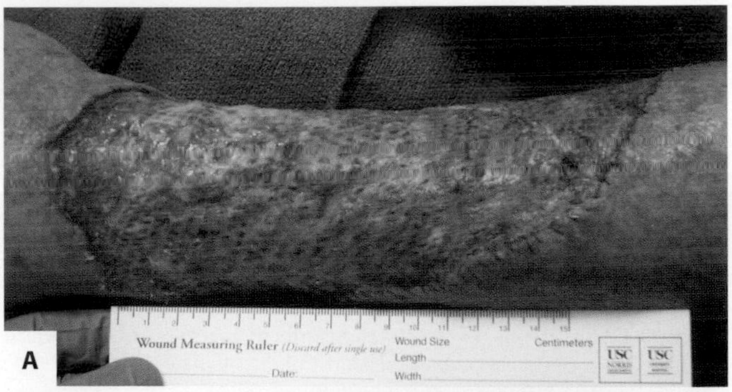

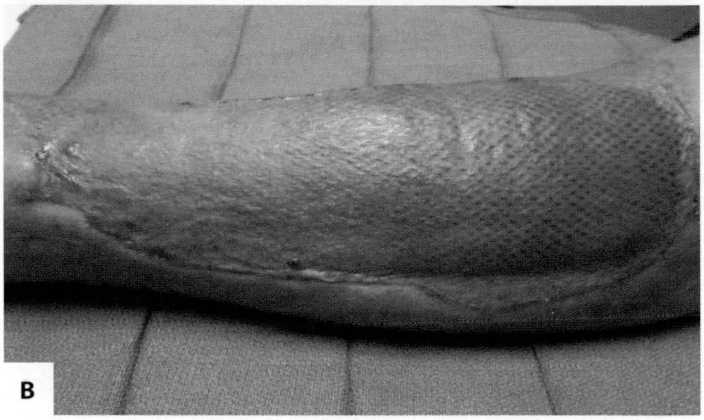

FIGURE 12-17 A. Effect of edema on wound healing. Edema impedes the healing of a wound regardless of etiology. This patient received extensive debridement of skin and subcutaneous tissue for necrotizing fasciitis, followed by extensive skin grafts. The ankle had less than a 30°-degree range of motion, combined with trauma to the lymphatic system. Compression was a vital component of the care plan in order for the skin graft to fully heal. **B. Healed skin graft.**

CASE STUDY

CONTINUED

Although the patient's lower extremity did not appear edematous, there was pitting with finger pressure and severe visible reflux upon standing for more than 60 seconds. Vascular studies revealed incompetent valves in the greater saphenous vein; therefore, compression was initiated using a multilayer compression system with a decrease in calf girth of 1 cm at which time he was transitioned to a 40 mmHg, Class II compression garment.

DISCUSSION QUESTIONS

1. What are the patient's risk factors for chronic venous insufficiency?
2. What mechanisms of edema interfere with this patient's ability to heal?

Cardiac Disease

The overall physical status of an organism, broadly defined as health and viability, is defined by the relative representation of cells in the five major categories set forth by a very comprehensive review by Haines et al.[43] The five categories are as follows:

1. Regenerative mitotic (stem) cells
2. Quiescent postmitotic cells
3. Transformed cells (cancers)
4. Senescent postmitotic cells
5. Apoptotic cells

Senescent postmitotic cells are defined as cells that are damaged in ways that disable their ability to proliferate but do not cause carcinogenic transformation. Apoptotic cells are defined as cells that execute a normal death program. One of the most sensitive tissue types to a balanced cell homeostasis is the cardiac tissue. Cardiac cells, termed cardiomyocytes, in healthy individuals represent a cell population that

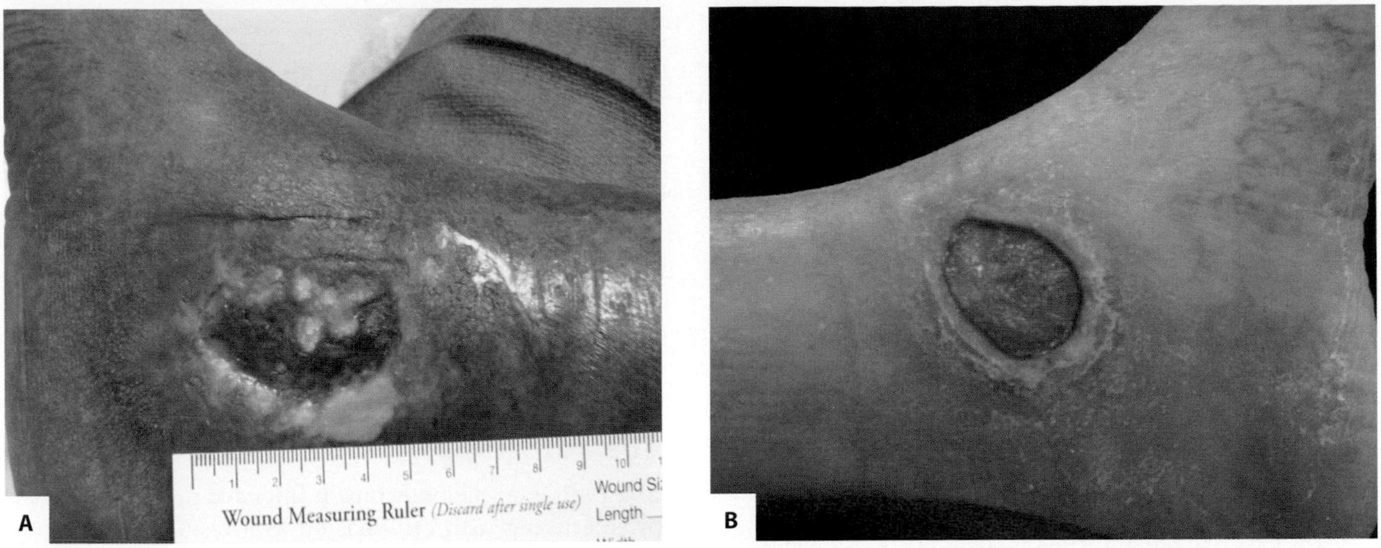

FIGURE 12-18 A and B. Wounds with cardiac insufficiency. Both of the ankle wounds were on patients whose healing potential was impaired by cardiac insufficiency. The wound in A was a 90-year-old lady with a known history that included coronary bypass surgery, mitral valve regurgitation, and pacemaker. The wound in B was on the ankle of a 65-year-old man who had no known history of heart disease. He had palpable pulses so the wound was thought to be more venous. However, after he had emergency cardiac bypass surgery, the wound healed in a timely sequence. Note that both wounds, while at first appearing to be venous by location, are actually on the ankle and not in the gaiter area. Also, the round even edges are typical of wounds that have hypoxia.

has terminally differentiated and is in a healthy state, ready to perform their specific function.[123,124]

Cardiac disease is a common comorbidity associated with poor wound healing which may be age-related or trauma-related tissue buildup of senescent cells, which in turn creates cytotoxic local environments. The accumulation of senescent cell types over time is a major contributor to age-associated pathologies characterized by dysregulated inflammation, including atherosclerosis and stroke.[66,125]

A study by Zhao et al. in 2012 sought to determine the effect of type 2 diabetes on the reparative function of endothelial progenitor cells (EPCs), which are responsible for maintaining microvascular integrity and angiogenesis.[126] They hypothesized that the elevated hemoglobin A1C levels found in patients with diabetes have a profound effect on both peripheral and cardiovascular systems. The lack of EPCs at a site requiring vascular repair results in delayed healing, increased fibrosis, and an overall decrease in tissue function.

Patients with a cardiovascular system that is repeatedly insulted by prolonged exposure to elevated proinflammatory stressors, including obesity and elevated blood glucose levels, are at risk for delayed wound healing. Obesity is a common denominator in both cardiac disease and diabetes. Adipokines, produced by the adipose tissue, are proinflammatory. Thus, the overall proinflammatory bias impairs cardiac function and contributes to an overall systemic state of chronic inflammation, which has the potential to delay wound healing.[125,127,128]

Clinically, poor healing is observed in infection and dehiscence of postsurgical incisions and in distal lower extremity wounds of patients who have wounds of other etiologies (eg, pressure) that do not heal because of poor cardiac output (**FIGURE 12-18A, B**). In addition, untreated congestive heart failure (CHF) can cause chronic lower extremity edema which in turn can cause skin failure. Wounds as a result of CHF have a different location than typical venous insufficiency wounds and usually begin as blisters.

A study by Rhou et al. to determine the independent predictors of failure to heal in patients with diabetic foot ulcers found that comorbid CHF was the only factor independently predictive of delayed or reduced rate of healing.[129] This reinforces the importance of performing a complete systems review, including the cardiovascular system, for a patient who has a hard-to-heal or surgical wound.[130]

CANCER/RADIATION

Three factors affect wound healing in patients who are being treated for any type of cancer: the use of radiation to target specific malignant cells, the use of chemotherapy to treat or prevent metastasis, and the overall decline in general health when a patient is in a catabolic state.

Radiation

Radiotherapy is the use of ionizing radiation given as daily fractions over a period of weeks to a field that includes the tumor tissue and the surrounding nodal stations.[131] While every effort is made to target only the malignant cells, damage to adjacent tissue cannot always be avoided. The effects of the radiation on the tissue can be immediate, acute, and chronic and are summarized in **TABLE 12-12**.[132,133] In addition to causing wounds, which are much like partial- and full-thickness burns, wounds that occur

TABLE 12-12 Immediate, Acute, and Chronic Effects of Radiation

Immediate (within 1 week)	Acute (days to weeks)	Chronic (months to years)
▪ Transient, faint erythema ▪ Dilated capillaries ▪ Epilation ▪ Dry skin	▪ Erythema localized to a radiation field ▪ Warm and tender skin ▪ Edema ▪ Arteriole obstruction by fibrin thrombi ▪ Small foci of hemorrhage ▪ Hyperpigmentation ▪ Dry desquamation ▪ Wet desquamation ▪ Ulceration	▪ Thin, dry, semitranslucent skin ▪ Lack of hair follicles and sebaceous glands ▪ Fibrosis of the skin ▪ Dyspigmentation ▪ Induration with loss of range of motion ▪ Accumulation of fibrinous exudate under the skin ▪ Telangiectasia ▪ Delayed ulceration due to ischemia ▪ Radionecrosis

long after the radiation has been discontinued (eg, trauma, pressure, neuropathic) will have impaired healing because of the histological changes that occur at the time of radiation.

The effects of radiation on the tissue are dependent on the following factors: dose, treatment volume, daily fraction size, energy and type of radiation, total treatment time, individual cellular differences, and host overall well-being.[134] Dosage is measured in mGrays. (One Gray is defined as the absorption of 1 joule of radiation energy by 1 kilogram of matter.) With low doses (up to 100 mGy), there may be single-strand DNA breaks in the cell; however, because of remaining DNA strands in the surrounding area, the damage may be repaired.[135] When medium doses (0.5–5 Gy) are used, cellular death occurs after one or more reproductive divisions as a result of irreparable double-strand DNA breaks. If more than 5 Gy are used, cellular death occurs immediately. The edema and occlusion of the small vessels prevent the influx of platelets to the injured tissue,[135] followed by an increased expression of matrix metalloproteinases, reduction in cytokines and fibroblast recruitment, and decreased angiogenesis.[131] Radiation also causes direct cell death to fibroblasts, which results in decreased tensile strength, altered collagen function, loss of normal tissue construction, and impaired wound healing. The lack of angiogenesis causes skin changes (eg, thin translucent appearance; absent hair follicles, ergo fewer stem cells; lower tensile strength), as well as poor healing of skin that is injured by trauma even after the radiation wound has resolved.[131]

Two therapies that have been reported as potentially beneficial for healing late radiation tissue injury include hyperbaric oxygen therapy[136,137] and stem cell therapy.[138,139] The purpose of both therapies is to increase tissue oxygenation with resulting revascularization of the injured tissue and thereby improve wound healing. As discussed in the case study, hair follicle transplants or pinch grafts have been used to replace hair follicles for dermal wounds occurring in skin damaged by radiation; the follicle bulges are a source of autologous stem cells.[140] Treatment of radiation wounds is much like the treatment of superficial- and deep-partial thickness burns (see Chapter 11, Burn Wound Management): manage the drainage with absorbent dressings, remove necrotic tissue in the least painful way for the patient, prevent infection, use nonadherent dressings such as silicone-backed foams, and optimize quality of life during a very difficult time for the patient.

Chemotherapy

Like radiation, chemotherapy is intended to kill cancer cells by interfering with cell division as a result of the chemical interaction with the DNA.[141] And like radiation, in the process chemotherapy also affects some of the normal cells. One of the most common systemic effects is myelosuppression, defined as decreased production of blood cells by the bone marrow. Myelosuppression results in three conditions that affect wound healing: anemia (decreased red blood cells) with fewer cells to deliver oxygen and nutrients to the injured tissue, neutropenia (decreased white blood cells, especially neutrophils) with decreased ability to phagocytose bacteria and increased risk for infection,[142] and thrombocytopenia (decreased platelets) with an increased risk of bleeding. Chemotherapy has also been reported to inhibit protein synthesis, decrease angiogenesis, decrease extracellular matrix formation, and ultimately delay surgical wound healing or impede healing in other wounds such as pressure ulcers.[142]

Chemotherapy-induced peripheral neuropathy (CIPN) is a side effect of chemotherapy treatment that can potentially result in neuropathic wounds or prevent a patient with a plantar foot wound from feeling the causative mechanical forces. CIPN can be either sensory and painful or sensorimotor and is often associated with nerve damage from diabetes, alcohol, or inherited neuropathy.[143]

Common categories of chemotherapeutic agents and their effects on wound healing are presented in **TABLE 12-13**.[115] The optimal time to deliver chemotherapy to patients requiring surgical removal of a tumor has been the focus of numerous human and animal studies. Historically, it was felt that impaired wound healing occurred most commonly when drugs were administered preoperatively or within 3 weeks postoperatively (specifically those such as adriamycin[144]). In an extensive discussion of wound healing in patients with cancer, Payne et al.[104] conclude that "delaying the initiation of chemotherapeutic regimes until 7–10 days postoperatively seems to have minimal effects on wound healing in this patient population."

Deptula et al. state that in order to minimize the side effects of preoperative radio- and chemotherapy, the best time for surgery is 4–6 weeks after neoadjuvant therapy.[142]

TABLE 12-13 Chemotherapies and Their Effects on Wound Healing

Chemotherapy Agents	Effect on Wound Healing	Recommendations
Alkylating agents Cyclophosphamide Chlorambucil Thiotepa Mechlorethamine Cisplatin	Inhibits fibroblast function Attenuates vasodilation and later neovascularization Delayed wound closure Decreased wound tensile strength	Use as low a dose as possible during the wound healing process
Antimetabolites Methotrexate 5-fluorouracil 6-mercaptopurine Azathioprine	Decrease in wound tensile strength especially in days 3–7	Administer leucovorin with methotrexate Optimize nutrition Begin administering the drug 1–2 weeks postoperatively
Plant alkaloids Vincristine Vinblastine	Transient early decrease in wound tensile strength	Administer preoperatively
Antitumor antibiotics Cleomycin Doxorubicin Actinomycin D Mitomycin C	Limits skin fibroblast production with delayed closure Decreased wound tensile strength	Delay administration 1–2 weeks postoperatively

Adapted from Payne WG, Naidu DK, Wheeler CK, Barkoe D, Mentis M, Salas RE, Smith DJ, Robson MC. Wound healing in patients with cancer. *ePlasty*. 2008;e9. Available at: https://www.ncbi.nlm.nih.gov/pmc/articles/pmc2206003. Accessed September 1, 2018.

The similarities of wound healing cellular processes and metastases of malignant cells are well-documented. Surgical removal of a tumor initiates the wound healing cascade in order to heal the incision; however, the inflammatory process that ensues involves cellular activity that forms "premetastatic niches" where tumor cells can successfully metastasize and develop into tumors.[145,146] Both of these reviews conclude that postponing chemotherapy until after the surgical wound has healed may facilitate the metastatic spread of cancer and that more studies are needed to determine the efficacy of pre- and perioperative chemotherapy.

Bevacizumab, a frequently used chemotherapeutic agent, is an antiangiogenesis drug that works by targeting vascular endothelial growth factor (VEGF). Tumors require high vascularity for survival, so by decreasing the blood supply, tumor growth is impeded. However, wound healing (eg, incisions or pressure ulcers) may also be impaired. The effects of chemotherapy on wound healing are sometimes considered in the sequence of cancer interventions.[147,148] For example, if a patient has radiation for a tumor, followed by surgery to remove the residual malignant tissue, chemotherapy may be delayed until after the surgical incision has healed. If a patient has an existing wound, for example, a pressure ulcer, chemotherapy may be delayed until the wound is healed. Optimizing the healing response for the overall benefit of treating cancer requires a team approach, including patient engagement and adherence.

In addition to delaying wound healing, chemotherapy may induce skin toxicity, manifested as skin rash, skin dryness, and hyperpigmentation[143] (**FIGURE 12-19A, B**). The symptoms will usually resolve when chemotherapy is discontinued. Whether the wound is caused by the chemotherapy or healing is delayed, optimizing the healing response for the overall benefit of treating the patient with cancer requires a team approach, including patient engagement and adherence.

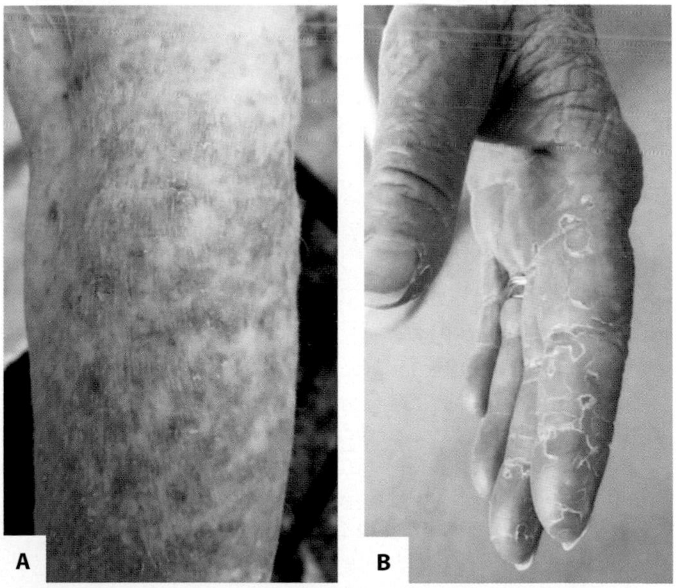

FIGURE 12-19 A and B. Dry scaly skin associated with oral chemotherapy. Even though the targeted cancer cells in this patient were not in the skin, a side effect of the oral chemotherapy was dry, scaly, pruritic skin on both arms. The condition resolved after chemotherapy was discontinued.

Decline in General Health

Short-term systemic side effects of cancer treatments discussed above include nausea and vomiting with decreased appetite, which in turn may lead to protein and calorie deficits for wound healing. Fatigue, depression, stress, and an overall decline in medical status are complications of dealing with cancer and may factor into poor wound healing.

AUTOIMMUNE DISORDERS

Autoimmune diseases such as rheumatoid arthritis, systemic lupus erythematosus, and polyarteritis nodosa present a conundrum in the medical management of associated wounds. The fluctuating state of inflammation of multiple organs, including small vessels to the skin, results in painful vasculitic wounds that are difficult to heal (**FIGURE 12-20**). Frequently, the patient is on steroid therapy to manage the systemic disorder, which may compromise the healing potential. However, if the inflammation is not controlled by medications, pain and wounding may progress.[149] Working closely with the rheumatologist who is managing the medications is required, especially in the acute phase.

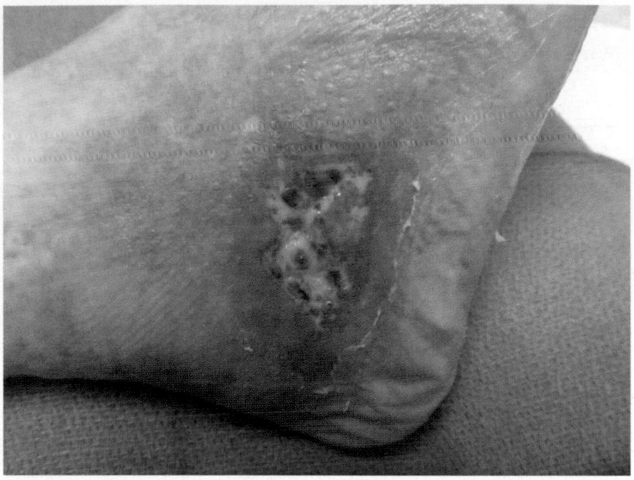

FIGURE 12-20 Wound associated with autoimmune disorder. Spontaneous wounds can occur in patients with autoimmune disorders, such as this one on the foot of a patient with systemic lupus erythematosus. They have a vasculitic presentation with skin necrosis, exquisite pain, and very slow healing because of the medications (eg, prednisone, methotrexate, and other anti-inflammatories).

AGING

In healthy older adults, wound healing may be delayed; however, the quality of healing is not impaired. Other than the delay, most problems with healing in older adults are related to comorbidities and other systemic factors. Delayed healing in the aged is associated with an altered inflammatory response (delayed T-cell infiltration to the wound, changes in chemokine production, and reduced macrophage phagocytic capacity).[144] Every phase of healing is affected by age-related changes, including the following: increased platelet aggregation, increased secretion of inflammatory mediators, delayed infiltration of macrophages and lymphocytes, impaired macrophage function, decreased secretion of growth factors, delayed re-epithelialization, delayed neovascularization, delayed collagen synthesis, delayed remodeling and decreased tensile strength.[150]

CASE STUDY

CONCLUSION

Although it was obvious that the patient's tissue had been irradiated (note the lack of hair on the periwound skin), it had been years since the treatment; however, the ability of the epithelial cells to replicate was destroyed. Because the wound did granulate and the edges were flat, electrical stimulation was initiated using a high-volt pulsed current, 100 pps, voltage sufficient to elicit a tingling response, and a positive active electrode (to attract epithelial cells). Although the response was slow, the wound did thinly epithelialize but would degenerate easily with the least amount of friction or edema.

The patient ultimately had dermatology intervention of transplanted hair follicles. Eight of the 32 transplanted follicles survived and were sufficient to enable the wound to fully epithelialize. The patient continued electrical stimulation at home and the wound remained closed. The key to success, in this case, was the patient's willingness to adhere to an intensive and changing care plan, as well as being proactive in managing the comorbidities (**FIGURE 12-21**).

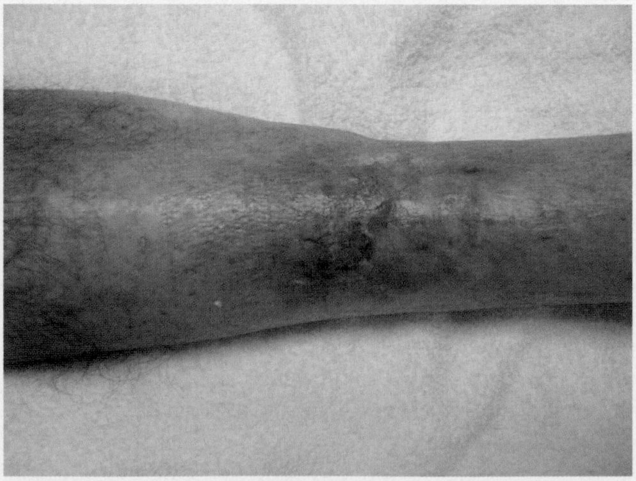

FIGURE 12-21 Case study wound, closed and remodeling.

One of the proven strategies to reduce age-related impairment of wound healing is exercise, which is thought to decrease the levels of proinflammatory cytokines by an exercise-induced anti-inflammatory response in the wound[151,152] (see Chapter 15, Exercise for the Patient with a Wound).

STRESS

Stress, both physical and psychological, has been shown to have a deleterious effect on wound healing. Closely associated with the stress response are fear, presurgical stress,[153] chronic wound-related pain, anticipatory pain (eg, with dressing changes), and anxiety.[154] Regardless of the cause of the stress, the mechanism is the same—stress modulates the immune system function which impairs wound healing.[155] The primary connection between stress and wound healing involves the activation of the hypothalamic–pituitary–adrenal axis in conjunction with the sympathetic–adrenal–medullary axis and the release of hormones. The interactive[144,156] effects of glucocorticoids (cortisol and corticosterone) with proinflammatory cytokines (interleukins and tumor necrosis factor-α) have a negative effect on the wound healing cascade.[157,158] The higher levels of cortisol and the diminished expression of proinflammatory cytokines have been shown to retard the initial inflammatory phase of healing.[153] In addition, the catecholamines (norepinephrine and epinephrine) released in response to stress result in vasoconstriction, decreased tissue perfusion, and decreased cellular response to injury.[144,159] This results in decreased fibroblasts and subsequent decreased granulation formation.

Strategies that help overcome the effect of stress on wound healing include education especially as it relates to anticipated pain, relaxation exercises, topical and systemic pain management, cognitive therapy that alters anxiety,[154] physical exercises,[160] and social support.[153]

PSYCHOSOCIAL BEHAVIORS

Stress can lead to higher levels of anxiety and depression, as well as increase the risk for negative health behaviors such as deprived sleep, poor nutrition, lack of exercise, smoking, and alcohol and drug abuse.[144] Psychosocial stress also leads to poor adherence to care plans, failure to keep medical appointments, and thus poorer clinical outcomes.[161] The effects of smoking and alcohol abuse on each of the phases of wound healing are listed in **TABLE 12-14**.

Smoking

Smoking adversely affects healing by several mechanisms, resulting in delayed and longer healing times, increased risk of the surgical site and chronic wound infections, increased skin necrosis, and increased incidence of dehiscence.[162–164] The primary effect of smoking is tissue hypoxia as a result of several mechanisms, including vasoconstriction.[165,166] As a result, cutaneous blood flow can be decreased by as much as 40%, thereby causing ischemia and impaired wound healing.[167] The vasoconstriction is caused by nicotine stimulating the sympathetic nervous system, resulting in the release of catecholamines that trigger peripheral vasoconstriction and decreased tissue perfusion.[166] Nicotine also decreases fibrinolytic activity and augments platelet adhesiveness, thus increasing blood viscosity and further decreasing the delivery of oxygen to peripheral injured tissue.[144,166] Two other substances in cigarettes that affect tissue perfusion are carbon monoxide, which binds to hemoglobin and thereby decreases the oxygen content of blood, and hydrogen cyanide, which impairs cellular oxygen metabolism.[144,166] As a result of these cellular effects, patients who smoke are also more likely to have higher rates of atherosclerosis, cardiovascular disease, PAD, chronic pulmonary disorders, and cancer, all of which have an impact on healing.

With the increased use of e-cigarettes that vaporize liquid nitrogen, the effect of these products on wound healing has been reported as well, with the following conclusions:

- E-cigarettes affect fibroblast proliferation and migration.
- E-cigarettes cause an increase in apoptosis.
- E-cigarettes prolong wound healing times.
- The adverse effects of cigarette smoke are greater than those of e-cigarettes.[168–170]

TABLE 12-14 Effects of Smoking and Alcohol Abuse on Wound Healing Phases

	Inflammation	Proliferation	Remodeling
Smoking	Impaired leukocyte activity Decreased macrophages Decreased neutrophil bactericidal activity Decreased IL-1 products Decreased phagocytosis of bacteria and debris Cytotoxicity of natural killer cells	Decreased fibroblast migration Decreased wound contraction Decreased epithelial regeneration Decreased extracellular production Increased proteases	
Alcohol abuse	Decreased neutrophil chemokines with decreased neutrophil infiltration Decreased IL-8 and TNF-α Decreased monocyte function Decreased macrophage response to microbes	Decreased endothelial cell response Decreased angiogenesis Increased tissue hypoxia Impaired cell signaling	Decreased production of Type 1 collagen Increased level of MMP-8 Degradation of epithelial ECM Decreased tensile strength of the skin

A study by Liu et al. demonstrated that e-cigarettes "induce endothelial dysfunction through excessive ROS production, resulting in decreased NO bioavailability, increased endothelial cell apoptosis, and impairment in angiogenesis and wound healing, especially under diabetic conditions."[171]

Fortunately, smoking has a transient effect on the tissue microenvironment, and cessation can restore the microenvironment rapidly. Recommendations are cessation at least 4 weeks prior to surgery; longer periods of smoking cessation will decrease the incidence of wound complications.[163,172–174] Abstinence until a surgical site has healed or at least 2 weeks has also been recommended.[164] Short-term cessation of less than 4 weeks does not appear to reduce postoperative complications. In summary, cessation of smoking can reverse some of the effects on wound healing, and patient education is a vital part of treating smokers who have wounds of any etiology.

Alcohol Abuse

Heavy alcohol abuse is defined as more than 4 drinks/day or 14 drinks/week for males and more than 3 drinks/day or 7 drinks/week for females.[175] Patients who are alcohol abusers have higher rates of hospital-acquired infections and surgical site infections.[175] Alcohol intake has been shown to increase insulin resistance and result in higher blood glucose levels.[62] In addition, alcohol abusers have a higher risk for malnutrition as a result of poor eating habits (**FIGURE 12-22A, B**).

Wound healing is inhibited in the inflammatory, proliferative, and remodeling phases by the mechanisms listed in **TABLE 12-14**. Studies have shown that acute ethanol intoxication, not just chronic abuse, has a detrimental effect on wound healing.[176,177] In summary, there is a decrease in the inflammatory and immune responses to injury that result in both delayed healing and increased risk of infection, a decrease in fibroblast migration and angiogenesis during the proliferation phase, and a decrease in Type 1 collagen production with a concurrent increase in protease activity during the remodeling phase, resulting in weaker extracellular matrix.[178,179] The clinical presentation will be slower healing with a tendency to recur with any mechanical force.

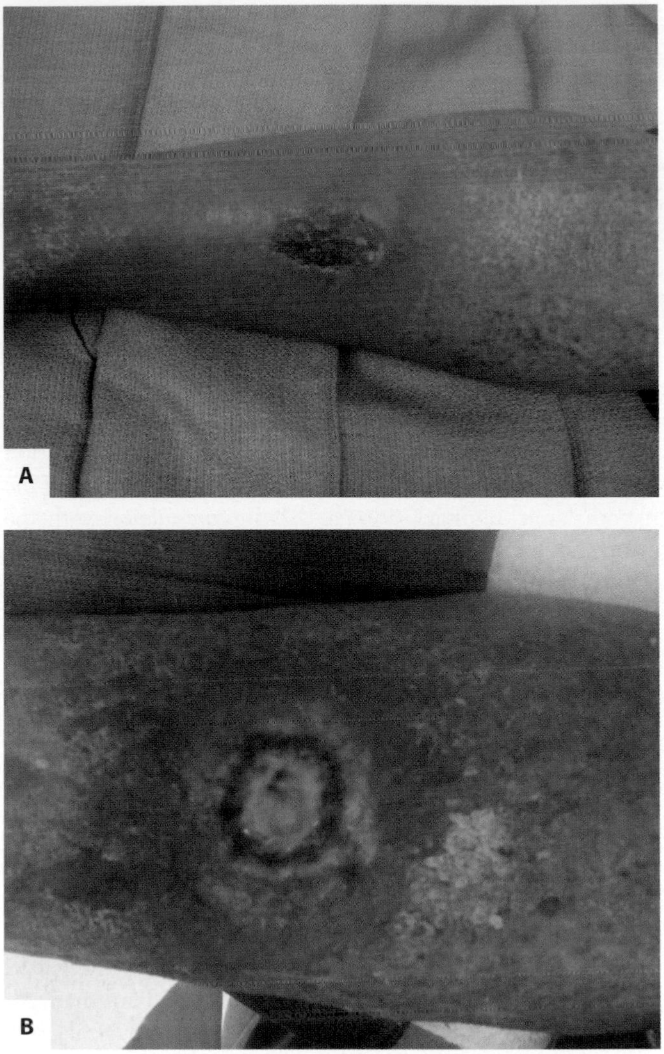

FIGURE 12-22 A. Wound associated with alcohol abuse. Nonhealing wound on the anterior shin of a 23-year-old male who sustained the injury playing recreational sports. The wound was treated with compression, noncontact low-frequency ultrasound, debridement, and collagen matrix dressings. **B. Eight weeks after initiation of treatment.** Although the wound has improved with the treatment, it is not what would be expected for a healthy, nondiabetic young male. This is a red flag of some inhibiting factor. Further discussion with the patient revealed a high alcohol intake, and once he eliminated the drinking, the wound closed and remained healed.

FOREIGN BODIES

Foreign bodies are detected by the body's immune system, thereby initiating or increasing an inflammatory state that can impede wound healing, cause granuloma formation, or increase infection risk. The foreign body may be an identifiable exogenous material or an endogenous material that has become altered in such a way that the body responds to it as a foreign body.[180] Examples include tattoo and cosmetic filler particles, biomaterials and synthetic materials associated with medical devices and prostheses,[181] foam remnants associated with negative pressure wound therapy,[182] suture materials,[183–185] infected orthopedic hardware, and objects as a result of trauma (eg, glass, nails, needles, metal shards). The latter is especially of concern in the neuropathic foot when the wound is in an area other than a bony weight-bearing surface.

The histological sequence of a foreign body reaction and granuloma formation is composed of macrophages and foreign body giant cells and is the end-stage response of the inflammatory and wound healing response.[180,181] Signs and symptoms of a foreign body in a wound include the following:

1. Failure of the wound to achieve full closure
2. Persistent drainage from a residual wound opening
3. Consistent epithelial breakdown of a closed wound
4. Subcutaneous tenderness
5. Palpable subcutaneous nodule

6. Periwound erythema and edema
7. Pain with weight-bearing (in the neuropathic foot)

Radiography can detect a metal foreign body; however, ultrasonography is recommended for a nonradiopaque foreign body.[186] Surface markers, multiple-projection radiographs, wire grids, fluoroscopy, or stereotaxic devices are also helpful in locating the embedded foreign body.[187] Removal of the foreign body is advised if possible, considering patient risk factors, followed by standard wound care to facilitate timely closure.

SUMMARY

Wounds will heal in a timely sequence if the cellular and tissue environment is healthy; however, there are numerous intrinsic, extrinsic, and local factors that can alter the injured tissue environment and impede the healing process. These factors are usually related to infection, nutrition, medications, other disease processes and necessary interventions, or psychosocial behaviors. Identification of these factors and addressing the implications as part of a comprehensive care plan are essential in order for wounds to progress through the phases of healing, achieve wound closure, and prevent recurrence.

STUDY QUESTIONS

1. A wound has pathogens on the surface that are replicating and interfering with the normal healing response. The wound is said to be
   a. Contaminated.
   b. Colonized.
   c. Locally infected.
   d. Systemically infected.
2. Which of the following disorders is most likely to result in a wound that bleeds easily with resulting loss of growth factors and failure to progress from inflammation to proliferation?
   a. Abnormally low platelets
   b. Protein energy malnutrition
   c. Increased neutrophil count
   d. Hyperglycemia
3. Which of the following conditions will require the highest calorie count for effective healing?
   a. Diabetic foot wound
   b. Postoperative incision with infection
   c. Traumatic skin tear
   d. 30% total body surface of burns
4. Which of the following symptoms is most likely to occur 6 weeks after initiation of radiation on the chest for a recurrent squamous cell carcinoma?
   a. Superficial erythema
   b. Wet desquamation
   c. Dyspigmentation
   d. Nonhealing traumatic wound
5. Chemotherapy affects healing by which of the following mechanisms?
   a. Destruction of the DNA of the affected tissue
   b. Lack of available neutrophils to migrate to the wound
   c. Myelosuppression, or decreased production of red blood cells in the bone marrow
   d. Dehydration as a side effect of the chemotherapy
6. Of the following factors that can impede wound healing, which one has effects that are reversible?
   a. Smoking
   b. Chemotherapy
   c. Radiation
   d. Autoimmune disorders
7. One of the primary reasons that obese patients have higher rates of surgical site infections is
   a. Higher rates of drug resistance.
   b. Adipose is poorly vascularized and more susceptible to necrosis.
   c. Poor absorption of antibiotics after surgery.
   d. Higher rate of presurgical exposure to bacteria.
8. A patient presents with a venous wound on the lateral leg that is not healing. The most likely cause for failure to close is
   a. Undetected diabetes.
   b. Vitamin A insufficiency.
   c. Chronic edema with poor skin perfusion.
   d. Protein energy malnutrition.

Answers: 1-c; 2-a; 3-d; 4-b; 5-c; 6-a; 7-b; 8-c

REFERENCES

1. Murphy K, ed. *Janeway's immunobiology*. 7th ed. New York, NY: Garland Science, Taylor & Francis Group, LLC; 2007.
2. Snyder RJ, Bohn G, Hanft J, et al. Wound biofilm: current perspectives and strategies on biofilm disruption and treatments. *Wounds*. 2017; 29(6):S1-S17.
3. Krahenbuhl JL, Adams LB. The role of the macrophage in resistance to the leprosy bacillus. *Immunol Ser*. 1994;60:281-302.
4. Sibbald RG, Elliott JA, Persaud-Jaimangal R, et al. Wound bed preparation 2021. *Adv Skin Wound Care*. 2021;34(4):183-195.
5. Bates-Jensen B, Schultz G, Ovington LG. Management of exudate, biofilms, and infection. In: Sussman C, Bates-Jensen B, eds. *Wound Care: A Collaborative Practice Manual for Health Professionals*. 4th ed. Baltimore, MD: Lippincott Williams & Wilkins; 2012:457-476.
6. Bessa LJ, Fazii P, Di Giulio M, Cellini L. Bacterial isolates from infected wounds and their antibiotic susceptibility pattern: some remarks about wound infection. *Int Wound J*. 2015;12(1):47-52.
7. Bibel DJ, Aly R, Bayles C, Strauss WG, Shinefield HR, Maibach HI. Competitive adherence as a mechanism of bacterial interference. *Can J Microbiol*. 1983;29(6):700-703.
8. Collette JR, Lorenz MC. Mechanisms of immune evasion in fungal pathogens. *Curr Opin Microbiol*. 2011;14(6):668-675.
9. Kuosjy BL. Infectious problems of the foot in diabetic patients. In: Fowker JH, Pfeifer MA, eds. *Levin & O'Neal's The Diabetic Foot*. 7th ed. Philadelphia, PA: Mosby/Elsevier; 2008:305-318.
10. Haalboom M, Blokhuis-Arkes MHE, Beuk RJ, et al. Wound swab and wound biopsy yield similar culture results. *Wound Repair Regen*. 2018. doi:10.1111/wrr.12629.

11. Haalboom M, Blokhuis-Arkes MHE, Beuk RJ, et al. Culture results from wound biopsy versu wound swab: does it matter for the assessment of wound infection? *Clin Microbiol Infect*. 2019;629.e7-629.e12.
12. Le L, Baer M, Briggs P, et al. Diagnostic accuracy of point-of-care fluorescence imaging for the detection of bacterial burden in wounds: results from the 350 patient fluorescence imaging assessment and guidance trial. *Adv Wound Care (New Rochelle)*. 2021;10(3):123-136.
13. Ehrlich HP, Hunt TK. Effects of cortisone and vitamin A on wound healing. *Ann Surg*. 1968;167(3):324-328.
14. Ehrlich HP, Tarver H, Hunt TK. Effects of vitamin A and glucocorticoids upon inflammation and collagen synthesis. *Ann Surg*. 1973;177(2):222-227.
15. Roberts AB. Transforming growth factor-beta: activity and efficacy in animal models of wound healing. *Wound Repair Regen*. 1995;3(4):408-418.
16. Mueller RV, Hunt TK, Tokunaga A, Spencer EM. The effect of insulinlike growth factor I on wound healing variables and macrophages in rats. *Arch Surg*. 1994;129(3):262-265.
17. Steenfos HH, Hunt TK, Scheuenstuhl H, Goodson WH 3rd Selective effects of tumor necrosis factor-alpha on wound healing in rats. *Surgery*. 1989;106(2):171-175; discussion 175-176.
18. Duman E, Ceylan KC, Akpınar D, et al. The effects of steroidal and non-steroidal anti-inflammatory drugs on tracheal wound healing in an experimental rat model. *Interact Cardiovasc Thorac Surg*. 2020;30(4):646-651.
19. Cerci C, Yildirim M, Ceyhan M, Bozkurt S, Doguc D, Gokicimen A. The effects of topical and systemic beta glucan administration on wound healing impaired by corticosteroids. *Wounds*. 2008;20(12): 341-6.
20. Khanna R, Dlouhy BJ, Smith ZA, Lam SK, Koski TR, Kahdaleh NS. The impact of steroids, methotrexate, and biologics on clinical and radiographic outcomes in patients with rheumatoid arthritis undergoing fusions at the craniovertebral junction. *J Craniovertebr Junction Spine*. 2015;6(2):60-64.
21. Tada M, Inui K, Sugioka Y, et al. Delayed wound healing and postoperative surgical site infections in patients with rheumatoid arthritis treated with or without biological disease-modifying antirheumatic drugs. *Clin Rheumatol*. 2016;35(6):147581.
22. Ito H, Kijima M, Nishida K, et al. Postoperative complications in patients with rheumatoid arthritis using a biological agent—a systematic review and meta-analysis. *Mod Rheumatol*. 2015;25(5):672-678.
23. Kubota A, Nakamura T, Miyazaki Y, Sekiguchi M, Suguro T. Perioperative complications in elective surgery in patients with rheumatoid arthritis treated with biologics. *Mod Rheumatol*. 2012;22(6):844-848.
24. Tsai DM, Borah GL. Implications of rheumatic disease and biological response—modifying agents in plastic surgery. *Plast Reconstr Surg*. 2015;136(6):1327-1336.
25. Gaucher S, Nicolas C, Piveteau O, Philippe H, Blanche P. Sarcoidosis and wound healing after cellulitis of the lower limb: is methotrexate responsible for skin graft failure? *Wounds*. 2017;29(8):229-230.
26. Chakravarty K, McDonald H, Pullar T, et al. BSR/BHPR guideline for disease modifying anti-rheumatic drug (DMARD) therapy in consultation with the British Association of Dermatologists. *Rheumatology (Oxford)*. 2008;47(6):924-925.
27. Ledingham J, Deighton C. Update on the British Society for rheumatology guidelines for prescribing TNFα blockers in adults with rheumatoid arthritis (update of previous guidelines of April 2001). *Rheumatology (Oxford)*. 2005;44(2):157-163.
28. Hwang JL, Weiss RE. Steroid-induced diabetes: a clinical and molecular approach to understanding and treatment. *Diabetes Metab Res Rev*. 2014;30(2):96-102.
29. Roberts A, James J, Dhatariya K; Joint British Diabetes Societies (JBDS) for Inpatient Care. Management of hyperglycaemia and steroid (glucocorticoid) therapy: a guideline from the Joint British Diabetes Societies (JBDS) for Inpatient Care group. *Diabet Med*. 2018;35(8):1011-1017.
30. Busti AJ, Hooper JS, Amaya CJ, Kazi S. Effects of perioperative anti-inflammatory and immunomodulating therapy on surgical wound healing. *Pharmacotherapy*. 2005;25(11):1566-1591.
31. Beitz JM. Pharmacologic impact (aka "breaking bad") of medications on wound healing and wound development: a literature-based overview. *Ostomy Wound Manage*. 2017;63(3):18-35.
32. Fairweather M, Heit YI, Rosenberg LM, Briggs A, Orgill DP, Bertagnoli MM. Celecoxib inhibits early cutaneous wound healing. *J Surg Res*. 2015;194(2):717-724.
33. Patrono C. The multifaceted clinical read-outs of platelet inhibition by low-dose aspirin. *J Am Coll Cardiol*. 2015;66(1):74-85.
34. Su WH, Cheng MH, Lee WL, et al. Nonsteroidal anti-inflammatory drugs for wounds: pain relief or excessive scar formation? *Mediators Inflamm*. 2010; 2010:413238.
35. Pasero C, Stannard D. The role of intravenous acetaminophen in acute pain management. *Pain Manag Nurs*. 2012;13(2):107-124.
36. Kragh AM, Walden M, Apelqvist A, Wagner P, Atroshi I. Bleeding and first-year mortality following hip fracture surgery and preoperative use of low-dose acetylsalicylic acid. *BMC Musculoskelet Disord*. 2011;12:254. Available at: http://www.medscape.com/viewarticle/757643. Accessed June 23, 2013.
37. Levine JM. The effect of oral medication on wound healing. *Adv Skin Wound Care*. 2017;30(3):137-142.
38. Limmer JS, Grotegut CA, Thames E, Dotters-Katz SK, Brancazio LR, James AH. Postpartum wound and bleeding complications in women who received peripartum anticoagulation. *Thromb Res*. 2013;132(1):e19-e23.
39. Choudhry S, Fishman PM, Hernandez C. Heparin-induced bullous hemorrhagic dermatosis. *Cutis*. 2013;91(2):93-99.
40. Amato L, Berti S, Fabbri P. Warfarin-induced skin necrosis. Available at: http://medscape.com/viewarticle/451073_2. Accessed May 7, 2017.
41. Smith SL. Immunosuppressive therapies in organ transplantation. Available at: http://www.medscape.com/viewarticle437182. Accessed June 3, 2013.
42. Smith SI. Immunosuppressive therapies in organ transplantation. Available at: http://medscape.com/viewarticle437182. Accessed May 7, 2017.
43. Haines DD, Juhasz B, Tosaki A. Management of multicellular senescence and oxidative stress. *J Cell Mol Med*. 2013;17(8):936-957.
44. DeVries JG, Collier RC, Niezgoda JA, et al. Impaired lower extremity wound healing secondary to sirolimus post kidney transplantation. *J Am Col Certi Wound Spec*. 2009;1(3):86-91.
45. Francis S, Berg D. Reducing skin malignancy in organ transplant recipients. *Skin Therapy Lett*. 2013;18(1). Available at: http://www.medscape.com/viewarticle/777623. Accessed May 3, 2013.
46. Hunt SA, Haddad F. The changing face of heart transplantation. *J Am Coll Cardiol*. 2008;52(8):587-598.
47. Patel S, Srivastava S, Singh MR, Singh D. Mechanistic insight into diabetic wounds: pathogenesis, molecular targets, and treatment strategies to pace wound healing. *Biomed Pharmacother*. 2019;112:108615.
48. Singer AJ, Clark RA. Cutaneous wound healing. *N Engl J Med*. 1999; 341(10):738-746.

49. Genco RJ, Grossi SG, Ho A, Nishimura F, Murayama Y. A proposed model linking inflammation to obesity, diabetes, and periodontal infections. *J Periodontol.* 2005;76(11 suppl):2075-2084.
50. Wetzler C, Kampfer H, Stallmeyer B, Pfeilschifter J, Frank S. Large and sustained induction of chemokines during impaired wound healing in the genetically diabetic mouse: prolonged persistence of neutrophils and macrophages during the late phase of repair. *J Invest Dermatol.* 2000;115(2):245-253.
51. Wong SL, Demers M, Martinod K, et al. Diabetes primes neutrophils to undergo NETosis which severely impairs wound healing. *Nat Med.* 2015;21(7):815-819.
52. Loots MA, Lamme EN, Zeegelaar J, Mekkes JR, Bos JD, Middelkoop E. Differences in cellular infiltrate and extracellular matrix of chronic diabetic and venous ulcers versus acute wounds. *J Invest Dermatol.* 1998;111(5):850-857.
53. Werner S, Krieg T, Smola H. Keratinocyte-fibroblast interactions in wound healing. *J Invest Dermatol.* 2007;127(5):998-1008.
54. Werner S, Breeden M, Hubner G, Greenhalgh DG, Longaker MT. Induction of keratinocyte growth factor expression is reduced and delayed during wound healing in the genetically diabetic mouse. *J Invest Dermatol.* 1994;103(4):469-473.
55. Liao H, Zakhaleva J, Chen W. Cells and tissue interactions with glycated collagen and their relevance to delayed diabetic wound healing. *Biomaterials.* 2009;30(9):1689-1696.
56. Deng L, Du C, Song P, et al. The role of oxidative stress and antioxidants in diabetic wound healing. *Oxid Med Cell Longev.* 2021;2021:8852759.
57. Dalton SJ, Whiting CV, Bailey JR, Mitchell DC, Tarlton JF. Mechanisms of chronic skin ulceration linking lactate, transforming growth factor-beta, vascular endothelial growth factor, collagen remodeling, collagen stability, and defective angiogenesis. *J Invest Dermatol.* 2007;127(4):958-968.
58. Ben-Porath I, Weinberg RA. The signals and pathways activating cellular senescence. *Int J Biochem Cell Biol.* 2005;37(5):961-976.
59. Tchaikovski V, Olieslagers S, Bohmer FD, Waltenberger J. Diabetes mellitus activates signal transduction pathways resulting in vascular endothelial growth factor resistance of human monocytes. *Circulation.* 2009;120(2):150-159.
60. Sari N. Physical inactivity and its impact on healthcare utilization. *Health Econ.* 2009;18(8):885-901.
61. American College of Endocrinology. Clinical Practice Guidelines for the Perioperative Nutritional, Metabolic, and Nonsurgical Support of the Bariatric Surgery Patient—2013 Update. Available at: https://www.aace.com/files/publish-ahead-of-print-final-version.pdf. Accessed May 4, 2013.
62. Markuson M, Hanson D, Anderson J, et al. The relationship between hemoglobin A1c values and healing time for lower extremity ulcers in individuals with diabetes. *Adv Skin Wound Care.* 2009;22(8):365-372.
63. Joseph JI. Anesthesia and surgery in the diabetic patient. In: Goldstein BJ, Müller-Wieland D, eds. *Type 2 Diabetes: Principles and Practice.* 2nd ed. New York, NY: Informa Healthcare; 2008:475-500.
64. Salazar JJ, Ennis WJ, Koh TJ. Diabetes medications: impact on inflammation and wound healing. *J Diabetes Complications.* 2016; 30(4):746-52.
65. Grada A, Phillips T. Nutrition and cutaneous wound healing. *Clin Dermatol.* 2022;40(2):103-113.
66. Rocha VZ, Libby P. Obesity, inflammation, and atherosclerosis. *Nat Rev Cardiol.* 2009;6(6):399-409.
67. Kahn SE, Hull RL, Utzschneider KM. Mechanisms linking obesity to insulin resistance and type 2 diabetes. *Nature.* 2006;444(7121): 840-846.
68. Kahn SE, Zinman B, Haffner SM, et al. Obesity is a major determinant of the association of C-reactive protein levels and the metabolic syndrome in type 2 diabetes. *Diabetes.* 2006;55(8):2357-2364.
69. Zajacova A, Dowd JB, Burgard SA. Overweight adults may have the lowest mortality—do they have the best health? *Am J Epidemiol.* 2011;173(4):430-437.
70. Lee MJ, Wu Y, Fried SK. Adipose tissue remodeling in pathophysiology of obesity. *Curr Opin Clin Nutr Metab Care.* 2010;13(4):371-376.
71. Ouchi N, Parker JL, Lugus JJ, Walsh K. Adipokines in inflammation and metabolic disease. *Nat Rev Immunol.* 2011;11(2):85-97.
72. Hirt PA, Castillo DE, Yosipovitch G, Keri JE. Skin changes in the obese patient. *J Am Acad Dermatol.* 2019;81(5):1037-1057.
73. Pence BD, Woods JA. Exercise, obesity, and cutaneous wound healing: evidence from rodent and human studies. *Adv Wound Care.* 2014;3(1):71-79.
74. Franz S, Ertel A, Engel KM, Simon JC, Saalbach A. Overexpression of S100A9 in obesity impairs macrophage differentiation via TLR4-NFkB-signaling worsening inflammation and wound healing. *Theranostics.* 2022;12(4):1659-1682.
75. Allama A, Ibrahim I, Abdallah A, et al. Effect of body mass index on early clinical outcomes after cardiac surgery. *Asian Cardiovasc Thorac Ann.* 2014;22(6):667-673.
76. Lemaignen A, Birgand G, Ghodhbane W, et al. Sternal wound infection after cardiac surgery: incidence and risk factors according to clinical presentation. *Clin Microbiol Infect.* 2015;21(7):674.e11-674.e18.
77. Stevens SM, O'Connell BP, Meyer TA. Obesity related complications in surgery. *Curr Opin Otolaryngol Head Neck Surg.* 2015;23(5):341-347.
78. Hu H, Mei J, Lin M, Wu X, Lin H, Chen G. The causal relationship between obesity and skin and soft tissue infections: a two-sample Mendelian randomization study. *Front Endocrinol (Lausanne).* 2022;13:996863.
79. Pierpont YN, Dinh TP, Salas RE, et al. Obesity and surgical wound healing: a current review. *ISRN Obes.* 2014:Article ID 638936.
80. Barber GA, Weller CD, Gibson SJ. Effects and associations of nutrition in patients with venous leg ulcers: a systematic review. *J Adv Nurs.* 2018;74(4):774-787.
81. Cottam DR, Mattar SG, Barinas-Mitchell E, et al. The chronic inflammatory hypothesis for the morbidity associated with morbid obesity: implications and effect of weight loss. *Obes Surg.* 2004;14(5):589-600.
82. Khalil H, Cullen M, Chambers H, Carroll M, Walker J. Elements affecting wound healing time: an evidence based analysis. *Wound Repair Regen.* 2015;23(4):550-556.
83. Tapking C, Houschyar KS, Rontoyanni VG, et al. The influence of obesity on treatment and outcome of severely burned patients. *J Burn Care Res.* 2019;40(6):996-1008.
84. Breen L, Phillips SM. Skeletal muscle protein metabolism in the elderly: interventions to counteract the "anabolic resistance" of ageing. *Nutr Metab.* 2011;8(68). Available at: http://www.medscape.com/viewarticle/754680. Accessed June 23, 2013.
85. Frost KR. Use of steroids for wasting and lipodystrophy syndromes in HIV/AIDs. *AIDS Read.* 2001;11(3):130-131.
86. Sam J, Nguyan GC. Protein-calorie malnutrition as a prognostic indicator of mortality among patients hospitalized with cirrhosis and portal hypertension. *Liver Int.* 2009;29(9):1396-1402.
87. Demling RH. Nutrition, anabolism, and the wound healing process: an overview. *ePlasty.* 2009;9:65-94.
88. Roberts S, Collins P, Rattray M. Identifying and managing malnutrition, frailty and sarcopenia in the community: a narrative review. *Nutrients.* 2021;13(7):2316.

89. Patterson GK, Martindate RG. Nutrition and wound healing. In: McCulloch JM, Kloth LC, eds. *Wound Healing: Evidence-Based Medicine*. 4th ed. Philadelphia, PA: FA Davis Company; 2010:44-50.
90. Huckleberry Y. Nutritional support and the surgical patient. *Am J Health Syst Pharm*. 2004:61(7):671-682.
91. Parrish CR. Serum proteins as markers of nutrition: what are we treating? *Pract Gastroenterol*. 2006;October:46-64. Available at: http://www.medicine.virginia.edu/clinical/departments/medicine/divisions/digestive-health/nutrition-support-team/nutrition-articles/BanhArticle.pdf. Accessed September 25, 2014.
92. Baeten JM, Richardson BA, Bankson DD, et al. Use of serum retinol-binding protein for prediction of vitamin a deficiency: effects of HIV-1 infection, protein malnutrition, and the acute phase response. *Am J Clin Nutr*. 2004;79(2):218-225.
93. Quain AM, Khardori NM. Nutrition in wound care management: a comprehensive overview. *Wounds*. 2015;27(12):327-335.
94. Collins N, Friedrich L. Appropriately diagnosing malnutrition to improve wound healing. *Wound Clin*. 2016;10(11):10-12.
95. Evans DC, Corkins MR, Mlone A, et al. The use of visceral proteins as nutrition markers: an ASPEN position paper. Available at: https://aspenjournals.onlinelibrary.wiley.com/doi/10.1002/ncp.10588. Accessed April 18, 2023.
96. Laporte M. The Canadian Nutrition Screening Tool. *Adv Skin Wound Care*. 2017;30(2):64-65.
97. Fulton J, Evans B, Miller S, et al. Development of a nutrition screening tool for an outpatient wound center. *Adv Skin Wound Care*. 2016;29(3):136-142.
98. A guide to completing the Mini Nutritional Assessment – Short Form (MNA®-SF). Available at https://www.mna-elderly.com/sites/default/files/2021-10/mna-guide-english-sf.pdf. Accessed August 30, 2023.
99. Kaiser MJ, Bauer JM, Ramsch C, et al. Validation of the mini nutritional assessment short-form (MNA®-SF): a practical tool for identification of nutritional status. *J Nutr Health Aging*. 2009;13:782-788.
100. Dong V. Karvellas CJ. Using technology to assess nutritional status and optimize nutrition therapy in critically ill patients. *Curr Opin Clin Nutr Metab Care*. 2021;24(2):189-194.
101. Russell MK. Functional assessment of nutrition status. *Nutr Clin Pract*. 2015 ;30(2):211-8.
102. Wu G, Bazer FW, Davis TA, et al. Arginine metabolism and nutrition in growth, health, and disease. *Amino Acids*. 2009;37(1):153-168.
103. Leigh B, Desneves K, Rafferty J, et al. The effect of different doses of arginine-containing supplement on the healing of pressure ulcers. *J Wound Care*. 2012;21(3):150-156.
104. Payne WG, Naidu DK, Wheeler CK, et al. Wound healing in patients with cancer. *ePlasty*. 2008;8:e9.
105. Zinder R, Cooley R, Vlad LG, Molnar JA. Vitamin A and wound healing. *Nutr Clin Pract*. 2019 ;34(6):839-849.
106. Polcz ME, Barbul A. The role of vitamin A in wound healing. *Nutr Clin Pract*. 2019;34(5):695-700.
107. Hourigan LA, Omaye ST, Keen CL, Jones JA, Dubick MA. Vitamin and trace element loss from negative-pressure wound therapy. *Adv Skin Wound Care*. 2016;29(1):20-25.
108. Bolton L. Evidence corner. *Wounds*. 2017;29(10):324-326.
109. Werdin F, Tennenhaus M, Schaller HE, Rennekampff HO. Evidence-based management strategies for treatment of chronic wounds. *ePlasty*. 2009;9:e19.
110. Hess CT. Arterial ulcer checklist. *Adv Skin Wound Care*. 2010; 23(9):432.
111. Grey JE, Harding KG, Enoch S. Venous and arterial leg ulcers. *BMJ*. 2006;332(7537):347-350.
112. Hopf HW, Ueno C, Aslam R, et al. Guidelines for the treatment of arterial insufficiency ulcers. *Wound Repair Regen*. 2006;14(6): 693-710.
113. Bergan JJ, Schmid-Schonbein GW, Coleridge PD, Nicolaides AN, Boisseau MR, Eklof B. Chronic venous disease. *N Engl J Med*. 2006;355:488-498.
114. de Araujo T, Valencia I, Federman DG, Kirsner RS. Managing the patient with venous ulcers. *Ann Intern Med*. 2003;138(4):326-334.
115. Falanga V, Eaglstein WH. The "trap" hypothesis of venous ulceration. *Lancet*. 1993;341(8851):1006-1008.
116. Browse NL, Burnand KG. The cause of venous ulceration. *Lancet*. 1982;2(8292):243-245.
117. Collins L, Seraj S. Diagnosis and treatment of venous ulcers. *Am Fam Physician*. 2010;81(8):989-996.
118. Pardes JB, Takagi H, Martin TA, Ochoa MS, Falanga V. Decreased levels of alpha 1(I) procollagen mRNA in dermal fibroblasts grown on fibrin gels and in response to fibrinopeptide B. *J Cell Physiol*. 1995;162(1):9-14.
119. Higley HR, Ksander GA, Gerhardt CO, Falanga V. Extravasation of macromolecules and possible trapping of transforming growth factor-beta in venous ulceration. *Br J Dermatol*. 1995;132(1):79-85.
120. Kobrin KL, Thompson PJ, van de Scheur M, Kwak TH, Kim S, Falanga V. Evaluation of dermal pericapillary fibrin cuffs in venous ulceration using confocal microscopy. *Wound Repair Regen*. 2008;16(4):503-506.
121. Shavit E, Alavi A. Compression therapy for non-venous leg ulcers: current viewpoint. *Int Wound J*. 2019;16(6):1581-1586.
122. McGuire J, Love E, Vlahovic TC, et al. The ABCESS system for chronic wound management: a new acronym for lower extremity wound management. *Wounds*. 2020 ;32(suppl 11):S1-S25.
123. Herrup K, Yang Y. Cell cycle regulation in the postmitotic neuron: oxymoron or new biology? *Nat Rev Neurosci*. 2007;8(5):368-378.
124. Farbehi N, Patrick R, Dorison A, et al. Single cell expression profiling reveals dynamic flux of cardiac stromal, vascular and immune cells in health and injury. *Elife*. 2019 ;8:e43882.
125. Buckley CD, Gilroy DW, Serhan CN, Stockinger B, Tak PP. The resolution of inflammation. *Nat Rev Immunol*. 2012;12(1):3.
126. Zhao CT, Wang M, Siu CW, et al. Myocardial dysfunction in patients with type 2 diabetes mellitus: role of endothelial progenitor cells and oxidative stress. *Cardiovasc Diabetol*. 2012;11:147.
127. Abrahamian H, Endler G, Exner M, et al. Association of low-grade inflammation with nephropathy in type 2 diabetic patients: role of elevated CRP-levels and 2 different gene-polymorphisms of proinflammatory cytokines. *Exp Clin Endocrinol Diabetes*. 2007;115(1):38-41.
128. Ouchi N, Walsh K. A novel role for adiponectin in the regulation of inflammation. *Arterioscler Thromb Vasc Biol*. 2008;28(7):1219-1221.
129. Rhou YJ, Henshaw FR, McGill MJ, Twigg SM. Congestive heart failure presence predicts delayed healing of foot ulcer in diaberes: an audit from a multidisciplinary high-risk foot clinic. *J Diabetes Complication*. 2015;29(4):556-562.
130. Hom DB, Morgan ED. Reducing risks for poor surgical wound healing. Facial Plastic *Surg Clin North Am*. 2023;31(2):171-181.
131. Subramania I, Balasubramanian D. Management of radiation wounds. *Indian J Plast Surg*. 2012;45(2):325-331.
132. Mendelsohn FA, Divino CM, Reis ED, Kerstein MD. Wound care after radiation therapy. *Adv Skin Wound Care*. 2002;15(5):216-224.
133. Haubner F, Ohmann E, Pohl F, Strutz J, Gassner HG. Wound healing after radiation therapy: review of the literature. *Radiat Oncol*. 2012;7:162-170.

134. Gosselin TK, Schneider SM, Plambeck MA, Rowe K. A prospective randomized, placebo-controlled skin care study in women diagnosed with breast cancer undergoing radiation therapy. *Oncol Nurs Forum*. 2010;37(5):619-626.
135. Tibbs MK. Wound healing following radiation therapy: a review. *Radiother Oncol*. 1997;42:99-106.
136. Bennett MH, Feldmeier J, Hampson NB, Smee R, Milross C. Hyperbaric oxygen therapy for late radiation tissue injury. *Cochrane Database Syst Rev*. 2016;4:CD0050555.
137. Borab Z, Mirmanesh MD, Gantz M, Cusano A, Pu LL. Systematic review of hyperbaric oxygen therapy for the treatment of radiation-induced skin necrosis. *J Plast Reconstr Aesthet Surg*. 2017;70(4):529-538.
138. Benderitter M, Caviggioli F, Chapel A, et al. Stem cell therapies for the treatment of radiation-induced normal tissue side effects. *Antioxid Redox Signal*. 2014;21(2):338-355.
139. Rigotti G, Marchi A, Varoni GM, et al. Clinical treatment of radiotherapy tissue damage by lipoaspirate transplant: a healing process mediated by adipose-derived adult stem cells. *Plast Reconstr Surg*. 2007;119(5):1409-1422.
140. Nuutila K. Hair follicle transplantation for wound repair. *Adv Wound Care (New Rochelle)*. 2021;10(3):153-163.
141. Goodman CC, Snyder TE. Problems affecting multiple systems. In: Goodman CC, Fuller KS, Boissonnault WG., eds. *Pathology: Implications for Physical Therapists*. Philadelphia, PA: Saunders; 2003;85-119.
142. Deptuła M, Zieliński J, Wardowska A, Pikuła M. Wound healing complications in oncological patients: perspectives for cellular therapy. *Postepy Dermatol Alergol*. 2019;36(2):139-146.
143. Quasthoff S, Hartung HP. Chemotherapy-induced peripheral neuropathy. *J Neurol*. 2002;249(1):9-17.
144. Guo S, DiPietro LA. Factors affecting wound healing. *J Dent Res*. 2010;89(3):219-229.
145. Harless WH. Revisiting perioperative chemotherapy: the critical importance of targeting residual cancer prior to wound healing. *BMC Cancer*. 2009;9:118.
146. Celeen W, Pattyn P, Marell M. Surgery, wound healing, and metastasis: recent insights and clinical implications. *Crit Rev Oncol Hematol*. 2013;89(1):16-26.
147. Gordon CR, Rojavin Y, Patel M, et al. A review of bevacizumab and surgical wound healing: an important warning to all surgeons. *Ann Plast Surg*. 2009;62(6):707-709.
148. Erinjeri JP, Fong AJ, Kemeny NE, Brown KT, Getrajdman GI, Solomon SB. Timing of administration of bevacizumab chemotherapy affects wound healing after chest wall port placement. *Cancer*. 2011;117(6):1296-1301.
149. Padovan M, Vincenzi F, Govoni M, et al. Adenosine and adenosine receptors in rheumatoid arthritis. *Int J Clin Rheumatol*. 2013;8(1):13-25.
150. Gosain A, DiPietro LA. Aging and wound healing. *World J Surg*. 2004;28(3):321-6.
151. Emery CF, Kiecolt-Glaser JK, Glaser R, Malarkey WB, Frid DJ. Exercise accelerates wound healing among healthy older adults: a preliminary investigation. *J Gerontol A Biol Sci Med Sci*. 2005; 60(11):1432-6.
152. Keylock KT, Vieira VJ, Wallig MA, DiPietro LA, Schrementi M, Woods JA. Exercise accelerates cutaneous wound healing and decreases wound inflammation in aged mice. *Am J Physiol Regul Integr Comp Physiol*. 2008;294(1):R179-84.
153. Gouin JP, Kiecolt-Glaser JK. The impact of psychological stress on wound healing: methods and mechanisms. *Immunol Allergy Clin North Am*. 2011;31(1):81-93.
154. Woo K. Exploring the effects of pain and stress on wound healing. *Adv Skin Wound Care*. 2012;25(1):38-44.
155. Lucas VS. Psychological stress and wound healing in humans. *Wounds*. 2011;22(4):76-83.
156. Gouin JP, Kiecolt-Glaser JK. The impact of psychological stress on wound healing: methods and mechanisms. *Crit Care Nurs Clin North Am* 2012;24:201-213.
157. Christian LM, Graham JE, Pdgett DA, Glser R, Keicolt-Glaser JK. Stress and wound healing. *Neuroimmunomodulation*. 2006:13(5-6):337-346.
158. Fayne RA, Borda LJ, Egger AN, Tomic-Canic M. The Potential Impact of Social Genomics on Wound Healing. *Adv Wound Care (New Rochelle)*. 2020;9(6):325-331.
159. Ennis WJ, Meneses P. Complications in repair. In: McCulloch JM, Kloth LC, eds. *Wound Healing: Evidence-Based Medicine*. 4th ed. Philadelphia, PA: FA Davis Company; 2010:51-64.
160. Saguie BO, Romana-Souza B, Martins RL, Monte-Alto-Costa A. Exercise prior to, but not concomitant with, stress reverses stress-induced delayed skin wound healing. *Wound Repair Regen*. 2017; 25(4):641-651.
161. Fayne RA, Borda LJ, Egger AN, Tomic-Canic M. The potential impact of social genomics on wound healing. *Adv Wound Care (New Rochelle)*. 2020;9(6):325-331.
162. Theocharidis V, Katsaros I, Sgouromallis E, et al. Current evidence on the role of smoking in plastic surgery elective procedures: a systematic review and meta-analysis. *J Plast Reconstr Aesthet Surg*. 2018;71(5):624-636.
163. Sorensen LT. Wound healing and infection in surgery. The clinical impact of smoking and smoking cessation: a systematic review and meta-analysis. *Arch Surg*. 2012;147(4):373-383.
164. Pluvy I, Panouilleres M, Garrido I, et al. Smoking and plastic surgery, part II. Clinical implications: a systematic review with meta-analysis. *Ann Chir Plast Esthet*. 2015;60(1):e15-e49.
165. Basnett AM. Cutaneous manifestations of smoking. 2018. Available at: http://emedicine.medscape.com/article/1075039. Accessed September 2, 2018.
166. McDaniel JC, Browning KK. Smoking, chronic wound healing, and implications for evidence-based practice. *J Wound Ostomy Continence Nurs*. 2014;41(5):415-423; quiz E1-E2.
167. Sorensen LT. Smoking and wound healing. *Eur Wound Manage Assoc J*. 2003;3:13-15.
168. Alanazi H, Park HJ, Chakir J, Semlali A, Rouabhia M. Comparative study of the effects of cigarette smoke and electronic cigarettes on human gingival fibroblast proliferation, migration, and apoptosis. *Food Chem Toxicol*. 2018;118:390-398.
169. Taub PJ, Matarasso A. E-cigarettes and potential implications for plastic surgery. *Plast Reconstr Surg*. 2016;138(6):1059e-1066e.
170. Agochukwu N, Liau JY. Debunking the myth of e-cigarettes: a case of free flap compromise due to e-cigarette use within the first 24 hours. *J Plast Reconstr Aesthet Surg*. 2018;71(3):451-453.
171. Liu Z, Zhang Y, Youn JY, Zhang Y, Makino A, Yuan JX, Cai H. Flavored and nicotine-containing E-cigarettes induce impaired angiogenesis and diabetic wound healing via increased endothelial oxidative stress and reduced NO bioavailability. *Antioxidants (Basel)*. 2022;11(5):904.
172. Sorensen LT. Wound healing and infection in surgery: the pathophysiological impact of smoking, smoking cessation, and nicotine replacement therapy: a systematic review. *Ann Surg*. 2012;255(6):1069-1079.
173. Mills E, Eyawo O, Lockhrt I, Kelly S, Wu P, Ebbert JO. Smoking cessation reduces postoperative complications: a systematic review and meta-analysis. *Am J Med*. 2011;124(2):144-154.

174. Wong J, Lam DP, Abrishami A, Chan MT, Chung F. Short-term preoperative smoking cessation and postoperative complications: a systematic review and meta-analysis. *Can J Anaesth.* 2012;59(3): 268-279.
175. deWit M, Goldberg S, Hussein E, Neifeld JP. Health care-associated infections in surgical patients undergoing elective surgery: are alcohol use disorders a risk factor? *J Am Coll Surg.* 2012;215:229-236.
176. Ranzer MJ, Chen L, DiPietro LA. Fibroblast function and wound breaking strength is impaired by acute ethanol intoxication. *Alcohol Clin Exp Res.* 2011;35(1):83-90.
177. Radek KA, Matthies AM, Burns AL, Heinrich SA, Kovacs EJ, DiPietro LA. Acute ethanol exposure impairs angiogenesis and the proliferative phase of wound healing. *Am J Physiol Heart Circ Physiol.* 2005; 289:H1084-H1090.
178. Radek KA, Ranzer MJ, DiPietro LA. Brewing complications: the effect of acute ethanol exposure on wound healing. *J Leukoc Biol.* 2009;86:1125-1134.
179. Jung MK, Callaci JJ, Lauing KL, et al. Alcohol exposure and mechanisms of tissue injury and repair. *Alcohol Clin Exp Res.* 2011; 35(3):392-9.
180. Molina-Ruiz AM, Requena L. Foreign body granulomas. *Dermatol Clin.* 2015;33:497-523.
181. Anderson JM, Rodrigues A, Chang DT. *Foreign body reaction to biomaterials.* Available at: https://doi.org/10.1016/j.smim.2007.11.004. Accessed September 2, 2018.
182. Mazoch M, Montgomery C. Retained wound vacuum foam in non-healing wounds: a real possibility. *J Wound Care.* 2015;24(6 suppl): S18-S20.
183. Chandorkar Y, Bhaskar N, Madras G, Basu B. Long-term sustained release of salicylic acid from cross-linked biodegradable polyester induces a reduced foreign body response in mice. *Biomacromolecules.* 2015;16(2):636-649.
184. Lambertz A, Schroder KM, Schob DS, et al. Polyvinylidene fluoride as a suture material: evaluation of comet tail-like infiltrate and foreign body granuloma. *Eur Surg Res.* 2015;55(1-2):1-11.
185. Sung KY, Lee SY. A chronic, nonhealing wound of the finger caused by polypropylene suture material. *Wounds.* 2015;27(7):E16-E19.
186. Turkcuer I, Atilla R, Topacoglu H, et al. Do we really need plain and soft-tissue radiographies to detect radiolucent foreign bodies in the ED? *Am J Emerg Med.* 2006;24(7):763-768.
187. Lammers RL. Soft tissue foreign bodies. *Ann Emerg Med.* 1988; 17(12):1336-1347.

PART THREE
Wound Bed Preparation

CHAPTER THIRTEEN

Wound Debridement

Dot Weir, RN, CWON, CWS and Pamela Scarborough, PT, DPT, MS, CWS, FAAWC

CHAPTER OBJECTIVES

At the end of this chapter, the learner will be able to:

1. **Discuss the critical importance of wound cleansing.**
2. **Verbalize the contribution of debridement to wound bed preparation.**
3. **Define the types of debridement currently used in wound care practice.**
4. **Differentiate selective from nonselective debridement.**
5. **Select the appropriate type of debridement for patients whose wounds would benefit from the procedure.**

INTRODUCTION

Debridement as a Component of Wound Bed Preparation

Wound bed preparation (WBP) restores physiological balance in an open wound in order to move the wound to a state of "readiness to heal" and incorporates management strategies in order to accelerate endogenous healing or to facilitate the effectiveness of other therapeutic measures. These strategies integrate proven concepts to build a platform for the treatment of hard-to-heal wounds and organize medical procedures into a holistic approach that can be used to evaluate and remove barriers to the wound healing processes. In addition, WBP addresses several barriers to healing including devitalized tissue and other detritus, bacterial load, and the management of exudate. The primary goal is the formation of good, quality granulation tissue leading to complete wound closure.

One component of WBP is effective wound cleansing, also termed wound hygiene, a fundamental aspect of care for all patients with an open wound. Because wound healing is a biologically preferred phenomenon, nonhealing should be regarded as a pathology that can be successfully addressed with the right tools, provided that the underlying etiology is managed with current practice standards to the extent possible. Appropriate and adequate cleansing is performed at every dressing change with a nontoxic pH-balanced cleanser and includes cleansing of the wound bed and the periwound area of 10–20 cm from the wound edge.[1]

Additionally, WBP is the global management of hard-to-heal wounds, which includes the following goals:

1. Removing necrotic tissue from the wound bed
2. Reducing the bacterial burden
3. Managing the moisture content, ensuring that the wound edges are conducive to cellular migration for resurfacing the wound (**FIGURE 13-1**)

These components of WBP contribute to the correction of abnormal wound repair with the goal of facilitating the processes of wound closure and subsequent healing. Adequate WBP is required prior to the use of advanced wound care therapies, such as cellular and tissue-based products, other biological wound interventions, collagen **dressings**, and negative pressure wound therapy.[2]

Debridement of necrotic tissue from a wound bed is a key component of preparing a hard-to-heal wound for closure and subsequent healing (**FIGURE 13-2**).[3–13] Numerous evidence-based wound care guidelines describe the importance of adequate and serial debridement as a fundamental intervention for hard-to-heal wounds. One of the well-known international documents is the European Pressure Injury Advisory Panel (EPIAP) and the National Pressure Injury Advisory Panel (NPIAP) guideline *Prevention and Treatment of Pressure Ulcers/Injuries: Clinical Practice Guidelines*, which states several reasons to debride a hard-to-heal wound (**TABLE 13-1**).[14]

Epibole (**FIGURE 13-3**) is defined as a condition in which the upper edges of the epidermis migrate down (sometimes with a rolled appearance) to envelop the basement membrane or lower edges of the epidermis. Thus, epithelial cells cannot migrate at wound edges and the wound is unable to resurface.[15]

During the normal cascade of events leading to wound repair, inflammatory cells such as neutrophils and macrophages are activated to remove microscopic debris, participate in microbial defense, and facilitate the beginning of the repair process. Any interruption in or impairment of the processes associated with the wound repair cascade may create an environment leading to wound chronicity and, ultimately, an environment of increasing necrotic burden.

> **CLINICAL CONSIDERATION**
>
> The presence of necrotic or devitalized tissue on the surface of a wound prevents accurate assessment of the extent of tissue destruction or depth of the wound.

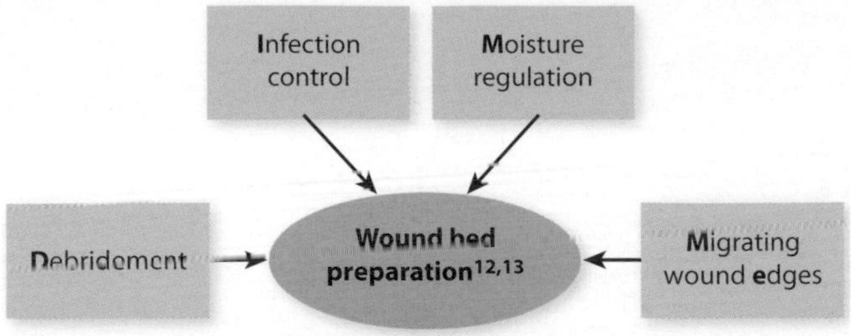

FIGURE 13-1 The components of wound bed preparation are expressed in this paradigm of DIME and can guide the clinician in the principles to facilitate wound healing.

The term *necrotic burden* refers to the following components:

- Dead or devitalized tissue
- Excess exudate
- Levels of bacteria sufficient to interfere with wound healing

Necrotic burden is found on the surface of many hard-to-heal wounds. In addition, resident cells such as fibroblasts and keratinocytes may be phenotypically altered and no longer responsive to certain signals, such as those from chemical mediators, including growth factors. This state of the cell being alive but impaired by its nonresponsive condition is termed *cellular senescence*.[8,16]

TABLE 13-2 lists processes by which necrotic or devitalized tissue impairs and impedes wound closure and healing.

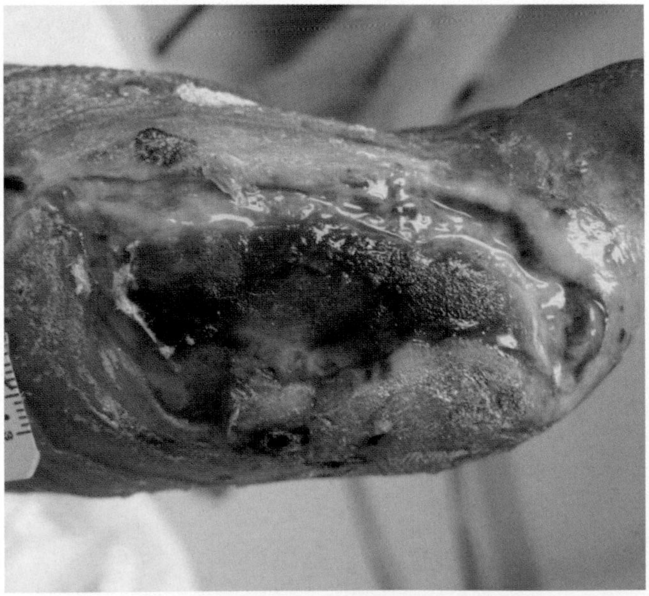

FIGURE 13-2 Wound with necrotic tissue. After a partial forefoot amputation, this foot wound has a large amount of necrotic tissue, both eschar and slough, that requires debridement in order for adjunctive therapies, biological dressings, or negative pressure to be successful in facilitating wound healing.

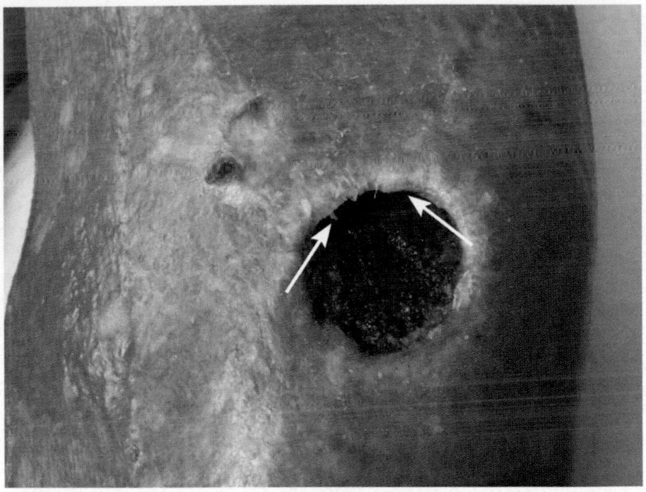

FIGURE 13-3 Epibole, as seen between the arrows, will impede wound closure and requires debridement of the edges to facilitate epithelial migration.

TABLE 13-1 Reasons to Debride Chronic Wounds[14]

- Remove necrotic tissue
- Decrease the bioburden
- Remove senescent cells
- Decrease stimulation of inflammatory cell production
- Remove callous, rolled edges (epibole[14])
- Facilitate angiogenesis
- Prepare wound bed for application of cellular/acellular matrix products
- Prepare wound bed for flap/graft
- Determine depth of tissue destruction

TABLE 13-2 Ways Necrotic or Devitalized Tissue Impairs and Impedes Wound Closure and Healing

- Masking or mimicking signs of infection
- Serving as a source of nutrients for bacterial cells, thereby contributing to the risk of critical colonization or infection
- Acting as a physical barrier to closure and impeding normal matrix formation, angiogenesis, or granulation tissue development
- Impairing contraction of the wound area and epidermal resurfacing
- Stimulating the incessant production of inflammatory cytokines, leading to the overproduction of matrix metalloproteases[3,6–12]

THE DECISION TO DEBRIDE

Many clinical and patient-centered factors need to be considered when making decisions about wound debridement (**TABLE 13-3**).

The overall condition of the patient and individual goals of care are two primary factors to be considered in the decision to debride.[14] For example, a terminally ill patient with intact, noninfected eschar may not be a candidate for debridement because of comorbidities, medication, and poor cardiac function. The result of

CLINICAL CONSIDERATION

Access to adequate anesthesia (topical, regional, or general) must be considered for the patient with intact sensation in the area to be debrided.

CASE STUDY

INTRODUCTION

A 62-year-old female resident of a long-term care facility with a past medical history of obsessive compulsive and anxiety disorders, hypertension, hyperlipidemia, congestive heart failure, coronary artery disease, chronic obstructive pulmonary disease, and urinary incontinence presents to the wound center with an 8-week history of pressure injury on the sacral/coccygeal area (**FIGURE 13-4**).

DISCUSSION QUESTIONS

1. What other information is needed about this patient in order to make a diagnosis?
2. What information is needed to determine the plan of care?

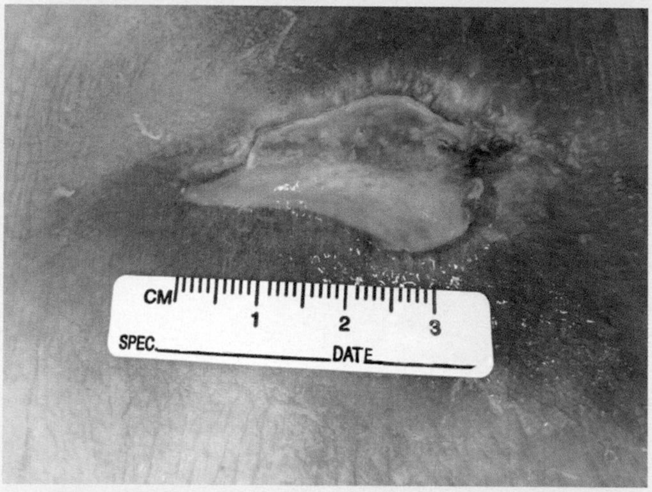

FIGURE 13-4 Sacral pressure ulcer at the time of initial assessment, prior to debridement.

TABLE 13-3 Factors for Consideration Before Debridement[3,13,14]

- Overall condition of the patient and their ability to achieve and sustain a closed wound
- Inclusion of the patient's and family's individualized goals for care
- The patient's ability to adhere to the plan of care
- Etiology of the wound
- Type/s of necrotic tissue (ie, slough, eschar)
- Potential of the wound to close and heal due to local factors (eg, blood flow, presence of infection)
- Potential of the wound to close and heal due to systemic factors (eg, nutrition, glucose control, immune status, medications)
- Ability to achieve adequate pain control during debridement
- Clinicians' knowledge, skills, and expertise
- Available resources to support wound care (eg, personnel, reimbursement, availability of equipment and supplies)

debridement may be a larger, potentially more painful wound requiring more extensive topical care with little or no opportunity for closure due to the patient's severely compromised medical status. The patient's general state of health, nutrition, hydration, medications, mobility, and activity status are other factors to be taken into consideration.[14] Patients who take anticoagulants may need a less-invasive debridement technique than sharp or surgical debridement. In addition, patients requiring more aggressive techniques are more safely debrided in a controlled setting, such as the operating room or hospital clinic, rather than at the bedside, in the home, or in the long-term care setting.

Hard-to-heal wounds often have underlying pathogenic abnormalities that can cause devitalized tissue to reaccumulate. Generally, debridement is not a singular event, but rather combines different methods and/or repeated interventions over time to achieve a clean, functional wound bed. Frequent serial debridements are often necessary to continually stimulate and refresh the surface cells, keeping the wound in a state of readiness to close.[16–18]

The decision to debride requires careful consideration in certain wound etiologies. Stable, noninfected heel or lower-extremity ulcers with impaired perfusion should not be debrided unless signs of infection are present (eg, erythema, fluctuance, separation of eschar from the edge with drainage, or purulence).[14,18,19] Best practice guidelines state that heel pressure injuries with stable dry eschar should not be debrided unless there is adequate perfusion[14]; however, in some instances, it may be clinically appropriate to remove stable black eschar on patients who have functional goals with good blood flow. When making the decision to debride stable heel eschar, documentation to justify this decision is important.

CLINICAL CONSIDERATION

- *Vascularity* must be assessed prior to performing any debridement of a lower extremity wound.
- Palpation *only* of lower extremity vasculature is *inadequate* for assessing blood flow in patients with hard-to-heal lower extremity wounds.

Patients with diabetes who have lower-extremity wounds need more extensive noninvasive vascular assessments (eg, toe pressures [**FIGURE 13-5**] and wave forms, transcutaneous oxygen tension, skin perfusion, or duplex arterial studies) to determine blood flow because of the propensity of the more proximal vessels to calcify in people with diabetes.[3,17,20,21] Guidelines for healing potential and for debridement are discussed in Chapter 4, Vascular Wounds.

Maintaining a dry, stable eschar often leads to slow eschar demarcation and separation as epithelial migration occurs from the edge, eventually closing the wound (**FIGURE 13-6**). This process has been reported in many cases when a patient is

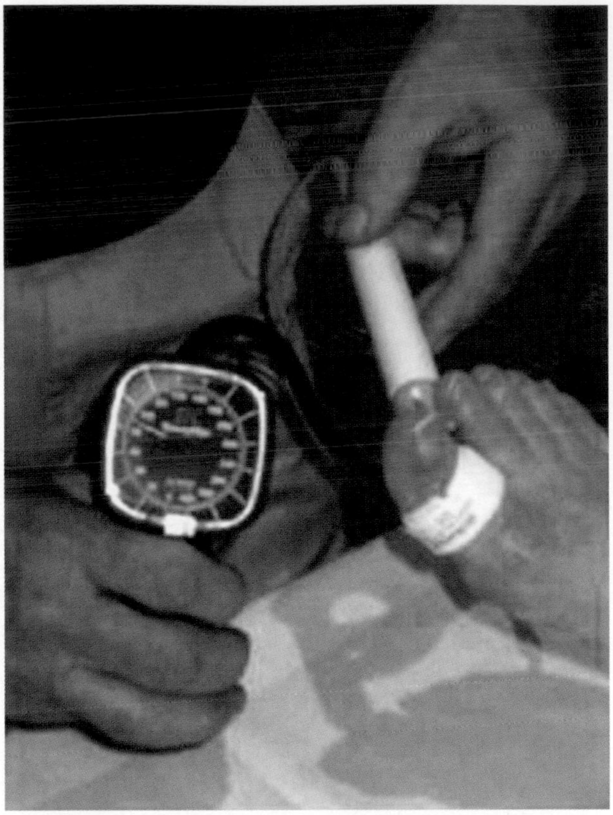

FIGURE 13-5 **Toe pressures in patients with diabetes are assessed before debridement.**

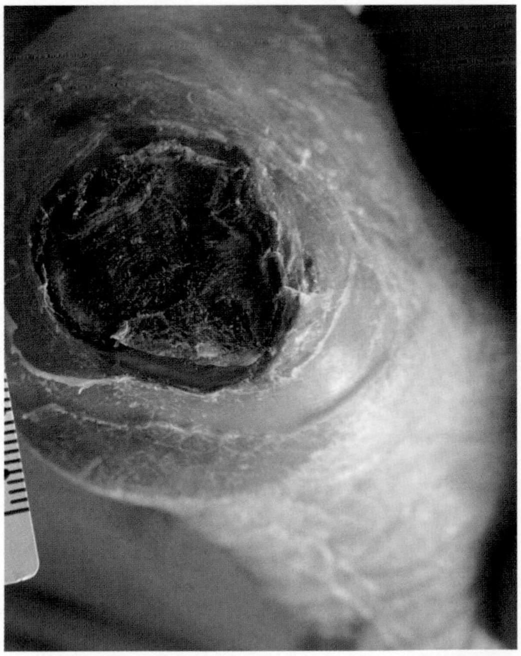

FIGURE 13-6 **Eschar demarcation and separation.** Dry eschar on a heel with compromised vascular status is sometimes best left in place and not debrided unless there are signs of infection. The epithelium may migrate from the edges under the eschar, which can then be trimmed as it releases. With meticulous care, these wounds will sometimes progress to full closure, albeit quite slowly.

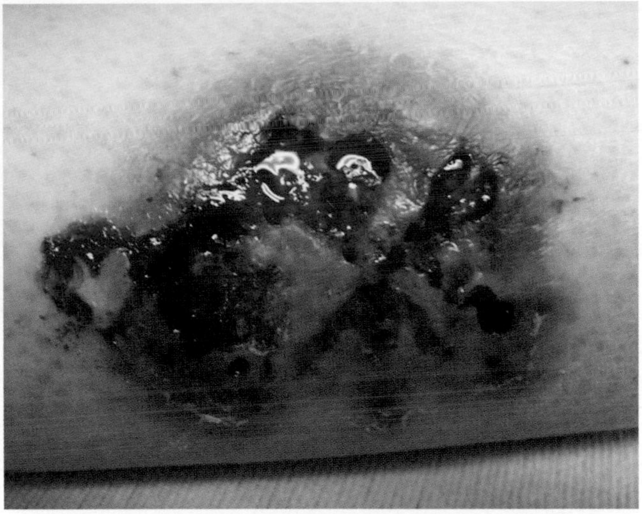

FIGURE 13-7 **Pyoderma gangrenosum.** Pyoderma gangrenosum has defining violaceous borders around the wound. Wound trauma (eg, aggressive scrubbing, sharp/surgical debridement) should be avoided with suspected pyoderma gangrenosum etiology because of the risk of *pathergy*.

not a candidate for debridement. In addition, diagnoses such as pyoderma gangrenosum may result in *pathergy* (defined as enlarging or worsening of the wound), with sharp or surgical debridement (FIGURE 13-7).[21,22]

The clinician who performs debridement must have knowledge of anatomy, understand the patient's overall medical condition, know the wound etiology, and have the technical skills and clinical judgment for debridement, especially when using the more invasive techniques (such as, sharp or surgical debridement) in order to have safe, successful outcomes. Clinicians must discriminate viable from nonviable tissue, recognize structures such as arteries and veins, recognize the difference between muscle and granulation tissue, identify fascia covering muscles, identify tendons and cartilage versus slough (which are sometimes similar in color), and identify bone, which when exposed heightens the risk of osteomyelitis (see FIGURES 13-8 to 13-18).

In addition to a thorough awareness of the patient's clinical conditions, knowledge of the different types of necrotic tissue is necessary to determine the most effective method of debridement. Devitalized tissue is generally categorized as slough or eschar; however, any tissue in or adjacent to the wound bed can become necrotic if it loses its blood supply (FIGURES 13-12 and 13-13). Therefore, reassessment of the wound is required at every debridement session.

Eschar may be soft or hard, depending on the amount of desiccation (extreme dryness), and is often described as leathery when completely dry. Slough (FIGURE 13-12) may be yellow, tan, gray, or brown; is generally moist; and may be loosely or firmly adhered to the wound bed.

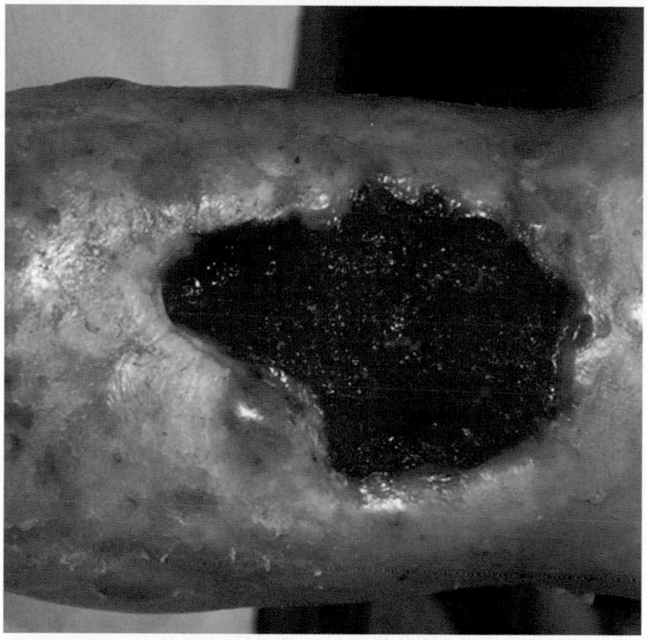

FIGURE 13-8 Healthy granulation. Granulation tissue is pink/red and moist; composed of new capillaries, extracellular matrix, fibroblasts, and inflammatory cells. The presence of granulation tissue indicates a full-thickness wound. Healthy granulation tissue has an irregular, bumpy, or granular surface.

The presence of granulation tissue is the hallmark of the proliferative phase of wound repair. Healthy granulation tissue most often appears bright or "beefy" red due to its rich vascular composition (**FIGURE 13-8**). Unhealthy granulation tissue, sometimes called *friable* or fragile granulation tissue, maybe a dull, dark red, or pale pink color.

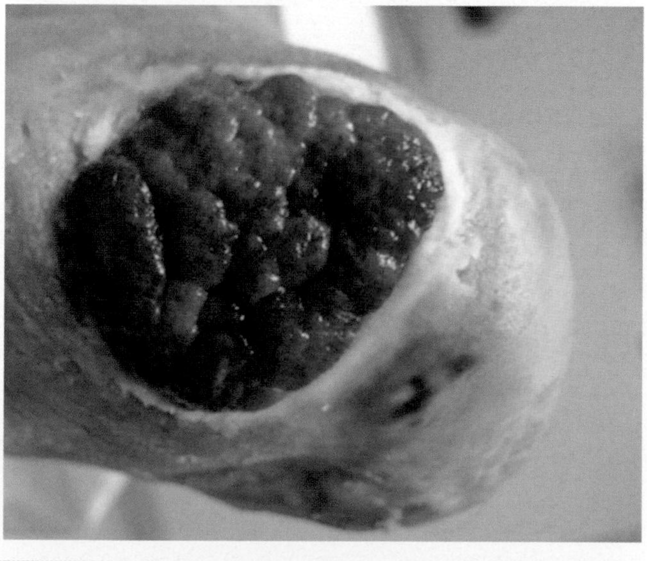

FIGURE 13-9 Hypergranulation tissue. Granulation tissue that is bulbous and friable suggesting heavy bacterial bioburden. Frequently raised above the level of the periwound skin, it may also be seen in wound base, below the periwound surface.

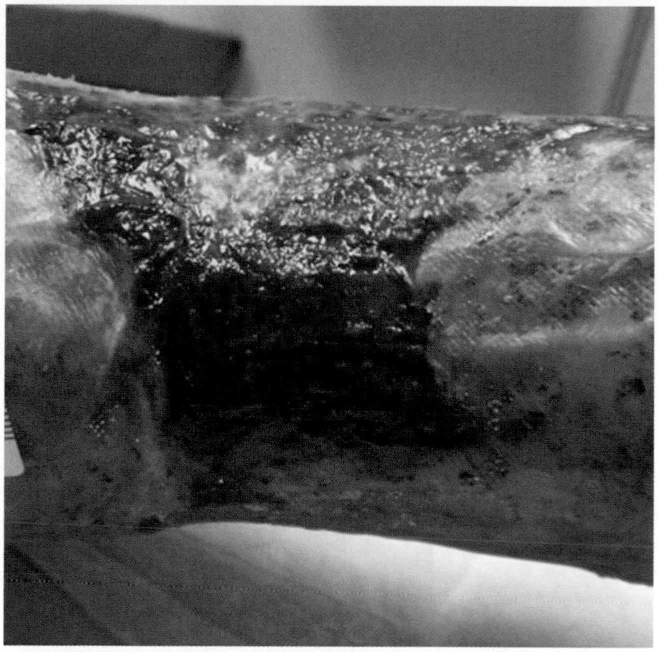

FIGURE 13-10 Friable granulation. A sign of critical contamination, infection, poor extracellular matrix quality, or overall edema.

Hypergranulation tissue (also known as "proud flesh," exuberant granulation tissue, hypertrophic granulation tissue, and hyperplasia of granulation tissue) is a condition that is characterized by overabundance of granulation tissue, resulting in the extension of this tissue above the level of the wound margins (**FIGURE 13-9**).[20–25] This condition may prevent migration of epithelial cells across the wound surface as these cells do not travel vertically, thereby delaying closure and making the wound more susceptible to infection. In addition, wounds with hypergranulation tissue have an increased risk for excessive scar formation by forcing the wound edges further apart.[25] Malignancies can also present with tissue resembling hypergranulation tissue; therefore, an appropriate referral, biopsy, or both may be indicated (**FIGURE 13-11**).[25]

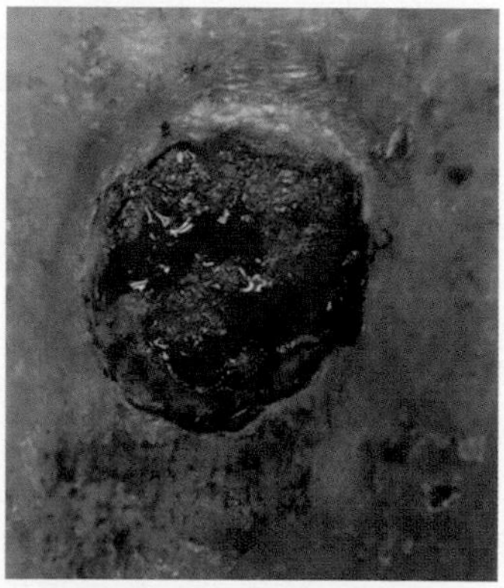

FIGURE 13-11 Skin cancer that resembles healthy granulation tissue. Note the bleeding and unusual periwound skin color, both signs of an atypical diagnosis.

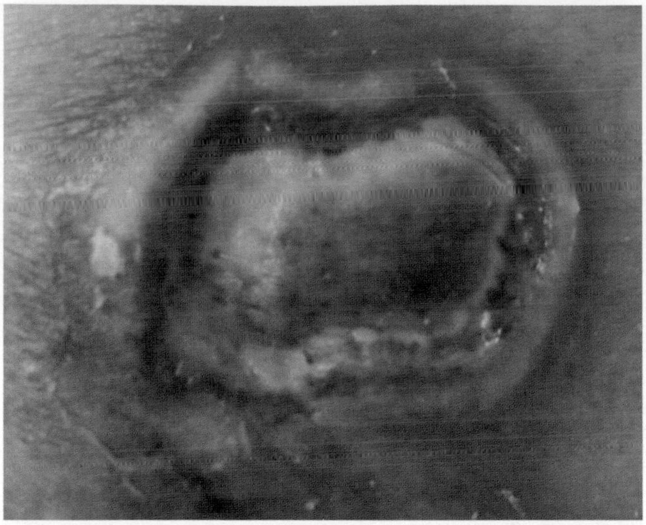

FIGURE 13-12 Slough. A metabolic by-product that is composed of serum and matrix proteins; may be white, yellow, tan, brown, or green. It may be loose or firmly adherent and it has a stringy or fibrous texture and appearance has either a soft mushy or stringy fibrous texture, depending on the tissue that has been autolyzed by the phagocytic cells.

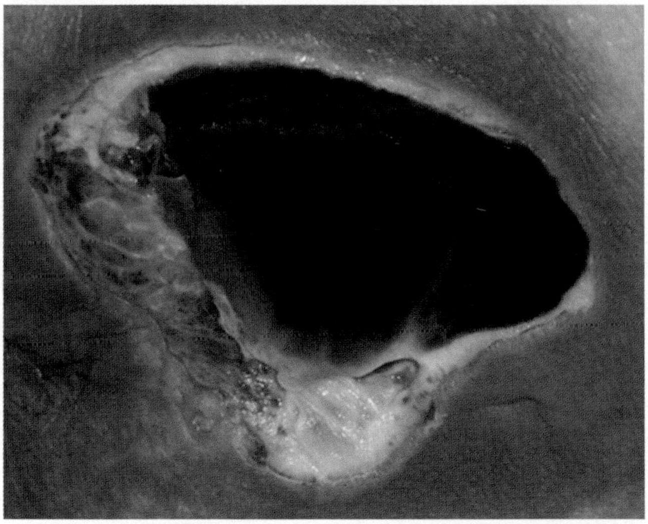

FIGURE 13-13 Eschar. Firmly adherent, hard, black, firm, leathery tissue, may be strongly or loosely attached to wound base and edges.

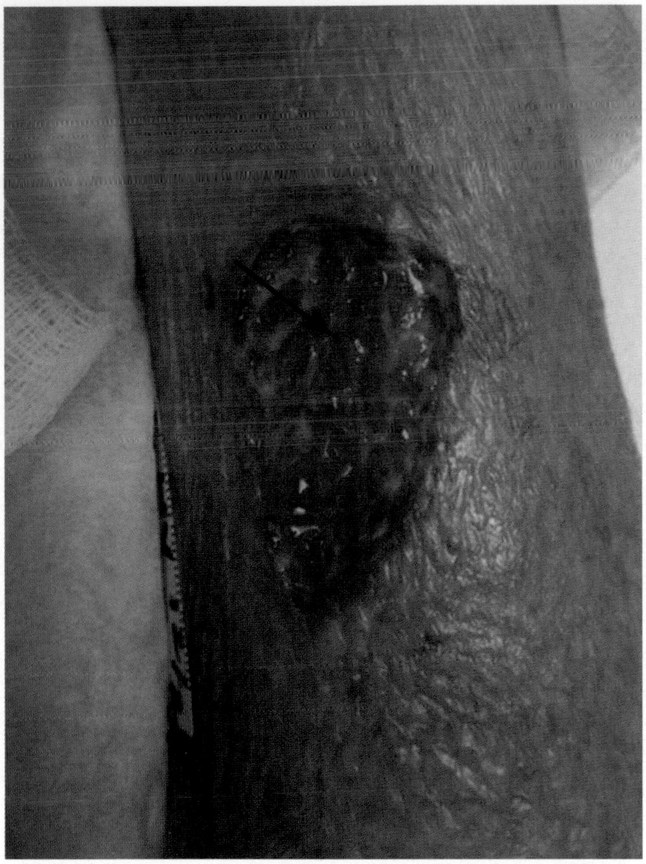

FIGURE 13-14 Vessel in wound bed. Any visible vessels, even if they appear coagulated, are to be avoided in order to prevent bleeding.

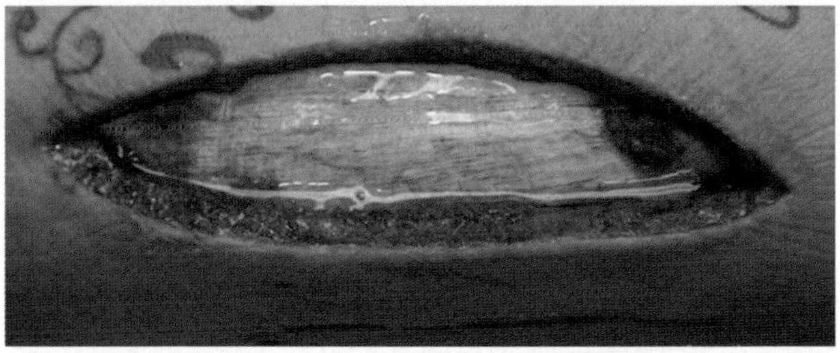

FIGURE 13-15 Muscle/fascia. Healthy muscle is bright red and sensate, bleeds when cut, and may twitch when stimulated. Conversely, necrotic muscle does not bleed when cut, is brown and stringy, and does not contract.

CLINICAL CONSIDERATION

Malignant tissue that resembles hypergranulation will bleed easily, have a darker red to purple color due to hypervascularity, and most frequently occurs when there has been a history of hyperplasia.

TABLE 13-4[3,20,23] provides examples of treatment to diminish or alleviate hypergranulation tissue. **FIGURES 13-19** and **13-20** illustrate the use of polyvinyl alcohol foam to treat hypergranulation tissue.

Chapter 3, Examination and Evaluation of the Patient with a Wound, provides more detailed information on tissue types in chronic wounds.

TABLE 13-4 Interventions to Reduce Hypergranulation Tissue[3,24,25]

- Compression with dressings such as foams
- Dressings to decrease moisture (eg, hypertonic dressings, calcium alginates, hydrofibers)
- Antimicrobial dressings (eg, silver-impregnated dressings, polyvinyl alcohol foam with organic pigments [**FIGURES 12-18** and **12-19**] cadexomer iodine)
- Mechanical debridement (eg, scrubbing, low-frequency ultrasound)
- Chemical cauterization with silver nitrate
- Sharp debridement
- Application of topical corticosteroids

CASE STUDY

CONTINUED

A review of the patient's medical history (available through records brought to the clinic with the patient) includes the following:

- Medications: Amlodipine, atorvastatin, furosemide, albuterol sulfate, and two antidepressants
- Vital signs (taken at the time of evaluation): BP—100/65; HR—78 bpm; O_2 saturation—94% on room air
- Function: The patient arrives in a wheelchair, records indicate that she is nonambulatory; transfers from bed to wheelchair with moderate assistance and sits in the chair 3–4 hours each morning and afternoon.
- In addition to regular meals, patient receives protein shakes.
- The patient's wound measurements, using the perpendicular method, are 3.8 cm × 1.7 cm × 0.1 cm deep.

There is minimal serous drainage on the dressing upon removal and no odor. The patient has visible changes in facial expression and verbal complaints of pain with any tactile sensation to the wound bed.

DISCUSSION QUESTIONS

1. What type of tissue is visible in the wound bed?
2. Describe the edges and the periwound skin.
3. Are any clinical signs of infection present?
4. Using the NPIAP Classification for Pressure Injury Staging, what stage would be appropriate for this wound?

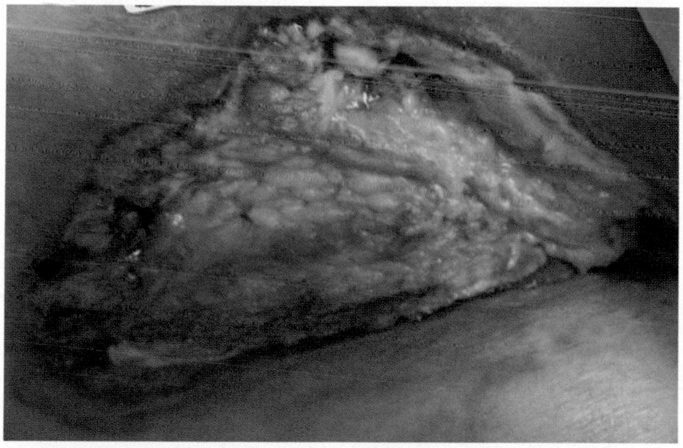

FIGURE 13-16 Subcutaneous fat. Fat is poorly vascularized and thus can become necrotic and desiccated easier than other tissue types; therefore, it can become a likely source of bacteria growth.

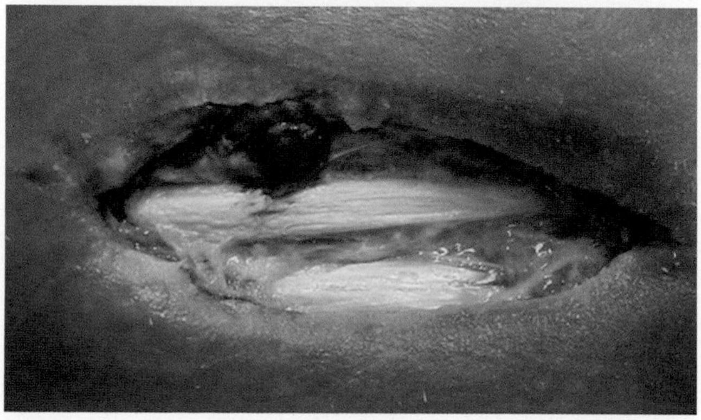

FIGURE 13-17 Tendons. A tendon that has the sheath with paratenon intact should be protected with a moist dressing to prevent desiccation. Stringy nonviable tendon can be debrided.

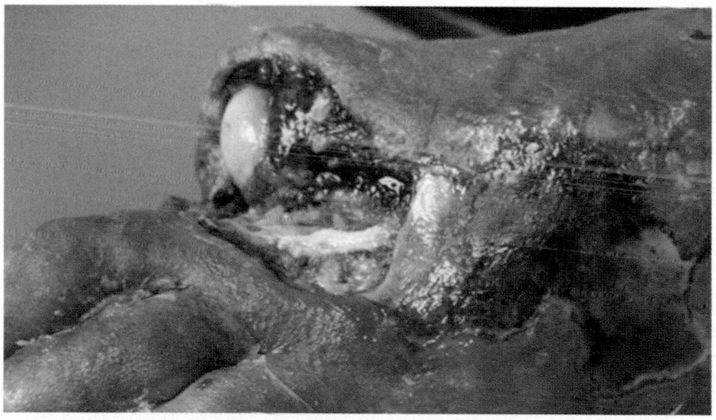

FIGURE 13-18 Bone in wound bed.

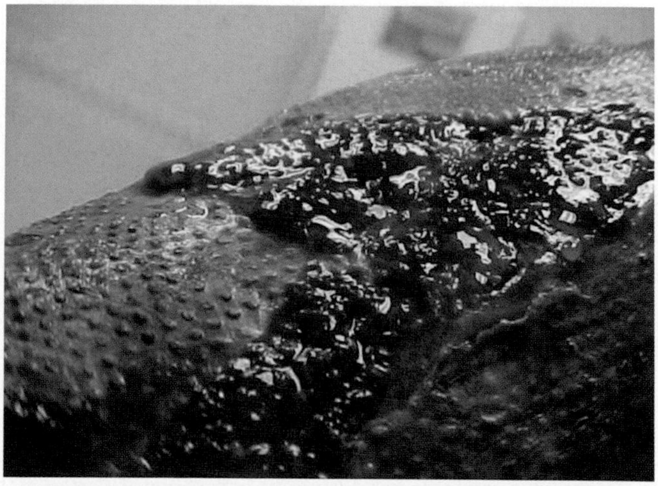

FIGURE 13-19 Hypergranulation tissue before treatment with PAV foam.

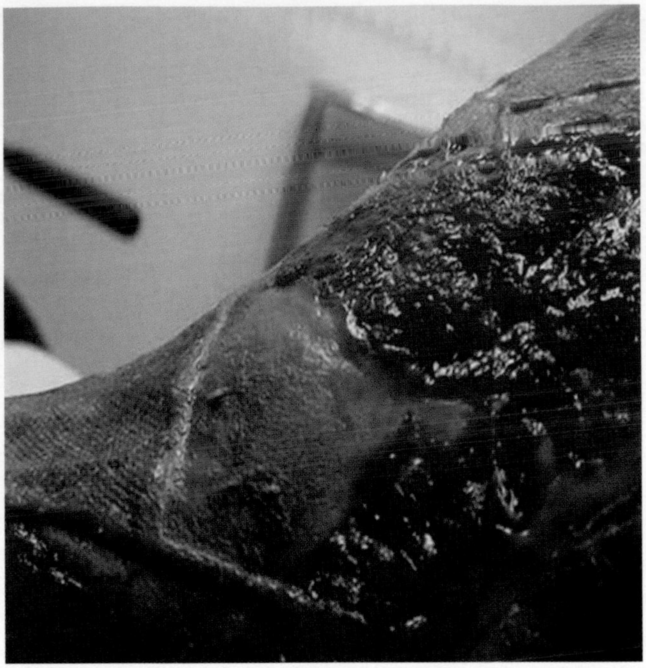

FIGURE 13-20 Hypergranulation tissue after treatment with PAV foam. Note that granulation tissue is more flush or even with wound edges, thereby allowing epithelial migration toward the center of the wound bed.

TYPES OF DEBRIDEMENT

Debridement falls into two general categories: selective and nonselective. With selective debridement, only nonviable tissue is removed; with nonselective techniques, both viable and nonviable tissues may be removed. Debridement is also classified by the method or the mechanism of action of the various techniques that are used to remove nonviable tissue.

The most common types of debridement used in clinical practice include:

- Autolytic
- Enzymatic
- Mechanical (ie, scrubbing, pulsed lavage/irrigation, and contact low-frequency ultrasound)
- Instrument (sharp, surgical, and hydrosurgical)
- Biotherapy, larval, or maggot debridement therapy

One or more types of debridement may be used synergistically to achieve and maintain a clean, functional wound bed.

Autolytic Debridement

Autolytic debridement is the removal of nonviable tissue by phagocytic cells and proteolytic enzymes that naturally break down necrotic tissue (**FIGURES 13-21** and **13-22**). Wound fluid contains these enzymes in addition to inflammatory cells, such as neutrophils and macrophages, and metalloproteases that enter the wound site during the normal inflammatory process to remove bacteria and debris.[4,16] It is a highly selective process whereby only necrotic tissue will be affected. Dressing categories customarily used to provide the optimal environment for autolytic debridement by retaining the patient's endogenous wound fluid in the wound bed include hydrogels, hydrocolloids, transparent films, foams, alginates, and medical-grade honey (see Chapter 14, Wound Dressings).[3,22,23]

CLINICAL CONSIDERATION

Clinicians working in home health or other settings where dressings are not readily available often ask, "What can I use instead?" For autolytic debridement of the dry eschar, a thin layer of petroleum jelly can be used instead of hydrogel, under an occlusive dressing (eg, transparent film) to facilitate autolytic debridement.

The process of autolytic debridement is slower than other methods, requires multiple dressing applications, and frequently takes several weeks to complete; therefore, it is most indicated on thin superficial eschar. Older or frail patients may have difficulty achieving a clean wound bed using autolytic debridement because of a possibly impaired immune system, aging, comorbidities, and nutrition and hydration deficits. This finding suggests that older patients may need more aggressive forms of debridement than the autolytic process alone.[26]

Autolytic debridement is frequently used in combination with other types of debridement, such as mechanical or instrument debridement. While slower, it may be the least painful type of debridement as long as the patient tolerates the dressing changes. The frequency of dressing changes depends on the amount of nonviable tissue to be removed and the amount of fluid that collects under the dressing.

Fluid collection beneath the selected dressing is monitored to prevent prolonged exposure of intact skin, which could lead to moisture-associated skin damage and ultimately create fragile skin that is at risk for further

CLINICAL CONSIDERATION

An adequate immune system and local vascular supply are necessary for autolytic debridement to proceed optimally.

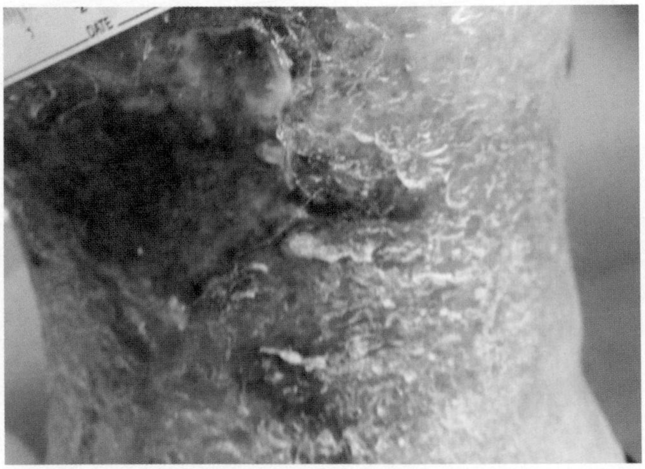

FIGURE 13-21 Wound before autolytic debridement.

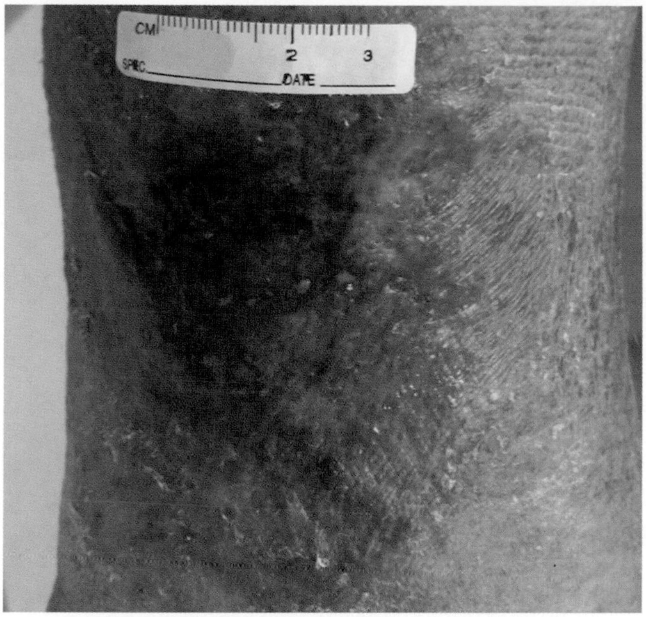

FIGURE 13-22 Wound after autolytic debridement. Note the preservation of periwound skin, flat edges, and lack of necrotic tissue, all a result of the patient's healthy cellular components and enzymes that could break down and phagocytose the nonviable tissue.

damage (**FIGURE 13-23**). Also, the fluid contains dead cells, cellular debris, and bacteria, frequently causing an odor that may lead to the assumption that the wound is infected, despite the absence of other clinical indicators of infection. Culture of the fluid would likely reveal bacteria that are present but not pathogenic to the wound or patient, possibly leading to unnecessary treatment with antibiotics. The wound surface and surrounding skin should be thoroughly and safely irrigated or cleansed after each dressing removal and before assessing for clinical signs of infection.[22]

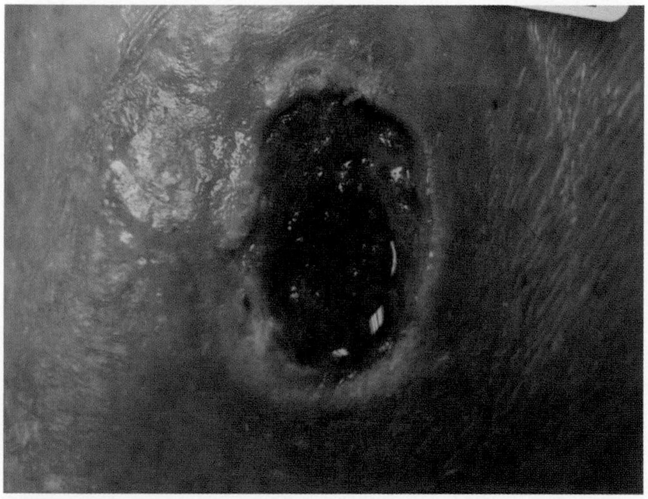

FIGURE 13-23 Maceration around the wound edges as a result of exposure to the fluids that collect under the dressing used for autolytic debridement.

Autolytic debridement can be employed to debride wounds of all types, regardless of etiology. However, wounds in the presence of peripheral arterial disease should be approached cautiously with autolytic debridement because of impaired blood supply not only resulting in a potential lack of moisture in the lower extremity skin, but also the heightened risk of infection.

Autolytic debridement is frequently the initial intervention in the home and long-term care setting where other, more aggressive forms of debridement may not be feasible or available. The only absolute contraindication to autolytic debridement is the infected wound, which needs to be debrided more urgently.[14] Also, the moisture under the dressing is an ideal environment for bacteria to thrive. Autolytic debridement can be accomplished with minimal technical skills on the part of the caregiver; however, knowledge and skills are required to know if the process is appropriate for a particular wound and patient.

Surfactant Debridement

A unique enhancement to autolytic debridement is the use of a water-soluble Concentrated Surfactant Gel (CSG; PluroGel Burn and Wound Dressing, Medline Industries, Inc., Northfield, IL). The surfactant, Poloxamer 188, is also often referred to as pluronic F68. Poloxamers are nonionic synthetic surfactants comprising one central hydrophobic chain and two outer hydrophilic chains. These molecules form loose (noncovalent) cross-links with water to form a micelle matrix (Plurogel micelle matrix or PMM). The matrix is surface active, and in a dynamic system creates a "rinsing" action at a molecular level on the wound bed. This surfactant-driven activity enables the product to disrupt the noncovalent bonds which are instrumental in keeping necrotic tissue and other undesirable elements adherent to the wound bed, thus impairing healing. The product adds moisture more efficiently via the surfactant activity and essentially solubilizes dried exudate and other matter, thereby helping to soften, loosen, and trap wound debris.[27] These undesirable elements can then be rather easily removed at dressing changes via simple rinsing or wiping with wet gauze or similar materials.[28] For thermodynamic reasons specific to the polymer poloxamer, the CSG has a low viscosity appearance when at ambient conditions, particularly in cool ambient conditions (it turns into a liquid in a refrigerator for example), but forms a thick gel as it warms in contact with living tissue. This differentiates it from other common gel-like preparations, which are generally viscous when cooled and "runny" when warmed to body temperature. Furthermore, because the surfactant micelles are easily water soluble, the debris-laden gel can be atraumatically washed away during dressing changes.[29]

Lastly, laboratory and clinical studies have demonstrated the ability of the CSG to sequester planktonic microbes and disrupt wound biofilm using the mechanism of action described above.[30,31] The ability of the surfactant to salvage damaged cells has also been extensively reported in the literature.[32–36]

Enzymatic Debridement

Enzymatic debridement uses a topical pharmaceutical preparation that is specifically designed to target and break down the devitalized collagen or other tissues in the wound bed.[15,26,37,38] As with autolysis, enzymatic debridement is an alternative to the more aggressive methods of debridement.

At present, there is only one commercially available enzymatic debriding agent in the United States, collagenase, marketed under the trade name Santyl (Smith & Nephew, London, UK).[39] In wound healing, endogenous collagenases belong to a family of extracellular matrix metalloproteases (MMPs) which are naturally occurring enzymes produced by activated inflammatory cells (neutrophils and macrophages) and in certain wound cells (epithelial cells, fibroblasts, and vascular endothelial cells).[9,10,38–41]

Topical collagenase is derived from the bacteria *Clostridium histolyticum*. Reported to be most active in a pH range of 6–8, topical collagenase is specific to native, denatured collagen.[9,16,39] Collagenase promotes debridement by selectively cleaving devitalized collagen strands anchoring necrotic cellular debris without harming viable collagen.[9,16,39] Clostridial collagenase differs in action from naturally occurring collagenase in that it cleaves the devitalized (and therefore unprotected triple helix collagen strands) in seven sites versus just one. As a result, the presence of the collagen fragments has been found to stimulate migration and proliferation of cells into the wound site.[42,43] Collagenase has no known effect on viable tissue and is not associated with increased patient discomfort.[16,39]

CLINICAL CONSIDERATION

A 2-mm layer of collagenase ointment is applied directly to the tissue and covered with an appropriate dressing. The collagenase enzyme is activated by moisture, so the application of a secondary dressing that maintains a moisture balance will allow the enzyme to be released from the ointment.

Collagenase is best applied daily (**FIGURES 13-24** and **13-25**). Cross-hatching of dry or dense eschar is recommended to facilitate penetration of the ointment into softer devitalized tissue and to hasten the debridement process (**FIGURE 13-26**).[21,38] Protection of the surrounding skin with a moisture barrier can prevent maceration and denudation of the intact skin from the increased exudate that results from the enzymatic debridement process. The ointment should not be used with products that could inactivate collagenase (such as detergents or products containing iodine or heavy metals such as lead, silver, or mercury as well as some antimicrobials and antibiotics).[39,41,44] If a wound infection is suspected, the use of an antimicrobial agent per manufacturer's recommendations should be considered for use on the wound surface prior to application of the collagenase ointment.[39]

While initial debridement is important to remove necrotic tissue as a barrier to healing, maintenance or ongoing debridement may be needed to prevent the reaccumulation of debris. Apoptosis, or programmed cell death, is a recurring process in wounds.[16] Continued use of collagenase may address this reaccumulation, thereby allowing the proliferation of healthier granulation tissue.[16,26]

Choosing between autolytic and enzymatic debridement is based on the following:

- Patient condition
- Speed at which debridement is desired
- Access to products
- Type of tissue to be debrided
- Ability of the patient's body to support the autolytic debridement process

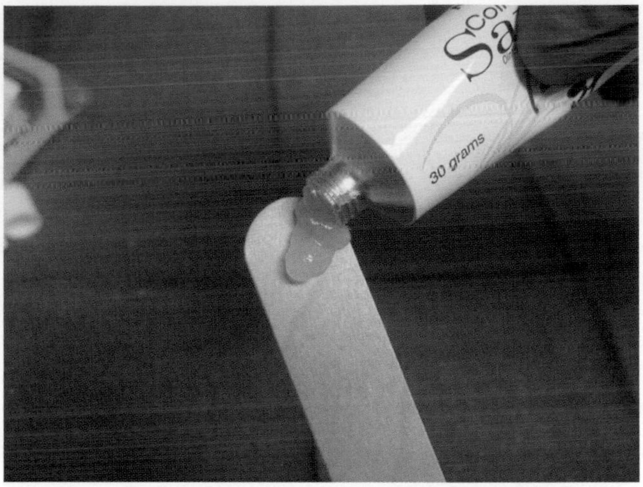

FIGURE 13-24 Enzymatic debridement. Collagenase, available in a thick ointment that is most effective when applied daily, is an enzyme that breaks down denatured protein, thereby releasing the necrotic tissue from the underlying healthy tissue.

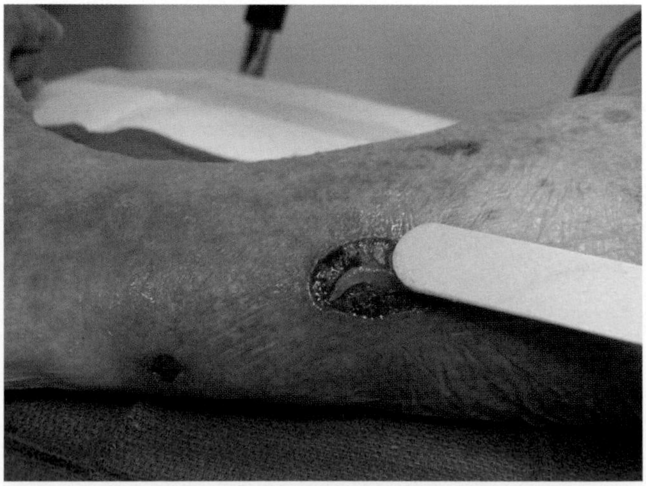

FIGURE 13-25 Application of collagenase.[40] The ointment is applied in a thin layer with a sterile applicator and secured with a moist occlusive dressing that will both provide moisture to activate the enzymes and contain the resulting exudates and debris.

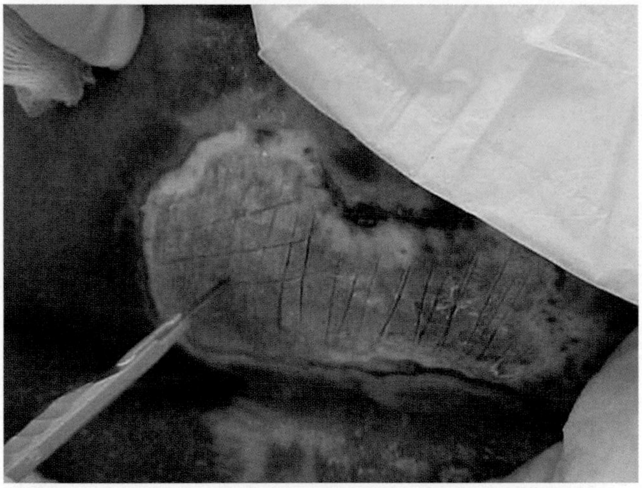

FIGURE 13-26 Cross-hatching of eschar. Both autolytic and enzymatic debridement of eschar is facilitated by cross-hatching the surface of the necrotic tissue with a scalpel prior to application of the dressings.

Autolytic debridement, while effective in some patients, is a more passive approach than enzymatic debridement. Milne et al.[45] conducted a randomized controlled trial of 27 patients with pressure ulcers with nonviable tissue, who had received no previous debridement or cross-hatching. The collagenase group was found to have statistical significance in achieving full debridement by day 42. Additionally, the collagenase group had a greater reduction in nonviable tissue on a weekly basis as compared to a control group receiving autolytic debridement with hyrogel.[45]

Bromelain

An emerging but not mainstream topical enzymatic debriding agent is the use of bromelain, an extract from the stems and fruit of pineapples. Pineapple is the leading edible member of the *bromeliaceae* family grown in several tropical and subtropical countries and has been used as a medicinal plant in several native cultures. An aqueous extract of the fruit contains various proteinases which exhibit fibrinolytic properties in vitro and in vivo, among other activities. Bromelain concentration is highest in the pineapple stem, and differs from that in the fruit. It is prepared from cooled juice by centrifugation, ultrafiltration and lyophilization, yielding a yellowish powder.[46] Clinical trials have been conducted primarily in burns, but more recently in lower extremity ulcers, including venous and diabetic ulcers.[47–49]

The use of bromelain for debridement at this time is primarily limited to acute care settings. The procedure includes significant need for analgesia due to the potential pain involved. In burn studies, topical analgesics are applied for up to 2 hours prior to the application. The powder is mixed with a gel, the periwound skin is protected with a barrier ointment,

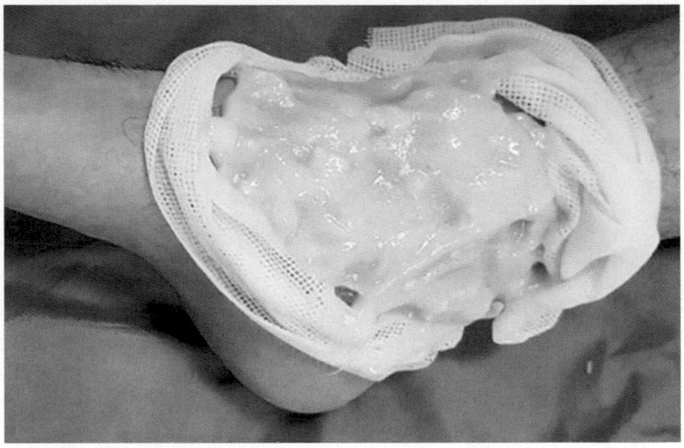

FIGURE 13-27 Bromelain on a foot wound for enzymatic debridement.

and the gel is applied for every 4 hours, then removed and the wound is redressed (**FIGURE 13-27**).

Mechanical Debridement

Mechanical debridement is the use of external forces or energy directly to the wound surface to dislodge and remove debris, bacteria, and necrotic burden. Depending on the method used, this type of debridement can be selective (nonviable tissue only) or nonselective (viable tissue included in the process). The most common types of mechanical debridement include the following:

- Soft abrasive debridement
- Various forms of hydrotherapy
- Wet-to-dry or wet-to-moist dressings
- Low-frequency contact ultrasound

Soft Abrasion Debridement Soft abrasion debridement uses dry gauze or a cotton- or alginate-tipped applicator to gently lift and remove nonadherent debris and congealed surface exudates.[3] Pain that sometimes occurs may be mitigated with the use of a topical anesthetic, which needs to be applied at least 15 minutes prior to treatment for maximum benefit. Abrading the wound edge of new advancing epithelial cells may be used to prevent the formation of epibole.[3] Other indications for soft abrasion are scales that result from chronic venous insufficiency, debris after autolytic or enzymatic debridement, coagulum in the wound bed, or any other loose devitalized tissue.

CLINICAL CONSIDERATION

A monofilament debridement pad (Debrisoft by Lohmann-Rauscher, Rengsdorf, Germany) is available in a 10 × 10 cm pad or a smaller pad on a stick and is excellent for mechanical debridement of wounds (**FIGURE 13-28**).

Hydrotherapy Historically, hydrotherapy for wound care was whirlpool; however,

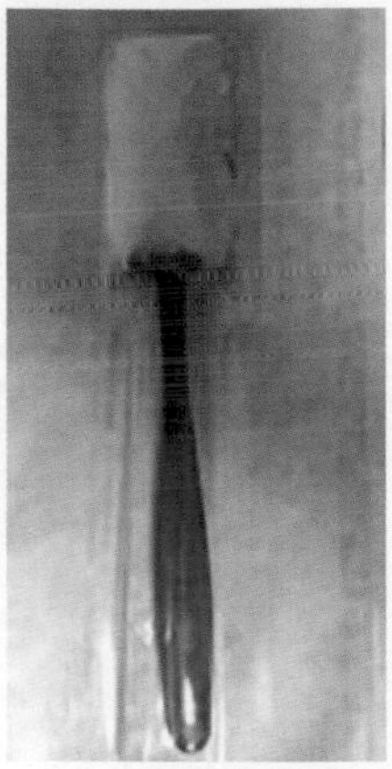

FIGURE 13-28 A monofilament debridement pad for mechanical debridement is especially useful for pediatric patients.

TABLE 13-5 Contraindications to Whirlpool Therapy for Debridement or Wound Cleansing[3,50–52]

- Potential for biofilm growth in WP and associated plumbing
- Potential cross-contamination by bacteria (eg, *Pseudomonas aeruginosa*)
- Inability to determine if WP pressure delivered to wound surface is damaging to granulation tissue
- Maceration of tissues from water (particularly detrimental to diabetic feet)
- Increased venous hypertension in presence of venous insufficiency

the development of pulsed lavage with suction (PLWS) essentially eliminated the use of whirlpool in wound care.[6,50,51] The documented contraindications for whirlpool are listed in **TABLE 13-5**, and the discussion of hydrotherapy is focused on PLWS.

PLWS uses a pulsating mechanical force delivering saline (or other desired solutions) to loosen debris and cleanse the wound bed, with or without simultaneous suction, depending on the equipment used (**FIGURE 13-29** and **TABLE 13-6**).[3,38] This biophysical energy is highly effective in dislodging slough and other detritus and can be a selective form of debriding necrotic tissue when the lavage force is targeting nonviable tissue only.

PLWS is one of the few debridement methods that can function in tracts, tunnels, and areas of extensive undermining using specialized tips.[38] Pressure settings are recommended to be below 15 pounds per square inch (psi) to prevent driving the bacteria into underlying soft tissue and to prevent damage to granulation tissue present in the wound bed.[3,14,38] See Chapter 19, Pulsed Lavage with Suction, for specific details on techniques, indications, and contraindications.

Personal protective equipment is necessary for the clinician performing PLWS. In addition, treatment should be delivered in an enclosed, private treatment area to avoid contamination by aerosolization.[3,38] The clinician must be experienced in using PLWS when treating complex wounds, such as those with fistulas, exposed cavity linings, and long tunnels into body cavities.[3,38]

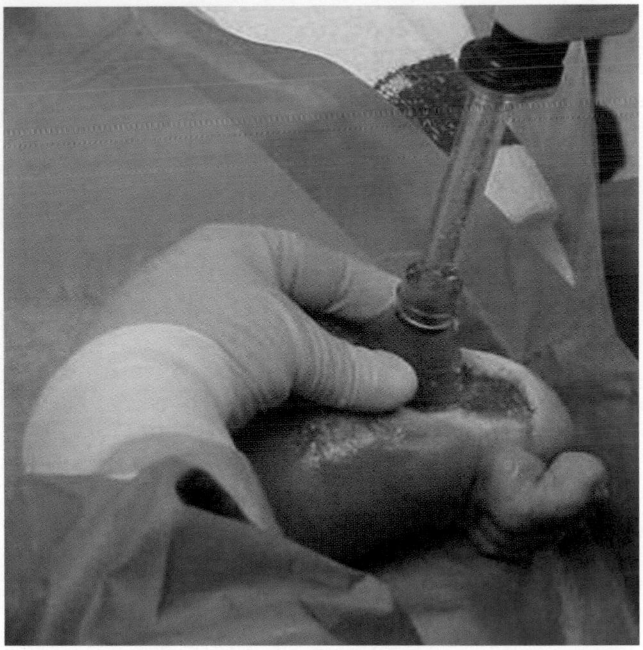

FIGURE 13-29 Pulsed lavage with suction. A flexible tip allows the clinician to mechanically debride and irrigate a variety of wound sizes and shapes with PLWS. The clinician uses the fingers to control the contact of the tip with the wound surface, thereby controlling pressure on the tissue, as well as preventing unnecessary splashing of contaminated saline. The technique requires practice and knowledge of wound healing in order to obtain optimal outcomes. (Used with permission from Harriett Loehne, PT, DPT, CWS, PLWS with splash shield.)

TABLE 13-6 Proposed Benefits of Pulsatile Lavage with Suction

- Provides controlled pressure below 15 psi guidelines for optimal cleansing and irrigation.
- Efficient removal of necrotic tissue, bacteria, and foreign material.
- Site-specific treatment avoids possible maceration of adjacent tissue or viable tissue.
- Portable; can take PLWS units to any care setting.
- Easy setup.
- Single patient use—eliminates sterilization and equipment maintenance.
- Minimizes potential for cross-contamination or staff injuries resulting from lifting and moving patients.
- Convenient premade kits available.
- Various application tips for use in different types of wound beds (ie, tunnels, tracts, fistulas).

Wet-to-Dry Dressings Wet-to-dry dressings are a nonselective method for debridement of devitalized tissue. This dressing technique, normally referred to as either wet-to-dry or wet-to-moist, unfortunately remains a common form of debridement in many care settings.[52–55] The name is somewhat misleading in that the gauze dressing is rarely placed into the wound bed in what would be considered a wet level of hydration. Rather, the most commonly discussed procedure is to wet open-weave gauze, squeeze or wring out the fluid until it is just moist, and then open and place the gauze into the wound bed such that a layer of the gauze is in intimate contact with all areas of the wound surface. The proposed mechanism of action is that as the gauze dries, it becomes adherent to the wound surface, and the surface debris is torn from the wound bed as the dressing is removed (**FIGURE 13-30**).[3,55]

This nonselective form of debridement, which can damage healthy granulation tissue and deeper structures in the wound bed, has many disadvantages that may overshadow any potential benefit. These disadvantages include, but are not limited to, the following:

- The procedure is nonselective as a form of debridement and indiscriminately removes any tissue, viable or nonviable, with which it is in contact.
- Gauze does not have to completely dry to cause trauma to the wound surface. The absorption of exudate from the wound surface causes gauze fibers to become embedded in the wound bed and consequently to adhere upon removal of the gauze.

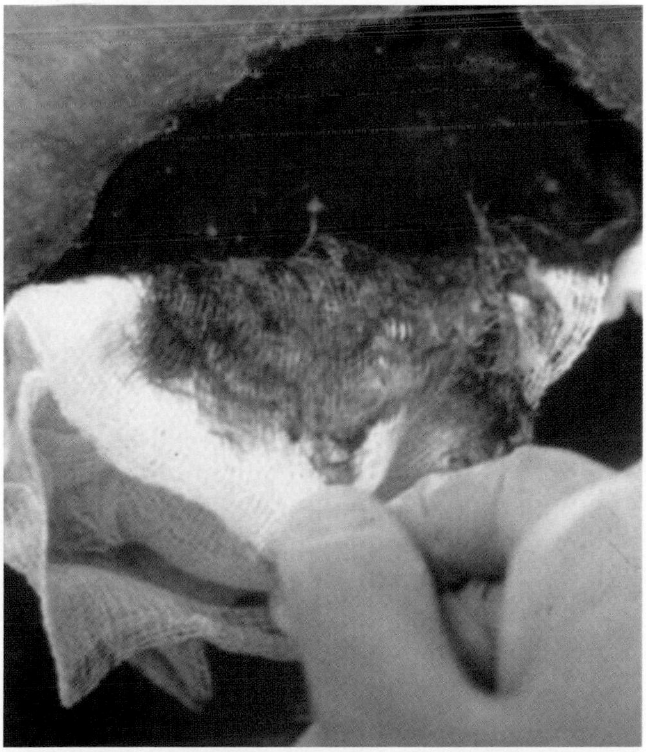

FIGURE 13-30 Wet-to-dry debridement. Removal of a wet-to-dry dressing over healthy granulation tissue disrupts fragile capillaries and damages new granulation tissue.

- Wet-to-dry dressings often cause pain upon removal.
- Gauze as a packing material is often over-packed, potentially causing increased pressure on the surface of the wound, thereby increasing the likelihood of further superficial tissue necrosis.
- Exposed structures such as bone, muscle, or tendon are likely to desiccate using a wet-to-dry procedure.[3,14,53–55]

Although the materials for wet-to-dry debridement are inexpensive and readily available, this procedure can actually be more expensive than current advanced dressing choices and debridement techniques. Wet-to-dry requires increased clinician time for each dressing change and more frequent dressing changes, as well as prolonged time to heal.[54]

Additionally, wet-to-dry dressings may impede wound healing due to local tissue cooling; disruption of granulation tissue by dressing removal; and increased infection risk from frequent dressing changes, strike-through drainage, and prolonged inflammation.[54,55] One study found that wet-to-dry dressings were inappropriately prescribed for wounds not needing debridement in more than 78% of the wounds for which they were ordered.[55]

CLINICAL CONSIDERATION

Wet-to-dry dressings are absolutely inappropriate for wounds with significant amounts of healthy granulation tissue in the wound bed.

All of the negatives aside, when performed properly, wet-to-dry debridement can be a relatively quick and often effective method for removing devitalized tissue from a wound bed that is predominately covered with necrotic tissue and has adequate blood flow. Caution is advised with anticoagulated patients as bleeding may occur with dressing removal. As with any wound dressing change, adequate pain control is necessary for successful treatment.[3,14] For large wounds, moistened gauze may be the only packing material that can reasonably and cost-effectively fill a large defect. However, once granulation tissue begins to form in the wound bed, the clinician should shift from the wet-to-dry technique to another intervention (eg, negative pressure wound therapy) that will not damage the new, fragile tissue and will facilitate faster closure. If negative pressure wound therapy is not available, a thin layer of hydrogel over the wound surface before filling with a moist gauze dressing will help prevent adherence to the viable tissue and decrease pain with removal.

Low-Frequency Ultrasound Energy in Debridement In recent years, low-frequency ultrasound (LFUS) energy has been employed to positively impact tissues in the hard-to-heal wound by performing debridement and facilitating wound closure and healing.[14,56] There are several devices, manufactured by various companies, which provide different methods of delivering ultrasound energy to the wound for bactericidal effects, and with the *contact* devices, immediate selective debridement of necrotic tissue is achievable. In addition, *noncontact* forms of low-frequency ultrasound are thought to facilitate wound closure and healing processes.[56–59] (See Chapter 18, Ultrasound, for a discussion of ultrasound energy in wound care.)

Use of low-frequency *contact* ultrasound for wound debridement has several advantages:

- Immediate results when using contact LFUS
- Pain management with only topical anesthesia
- Selective debridement of necrotic tissue; nonselective debridement of *unhealthy* viable tissue, and undesirable tissues such as rolled or thickened nonmigrating edges (**FIGURES 13-31** and **13-32**)

A recent meta-analysis found that LFUS used with diabetic foot and venous leg ulcers had significantly lower nonhealed wounds at ≥3 months, with a higher percentage of wound area reduction compared with the standard of care.[60]

As mentioned earlier, LFUS is bactericidal at the surface and penetrates several millimeters into deeper tissues directly beneath the probe tip. It can be performed in a variety of settings by trained personnel, permitting energy delivery at the bedside, in the outpatient setting, or during operative procedures. In addition to separating dead tissue from the wound bed, contact LFUS has the following positive effects that contribute to wound closure and healing:

- Increased local tissue perfusion via vasodilation and resolution of vasospasm (thermal effect)
- Decreased bacterial load
- Stimulation of fibroblasts, macrophages, and endothelial cells to promote healing[56–59,61–63]

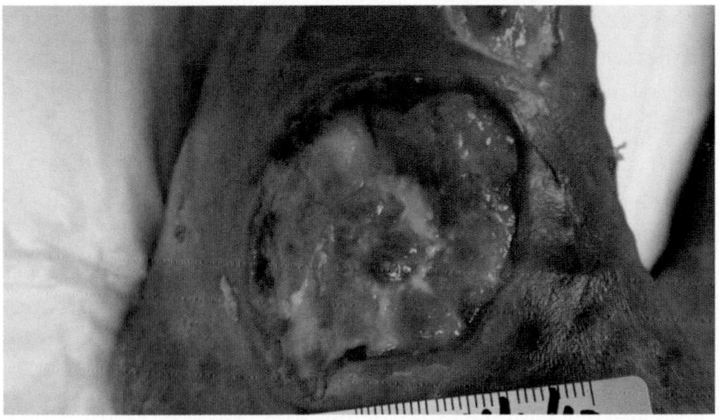

FIGURE 13-31 Ankle wound before contact LFUS debridement.

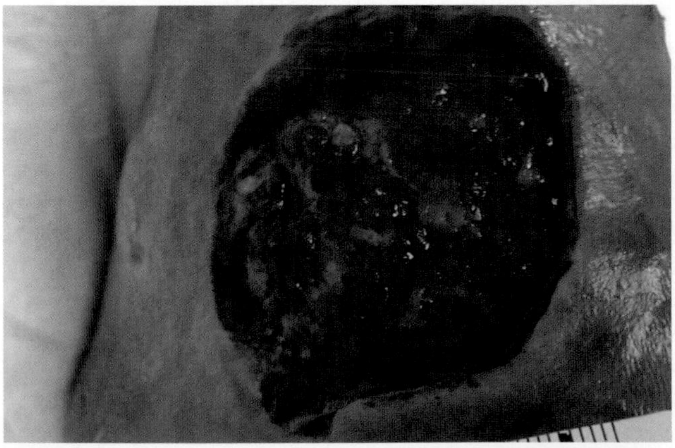

FIGURE 13-32 Wound after contact LFUS debridement. Note wound edges are debrided to fresh tissue to facilitate keratinocyte migration for wound re-epithelialization.

Sharp/Surgical Debridement

Sharp/surgical debridement refers to the use of instruments or devices capable of excising or cutting away necrotic tissue and surface debris. The instruments include, but are not limited to, forceps, scalpels, curettes, and scissors (**FIGURES 13-33** to **13-36**).

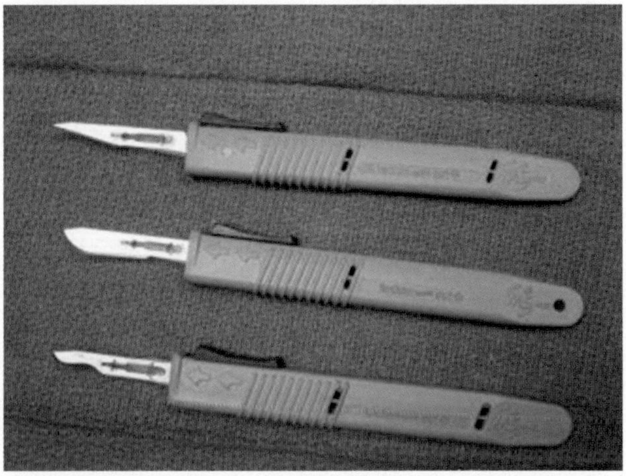

FIGURE 13-33 Scalpels. Each numbered blade has a different shape that makes it useful for different types of tissue and wound shapes.

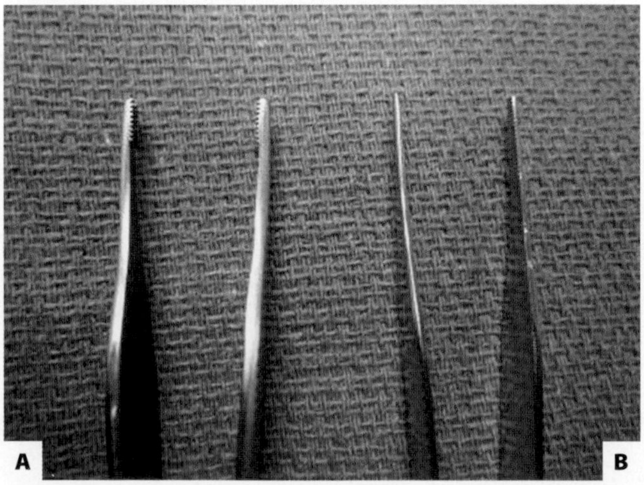

FIGURE 13-34 Example of serrated (A) and standard forceps (B).

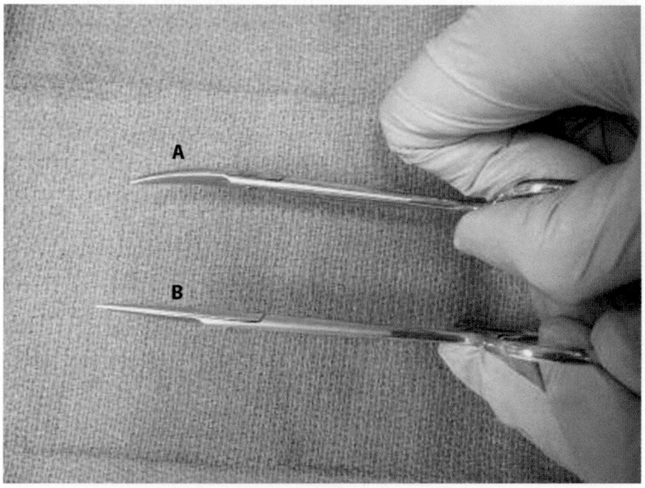

FIGURE 13-35 Examples of curved (A) and straight iris (B) scissors. The small pointed tip allows for precise cutting of necrotic tissue in small areas.

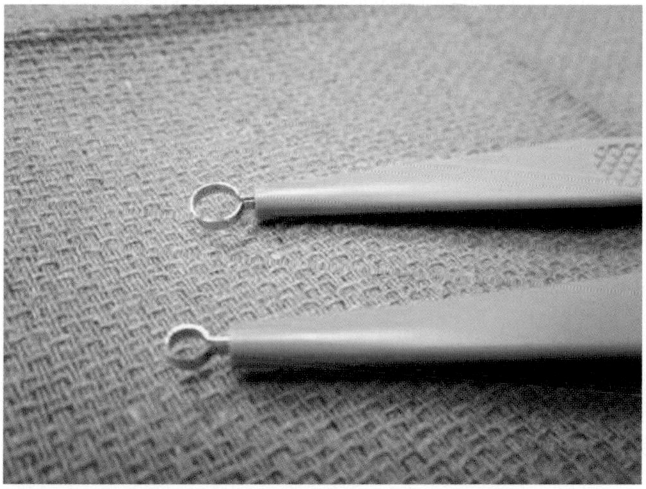

FIGURE 13-36 Curettes. Examples of disposable curettes useful for sharp debridement of slough and devitalized adipose tissue.

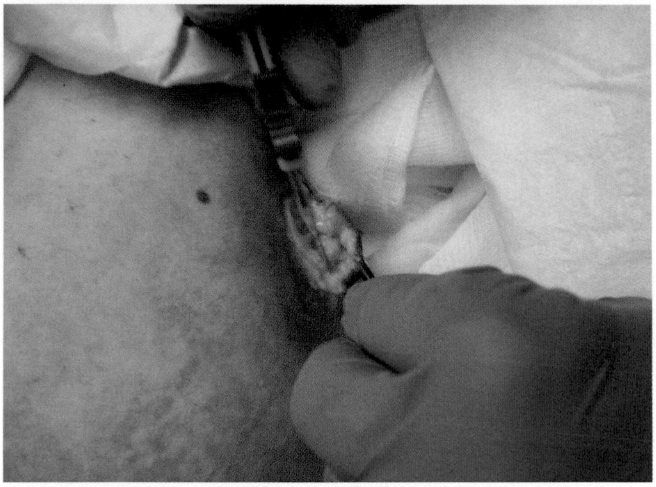

FIGURE 13-37 Sharp debridement of pressure ulcer eschar. Performing sharp debridement of a pressure ulcer using the lift and cut technique. The forceps are used to lift the edge of the eschar so the scalpel or scissor cut can be made precisely between nonviable and viable tissue.

CLINICAL CONSIDERATION

Prior to mechanical or sharp/surgical debridement, a review of the medications for anticoagulant therapy is imperative. Excessive, potentially dangerous bleeding can occur with patients on blood thinners or with low platelet counts, thereby creating an emergency situation.

The instruments used for sharp/surgical debridement may be reusable or disposable; however, those found in the average suture removal kit are generally not strong nor sharp enough to adequately accomplish wound debridement. (An exception is the suture removal kit that contains scissors that are pointed and sharp enough to be termed iris scissors.) In addition, surgical debridement may be accomplished using a device such as the high-powered parallel waterjet.

Sharp/surgical instrument debridement (**FIGURE 13-37**) is a rapid method of removing necrotic tissue. Conservative sharp debridement may also be performed in serial sessions, potentially combined with another form of debridement, to create a functional clean wound bed. Callous debridement on diabetic feet is critical to prepare the wound bed for closure and is performed with a scalpel using a shaving motion, a curette, or with forceps and scissors to lift and cut (**FIGURE 13-38**).

CLINICAL CONSIDERATION

Knowledge of one's scope of practice as defined by the state practice act is paramount before performing sharp debridement. In general, nurses and physical therapists perform sequential or serial conservative sharp instrument debridement, ensuring that only nonviable tissue is removed, whereas physicians, podiatrists, nurse practitioners, and physician assistants may perform both conservative sharp and surgical/excisional debridement that may or may not extend into unhealthy viable tissue.[22]

The clinician performing instrument debridement should have adequate training and skill competency validation. Physicians, especially surgeons and podiatrists, are well prepared as a result of their education and training. Other providers (nurses, physical therapists, physician assistants) require additional didactic and skills lab training followed by hands-on preceptorship before performing sharp debridement. Even if the training is part of the educational curriculum, validation of skills and competencies according to facility procedure is required, and evidence of completion of such training should be maintained in the clinician's employee file.[22]

The patient must be adequately prepared for sharp/surgical debridement. Informed consent is required for surgical/excisional debridement. The facility or agency protocol dictates consent policies, and the clinician should carefully adhere to these policies. Prior to sharp/surgical debridement, the wound site is prepared by adequate cleansing to remove exudate, residue, and any loose debris that may have accumulated

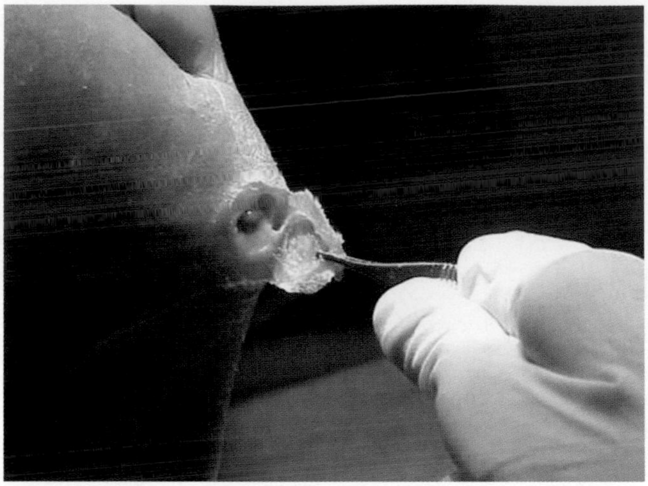

FIGURE 13-38 Callus debridement. Removal of callus from a plantar metatarsal head. Note the wound under the debrided callus.

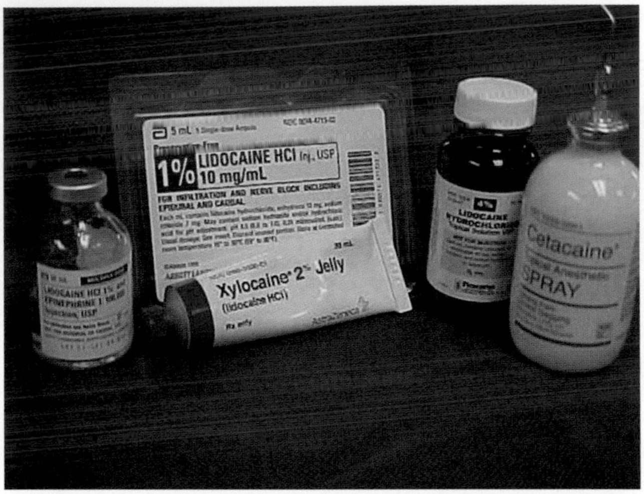

FIGURE 13-39 Examples of analgesics. Topical analgesics are used to decrease pain during debridement of sensitive wounds. A thin layer is applied to the wound bed and edges and allowed to sit for 10–15 minutes before beginning the procedure. Two percent Lidocaine sprays are now available without a prescription.

since the previous dressing change. This is a necessary step to avoid contamination of the wound bed with the flora present on periwound skin. Additionally, wound cleansing should be performed after debridement to remove any devitalized material that may remain on the wound surface as part of infection control practices.

Adequate pain management both during and after the procedure is essential for patient-centered care.[13,22,64] Although devitalized tissue is devoid of sensation, the actual procedure may induce discomfort of various degrees especially if the wound/periwound tissue is inflamed. Preprocedure instructions include advising the patient to inform the practitioner when they feel discomfort, thus giving the patient a sense of control during the debridement process. Debridement is stopped as soon as the patient expresses unacceptable discomfort. This level varies greatly among patients, and strategies for pain management are individualized. Premedication can help reduce the patient's anxiety and minimize discomfort related to cleansing, preparing the wound for debridement, and performing the debridement procedure. Oral or intravenous medications can be prescribed by the physician and administered by the nurse in an inpatient setting. Additionally, topical or local anesthetics (**FIGURE 13-39**) may be employed after adequate cleansing to reduce or eliminate procedural pain in sensate tissues. Finally, there should be a plan for adequate pain management once the procedure is completed.

The decision to perform surgical debridement in the operating room is based largely on the extent and depth of the required debridement and the need to accomplish the procedure under controlled conditions (eg, due to pain, bleeding, sepsis). Other factors may include the following:

- The need for emergent procedures such as in the case of infected wounds or patient sepsis
- The need for a higher degree of asepsis, such as the potential exposure of tendon, bone, or joints
- The need for extensive bone debridement
- The need for adequate anesthesia
- The presence of extensive undermining, sinus tracts, or tunneling
- The potential for excessive bleeding
- The patient's anxiety or stress related to the procedure[22]

In addition to the use of instruments, the operating room provides an environment for the use of devices that accomplish debridement into deeper tissues more rapidly than with instruments, including the use of the high-powered waterjet, as well as electrocautery equipment in the case of excessive bleeding.

Hydrosurgical Debridement

The high-powered parallel waterjet (Versajet, Smith Nephew, Largo, FL), a device for performing surgical debridement, precisely removes nonviable tissue using a high-energy water stream. It is used only by a skilled surgeon in an operating room environment (**FIGURES 13-40** and **13-41**). The waterjet is a Food and Drug Administration–approved medical device that can focus a high-powered stream of water into a high-energy cutting implement. The saline used in the waterjet is enclosed in a sterile circuit that passes through a small but powerful pump. This cutting action provides the surgeon precise control over the wound surface.[65,66]

This form of surgical debridement is reported to be less effective in pressure ulcers that are covered with dry eschar.[66] The preferred strategy is to remove the eschar by sharp debridement and follow with the use of waterjet to debride the underlying necrotic tissue. Consequently, all of the necrotic tissue, fibrinous debris, and unhealthy tissue can be removed

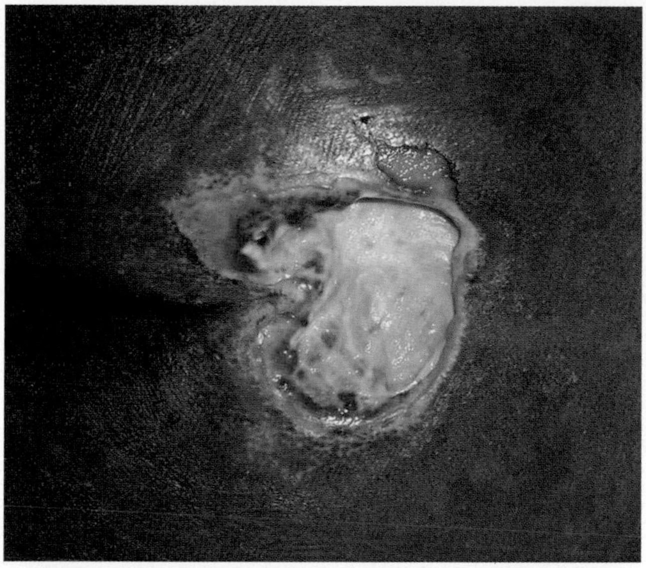

FIGURE 13-40 Hydrosurgical debridement. Wound with a large amount of slough is appropriate to be debrided with Versajet. (Used with permission from Greg Patterson, MD, FACS, CWS, FASA.)

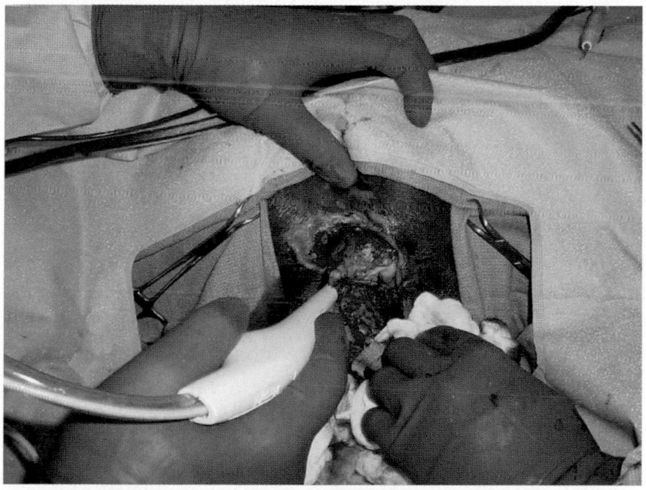

FIGURE 13-41 Clean, healthy wound bed after debridement with Versajet. (Used with permission from Greg Patterson, MD, FACS, CWS, FASA.)

with no injury to the healthy underlying collateral tissue.[66] Surgeons can perform more aggressive wound debridement while simultaneously removing less surrounding healthy tissue.[65,66]

Bleeding in Mechanical and Sharp/Surgical Debridement

Bleeding is always a possibility as a result of debridement by mechanical means or with the use of instruments. Small amounts of punctate bleeding are expected and easily controlled with either time or gentle pressure. If bleeding continues, the site is elevated and firm pressure is applied to the wound with gauze or a gloved finger for 5–10 minutes *without lifting the gauze to look because this may dislodge the clot and cause more bleeding to occur*. If there is one small site of bleeding, using a sterile applicator to apply direct pressure at the specific location may be effective. If bleeding continues, hemostatic agents may be applied, including calcium alginates, silver nitrate, dressings containing chitosan, or thrombin agents such as Gelfoam (Pfizer, Inc., New York, NY), Surgicel (Ethicon, Inc., Somerville, NJ), or QuikClot (Z-Medica Corporation, Wallingford, CT). If bleeding does not stop with the methods above, the physician should be notified for further intervention such as sutures or electrocautery.[3,22] If the bleeding is pulsatile, indicating that it is coming from an artery, a physician should be called immediately as only suturing will halt arterial bleeding. Pressure is maintained while waiting for the sutures to be applied.

> **CLINICAL CONSIDERATION**
> Bleeding is always a concern when performing sharp or surgical debridement and is managed by having a hemostatic agent readily available during the procedure.

Checking the patient's medication list prior to debriding is imperative. Often people needing debridement are on anticoagulant therapy, which causes longer clotting times, thereby creating potential for excessive bleeding with sharp/surgical or mechanical debridement. Low platelets can also cause excessive bleeding, therefore checking lab values is an integral part of the predebridement assessment especially in the acute care setting. Conservative types of debridement are preferred for these patients. If large amounts of tissue need to be removed, surgical debridement by a physician in the operating room is advised.

Maggot Debridement Therapy

Maggot debridement therapy (MDT) (also known as larval therapy, biotherapy, biosurgery, and biodebridement) is the purposeful use of maggots in wound care (**FIGURE 13-42**).[67,68]

The benefits of maggot therapy have been documented as far back as the 16th century.[3,67] Military surgeons noted that soldiers whose wounds became infested with maggots had a much lower mortality rate and exhibited cleaner, faster-healing wounds than did soldiers with similar wounds that were not infested. During the late 1920s, William Baer, an orthopedic surgeon at Johns Hopkins University, began to systematically treat, study, and publish case studies of patients using MDT.[67] Weil et al.[68] suggested using the term *larval therapy* in 1933, and up to 1936, there was a massive growth in popularity. With the introduction of penicillin in the 1940s, larval therapy was relegated to the archives of "old-fashioned" treatments.[67] In the 1980s, Sherman[69,70] began to reintroduce larval therapy following his research in the treatment of pressure ulcers, and later, Dumville et al.[71] reported use with chronic venous ulcers on the lower extremity. The rationale, application, and benefits reported were no different than those of Baer 64 years earlier. The positive results sparked a new wave of interest in

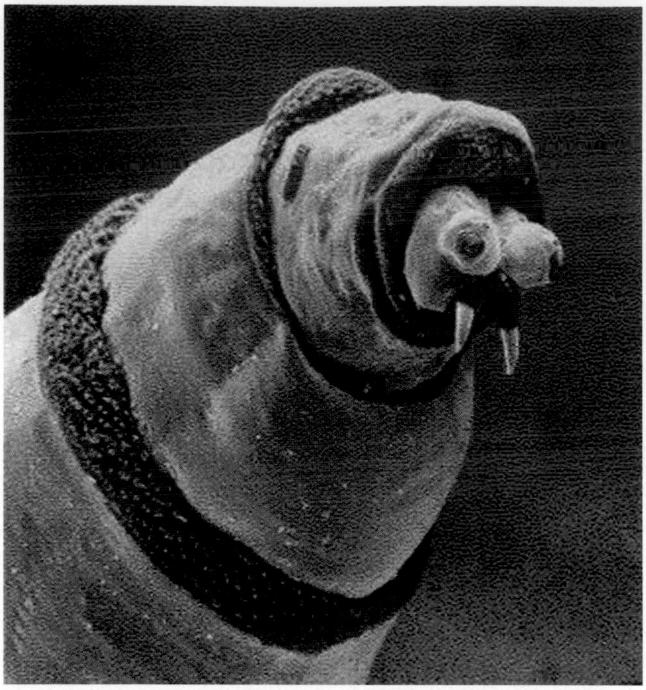

FIGURE 13-42 Maggot used for debridement. Photo of maggot under color scanning electron micrograph (SEM). Maggots feed on necrotic tissue only creating a debridement effect and have antibacterial chemicals in their saliva and excrement to help fight infection.

this historical treatment, and a surge in research followed. By the mid-1990s, there were reports of approximately 60 centers in the United Kingdom using maggots to treat intractable wounds. Larvae were being used to treat hard-to-heal necrotic wounds with significant slough that were not responsive to conventional treatment such as hydrogel dressings and surgical debridement.[72] A resurgence of maggot therapy has occurred in recent years, as more widespread acceptance among the medical community, as well as patients, has occurred.

Maggots have three proposed actions: debridement of necrotic tissue, antimicrobial activity, and facilitation of wound healing. They are indicated for debriding nonhealing necrotic skin and soft tissue wounds including pressure ulcers, chronic venous insufficiency ulcers, neuropathic foot ulcers, and nonhealing traumatic or postsurgical wounds.[69–76] Maggots selectively debride by feeding on the necrotic tissue, cellular debris, and exudate in wounds. The maggot secretes trypsin-like collagenases and chymotrypsin-like enzymes, which lyse the necrotic tissue into a semiliquid form that the creatures can ingest.[77]

CLINICAL CONSIDERATION

Maggots have been used successfully to debride:

- Pressure ulcers[69,70]
- Venous insufficiency ulcers[71]
- Diabetic foot ulcers[72,73]
- Infections including necrotizing soft tissue infections[74–76]

Maggots use a pair of mandibles or hooks to attach to tissue and provide locomotion. The maggot also uses these hooks during feeding to disrupt membranes and thus facilitate the penetration of its proteolytic enzymes.[67] Additional debridement may be facilitated by the maggots crawling about within the wound, dislodging small amounts of necrotic material.

The ability of maggots to kill or prevent the growth of potentially pathogenic bacteria has been the subject of a number of studies. Marked antimicrobial activity has been detected against *Streptococcus* A and B and *Staphylococcus aureus*, with some activity detected against *Pseudomonas* and a clinical isolate of a resistant strain of *S. aureus* (MRSA).[74,76]

Growth of granulation tissue has been reported to be faster with better wound healing rates using maggot therapy. One study suggests that a possible mode of action for facilitating wound healing is the increase in tissue oxygenation that takes place when using MDT.[78]

In 2004, the United States Food and Drug Administration approved the production and marketing of medical grade maggots in the United States as a medical device. The technique for application and use of MDT is not difficult but is specific; there are two methods of delivery of the larvae to the wound bed. In the original method, the wound bed is cleansed and prepared, and the surrounding skin is dried thoroughly and protected with a skin barrier wipe. A combination dressing supplied by the manufacturer to secure and trap the larvae may be used or the clinician may create an appropriate dressing. The wound is "picture framed" by building one or two layers of hydrocolloid or pectin skin barrier strips along the wound edges. Commonly, practitioners also apply skin contact cement to the edges. The maggots are applied to the wound with five to eight maggots per square centimeter of wound surface area. A closed-mesh or veil dressing is applied and adhered to the cement-edged barrier, thus preventing migration of the maggots outside of the wound area. The wound is further covered with an absorbent dressing to adequately manage the increased exudate that generally accumulates. The dressing is left in place for 48–72 hours and the maggots are removed as they become satiated and move to the surface of the dressing. A newer delivery system utilizes a "bagged" system where the larvae are delivered to the wound bed in a sealed bag sized appropriately to the wound, and if needed using more than one bag. The activity and mechanism of action of the maggots are unchanged; however, the ease of use is enhanced by one-step application and removal. One or two cycles of MDT are applied each week. The total duration of treatment depends on the size and character of the wound, the clinical response, and the goals of therapy. Instrument debridement of thick, dry eschar or tough, fibrous tissue prior to initiation of MDT hastens the effect and shortens the treatment time (**FIGURES 13-43** to **13-48**).

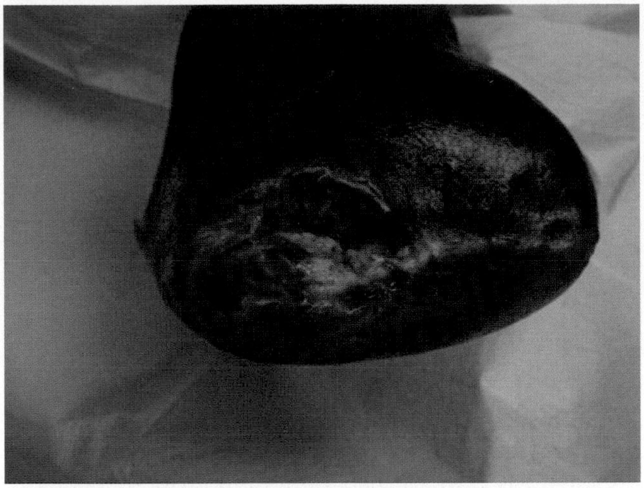

FIGURE 13-43 Maggot debridement therapy: clinical series. Dehisced transmetatarsal amputation before treatment with maggot therapy to debride the necrotic tissue.

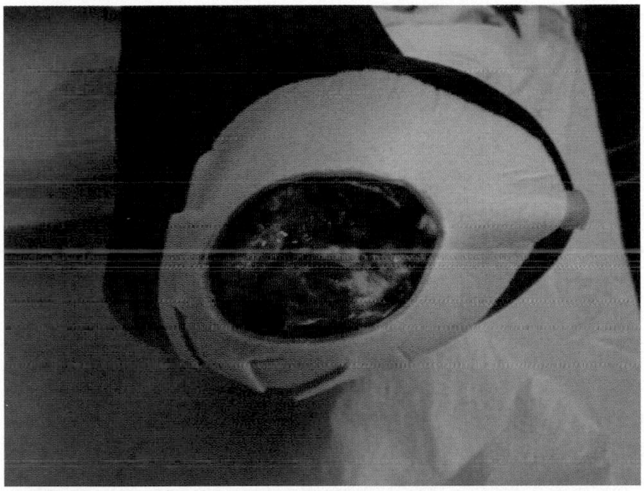

FIGURE 13-44 Step 1. A barrier and "trough" made from hydrocolloid and hydrocolloid paste, onto which skin cement will be painted.

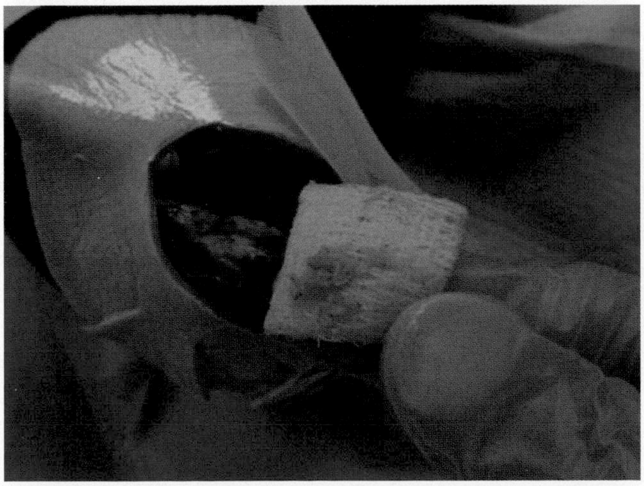

FIGURE 13-45 Step 2. Wound veil preattached to barrier at the top, disinfected larvae applied using gauze containing nutrient that is included in the package with the larvae.

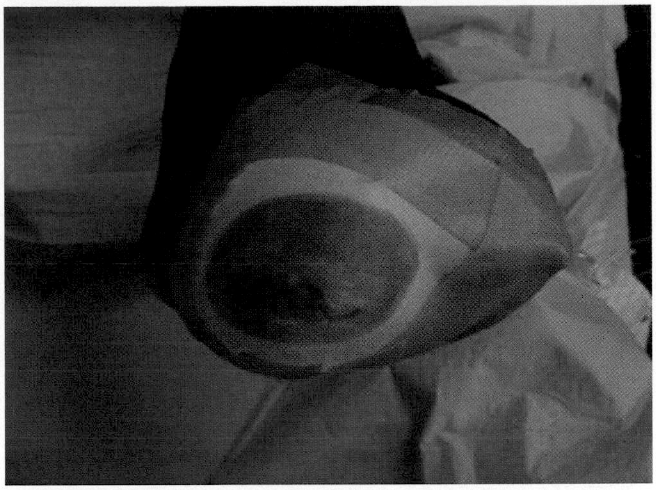

FIGURE 13-46 Step 3. Larvae in place with veil attached to the hydrocolloid barrier and reinforced with waterproof tape.

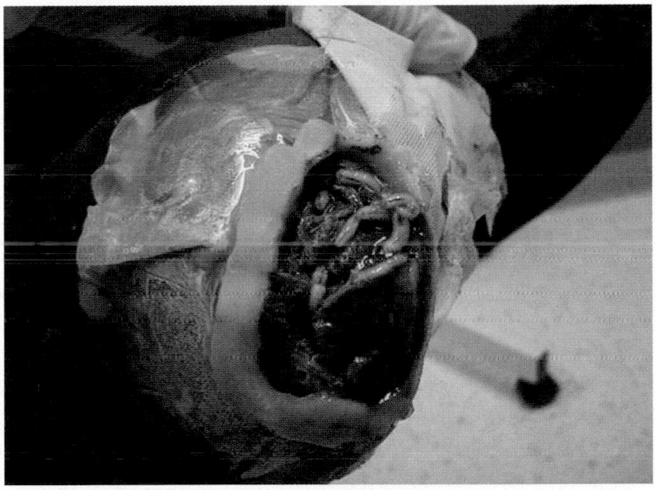

FIGURE 13-47 Veil removed after 4–5 days of therapy to expose maggots. Note the visible change in size after ingestion of necrotic debris.

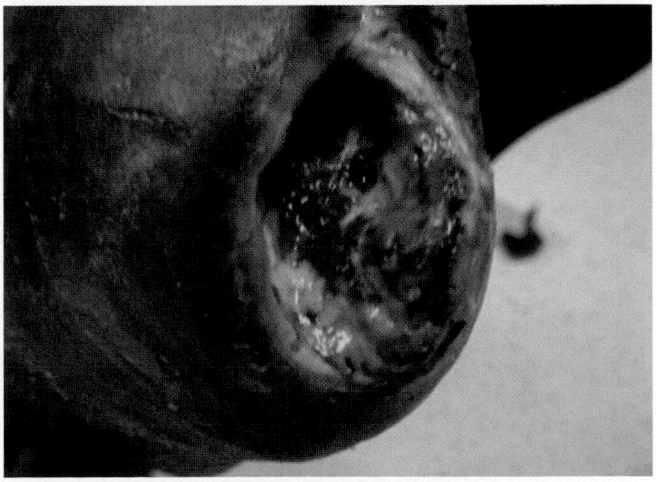

FIGURE 13-48 Wound after cleansing of slough and debris.

CASE STUDY

CONCLUSION

A topical anesthetic gel was applied for pain management, and debridement was attempted with a curette. The patient was unable to tolerate the instrument debridement due to pain assessed as severe. Contact LFUS was initiated and 50% of the nonviable tissue was removed. The ulcer was then assessed as a Stage 3 (FIGURE 13-49). The patient began to get very anxious and agitated, both indications to terminate this treatment session. Collagenase ointment was ordered for the nursing staff to apply daily and cover with a foam dressing. The patient returned to the long-term care facility with an appointment to return to clinic in 1 week. Because of the patient's anxiety disorder, the goal was to get the wound debrided as quickly as possible and reduce the frequency of visits to the wound center.

Goals:

1. Wound will be debrided of all necrotic tissue and progress to the proliferative phase of wound healing.
2. Patient pain levels will be less than 4 on the Faces Pain Scale.
3. The nursing staff will be consistent in repositioning patient in both supine and sitting positions.

Second visit (after 1 week of treatment)

At the time of the second visit 1 week later, the wound measured 3.1 cm × 1.6 cm × 0.1 cm. Scattered slough and fibrinous debris remained on the wound surface. A topical anesthetic was applied for 15 minutes, a curette was used to release the edges of the wound, which were beginning to roll with epibole; however, the patient complained of pain and became agitated, thus the debridement process was stopped. Orders were written for the nursing staff to continue the collagenase ointment, and an appointment was made for 1 week later.

DISCUSSION QUESTIONS

1. Describe the tissue, edges, and periwound skin in FIGURE 13-50.
2. What is the wound healing phase?
3. What is the wound stage (based on the information provided in Chapter 6, Pressure Injuries and Ulcers)?

Third visit (after 2 weeks of treatment)

The wound is now cleaner as the enzymatic debriding agent continues to lyse and clean the wound bed. The patient tolerates the cleansing and reassessment with no complaints of pain. The wound now measures 2.7 cm × 1.1 cm × 0.1 cm. The nursing staff is to continue the same plan of care. Goals are revised to full closure by secondary intention. The nursing staff is to continue repositioning and monitoring of nutritional status to ensure no recurrence.

DISCUSSION QUESTIONS

1. Describe the tissue, edges, and periwound skin in FIGURE 13-51.
2. What phase of wound healing is evident?

Fourth visit (after 3 weeks of treatment) (FIGURE 13-52)

The wound has made excellent progress in the last week presenting with a small open area, mostly covered with newly formed epithelium. Scant drainage is noted on the dressing after removal and the patient expresses no pain during the treatment session. A foam dressing is ordered for protection

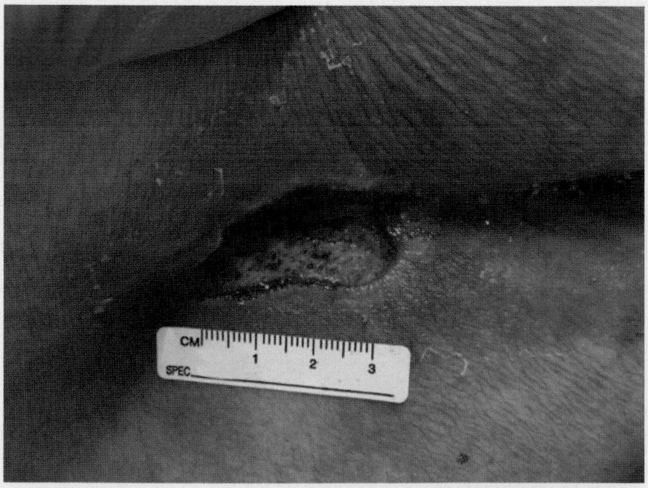

FIGURE 13-49 Case study wound on the first visit after debridement with contact, low-frequency ultrasound.

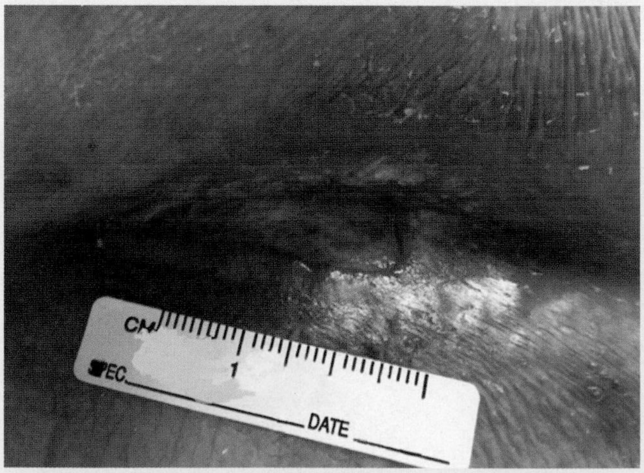

FIGURE 13-50 Presentation of the wound at the time of the second visit, after removal of the dressing and before treatment was attempted. Debridement was aborted due to patient complaint of pain and increasing agitation.

CASE STUDY (Continued)

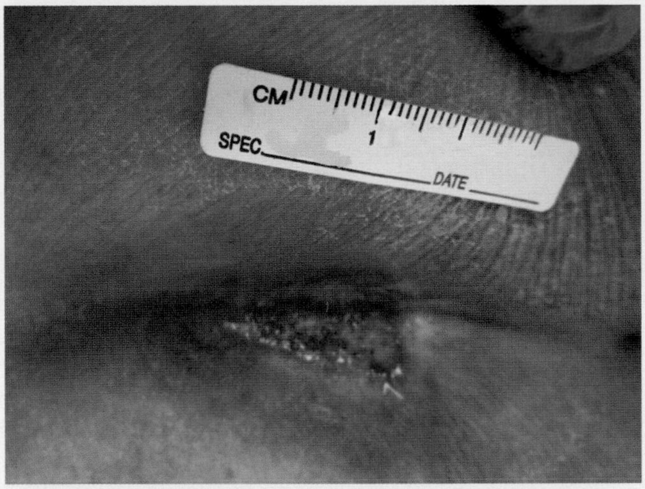

FIGURE 13-51 Presentation of the wound after 2 weeks of treatment with enzymatic debridement.

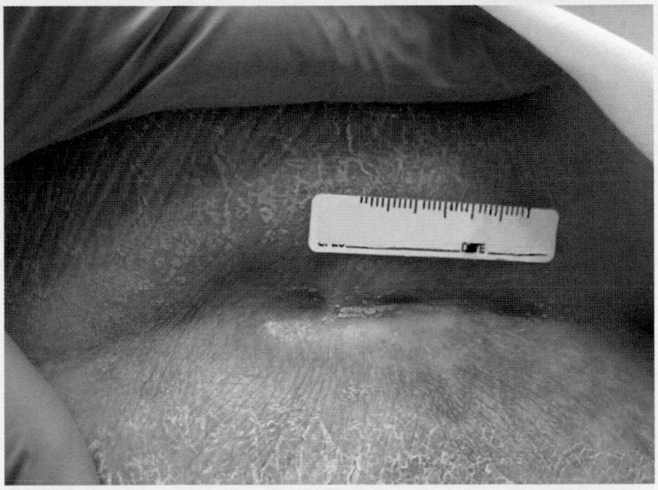

FIGURE 13-53 At the time of the fifth visit, the newly closed wound has fragile epithelial tissue and is in the remodeling phase of healing.

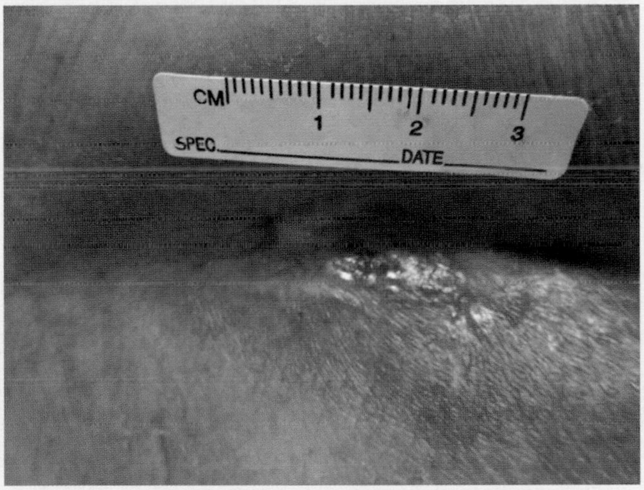

FIGURE 13-52 At the time of the fourth visit, the wound is covered with new epithelial tissue.

from friction and incontinence moisture. The patient is scheduled to return for a final assessment in 1 month.

Fifth visit (after 4 weeks of treatment)

At the time of the final visit, the wound is fully re-epithelialized. Nursing staff will continue to provide pressure redistribution in both sitting and supine positions and will cover the new fragile epithelial tissue with a foam dressing for protection from incontinence and friction. The patient will return to the clinic only if needed.

DISCUSSION QUESTIONS

1. What phase of healing is used to describe the wound in FIGURE 13-53?
2. What is the wound stage (using NPIAP Staging guidelines)?
3. Were all of the goals met?

SUMMARY

Effective wound debridement is paramount to achieving adequate wound bed preparation leading to wound closure and subsequent healing, and has become a standard of care among wound care practitioners. Once the decision to debride is made, selection of the preferred method depends on the overall goals of therapy, the urgency of need, the setting in which the care is being provided, the availability of the debridement modalities, and the skill level of the care providers. Adequate wound debridement is essential to the realization of successful outcomes in the management of hard-to-heal wounds, and creating a clean wound environment free of necrotic tissue is essential prior to using modern, advanced wound therapies such as collagen dressings, growth factors, and cellular, acellular and matrix-like products (CAMPS).[79]

STUDY QUESTIONS

1. Which class of medications requires that extreme caution be used when debriding with sharp instruments or mechanical techniques?
   a. β-blockers
   b. Corticosteroids
   c. Anticoagulants
   d. Antipsychotics

2. Which of the following is a contraindication for sharp debridement?
   a. Diabetic foot ulcers
   b. Pressure ulcers
   c. Venous insufficiency
   d. Severe arterial insufficiency
3. Autolytic debridement is
   a. The application of a topical pharmaceutical preparation that is specifically designed to target and break down the devitalized collagen.
   b. Use of an outside force or energy directly to the wound surface to remove necrotic tissue.
   c. The process by which the body's endogenous enzymes loosen and liquefy necrotic tissue.
   d. The use of maggots to digest and debride necrotic tissue.
4. Which of the following procedures is a method of nonselective debridement?
   a. Wet-to-dry debridement
   b. Sharp debridement
   c. Enzymatic debridement
   d. Autolytic debridement
5. Which of the following debridement techniques is an absolute contraindication for removing necrotic tissue in a venous insufficiency leg ulcer?
   a. Autolytic debridement
   b. Whirlpool
   c. Enzymatic debridement
   d. Low-frequency ultrasound
6. Which group of patients is more inclined to have difficulty with autolytic debridement, often requiring more aggressive forms of debridement to clean the wound bed of necrotic tissue?
   a. Older adults
   b. Children
   c. Immobilized patients
   d. Patients who smoke
7. Maggot debridement proposed actions include all of the following except
   a. Debridement of necrotic tissue.
   b. Antimicrobial activity.
   c. Facilitation of wound healing.
   d. Improved arterial blood flow.
8. Which of the following is not required in order to perform any type of debridement safely?
   a. Thorough knowledge of anatomy
   b. Knowledge of the patient's financial status
   c. An accurate diagnosis of the wound etiology
   d. Technical skills and clinical judgment for debridement
9. Hypergranulation tissue is defined as
   a. An overabundance of granulation tissue, resulting in the extension of this tissue above the level of the skin.
   b. Dried secretions, exudates, and dead cells covering a wound.
   c. Rolled upper edges of the epidermis that envelop the basement membrane or lower edges of the epidermis, thus preventing epithelial migration at wound edges.
   d. Pink/red and moist tissue that is composed of new blood vessels, connective tissue, fibroblasts, and inflammatory cells.
10. Which of the following types of tissue should not be debrided or have some intervention to decrease its negative impact on the wound?
   a. Slough
   b. Eschar
   c. Hypergranulation tissue
   d. Granulation tissue

Answers: 1-c; 2-d; 3-c; 4-a; 5-b; 6-a; 7-d; 8-b; 9-a; 10-d

REFERENCES

1. Murphy C, Atkin L, Swanson T, et al. International consensus document. Defying hard-to-heal wounds with an early antibiofilm intervention strategy: wound hygiene. *J Wound Care* 2020; 29(Suppl 3b):S1-28.
2. European Wound Management Association (EWMA). Position Document. Debridement. London: MEP Ltd. Available at: https://ewma.org/fileadmin/user_upload/EWMA.org/Project_Portfolio/EWMA_Documents/EWMA_Debridement_Document_JWCfinal.pdf. Accessed April 16, 2023.
3. Albaugh K, Loehne H. Wound bed preparation/debridement. In: McCulloch JM, Kloth LC, eds. *Wound Healing: Evidence-Based Management*. 4th ed. Philadelphia, PA: FA Davis Co; 2010:155-179.
4. Enoch S, Harding K. Wound bed preparation: the science behind the removal of barriers to healing. *Wounds*. 2003;15(7):213-229.
5. Myers B. Debridement. In: Myers B, ed. *Wound Management: Principles and Practice*. Upper Saddle River, NJ: Prentice Hall; 2004:65-87.
6. Ramundo JM. Wound debridement. In: Bryant RA, Nix DP, eds. *Acute and Chronic Wounds: Current Management Concepts*. 4th ed. St Louis, MO: Mosby Elsevier; 2012:270-288.
7. Calianno C, Jakubek P. Wound bed preparation: laying the foundation for treating chronic wounds, part 1. *Nursing*. 2006; 36(2):70-71.
8. Ayello EA, Dowsett C, Schultz GS, et al. TIME heals all wounds. *Nursing*. 2006;34(4):36-42.
9. Sibbald GR, Williamson D, Orsted HL, et al. Preparing the wound bed—debridement, bacterial balance and moisture balance. *Ostomy Wound Manage*. 2000;46:14-35.
10. Falanga V. Classifications for wound bed preparation and stimulation of chronic wounds. *Wound Repair Regen*. 2000;8(5):347-352.
11. Sibbald RG, Orsted H, Schultz G, et al. Preparing the wound bed 2003: focus on infection and inflammation. *Ostomy Wound Manage*. 2003;49(11):24-51.
12. Sibbald RG, Orsted HL, Coutts PM, et al. Best practice recommendations for preparing the wound bed: update 2006. *Adv Skin Wound Care*. 2007;20:390-405.
13. Sibbald RG, Goodman L, Woo KY. Special considerations in wound bed preparation 2011: an update. *Adv Skin Wound Care*. 2011;24(9): 415-436.
14. National Pressure Injury Advisory Panel, European Pressure Ulcer Advisory Panel, and Pan Pacific Pressure Injury Alliance. *Prevention and Treatment of Pressure Ulcers/Injuries: Clinical Practice Guideline. The International Guideline*. Washington, DC: National Pressure Injury Advisory Panel; 2019.
15. Luo S, Yufit T, Carson P. Differential keratin expression during epiboly in a wound model of bioengineered skin and in human chronic wounds. *Int J Low Extrem Wounds*. Available at: https://doi.org/10.1177/1534734611418157. Accessed April 16, 2023.

16. Falanga V. Wound bed preparation and the role of enzymes: a case for multiple actions of therapeutic agents. *Wounds*. 2002;14(2):47-57.
17. Steed DL, Donohoe D, Webster MW, Lindsley L, Diabetic Ulcer Study Group. Effect of extensive debridement and treatment on the healing of diabetic foot ulcers. *J Am Coll Surg*. 1996;183:61-64.
18. Ayello EA, Cuddigan JE. Debridement: controlling the necrotic/cellular burden. *Adv Skin Wound Care*. 2004;17(2):66-75.
19. Haesler E, Swanson T, Ousey K, et al. Establishing a consensus on wound infection definitions. *J Wound Care*. 2022;31(Suppl 12):S48-S59.
20. Myers BA. *Wound Management: Principles and Practice*. 3rd ed. Upper Saddle River, NJ: Pearson Education, Inc; 2012:114-149.
21. Barbe M, Batra A, Golding S, et al. Pyoderma gangrenosum: a literature review. *Clin Podiatr Med Surg*. 2021;38(4):577-588.
22. Weir D, Scarborough P, Niezgoda JA. Wound debridement. In: Krasner DL, Rodeheaver GT, Sibbald GR, eds. *Chronic Wound Care: A Clinical Sourcebook for Healthcare Professionals*. 4th ed. Malvern, PA: HMP Communications; 2007:343-355.
23. Sussman C, Bates-Jensen B. *Wound Care: A Collaborative Practice Manual for Health Professionals*. 4th ed. Philadelphia, PA: Lippincott, Williams and Wilkins; 2012:17-52, 96.
24. Vuolo J. Hypergranulation: exploring possible management options. *Br J Nurs*. 2010;19(6):s4-s8.
25. Young T. Common problems in wound care: overgranulation. *Br J Nurs*. 1995;4(3):169-170.
26. Romundo J, Gran M. Enzymatic wound debridement. *J Wound Ostomy Continence Nurs*. 2008;35(3):273-280.
27. Percival SL, Mayer D, Malone M, Swanson T, Schultz G. Surfactants and their role in wound cleansing and biofilm management. *J Wound Care*. 2017;26(11):680-690.
28. Percival SL, Mayer D, Salisbury AM. Efficacy of a surfactant-based wound dressing on a biofilm control. *Wound Repair Regen*. 2017;25(5):767-773.
29. Palumbo FP, Harding KG, Abbritti F. New surfactant-based dressing product to improve wound closure rates of non-healing wounds: a multicentre study including 1036 patients. *Wounds*. 2016;28(7):233-240.
30. Yang Q, Larose C, Porta AD, Schultz GS, Gibson DJ. A surfactant-based wound dressing can reduce bacterial biofilm in a porcine skin explant model. *Int Wound J*. 2017;14(2):408-413.
31. Yang Y, Schultz GS, Gibson DJ. A surfactant-based dressing to treat and prevent *Acinetobacter baumannii* biofilms. *J Burn Care Res*. 2018;39(5):766-770.
32. Maskarinec SA, Wu G, Lee KY. Membrane sealing by polymers. *Ann N Y Acad Sci*. 2005;1066:310-320.
33. Wu G, Majewski J, Ege C, Kjaer K, Weygand MJ, Lee KY. Lipid corralling and poloxamer squeeze-out in membranes. *Phys Rev Lett*. 2004;93(2):028101.
34. Mayer D, Armstrong D, Schltz G, et al. Cell salvage in acute and chronic wounds: a potential treatment strategy. Experimental data and early clinical results. *J Wound Care*. 2018;27(9):594-605.
35. Weigelt MA, McNamara SA, Sanchez D, Hirt PA, Kirsner RS. Evidence-based review of antibiofilm agents for wound care. *Adv Wound Care (New Rochelle)*. 2021;10(1):13-23.
36. Percival SL, Mayer D, Kirsner RS, et al. Surfactants: role in biofilm management and cellular behaviour. *Int Wound J*. 2019;16(3):753-760.
37. Smith J, Thow J. Update of systematic review of debridement-wound care. *Diabetic Foot*. 2003;6:12-16.
38. Sussman C, Bates-Jensen B. *Wound Care: A Collaborative Practice Manual for Health Professionals*. 4th ed. Philadelphia, PA: Lippincott, Williams and Wilkins; 2011:17-433, 456,754.
39. https://santyl.com/hcp. Accessed April 16, 2023.
40. Gibson D, Cullen B, Legerstee R, Harding KG, Schultz G. MMPs made easy. *Wounds Int*. 2009;1(1). Available at: http://www.woundsinternational.com. Accessed April 13, 2013.
41. Jovanovic A, Ermis R, Mewaldt R, Shi L, Carson D. The influence of metal salts, surfactants, and wound care products on enzymatic activity of collagenase, the wound debriding enzyme. *Wounds*. 2012; 24(9):242-253.
42. Shi L, Ermis R, Garcia A, Telgenhoff D, Aust D. Degradation of human collagen isoforms by clostridium collagenase and the effects of degradation products on cell migration. *Int Wound J*. 2010;7(2):87-95.
43. Sheets AR, Demidova-Rice TN, Shi L, Ronfard V, Grover KV, Herman IM. Identification and characterization of novel matrix-derived bioactive peptides: a role for collagenase from Santyl® ointment in post-debridement wound healing? *PLoS One*. 2016; 11(7):e0159598.
44. https://santyl.com/hcp/compatibility. Accessed April 16, 2023.
45. Milne CT, Ciccarelli AO, Lassy M. A comparison of collagenase to hydrogel dressings in wound debridement. *Wounds*. 2010;22:270-274.
46. Pavan R, Jain S, Shraddha KA. Properties and therapeutic application of bromelain: a review. *Biotechnol Res Int*. 2012;2012:976203.
47. Pertea M, Poroch V, Ciobanu P, et al. Efficiency of Bromelain-enriched enzyme mixture (nexobrid™) in the treatment of burn wounds. *Appl Sci*. 2021;11(17):8134.
48. Shoham Y, Krieger Y, Tamir E, et al. Bromelain-based enzymatic debridement of chronic wounds: a preliminary report. *Int Wound J*. 2018;15(5):769-775.
49. Snyder RJ, Dove C, Driver V. Introducing bromelain-based enzymatic debridement. *Podiatry Management*, November/December 2022.
50. Hanz T, Butler I, Luttrell T. The role of whirlpool in wound care. *J Am Coll Clin Wound Spec*. 2013;4(1):7-12.
51. McCulloch JM, Boyd VB. The effects of whirlpool and the dependent position on lower extremity volume. *J Orthop Sports Phys Ther*. 1992; 16(4):169-173.
52. American Diabetes Association. *Consensus Development Conference on Diabetic Foot Wound Care*. Boston, MA: American Diabetes Association; 1999:7-8.
53. Armstrong MH, Price P. Wet-to-dry gauze dressings: fact and fiction. *Wounds*. 2004;16(2):56-62.
54. Ovington LG. Hanging wet-to-dry dressings out to dry. *Home Healthc Nurse*. 2001;19(8):28-34.
55. Cowan LJ, Stechmiller J. Prevalence of wet-to-dry dressings in wound care. *Adv Skin Wound Care*. 2009;22:567-573.
56. Stanisic MM, Provo BJ, Larson DL, Kloth LC. Wound debridement with 25 kHz ultrasound. *Adv Skin Wound Care*. 2005;18:484-490.
57. Voigt J, Wendelken M, Driver V, Alvarez O. Low-frequency ultrasound (20-40 kHz) as an adjunctive therapy for chronic wound healing: a systematic review of the literature and meta-analysis of eight randomized controlled trials. *Int J Low Extrem Wounds*. 2011;10(4):190-199.
58. Altland OD, Dalecki D, Suchkova VN, Francis CW. Low-intensity ultrasound increases endothelial cell nitric oxide synthase activity and nitric oxide synthesis. *J Thromb Haemost*. 2004;2:637-643.
59. Suchkova VN, Baggs RB, Sahni SK, Francis CW. Ultrasound improves tissue perfusion in ischemic tissue through a nitric oxide dependent mechanism. *Thromb Haemost*. 2002;88:865-870.
60. Chen, H, Yu, Z, Liu, N, et al. The efficacy of low-frequency ultrasound as an added treatment for chronic wounds: a meta-analysis. *Int Wound J*. 2023;20(2):448-457.
61. Pierson T, Niezgoda JA, Learmonth S, Blunt D, McNabb K. Effects of low frequency ultrasound applied in vitro to highly antibiotic

resistant *Acinetobacter* isolates recovered from soldiers returning from Iraq. Presented at the 18th Annual Symposium on Advanced Wound Care, San Diego, CA, April 21–24, 2005.

62. Breuing KH, Bayer L, Neuwalder J, Arch M, Orgill DP. Early experience using low frequency ultrasound in chronic wounds. *Ann Plast Surg*. 2005;55:183-187.
63. Ennis WJ, Foremann P, Mozen N, Massey J, Conner-Kerr T, Meneses P. Ultrasound therapy for recalcitrant diabetic foot ulcers: results of a randomized, double-blind, controlled, multi-center study. MIST Ultrasound Diabetic Study Group. *Ostomy Wound Manage*. 2005;51:24-39.
64. Baranoski S, Ayello EA. *Wound Care Essentials: Practice Principles*. 3rd ed. Philadelphia, PA: Wolters Kluwer/Lippincott Williams & Wilkins; 2012:295-321.
65. Granick MS, Jacoby M, Noruthrun S, Datiashvili RO, Ganchi PA. Clinical and economic impact of hydrosurgical debridement on chronic wounds. *Wounds*. 2006;18(2):35-39.
66. Mosti G, Mattaliano V. The debridement of chronic leg ulcers by means of a new, fluidjet-based device. *Wounds*. 2006;18(8):227-237.
67. Sherman RA. Maggot debridement in modern medicine. *Infect Med*. 1998;15:651-656.
68. Weil GC, Simon RJ, Sweadner WR. A biological, bacteriological and clinical study of larval or maggot therapy in the treatment of acute and chronic pyogenic infections. *Am J Surg*. 1933;19:36-48.
69. Sherman RA. Maggot versus conservative debridement therapy for the treatment of pressure ulcers. *Wound Repair Regen*. 2002;10:208-214.
70. Sherman RA, Wyle FA, Vulpe M. Maggot debridement therapy for treating pressure ulcers in spinal cord injury patients. *J Spinal Cord Med*. 1995;18:71-74.
71. Dumville JC, Worthy G, Bland JM, et al. Larval therapy for leg ulcers (VenUS II): randomised controlled trial. *BMJ*. 2009;338:b773.
72. Knowles A, Findlow A, Jackson N. Management of a diabetic foot ulcer using larval therapy. *Nurs Stand*. 2001;16(6):73-76.
73. Sherman RA. Maggot therapy for treating diabetic foot ulcers unresponsive to conventional therapy. *Diabetes Care*. 2003;26:446-451.
74. Thomas S, Andrews AM, Hay NP, Bourgoise S. The anti-microbial activity of maggot secretions: results of a preliminary study. *J Tissue Viability*. 1999;9:127-132.
75. Dunn C, Raghavan U, Pfleiderer AG. The use of maggots in head and neck necrotizing fasciitis. *J Laryngol Otol*. 2002;116(1):70-72.
76. Nigam Y, Bexfield A, Thomas S, et al. Maggot therapy: the science and implications for CAM-history and bacterial resistance. *Evid Based Complement Alternat Med*. 2006;3(pt 1):223-227.
77. Armstrong DG, Mossel J, Short B, et al. Maggot debridement therapy: a primer. *J Am Podiatr Med Assoc*. 2002;92:398-401.
78. Wollina U, Liebold K, Schmidt WD, Hartmann M, Fassler D. Biosurgery supports granulation and debridement in chronic wounds—clinical data and remittance spectroscopy measurement. *Int J Dermatol*. 2002;41:635-639.
79. Wu S, Carter M, Cole W et al. Best practice for wound repair and regeneration: use of cellular, acellular and matrix-like products (CAMPs). *J Wound Care*. 2023;32(4 Suppl B):S1-S32.

CHAPTER FOURTEEN

Wound Dressings

Dot Weir, RN, CWON, CWS

CHAPTER OBJECTIVES

At the end of this chapter, the learner will be able to:

1. **Define the function of primary and secondary dressings.**
2. **Describe the role of dressings in moist wound healing.**
3. **Select the appropriate primary dressing based on wound characteristics.**
4. **Select the appropriate secondary dressing based on patient function.**
5. **Determine when an antimicrobial dressing is needed for wound healing.**
6. **Describe the mechanism by which different antimicrobial dressings reduce bacterial burden.**

WOUND DRESSINGS: A HISTORICAL PERSPECTIVE

Chronicles about the care and management of open wounds go back to early civilization's use of natural remedies to treat injuries of unfathomable causes. One of the oldest medical manuscripts known to man is a clay tablet dated circa 2100 BC that contains a collection of prescriptions described as "three healing gestures," which even in modern times is the basis for wound treatment.[1,2] These gestures were washing the wound, making plasters, and bandaging the wound.

The Ebers Papyrus, circa 1500 BC, detailed the use of lint, animal grease, and honey for the management of open wounds. The lint provided a fibrous base that promoted wound site closure, the animal grease provided a barrier to environmental pathogens, and the honey served as an antimicrobial agent. The Egyptians believed that closing a wound preserved the soul and prevented the exposure of the spirit to "infernal beings," as was noted in the Berlin papyrus. The Greeks, who had a similar perspective on the importance of wound closure, were the first to differentiate between acute and chronic wounds, calling them "fresh" and "nonhealing," respectively. Galen of Pergamum, a Greek surgeon who served Roman gladiators circa AD 120–201, made many contributions to the field of wound care. The most important was acknowledgment of the importance of maintaining wound-site moisture to ensure successful wound closure.

Limited advances were made throughout the Middle Ages and the Renaissance; however, the most profound advances, both technological and clinical, came with the development of microbiology and cellular pathology. In the 19th century, Pasteur advocated that wounds be covered and kept dry because he believed this would keep them "germ" free. The dressings developed at this time (made from cloth, cotton, and gauze) have dominated wound management in recent history, and in some countries, continue to be the main products used.

The first manufactured dressings were probably Gamgee wadding and tulle gras. Gamgee discovered that degreased cotton wrapped in bleached lint would absorb fluids, and he introduced his first dressing in the 19th century. During the 1914–1918 war, Frenchman Lumiere developed cotton gauze that was impregnated with paraffin to prevent the dressing from sticking to the wound. Wound management technology did not progress significantly beyond these early developments until the 1960s when comparisons were made of wound healing in dry and moist environments.[3]

In 1962, Winter[4] published his landmark paper about the effect of occlusion on wound healing. He made experimental wounds on the backs of domestic pigs, covered half of the wounds with an occlusive film, and left the other half exposed to the air. The occluded, and hence moist, wounds had an epithelialization rate twice that of those left open to form a scab. The concept of moist wound healing was accepted, and a plethora of dressings have become available since the late 1970s to deliver and maintain a moist healing environment. Although six plus decades have passed since this historical work documenting the benefits of moist wound healing and managing exudate, too often topical wound care is still based on "how we've always done it", ie, how one was previously taught, on previous concepts, or on the way it has always been done.

Maintaining a moist wound bed is the evidence-based standard of care for the management of open wounds; however, the "wet-to-dry" dressing (ie, packing a wound space with moist gauze and removing it after it has adhered to the wound bed) is a common treatment still used today.[5,6] Wet-to-dry dressings are considered substandard, outdated care for debriding wounds, given the evidence that they delay healing and increase wound pain and the incidence of infection when compared to alternative modern therapies.[7] Wet-to-dry debridement is not selective (see Chapter 13, Wound Debridement); in fact, it often removes healthy tissues, thereby causing further tissue trauma and potentially significant pain upon removal (**FIGURE 14-1**).

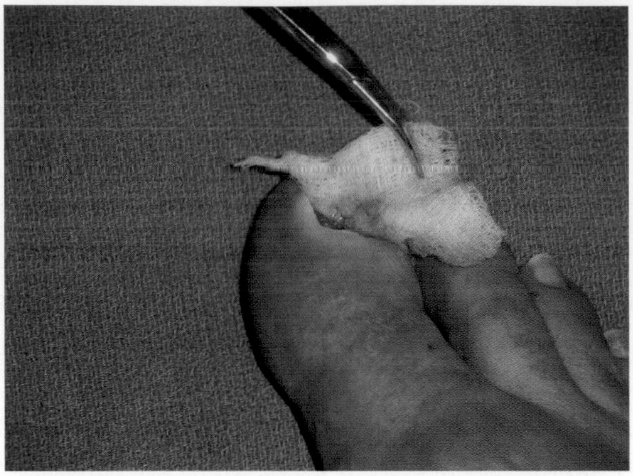

FIGURE 14-1 Wet-to-dry dressings. Wet-to-dry dressings adhere to healthy granulation tissue and can cause capillary destruction upon removal. In addition to causing the wound to bleed, removal of dry adhered dressings can be very painful for the patient.

The concept of using a wet-to-*moist* dressing to avoid this trauma may still cause injury. The dressing is prepared in the same manner as a wet-to-dry dressing except the gauze is applied with more moisture with the intent that it will remain moist until removal. Nevertheless, it may become a wet-to-dry dressing in practice. A study of the mechanism of action of saline dressings suggests that they function as an osmotic dressing. Normal saline is isotonic. As water evaporates from the saline dressing, it becomes hypertonic and fluid from the wound tissues is drawn into the dressing in an attempt to reestablish isotonicity. However, wound fluid is not merely water; it contains blood and proteins that may begin to form an impermeable layer on the dressing's surface. At this point, fluid from the wound is unable to replace the fluid lost from the dressing by evaporation and the dressing dries out completely. Consequently, unless the dressing is changed frequently, or remoistened between dressing changes, it will still function as a wet-to-dry dressing.

Additionally, cooling of the tissues at dressing changes may impede healing. Evaporation of water from a surface results in a reduction of temperature at that surface. Reduction in tissue temperature has multiple physiologic effects, including local reflex vasoconstriction and hypoxia, impairment of leukocyte mobility and phagocytic efficiency, and increased affinity of hemoglobin for oxygen—all of which not only impede healing but increase susceptibility to infection.[6]

Gauze dressings do not present a physical barrier to the entry of exogenous bacteria. An in vitro study showed that bacteria were capable of penetrating up to 64 layers of dry gauze, and moistened gauze provides even less of a barrier to bacterial penetration, again increasing the risk of infection. In a literature review of 3047 wounds, the overall infection rate for wounds dressed with moisture-retentive dressings was 2.6%, whereas the infection rate for gauze-dressed wounds was 7.1%.[6]

Wet-to-dry dressings may incur more labor for the clinician or caregiver and more costs for the healthcare system. In order for gauze to remain continuously moist to support optimal healing, it must be either changed frequently or remoistened with additional saline. This requires additional labor on the part of the clinician or the lay caregiver. Dressing changes two or three times a day used to be common. In today's reimbursement climate, this practice is no longer feasible, not only from a reimbursement perspective, but also from the standpoint of best patient outcomes. In home healthcare, multiple dressing changes a day require the expense of extra travel, home visits, and post-visit time for documentation. Even without the expense of travel in acute or long-term care settings, frequent dressing changes still require time that could be used for other patient care tasks.

GOAL-BASED WOUND MANAGEMENT[8]

Assessment of the patient with an open wound involves a holistic approach and many facets of the evaluation go beyond purely the physical makeup of the wound, for example, the appropriate diagnosis of the wound etiology, patient comorbidities, nutrition, tissue oxygenation, and patient function. Open wounds are dynamic and are continuously changing; therefore, dressing selection for optimal healing must also change as the wound progresses or regresses. Rarely does a singular treatment plan for any given wound remain the same throughout the healing process.[9] Decision-making relative to treatment is based on a thorough assessment of the patient and the wound at regular intervals so that timely changes in the care plan can be made. Specific wound and patient characteristics to be assessed that will drive treatment decisions are presented in **TABLE 14-1**.

Location

The location of the wound on the patient has less to do with the primary dressing (the dressing that is in contact with the wound bed) and more to do with how the dressing is secured. Wounds located on the torso require a dressing that is self-adhering, has an incorporated adhesive border, or is secured with additional tape. Wounds on the extremities can be secured with self-adhering dressings, gauze rolls, tubular bandages, stretch net, or compression bandages. The skin condition, patient activity level, potential pain and trauma with dressing removal, possible contamination, and the desire to bathe or shower are also factors to be considered when selecting the secondary dressing.

CLINICAL CONSIDERATION

The nonwoven, hypoallergenic, self-adhesive fabric fixation tape is a good tape for "picture-framing" a dressing to maintain the peripheral seal.

Size

The size of the wound determines the size of the dressing required to adequately fill any cavity and cover the wound surface. Undermining or sinus tracts need to be loosely packed or filled with a primary dressing that can be removed without leaving dressing fragments in the wound. All categories

TABLE 14-1 Assessment of the Wound and the Patient for Dressing Selection

Location: The location of the wound helps determine the secondary dressing that will best secure the primary dressing.	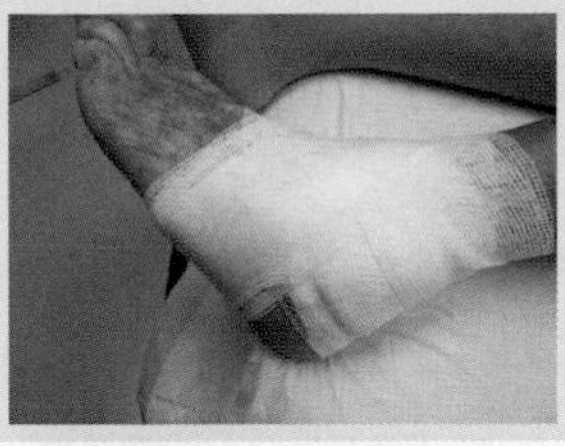	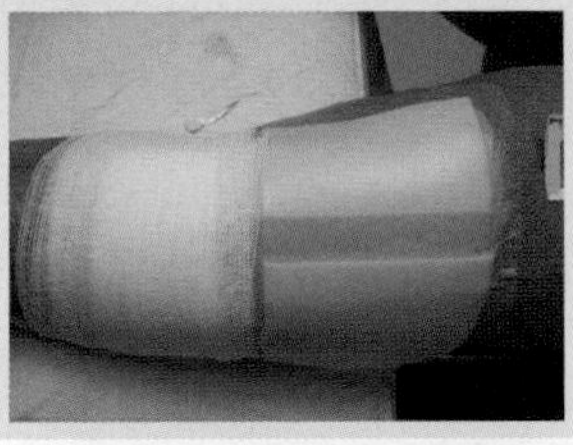	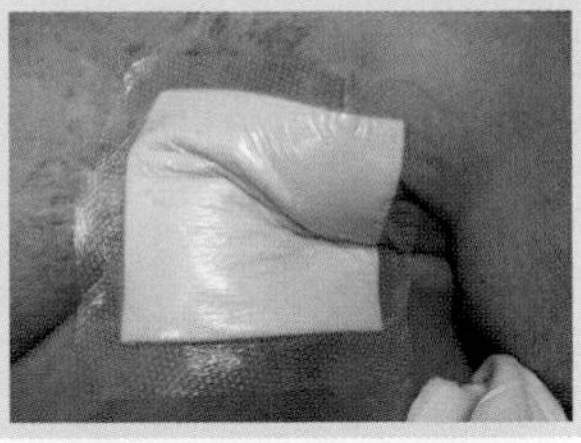
Size: The wound size determines the size and amount of the primary dressing that is required to adequately fill and cover the wound surface.	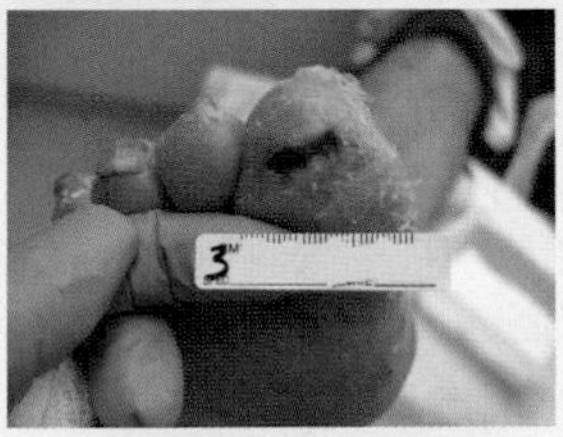	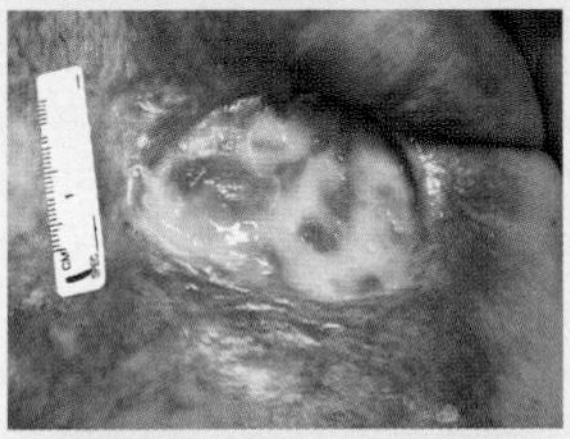	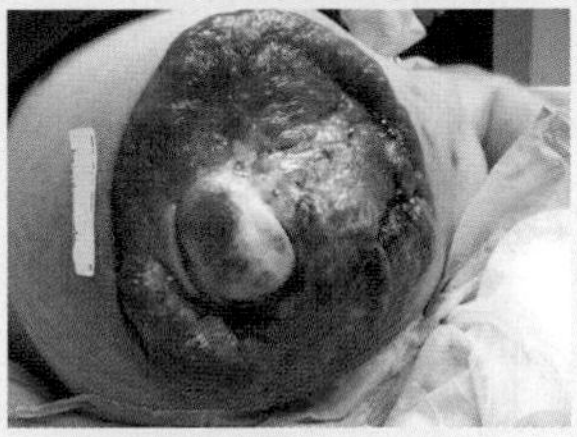
Tissue Type: The tissue appearance and predominant tissue type, as well as the presence of any exposed structures, are key determinants of primary dressing selection.	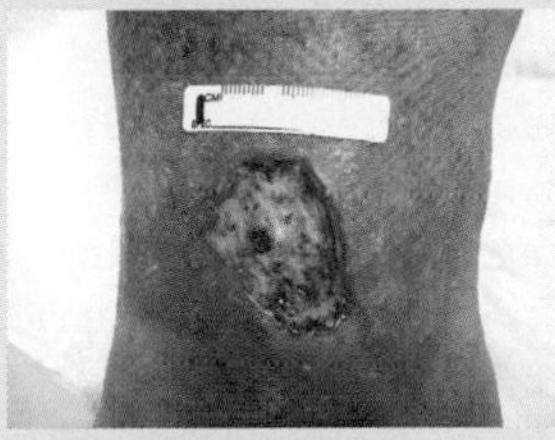	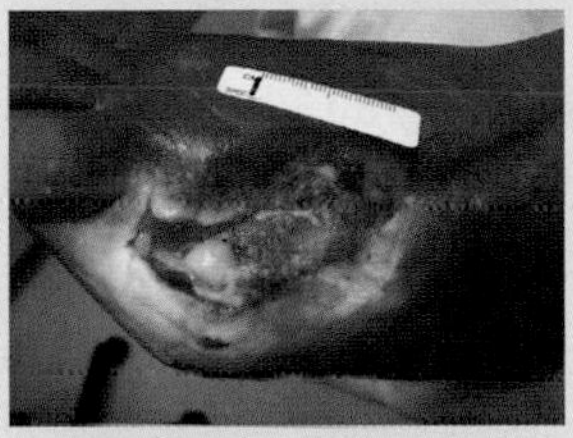	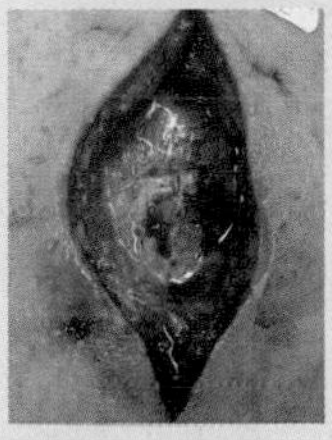
Exudate: The amount and type of exudate is a fundamental consideration in both primary and secondary dressing selection.	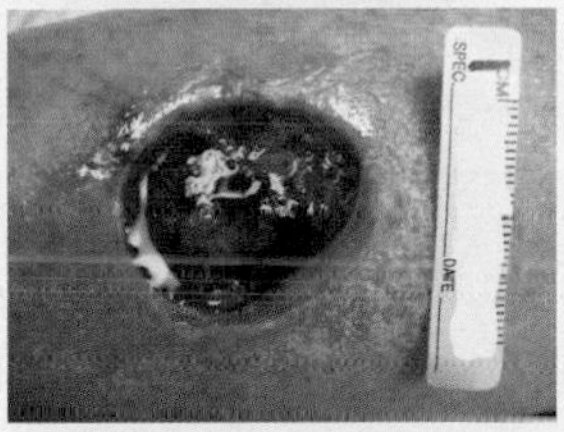	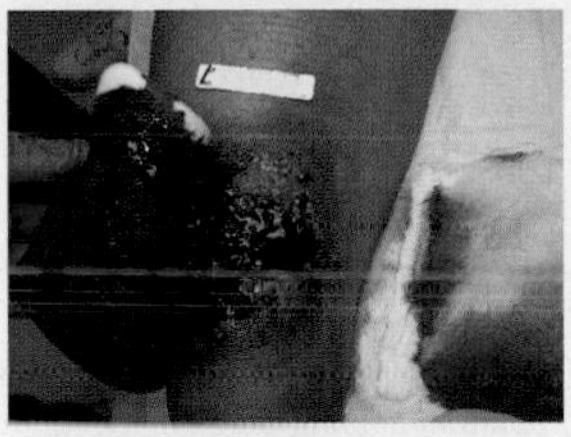	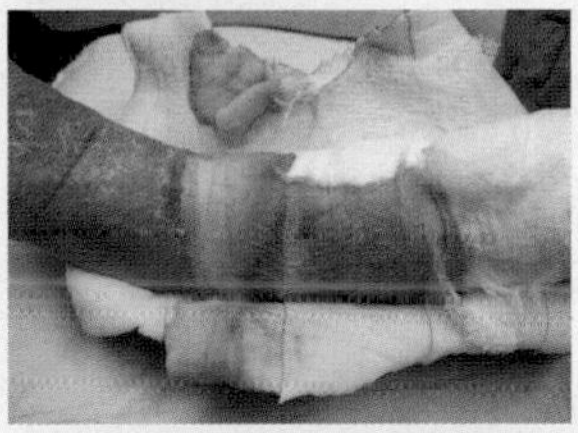
Periwound Condition: A key goal of the total dressing is to maintain the periwound skin integrity, which reduces pain and risk of infection.	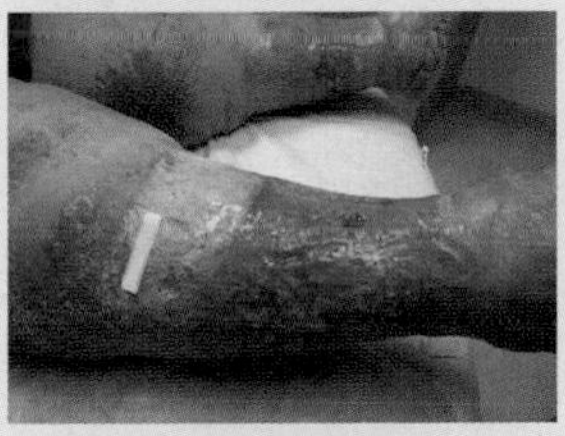	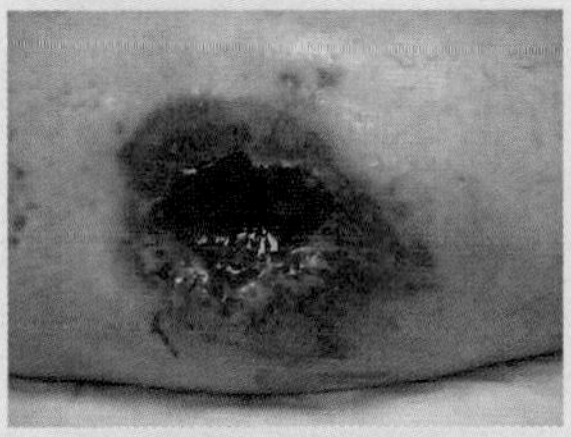	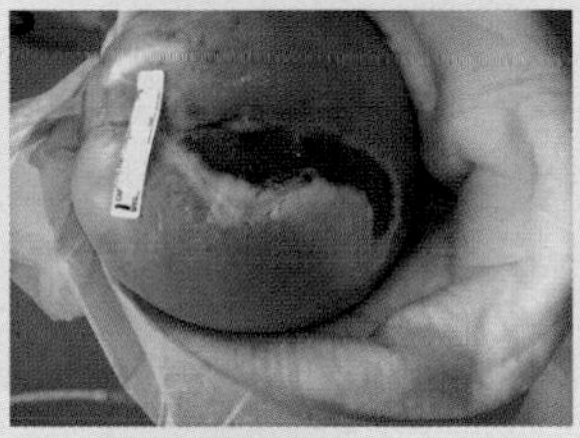
Bacterial Burden: The use of topical agents and dressings to reduce local bioburden can reduce the number of bacteria before they replicate to a critical level.	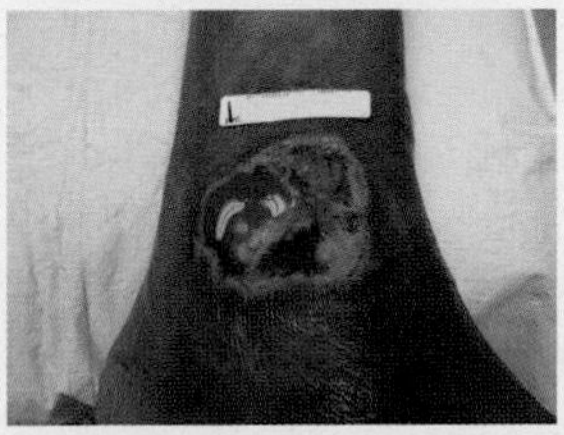	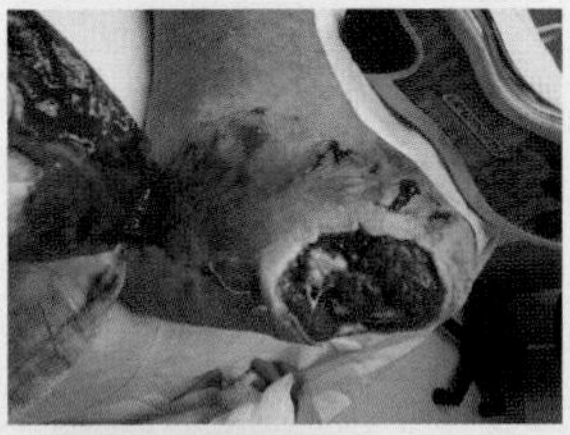	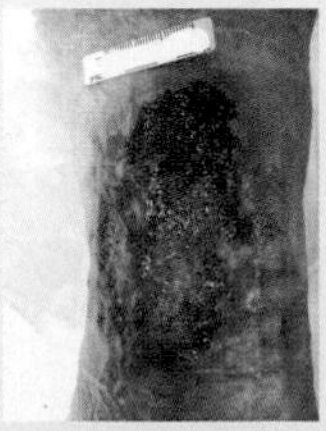
Support Needs: Compression for venous wounds, off-loading for diabetic foot ulcers, and visualization for infected wounds are examples of needs that may require special dressings.	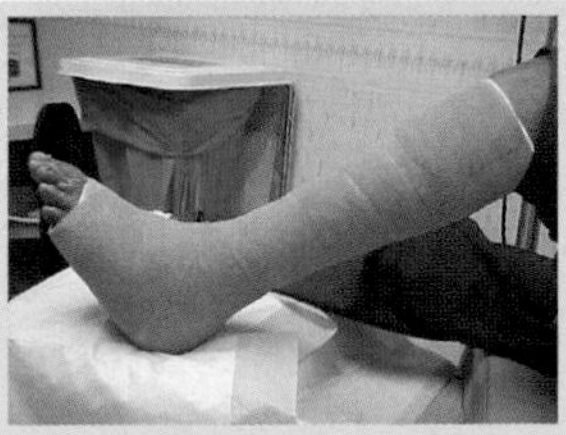	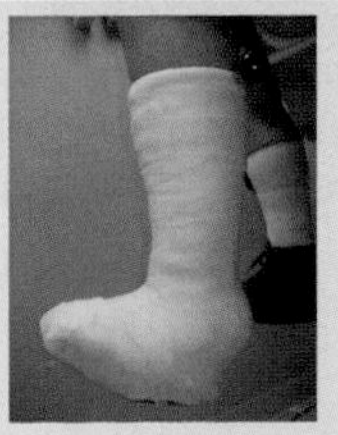	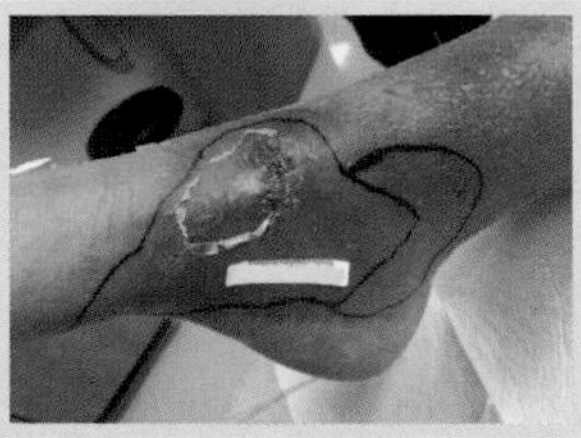

Optimal dressing selection depends on a thorough assessment of the wound, especially for the primary dressing that will interact with the wound bed to facilitate healing, as well as assessment of the patient. Activity levels and patient goals are important for selection of the secondary dressings and interventions such as negative pressure wound therapy that may affect activities of daily living and work demands.

CLINICAL CONSIDERATION

In dressing selection, the drier the wound, the more moisture the dressing will need to provide or create; and the wetter the wound, the more absorbent the dressing needs to be. The primary goal is to maintain a balanced moist wound environment to facilitate healing without causing periwound skin maceration. A secondary goal is to select a dressing absorbent enough to manage exudate and still minimize dressing changes.

of dressings are available in a variety of sizes and shapes to accommodate the dimensions of most wounds. The outlier in the size consideration is the very large wound requiring frequent dressing changes (eg, a large surgical wound) in which case negative pressure wound therapy (NPWT) may accomplish more rapid reduction in wound size and allow more patient activity (see Chapter 17, Negative Pressure Wound Therapy). If wound healing is not the immediate or long-term goal, a better dressing selection is cost-effective; requires less frequent changes; and manages exudate, odor, and pain.

Tissue Type

The predominant tissue type and the exposure of vital structures such as bone, tendon, and muscle are key determinants of dressing selection. Healthy granulating wound beds and exposed viable structures need to be kept moist and protected from trauma. The presence of necrotic tissue requires a decision about appropriateness and type of debridement.

Exudate

The amount and type of exudate are fundamental considerations in dressing selection. The optimal dressing material adequately manages the wound by wicking the exudate into a secondary dressing. This prevents pooling of exudate on the wound surface, which can become a nidus for bacterial growth as well as a source of leakage and maceration of the surrounding skin (**FIGURE 14-2**). A dry tissue bed requires hydration, a moist bed needs to be maintained, and a wet surface with large amount of exudate requires absorption. The exudate levels will also determine the frequency of the dressing change.[10]

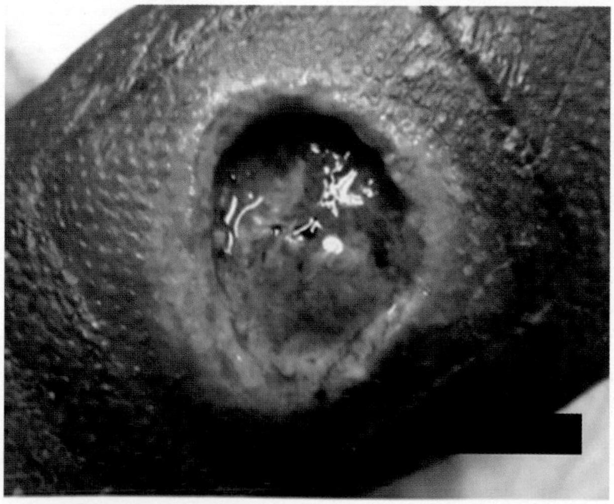

FIGURE 14-2 Wound with pooled exudate requiring an absorbent dressing.

Periwound Condition

A dressing that adequately manages exudate is the primary strategy for maintaining intact skin. The use of a barrier wipe or cyanoacrylate protects the skin from moisture as well as from trauma during tape removal. Silicone-backed dressings help prevent pain and trauma at dressing changes and prevent injury of the wound areas that have re-epithelialized. A rash or blistering of the periwound area may be an indication of an allergic reaction to a particular dressing or tape; the location and distribution of the rash or blisters are a clue to the etiology. A true allergic reaction usually results in the presence of rash or blistering where the tape or irritating agent was in contact with the skin.

Blistering, especially on one side of the dressing edge, is usually indicative of tape being applied with tension, thus resulting in a separation of the epidermis and dermis that subsequently fills with fluid, hence the blister (**FIGURE 14-3**).[11] Blistering can be prevented by applying tape without tension which is achieved by anchoring the tape in the middle and smoothing outward.

CLINICAL CONSIDERATION

When removing tape, think of taking the skin off of the tape, not the tape off of the skin. Hold the tape in one hand and gently push the skin away from the tape, possibly with moistened gauze. This technique prevents skin tears and is much more comfortable for the patient. If removing adhesives from skin with significant hair, pull in the direction of the hair growth, and not against the direction of growth. This technique does not activate the pain receptors located around the hair follicles in the dermis and is therefore less painful. Another strategy to minimize pain and trauma to the skin under the tape is to use adhesive tape remover wipes to release the bond between the adhesive and the skin as the dressing is removed. Allowing the patient to assist in dressing removal can sometimes produce less anxiety and therefore less pain by providing them control. The availability of tapes with silicone adhesion has vastly improved the avoidance of pain and injury to the skin with dressing removal.

Bacterial Burden

All wounds are contaminated. As bacterial levels rise, the potential for infection in the deeper tissue increases. Even in the absence of gross infection, wound healing can be affected by the increase of proteases, toxins, and other consequences of bacteria such as biofilm. The use of topical agents and dressings

CLINICAL CONSIDERATION

The following guidelines for pain medications to take effect are helpful in minimizing pain during dressing changes:

- Oral medications—30 minutes before treatment
- IM injections—10 minutes before treatment
- IV injections—immediately before treatment
- Topical anesthetics—5–20 minutes before treatment
- Injectable anesthetics—only by licensed provider, effective within seconds to minutes
- TENS—place proximal to wound during debridement

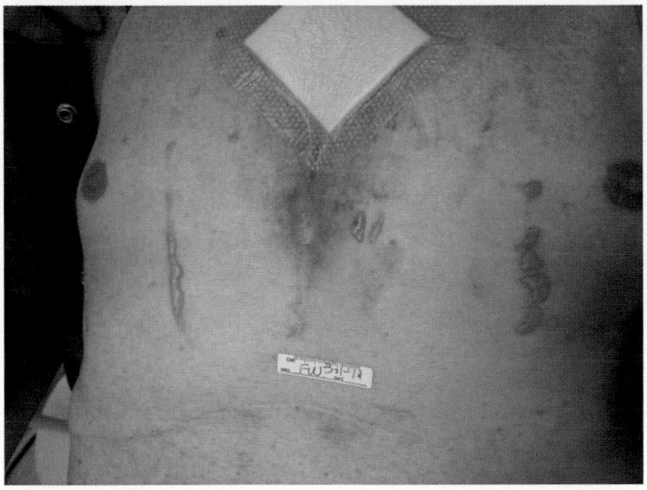

FIGURE 14-3 The blisters on this patient's chest are a result of adhesive tape. The silicone-backed dressing above the blisters is one strategy to prevent blisters and skin tears with dressing removal.

to reduce local bioburden can reduce the number of bacteria before they rise to a critical level and negatively influence wound healing. Multiple dressing options exist to address bacteria while still meeting the environmental needs of the wound (see "Antimicrobial Dressings" section).

Pain

Every patient has an acceptable level of pain, and every treatment plan should include strategies to mitigate or eliminate pain to the extent possible, or at least to the patient's acceptable level. A survey conducted in 2002 in 11 European and North American countries identified the top issues in wound healing as (1) preventing trauma to the wound surface and periwound skin and (2) preventing pain to the patient during dressing changes.[12] Dressing changes cause moderate to severe pain in 74% of patients, nearly half (36%) of whom experience severe pain (rated 8 to 10 on a 10-point numeric rating scale). Further, experiencing pain at a dressing change can elevate anticipatory pain, making future procedures even more painful.[13] Maintaining a moist wound bed, selecting a nonadherent dressing that is easy to remove, gentle cleansing, administering oral and IV pain medications at the optimal times, and using a topical anesthetic for procedures such as wound cleansing, dressing changes and debridement, are strategies that reduce the pain associated with both acute and chronic wound care. In some cases, having the patient don gloves and assist in the dressing removal can help minimize pain and reduce anxiety.

Support Needs

Topical care is only a part of the multifaceted approach to achieving wound healing. A thorough patient assessment to determine wound etiology and the appropriate supportive management is an integral part of the treatment plan. To that end, dressing choices are also determined by the supportive care or other medical interventions required to manage the underlying etiology and comorbidities. Examples include but are not limited to the following:

- Patients with venous disease requiring compression wraps or patients with diabetic foot ulcers (DFUs) offloaded with total contact casts require dressings that may be left in place until the compression or casts are removed and changed.
- Patients with suspected or confirmed infection may require frequent observation of the wounds, as well as more frequent dressing changes, depending on the topical antimicrobial being used.
- Patients with periwound dermatitis being treated with topical agents require dressing changes at the frequency needed for the reapplication of medications.

Quality of Life

Optimal wound management involves a holistic approach that considers patient wishes and lifestyle, work requirements, and activities of daily living. An important first consideration is the overall goal for the wound, for example, can it be healed? In the case of a patient with a terminal illness or a wound of the lower extremity with inadequate circulation, the goal may not be healing but pain and odor control, prevention of infection, prevention of wound deterioration, and maintenance of a dressing that allows family to be with the patient without wound concerns. The patient who desires or requires showering needs a waterproof dressing. The working patient needs a treatment plan that accommodates the working schedule and environment, as well as a dressing that can be camouflaged, hidden, or at least presentable. In a study undertaken to understand the personal impact of VLUs from the perspective of patients, the impact of exudate (eg, leakage) and malodor was described as devastating, causing embarrassment, shame, and stress. Some patients reported trying to manage this situation by limiting their contact with others and creating self-imposed isolation.[14] In summary, the patient needs a dressing that will prevent the wound from interrupting daily life as much as possible.

CLINICAL CONSIDERATION

Decision-making based on wound assessment includes the following:

- If the wound is dry, add moisture.
- If the wound is exudating, absorb.
- If there is space, fill it.
- If the wound is filled in and healing, cover and leave it undisturbed.

CHARACTERISTICS OF THE IDEAL WOUND DRESSING[15–20]

There is no "one size fits all" for dressing selection for open wounds. There are literally thousands of dressings available considering the various categories, shapes, and sizes. Although the *form* (ie, the ingredients) of the dressing is important, the

TABLE 14-2 Characteristics of the Ideal Wound Dressing

Provides a moist wound environment	By either donating or removing moisture from the wound bed, the dressing maintains the optimal moisture level, thereby preventing desiccation of the cells.
Manages exudate appropriately	The dressing adequately absorbs or manages the wound exudate so that it is sequestered in the dressing and does not exude onto the intact periwound skin, thus causing maceration or denudation.
Facilitates autolytic debridement	In the presence of necrotic tissue, the dressing creates an environment so that ambient wound fluid containing phagocytic cells and endogenous enzymes is in contact with the tissue, thus facilitating autolysis.
Provides antimicrobial properties if needed	If a wound is highly colonized or infected, the antimicrobial dressing will aid in sequestering wound fluid or providing active antimicrobial activity to reduce or eliminate bacteria.
Minimizes pain	The selected dressing material does not adhere to the wound bed and cause disruption of the surface, thus harming healthy cells. By not adhering, the dressing lifts from the wound and periwound easily, and as a result, does not cause the patient undue discomfort.
Prevents contamination by being impermeable to environmental bacteria	On all wounds (especially those in the sacral, coccyx, and ischial area where contamination is likely), the dressing surface is impermeable to bacteria and contamination from the environment. This is especially important for the incontinent patient.
Is compatible with support needs	The dressing can be used under support treatments such as contact casts and compression wraps that are often left in place for a full week.
Insulates and maintains optimal temperature	The dressing allows maintenance of constant temperature without frequent cooling of the tissues that can impact healing. Frequent dressing changes can negatively impact wound healing more than the dressing selection itself.
Prevents particulate contamination or allergens from coming in contact with the wound surface	The dressing does not leave threads or pieces of adherent dressing in the wound bed, which could act as a foreign body in the tissue. Also, the dressing does not contain common allergens such as latex.
Is easily applied and removed (user friendly)	The dressing can be used by the care providers in the patient's setting, including by family members at home.
Is available and cost-effective	The dressing must be available in the healthcare setting in which the patient resides. Choices available in a hospital or clinic may not be reimbursable for the patient at home, or they may not be on the formulary of a particular home care agency or skilled nursing facility. Flexibility in dressing selection by the prescriber is required as long as the selection meets the needs of the wound.

function, or how it will optimize the wound environment, is more essential in decision-making. That being said, there is almost always more than one option available to meet the assessed needs of any wound. **TABLE 14-2** describes the desired characteristics of an ideal wound dressing.

WOUND DRESSING CATEGORIES[15–20]

A myriad of dressing materials are available to meet the ever-changing needs of the open wound, and the task of selecting the appropriate dressing can at times be daunting. Numerous specialty dressings create or enhance the wound environment to promote healing. Some have a singular function while others are combinations or composites possessing attributes of more than one category. Familiarity with the basic categories enables the clinician to understand the combination products and make appropriate decisions for optimal outcomes.

Skin Protectants

Although they are not dressings per se, skin protectants are formulations designed to protect the skin from the effects of mechanical injury due to tapes and adhesives. Composed of a polymer or a cyanoacrylate adhesive plus a solvent, when applied to the skin, the solvent evaporates and the polymer/cyanoacrylate dries, thereby forming a visible transparent protective coating on the skin. When tapes or adhesives are applied over this coating, mechanical injury to the epidermis is avoided because the protective layer is lifted instead of layers of skin cells. Skin protectants are available with and without alcohol, an important distinction when considering an application to broken or irritated skin that is painful with alcohol exposure. Skin protectors are available in foam applicators, wipes, and sprays (**FIGURES 14-5** and **14-6**).

Contact Layer Dressings

Contact layers are single-layer primarily nonwoven dressings that act as a barrier between the wound surface and a secondary dressing. Contact layers protect the wound bed from trauma while allowing wound exudate to pass through into a secondary or negative pressure wound dressing. Alternatively, contact layers may be used over-medicated creams, ointments, or biologics such as growth factors or cellular- and tissue-based products in order to protect them from the secondary dressing. Contact layers are made from nonadherent fabrics such as polyethylene and can be coated with silicone, an oil emulsion, or petrolatum to prevent or minimize adherence (**FIGURES 14-7** to **14-10**).

Contact layers may be cut to fit any wound or allowed to overlap onto the adjacent skin. They are usually removed and reapplied with each dressing change; however, they can be left in place to avoid skin/wound trauma when only changing the secondary dressing in the presence of larger amounts of exudate (eg, with radiation burns). Contact layers can be

CASE STUDY

INTRODUCTION

A 59-year-old man presents with a Charcot foot deformity and a recurrent Wagner Grade 3 ulcer on the right plantar foot (FIGURE 14-4). The patient is morbidly obese and has type 2 diabetes, which is well controlled with an A1C of 6.9. Blood flow is adequate for healing based on the results of an arteriogram done 3 weeks prior to wound assessment. An MRI has confirmed the presence of osteomyelitis. The patient is receiving IV antibiotics based on tissue culture and is receiving daily hyperbaric oxygen treatments. Surgical debridement of the wound is planned; however, appropriate dressings will be used until then.

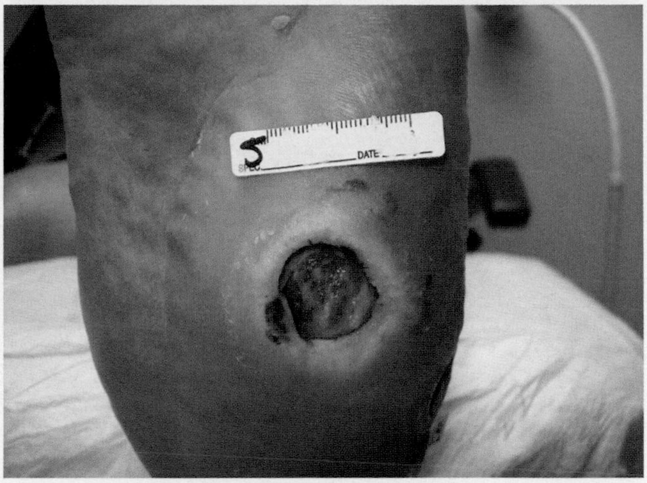

FIGURE 14-4 Case study—initial evaluation.

DISCUSSION QUESTIONS

1. Describe the wound characteristics that will influence the dressing selection.
2. What are the immediate goals for wound care?
3. What are the purposes of the primary dressing and the secondary dressings for this patient?

CLINICAL CONSIDERATION

Dressings used to fill space in deeper wounds, sinus tracts/tunnels, or undermined areas should be placed so that the dressing will be evident at the next dressing change. Ideally, one continuous dressing is used to fill the entire wound for ease of removal and to avoid residual dressing fibers in the deeper wound bed. Residual dressing fibers can lead to granuloma formation, fluid collection, and potential infection. Both the type of dressing and number of pieces used need to be documented in order to inform the next person changing the dressing of the materials that need to be removed.

used for wounds of all types and any amount of exudate. Advantages and disadvantages are listed in TABLES 14-3 and 14-4, respectively.

Film Dressings

Film dressings, also referred to as transparent film dressings because of the ability to see through them, are polyurethane self-adhering membranes that are moisture vapor permeable. Moisture vapor permeable dressings allow for the passage of water vapor but maintain an impermeable barrier to liquid water and bacteria. These dressings help create a moist wound-healing environment while preventing excessive fluid accumulation and protecting the wound from external contaminants. Film dressings are waterproof and thereby prevent contamination of the wound bed; however, they are vapor permeable so that some moisture can evaporate from the wound bed.

Film dressings are transparent, thin, and flexible and therefore allow visualization of the wound and surrounding skin. They are frequently used on intact skin for protection from friction and moisture and to reduce shear. Placing transparent films over early skin changes such as Stage 1 pressure injuries or deep tissue pressure injuries allow the clinician to frequently assess the site for progression or changes. Standard film dressings cannot absorb exudate, thus they are not indicated for draining wounds. There is, however, a film dressing

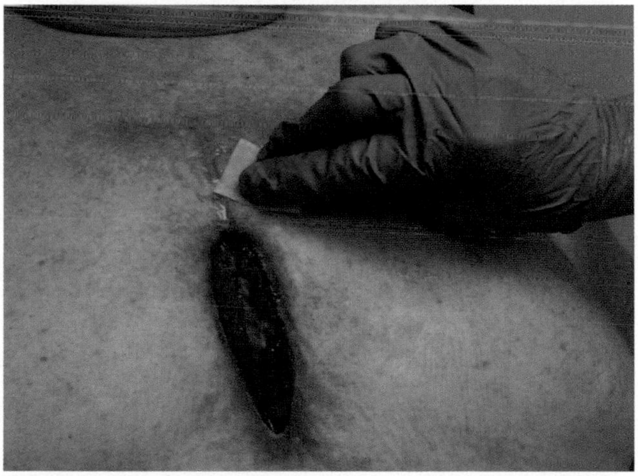

FIGURE 14-5 Skin protector wipes. Skin protectors, also called moisture barriers, can help prevent skin maceration and tearing upon removal of a dressing. This is especially helpful if the dressing has an adhesive backing such as transparent film. The protector agent can be with or without alcohol, a consideration if the periwound is inflamed which causes the alcohol to burn or sting.

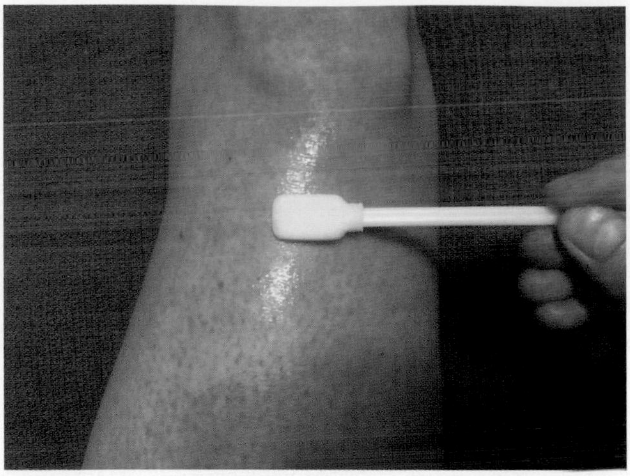

FIGURE 14-6 Skin protector wand. Skin protectors are available in wands that are helpful when treating large areas.

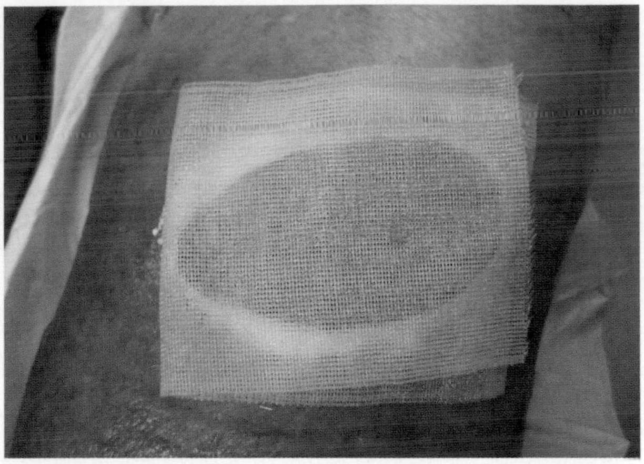

FIGURE 14-8 Protective covering. A nonadherent mesh over moistened PVA foam prevents the dressing from drying out, maintains a moist wound environment, and decreases the need to disrupt the dressing to add moisture.

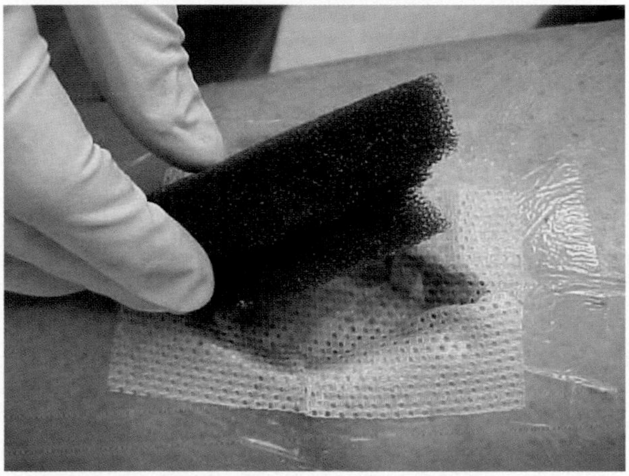

FIGURE 14-7 Contact layers used to protect fragile tissue. A nonadherent contact layer used under the foam of a negative pressure foam dressing can prevent tearing of fragile tissue and bleeding when removing the dressing, protect tissue such as bone and tendon that can be desiccated by the foam, and decrease the pain of dressing changes. If the wound bed does not need protection, using strips of a contact layer or petrolatum gauze over the edges will decrease pain with dressing removal, especially if the edges are inflamed.

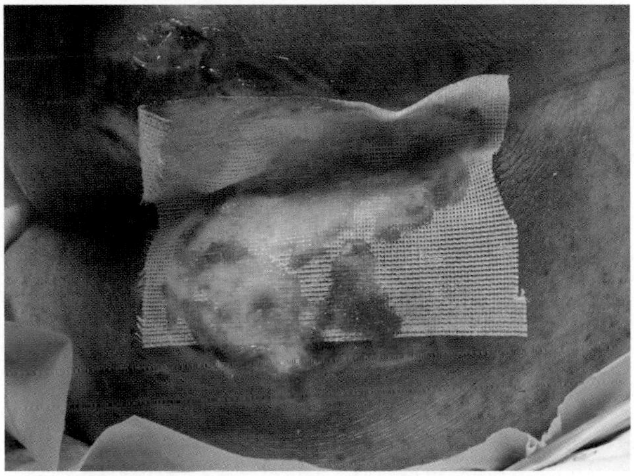

FIGURE 14-9 Contact layer over enzymatic debrider. A nonadherent contact layer over an enzymatic debrider ointment keeps the topical in contact with the wound bed, prevents it from drying out, and maximizes the action of the enzymes.

CLINICAL CONSIDERATION

The frequency of dressing changes is determined by the amount of exudate. Collection of exudate causes maceration of the surrounding skin and potential leakage out of the edge of the dressing. Therefore, selection of a dressing adequate for the amount of drainage is critical for optimal healing outcomes.

that incorporates an acrylic polymer pad so that exudate transfers through perforations and into the absorbent pad and away from the wound surface (**FIGURES 14-11** to **14-13**).

Film dressings create an environment conducive to autolytic debridement by holding the body fluid onto the necrotic tissue. The natural enzymes in the fluid emulsify only the necrotic tissue so that it can be easily removed, usually after only 24 hours (refer to Chapter 13) (**FIGURES 14-11** to **14-13**).

Care is required when removing film dressings from intact fragile skin in order to avoid mechanical stripping. The use of a skin barrier wipe before applying the film helps protect the skin as well as increases the adherence of the dressing. Films are often used as secondary dressings to waterproof and allow showering, and are the dressing materials used with most NPWT devices. See **TABLES 14-5** and **14-6** for advantages and disadvantages of transparent film dressings, respectively.

CLINICAL CONSIDERATION

To safely remove transparent film (or any adhesive dressing) from the skin, begin by lifting one corner, then pushing the skin away from the dressing. This minimizes both the pain and the risk of tearing the skin.

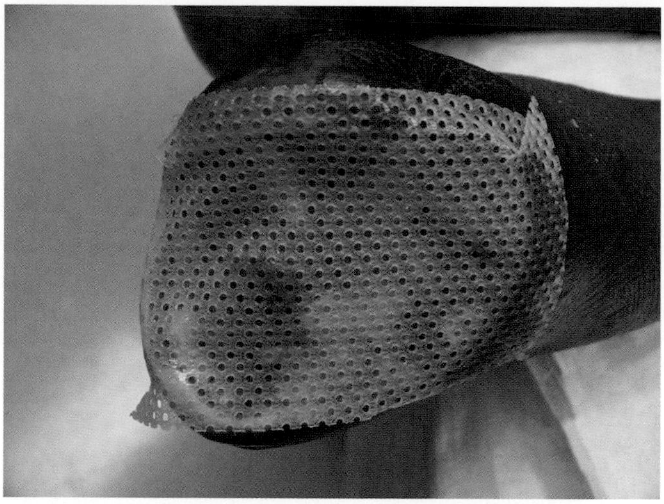

FIGURE 14-10 Contact layer for protection of wound bed. A contact layer over a recent surgical wound, such as the transmetatarsal amputation in this photo, protects the healthy tissue, prevents desiccation, and decreases pain with dressing changes.

TABLE 14-3 Advantages of Contact Layer Dressings

- Protect the wound bed from trauma with dressing removal
- Maintain contact of medicated creams, ointments, and gels, cell-based therapies, matrix devices, and skin grafts against the wound bed and thereby maximize their actions
- Prevent absorption or removal of medications when the secondary dressing is removed
- Prevent in-growth of granulation tissue into the foam when incorporated into negative-pressure wound therapy
- Prevent pain and bleeding upon removal of the foam
- Protect partial-thickness wounds such as skin tears, skin graft donor sites, and radiation burns

TABLE 14-4 Disadvantages/Considerations with Contact Layer Dressings

- Not recommended for dry wounds, third-degree burns, or other wounds that need contact moisture
- May leave "dead spaces" if good contact is not achieved upon application, thereby allowing exudate to collect on the wound surface

TABLE 14-5 Advantages of Film Dressings

- Allows visualization of the wound bed and the wound exudate
- Protects skin in high trauma areas (heels, sacrum)
- Is impermeable to fluids and bacteria
- Conforms to body contours
- Facilitates autolytic debridement
- Serves as a secondary dressing
- Is cost-effective

Hydrogels and Hydrogel Dressings

Hydrogels are water- or glycerin-based products that are either amorphous (defined as dispensed from a tube or impregnated into gauze dressings) or cross-linked polymers formed into

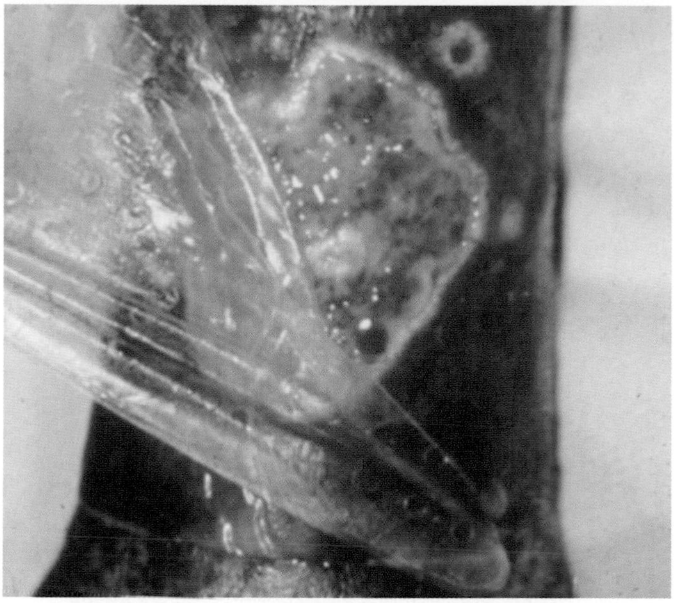

FIGURE 14-11 Transparent film. Transparent film over a venous wound illustrates that it has little or no absorption. Fluid has collected under the film and created a layer of clear exudate that is sometimes termed gelatinous edema.

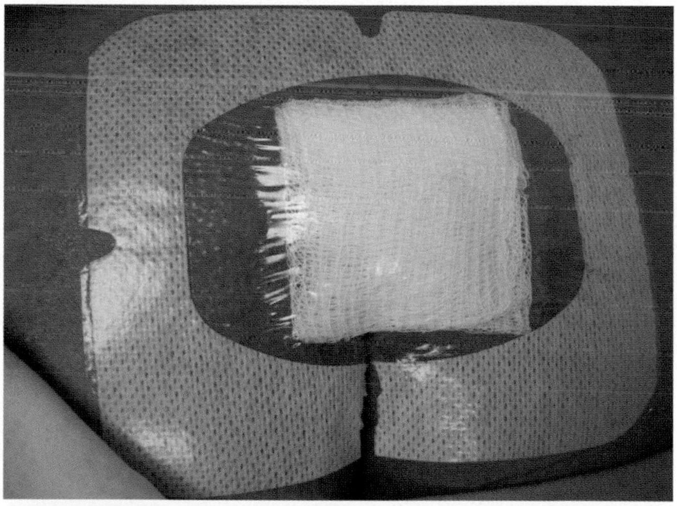

FIGURE 14-12 Transparent film as secondary dressing. Transparent film with an adhesive border is useful as a secondary dressing to cover and protect a primary dressing. The ability to allow vapor to evaporate while keeping environmental contaminants out of the wound is an advantage of transparent films, which have different moisture evaporation rates.

TABLE 14-6 Disadvantages/Considerations with Film Dressings

- May tear fragile skin upon removal
- Does not absorb exudate
- May not adhere well to dry, flaky skin
- May macerate skin if fluid collects underneath the film
- May exacerbate fungal growth if present on skin
- Tends to roll at the edges in areas of high friction

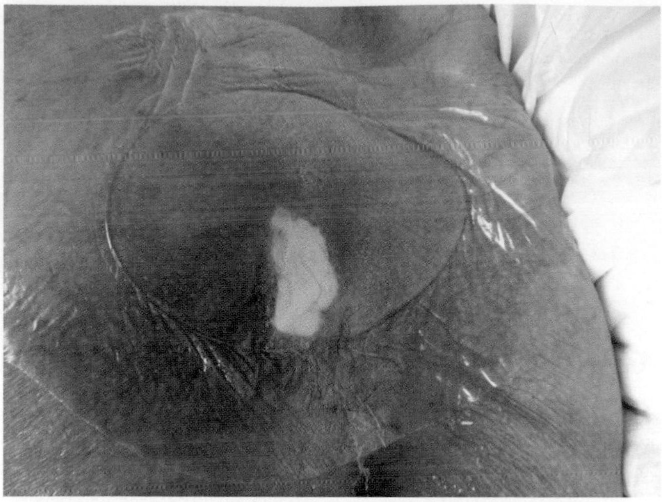

FIGURE 14-13 Transparent film. Transparent film with an acrylic center is used as a secondary dressing over a calcium alginate primary dressing. The film forms a waterproof protector for the underlying dressing and tissue.

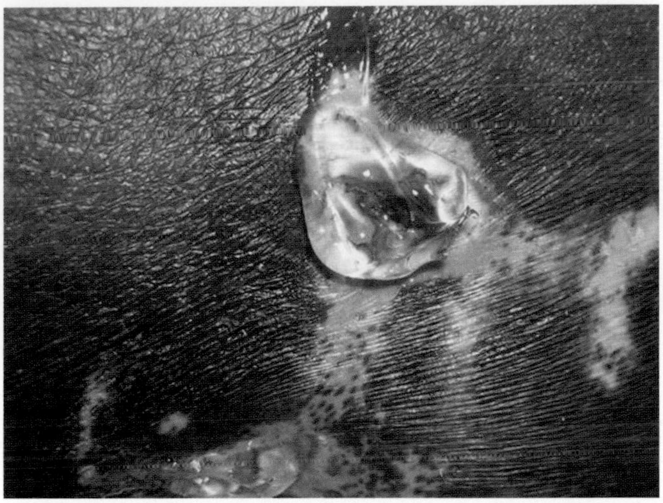

FIGURE 14-15 Amorphous gel on a wound. An example of a wound appropriate for an amorphous gel. When covered with an occlusive or semiocclusive dressing, the gel will facilitate autolytic debridement.

three-dimensional sheets. Hydrogels are moisture-donating products that enable the most rapid hydration of a wound surface as compared to other categories of wound dressings. They may contain other ingredients such as surfactants to enhance cleansing, alginate to increase viscosity or allow for small amounts of absorption, antimicrobial agents to address bioburden, and collagen or growth factors to enhance wound healing (**FIGURES 14-14** to **14-17**).

Amorphous gels are reapplied daily; sheet forms may offer extended wear time depending on the amount of exudate that collects beneath them. The periwound skin of a wound treated with hydrogels may need protection with a moisture barrier film or ointment to prevent over-hydration or maceration. Hydrogels are used for dry wounds and are contraindicated for wounds that have visible exudate. See **TABLES 14-7** and **14-8** for advantages and disadvantages of hydrogels.

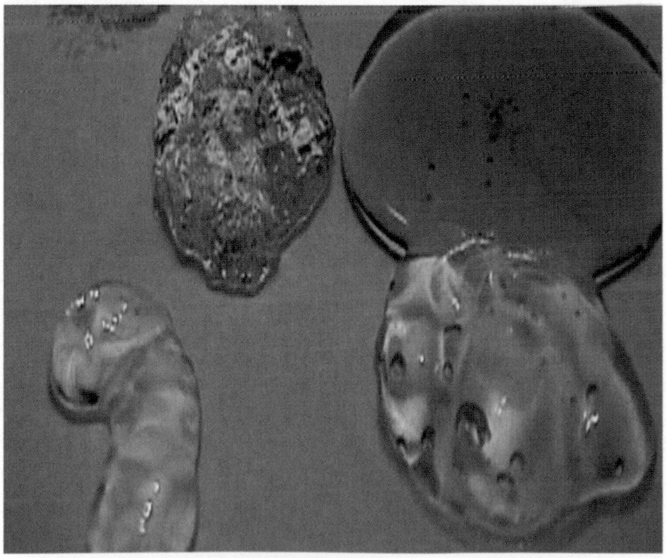

FIGURE 14-14 Examples of amorphous gels. Amorphous gels are hydrating primary dressings that are water- or glycerin-based. The consistency allows the gel to conform to the shape of the wound and maintain contact with the entire wound bed; thus, they require a secondary dressing. Gels come in a variety of containers, from squeeze tubes to sprays, and may contain other agents such as growth factors, lidocaine, or silver.

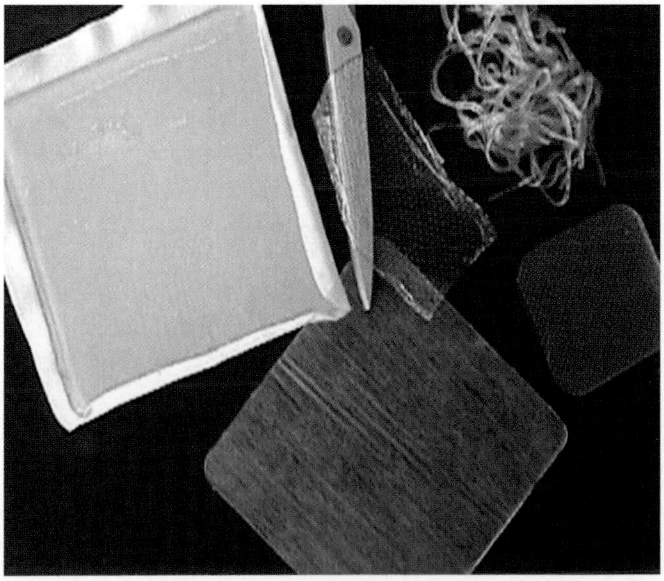

FIGURE 14-16 Hydrogel sheet. Sheet hydrogels, available in different sizes and thicknesses, are useful for partial-thickness, superficial, and flat wounds, such as partial-thickness burns and skin tears.

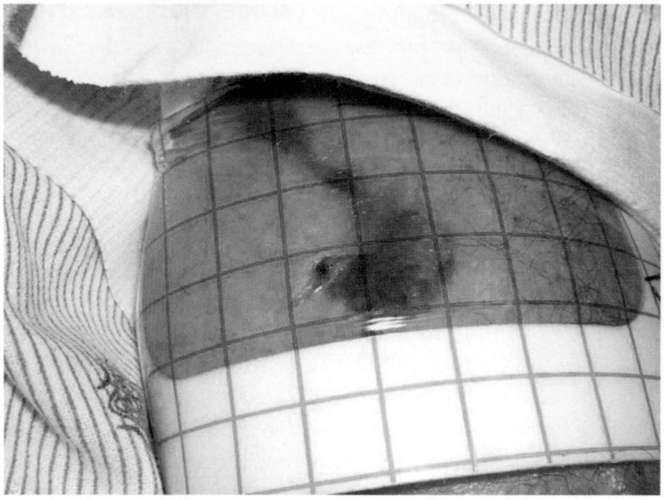

FIGURE 14-17 Hydrogel sheet on a wound. Example of a hydrogel sheet on a wound. The grid is in centimeters, which allows measurement of the wound surface area. The grid intersections that are within the wound bed are an estimate of the total surface area; in this case, 4 would indicate a surface area of approximately 4 cm^2. This technique of measuring surface area is useful for wounds that have irregular borders, which makes the perpendicular method less accurate.

TABLE 14-7 Advantages of Hydrogels

- Hydrate dry wound beds
- Facilitate autolytic debridement when used under an occlusive dressing
- Rinse or clean easily from the wound surface
- Conform to the shape of the wound and fills all spaces
- Soothe "hot" wounds and reduce pain
- Serve as a delivery system for other agents such as silver, collagen, growth factors, or lidocaine
- Are available in saturated gauze pads for flat wounds

TABLE 14-8 Disadvantages/Considerations with Hydrogels

- Macerate the periwound skin if wound becomes too wet
- Do not absorb drainage
- Dry out if not covered adequately
- Require a secondary dressing
- Usually require daily dressing changes

Hydrocolloid Dressings

Hydrocolloids are wafer-type dressings composed of three layers: an inner slightly adhesive layer, a middle absorbent layer, and an outer semiocclusive layer. The middle absorbent layer contains combinations of gelatin, pectin, and carboxymethylcellulose with hydrophilic particles that interact with wound fluid to form a gel mass over the wound bed. The gel conforms to the wound surface and functions to maintain a moist environment, support autolytic debridement, and prevent trauma upon removal. The resulting gel is reported to be acidic, therefore, not conducive to bacterial growth; however, caution is advised in suspected or known wound infection as the resulting gelled dressing becomes occlusive in nature and may support bacterial proliferation. The outer layer of the hydrocolloid dressings is either film- or foam-based and does not allow contamination from the outside environment to reach the wound, nor does it allow exudate to strike through from beneath the dressing. Dressings that become soiled from incontinence may be cleaned but care should be taken to ensure that residual stool or urine does not remain trapped at the edge of the dressing (**FIGURES 14-18** to **14-21**).

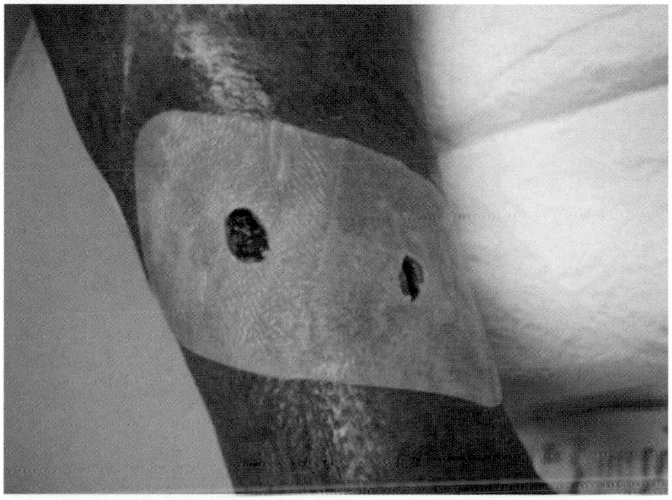

FIGURE 14-18 Hydrocolloid dressing. Hydrocolloids contain absorbent hydrophilic particles that make the dressing versatile for both minimal exudate and skin protection. In this photo, the hydrocolloid sheet is placed over the periwound skin to prevent maceration. It can also be the base for applying the adhesive secondary dressing, thus preventing the adhesive from causing further tissue damage with removal. Hydrocolloids are also the contact layer for many of the ostomy appliances.

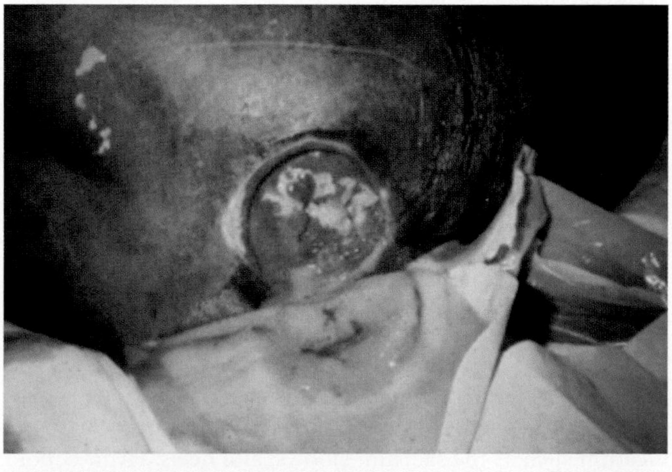

FIGURE 14-19 Hydrocolloid gelling. The hydrocolloid interacts with the exudate to form a gel that conforms to the wound bed and maintains a moist wound environment.

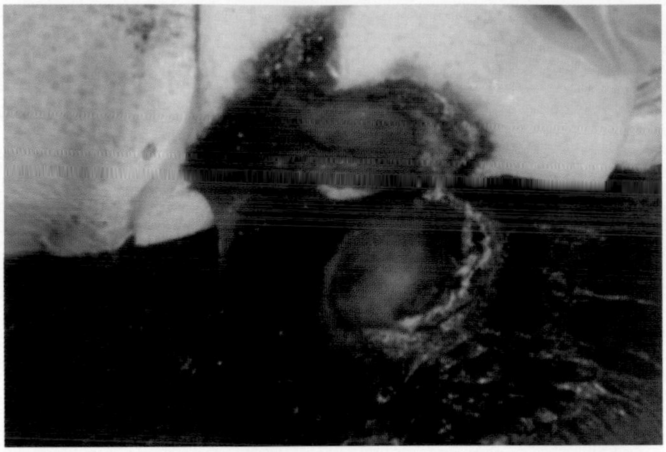

FIGURE 14-20 Discoloration of hydrocolloid. Exudate, especially if it contains any red blood cells, will cause the hydrocolloid to be discolored upon removal. Hydrocolloids can also release an odor upon removal that is not to be confused with infection.

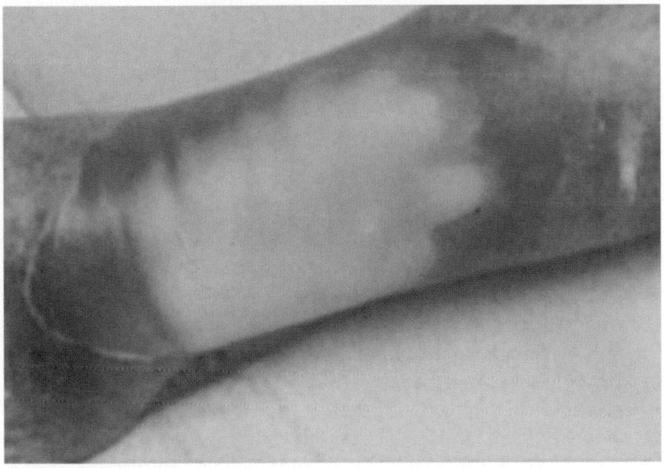

FIGURE 14-21 Hydrocolloid appearance after gelling. When the hydrocolloid absorbs exudate and forms the gel, it has a blister appearance from the outside. This allows the clinician to assess when a dressing change is indicated.

As the middle layer of the dressing gels, the contained moisture is observable from the top of the dressing, thus enabling the clinician to assess the amount of exudate and determine the need for a dressing change. The gel will ultimately migrate toward the edge of the dressing and may leak out from the edge unless it has an adhesive border. The gelatinized exudate is fairly tenacious and sticky, thus can be challenging to remove without tearing the skin. Particles of the gel may adhere to the wound surface or periwound skin and need to be removed prior to applying a new dressing.

Hydrocolloid dressings are available in various shapes and sizes designed to fit and adhere to almost any anatomic location such as the sacrum, elbows, and heels. Hydrocolloid material is also available in pastes, rings, strips, and powders to fill cavities and creases, as well as for use under pectin ostomy appliances. The frequency of dressing changes is dependent on the particular manufacturers' instructions for use but is generally between 3 and 7 days. Shearing forces over areas such as the sacrum and coccyx may cause dressing edges to roll and require more frequent changes, although many versions have thin borders that adhere better without rolling. In addition, the dressing can be picture framed with tape (**FIGURE 14-22**). Hydrocolloid dressings can be used as protection from friction and trauma; however, they are not recommended to use over a deep tissue pressure injury (DTPI) because the opaqueness prevents visualization of the skin beneath the dressings. Consequently, the evolution of the DTPI cannot be observed frequently. **TABLES 14-9** and **14-10** list the advantages and disadvantages of hydrocolloid dressings, respectively.

CLINICAL CONSIDERATION

Hydrocolloids are effective in protecting periwound skin when other dressings are likely to cause maceration, for example, in conjunction with NPWT systems or when using moist dressings to fill large cavity wounds.

Foam Dressings

Foam dressings, generally made from polyurethane with or without a film outer layer, are very absorbent and help prevent "strike-through" or leakage of exudate. There are many differences between the various foam dressings, including thickness, fluid-handling capability, and ability to hydrate or absorb moisture. Foams are available with or without adhesive borders, as well as with standard adhesive or silicone as the adhesion material. The frequently used silicone adhesion facilitates painless and atraumatic removal. Foam dressings are semiocclusive, thus allowing for gas and vapor exchange (**FIGURES 14-23** to **14-25**).

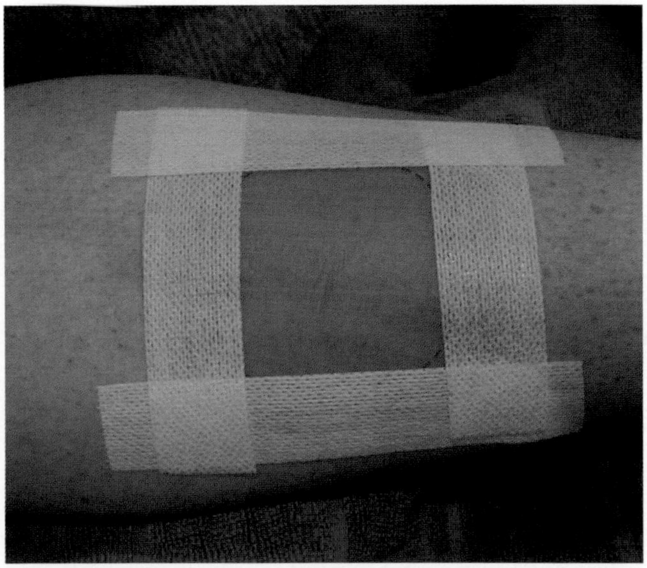

FIGURE 14-22 Securing dressing with tape. Dressings that have a tendency to roll at the edges can be secured with tape in a "picture-frame" technique.

TABLE 14-9 Advantages of Hydrocolloids

- Maintain moist wound environment
- Keep bacteria, moisture, and contamination from incontinence out of the wound bed
- Absorb minimal to moderate exudate
- Facilitate autolytic debridement
- Provide thermal insulation to maintain optimal wound temperature
- Stay in place up to 7 days
- Are effective under compression wraps
- Are self-adhering; do not need a secondary dressing if the borders are adhesive
- Conform to the surface of a flat wound
- Come in various shapes, sizes, and thicknesses

TABLE 14-10 Disadvantages/Considerations with Hydrocolloids

- Prevent visualization of the wound bed
- Do not absorb heavy exudate
- Are not recommended for covering exposed structures (tendon, bone)
- Are contraindicated for infection
- Are difficult to remove from fragile skin
- May leak, leaving sticky residue on the skin
- Require a different primary dressing to fill spaces such as fissures or undermining (paste, powders, etc.)

CLINICAL CONSIDERATION

Foam dressings have varying amounts of absorptive capacity, mechanism of fluid movement, and moisture vapor permeability which will allow moisture to escape to prevent skin maceration. Knowing the capabilities of a particular foam dressing will drive the decision on frequency of dressing changes.

Foam dressings may be used for all wound types, both as a filler and as a secondary dressing, and while indicated for wounds with moderate to large amounts of exudate, they are also suitable for wounds with little to no exudate, especially when used as a secondary dressing. The frequency of dressing change is 3–7 days depending on the amount of exudate, or the frequency of change required for the primary dressing when the foam is being used as the secondary. The moist environment created under the foam dressing can facilitate autolytic debridement. Foams may be used on infected wounds; however, they should be changed daily or according to manufacturer recommendations, especially if the foam contains an antimicrobial. Newer, multilayer foams have increased the absorption capacity significantly, allowing for less-frequent changes (**FIGURE 14-26**).

Foam dressings are available in anatomical shapes appropriate for problematic areas such as the sacrum, heels, and elbows. Bordered sacral foam dressings, specifically multilayered silicone-backed dressings, have been used successfully for prevention of sacral pressure injuries when used in conjunction with other standard prevention protocols.[21–26] See **TABLES 14-11** and **14-12** for the advantages and disadvantages of foam dressings, respectively.

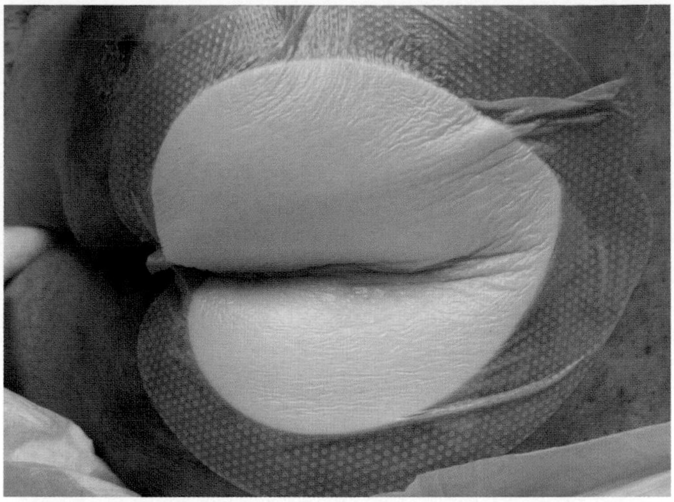

FIGURE 14-23 Foam dressing on a sacral wound. Foam dressings are available in a variety of shapes and sizes to accommodate almost any anatomical part, for example, this heart-shaped foam with an adhesive border on the sacrum. Note that the foam has to be applied so that the surface of the dressing is in contact with the skin and not just lying across a crease or empty space.

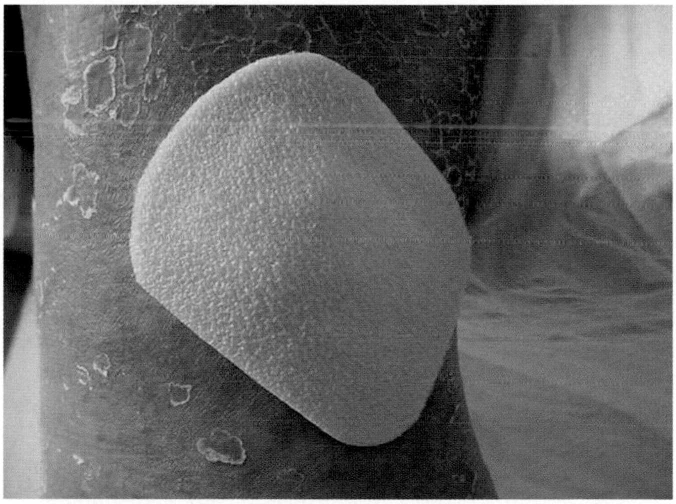

FIGURE 14-24 Foam dressing as a secondary dressing. Foams can be used as both primary or secondary dressings, as in this photo. Some foams have a silicone backing with or without an adhesive border. If placed on an area that gets a lot of friction, such as an extremity, the foam without an adhesive border will need to be anchored with a gauze roll, compression wrap, or hypoallergenic tape.

TABLE 14-11 Advantages of Foam Dressings

- Create and maintain a moist environment
- Are easy to apply
- Are effective under compression wraps
- Absorb light to heavy amounts of exudate
- Conform well to the wound bed and anatomical area
- Do not adhere to a moist wound surface
- Are available with antimicrobial agents
- Protect the skin against mechanical trauma

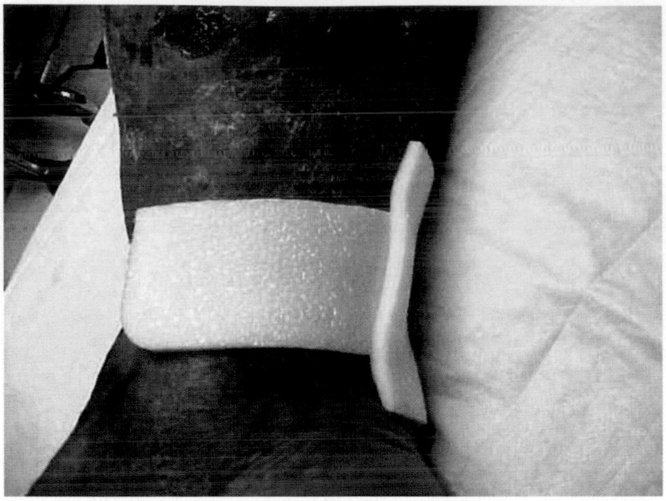

FIGURE 14-25 **Foam for skin protection.** Foams, especially those with silicone backings, prevent skin damage from compression wraps in areas where wrinkles are hard to avoid.

TABLE 14-12 Disadvantages/Considerations with Foam Dressings

- Require a secondary dressing if nonbordered
- Are not effective for dry eschar
- May macerate periwound skin if the foam becomes saturated
- Are costly if daily dressing changes are required

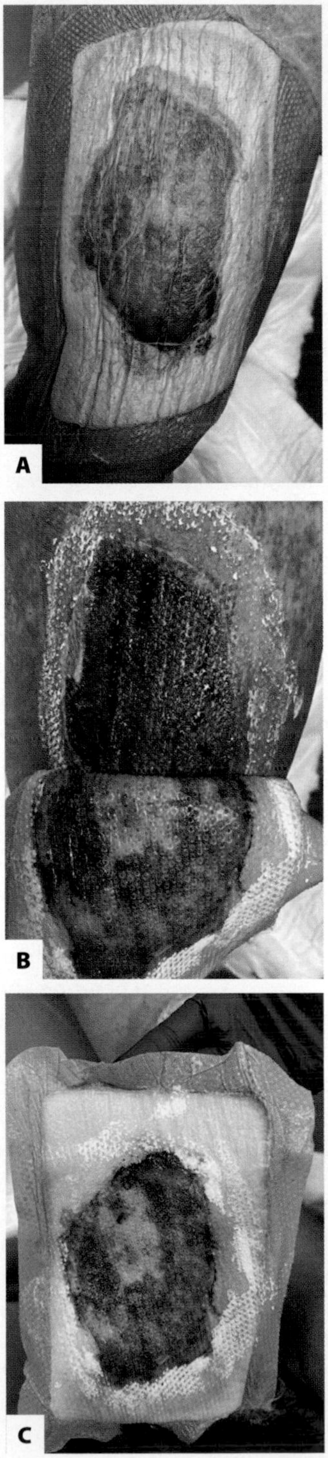

FIGURE 14-26 **A–C. Multilayer foam illustrating high absorption capacity without exudate pooling on the wound bed.**

Absorbent Dressings

Calcium Alginates Calcium alginate dressings are absorbent, biodegradable, nonwoven fibers that are derived from seaweed and composed of calcium/sodium salts of alginic acid and mannuronic and guluronic acids. Alginate dressings are available in fiber sheets or packing ribbon/strips and reportedly absorb 15–20 times their weight in wound fluid. When applied to a wound with adequate ambient wound exudate, the sodium ions in the exudate are exchanged for the calcium ions in the dressings, thereby forming a sodium alginate gel. This soft gel mass conforms intimately to the wound surface and creates a moist wound environment while continuing to absorb exudate until the dressing is saturated. As long as they remain moist, alginate dressings are atraumatically and painlessly removed from the wound bed. Occasionally, fibers from the alginate will adhere to the wound bed and require removal with soft debridement or sterile forceps, in which case another dressing may be more appropriate.

Calcium alginates are indicated for moderate to highly exudating wounds of all types. The frequency of dressing change is dependent on the amount of exudate. Copiously draining wounds may need daily changes while wounds with less drainage may be left in place up to 7 days. Calcium alginate dressings tend to wick fluid laterally; therefore, protection of the skin immediately adjacent to the wound is necessary if the alginate dressing extends beyond the wound edge (FIGURE 14-27). Calcium is known to act as a clotting factor (factor IV); therefore, alginate dressings may be used as a hemostatic agent for minimally bleeding wounds, for example, after debridement or in the case of low platelets. Alginate dressings require a secondary dressing to manage excess drainage, to hold the dressing against the wound bed, and to protect from external contaminants.

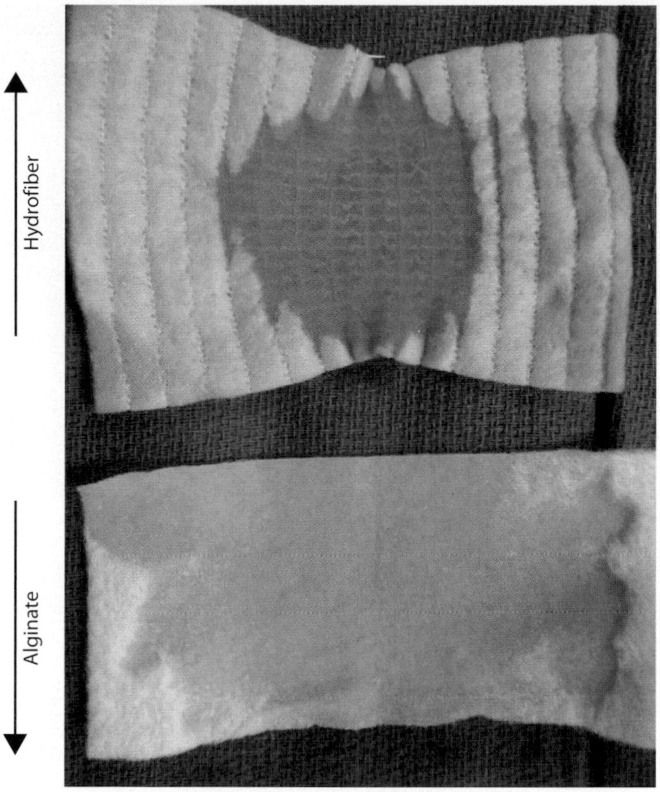

FIGURE 14-27 Wicking characteristics of different dressings. Alginates absorb, or wick, exudates horizontally, meaning that the fluid will spread throughout the entire dressing, as seen in the lower dressing. Gelling fibers (eg, cellulose) wick vertically, meaning the fluid is absorbed only by the dressing that is in contact with the wound bed. In order to avoid periwound maceration, an alginate dressing needs to be placed in the wound bed only, whereas a gelling fiber can extend over the wound edges without harming the periwound skin.

Gelling Fiber Dressings ***Gelling fiber*** dressings are soft, sterile dressings composed either of sodium carboxymethylcellulose or polyvinyl alcohol (PVA) fibers; they are also available as sheets or packing ribbons/ropes. Gelling fibers absorb large amounts of wound exudate, which transforms the dressing into a soft gel that creates a moist wound-healing environment and supports autolytic debridement. Gelling fibers are used in similar wounds as calcium alginates but are technically in a category by themselves due to their composition, features, and mechanism of action. They do tend to wick only vertically so that any excess dressing overlapping onto the periwound skin does not become wet with exudate. The nature of the dressing creates a soft, conformable gel mass that maintains intimate contact with the wound bed. Thus, if they adhere to a dry wound bed, they can be rehydrated and fairly easily removed. See TABLES 14-13 and 14-14 for advantages and disadvantages of these absorbent dressings (FIGURES 14-28 to 14-33).

CLINICAL CONSIDERAION

Gauze and gauze products are not covered specifically in this chapter because they are rather generic in nature. One example is the abdominal pad, a larger absorbent dressing used as a secondary wound cover over filler products to absorb exudate and provide padding for the wound (FIGURE 14-34).

TABLE 14-13 Advantages of Calcium Alginate and Hydrofiber Dressings

- Absorb large amounts of fluid
- Provide a moist environment once hydrated
- Facilitate autolytic debridement
- Conform to the wound bed; fill spaces, tracts, and undermined areas
- Provide protection from contamination
- Available in multiple flat sizes and ribbons/ropes
- Available with silver and honey for bioburden management

TABLE 14-14 Disadvantages/Considerations with Calcium Alginate and Hydrofiber Dressings

- Adhere to wound bed if exudate is inadequate to create gel effect
- Are not suitable for dry eschar or low exudating wounds
- Are not indicated for third-degree burns
- Require daily changes for an infected wound if the dressing is non-antimicrobial
- Require a secondary dressing

Super Absorbent Dressings

Superabsorbent dressings are multilayer wound covers that provide either a semiadherent or a nonadherent layer, combined with highly absorptive layers of fibers, such as cellulose, cotton, or rayon. Designed to minimize adherence to the wound and manage exudate, they may be used as a primary or secondary dressing to manage surgical incisions, lacerations, abrasions, burns, donor or skin graft sites, or any other type of exudating wound.

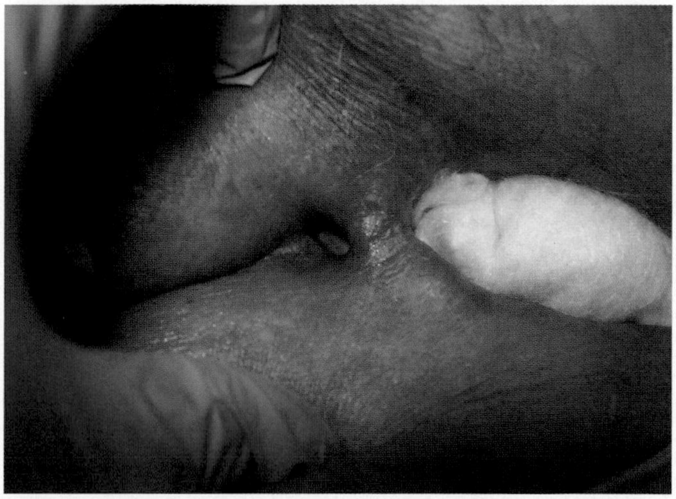

FIGURE 14-28 Calcium alginate. Calcium alginate dressings are excellent fillers for cavity wounds. They conform to the wound surface and do not tear easily upon removal.

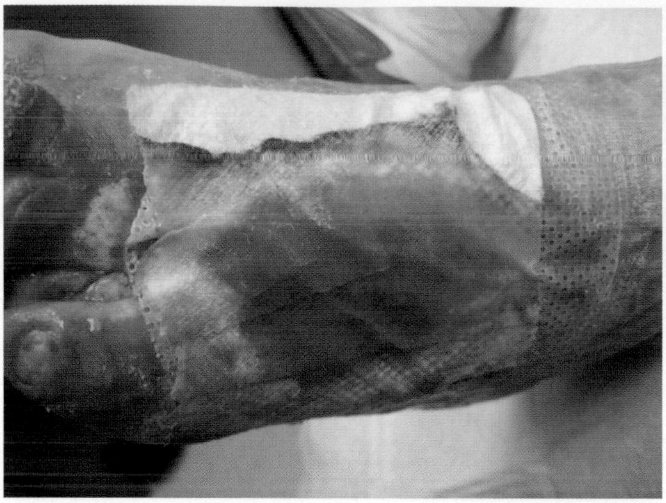

FIGURE 14-29 Calcium alginate with exudate. Calcium alginate on a wound with moderate exudate that is locked into the dressing fibers. Fluids on alginate dressings will wick laterally, meaning that the exudate will spread throughout the dressing. Thus, it is recommended that the dressing only touch the wound surface in order to protect the periwound skin.

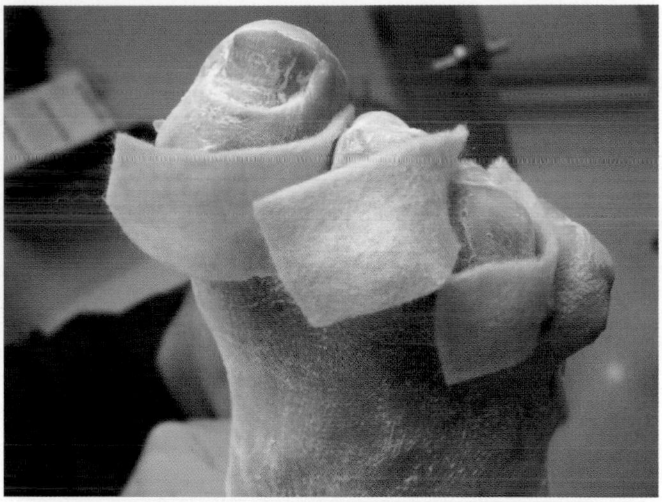

FIGURE 14-31 Gelling fiber used as a protective dressing. Strips of gelling fiber dressings are placed between toes to protect them from friction and to absorb any moisture, thereby preventing skin breakdown.

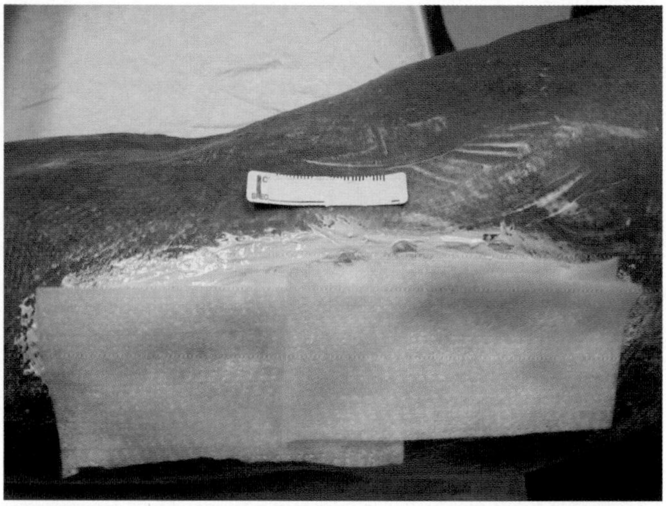

FIGURE 14-30 Gelling fiber dressing. Gelling fiber dressing on a wound with large amount of exudate. Gelling fibers tend to wick vertically, meaning the exudate will remain in the part of the dressing that covers the wound bed. A moisture barrier, as seen on the skin, will also help protect the periwound skin from maceration.

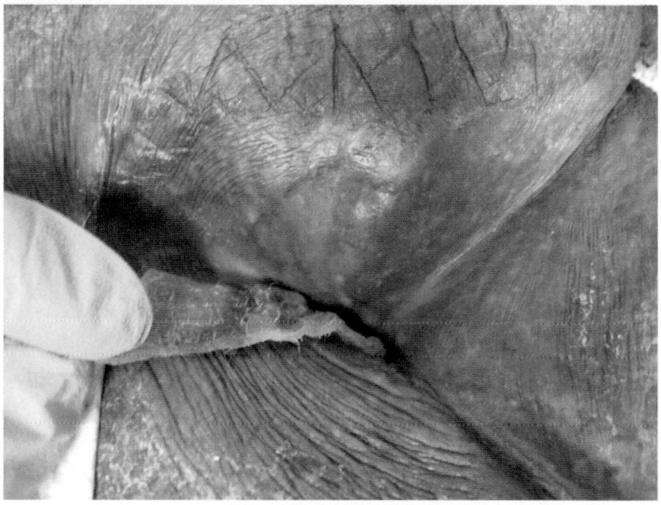

FIGURE 14-32 Removal of gelling fiber. Gelling fiber dressings come in ribbons (sometimes with threads interwoven to prevent tearing upon removal) that are ideal for wicking into tracking wounds.

Collagen Dressings

Collagen is the primary protein in human tissues and is necessary for wound healing and repair. Research about and evidence for the use of collagen dressings in wound healing has proliferated in recent years as the role of topically applied collagen has been better understood.[27] Because of its chemotactic effects, collagen plays an important role in each of the wound healing phases. It attracts cells needed for healing (eg, fibroblasts and keratinocytes) to the wound and then provides temporary scaffolding for these cells. Additionally, chronic wounds are known to have higher levels of matrix metalloproteases (MMPs) and a reduced number of MMP inhibitors (TIMPs). When MMPs are present in a wound bed at too high a level, for too long a time, and in the wrong places, they begin to degrade proteins that are not their normal substrates. This can result in "off-target" destruction of proteins (eg, growth factors, receptors, and ECM proteins that are essential for healing) and thus impair the healing process.[28,29] Adding topical collagen to a wound provides an alternate collagen source that can be degraded by the high levels of MMPs as a sacrificial substrate, leaving the endogenous native collagen to continue normal wound healing and to protect other proteins such as growth factors (**FIGURES 14-35** to **14-37**).[28,29]

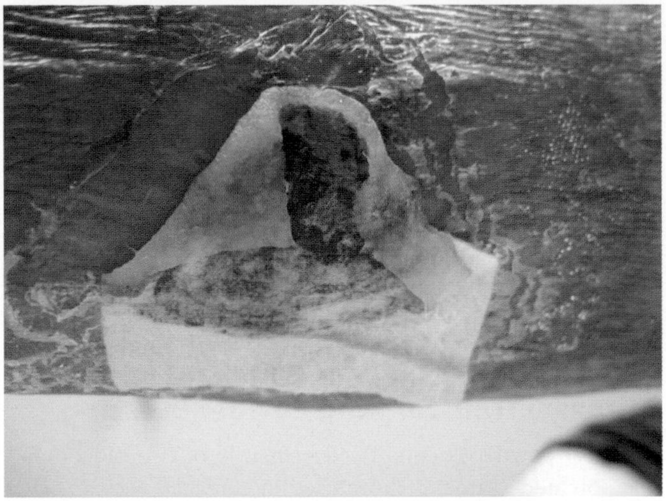

FIGURE 14-33 Removal of dry gelling fiber. Gelling fiber dressings that are allowed to dry onto the wound bed may cause tissue damage upon removal. Moistening the dressing before removal can prevent tissue damage as well as minimize pain with dressing changes.

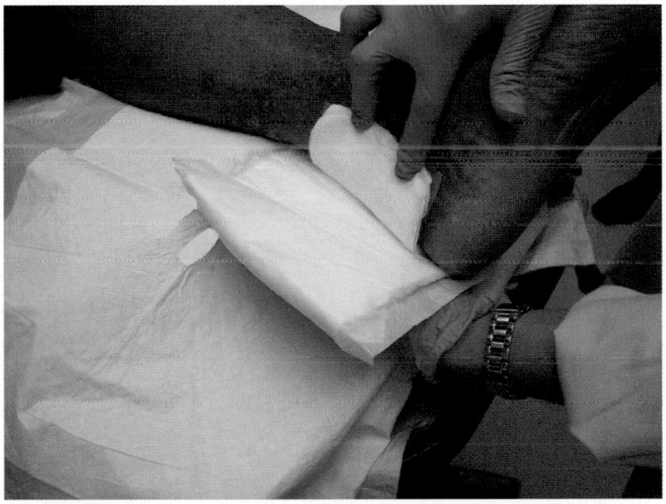

FIGURE 14-34 Absorptive pad. Thick cotton pads, commonly called abdominal or abd pads, are used for extra absorbency or padding over primary dressings. The outer layer is not appropriate to be in direct contact with any wound that has skin loss because it will adhere and tear tissue with removal. The abd pad may also be used under compression systems to pad bony prominences such as the tibia. Newer pads use construction similar to baby diapers in which the outer layer wicks to an inner absorbent layer without having any residual moisture on the skin.

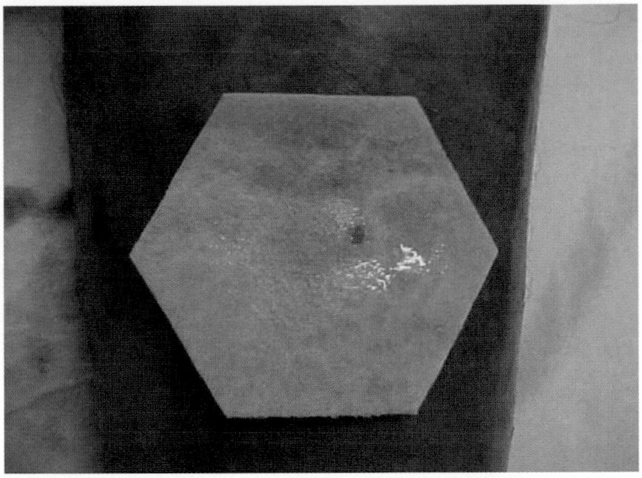

FIGURE 14-35 Collagen dressing. Collagen dressings may be 100% collagen or collagen combined with other materials such as calcium alginate or ORC. The collagen attracts cells needed for each phase of tissue repair and serves as temporary scaffolding for those cells to function.

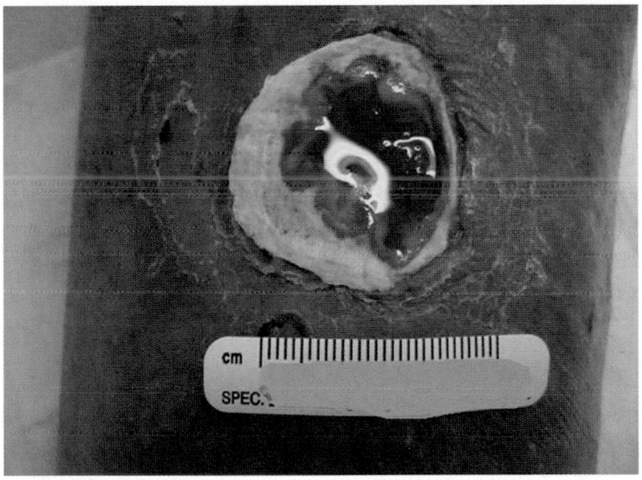

FIGURE 14-36 Collagen on a granulating wound bed. As the cells migrate to the wound and new tissue is synthesized, the collagen dressing is biodegraded, as visible in the center of this wound bed. The collagen attracts cells with which it is in contact; therefore, if epithelialization is the desired effect, the collagen needs to overlap the edges of the wound bed. Manufacturer's recommendations are advised when using any of the collagen products.

There are variations in collagen dressings, including the source from which the collagen is harvested. Collagen is basically the same regardless of the source; it can be derived from any animal source because there is no difference between species. Current collagen dressings are derived from bovine, porcine, ovine, or piscine sources and have been treated to make it nonantigenic. While most of the other categories of dressings are used to interact with wound fluid and impact moisture balance in some way, collagen dressings are not designed to manage moisture. Although some collagen dressings are powdered[30] and/or combined with additional material (eg, alginate) to provide some absorption, collagen dressings are intended to interact with the wound at the cellular level and are biodegradable; therefore, most have a minimal impact on fluid balance. Frequency of dressing change, which varies from 2 to 7 days, is dependent on the formulation of the collagen product and the amount of wound exudate. *Collagen*

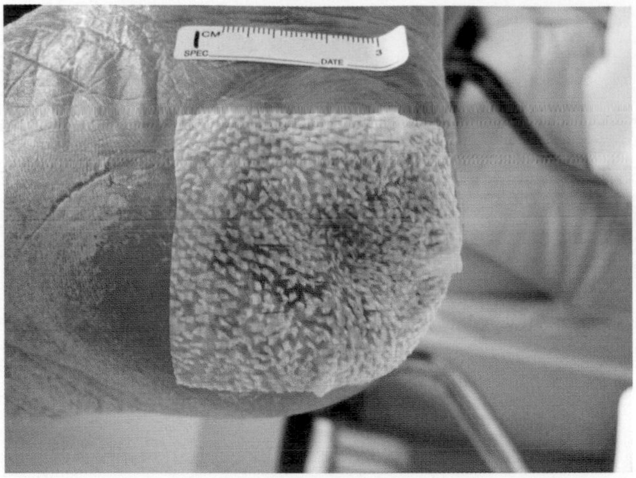

FIGURE 14-37 Collagen matrix on a wound bed. Products that are 100% collagen may not be visible when dressings are changed; however, collagen matrices that contain other products, for example, calcium alginate or ORC, will leave a residual that is removed with each dressing change.

products are used on clean wounds with minimal or no necrotic tissue. The collagen attracts the cells to which it is adjacent, so if epithelial migration is the goal, the dressing needs to connect with the skin at the edge of the wound. Most products are more effective if moistened with normal saline at the time of application and are covered with a secondary dressing that will prevent desiccation of the material. Manufacturers' instructions are advised for optimal results with each product. Advantages and disadvantages of collagen dressings are listed in **TABLES 14-15** and **14-16**, respectively.

Miscellaneous Dressings

The previously described dressing categories are the more standard, with multiple sizes, types, and brands within each category. Knowledge of the category functions enables the clinician to understand combination dressings (also referred to as *composites*), which have attributes of more than one dressing type and serve to be all inclusive. Combination dressings manage exudate as well as provide absorption, coverage, and security. They may be as simple as a transparent film or adhesive sheet with a central pad for coverage and minimal exudate absorption, or as complex as an antimicrobial gelling fiber with a bordered foam covering. These dressings tend to be more expensive, but can be cost-effective if both the frequency of changing the dressing and the time for wound closure are reduced.

Other dressings fall into "stand-alone" categories and are unique in their attributes and mechanism of action. The following are a few of these specialty dressings.

TABLE 14-15 Advantages of Collagen Dressings

▪ Bind MMPs, thereby potentially impacting wound healing, providing temporary scaffolding, and attracting cells to wound site
▪ Create moist environment after interaction with wound fluid
▪ Are easy to apply
▪ Provide cost-effective advanced wound care

TABLE 14-16 Disadvantages/Considerations with Collagen Dressings

▪ Are not recommended for third-degree burns
▪ Are not effective on necrotic tissue; require a clean wound bed
▪ May not be appropriate for patients with sensitivity or cultural restrictions relative to the use of bovine or porcine products.
▪ Require a secondary dressing

Altrazeal Transforming Powder Dressing

Altrazeal powder is comprised primarily of two biocompatible polymers (same as those used in contact lenses).[31] Upon hydration, Altrazeal granules aggregate to form a moist, oxygen-permeable barrier that protects the wound from contamination while helping to manage excess exudate through vapor transportation. Once applied, Altrazeal may be left in place for up to 30 days. Additional powder may be added ("topped off") as needed without requiring primary dressing changes. Simple secondary dressings may be used in areas of high friction or exudation. If clinically necessary, the dressing may be removed atraumatically by lifting off with a pair of forceps. As the wound heals, Altrazeal dries and flakes off (**FIGURE 14-38**).

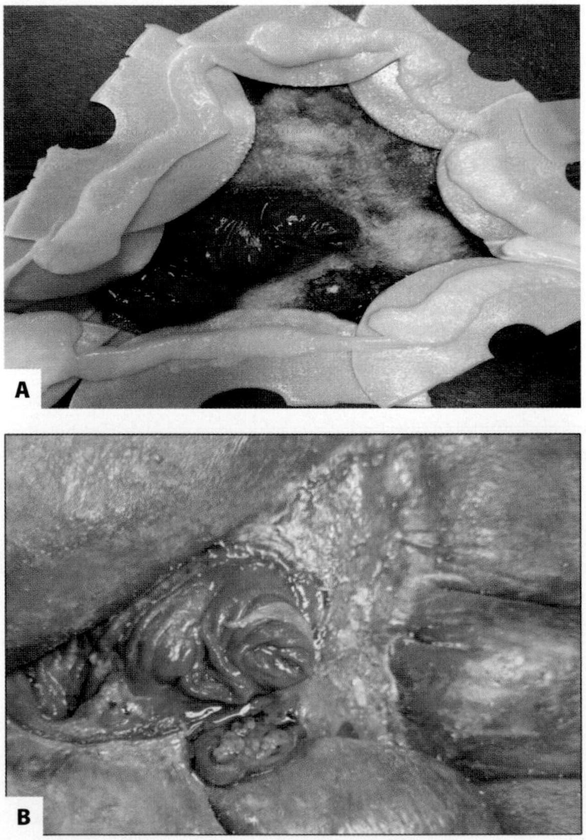

FIGURE 14-38 A. Initial application transforming powder dressing (TPD). B. 61 Days post initial TPD application.

Procellera[32] Numerous physical modalities have been used in attempts to augment the healing process, including ultrasound, low-energy light therapy, and electrical stimulation. There is good clinical evidence supporting the use of electrical stimulation; it has been shown to benefit tissue repair in a variety of wound types and is used extensively for multiple indications in the practice of physical therapy (see Chapter 16, Electrical Stimulation). Procellera (Vomaris Wound Care, Inc., Chandler, AZ) is a unique antimicrobial wound dressing with wireless microcurrent technology that provides an advanced wound healing solution for the management of wounds. Silver and zinc are applied on the device surface in a dot matrix pattern, creating multiple microbatteries.[32] In the presence of moisture, which may come from wound exudate or exogenously applied saline or hydrogel, low-level microcurrents are generated at the device surface. These reactions occur without an external power source or accessories. Procellera antimicrobial dressing is indicated for partial- and full-thickness wounds such as pressure injuries, venous ulcers, diabetic ulcers, burns, surgical incisions, donor and/or recipient graft sites, and so forth.[33,34] The dressing may be left in place for up to 7 days; more frequent dressing changes may be needed with high exudate levels (**FIGURES 14-39** and **14-40**).

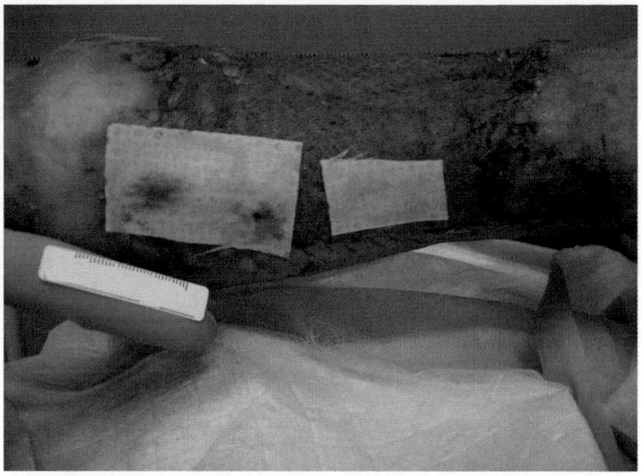

FIGURE 14-40 The Procellera dressing needs moisture to activate the microcurrent mechanism; thus, it can be moistened prior to application or placed on a wound with some fluid. In this photo, it is moistened and placed on a split thickness skin graft that has small areas of nontake that need re-epithelialization. The microcurrent will attract epithelial cells by electrotaxis.

Enluxtra Self-Adaptive Dressing[35] The Enluxtra Self-Adaptive Wound Dressing (Osnovative Systems, Inc., Santa Clara, CA) adapts to continuously changing wound conditions and emerging requirements that may have been unknown or unpredictable when the dressing was first applied. The dressing material is designed to change its properties according to the feedback from underlying wound tissues. Thus, the dressing dynamically balances the evolving moist wound environment and provides hydration or absorption depending on the instantaneous needs of wound and periwound skin. Dry areas of the wound stay properly hydrated, fluid from exuding areas is absorbed and locked in, and periwound skin is protected from maceration. The dressing is indicated for all wound types and all exudate levels and is changed based on the amount of exudate; however, it may be left in place for up to 7 days (**FIGURE 14-41**).

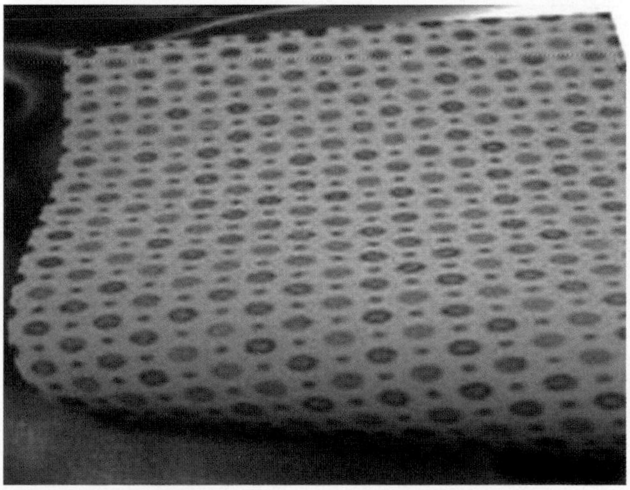

FIGURE 14-39 Procellera. Procellera, a dressing that provides electrical microcurrent stimulation to the wound bed, has small dots of silver and zinc that create the microbatteries when they are activated by moisture.

Biologics

The field of wound care began a journey into the use of biological devices beginning in the late 1990s, and there has been a significant expansion in options for actively enhancing the wound healing process. The plethora of available wound dressings balance the local wound milieu to create an ideal environment for wound healing, but with the exception of collagen,[28,29] these specialty dressings do not directly interact with cells or impact cellular activity.

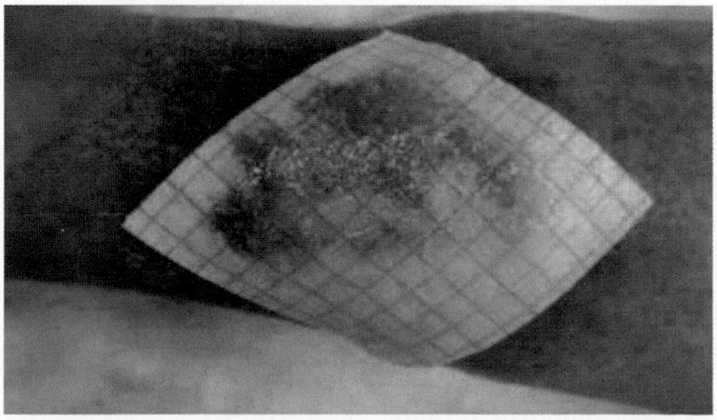

FIGURE 14-41 Enluxtra. Enluxtra is a specialty primary dressing that can both absorb excess moisture and rehydrate dry tissue. Note it also had a centimeter grid that can be used to measure the wound surface area.

A biologic is defined as a device or product that in its natural state is a contributor to the wound healing process and thereby manipulates the process when applied topically to an open wound. A consensus document to provide universal guidelines for the use of CTPs proposes a new name: cellular, acellular and matrix-like products (CAMPs) which are defined as "a broad category of biomaterials, synthetic materials, or biosynthetic matrices which support repair or regeneration of injured tissues through their influence on and modulation of the cellular and acellular activity within the host tissue."[36] This proposed name and definition reflects the innovations of the past two decades in biomaterial technology and distinguishes them from wound dressings.

The CAMP mechanisms of cellular influence on tissue healing include intracellular signaling, extracellular communication, and extracellular matrix activities, all of which are discussed in detail in Chapter 2, Healing Response in Acute and Chronic Wounds, and summarized in the consensus paper. Some of the products contain human cells or tissue in a variety of matrices and are used for soft tissue coverage and to facilitate wound closure. These products are derived from autologous (from the patient's own body), allogeneic (from a donor of the same species), synthetic, xenogeneic (from a different species), or a combination of these sources.

The materials used to produce CAMPs are derived from human (autograft or allograft) or animal (xenograft) tissue. The products, which may or may not include viable cells, undergo minimal to extensive processing to manufacture the finished product. Consequently, the extent of processing and the source of the material used in the product also determine the regulatory pathway required before the product can be marketed.[37]

There are over 80 CAMPs currently available, each with its own trade name and marketed for specific indications. These products can be used in any clinical settings and are indicted for hard-to-heal wounds, surgical wounds, reconstructive surgery, burns, traumatic wounds, and cosmetic procedures.[36] The bioengineered construct should meet the following essential criteria to be considered as optimal[38]:

- Provide protective functions: protect the wound from infectious agents, prevent fluid loss and accumulation by transmitting water in a way similar to normal skin, and help to withstand mechanical tensions and sheer forces.
- Provide an ideal environment for cell proliferation, differentiation, migration, and proper functions according to their porosity and morphological features.
- Carry minimal risk of adverse reactions.
- Be pliable and clinician friendly.
- Be stable and biodegradable.
- Have long shelf life and be easily stored.

Examples of CAMPs include acellular dermal matrix (ADM), which is derived from human or animal skin and used for soft tissue reconstruction, and platelet-rich plasma (PRP), which is derived from the patient's own blood and applied to the wound surface to facilitate wound healing and tissue regeneration. Other CAMPs include various types of collagen matrices, skin substitutes, and amniotic membrane products. Some of the more commonly used products are illustrated in **FIGURES 14-42** to **14-47**. General guidelines for the use of any CAMP are listed in **TABLE 14-17**. The early use of CAMPs has been shown to reduce hospital stays, reduce cost of care, and promote faster wound closure; thus, their use in wound care is becoming standard care in many cases.[39,40]

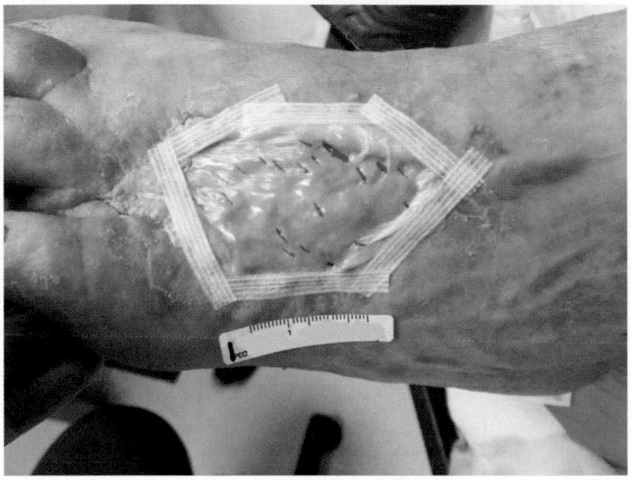

FIGURE 14-42 Apligraf. Apligraf is composed of bovine type 1 collagen with living fibroblasts and keratinocytes as well as structural proteins. It can be fenestrated to allow exudate to escape into a secondary dressing. Apligraf is applied to clean wound bed to create an environment where the living cells can deliver cytokines and growth factors that stimulate a healing response from the recipient tissue.

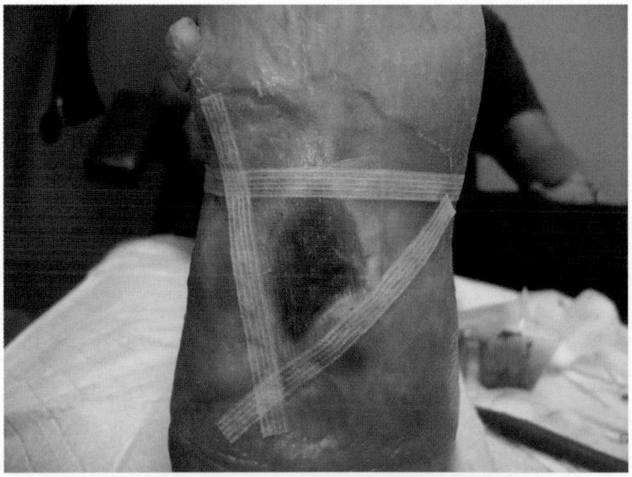

FIGURE 14-43 Dermagraft. Dermagraft is a dermal substitute that contains living fibroblasts, extracellular matrix, and a bioabsorbable polyglactin mesh scaffold. It is applied to a clean wound bed, anchored with Steri-Strips, a nonadherent contact layer, and a bolster dressing. Dermagraft is approved for diabetic foot ulcers and is used in conjunction with off-loading strategies and blood glucose control.

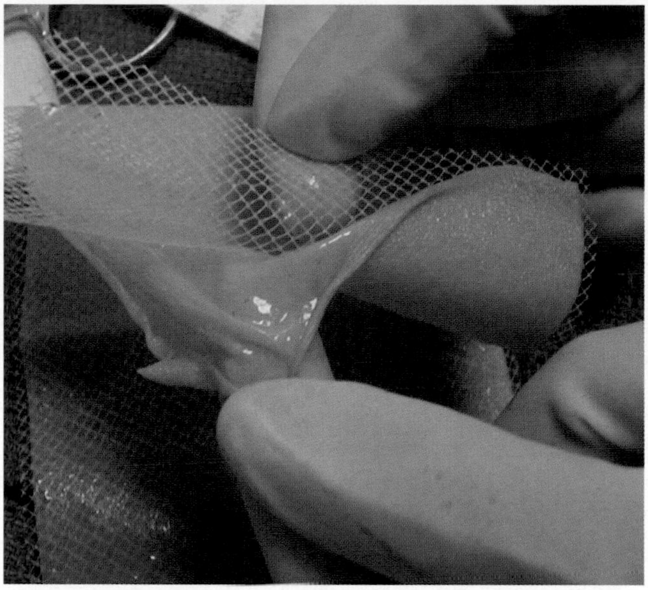

FIGURE 14-44 Allograft dressing. Allograft dressings are skin harvested from cadavers and are used to protect the wound bed and facilitate granulation while awaiting the optimal time for autologous skin grafting.

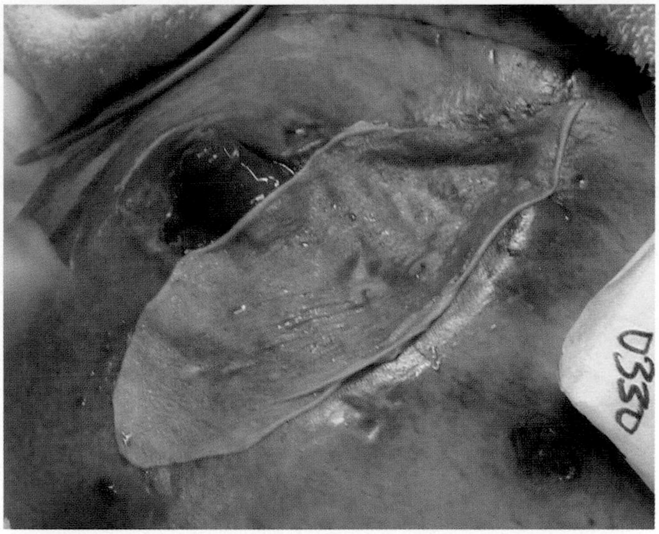

FIGURE 14-45 Allograft on a wound. Allograft has been placed on the abdominal wound with a fistula. When the patient is medically ready for resection of the fistula, an STSG will be used to cover the wound. In the meantime, the allograft helps protect the wound bed from fistula drainage.

Growth Factors

Growth factors (GFs) are small proteins produced by multiple cells and act as signals for intracellular communication. GFs specifically stimulate the migration and proliferation of cells, and thus the formation of new tissue.[41–43] Many cell types are involved in wound healing, including platelets, macrophages, and fibroblasts. Platelets are the first cellular components to invade the wound site and initiate the wound-healing process by releasing stored growth factors.

REGRANEX Gel[44] (Smith & Nephew, Fort Worth, Texas) is formulated with 0.01% becaplermin, a recombinant human platelet-derived growth factor (rh PDGF-BB), in aqueous sodium carboxymethylcellulose-based gel for topical application on a clean wound bed. REGRANEX i (the only FDA-approved topical agent with PDGF) promotes the recruitment and proliferation of chemotactic cells, thereby stimulating the wound-healing process and aiding formation of granulation tissue.

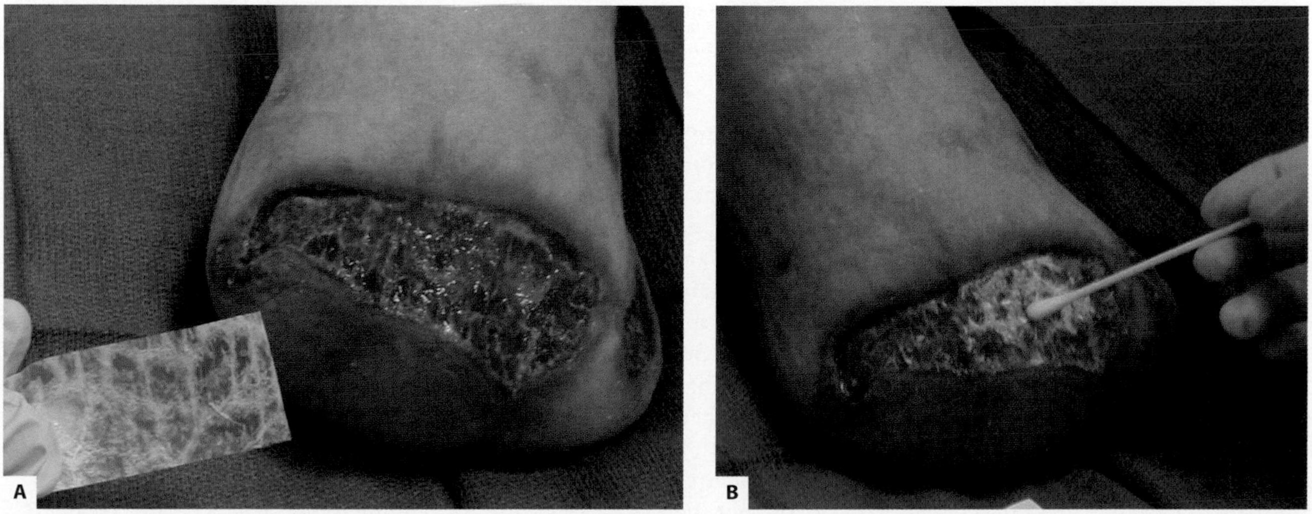

FIGURE 14-46 Oasis. Oasis (Smith & Nephew, Fort Worth, Texas) is a biological collagen dressing derived from porcine small intestine submucosa. **A.** The wound bed on a below-knee amputation stump is prepared, free of bacteria, and granulating. The patient is not a candidate for a skin graft because of impaired circulation in the stump; therefore, a collagen matrix is appropriate to facilitate granulation and epithelial migration. **B.** The collagen matrix is applied to the wound bed and moistened with sterile water, and covered with a secondary dressing.

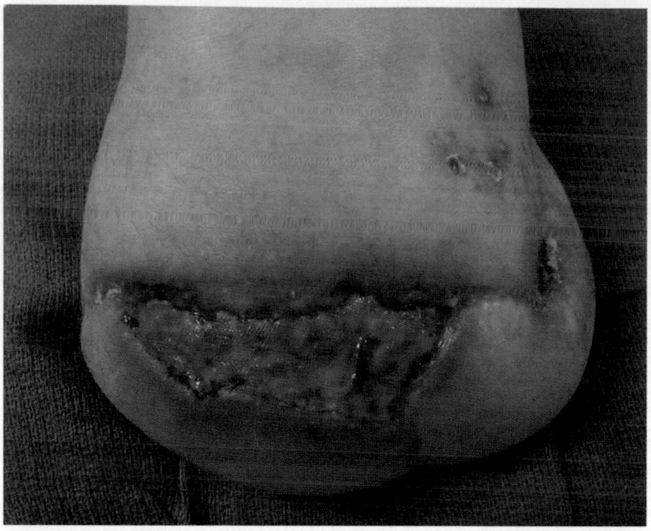

FIGURE 14-47 Oasis on the wound bed after 1 week. After 1 week, the dressing is removed, and although the wound bed appears to be covered with a thin layer of sloughs, it is actually the collagen matrix being resorbed by the wound bed and producing a scaffolding for the extracellular matrix. Note the re-epithelialization that has occurred at the proximal edge of the wound.

TABLE 14-17 Guidelines for the Use of Biologic Products[36]

▪ Complete a thorough patient assessment
▪ Manage any underlying comorbidities
▪ Complete a thorough wound assessment
▪ Achieve adequate wound bed preparation, including debridement of all non-viable tissue
▪ Adequately manage the bacterial load to prevent wound and product infection
▪ Include standard of care based on wound etiology (eg, off-loading the diabetic foot ulcer, revascularization of an arterial wound, compression of a venous wound, and pressure redistribution of a pressure injury)
▪ Provide patient/caregiver education on postapplication care, restrictions, and expectations

REGRANEX Gel[44] is indicated for the treatment of lower extremity diabetic ulcers that extend into the subcutaneous tissue or beyond and *have an adequate blood supply*.[45] It is an adjunct to, and not a substitute for, good wound care practices, and is contraindicated in patients with known neoplasm(s) at the site(s) of application. Additionally, malignancies distant from the site of application have been reported in both a clinical study and postmarketing use. Therefore, REGRANEX Gel should be used with caution in patients with known malignancy. Available by prescription only, REGRANEX is applied daily in a thin layer to a clean wound bed and covered with a moist dressing. Based on the clinical trials, the manufacturer recommends a second dressing change daily to reapply the moist dressing. In this author's experience, the second dressing change is not necessary as long as the wound bed can remain moist; however, this is considered off-label use and must be determined by the prescriber.

ANTIMICROBIAL DRESSINGS

Acute wounds in healthy patients with low comorbidities will usually progress through the wound healing cascade in a timely manner; however, a delay in healing and subsequent development of a chronic wound requires complex wound assessment and intervention. The changes associated with chronic wound development often involve alterations in one of the three primary categories: systemic and cellular changes, macrovascular or microvascular ischemia, and the negative effects of bacterial bioburden. These challenges highlight the fact that selection of one antimicrobial dressing, or any single therapeutic intervention, will not result in wound healing alone.[46] Instead, systemic management of known comorbidities and wound bed preparation are necessary to ready the wound bed for healing.

Sibbald et al.[47] first described the TIME model for wound bed preparation, which involves removal of devitalized **T**issue, reduction of **I**nfection/inflammation, **M**oisture management, and prevention of **E**dge rolling or epibole. There have since been new iterations of the TIME model. TIMERS is an acronym that stands for the six critical components of comprehensive care for patients with hard-to-heal wounds.[48] These components are:

- **T**issue refers to the quality and quantity of the tissue surrounding the wound.
- **I**nflammation/Infection refers to the presence of inflammation and/or infection in and around the wound.
- **M**oisture Balance refers to the proper balance of moisture in the wound bed.
- **E**dges refers to the condition of the wound edges, which should be free from any signs of maceration or necrosis, and the removal of senescent cells.
- **R**epair/Regeneration refers to the body's ability to repair and regenerate the tissue around the wound.
- **S**ocial Factors refer to the social, emotional, and economic factors that may impact the patient's ability to care for their wound and/or their overall health.

By considering all of these components, healthcare providers can develop a comprehensive and effective care plan for patients with hard-to-heal wounds.

The wound clinician approaches wound bed preparation holistically and determines the amount and type of debridement necessary, the methods by which to reduce bioburden and proinflammatory local wound mediators, and the optimal dressings to maintain adequate moisture levels and normothermia as well as to provide adequate wound filling. Each decision involves an evaluation of the available evidence, professional experience, and availability of the patient resources to obtain and provide the necessary care.

The use of antimicrobial wound care products has received a great deal of scrutiny with some literature suggesting there is no evidence for the use of these products in wound care. However, it is important to understand that the selection of an antimicrobial agent is *not* meant to bring about wound healing.[49] An antimicrobial dressing may be selected for treatment or palliation in order to accomplish any of the following:

- Reduce the bacterial burden of a wound.
- Decrease pain associated with care.
- Diminish wound odor.
- Potentially prevent the formation of bacterial biofilm.

An important potential benefit of antimicrobial dressings is to reduce the use of systemic antibiotic therapy that is prone to bacterial resistance. Landis et al.[50] state that one in four persons with a chronic wound receives antibiotic therapy at any given time and that over 60% have received these medications in the last 6 months. The overuse and abuse of antibiotics reflect the lack of practitioner knowledge surrounding proper management of complex chronic wounds. With these concepts in mind, it is necessary to examine the levels of bacterial influence in the wound milieu, the products available for bacterial control, and how topical antimicrobial agents can be utilized appropriately.

Infection in humans is generally the result of bacteria, fungi, viruses, or protozoa.[51] The term bioburden is utilized in varying connotations to refer to the effect of organisms within a wound bed that influence wound healing. All chronic wounds have some level of bacterial bioburden; however, the presence of bacteria does not indicate infection. Historically levels of bacterial presence on a wound surface have been described as contaminated, colonized, critically colonized, and then infected. Newer terminology has eliminated the term critical colonization to more accurately describe bacterial growth on and in a wound. The International Wound Infection Institute published an updated Consensus document (**IWII CD**) more explicitly describing the wound infection continuum.[52]

The updated terms used to describe the continuum of bacterial growth in and on wounds include contamination, colonization, local infection, spreading infection, and systemic infection. The definitions of these terms are presented in **TABLE 14-18** and illustrated in **FIGURE 14-48**.

Wounds are assessed for etiology, quality, and amount of granulation tissue, percentage of nonviable tissue present, condition of the wound edges, presence and amount of exudate, total surface area, and presentation of the surrounding intact skin. While acute infection in a healthy individual displays the classic signs and symptoms of erythema, induration, edema, pain, suppuration, and fever, these findings are often either reduced or absent in the patient with poor perfusion or an incompetent immune system.[50] However, the clinician again must utilize keen assessment skills because subtle changes in wound bed appearance may represent alterations in nutrition, inappropriate systemic or local inflammatory states, inadequate perfusion, or medications, all of which may mimic changes seen with an increase in bioburden.

Biofilm

For years topical application and systemic administration of antibiotics have been utilized because of their bactericidal effects on planktonic bacteria, defined as free-living bacteria that grow independently in a laboratory flask or dish. They are hydrophilic and have cell walls that can be eliminated by the host's immune system or targeted antimicrobial dressing. However, some bacteria and fungi have the capability of inducing a radical change in their phenotype following attachment to the wound surface. Biofilms are complex microbial communities consisting of multiple species of bacteria and fungi. Unlike planktonic bacteria, biofilm microorganisms attach firmly to surfaces using a matrix composed mainly of polysaccharide chains and bacterial DNA. Biofilms are dynamic and constantly changing in response to the surrounding environment and begin with reversible attachment of free-floating bacteria to a surface. As they multiply, they become firmly attached and produce quorum molecules. When the concentration of quorum molecules reaches a certain threshold, it triggers gene expression changes which in turn lead to the synthesis and secretion of the protective exopolymeric matrix, distinguishing biofilm bacteria from planktonic bacteria. Bacteria in biofilms have protective advantages provided by the polymicrobial community. The biofilm matrix defends against predators, such as viruses and amoebae, and reduces the impact of neutrophils, macrophages, antibodies, reactive oxygen species, and disinfectants. Metabolically quiescent bacteria in biofilms, called persister bacteria, are highly tolerant to antibiotics that target actively dividing bacteria.

TABLE 14-18 Classification of Bacterial Burden on a Wound[52]

Contamination—microorganisms are present not actively multiplying; they do not interfere with healing nor activate a host reaction. Innate phagocytosis helps eliminate the microorganisms.
Colonization—the presence of microorganisms in a wound without causing a significant host reaction or delaying wound healing. Virulence is low even though there may be some replication. These microorganisms can come from the external environment or be introduced through exogenous sources.
Local infection—microorganisms are present and multiplying within a wound, causing a response from the host and potentially delaying wound healing. Local infection is confined to the wound and the immediate area around it (within 2 cm); may have subtle signs and symptoms that are not immediately recognized as indications of infection.
Spreading infection—(also known as cellulitis) infective microorganisms from a wound invade and proliferate in the surrounding tissue, extending beyond the wound border; may involve deep tissue, muscles, fascia, organs, or body cavities.
Systemic infection—microorganisms from a localized infection spread throughout the body via the bloodstream or lymphatic system triggering a host response that affects the entire body. In the case of wound infection, microorganisms can spread from the infected wound to cause a systemic infection. A systemic inflammatory response can also be triggered by a local wound infection through other pathways, such as the release of toxins or an impaired immune system.

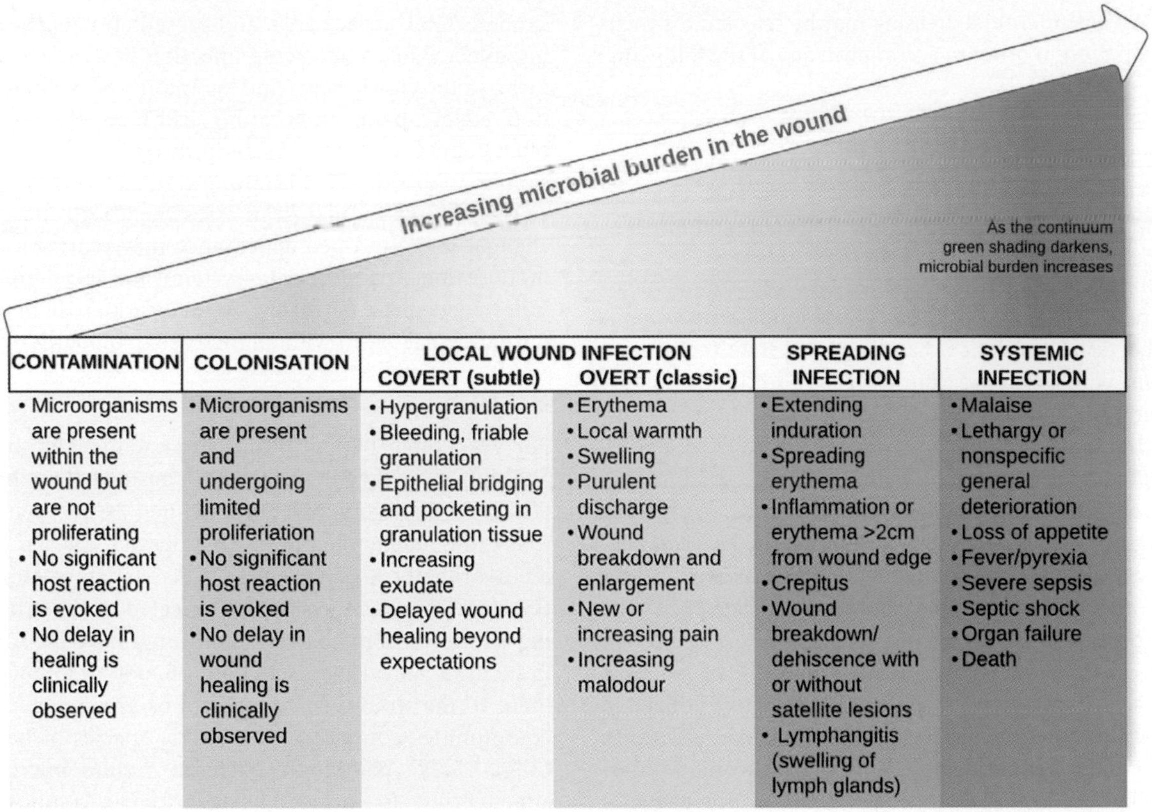

FIGURE 14-48 Illustration of bacterial continuum on a wound.

The formation of polymicrobial biofilms allows bacteria to survive in conditions that typically kill planktonic bacteria. Bacterial biofilms can form both on the surface and beneath the surface of chronic wound beds. Scanning electron microscopy (SEM) shows the presence of biofilm communities on the surface of punch biopsies taken from chronic wounds. Measurements reveal that Pseudomonas aeruginosa biofilm aggregates form at an average depth of 50–60 μm, while *Staphylococcus aureus* aggregates form at an average depth of 20–30 μm beneath the surface of wound beds. It is important to note that biofilms are not evenly distributed across the wound bed. Effective removal of biofilms from chronic wounds requires procedures that address both surface and subsurface biofilm aggregates.[53]

The development of bacterial biofilm results in a chronic state of inflammation for the host and cannot be removed with the routine use of wound cleansing or antibiotics. In fact, the minimum concentrations of many antibiotics needed to eliminate a biofilm may be thousands of times the standard dose and exceeds the maximum prescription dose available.[54,55] While biofilms are microscopic in size, the bedside clinician may suspect the presence of biofilm-encased bacterium in 90% of nonhealing chronic wounds.[56,57] Additionally, when the biofilm grows undeterred it may exhibit surface changes further causing suspicion, such as a slimy surface indicating the biofilm contribution to sustained, chronic inflammation (**FIGURE 14-49**).

The inability to remove biofilms through systemic antibiotics and topical antimicrobial therapies highlights the need for wound hygiene at each dressing change, including

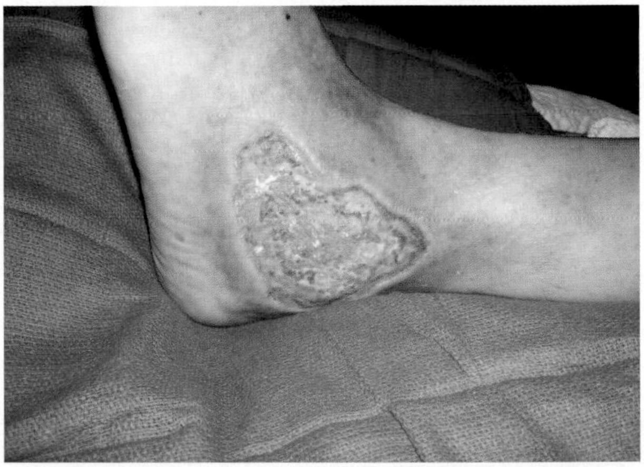

FIGURE 14-49 Biofilm on a chronic wound. The yellow layer on a chronic wound (present more than 3 years on this patient) is an indication of critical colonization and the presence of biofilm. The film cannot be removed with normal cleansing and requires some type of debridement to remove. Other signs that indicate the presence of biofilm are pain, drainage, and periwound erythema, all a result of the chronic inflammatory state that is caused by the biofilm.

cleansing of the wound bed and 10–20 cm of the periwound skin,[58] as well as repetitive and multimodal debridement.[57,59] Components of wound hygiene are illustrated in **TABLE 14-19**.

With specific biofilm-based infections, such as chronic osteomyelitis or prosthetic implant infection, wound healing may not be possible with surface debridement and antimicrobial agents alone. While acute osteomyelitis may resolve

TABLE 14-19 Wound Hygiene at Each Dressing Change

Activities of Wound Hygiene	
Cleanse the wound and periwound skin	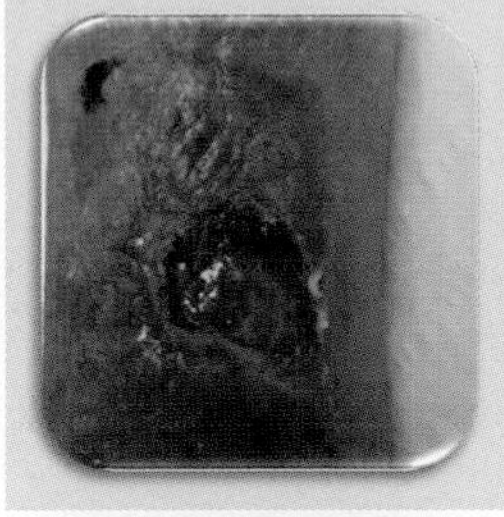 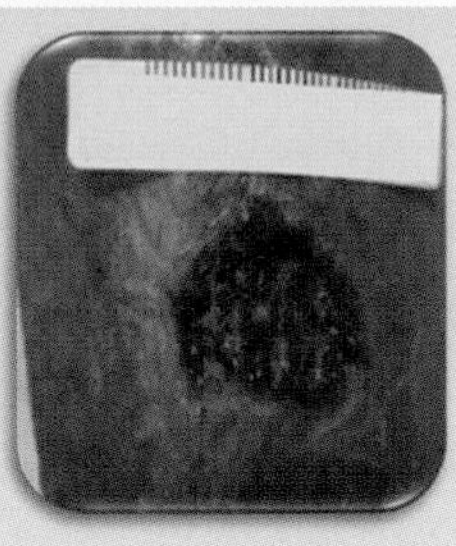
Debride	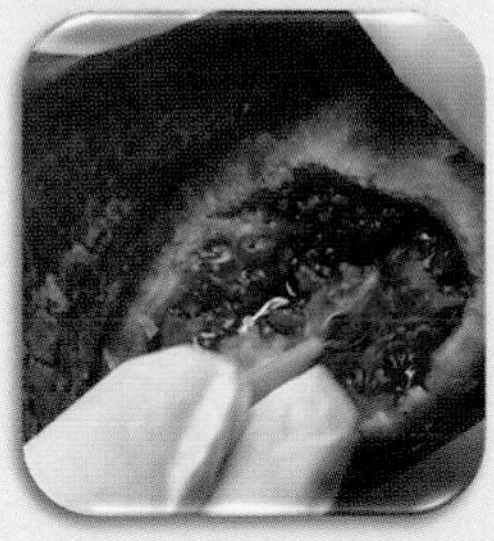
Refashion the wound edges	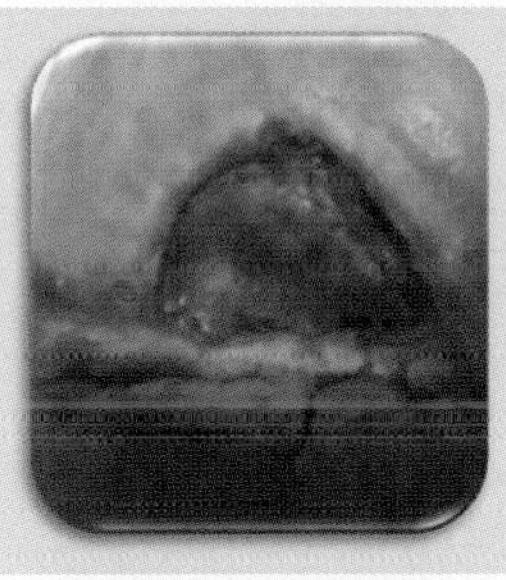 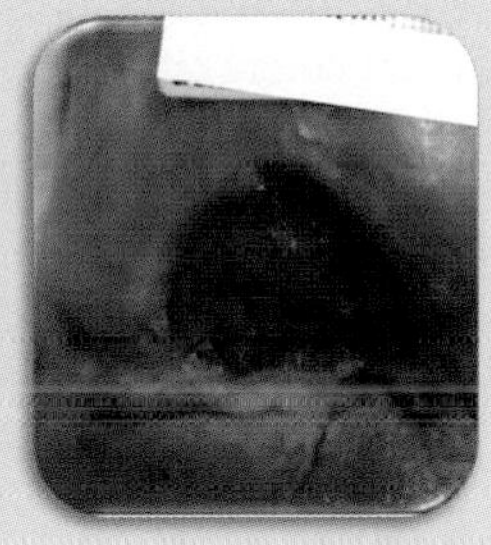
Dress the wound	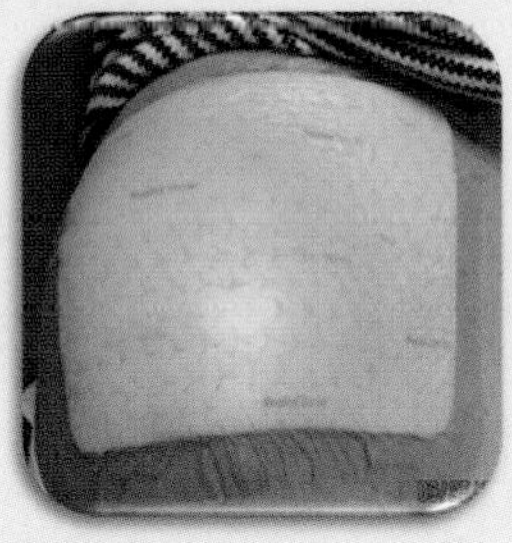

with early identification and antibiotic therapy, recalcitrant osteomyelitis results from poor tissue perfusion that fails to supply antibiotics, as well as biofilm formation. Removal of the infected bone and/or the prosthetic implant is necessary, as described in detail by Roy and colleagues.[60] Exposed bone in a hard-to-heal wound has been shown to have a positive likelihood ratio (LR) of 9.2 for osteomyelitis, and the finding of a jagged feel to the bone when probed has been shown to carry a prevalence of over 60%.[61] While imaging studies remain the primary diagnostic, laboratory data including erythrocyte sedimentation rate (ESR) can be used to diagnose osteomyelitis in DFUs, especially when the result is over 70 mm/h.[61] However, the clinical finding of exposed bone in an open wound indicates the need for more vigilance (**FIGURE 14-50A–C**).

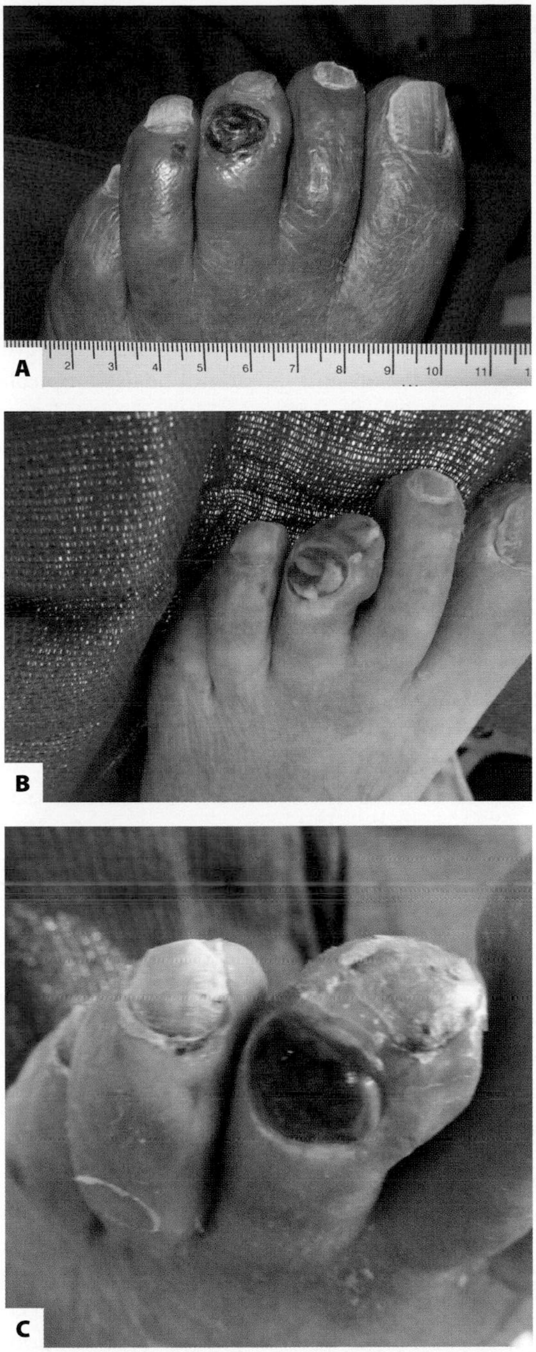

FIGURE 14-50 Wounds with osteomyelitis. A. The arterial wound on the digit is treated first with revascularization by a stent in the femoral artery. The ischemic wound at this point is suspected for osteomyelitis by the sausage appearance of the toe and palpation of bone in the eschar. Topical antimicrobial dressings are indicated while tests to confirm the diagnosis are planned. **B.** Two weeks after receiving the stent, the eschar has been debrided and exposed bone is visible, along with loss of the joint stability, resulting in rotation of the distal phalanx. Osteomyelitis has been confirmed and treatment with antibiotics was initiated. **C.** As a result of the osteomyelitis and the resulting inflammation in the bone, shards of cortical bone have been removed from the open wound with resulting granulation of the soft tissue. The distal phalanx will probably need amputation in order for the patient to fully close and resume wearing adaptive shoes.

Categories and Considerations for Antimicrobial Use

The term antimicrobial is an umbrella term that refers to disinfectants, antibiotics, antiseptics, antivirals, antifungals, and antiparasitics.[62]

Disinfectants

Disinfectants are chemicals that are used primarily to kill microorganisms on surfaces or devices and are an integral part of infection control in medical facilities; however, they are harmful to humans and should not be used topically or in open wounds. While the active agents in these solutions may be familiar to other topical antiseptics, the pH, concentration, and chemical additives warrant that they should never be used for wound care.

Antibiotics

Antibiotics have decreased in popularity as first-line treatments for management in wound care secondary to the rise of bacterial resistance. While the method of action varies, antibiotics generally have one defined target, thereby limiting their effectiveness against multiple pathogens.[63] Systemic antibiotics should be avoided unless there is evidence of true clinical infection; topical antibiotics are similarly avoided when treating infections because they may cause hypersensitivity reaction, lead to super infections, and encourage resistance.[64] Antibiotics are not to be abandoned, rather reserved for situations where advancing clinical infection is present, highly virulent organisms exist in the wound bed, or the host's immune response is severely compromised, such as in diabetic foot infections.

Antiseptics

Topical antiseptics are antimicrobial agents that reduce the number of microorganisms and are an adjunct to infection control. Whereas antibiotics have a specific method of action, antiseptics utilize multiple targets to inhibit or kill organisms and have a larger spectrum of activity against bacteria, fungi, and viruses. Categories of antiseptics include alcohols (ethanol), anilides (triclocarban), biguanides (chlorhexidine), bisphenols (triclosan), choline compounds, iodine compounds, silver compounds, peroxygens, and quaternary ammonium compounds.[46] These compounds may be in hand soaps, presurgical skin preparations, and some wound cleansers. The use of antiseptics in the open wound has previously been viewed with great scrutiny due to the risks of cytotoxicity and the potential for repetitive tissue trauma during their use[65]; however, this greatly depends on which product is used and more importantly, *how* it is used. For example, most experts agree that continuously packing a wound with dressing materials saturated in cytotoxic antiseptics is not appropriate wound care; however, the short-term use of an antiseptic as part of wound irrigation is often found to be very effective in decreasing the bacterial load so that healing can progress. Cytotoxic effects can occur with many approved topicals, including silver, but detrimental effects are generally a result of exposure time and overall concentration.[66] Generally, antiseptics are used when the clinician perceives the need to reduce the level of bioburden as a priority or visualizes signs of infection; however, discontinuing the solution is advised as soon as granulation tissue is visible in the wound bed.

CLINICAL CONSIDERATION

Antiseptics with high potential for cytotoxicity include dyes (scarlet red and proflavine), sodium hypochlorite (Dakin solution), hydrogen peroxide, and quaternary ammonia-centrimide. Hydrogen peroxide is associated with air emboli if used in deep cavities, and quaternary ammonium compounds have the most tissue toxicity.[67]

CLINICAL CONSIDERATION

The ideal wound cleansing agent has the following characteristics: is nonirritating, is noncytotoxic, has a slightly acidic pH (3.5–5.5), and if effective, controls odor.

Antiseptics may also be utilized for specific wounds, such as large total body surface area burns that are prone to detrimental colonization from a variety of organisms that can lead to sepsis, a leading cause of morbidity and mortality. However, guidelines by the US Health and Human Services historically recommend these products not be used in pressure injuries and suggest alternatives such as normal saline.[68] Compromise can be reached in these differing opinions as newer noncytotoxic antiseptics are available, such as superoxide water solutions, polyhexamethylene biguanide (PHMB) solutions, diluted and stabilized sodium hypochlorites, and hypochlorous acid. These products provide the benefits of bioburden reduction without injury to the host cells.

Systematic reviews have failed to identify evidence to recommend one specific cleansing solution or technique for wound management over another;[69] however, a best practice statement for the use of topical antiseptics and antimicrobial agents in wound care[49] agreed that there are clinically justified circumstances when antiseptics can be utilized for well-defined, short-term periods, and as part of a wound care plan that involves serial debridement and biofilm prevention/removal strategies. *How* a wound is irrigated

CLINICAL CONSIDERATION

Syringe/Needle Combination Pressures

Syringe Size	Needle/ Anglo (gauge)	Pressure (psi)
35	25	4
35	21	6
35	19	8
20	18	12
12	22	13
12	19	20
6	19	20

Data from Stevenson TR, Thacker JG, Rodeheaver GT, Bacchetta C, Edgerton MT, Edlich RF. Cleansing the traumatic wound by high pressure syringe irrigation. *JACEP*. 1976;5(1):17-21; Shetty R, Paul MK, Barreto E, Sreekar H, Dawre S. Syringe-based wound irrigating device. *Indian J Plast Surg*. 2012;45(3):590-591; White W, Asimus M. Chapter 8: Assessment and management of nonviable tissue. In: Swanson T, Asimus M, McGuiness W, eds. *Wound Management for the Advanced Practitioner*. 2014, IP Communications.

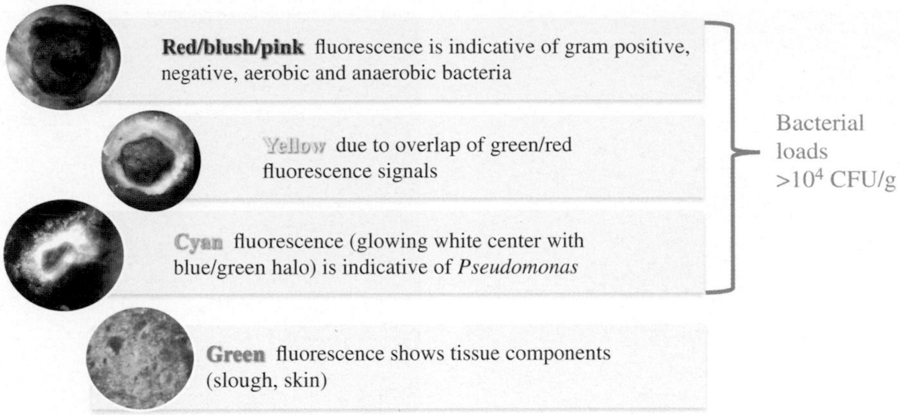

FIGURE 14-51 Understanding fluorescent signals.

and cleansed needs careful attention, and not just with *what* it is cleansed. Simply dripping any solution onto a wound bed does not disrupt bacteria and detritus from the wound surface. Enough force, either through the use of scrubbing with gauze or a cleansing pador through irrigation with an adequate pounds per square inch (PSI) force, is required to dislodge unwanted elements from the wound surface. A common recommendation for effective wound irrigation involves the use of a 35 ml syringe and a 19-gauge angiocath combination to result in a PSI of 8.[70]

Fluorescence imaging has demonstrated the following concepts about wound cleansing:

- Significant levels of bacteria contaminate the periwound skin; therefore, it is recommended to cleanse 10–20 cm outside of the wound bed, or at least where the previous dressing was covering the skin.
- Callus and macerated skin harbor significant levels of bacteria.
- Gauze pads quickly become contaminated with bacteria from cleansing and thus should be changed out frequently.

FIGURES 14-51 to **14-54** illustrate these points with fluorescence imaging.

Topical-Antimicrobial Wound Dressings

Selection of a wound care dressing is based on criteria other than reduction of bioburden. The decision and selection are multifactorial, with the clinician asking these questions:

- Which dressing will best manage the exudate or moisture level?
- Which dressing will require the least frequent changes?
- Which dressing will minimize patient pain with removal?
- Which dressing will cause the least amount of trauma to the wound bed?
- Which dressing will most adequately fill the wound dead space?
- Does the patient have any history of allergic reactions?
- Is an antimicrobial necessary?

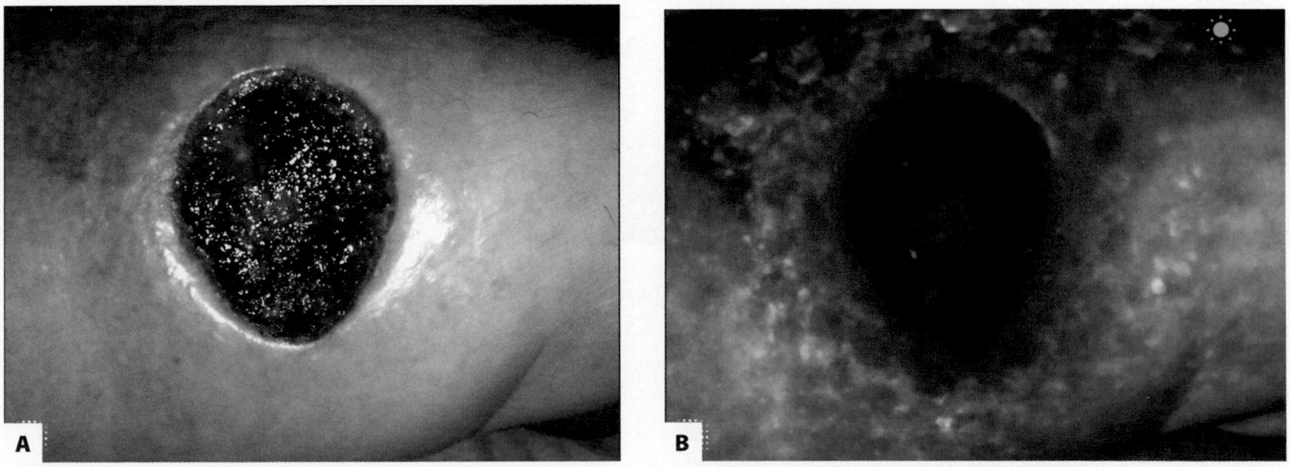

FIGURE 14-52 A, B. Contamination of the periwound skin.

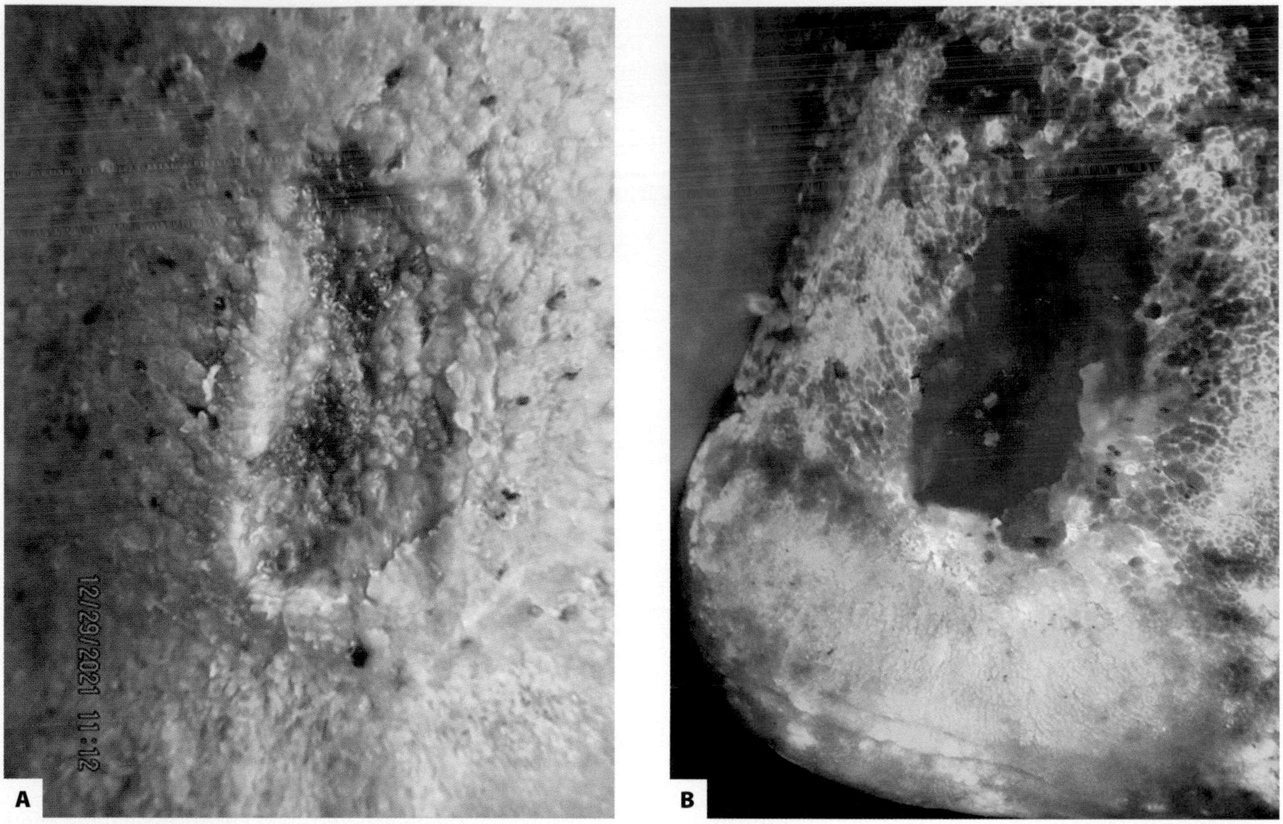

FIGURE 14-53 A, B. Macerated skin harbors a great deal of bacteria.

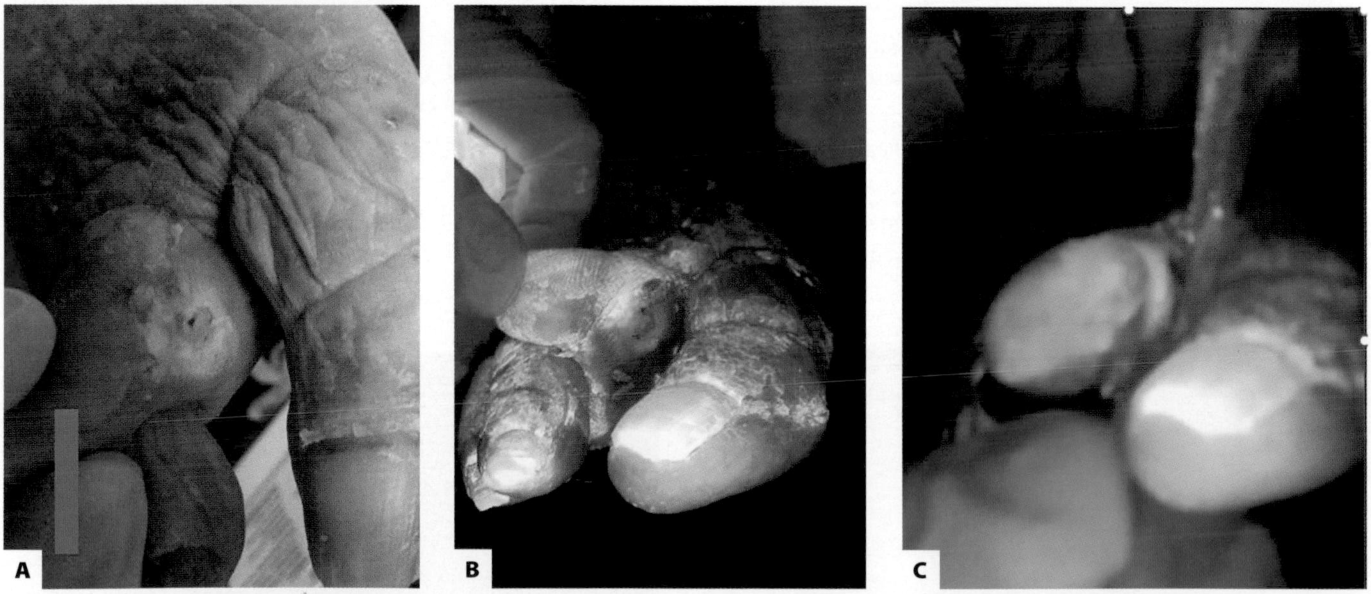

FIGURE 14-54 A–C. Cleansing between toes, showing contamination of gauze. Fluorecence imaging illustrates the bacterial contamination on gauze used to clean between the patient's toes.

- Can the patient afford these dressings after discharge if they are not covered by insurance?
- Can the patient return to the clinic for routine dressing changes and wound assessment?
- What has been the wound response to previously used dressings?
- Which dressing is needed to fill undermining and sinuses?

In some cases, the antimicrobial selected is related to its known effect against certain pathogens. In other cases, selection is more related to the dressing construct and delivery method of the agent into the wound, and how it manages the other considerations listed above. The decision may be made based on the clinician's personal experience with a particular agent in the specific wound type that is being assessed. Finally, any patient allergies need to be factored into the selection.

Given the number of dressings available and the research about the different categories, the wound care practitioner has to use keen assessment skills, history and physical assessment, laboratory data, experience, and craftsman-like creativity

CASE STUDY

CONTINUED

The patient received surgical debridement of nonviable soft tissue and infected bone (**FIGURE 14-55A–D**). Interventions included antimicrobial absorbent dressings and total contact casting for off-loading. In addition, the patient is receiving daily hyperbaric oxygen therapy to increase oxygenation of the wound and periwound tissue.

DISCUSSION QUESTIONS

1. Have the goals for treatment changed? If so, what are the new goals?
2. Which of the dressings discussed would be appropriate for this patient?
3. Are there signs of active infection in any of the photos? If so, what are they?

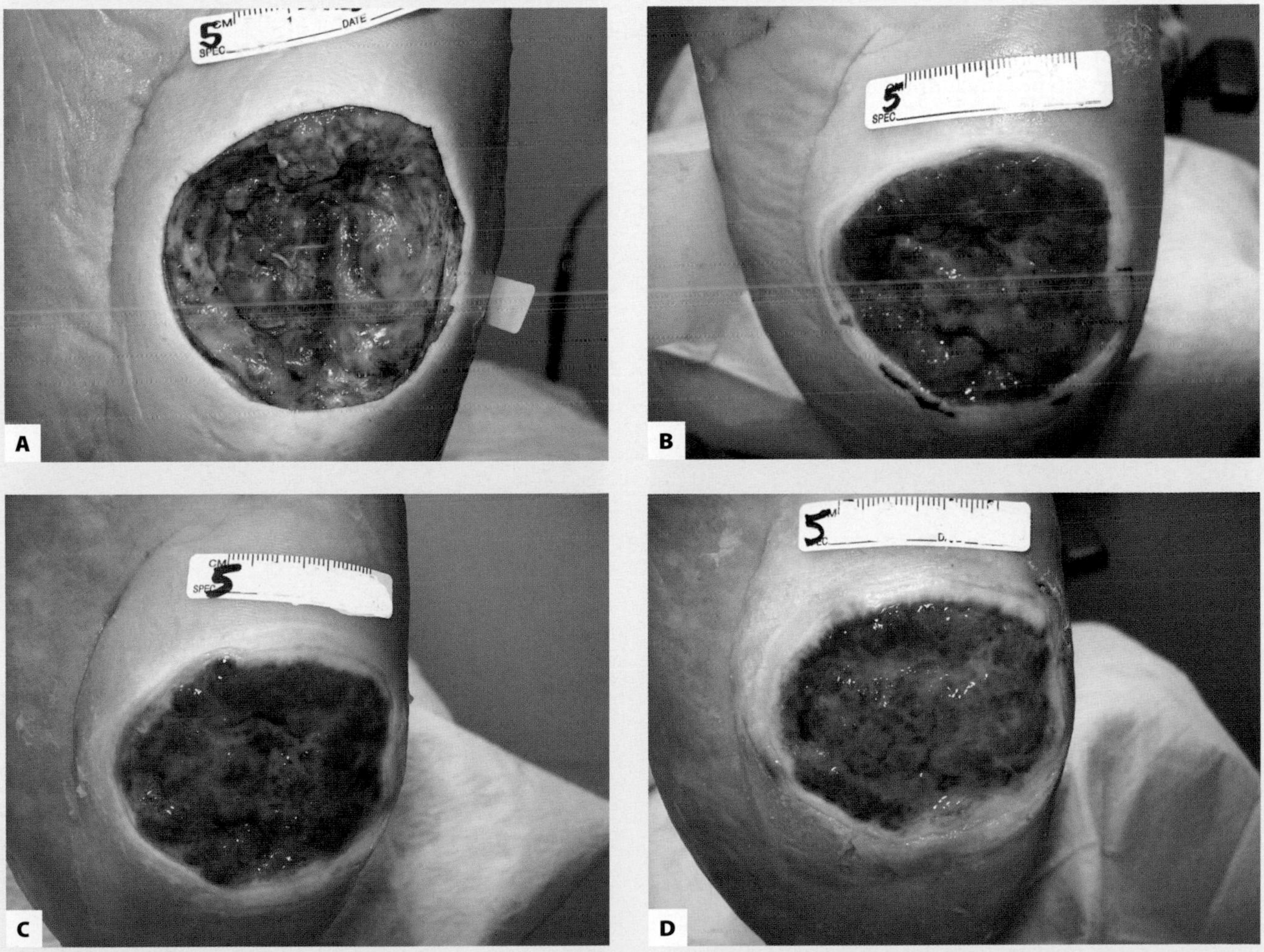

FIGURE 14-55 Case Study—continued. A. The wound after surgical debridement. Initially dressing changes, including the TCC, were performed twice weekly. As the drainage abated, dressings were decreased to weekly. The patient continues to receive hyperbaric oxygen therapy. **B.** In addition to the TCC and hyperbaric oxygen therapy, selective debridement, and bilayered cell therapy dressings were added to the care plan. A contact layer and silver gelling fiber dressing were the secondary dressings. **C.** Two weeks postcellular therapy, there is increased granulation, slightly smaller surface area, and less exudate. The film visible over the granulation tissue is sometimes a result of cell therapy. **D.** Two weeks after initiation of cellular therapy.

to select the dressing that will result in optimal outcomes. Further, in vitro data are not real-world clinical reality and nonclinical parameters such as availability and affordability also influence practice. According to Gethin,[51] dressings should be selected per the specificity and efficacy of the agent, potential cytotoxicity to human cells, effect on resistant bacterial strains, allergenicity, cofactors of the wound based on size and exudate, and total bacterial load.

With that in mind, the most commonly used antimicrobials will be evaluated based on their mechanism of action to reduce bacterial bioburden as well as the practical considerations that influence their use.[71]

Silver Silver dressings may be the most popular selection for the reduction of wound bioburden, in large part due to its history. The first reports of silver being used as an antimicrobial agent were in the days of Hippocrates, until it lost favor with the advent of antibiotics during World War II.[72] With increasing resistance to antibiotics, silver provides a viable option for the reduction of bioburden and the control of localized infection. Silver is readily available in a wide variety of dressing delivery types, including amorphous hydrogels, sheet hydrogels, alginates, gelling fibers, foams, silicones, contact layers, wound powders, ointments, negative pressure foams, and irrigations in the form of silver nitrate solutions (**FIGURE 14-56A–C**). As described by Mooney et al.,[72] silver's broad-spectrum antimicrobial ability is not in question, but the choice of dressing is more dependent on the characteristics of the particular carrier dressing, the way silver is delivered to the wound bed, and the needs of the wound based on tissue and exudate. An International Consensus Document[77] which discusses the appropriate use of silver in wound care and describes the function of various silver forms, states that the metallic form of silver is unreactive and does not have a bactericidal effect but must ionize to its active form, usually through contact with wound exudate. The silver must either be in contact with the wound bed to kill organisms on the surface or be in an absorbent dressing that will reduce the bioburden by destroying bacteria absorbed into the dressing through the wound exudate. It is critical to note that the amount of silver concentration in a particular dressing does *not* correlate to the amount of silver delivered to the wound bed. The discrepancy is a result of inactivation by levels of wound chloride and proteins.

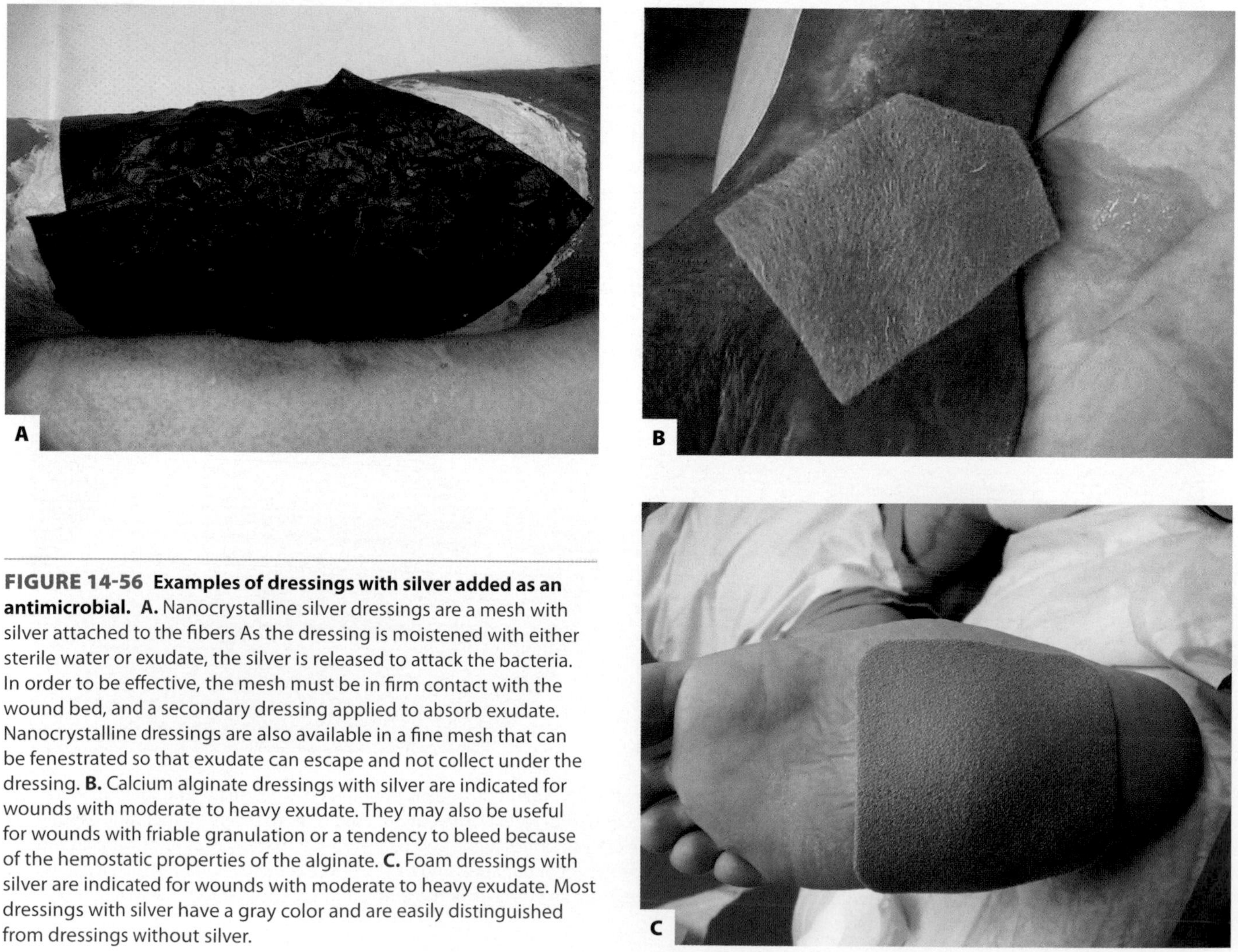

FIGURE 14-56 Examples of dressings with silver added as an antimicrobial. A. Nanocrystalline silver dressings are a mesh with silver attached to the fibers As the dressing is moistened with either sterile water or exudate, the silver is released to attack the bacteria. In order to be effective, the mesh must be in firm contact with the wound bed, and a secondary dressing applied to absorb exudate. Nanocrystalline dressings are also available in a fine mesh that can be fenestrated so that exudate can escape and not collect under the dressing. **B.** Calcium alginate dressings with silver are indicated for wounds with moderate to heavy exudate. They may also be useful for wounds with friable granulation or a tendency to bleed because of the hemostatic properties of the alginate. **C.** Foam dressings with silver are indicated for wounds with moderate to heavy exudate. Most dressings with silver have a gray color and are easily distinguished from dressings without silver.

The benefit of silver is its ability to affect multiple sites within the bacterial cells, such as binding to bacterial cell membranes, interfering with binding proteins and energy production within the cell, decreasing enzyme function, and providing DNA and RNA transcription inhibition.[73] The multimodal approach to bacterial death makes silver effective, but also at very low risk to bacterial resistance.[74] Additionally, silver may increase the sensitivity of a biofilm to antibiotics as well as alter its adhesion to the wound bed.[75]

Silver must have a controlled and sustained release in order to obtain its total bactericidal potential. so that the bacteria is exposed to a sufficient concentration of silver ions over time without causing tissue toxicity.[76] The ability for the dressing to conform, remain in place, and provide consistent coverage of the wound bed is necessary in order to achieve antimicrobial reduction. Silver appears in many dressings; however, its quantity, chemical form, delivery, release, and ability to conform influence the outcomes observed at the wound site.[77,78]

Silver also has the potential to reduce inflammation. Hoekstra et al.[79] reported a histological comparison between two dressings and showed a reduction in inflammation between the silver hydrofiber group and a tulle gauze control. This finding has similarly been reported in burn management[80] and via review of literature by an expert panel.[73] It is unclear, however, whether the anti-inflammatory effects of silver are directly related to the resultant reduction in wound bioburden or through some additional unknown mode of action.

The impact of pain and stress on wound healing is of concern, and dressings capable of delivering silver to the wound bed without adhering to the wound surface are advised in order to decrease pain and prevent trauma to the surface. Dressings that minimize pain can interrupt the cycle of repetitive trauma and wound pain, as described by Krasner.[81] The use of silicone dressings, especially those impregnated with silver, has become very advantageous for these reasons. When compared to topical silver sulfadiazine, a silver-impregnated silicone foam dressing showed a reduction in patient experience of pain at application ($p = 0.02$) and during wear ($p = 0.048$), decreased frequency of dressing changes (2.2 vs. 12.4), and significantly reduced costs ($309 vs. $513) in a multicenter randomized comparative trial.[82] The reduction of cost and dressing change frequency was also noted to depend on dressing type in an RCT by Muangman et al.[83] However, when levels of silver content and dressing construction type are similar, outcomes may be more comparable, as described in a study looking at silver alginates versus silver carboxymethylcellulose dressings.[84]

A study by Glat et al.[85] showed no statistically significant difference in the rate of infection or time of re-epithelialization in partial-thickness burn wounds between silver sulfadiazine ointment and a silver hydrogel; however, the author identified less pain and increased patient satisfaction in the hydrogel group. Additional benefits of silver include odor reduction, decreased wound exudate, and prolonged wear time.[86]

Despite all of its benefits, silver is not intended to be utilized for the entire duration of the healing process. In fact, the use of silver is recommended for a limited time due to potential apoptosis of keratinocytes, fibroblasts, and leukocytes.[87,88] Silver can become cytotoxic to host cells if the dressing delivers large quantities of the ion to the wound and is used over extended periods of time; therefore, silver dressings should be discontinued when signs of inflammation and localized infection have resolved. Symptoms indicative of resolution include improved color and quality of granulation tissue, disappearance of periwound hyperemia, reduction in surrounding erythema, absence of purulence, decrease in pain, and decrease in purulent exudate. Similarly, when new epithelium appears along the wound edge with increasing granulation and contraction of the wound, proliferation should be supported with moist wound therapy. Most experts suggest a 2-week period of antimicrobial use, at which point the wound should be assessed and the determination made about continuation of current therapy, the need of further wound bed preparation, or the need for a different topical product.[49,63,66]

Although silver is not indicated for use in wounds that show no evidence of increased bioburden or infection, a 2-week window may be considered for patients who are severely immunocompromised, wounds near contaminated areas such as the genitals, wounds with exposed bone, or wounds on extremities with poor circulation.[89]

Surgical site infections (SSI) may occur within the organ space or as a deep SSI, in which cases antimicrobial dressings have little effect when applied topically. However, superficial SSI may also occur, especially in patients with systemic comorbidities that impair wound healing, and thereby increase the risk of deeper tissue infection. While SSIs are multifactorial, an RCT by Siah and Yatim[90] showed a statistically significant difference in the amount of bioburden on postoperative incisions 5–7 days after surgery when using nanocrystalline silver compared with control. Studies of the incidence of SSIs with the postoperative use of silver-impregnated dressings are inconclusive and suggest that further randomized controlled trials are needed in order to make strong recommendations.[91–94] Safety concerns for the use of silver dressings in the pediatric population need consideration. A child's skin is at risk for absorption of topical products which can lead to systemic toxicity.[95] Although silver has been reported in the literature as safe to use in pediatrics,[85,96] many studies focused on the endpoint of wound healing, decrease in pain, or length of stay rather than the risk of harm. The concern for toxicity as seen in in vitro studies has warranted further research in this vulnerable population.[97,98] Wang et al.[99] showed that silver toxicity was a concern when examining pediatric burn patients and the use of nanocrystalline silver dressings. Not only were serum levels elevated, but the levels were closely proportional to the surface area of the wounds treated. An animal model raised question over deposition of silver in the major organs. In some cases, serum levels of silver have been noted to be 800 times greater than normal.[100] Dressings or topical agents providing adult dosages are not suitable for children; however, more research is necessary to determine the amount, length of use, and type of silver dressings that may or may not be safe for the pediatric population. Therefore, the patient's age, the surface area of the wound, the amount of silver in the dressing, and its delivery are factors to be considered. Silver dressings are not advised for neonates, and the usage of such products in the pediatric population is limited to no more than 2 weeks.[63] A product with lower parts per million (ppm) concentration of silver and slow active release from the dressing, instead of high parts per million dressing that actively releases silver ions into the wound bed, are a better selection. These qualities are very product specific and overall caution is advised when considering these products for the pediatric population.

Controversy also exists regarding the use of silver wound dressings on patients having magnetic resonance imaging (MRI) studies. There are concerns regarding the effect of MRI on medical products as metallic devices should never enter the MRI machine. However, wound care products are often not tested for MRI safety. Because silver is a metallic substance, many manufacturers will often issue warnings regarding its use near MRIs even if no testing has been performed. The concerns are for burns associated with response of the dressing to a magnetic field as well as for image disturbances. A recent study[101] assessed silicone wound dressings with silver (Mepilex AG+ and Mepilex Border AG+, Molnlycke Healthcare, LLC, Norcross, GA) under 3-Tesla and found both dressings to be MRI safe. However, the authors caution that they only tested these two specific dressings, and therefore the results cannot be generalized across all product types. Another study by Bailey et al.[102] looked at both heating and image distortion when five different silver dressings were left intact during MRI imaging on a porcine model. They found that heating was no more than 0–0.2°C and there was no image distortion with either dry or hydrated dressings, leading them to conclude that it was acceptable to leave the dressings in place. Clinicians are advised to follow manufacturer's recommendations for use before allowing patients to undergo an MRI with silver dressings in place. These same concerns need to be addressed with an oncology radiologist before having a patient undergo radiation with silver dressings in place.

Honey The use of medicinal honey has increased in popularity over the last several years; however, it is by no means the new-kid-on-the-block. The use of various forms of honey dates back thousands of years to the time of Dioscrodies,[103] Hippocrates,[104] and descriptions on medical papyrus from 1325 BC.[105] However, the form of medical grade honey used today differs greatly from that of natural or culinary versions. Medical grade honey has two general sources: *Leptospermum scoparium* (manuka), which is derived from tea plants, and *Leptospermum polygalifolium,* which is jelly bush honey.[106] Both forms have specific qualities related to their processing that affect the bacterial count, pH, enzyme activity, and overall benefit in wound care.

Pieper[106] reports that while culinary honey uses heat to prepare the product for consumption, this invariably reduces the enzyme responsible for hydrogen peroxide production, whereas medicinal honey's gamma radiation sterilization process allows it to retain its biologic activity. This biologic activity is multifactorial and relates to the unique blend of glucose, fructose, sucrose, water, amino acids, vitamins, minerals, and enzymes found in the final product.[107] Honey is used for its many capabilities, including antimicrobial action, debridement action, anti-inflammatory properties, moist wound maintenance, low pH, and exudate absorption.

Honey is known to be an effective antimicrobial agent.[108,109] However, its ability to reduce wound bioburden is directly dependent on the geographical, seasonal, and botanical source, as well as manufacturer processing and storage.[110] Honey has been shown to have a polyantimicrobial effect on a broad spectrum of viruses, fungi, protozoa, and over 50 species of bacteria, including organisms such as *Pseudomonas aeruginosa*, *Staphylococcus aureus*, methicillin-resistant *Staphylococcus aureus* (MRSA), and vancomycin-resistant *Enterococcus* (VRE).[64,111] Honey has no risk of bacterial resistance and has been shown to be equal to antibiotics in the prevention of infection following eye surgery[110] as well as capable of providing wound healing in pressure injuries.[112] This versatility is enhanced through its availability in many forms, including gels, alginates, hydrocolloids, and solutions.

The antimicrobial action of honey is a result of its ability to kill bacteria, as well as the capacity to regulate biologic activity within the wound. A major benefit is its low pH (3.5–4), which may move a chronic wound from a normally alkaline to an acidic environment, thereby producing a shift in the oxygen–hemoglobin disassociation curve. As described by Gethin and Cowman,[111] this drop in wound pH leads to increased oxygen release, reduced toxicity of bacterial end products, enhanced removal of abnormal wound collagen, decreased protease activity, increased angiogenesis, increased macrophage and fibroblast activity, and enzyme regulation. Further, the biologic activity includes the regulation of the immune response because honey stimulates monocytes to release cytokines, stimulates B and T lymphocytes to activate phagocytes, contributes to therapeutic levels of hydrogen peroxide production, and reduces edema, thereby facilitating improved microcirculation of oxygen and nutrients.[106] Although these effects may not be visible, the actions likely explain the experience of seeing honey "jump start" a recalcitrant wound in clinical practice.

Honey has also been shown to enhance debridement of necrotic tissue. A study by Gethin and Cowman[113] showed that honey was more effective in desloughing wounds with greater than 50% necrotic tissue than standard hydrogel, leading to statistically significant faster healing rates and decreased time to epithelialization. Moreover, the authors state that while sharp and biologic debridement may be faster, honey may be superior to the autolytic or enzymatic debridement seen with hydrogel, collagenase, or cadexomer iodine.

Although the benefits of honey have been described in many studies, there remains conflicting evidence as to where honey fits in best practice. This is largely related to RCTs and Cochrane reviews that have pointed out that honey did not show any significant differences versus standard care, thus questioning its efficacy.[114,115] Some studies may limit the potential benefits of honey dressings through the selection of study samples. Often the wounds evaluated are nonnecrotic or without signs of infection and therefore the use of time-to-healing parameters negates the many potential benefits of honey. Additionally, secondary symptoms such as pain, odor, and frequency of changes are not factored in. Rodgers and Walker[114,115] point out this discrepancy as they do not find sufficient evidence for the use of honey in leg ulcers, pressure injuries, or Fournier gangrene due to lack of available studies; however, they do support honey's benefit in the management of partial-thickness burns. This underlines the need for, as well as the difficulty of, proper research to test honey's potential methods of action in wound healing.

Potential adverse effects of using honey include stinging or burning pain after initial application of the dressing to the wound bed, most likely because of the osmotic and pH-lowering action of the dressing. These symptoms will often be transient; however, in some cases, they persist and warrant a change in therapy. Unlike silver, Pieper[106] describes many studies showing safe and effective use of honey in children, but the author indicates the need to avoid its use in wounds requiring surgical debridement, following incision and drainage of an abscess, or when sensitivity to bee stings is present. Although allergy to bee venom is a common fear with the use of honey products, and most clinicians will not select honey with a known bee allergy, no reports of anaphylaxis have currently been described with the use of medicinal honey.[116]

Honey is increasing in its popularity because of its excellent debridement properties, especially following the lack of availability of papain-based enzymatic debriding agents. Whether the wound is dry or has copious exudate, honey may be utilized with a proper secondary dressing. The osmotic structure of the dressing acts to bathe the wound bed by drawing out peripheral edema in exudative wounds, by adding moisture with the gel form, or by trapping ambient moisture in the hydrocolloid version. Because of this balance, the absorptive alginate dressing can be used in dry wounds. The alginate may be easier to apply and thus preferable to gel forms that may drip out of the wound in response to gravity or cause periwound maceration. Additionally, because of its theoretical benefits of anti-inflammatory/cytokine-regulating properties, honey may be preferable to a more expensive biologic dressing when treating hard-to-heal wounds. However, the actual clinical significance of this has not been tested (**FIGURE 14-57A–C**).

CLINICAL CONSIDERATION

Cadexomer iodine helps prevent a separating surgical incision from progressing to a dehisced incision. A small amount placed on the separation will decrease the bioburden and thereby facilitate re-epithelialization of the incision edges.

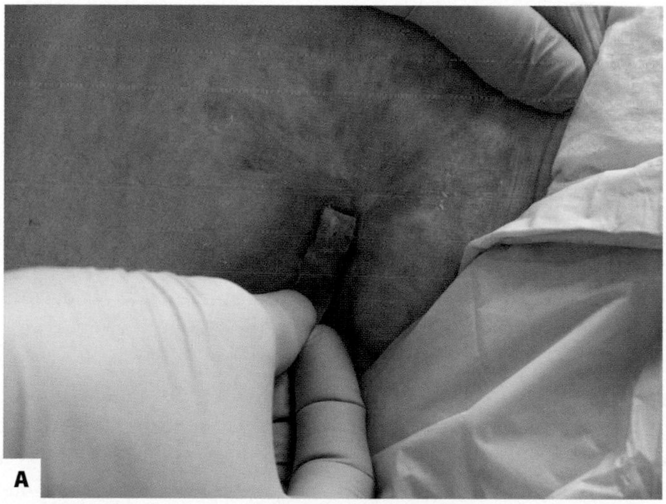

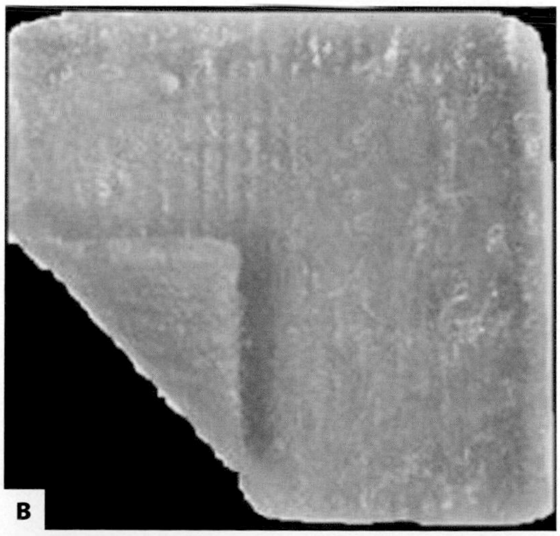

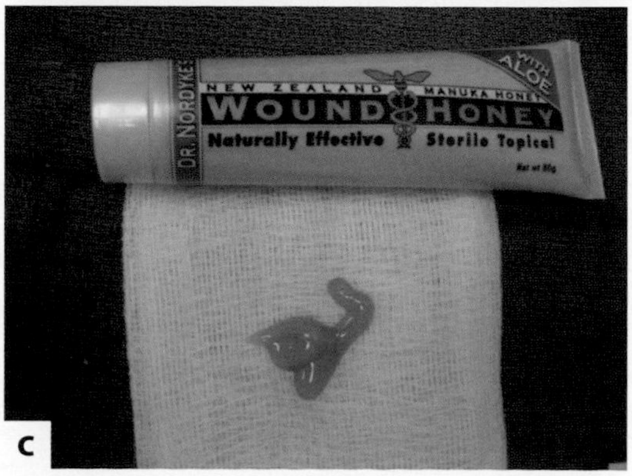

FIGURE 14-57 Honey dressings. A. Honey dressings are applied directly onto the wound base and covered with an appropriate secondary dressing. The honey is pliable and conforms to the wound surface without any empty spaces, thus maintaining moisture balance. **B.** Alginate permeated with honey provides both the properties of honey and the absorbency of alginate fibers. The dressing can be cut into strips for undermining and sinuses, but care must be taken to have the dressing fully in contact with the wound surface. **C.** Honey in a gel form is not absorbent, but does hydrate a dry wound and aids autolytic debridement. Its viscosity allows the honey to conform to irregular wound surfaces. An absorbent dressing with adhesive borders is recommended to prevent leakage.

Cadexomer Iodine Iodine was first discovered by Coutoius in 1811 and it took less than 50 years for it to be utilized in wound care.[117] Iodophors were well regarded for their ability to provide both bactericidal and bacteriostatic effects on a broad spectrum of bacterial species. Although many iodine preparations exist, not all of them are appropriate for wound care because of the cytotoxicity that may occur relative to the concentration, release, and solubility. Mertz et al.[118] stated that while iodine has traditionally been seen as an inhibitor of normal wound healing due to results of both in vitro and in vivo toxicity studies, the difference may lie in the components of iodine delivery. For example, povidone iodine includes active agents that improve its solubility and make the solution less damaging to host cells, and thus has been approved by the FDA for short-term use in the treatment of superficial and acute wounds.[80] However, its interaction with the wound environment results in fast consumption, requiring the clinician to reapply the solution multiple times daily for the full antimicrobial effect.[117,118] This results in many undesirable consequences for the wound environment, including the need for frequent dressing changes that negatively affect normothermia; the potential for repetitive, rapid release of large concentrations of iodine into the wound bed; and secondary symptoms such as pain and wound trauma. In other words, iodine itself is not the destroyer of the wound bed; however, the beneficial antimicrobial action of iodine needs to be controlled by the speed and amount of its release into the tissue while maintaining its bactericidal action without inducing cytotoxicity, and it needs to be in a delivery vehicle that allows for less-frequent dressing changes by adequately managing exudate.

Cadexomer iodine (CI) solves this dilemma. Available in a paste or sheet dressing (Iodosorb, Iodoflex, Smith & Nephew, Andover, Massachusetts), CI products have a three-dimensional, microspherical shape similar to a whiffle ball, with dextrin-based beads that allow controlled release of 0.9% iodine.[117] This structure can be thought of as an exchange system. As wound exudate is absorbed into the dressing, the starch carrier degrades and iodine is released into the wound bed. By doing so, CI does not inhibit or impair fibroblast function and is extremely effective in killing broad-spectrum organisms. Danielsen et al.[119] studied the bacteriological efficacy of CI on VLUs colonized with *P. aeruginosa* in an uncontrolled multicenter pilot study and found that 65% of the wounds had negative cultures for *P. aeruginosa* at 1 week and over 75% had negative cultures at 12 weeks.

In addition to improving wound healing potential by reducing bioburden, multiple researchers have found that CI has the ability to modulate the effects of macrophages to impact cytokine release and to increase growth factor production and activation in the chronic wound.[120] Specifically, CI was found to significantly increase the expression of interleukin-1-β, tumor necrosis factor alpha (TNF-α), vascular endothelial growth factor (VEGF), and microRNA, thereby enhancing the inflammatory response to support angiogenesis.[121] The combination of reducing wound pathogens and directly stimulating a refractory wound underscores the advantages of CI.

As previously discussed, biofilm phenotype bacteria (such as *S. aureus* and *P. aeruginosa*) pose a real threat to wound healing and infection. Almost all topical antimicrobials (including antibiotics, antiseptics, and concentrations of disinfectants) are unable to penetrate the polysaccharide matrix protecting the underlying pathogens; however, cadexomer iodine is the exception.[117] Recent studies[122] investigated the ability for a wide variety of topical antimicrobials to penetrate biofilm inoculated on pigs' ears. Of those tested, only CI was capable of penetrating the matrix and thus impact the bacteria present below the surface. Routine and frequent debridement is still necessary to ensure adequate removal; however, CI is useful in biofilm-based wound care, or in cases where a biofilm is suspected but aggressive debridement is not possible, for example, on a heavily anticoagulated patient.

Contraindications for CI include use on patients with a known allergy to iodine, dyes, or shellfish. Additionally, the starch-encased structure of CI necessitates an adequate amount of exudate or moisture to stimulate breakdown and release of the iodine, therefore dry wounds without exudate may not activate the dressing. Also, CI negatively interacts with exogenously applied collagenase for debridement so those two agents should not be used simultaneously. Caution is advised for use on children, patients with known thyroid dysfunction, and pregnant or lactating women. In addition, the amount of CI used relative to the size of the wound, the frequency of the application, and overall systemic absorption necessitate caution when considering its use in large surface area wounds, such as burns or surgical incisions (**FIGURE 14-58A, B**).

Polyhexamethylene Biguanide Polyhexamethylene biguanide (PHMB) has been used for its antimicrobial effects as an environmental disinfectant, swimming pool additive, and contact lens irrigation; however, because of its high biocompatibility PHMB is also used in wound care products. PHMB is described as a heterodisperse mixture of polymers with a structure similar to those found in naturally occurring AMPs and with a similar effect on bacterial cytoplasmic membranes.[123] The structure induces cell lysis by its mechanism of attaching and impairing the cell membrane, similar to the mechanism of some antibiotics. It is comparable to its closest chemical cousin chlorhexidine, having similar effects against bacteria such as *P. aeruginosa*, while lacking the potentially damaging chlorobenzene group.[124]

PHMB is effective on both common wound pathogens and resistant organisms. Cazzinga et al.[125] found that PHMB-impregnated foam showed a significant log reduction of *P. aeruginosa* within the wound compared to standard gauze, and did not allow *Pseudomonas* to colonize the PHMB-impregnated foam nor result in a reduction of normal flora. These results support the use of PHMB as a preventative barrier dressing against infection in high-risk individuals.

An RCT by Wild et al.[126] investigated the effect of PHMB delivered by a constantly applied cellulose dressing versus intermittent use of impregnated swabs for the eradication of MRSA in pressure injuries. Their results showed both applications of

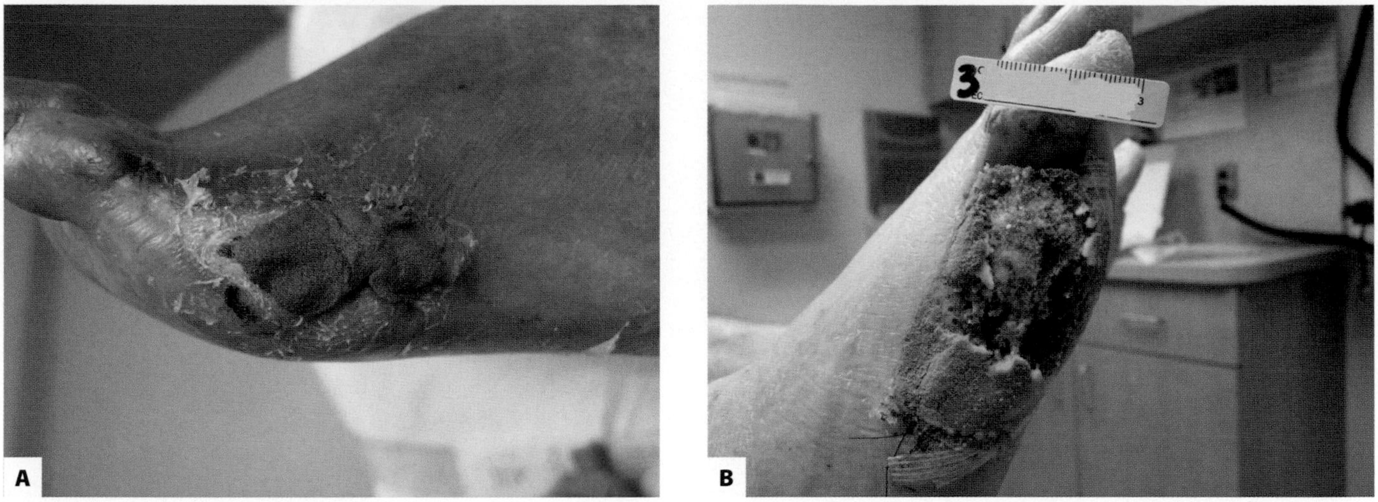

FIGURE 14-58 Cadexomer iodine dressings. A. Cadexomer iodine in paste form is pliable and can be molded to fit and fill almost any wound. A secondary dressing sufficient to manage any exudate is required. The iodine is slowly released over a period of approximately 72 hours so that 0.9% concentration is maintained at the wound bed. This concentration is effective against microbes without being cytotoxic. **B.** Residual iodine on a wound bed at dressing change may have changed color. The active form of iodine is brown, and as the iodine is inactivated (as it destroys bacteria) it becomes iodide which is colorless. This is an indication that all the active iodine has been used and the dressing needs to be changed. When initially used to treat an infected wound, the dressing may need to be changed daily. As the bacteria count decreases, dressings can stay in place longer, and when the dressing remains brown with no change in color, it is no longer indicated because bacteria are no longer being killed.

PHMB lowered the amount of MRSA present; however, the continuously applied cellulose dressing was more effective with a 100% reduction of MRSA on day 14 versus 67% reduction in the control. Both of these studies highlight the potential benefit of PHMB to reduce bioburden, but also focus on the fact that this substance is not released out of its delivery dressing.

Unlike some silver and iodine dressings, PHMB must be exposed to and in direct contact with the organisms for which it is intended to kill. Once it is bound to a dressing material such as gauze, foam, or alginate, it can only affect bacteria that have been absorbed into the dressing construct.[123] In the case of wound irrigations and solutions, time of exposure is the key determinant. Werner and Kramer[127] indicate that at least 10–15 minutes of exposure is necessary to induce the most antimicrobial effect. Therefore, PHMB in solution form is advised to stay in the wound bed during the cleansing process, or provide the agent as a continuous irrigation, for example, through the use of NPWT with instillation.[128]

Newer applications of PHMB into biosynthetic cellulose fibers have proven beneficial in managing the problem of PHMB binding as well as the moisture balance of the wound both in dry and wet environments. Biocellulose dressings provide unbound PHMB that is released into the surrounding wound fluid, rendering its antimicrobial action both within the dressing and at the wound interface.[129,130] The results further demonstrate that the qualities of the dressing may be as important as the antimicrobial agent contained in the dressing. For biofilm-based wound care, PHMB may be utilized as a method to prevent reattachment of bacteria to the wound bed following debridement, but it is not the frontline choice for biofilm disruption.

PHMB dressings are used to reduce bioburden and secondary symptoms such as wound pain. Many dressing types contain PHMB, including gauzed-based systems (rolled gauze, drain sponges, island dressings, etc.), foams, biocellulose dressings, and alginates. Most gauze-based NPWT systems utilize PHMB-impregnated gauze to provide antimicrobial benefits without the risk of cytotoxicity.

PHMB-impregnated gauzes should be saturated with normal saline, sterile water, or potable water. Other antiseptic solutions such as sodium hypochlorite may cause a chemical reaction that inactivates the PHMB and results in a nontoxic yellow stain. Patients with known adverse reactions to PHMB or chlorhexidine are excluded from use. Finally, because of the method of action of PHMB, it is generally recommended that it be used for prophylaxis or on critically colonized wounds, but *not* as the primary treatment in active wound infections (**FIGURE 14-59A, B**).[123]

CLINICAL CONSIDERATION

PVA foam with gentian violet and methylene blue is an antimicrobial that can be safely used with the enzyme collagenase without affecting its debriding action.[131]

PVA Foam with Gentian Violet and Methylene Blue

The antimicrobial action of methylene blue and gentian violet has long been described in the annals of science.[132,133] Due to their bactericidal, antifungal, and broad-spectrum bacteriostatic effects, these components are used to treat fungal infections, prevent infection, and assist with bacterial staining in laboratory studies. When combined with PVA foam, it becomes a versatile wound care dressing termed methylene blue–gentian violet polyvinyl alcohol (MBGV-PVA) foam.

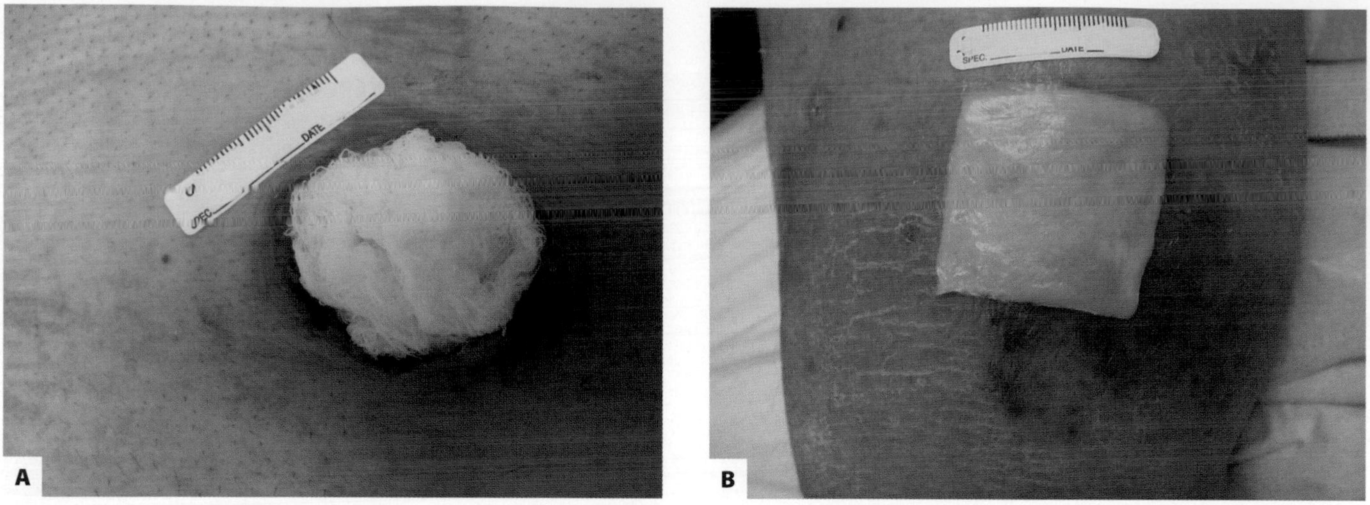

FIGURE 14-59 Polyhexamethylene biguanide (PHMB) dressings. A. PHMB, an antimicrobial similar to chlorhexidine (used as a surgical skin prep) without potentially harmful chlorobenzenes, can be impregnated in a variety of delivery dressing products, including gauze, foam, and gelling fibers. The active ingredient must be in contact with the bacteria to be effective; therefore, the dressing needs to be in full contact with the wound bed. **B.** A cellulose dressing containing PHMB is indicated for flat, superficial wounds as either a bacterial barrier for high-risk patients or an antimicrobial primary dressing.

This dressing removes exudate from the wound bed while creating singlet oxygen and free radicals that directly impact the plasma membrane causing bacteriolysis.[78] Other clinical benefits reported on the effect of MBGV-PVA in treating hard-to-heal wounds include decreased inflammation and pain, reduced fibrin wound covering, improved granulation tissue, and intriguingly, reduced wound edge epibole.[134–137] Unlike some products (antiseptics, silver, and iodine) that may inhibit the effect of exogenous collagenases, MBGV-PVA does not.[131] This permits combination therapy including reduction of necrotic tissue, entrapment of bacterial endotoxins, and decreased risk for infection.

The PVA foam itself is versatile and capable of being used in a variety of situations. The highly absorptive foam may be used in dry wounds, moist wounds, and excessively exudative wounds when a properly selected secondary dressing is applied. The moist foam will hydrate a dry wound bed when covered with a transparent film, will maintain moisture in a mildly exudative wound, and will achieve maximum absorption in exudative wounds when applied dry. Another benefit of MBGV-PVA foam is the ability to reduce hypergranulation tissue by the removal of excessive moisture from the wound base. Because the foam becomes rigid and hard when dry, it can be used to provide antimicrobial protection as well as mild joint splinting, such as in the case of partial-thickness burns over the fingers. By applying the moist foam with a secondary dressing after debridement, the foam at the wound surface stays moist enough for autolysis, while becoming rigid to support immobilization of the joint. The dressing can be subsequently rehydrated daily to maintain a moist wound bed. Additionally, chronic wounds with rolled wound edges (epibole) have been shown to smooth out and elicit epithelialization in recalcitrant wounds.[138] Again, the lack of research in these areas questions the actual clinical benefit of this dressing over standard care, but clinical results and its use with debriding enzymes are promising (**FIGURE 14-60A, B**).

Dialkylcarbamoylchloride Dialkylcarbamoylchloride (DACC) is a recently discovered antimicrobial dressing. The principles of hydrophobic interaction can be seen in daily life, such as how drops of oil aggregate into one larger grouping when dropped into water, or how a pathogenic bacteria may grab hold of exposed and damaged collagen in an open wound.[139] Microorganisms have the ability to attach to a denatured extracellular matrix through the interaction of their hydrophobic covering with cell surface proteins in the collagen known as hydrophobins.[140] This method of surface attachment is harnessed in the form of applying DACC, a naturally occurring hydrophobic fatty acid, to various dressing constructs in order to utilize the principles of hydrophobic binding by allowing bandage fibers to stick to the hydrophobic covering of potential microbes in the wound bed.

Dressings containing DACC, also known generically as pathogen-binding mesh, are not technically antimicrobial, but they have a decided advantage over some of the other products—they have no chemical, pharmacological, or antimicrobial agents, thus erasing the concern for bacterial resistance or sensitivity. Silver, iodine, and other antimicrobials utilize multiple pathways to induce bacterial cell lysis (eg, binding to DNA, affecting efflux pumps, disrupting the cell membranes of microbes, denaturing proteins, and displacing metallic cations in the bacterial cell wall).[78] In all of these cases, the bacteria are killed, and a resulting dump of endotoxins and cellular debris is released into the wound bed. This

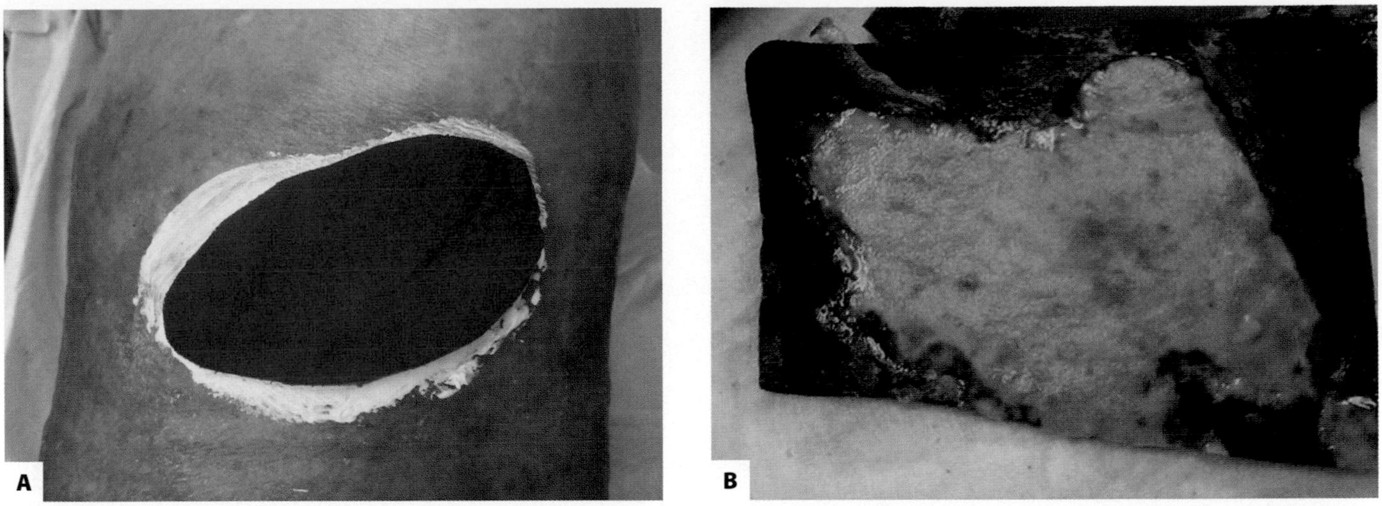

FIGURE 14-60 PVA foam with gentian violet and methylene blue. A. Polyvinyl alcohol (PVA) foam is combined with methylene blue and gentian violet for an absorbent antimicrobial dressing with distinctive versatility. The dressing absorbs exudate and creates an environment for bacteriolysis. The foam is available in both sheets and ropes and can be cut to fit any size wound, undermining, or sinus tract. **B.** As the foam absorbs drainage and the bacteria are lysed, the foam blanches in color. The foam allows adherence of wound debris, which assists in debridement at dressing changes. Note that the exudate stays in the foam that is in direct contact with the wound bed and does not wick laterally over the periwound skin, thus preventing maceration.

adds to the inflammatory response, risking the increase in inappropriate polymorphic neutrophil activation of MMPs.[141] To avoid these potentially disruptive insults to the wound environment, DACC covered dressing fibers work instead to bind the microbes to the dressing, render them inactive, and then remove them *whole*. This concept of repetitive removal of microbes with each dressing change is similar to the concept of sequestration. The principle of trapping and removing bacteria in their intact state is one of the reasons that gelling fibers and alginates are effective in the reduction of wound bioburden.[142] In the case of dressings with DACC, however, there is no risk of bacteria re-release from an oversaturated dressing, and the dressing is capable of showing a large log reduction in bacterial load with subsequent dressing changes. A study by Gentili et al.[143] used real-time PCR evaluations to study the bacterial bioburden in wounds with subsequent changes using DACC-coated dressings. The authors note that the bacterial load at the beginning of wound treatment was 4.41×10^7 per milligram of tissue and at the end of therapy 1.73×10^5 per milligram of tissue, or a 254-fold reduction in the bacteria present ($p = 0.0243$). More recent studies have supported the evidence that DACC is effective in reducing the bioburden of hard-to-heal wounds without having any negative side effects.[144–147]

The ability of the dressing to bind to aerobic bacteria, fungi, and often pathogenic anaerobes is determined by the organism's cellular surface hydrophobicity (CSH). The expression of CSH is often increased during periods of wound stress or as a result of the colonization of the wound environment.[148] This is an important concept when DACC dressings are used for wound care because irrigation must be properly performed and the wound environment assessed for appropriate levels of moisture. Common antiseptics and analgesics have the ability to reduce CSH expression, including eucteric mixture of local anesthetic (EMLA), which can eradicate CSH expression completely.[148] If CSH expression falls or is removed, DACC-coated dressings will lose their efficacy. Similarly, principles of hydrophobic binding require moisture to encourage the interaction between two hydrophobic surfaces. Thus, if a wound is dry and nonexudative, moisture may need to be added in the form of a hydrogel or the use of a secondary dressing that traps ambient moisture.[149]

Another consideration for the use of hydrophobic-binding dressings includes the frequency of wound changes. As the dressings remove bacteria with each change, wounds with clinical signs of critical colonization or infection may require dressing changes every 12–24 hours in order to achieve a necessary reduction in wound bioburden with a concurrent application of an appropriate absorptive secondary dressing to manage exudate.[150] In cases of prophylaxis or no clinical signs of infection, a change in frequency of up to 4 days has been described.[139] Because of the lack of chemical agents in this dressing, safe use in children has been reported. Meberg and Schoyen[151] performed a prospective randomized study on umbilical cord disinfection comparing a group using DACC ($n = 1{,}213$) with daily cleansing with 0.5% chlorhexidine in 70% ethanol ($n = 1{,}228$) and found no differences between the rate of infections in each group. No adverse reactions were reported in the DACC group.

As with other antimicrobial dressings, the selection of DACC is dependent on the wound size, depth, tissue type, exudate amount, pathogen detected in the wound, extent of infection if present, and host immunity (**FIGURE 14-61A, B**).

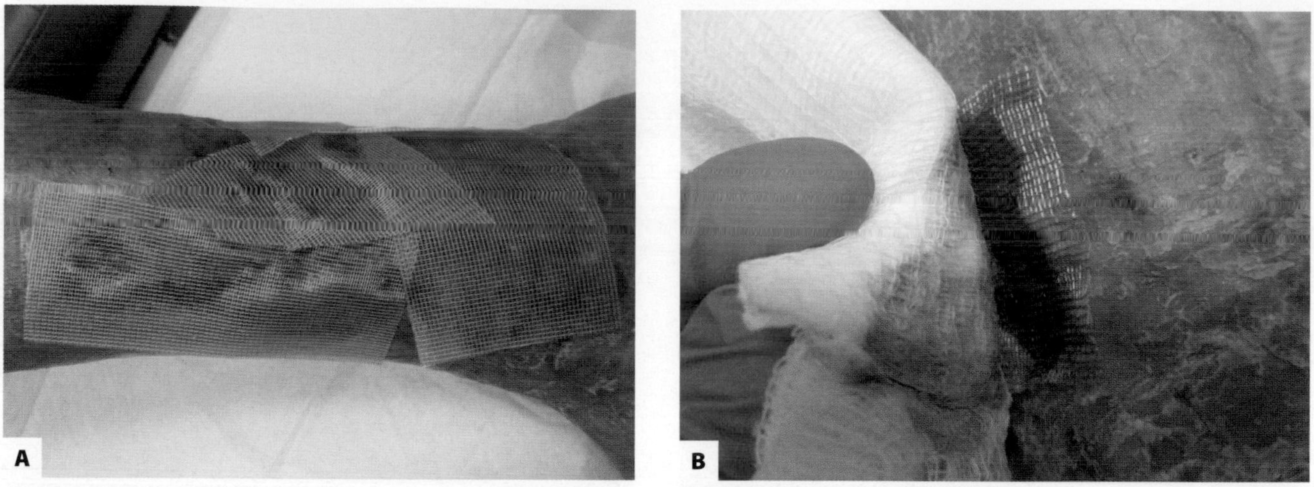

FIGURE 14-61 Dialkylcarbamoylchloride (DACC). A. Dialkylcarbamoylchloride (DACC) is a naturally occurring hydrophobic fatty acid that is attached to the dressing, in this case a nonadherent mesh. The bacteria load is decreased by the binding action of the microbes to the fatty acid on the dressing. The microbes are bound whole, rendered inactive, and removed in entirety with each dressing change. **B.** Evidence of bacteria, specifically *Pseudomonas aeruginosa* by the greenish tint, is visible in the secondary dressing over the DACC mesh.

CASE STUDY

CONCLUSION

Increased exudate, green tint to periwound tissue, mild odor, and macerated edges were observed after 2 weeks of cellular therapy. Nanocrystalline silver 7-day dressing, fenestrated to allow the exudate to escape, was covered with calcium alginate. TCC was continued and changed on weekly basis. The wound responded to the change in care plan, and after signs of infection were diminished, the wound was debrided with contact ultrasound and cellular therapy reapplied. Collagen matrix dressings were used at the weekly dressing changes, and after 2 months cellular therapy was applied again to obtain full closure. Total time from surgical debridement to full closure was 21 weeks (**FIGURE 14-62A–E**).

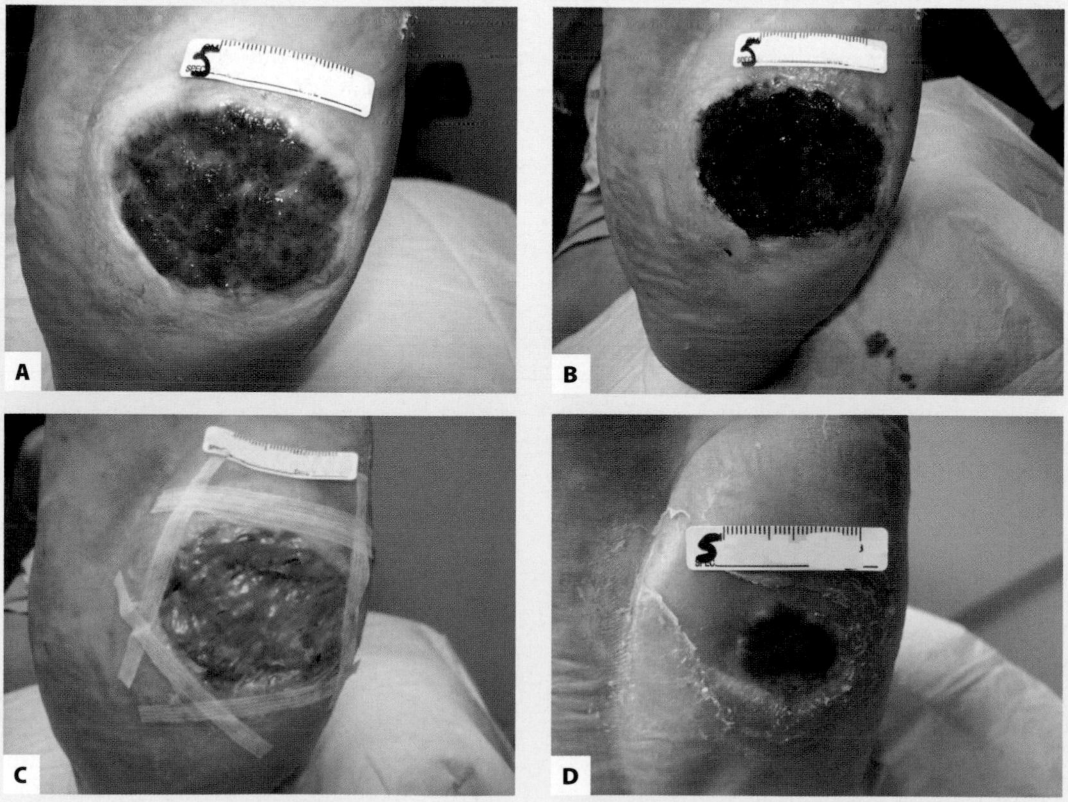

CASE STUDY (Continued)

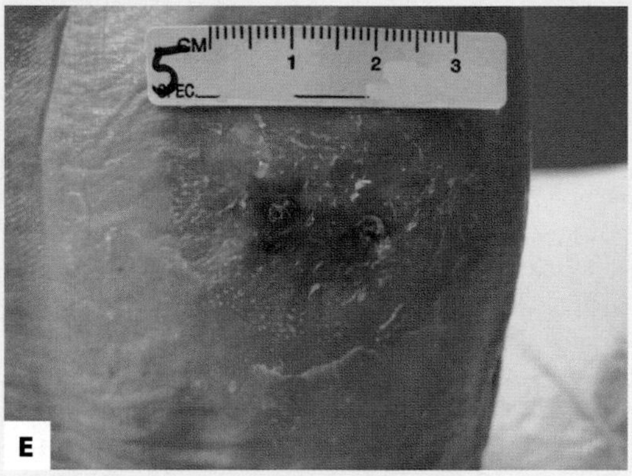

FIGURE 14-62 Case Study—conclusion. A. Wound after treatment with nanocrystalline silver, before debridement with low-frequency contact debridement. **B.** Wound bed after debridement with ultrasound. **C.** Wound with cellular therapy secured with Steri-Strips. **D.** Wound after 8 weeks of TCC and collagen matrix dressings to promote healing and reduce proteases. **E.** After 21 weeks of changing therapy at each session to meet the needs of the wound as it progressed through healing, the wound is fully epithelialized. Healing will continue as it progresses through the remodeling phase and the tissue regains its tensile strength. The patient was also able to have reconstructive surgery for the Charcot deformity.

SUMMARY

The use of topical antimicrobials demonstrates clear advantages over the misuse of antibiotic therapy in colonized and locally infected wounds. Due to the varying methods of action, the functional construction of the dressings selected, and the abundance of competitive products on the market, selecting one product over another can be difficult in the clinical setting. Some products are known to be more efficacious on specific organisms, while others are more adept in dry versus moist wounds. However, the clinician should avoid the temptation of mixing these products together for any perceived benefit that may come from an antimicrobial cocktail. Cowan et al.[152] described that in some cases mixing products can lead to problematic chemical reactions and inactivation of the dressings' properties, essentially stating, more is not necessarily better.

Certain dressings are known to be harmful to the wound bed, for example, those containing disinfectants or heavy antiseptics with severely cytotoxic concentrations. Clinical considerations are a dressing's intended use, its chemical makeup, the expected reaction by the host tissue, the frequency of changes, and the total time of safe usage.

Management of all wounds is complicated by the exponentially growing base of knowledge found in the science of acute and chronic wound healing.

Until dissemination of new knowledge occurs within the healthcare community, the inappropriate use of dressings such as wet-to-dry gauze (which are known to inhibit wound healing, increase the costs of care, and increase pain) is still prescribed.[153] Moreover, the lack of wound care knowledge by the nonwound clinician may also lead to the inappropriate selection and use of antimicrobial dressings, when in fact they are not indicated.

The IWII Consensus Guidelines state that the risk of infection is elevated when there are any conditions that compromise the immune response or perfusion. Once those factors are identified, the proper management of infection requires much more than a dressing. Optimal care also treats systemic comorbidities, tracks necessary markers of inflammation, and assesses the reduction of wound bioburden as a necessary holistic approach. The duration of topical antiseptic use should be personalized and based on regular wound assessment. A 2-week trial period is commonly recommended to allow for observation of the antiseptic's effectiveness. However, treatment may be needed for up to 4 weeks to achieve desired results in biofilm-based wound care. Alternating or rotating topical antiseptic treatments is a popular approach, where different antiseptics are used in a 2- or 4-week cycle to target a range of microorganisms. This strategy, along with cleansing and debridement, may help restore microbial balance, but further research is needed to support its clinical use.[52]

Silver, PHMB, CI, DACC, PVA-GVMB dressings, and honey are relatively safe to use with lower risks of resistance and cytotoxicity than antibiotics or antiseptics. However, there is a time and a place for all of these therapies to be utilized, and it is the responsibility of the clinician to make the best selection based on evidence-based guidelines.

STUDY QUESTIONS

1. An example of a "support need" when selecting a wound dressing is
   a. Amount of exudate.
   b. Size of the wound.
   c. Compression for concomitant edema.
   d. Quality of life issues.
2. Contact layers are used to
   a. Absorb exudate.
   b. Protect wound bed from trauma.
   c. Eliminate epibole.
   d. Trap bacteria.

3. Hydrocolloid dressings are contraindicated for which of the following wound type?
   a. Stage 3 pressure injury
   b. Venous leg ulcer
   c. Deep tissue pressure injury
   d. Diabetic foot ulcer
4. Which of the following growth factors is currently available for topical wound care?
   a. Epidermal growth factor (EGF)
   b. Fibroblast growth factor (FGF)
   c. Platelet-derived growth factor (PDGF)
   d. Vascular endothelial growth factor (VEGF)
5. Which of the following is not a category or consideration for reducing wound bioburden?
   a. Antibiotics
   b. Topical antimicrobial dressings
   c. Collagen dressings
   d. Antiseptics
6. The dressing most appropriate for promoting autolytic debridement is
   a. Petrolatum gauze and adhesive foam.
   b. Hydrogel and transparent film.
   c. Calcium alginate and foam.
   d. Becaplermin and transparent film.
7. Which of the following antimicrobial dressings must be in direct contact with the microbes in order to be effective?
   a. Polyhexamethylene biguanide
   b. Iodine
   c. Silver
   d. Honey
8. A patient presents with a draining sinus wound that is 1 cm × 0.7 cm × 8 cm deep. Which of the following dressings would be most appropriate?
   a. Honey-impregnated calcium alginate
   b. Silver hydrogel
   c. Tightly rolled DACC mesh
   d. PVA foam rope with gentian violet and methylene blue

Answers: 1-c; 2-b; 3-c; 4-c; 5-c; 6-b; 7-a; 8-d

REFERENCES

1. Shai A, Maibach HI. Milestones in the history of wound healing. In: *Wound Healing and Ulcers of the Skin: Diagnosis and Therapy—The Practical Approach*. Berlin, Heidelberg: Springer-Verlag; 2005:20.
2. Brown H. *A Brief History of Wound Healing*. Yardley, PA: Oxford Clinical Communications; 1998:8-9.
3. Bradley M, Cullum N, Nelson EA, Petticrew M, Sheldon T, Torgerson D. Systematic reviews of wound care management: (2) Dressings and topical agents used in the healing of chronic wounds. *Health Technol Assess*. 1999;3(17, pt 2):1-35.
4. Winter GD. Formation of the scab and the rate of epithelization of superficial wounds in the skin of the young domestic pig. *Nature*. 1962;193(4812):293-294.
5. Cowan LJ, Stechmiller J. Prevalence of wet-to-dry dressings in wound care. *Adv Skin Wound Care*. 2009;22(12):567-573.
6. Ovington LG. Hanging wet-to-dry dressings out to dry. *Home Healthc Nurse*. 2001;19;8:1-11.
7. Wound Healing and Management Node Group, *Evidence summary: Wound management: debridement - wet to dry moistened gauze*. Wound Practice and Research, The Joanna Briggs Institute, August 2013.
8. Weir D. How to … top tips for dressing selection. *Wounds Int*. 2012;3(4). Available at: http://www.woundsinternational.com. Accessed October 4, 2013.
9. Broussard KC, Powers JG. Wound dressings: selecting the most appropriate type. *Am J Clin Dermatol*. 2013;14(6):449-459.
10. Obagi Z, Damiani G, Grada A, Falanga V. Principles of wound dressings: a review. *Surg Technol Int*. 2019;35:50-57.
11. Ratliff CR. Descriptive study of the frequency of medical adhesive-related skin injuries in a vascular clinic. *J Vasc Nurs*. 2017;35(2): 86-89.
12. Moffatt CJ, Franks PJ, Hollinworth H. Understanding wound pain and trauma: an international perspective. *EWMA Position Document: Pain at Wound Dressing Changes*. 2002:2-7.
13. Gardner SE, Abbott LI, Fiala CA, Rakel BA. Factors associated with high pain intensity during wound care procedures: A model. *Wound Repair Regen*. 2017;25(4):558-563.
14. Green J, Jester R, McKinley R, Pooler A. Patient perspectives of their leg ulcer journey. *J Wound Care*. 2013;22(2):58-66.
15. Hess CT. *Skin & Wound Care*. 7th ed. Baltimore, MD: Lippincott Williams & Wilkins; 2013.
16. Baranoski S, Ayello EA, McIntosh A, Montoya L, Scarborough P. Wound treatment options. In: Baranoski S, Ayello EA, eds. *Wound Care Essentials*. 3rd ed. Philadelphia, PA: Lippincott Williams & Wilkins; 2012:181-239.
17. Ovington LG. Dressings and skin substitutes. In: McCulloch JM, Kloth LC, eds. *Wound Healing Evidence-Based Management*. 4th ed. Philadelphia, PA: FA Davis Company; 2010:180-200.
18. Sussman G. Management of the wound environment with dressings and topical agents. In: Sussman C, Bates-Jensen B, eds. *Wound Care: A Collaborative Practice Manual for Health Professionals*. 4th ed. Philadelphia, PA: Lippincott Williams & Wilkins; 2012:502-521.
19. Fletcher J, Moore Z, Anderson I, Matsuzaki K. Pressure ulcers and hydrocolloids made easy. *Wounds Int*. 2011;2(4). Available at: http://www.woundsinternational.com. Accessed October 4, 2013.
20. Romanelli M, Vowden K, Weir D. Exudate management made easy. *Wounds Int*. 2010;1(2). Available at: http://www.woundsinternational.com. Accessed October 4, 2013.
21. Santamaria N, Gerdtz M, Sage S, et al. A randomized controlled trial of the effectiveness of soft silicone foam multi-layer dressings in the prevention of sacral and heel pressure ulcers in trauma and critically ill patients: the border trial. *Int Wound J*. 2013; 12(3): 302-308.
22. Kalowes P, et al. Five-layered soft silicone foam dressing to prevent pressure ulcers in the intensive care unit. *Am J Crit Care*. 2016;25(6): e108-e119.
23. Tayyib N, et al. Effectiveness of pressure ulcer prevention strategies for adult patients in intensive care units: a systematic review. *Worldviews Evid Based Nurs* 2016;13(6):432-444.
24. Levy, A., Gefen, A. Assessment of the biomechanical effects of prophylactic sacral dressings on tissue loads: a computational modeling analysis. *Ostomy Wound Manage*. 2017;63(10):48-55.
25. World Union of Wound Healing Societies (WUWHS). *Consensus Document: Role of dressings in pressure ulcer prevention*. London, UK: Wounds Int; 2016.
26. Forni C, D'Alessandro F, Gallerani P, et al. Effectiveness of using a new polyurethane foam multi-layer dressing in the sacral area to prevent the onset of pressure ulcer in the elderly with hip fractures: a pragmatic randomised controlled trial. *Int Wound J*. 2018;15(3):383-390.

27. Chowdhry SA, Nieves-Malloure Y, Camardo M, Robertson JM, Keys J. Use of oxidised regenerated cellulose/collagen dressings versus standard of care over multiple wound types: a systematic review and meta-analysis. *Int Wound J*. 2022;19(2):241-252.
28. Gibson D, Cullen B, Legerstee R, Harding KG, Schultz G. MMPs made easy. *Wounds Int*. 2009;1(1). Available at: http://www.woundsinternational.com. Accessed October 4, 2013.
29. Brett D. A review of collagen and collagen-based wound dressings. *Wounds*. 2008;20(12):347-356.
30. Kallis PJ, Friedman AJ. Collagen powder in wound healing. *J Drugs Dermatol*. 2018;17(4):403-408.
31. Altrazeal® Transforming Powder Dressing. Available at: https://www.woundsource.com/product/altrazeal-transforming-powder-dressing. Accessed May 22, 2023.
32. Kim H, Park S, Housler G, Marcel V, Cross S, Izadjoo M. An overview of the efficacy of a next generation electroceutical wound care device. *Mil Med*. 2016;181(5 Suppl):184-190.
33. Kim H, Izadjoo MJ. Antibiofilm efficacy evaluation of a bioelectric dressing in mono- and multi-species biofilms. *J Wound Care*. 2015; 24(Suppl 2):S10-S104.
34. Ghatak PD, Schlanger R, Ganesh K, et al. A wireless electroceutical dressing lowers cost of negative pressure wound therapy. *Adv Wound Care (New Rochelle)*. 2015;4(5):302-311.
35. Self-adaptive wound care technology. Available at: http://www.cnluxtrawoundcare.com/. Accessed May 23, 2023.
36. Wu S, Carter M, Cole W, et al. Best practice for wound repair and regeneration: Use of cellular, acellular and matrix-like products (CAMPs). *J Wound Care*. 2023;32(Sup4b):S1-S31.
37. Snyder DL, Sullivan N, Schoelles KM. Skin substitutes from treating chronic wounds. Technology Assessment: Final Report. Prepared for the Agency for Research and Quality. December 18, 2012. Available at: http://www.ahrq.gov/research/findings/ta/skinsubs/HCPR0610_skinsubst-final.pdf. Accessed October 4, 2013.
38. Goodarzi P, Falahzadeh K, Nematizadeh M, et al. Tissue engineered skin substitutes. *Adv Exp Med Biol*. 2018;1107:143-188.
39. Armstrong DG, Tettelbach WH, Chang TJ, et al. Observed impact of skin substitutes in lower extremity diabetic ulcers: lessons learned from medicare database (2015-2018). *J Wound Care*. 2021;30(S7):S5-S16.
40. Tettelbach WH, Armstrong DG, Chang TJ, et al. Cost-effectiveness of dehydrated human amnion/chorion membrane allografts in lower extremity diabetic ulcer treatment. *J Wound Care*. 2022; 31(S2):S10-S31.
41. Ridiandries A, Tan JTM, Bursill CA. The role of chemokines in wound healing. *Int J Mol Sci*. 2018;19(10):3217.
42. Zubair M, Ahmad J. Role of growth factors and cytokines in diabetic foot ulcer healing: a detailed review. *Rev Endocr Metab Disord*. 2019;20(2):207-217.
43. Dolati S, Yousefi M, Pishgahi A, Nourbakhsh S, Pourabbas B, Shakouri SK. Prospects for the application of growth factors in wound healing. *Growth Factors*. 2020;38(1):25-34.
44. Regranex. Available at: https://smith-nephew.com/en-us/health-care-professionals/products/advanced-wound-management/regranex. Accessed May 23, 2023.
45. Waycaster CR, Gilligan AM, Motley TA. Cost-effectiveness of becaplermin gel on diabetic foot ulcer healingchanges in wound surface area. *J Am Podiatr Med Assoc*. 2016;106(4):273-282.
46. Atiyeh BS, Dibo SA, Hayek SN. Wound cleaning, topical antiseptics and wound healing. *Int Wound J*. 2009;6:420-430.
47. Sibbald RG, Williamson D, Orsted HL, et al. Preparing the wound bed—debridement, bacterial balance and moisture balance. *Ostomy Wound Manage*. 2000;46(11):14-35.
48. Atkin L, Bucko Z, Montero EC, et al. Implementing TIMERS: the race against hard-to-heal wounds. *J Wound Care*. 2019;28(3S3):S1-S49.
49. Best Practice Statement: The use of topical antiseptic/antimicrobial agents in wound management. Wounds UK, Aberdeen, 2013. Available at https://www.wounds-uk.com/resources/details/best-practice-statement-use-topical-antimicrobial-agents-wound-management. Accessed May 23, 2023.
50. Landis S, Ryan S, Woo K, Sibbald RG. Infections in chronic wounds. In: Krasner DL, Rodeheaver GT, Sibbald RG, eds. *Chronic Wound Care: A Clinical Source Book for Healthcare Professionals*. 4th ed. Malvern, PA: HMP Communications; 2007:299-321.
51. Gethin G. Role of topical antimicrobials in wound management. *J Wound Care, Activa Healthcare*. 2009;(Supplement):s4-s8.
52. International Wound Infection Institute (IWII) Wound Infection in Clinical Practice. *Wounds International. 2022*. Available at https://woundinfection-institute.com/wp-content/uploads/IWII-CD-2022-web-1.pdf. Accessed May 24, 2023.
53. Weir D, Schultz G. Assessment and management of wound-related infections. In: McNichol, L; Ratliff, C; Yates, S. *Wound, Ostomy and Continence Nurses Society Core Curriculum: Wound Management*. Wolters Kluwer Health, Kindle Edition; 2021.
54. Phillips P, Sampson E, Qingping Y, Antonelli P, Progulske-Fox A, Schultz G. Bacterial biofilms in wounds. *Wound Healing Southern Africa*. 2008;1(2):10-12.
55. Kirketerp-Moller K, Zulkowski K, James G. Chronic wound colonization, infection, and biofilms. In: Bjarnsholt TH, Jensen P, Hoiby N, eds. *Biofilm Infections*. 2011. Available at: http://www.springer.com/978-1-4419-6083-2. Accessed September 19, 2018.
56. Attinger C, Wolcott R. Clinically addressing biofilm in chronic wounds. *Adv Wound Care*. 2012;1(3):127-132.
57. Wolcott RD, Rumbaugh KP, James G, et al. Biofilm maturity studies indicate sharp debridement opens a time-dependent therapeutic window. *J Wound Care*. 2010;19(8):320-328.
58. Murphy CA, Atkin L, Swanson T, et al. International consensus document. Defying hard-to-heal wounds with an early antibiofilm intervention strategy: wound hygiene. *J Wound Care*. 2020;29(3 Suppl 1):S1-S28.
59. Kim P, Steinberg J. Wound care: biofilm and its impact on the latest treatment modalities for ulcerations of the diabetic foot. *Semin Vasc Surg*. 2012;25:70-74.
60. Roy M, Somerson JS, Kerr KG, Conroy JL. Osteomyelitis: pathophysiology and pathogenesis. In: Baptista MS, ed. *Osteomyelitis*. Rijeka: InTech Press; 2012.
61. Lipsky BA, Peteres EJG, Senneville E, et al. Expert opinion on the management of infection in the diabetic foot. *Diabetes Metab Res Rev*. 2012;28(suppl 1):163-178.
62. Edwards-Jones V. Antimicrobial stewardship in wound care. *Br J Nurs*. 2020;29(15): S10-S16.
63. International Consensus. *Appropriate Use of Silver Dressings in Wounds. An Expert Working Group Consensus*. London: Wounds International; 2012. Available at: www.woundsinternational.com. Accessed December 10, 2018.
64. Lipsky BA, HOey C. Topical antimicrobial therapy for treating chronic wounds. *Clin Infect Dis*. 2009;49(10):1541-1549.
65. Rodeheaver GT, Ratliff CR. Wound cleansing, wound irrigation, wound disinfection. In: Krasner DL, Rodeheaver GT, Sibbald RG, eds. *Chronic Wound Care: A Clinical Source Book for Healthcare Professionals*. 4th ed. Malvern, PA: HMP Communications; 2007:323-330.
66. Fife C, Carter MH, Walker D, Thomson B. A retrospective data analysis of antimicrobial dressing usage in 3,084 patients. *Ostomy Wound Manag*. 2010;56(3):28-42.

67. Sibbald RG, Elliott JA, Ayello EA, Somayaji R. Optimizing the moisture management tightrope with wound bed preparation 2015. *Adv Skin Wound Care*. 2015;28(10):466-476.
68. Bergstrom N, Bennet MA, Carlson CE, et al. *Clinical Practice Guideline Number 15: Treatment of Pressure Ulcers*. Rockville, MD: U.S. Department of Health and Human Services, Agency for Health Care Policy and Research; 1994. AHCPR Publication 95-0652.
69. Moore Z, Cowman S. A systematic review of wound cleansing of pressure ulcers. *J Clin Nurs*. 2008;7:1963-1972.
70. Shetty R, Kingsly PM, Barreto E, Sreekar H, Dawre S. Wound Irrigation, Letter to the Editor. *Indian J Plast Surg*. 2012;45(3):590.
71. Dai T, Huang YY, Sharma S, Hashmi J, Kurup D, Hamblin M. Topical antimicrobials for burn wound infections. *Recent Pat Antinfect Drug Discov*. 2010;5(2):124-151.
72. Mooney EK, Lipitt C, Friedman J. Safety and efficacy report—silver dressings. *Plast Reconstr Surg*. 2006; 117:666-669.
73. Lansdown AB. A review of the use of silver in wound care: facts and fallacies. *Br J Nurs*. 2004;13(6 suppl):s6-s19.
74. Aramwit P, Maungman P, Namviriyachote N, Srichana T. In vitro evaluation of the antimicrobial effectiveness and moisture binding properties of wound dressings. *Int J Mol Sci*. 2010;11:2864-2874.
75. Kostenko V, Lyczak J, Turner K, Martinuzzi RJ. Impact of silver-containing dressing on bacterial biofilm viability and susceptibility to antibiotics during prolonged treatment. *Antimicrob Agents Chemother*. 2010;5120-5131.
76. Cutting K, White R, Hoekstra H. Topical silver-impregnated dressings and the importance of the dressing technology. *Int Wound J*. 2009;6:396-402.
77. Jones S, Bowler PG, Walker M. Antimicrobial activity of silver-containing dressings is influenced by dressing conformability with a wound surface. *Wounds*. 2005;17:263-270.
78. Hamm R. Antibacterial dressings. In: Sen C, ed. *Advances in Wound Care*. Vol 1. New Rochelle, NY: Mary Ann Libert; 2010.
79. Hoekstra MJ, Hermans MH, Richters CD, Dutriex RP. A histological comparison of acute inflammatory responses with a hydrofibre or tulle gauze dressing. *J Wound Care*. 2002;11:113-117.
80. Atiyeh BS, Costagliola M, Hayek SN, Dibo SA. Effect of silver on burn wound infection control and healing review of the literature. *Burns*. 2007;33:139-148.
81. Krasner D. The chronic wound pain experience: a conceptual model. *Ostomy Wound Manage*. 1995;41:20-27.
82. Silverstein P, Heimbach D, Meites H, et al. An open parallel randomized comparative multicenter study to evaluate the cost-effectiveness, performance, tolerance, and safety of a silver-containing soft silicone foam dressing (intervention) vs. sulfadiazine cream. *J Burn Care Res*. 2011;32(6):617-626.
83. Muangman P, Pundee C, Opasanon S, Muangaman S. A prospective, randomized trial of silver containing hydrofiber dressing versus 1% silver sulfadiazine for the treatment of partial thickness burns. *Int Wound J*. 2010;7(4):271-276.
84. Hooper SJ, Williams DW, Thomas DW, Hill KE, Percival SL. An in vitro comparison of two silver-containing antimicrobial wound dressings. *Ostomy Wound Manage*. 2012;58 (1):16-22.
85. Glat PM, Kubat WD, Hsu JF, et al. Randomized clinical study of Silvasorb gel in comparison to Silvadene silver sulfadizine cream in the management of partial thickness burns. *J Burn Care Res*. 2009;30(2):262-267.
86. Carter MJ, Tingley-Kelley K, Warriner RA. Silver treatments and silver-impregnated dressings for the healing of leg wounds and ulcers: a systematic review and meta-analysis. *J Am Acad Dermatol*. 2010; 63:668-679.
87. Fredriksson C, Kratz G, Huss F. Accumulation of silver and delayed re-epithelialization in normal human skin: an ex-vivo study of different silver dressings. *Wounds*. 2009;21(5):116-123.
88. Van Den Plas D, De Smet K, Lens D, Sollie P. Differential cell death programmes induced by silver dressings in vitro. *Eur J Dermatol*. 2008;18 (4):416-421.
89. Cutting KF. Honey and contemporary wound care: an overview. *Ostomy Wound Manage*. 2007;53(11):49-54.
90. Siah CJ, Yatim J. Efficacy of total occlusive ionic silver-containing dressing combination in decreasing risk of surgical site infections: an RCT. *J Wound Care*. 2011;20(12):561-568.
91. NICE Guidelines. National Institute for Health and Clinical Excellence 2008. Available at: http://www.nice.org.uk/nicemedia/live/11743/42379/42379.pdf. Accessed October 4, 2013.
92. Anderson PA, Savage JW, Vaccaro AR, et al. Prevention of Surgical Site Infection in Spine Surgery. *Neurosurgery*. 2017 Mar 1;80(3S):S114-S123.
93. Staveski S, Abrajano C, Casazza M, et al. Silver-impregnated dressings for sternotomy incisions to prevent surgical site infections in children. *Am J Crit Care*. 2016;25(5):402-408.
94. Dumville JC, Gray TA, Walter CJ, et al. Dressings for the prevention of surgical site infection. *Cochrane Database Syst Rev*. 2016;12(12):CD003091.
95. Barrett DA, Rutter N. Transdermal delivery and the premature neonate. *Rev Ther Drug Carrier Syst*. 1994, 11:1-30.
96. Jester I, Bohn I, Hannmann T, Waag KL, Loff S. Comparison of two silver dressings for wound management in pediatric burns. *Wounds*. 2008;20(11):303-308.
97. Poon VKM, Burd A. In vitro cytotoxicity of silver: implication for clinical wound care. *Burns*. 2004;30: 140-147.
98. Treadwell TA, Fuentes ML, Walker D. Treatment of second degree burns with deyhdrated, decellularized amniotic membrane (biovance) vs. a silver dressing (acticoat). *Wound Rep Regen*. 2008;16:A39.
99. Wang XQ, Kempf M, Mott J, et al. Silver absorption on burns after the application of acticoat: data from pediatric patients and a porcine burn model. *J Burn Care Res*. 2009;30(2):341-348.
100. Treadwell TA. Children and wounds. *Wounds*. 2011. Available at: http://www.woundsresearch.com/article/children-and-wounds?page=0,0. Accessed October 4, 2013.
101. Escher KB, Shellock FG. An in vitro assessment of MRI issues at 3-Tesla for antimicrobial silver-containing wound dressings. *Ostomy Wound Manage*. 2012;58(11):22-27.
102. Bailey JK, Sammet S, Overocker J, et al. MRI compatibility of silver-based wound dressings. *Burns*. 2018;44(8):1940-1946.
103. Riddle JM. *Dioscorides on Pharmacy and Medicine*. Austin, TX: University of Texas Press; 1985.
104. Adam F. *The Genuine Works of Hippocrates*. Baltimore, MD: Williams and Wilkins; 1939.
105. Trevisanto SI. Treatments for burns in the London Medical Papyrus show the first seven biblical plagues of Egypt are coherent with Santorini's volcanic fallout. *Med Hypotheses*. 2006;66:193-196.
106. Pieper B. Honey-based dressings and wound care. *J Wound Ostomy Continence Nurs*. 2009;36(1):60-66.
107. Moore ZEH. Honey as a topical treatment for wounds. In: Sen C, ed. *Advances in Wound Care*. Vol 1. New Rochelle, NY: Mary Ann Libert; 2010.
108. Molan P, Rhodes T. Honey: a biologic wound dressing. *Wounds*. 2015;27(6):141-151.
109. Watson D, Bergquist S, Nicholson J, Norrie DH. Comprehensive in situ killing of six common wound pathogens with Manuka honey dressings using a modified AATCC-TM100. *Wounds*. 2017 Sep;29(9):262-268.

110. Cernak M, Majonova N, Cernak A, Majtan J. Honey prophylaxis reduces the risk of endophthalmitis during perioperative period of eye surgery. *Phytother Res*. 2012;26:613-616.
111. Gethin G, Cowman S. Bacteriological changes in sloughy venous leg ulcers treated with manuka honey or hydrogel: an RCT. *J Wound Care*. 2008;17(6):241-244, 246-247.
112. Biglari B, Linden PH, Simon A, Aytac S, Gerner HJ, Moghaddam A. Use of medihoney as a non-surgical therapy for chronic pressure ulcers in patients with spinal cord injury. *Spinal Cord*. 2012;50: 165-169.
113. Gethin G, Cowman S. Manuka honey vs. hydrogel—a prospective, open label, multicenter, randomized controlled trial to compare desloughing efficacy and healing outcomes in venous ulcers. *J Clin Nurs*. 2008;(18):466-474.
114. Jull A, Walker N, Parag V, Molan P, Rodgers A. Randomized clinical trial of honey-impregnated dressings for venous leg ulcers. *Br J Surg*. 2008;95:175-182.
115. Jull AB, Cullum N, Dumville JC, Westby MJ, Deshpande S, Walker N. Honey as a topical treatment for wounds. *Cochrane Database Syst Rev*. 2015 Mar 6;2015(3):CD005083.
116. Simon A, Sofka K, Wiszniewsky G, Blaser G, Bode U, Fleischhack G. Wound care with antibacterial honey (Medihoney) in pediatric hematology-oncology. *Support Care Cancer*. 2006;14:91-97.
117. Leaper DJ, Durani P. Topical antimicrobial therapy of chronic wounds healing by secondary intention using iodine products. *Int Wound J*. 2008;5:361-368.
118. Mertz PM, Oliveira-Gandia MF, Davis SC. The evaluation of a cadexomer iodine wound dressing on methicillin resistant *Staphylococus aureus* (MRSA) in acute wounds. *Dermatol Surg*. 1999;25:89-93.
119. Danielsen L, Cherry GW, Harding K, Rollman O. Cadexomer iodine in ulcers colonized by *Pseudomonas aeruginosa*. *J Wound Care*. 1997;6(4):169-172.
120. Moore K, Thomas A, Harding KG. Iodine released from the wound dressing iodosorb modulates the secretion of cytokines by human macrophages responding to bacterial lipopolysaccharide. *Int J Biochem Cell Biol*. 1997;29(1):163-171.
121. Ohtani T, Mizuashi M, Yumiko I, Aiba S. Cadexomer as well as cadexomer iodine induces the production of proinflammatory cytokines and vascular endothelial growth factor by human macrophages. *Exp Dermatol*. 2007;16:318-323.
122. Phillips PL, Yang Q, Sampson E, Schultz G. Effects of antimicrobial agents on an in-vitro biofilm model of skin wounds. In: Sen K, ed. *Adv Wound Care*. New Rochelle, NY: Mary Ann Liebert; 2010.
123. Barrett S, Battacharyya M, Butcher M, et al. PHMB and its potential contribution to wound management. *Wounds UK*. 2010;6(2):40-46.
124. Hubner N, Matthhes R, Koban I, et al. Efficacy of chlorhexidine, Cadexomer and pseudomonas aeruginosa biofilms grown on polystyrene and silicone materials. *Skin Pharmacol Physiol*. 2010;23(suppl 1):28-34.
125. Cazzinga A, Serralta V, Davis S, Orr R, Eaglstein W, Mertz PM. The effect of an antimicrobial gauze dressing impregnated with 0.2-percent polyhexamethylene biguanide as a barrier to prevent Pseudomonas aeruginosa wound invasion. *Wounds*. 14(5): 169-176.
126. Wild T, Bruckner M, Payrich M, Schaarz C, Eberlein T, Andreissen A. Eradication of methicillin-resistant *Staphylococcus aureus* in pressure ulcers comparing a polyhexanide-containing cellulose dressing with polyhexanide swabs in a prospective randomized study. *Adv Skin Wound Care*. 2012;25(1):17-22.
127. Werner HP, Kramer A. Local microbiological requirements with special emphasis on anti-infectives, anti-infective treatment of wounds. In: Kramer A, Wendt M, Werner HP, eds. *Possibilities and Perspectives of Clinical Antisepsis*. Wiesbaden, Germany: MHP-Verlag. 2005:26-30.
128. Butcher M. PHMB: an effective antimicrobial in wound bioburden management. *Br J Nurs*. 2012;21(12):s16-s21.
129. Kingsley A, Tradej M, Colbourn A, Kerr A, Bree-Aslan C. Suprasorb X + PHMB: antimicrobial and HydroBalance action in a new wound dressing. *Wounds UK*. 2009;5(1):72-77.
130. Nygaard R, Jorgensen S. New HydroBalance concept tested in the primary health care sector. *EWMA J*. 2009;9(2):15-22.
131. McCallon S, Hurlow J. Clinical applications for the use of enzymatic debriding ointment and broad-spectrum bacteriostatic foam dressing. *J Wound Ostomy Continence Nurs*. 2009;36(65):517-524.
132. Churchman J. The selective bactericidal action of methylene blue. *J Exp Med*. 1913;18(2):187-189.
133. Hoffmann CE, Rahn O. The bactericidal and bacteriostatic action of crystal violet. *J Bacteriol*. 1944;47(2):177-186.
134. Applewhite AJ, Attar P, Liden B, Stevenson Q. Gentian violet and methylene blue polyvinyl alcohol foam antibacterial dressing as a viable form of autolytic debridement in the wound bed. *Surg Technol Int*. 2015;26:65-70.
135. Edwards K. New twist on an old favorite: gentian violet and methylene blue antibacterial foams. *Adv Wound Care (New Rochelle)*. 2016;5(1):11-18.
136. Boyar V. Successful management of complex pediatric and neonatal wounds with methylene blue and gentian violet foam dressings. *Wounds*. 2021;33(10):253-259.
137. Coutts PM, Ryan J, Sibbald RG. Case series of lower-extremity chronic wounds managed with an antibacterial foam dressing bound with gentian violet and methylene blue. *Adv Skin Wound Care*. 2014;27(3 Suppl 1):9-13.
138. Alvarez J. The versatility of PVA foam dressing impregnated with methylene blue and genetian sic violet on acute and chronic wounds. Available at: http://www.hanstronics.com/pdf/hydroferablue_versatility_Sty_18x24_hires.pdf. Accessed May 27, 2023.
139. Probst A. Chronic arterial leg ulcer with MRSA. BSN Medical. Hands-on Case Report 6. Available at: http://www.cutimed.nl/sites/all/themes/cutimed/case-studies/112310.pdf. Accessed December 22, 2018.
140. Doyle RJ. Contribution of the hydrophobic effect to microbial adhesion. *Microbes Infect*. 2000;2(4):391-400.
141. Butcher M. Catch or kill. How DAC technology redefines antimicrobial management. *Br J Comm Nurs*. 2011 (suppl). Available at file:///C:/Users/Owner/Downloads/wuwhs_biofilms_web.pdf. Accessed August 4, 2023.
142. Wysocki AB. Evaluating and managing open skin wounds: colonization versus infection. *AACN Clin Issues*. 2002;13(3): 382-397.
143. Gentili V, Gianesini S, Balboni PG, et al. Panbacterial real-time PCR to evaluate bacterial burden in chronic wounds treated with Cutimed Sorbact. *Eur J Clin Micorbiol Infect Dis*. 2012;31:1523-1529.
144. Totty JP, Bua N, Smith GE, et al. Dialkylcarbamoyl chloride (DACC)-coated dressings in the management and prevention of wound infection: a systematic review. *J Wound Care*. 2017; 26(3):107-114.
145. Rippon MG, Rogers AA, Ousey K. Antimicrobial stewardship strategies in wound care: evidence to support the use of dialkylcarbamoyl chloride (DACC)- coated wound dressings. *J Wound Care*. 2021 Apr 2;30(4):284-296.

146. Husmark J, Morgner B, Susilo YB, Wiegand C. Antimicrobial effects of bacterial binding to a dialkylcarbamoyl chloride-coated wound dressing: an in vitro study. *J Wound Care*. 2022;31(7):560-570.
147. Susilo YB, Mattsby-Baltzer I, Arvidsson A, Husmark J. Significant and rapid reduction of free endotoxin using a dialkylcarbamoyl chloride-coated wound dressing. *J Wound Care*. 2022;31(6):502-509.
148. Ljungh A, Yanagisawa N, Wadstrom T. Using the principle of hydrophobic interaction to bind and remove wound bacteria. *J Wound Care*. 2006;15(4):175-180.
149. Hampton S. An evaluation of the efficacy of Cutimed Sorbact in different types of non-healing wounds. *Wounds UK*. 2007;3(4):1-6.
150. Von Hallern B, Lang F. Has Cutimed Sorbact proved its practical value as an antibacterial dressing? *Medizin und Praxis*. 2005; 8-11. Available at: http://cutimed.com/fileadmin/templates/PDF/Practical.pdf. Accessed October 16, 2014.
151. Meberg A, Schoyen R. Hydrophobic material in routine umbilical cord care and prevention of infections in newborn infants. *Scand J Infect Dis*. 1990;22(6):729-733.
152. Cowan L, Phillips P, Liesenfeld B, et al. Caution: when combining topical wound treatments, more is not always better. *Wound Prac Res*. 2011;19(2): 60-64.
153. Wodash J. Wet-to-dry dressings do not provide moist wound healing. *J Am Coll Clin Wound Spec*. 2012;4(3):63-66.

PART FOUR

Adjunctive Therapies

CHAPTER FIFTEEN

Exercise for the Patient with a Wound

Stephanie L. Woelfel, PT, DPT, CWS and Deborah M. Wendland, PT, DPT, PhD, CPed

CHAPTER OBJECTIVES

At the end of this chapter, the learner will be able to:

1. **Identify the benefits of exercise, including in the presence of chronic wounds.**
2. **Identify any precautions and/or contraindications to exercise based on patient and wound status.**
3. **Select exercise and supervision techniques based on special considerations related to medication.**
4. **Utilize exercise to facilitate wound healing, prevention, or delay in recurrence for at-risk populations.**
5. **Facilitate exercise adoption through the use of motivational interviewing, action and coping planning, and/or brief action planning.**

INTRODUCTION

Exercise as a therapeutic intervention is a well-documented concept with a multitude of participation options. The addition of exercise into one's lifestyle can be challenging, even with a direction that is available through apps, classes, or trained providers, eg, physical therapists, exercise physiologists, or personal trainers.

For the patient with a wound, especially in the presence of additional medical co-morbidities, it is critical to involve a professional who can individualize a safe and effective exercise prescription that takes into consideration all aspects of the patient's health and lifestyle. The training of physical therapists as movement experts makes them uniquely qualified to provide exercise prescriptions to patients at risk for, with, or recovering from wounds of various etiologies. The APTA Guide to Physical Therapist Practice describes the physical therapist's role in the integumentary practice as one who identifies and responds to components, including impairments to function, that promote the development of wounds or slow their healing. In response to risk and impairments, physical therapists educate patients to reduce risk by modifying or removing contributing factors.[1] Addressing these factors and functional impairments often incorporates exercise as a key management strategy.

Joint and Body Mobility: Effect on Wound Healing and Skin Health

Skin health, to some extent, is a movement issue. Movement is necessary to maintain good skin pliability, and limitations to movement can place individuals at increased risk for loss of skin health (eg, reduced mobility increases the risk for pressure injuries).[2] Furthermore, restriction in motion at a specific joint can affect the risk of skin injury.[3] The presence of a fixed deformity can alter weight-bearing and skin-loading in such a way that excessive overloading occurs, resulting in skin breakdown. When a restriction is present in a joint, other joints must increase movement to complete body motion for functional mobility. Movement pattern changes that accompany joint motion changes can affect the loading of both joints and skin. At other times, the wounds themselves can cause limitations in mobility (eg, diabetic foot ulcer and subsequent off-loading can result in limited weight-bearing activity; a venous leg ulcer with edema can restrict the range of motion making movement difficult). It is important to recognize that movement through exercise may support positive skin health changes.

Benefits of Exercise

Physical activity and exercise are associated with many health benefits across the lifespan. These benefits are varied and include:

- Reduced all-cause mortality
- Improved cardiovascular fitness
- Improved musculoskeletal health including muscular fitness (ie, strength, endurance, power, flexibility) and bone health
- Lowered disease risk (eg, cardiovascular disease, hypertension, diabetes, and cancer)
- Improved cognitive and mental health status (eg, improved cognitive function, lowered dementia risk, reduced feelings of anxiety and depression, lowered risk for depression)
- Improved weight management
- Reduced falls risk
- Improved physical function
- Improved quality of life[4]

Although data continues to increase regarding the benefit of physical activity and exercise, few people meet the guidelines for physical activity and exercise engagement (**TABLE 15-1**).[5] Changes in work habits and chronic conditions may make exercise even more challenging despite the direct benefits that can be seen in populations with these conditions.

TABLE 15-1 Exercise Guidelines for Adults

Aerobic exercise (eg, walking, running, swimming)	▪ 150+ minutes per week of moderate intensity physical activity or vigorous intensity physical activity for 75+ minutes per week ▪ At least 3 days/week
Resistance exercise (eg, multijoint exercises like push-ups; single joint exercises like biceps curls; core exercise like planks)	▪ All major muscle groups ▪ Moderate intensity+ ▪ 2+ days/week
Flexibility exercise (stretches)	▪ All major muscle-tendon units ▪ Performed to point of tightness ▪ 2–3 days+/week
Avoidance of sedentary behavior	▪ Move more, sit less

General guidelines combined from Piercy KL, Troiano RP, Ballard RM, et al. The physical activity guidelines for Americans. *JAMA*. 2018;320(19):2020; Liguori G. *ACSM's Guidelines for Exercise Testing and Prescription*. 11th ed. Wolters Kluwer; 2022.[5,6]

TABLE 15-2 Options for Estimation of Exercise Intensity

Exercise Intensity	Rating of Perceived Exertion (6–20)	Percent Heart Rate Reserve[a]	Percent Heart Rate Max[b]
Very light	<9	<30	<57
Light	9–11	30–39	57–63
Moderate	12–13	40–59	64–76
Vigorous	14–17	60–89	77–95

[a]Percent HRR calculated as $[(HR_{max} - HR_{rest}) \times \text{desired\%}] + HR_{rest}$.

[b]HR_{max} is commonly calculated as (220 – age).

Most common RPE targets on the regular Borg scale for cardiac rehabilitation were 11–13 and 12–15. With the 1–10 Borg scale, 3–4 was consistently the target intensity.

From Pack QR, Shea M, Brawner CA, et al. Exercise prescription methods and attitudes in cardiac rehabilitation: a national survey. *J Cardiopulm Rehabil Prev*. 2022;42(5):359-365.[7] Modified from Table 5.2 in Liguori G. *ACSM's Guidelines for Exercise Testing and Prescription*. 11th ed. Wolters Kluwer; 2022.[6]

Exercise is critically important; however, it can be accompanied by risks, especially for someone new to exercise or in a chronic disease state.[6] To mitigate risk, an important practice for exercise safety is the monitoring of vital signs. Students in all health care disciplines are taught to perform vital signs as an indication of the patient's health status. Thus, vital signs are important to assess an individual's readiness to participate in an activity as well as their response to the activity. Given the chronic conditions that many patients with wounds have, assessment of the body's response to exercise (eg, blood pressure, heart rate, and respiratory rate) is a critical component of every exercise session. Moreover, patients need to be instructed on how to monitor their vital signs to ensure the performance of safe exercise.

Some chronic diseases affect one's ability to exercise. In cases where cardiovascular function is limited, specific parameters may be required for safety during exercise. Exercise targets remain important for patient exercise adoption and performance, for example, a prescribed target heart rate to match the desired exercise intensity. In the presence of certain medications (eg, beta blockers), heart rate response to exercise may be blunted and an appropriate assessment for exercise intensity is a Rating of Perceived Exertion (RPE) (**TABLE 15-2**).[6]

A patient's physical activity needs to be considered along with any prescribed exercise. Studies of the relationship between sedentary behavior and all-cause mortality indicate that health risk increases with increased sedentary time.[8] In response, the Physical Activity Guidelines for Americans (2018) recommends "moving more and sitting less."[5] Furthermore, the World Health Organization (WHO) strongly recommends that both adults and older adults "limit the amount of time spent being sedentary."[9]

CLINICAL CONSIDERATION

A patient who is 50 years old and at risk for skin breakdown is encouraged to meet the Physical Activity Guidelines for Americans. To better understand how hard the patient should work during aerobic exercise, consider what moderate intensity exercise means, eg, for a patient who has a resting heart rate of 80 beats per minute (**TABLE 15-3**).

Sedentary time can be replaced with any intensity of physical activity. While the Physical Activity Guidelines for Americans does not specify beyond "sitting less," the Standards of Care in Diabetes recommends that extended bouts of "sitting should be interrupted every 30 min for blood glucose benefits."[10] Increasing amounts of moderate to vigorous activity beyond that recommended can also serve to mitigate the risk associated with poorer health outcomes related to sedentary behavior.[8]

The challenge for people with chronic illnesses is that physical activity may be difficult. For example, people with type 2 diabetes commonly present with hypertension, dyslipidemia, peripheral neuropathy, renal disease, retinal disease, and peripheral vascular disease which may make certain exercises challenging in terms of practice and volume. Additionally, medications can impact the safety of exercise (**TABLE 15-4**). Therefore, it is important to consider the breadth of exercise that can be included for positive health outcomes.[25]

In wound management, chronic diseases such as diabetes, peripheral vascular disease, and venous insufficiency are

TABLE 15-3 Sample Moderate Intensity Exercise Targets for 50-Year-Old Patient with Resting HR 80 Beats Per Minute

%Heart Rate Reserve (HRR)	%Heart Rate (HR) Max	Rating of Perceived Exertion (RPE)
Moderate intensity = 40–59% HRR	Moderate intensity = 64–76% HR_{max}	Moderate intensity = 12–13 on 6–20 scale
40% HRR = $(H_{Rmax} - H_{Rrest}) \times .40 + HR_{rest}$	$HR_{max} = 220 - \text{age}$	
40% HRR = 36 + 80 = 116 bpm	$HR_{max} = 220 - 50 =$ 170 bpm	
59% HRR = $(HR_{max} - HR_{rest}) \times .59 + HR_{rest}$	64% $HR_{max} = 170 \times .64 =$ 109 bpm	
59% HRR = 53 + 80 = 113 bpm	76% $HR_{max} = 170 \times .76 =$ 129 bpm	
Moderate intensity = 116–133 bpm	Moderate intensity = 109–129 bpm	

TABLE 15-4 Medications to Consider with Exercise for People with Chronic Wounds or Disease

Drug Class	Condition	Example Medications	Consideration	Response
Insulin	Diabetes[11]	Insulin aspart (Novolog); insulin glargine (Lantus); Insulin lispro (Humalog); insulin regular (Novolin)	▪ Risk for hypoglycemia[10] ▪ Risk at time of peak insulin action ▪ Risk at location of insulin injection	▪ Ask patient to monitor blood glucose levels ▪ Avoid exercise during time of peak insulin action[12] ▪ Avoid exercise in the immediate area following injection
Sulfonylureas, Meglitinides	Diabetes[11]	Glipizide (Glucotrol); glyburide (Diabeta); nateglinide (Starlix); repaglinide (Prandin)	▪ Increased secretion of insulin which increases risk for hypoglycemia with exercise[10,11]	▪ Ask patient to monitor blood glucose levels
Beta Blockers	Heart/circulatory conditions, eg, hypertension and heart failure[13]	Atenolol (Tenormin); bisoprolol (Zebeta); metoprolol (Lopressor, Toprol XL); propranolol (Inderal LA)	▪ Decreased heart rate (HR) and blood pressure (BP) both at rest and with exercise ▪ Masked signs of hypoglycemia during exercise possible[14]	▪ Monitor vital signs ▪ Ask patient to monitor blood glucoe levels
Calcium Channel blockers	Hypertension; arrythmias[15]	Amlodipine (Norvasc); diltiazem (Cardizem); nifedipine (Procardia); nisoldipine (Sular); verapamil (Verelan)	▪ Decreased BP at rest and with exercise ▪ Decreased HR at rest and with exercise with dihydropyridines (bolded examples)[6]	▪ Monitor vital signs
ACE inhibitors and angiotensin II receptor blockers	Hypertension, heart failure, acute coronary syndrome, renal dysfunction due to diabetes, nephrotic syndrome[16,17]	Benazepril (Lotensin); enalapril (Vasotec); lisinopril (Zesteril); losartan (Cozaar); Olmesartan (Benicar); telmisartan (Micardis); valsartan (Diovan)	▪ Decreased BP at rest and with exercise[6]	▪ Monitor vital signs
Anticoagulants, Antiplatelets, and Thrombolytics	Prevent clot formation, platelet aggregation, and dissolve clots, respectively[18]	Clopidogrel (Plavix); dabigatran (Pradaxa); Heparin; LMWH (Lovenox); meloxicam (Mobic); Warfarin (Coumadin)	▪ Increased risk for bleeding[18]	▪ Monitor for signs and symptoms of bleeding with fall or injury during exercise ▪ Select exercise with reduced risk for injury
NSAIDS	Anti-inflammatory; pain control[19]	Ibuprofen (Advil, Motrin); naproxen (Alleve);	▪ Increased risk for bleeding[20,21]	▪ Monitor for signs and symptoms of bleeding with fall or injury during exercise ▪ Select exercise with reduced risk for injury
HMG-CoA Reductase Inhibitors (statins)	High cholesterol; dyslipidemia[22]	Atorvastatin (Lipitor); fluvastatin (Lescol); lovastatin (Altoprev); pitavastatin (Livalo); pravastatin (Pravachol); rosuvastatin (Crestor); simvastatin (Zocor)	▪ Risk for skeletal muscle symptoms ranging from myalgia to elevation in creatine kinase and rhabdomyolysis can be exacerbated with exercise[22]	▪ Monitor for musculoskeletal complaints
Fluoroquinolones	Antibiotic for bacterial infections like sinusitis[23]	Ciprofloxacin (Cipro); gemifloxacin (Factive); levofloxacin (Levaquin); moxifloxacin (Avelox); norfloxacin (Noroxin); ofloxacin (Floxin)	▪ Risk for tendinitis, tendinopathy, or tendon rupture. (Higher risk with >60 years old, corticosteroid therapy, renal failure, diabetes, and history of musculoskeletal problems[23])	▪ Monitor for musculoskeletal complaints
Fibric Acid Derivatives (Fibrates)	Dyslipidemia[24]	Fenofibrate (Tricor, Trilipiz); gemfibrozil (Lopid)	▪ Risk for myopathy[24]	▪ Monitor for symptoms

common causes of ulceration. Depression is also common among those with chronic wounds.[26] Anxiety and depression have been linked to an elevated risk of developing ulceration.[26] Depression has also been shown to be predictive of decreased rates of wound closure for venous leg ulcers.[27] Exercise is an important avenue to address the common comorbidities associated with chronic wounds, including depression, in a way that can mitigate risk and support positive healing outcomes.

Exercise for Patients with Arterial Wounds

Peripheral arterial disease (PAD) is arteriosclerosis of the extremities. The clinical manifestations of PAD can vary greatly from being asymptomatic, to experiencing intermittent claudication (IC), to developing chronic limb-threatening ischemia (CLTI). Please refer to Chapter 4, Vascular Wounds, for additional information.

There are several other conditions with lower extremity symptoms that may masquerade as or be present in addition to PAD, including spinal stenosis, osteoarthritis, chronic venous insufficiency, and neuropathy.[28] Differential diagnose of the correct condition is critical in order to treat the patient safely and effectively.

IC is the most common symptom of moderate PAD and occurs in 20% of the population over 70 years old. This ischemic muscle pain that occurs with a predictable amount of exertion is commonly associated with decreases in walking ability, quality of life, balance, and overall physical function and activity.[29] Exercise is one of the primary interventions for IC and may help to alleviate symptoms by increasing and more effectively distributing blood flow to the lower extremities, improving rheological characteristics of the blood, increasing the use of oxygen, and decreasing reliance on anaerobic metabolism. Exercise is also suggested to increase angiogenesis and thus improve walking in people with claudication. Improvements in both pain-free and maximum walking distance were demonstrated after 3 months of supervised exercise, with effects sustained for up to 2 years.[30] Current guidelines recommend an exercise program as first-line treatment for IC, yet adherence to these recommendations remains low in general.[30]

Studies have investigated the differences between supervised exercise therapy (SET), home-based exercise therapy (HBET), and walking advice (WA).[30] Both HBET and WA are unsupervised exercise interventions with the latter consisting primarily of advice to "go home and walk" (at times combined with an instructional handout). SET programs assessed included three exercise sessions per week for a duration of at least 6 weeks. Exercise sessions involved walking on a treadmill at varying intensities until the patient experienced moderate to intense pain (**FIGURE 15-1**). Patients were then allowed a short period of rest for pain symptoms to subside; the cycle was continued for at least 30 minutes. The increasing incline is the parameter that stimulates the development of collateral circulation by the increased work load placed on the lower extremity muscles. Patients participating in SET showed significant improvement in maximum walking distance/time and pain-free walking distance/time compared with both HBET and WA groups. SET was also more beneficial for self-reported functional impairment and quality of life parameters (physical functioning and pain) than WA.[31]

There is also evidence to support alternative modes of exercise in the treatment of IC for patients for whom walking may not be ideal, or for patients who have an affinity for another type of activity. Alternative modes studied include upper extremity (UE) ergometry, strength training, cycling, and Nordic walking. These interventions were compared against the "traditional" IC walking program with all supervised exercise programs occurring at least twice a week during six consecutive weeks. There was no significant difference in pain-free walking distance or maximum walking distance between any of the alternative modes of exercise and traditional walking.[32] This gives clinicians additional options for selecting an exercise program that will fit the patient's interests and lifestyle (**TABLE 15-5**).

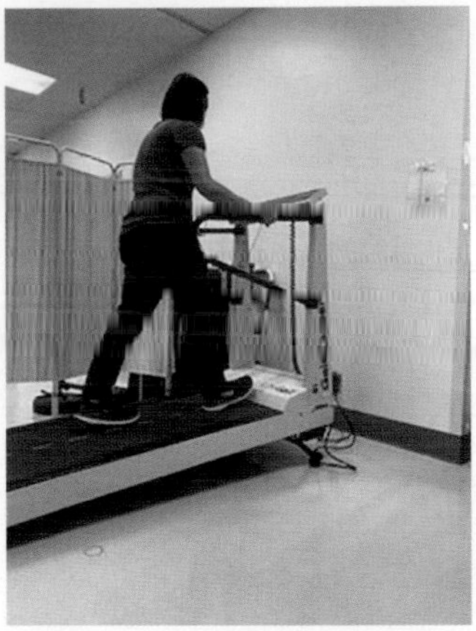

FIGURE 15-1 Walking on a treadmill with incline as part of supervised exercise therapy for intermittent claudication. (Photo courtesy of Stephanie Woelfel; used with permission.)

Strength training in particular may have additional benefits for patients with IC. Basic resistance training resources are provided in **TABLES 15-6** and **15-7**.

Patients participating in a 12-week supervised strength training program not only demonstrated significant improvement in maximum and pain-free walking distances but also in quality of life measures.[29] Muscle strength and endurance markers of 1-repetition max (1-RM) and 40% of 1-RM for endurance also demonstrated significant improvement (mean increase in leg strength of 26 kg and mean increase in number of repetitions from 21 to 32).[29] These changes translate directly to the patient's functional improvements for activities such as rising from a chair or toilet, walking, and maintaining balance. This study also found that lung capacity was significantly improved in patients following supervised strength training. Analyzing data collectively, patients who were the least fit initially demonstrated the most improvement following the strength training intervention and these improvements were sustained up to the 3-month follow-up (**TABLE 15-8**).[29]

TABLE 15-5 Exercise Considerations for Patients with Arterial Insufficiency

Precautions	Appropriate Exercise Interventions	Sample Exercises	Objective Tests/ Measures	Other Exercise Options
Do ***not*** exercise patients with rest pain until *after* revascularization	Supervised exercise therapy (SET)	Treadmill/Ambulation training INTO at least moderate pain with tracking of time and distance to onset of pain, percent of treadmill incline, and time to recovery (increasing incline does most to assist sprouting of collaterals)	6-Minute Walk, short physical performance battery (chair stand, balance, gait speed)	Cycling, strength training, UE ergometry, Nordic walking

TABLE 15-6: 1 Repetition Max (1RM) Calculation

# Repetitions Performed	Percent of 1-Repetition Max (%1RM)	Multiply Weight Lifted By
1	100	1.00
2	95	1.05
3	93	1.08
4	90	1.11
5	87	1.15
6	85	1.18
7	83	1.20
8	80	1.25
9	77	1.30
10	75	1.33

In addition to the benefits for patients with IC, exercise reduces cardiovascular risk factors such as diabetes, hypertension and hypercholesterolemia—all of which often occur concomitantly in patients with PAD. Patients with PAD who participated in an exercise program also demonstrated a lower rate of death and better long-term clinical outcomes.[31]

For patients with PAD or IC with an active arterial wound, care must be taken to protect the wound area and affected limb so the exercise intervention itself does not cause any additional trauma. Alternative modes of exercise, such as UE ergometry, may be especially useful in avoiding lower extremity weight-bearing while still providing benefits.

Patients with PAD who are experiencing rest pain need to have exercise limited to necessary activities of daily living (ADLs) until revascularization is achieved. Rest pain is a sign that the tissue oxygen demands cannot be met at baseline, thus increasing tissue oxygen demands by introducing exercise only worsens the patient's ischemia. Identifying the severity of a patient's PAD is vital to developing an appropriate exercise prescription.

Exercise for Patients with Venous Wounds

Venous leg ulceration (VLU) is a common ulceration that occurs as a result of chronic venous insufficiency. Best practice for the treatment of VLU includes the use of compression to help facilitate venous return along with appropriate wound care.[33]

The physiology of chronic venous insufficiency results in venous hypertension, and dysfunction of the lower extremity muscle pump may contribute to the pathophysiology[34] (see Chapter 4 for more information). Exercise to strengthen the gastrocsoleus muscles facilitates the return of blood to the heart, thus mitigating the calf muscle pump dysfunction that is contributory to chronic venous insufficiency. By promoting venous return and good functioning of the calf muscle pump, venous leg ulcer risk could be lowered.[35]

TABLE 15-8 Sample Strength Training Program for Intermittent Claudication[29]

3 exercise sessions/week, ~ 60-minutes per session

- 10-minute warm-up
- 6 exercise stations (below) performed for 2 minutes and separated by a 2-minute walking interval
- 5-minute cool down

Exercise stations

1. Step-ups
2. Double heel raises
3. Knee extension
4. Exercise bicycle
5. Elbow flexion
6. Sit-to-stand

12-week program

- Weeks 1–6 = 6 stations
- Week 7 = 6 stations
- Week 8 = 8 stations
- Week 9 = 9 stations
- Week 10 = 10 stations
- Week 11 = 11 stations
- Week 12 = 12 stations

In the presence of VLU associated with venous insufficiency, both resistance exercise and aerobic training have been shown to facilitate wound healing at 12 weeks as well as 12 months.[36] Rate of change of ulcer size was improved with range of motion exercises at the foot and ankle.[36] Compression therapy for VLUs often includes multilayer bandaging that contains a short stretch bandage that benefits venous return when the gastrocsoleus contracts and places pressure on the veins. These patients need to be instructed in their exercise routines after the bandages are applied in order to maximize efficacy and adherence (**TABLE 15-9**).

Individuals with VLUs may have been less active during the time of ulceration; therefore, it is critical to begin activity at a light intensity and progress to higher intensities as cardiorespiratory fitness improves and strength increases. This approach to exercise is a helpful strategy for adherence and advancement toward physical activity guidelines. Patients with VLU-associated edema may have decreased ankle ROM

TABLE 15-7 Basic Resistance Training Principles

Goal	%1RM	Sets	Reps	Rest	Recovery
Strength	≥85%	2–6	≤6	2–5 minutes	48 hours
Power	75–90%	3–5	1–5	2–5 minutes	
Hypertrophy	67–85%	3–6	6–12	30–90 seconds	
Endurance	≤67%	2–3	≥12	≤30 seconds	

Note: Need to monitor Rest because a decrease in rest time is an indication of progress.

TABLE 15-9 Exercise Considerations for Patients with Venous Leg Ulcers

Precautions/ Contraindications	Appropriate for Interventions	Sample Exercise	Objective Tests/ Measures	Other Considerations
Exercise is used in conjunction with compression therapy[37]	Progressive resistance exercise (may be endurance or strength training)[36]	Progression from seated to standing to single leg heel raises; ankle plantarflexion with elastic bands[36]	Circumferential measurements of the foot and leg to determine presence or extent of edema	Pain considerations; range of motion limitations; need for an assistive device for safe ambulation
	Aerobic exercise including walking; stress heel/toe gait	Walking on ground or treadmill; cycling		
	Foot/ankle range of motion exercise	Ankle pumps, ankle rotation, ankle ABC's		
	Combined exercise (resistance + walking or resistance + foot/ankle range of motion)[37]	Any combination of the above		

which can lead to a more inefficient, "waddling" walking pattern. These patients benefit from gait training activities to reintroduce a heel-toe gait sequence which activates the venous pump and aids in reducing edema (**FIGURES 15-2** to **15-4**).

Patients with venous disease have a high rate of recurrence; however, there is some support for exercise, like walking, to mitigate impaired calf muscle pump functioning to lower VLU recurrence. Movement specialists (ie, physical therapists) can be invaluable providers to prescribe and facilitate exercise adoption.[35]

Exercise for Patients with Pressure Injuries

Pressure injuries are typically located over bony prominences; however, with continued advances in technology, medical device-related pressure injuries (MDRPIs) to other parts of the body—including areas of predominantly soft tissue—are occurring more frequently. Patients with pressure injuries that are full thickness and extend into or through the musculature are those most in need of exercise. The focus should be on strengthening the surrounding muscles for adequate compensatory movement strategies.

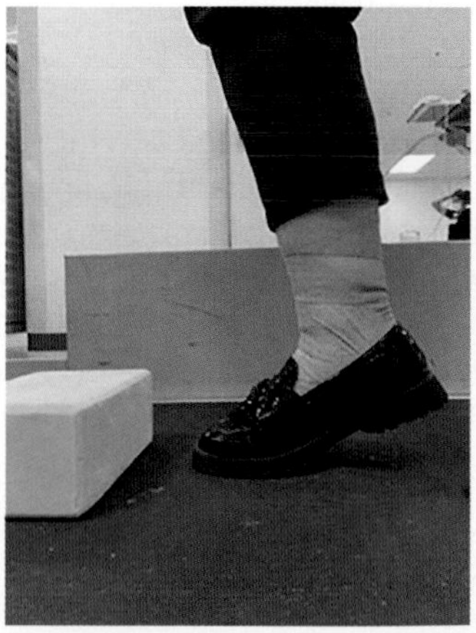

FIGURE 15-2 Standing heel raise exercise to retrain push off during gait. Patients can begin working on ankle ROM in supine and seated positions and progress to standing to benefit from body-weight resistance as a pregait activity. (Photo courtesy of Stephanie Woelfel; used with permission.)

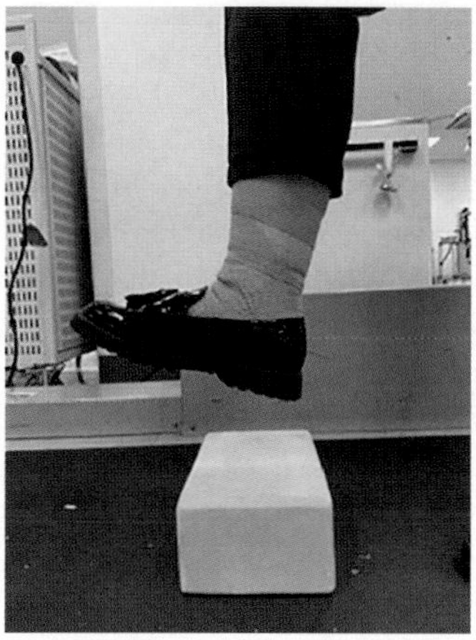

FIGURE 15-3 Stepping over an object to enhance ROM and foot clearance. (Photo courtesy of Stephanie Woelfel; used with permission.)

Because pressure injuries can occur in a multitude of locations, appropriate exercise interventions are best determined by a function-based approach which assesses the specific musculature that has been impacted, based on the underlying anatomy of the wound location as well as the severity of the wound. Identifying the muscles impacted provides detail on the muscle actions that are absent or impaired. Therefore,

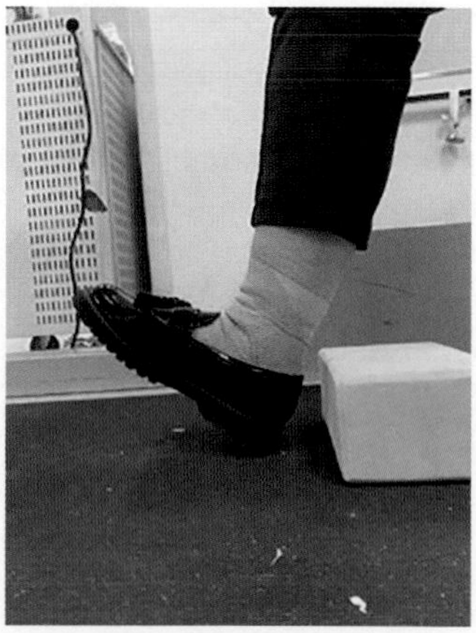

FIGURE 15-4 Exaggerated heel strike as part of pregait training. (Photo courtesy of Stephanie Woelfel; used with permission.)

CASE STUDY

INTRODUCTION

A 91-year-old white male presents to the outpatient wound care clinic with a Stage 4 sacral pressure injury. Medical history includes hypertension, type 2 diabetes, and coronary artery disease with surgical history including open heart surgery and gallbladder surgery.

The patient suffered a left hip fracture and was hospitalized for several weeks. During his hospitalization, he developed pressure injuries to bilateral heels. He was discharged to a rehabilitation facility where he developed a clostridium difficile infection and was rehospitalized and bed-bound for several weeks. This caused a significant setback in his rehabilitation, and he also developed a sacral pressure injury (**FIGURE 15-5**).

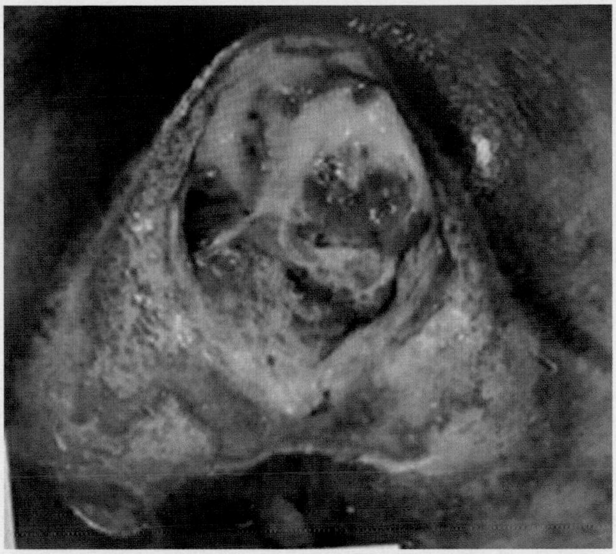

FIGURE 15-5 Case study. Stage 4 sacral pressure injury. (Photo courtesy of Stephanie Woelfel; used with permission.)

DISCUSSION QUESTIONS

1. What muscles are impacted by this patient's pressure injury?
2. What actions do those muscles typically perform?
3. What functional activities are likely impacted for this patient?
4. What would be an appropriate exercise prescription for this patient?

the functional activities impacted are also highlighted. This knowledge can help drive focused testing and subsequent intervention to assist the patient in rehabilitating to their maximum functional level.

Exercise prescription can assist patients with pressure injuries in more global ways. Physical activity and exercise are effective in the prevention and treatment of a multitude of chronic co-morbidities that often exist in patients with pressure injuries, including sarcopenia, diabetes, cardiovascular disease, hypertension, osteoarthritis, depression, and dementia.[25] Improving these underlying conditions can have a positive impact on pressure injury healing as well as prevention (**FIGURE 15-6**).

One of the main risk factors for pressure injury development is activity/mobility limitations.[38] Basic strengthening exercises help to improve patient independence with bed mobility and transfers and thereby decrease the risk of pressure injury development. For patients with an existing pressure injury, these same interventions can assist them in off-loading the injured tissue which in turn can help prevent the progression of the pressure injury to a more severe stage, as well as assist in the healing process.

Patients with a healed full-thickness pressure injury will always be at risk for recurrence of their wounds, as the new tissue reaches a tensile strength of about 80% of the original tissue.[39] Improving functional mobility in these patients can help prevent recurrence and avoid additional tissue damage (**TABLE 15-10**).

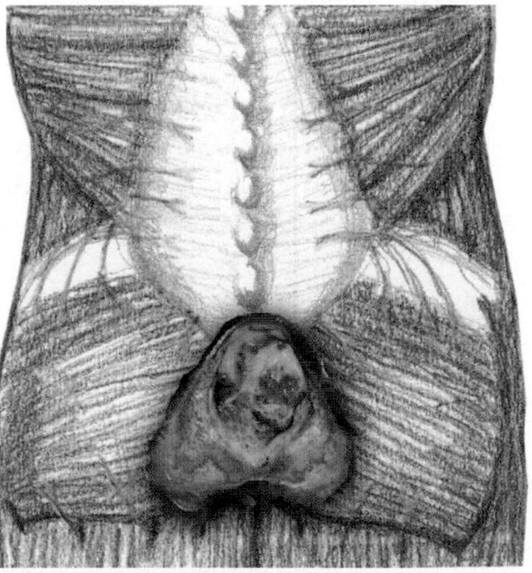

FIGURE 15-6 Case study. Wound image with underlying musculature. (Courtesy of Neil T. Woelfel; used with permission.)

TABLE 15-10 Pressure Injury-Associated Wounds and Exercise Considerations

Precautions	Appropriate Exercise Interventions	Objective Tests/Measures	Other Considerations
Avoid additional loading/pressure to area of pressure injury	Will vary based on wound location and muscles impacted	Varies	Off-loading, minimizing shear/friction, identifying compensatory strategies

CASE STUDY

CONTINUED

The patient was discharged home at wheelchair level for his mobility. His family was instructed in 1) assisting the patient with supine bed-level lower extremity exercises daily and 2) encouraging short standing bouts with a front-wheeled walker throughout the day.

DISCUSSION QUESTIONS

1. How should the patient's exercise program be progressed as he improves?
2. What is the appropriate intensity for the exercises?

Exercise for Patients with Diabetes

Diabetes is associated with multiple complications including cardiovascular disease, dyslipidemia, nephropathy, retinopathy, peripheral neuropathy (PN), foot ulcerations, and amputations. Less recognized complications associated with diabetes are related to the musculoskeletal system and can influence an individual's ability to participate in physical activity and exercise. Among the reported musculoskeletal complications are limited joint mobility; thickening, weakening, and stiffening of the tendons and ligaments; muscle weakness and sarcopenia; and increased musculoskeletal pain complaints. Such complications may be more likely in those with longer duration diabetes as well as people with poor glycemic control.[40] An individual with these complications may present with reduced function, specifically demonstrating lower 6-minute walk distances and reduced ability to generate power when climbing stairs.[41] The importance of lifestyle behaviors, including exercise, for improved diabetes management is well-reported.[10] Exercise can modulate the mechanisms associated with nephropathy, retinopathy, neuropathy, and cardiovascular disease.[42] Exercise is critical to improve function and facilitate good diabetes management; healthcare providers play a key role in encouraging patients, both with diabetes or at risk for diabetes, to exercise.

Challenges for exercise relate to the presence of diabetes-related complications within an individual. Musculoskeletal complaints must be considered when exercise or activity is prescribed. For example, patients with knee and hip pain may avoid high impact activities to minimize pain. Patients with PN are at a higher risk for skin breakdown as well as falls and may have additional challenges with exercise because of a lack of proprioception, kinesthesia, and strength.[41] Patient education needs to include foot inspection for skin safety, strengthening exercises, balance activities to mitigate fall risk, and appropriate shoe wear[10] (refer to Chapter 7, Diabetes and the Diabetic Foot).

For patients with a chronic disease and intact skin, exercise recommendations need to be close to the individual's ability to perform.[5,6,10] Such exercise, even in the presence of PN and other complications, has not been shown to increase risk for skin breakdown.[43] Rather, exercise has been shown to support good diabetes management which may help mitigate complications.[10,42] However, in the presence of complications, it is important to ensure that safety is maintained (**TABLE 15-11**).[10] Exercise can be varied but is recommended to be moderate to vigorous in intensity for 150 minutes per week.[10] This may include walking, interval training, dancing, athletics, or another mode that an individual enjoys.[45–51] More than 2 days without exercise should be avoided for optimal blood glucose control.[6,10,12] In addition to aerobic training, resistance training is important for glycemic control and balance, and flexibility activities are important for safety.[6,10,12]

When exercise and lifestyle choices help an individual maintain good glycemic control, skin may be at a lower risk for breakdown. Maluf and Mueller[52] report that people with diabetes and a plantar ulcer history accumulated less daily stress than those with diabetes without a history of plantar ulcers. This finding is consistent with the theory regarding the susceptibility of skin breakdown with low levels of accumulated stress in a population with diabetes and plantar ulcer history.[52] Exercise may help facilitate wound prevention by providing a "just right" challenge for tissue loading.[53]

Wound healing in people with diabetes is protracted which presents additional considerations for an exercise program (**TABLES 15-11** and **15-12**). Off-loading is critical for injured tissue on the plantar foot to heal, and typically takes at least 6 weeks.[54] Exercise needs to be encouraged concurrently to support good glycemic control and facilitate wound healing. Xiang et al.[55] suggested that maintaining a target HbA1C between 7% and 8% may facilitate healing without an increased risk of death.[55] Although more challenging, exercise can still be performed with adequate off-loading. Lindberg et al.[56] reported a safe and feasible exercise program for people with severe PN and diabetic foot ulcers (DFUs). This program provides examples of exercises that minimize or maintain non-weight bearing (NWB) on the plantar foot but still improve circulation, by using range of motion, seated activity (cycling on a stationary bicycle), and resistance training.[56] Exercise precautions or contraindications need to be observed, especially relative to risk for cardiovascular events.

Reloading/Reintroduction of Function (Activity titration)

Once a wound has closed, the skin is in a weakened state and requires controlled loading during the remodeling phase so that collagen and the extracellular matrix make a strong repair.[39] During this time, the weakened skin is vulnerable to wound recurrence.[57] Therefore, appropriate footwear and activity dosing (titration) are required so that forces are not applied too early, too much, or too fast resulting in disordered wound healing, including underhealing.[39,58] Tissue protection is balanced with progressive exercise, return to activity, and appropriate footwear (refer to Chapter 7). The overall goals are to improve tensile strength, to promote long-term health and disease management, and to optimize physical function. Multiple authors suggest that reloading occur over the first 1 to 3 months postclosure to mitigate risk for reulceration.[59–61] Little data is available regarding dosing of exercise during this time period.[62]

TABLE 15-11 Exercise Considerations for Patients with Diabetes

Guidelines:

- 150 minutes of moderate to vigorous aerobic activity at least 3 days/week with ≤2 consecutive days without activity.
- Shortened times are reasonable if performing vigorous aerobic activity.
- Resistance training for 2–3 nonconsecutive-day sessions/week.
- Decrease sitting time and interrupt sitting ≥30 minutes.
- For older adults include balance and flexibility training 2–3 times/week.
- Increase nonsedentary time.[6,10,12]

Precautions/ Contraindications	Appropriate for Interventions	Sample Exercises	Objective Tests/ Measures	Other Considerations
▪ *Glycemic management* (exercise within a safe glycemic level) ▪ *Uncontrolled hypertension* (monitor vital signs and exercise within safe limits) ▪ *Proliferative retinopathy, untreated or severe nonproliferative retinopathy* (avoid vigorous aerobic and resistance exercise without consulting ophthalmologist) ▪ *Autonomic neuropathy* (obtain cardiac assessment before engaging in physical activity at higher intensity than they are accustomed) ▪ *Peripheral neuropathy* (assess for safety, educate on and perform a foot examination, and utilize proper footwear) ▪ *Charcot foot history* (assess for safety, educate on foot care and perform a foot examination; advise on proper footwear)[10]	▪ Blood glucose levels >90 mg/dL before exercise, otherwise consume 15–30 g carbohydrates before exercise and recheck blood sugar levels ▪ Blood glucose levels 90–150 mg/dL may need to consume carbohydrates with exercise depending on exercise intensity ▪ Blood glucose levels 150–250 mg/dL, start exercise and may consume carbohydrates if blood glucose falls below 150 mg/dL ▪ Blood glucose levels >250 mg/dL, check for ketones and do not perform exercise if moderate to large amounts of ketones present, manage blood sugar ▪ Blood glucose levels >350 mg/dL, check for ketones and manage blood sugar—delay exercise[10,12]	▪ Aerobic activity (swimming, cycling, walk) ▪ Resistance training (may use resistance bands, weight machines, or free weights) ▪ Flexibility and balance activity (Tai chi, yoga) ▪ Perform NWB activities when weight-bearing is contraindicated[10]	▪ Check blood glucose levels prior to and following exercise ▪ Monitor vital signs and patient response to exercise ▪ Perform tests like 6-Minute Walk Test, 30 Second Chair Stand, and gait speed as outcome measures	▪ Perform careful history and assessment when patient has cardiovascular risks; important for safe exercise ▪ If on insulin or insulin secretagogues, carbohydrates may need to be consumed to avoid hypoglycemia[10,12] ▪ Patient may need to adjust timing of insulin medication in relation to when exercise is performed[10,11] ▪ Educate patient on response[6,10] ▪ Avoid exercises that increase shear loading on the plantar surface of the foot ▪ Be aware of anginal equivalents (eg, symptoms associated with exertion that go away with rest like shortness of breath, lightheadedness, or GI symptoms) during exercise[6,44] ▪ Consider medications that may mask hypoglycemia during exercise (beta-blockers)[14] ▪ Monitor vital signs during exercise if patient is on ACE inhibitors and calcium channel blockers[6,15,16] ▪ Be aware of other medications that can affect safety with exercise, eg, anticoagulants[19–21] ▪ Consider location of insulin injection regarding exercising muscle ▪ Consider timing and type of insulin administration (fast-acting) to avoid peak action during exercise[45] (refer to Chapter 7, Diabetes and the Diabetic Foot)
▪ *In the presence of neuropathic ulcer*: • Off-loading of wound area, especially if wound located on plantar surface (nonweight-bearing (NWB) activity only)[10]	▪ In addition to the standard considerations above, Resistance training in NWB position; NWB aerobic exercise (seated activity); chair yoga maintaining NWB position	▪ Rhythmic activity: Seated marching or knee extensions with accompanying upper extremity (UE) motions ▪ Resistance training with at least one set of ≥5 different exercises incorporating large muscle groups (may use resistance bands, weight machines, or free weights)	▪ Monitor blood sugar and vital signs	▪ Exercise and physical activity recommendations are important for glycemic management and general health. Progress activity (intensity, frequency, and/or time) to meet guidelines for individuals unable to meet guidelines initially

TABLE 15-12 Sample Exercise Prescription While Off-Loading the Foot with a Diabetic Ulcer

	Classification of Exercise	Frequency	Intensity	Time	Type	Volume	Progression
Goal guideline[6] (pp. 279–285)	Aerobic	3 or more days/week, avoiding more than 2 days consecutively without activity	Moderate to vigorous (TABLE 15-1)	Sessions of 10–30 minutes accumulating to 150 min/week of moderate to vigorous intensity. Shorter sessions can be used if needed	Repetitive, rhythmic activities with major muscle groups (eg, seated marching, cycling); continuous or interval	Goal of 150 min/week of moderate intensity exercise something is better than nothing. At start, unlikely to meet guideline goal volume	Maximizing caloric expenditure will be a high priority. Increase exercise duration Increase intensity if tolerated
	Resistance	At least 2 nonconsecutive days/week	"Moderate (50–69% of 1-RM) to vigorous (70–85% of 1-RM) to improve strength"[6]	Work toward 8–10 exercises with 10–15 reps; can start with 5. Consider starting with 1 set and progress to 3	Use patient preferred mechanism to add resistance (eg, exercise machines, weights, bands, or body weight) to major muscle groups in NWB position like seated (eg, bicep curls, triceps curls, supine straight leg raise, supine or side-lying hip abduction)	Goal of 8–10 exercises with 1–3 sets (repetitions per set dependent on intent of exercise)	Progression to heavier weight with fewer reps can be made when target number of repetitions per set are consistently exceeded. Can also increase the number of sets or exercises or frequency of resistance training
	Flexibility	At least 2–3 days/week	Should feel tightness or mild discomfort with stretch	2–4 reps of static stretching held for 10–30 seconds each	Patient-preferred is most likely static stretching; could include yoga. Seated approach should be used with off-loading	90 seconds accumulated stretch for major muscle groups	Continue to stretch to tightness/ mild discomfort
	Balance	At least 2–3 days/week	Light to moderate intensity balance exercises	Any amount of balance activity	Yoga; Tai chi; other balance exercises requiring motor skill and proprioceptive training. Seated position should be used with off loading	60 min/week (optimal volume not known)	Could progress length or frequency

Recurrence Prevention

Progressive loading continues to be important after wounds are closed. Feet need to be inspected daily and appropriate footwear must be worn. Assessing skin temperature on bilateral feet helps improve the safety of exercise.[63,64] If above-threshold variances in temperature (2.2°C/4° F) are present on consecutive days, the individual should be encouraged to decrease ambulation to decrease reulceration risk or revert to the previously worn footwear.[65]

Exercise Considerations for the Person with Diabetes with or without Ulceration

Exercise can pose an elevated risk for cardiac events for patients with diabetes. Silent ischemia can occur in people with diabetes resulting in these individuals not detecting or reporting atypical symptoms of myocardial infarction. Anginal equivalents may include symptoms, albeit atypical, that are linked to exertion or stress and resolve with rest. Such symptoms may include shortness of breath, fatigue, symptoms of the gastrointestinal system, or back pain. In some cases, patients should have stress tests performed prior to beginning an exercise program.[6,44]

Exercise for Patients with Surgical Wounds

Exercise and positioning interventions for patients undergoing surgery can occur at multiple times with each having a specific focus for assisting in the overall healing process. Prior to undergoing surgery, most patients will benefit from prehabilitation to optimize their surgical outcomes.[66] Patients who require urgent or emergent surgical intervention would be an exception for obvious reasons.

Many patients who have difficulty healing wounds are elderly and have comorbidities such as diabetes, perhaps due to sarcopenia and frailty. Sarcopenia is an age-associated change in skeletal muscle characterized by loss of muscle mass and strength. This, in turn, is associated with a myriad of age-related mobility disorders, falls, fractures, impairment in ADLs,

CLINICAL CONSIDERATION

Presurgical candidates benefit from any aerobic and/or resistance exercises that aid overall mobility and strengthen muscle groups that may be impacted by the surgical procedure. If a patient is going to have postoperative weight-bearing or other precautions, presurgical training can assist in safety and carry-over postprocedure.

decreased independence, and increased risk of death. Sarcopenia is also a component of *frailty* which is a state in which there is high vulnerability to stressors that lead to disability, dependency, and mortality with diminished physical reserves.[67]

The frailty phenotype developed by Fried et al.[68] has the following five components: exhaustion, physical inactivity, muscle weakness, slow walking speed, and weight loss. The components of slow walking speed and muscle weakness relate directly to sarcopenia, and weight loss has a known detrimental effect on wound healing as well.[69] Preoperative screening for frailty in patients undergoing major vascular surgery found that a significantly higher proportion of patients living independently were discharged to nonhome locations, required mobility assistance, or died within 30 days of surgery if they were categorized as frail prior to surgery.[70]

Fortunately, frailty is a reversible condition—patients may transition between prefrail, frail, and nonfrail states throughout their life span. Resistance training is one exercise intervention that may help move patients out of a frail condition. It has beneficial effects on sarcopenia as well as the loss of muscle performance often seen in older patients with type 2 diabetes.[67] There may be a place for structured, systematic preoperative rehabilitation programs to address frailty in affected patients.[70]

Another intervention time for exercise and positioning is in the immediate postoperative period. The stress of surgery itself can have a major physiologic impact on patients. The demand for protein synthesis increases significantly to meet the needs of immune function, wound healing, and acute phase reactants. Amino acid requirements may be as much as four times greater than what patients normally require.[71] To promote healing and avoid incisional dehiscence, factors that need to be optimized include fluid balance, nutrition, pain management, oxygen levels, and blood glucose levels. Positioning and interventions to avoid mechanical stress on the incision line are advised to prevent separation or dehiscence. Patients who are malnourished, have compromised perfusion, have a history of prolonged steroid use, or have factors that predispose them to incisional stress need to be identified and provided incisional support prior to initiating exercise.[72] Types of support may include the following:

- Modified compression to reduce edema tension on a lower extremity bypass incision line
- Mastectomy bra for a patient with large breasts following a sternal surgery
- Bed mobility and transfer modifications for a patient following abdominal surgery

Incisional dehiscence usually occurs between postoperative days five and eight which is the most critical time for strict adherence to incisional support and positioning interventions. Normal healing progression can be assessed by palpating perpendicular to the incision line for a "healing ridge" beginning on postoperative day five. The healing ridge is a result of the granulation tissue that forms underneath the incision to support closure and eventual remodeling. Absence of this healing ridge by postoperative days five to nine indicates delayed healing and risk for dehiscence.[72]

TABLE 15-13 Postoperative Exercise Considerations

Surgical Procedure	Exercise Considerations[a]
Sternal/abdominal wounds	Thoracic/lumbar spine posture, upper extremity/scapular mobility, chest expansion and lung capacity
Lower extremity amputations	Cardiopulmonary endurance, metabolic demand, core strength, balance, stump edema
Sacral/ischial flaps	Hip flexion ROM, progressive sitting regimen, weight shift strategies in patients with spinal cord injury (SCI)

[a]Discussion of the individual patient with the surgeon is of paramount importance prior to beginning any exercise interventions.

As patients move into more active postoperative recovery, additional exercise options become appropriate. Due to the wide variety of surgical procedures and anatomic locations for these interventions, exercise prescription for the patient with a surgical wound is based on the individual patient case. Additionally, certain surgical procedures have their own inherent postoperative precautions that need to be followed. Examples might include splinting during coughing or sneezing following a median sternotomy[73] or avoidance of prolonged lower extremity dependency immediately following a free flap to the leg. (refer to Chapter 10, Skin Grafts and Flaps, for additional information). Communication with the surgeon is advised prior to developing an exercise program for ANY postoperative patient in order to minimize the risk of complications and dehiscence (**TABLE 15-13**).

CLINICAL CONSIDERATION

- Following sacral/ischial flap surgery, affected tissue must be appropriately stretched and mobilized prior to initiating sitting protocols (**TABLE 15-14**).
- Specialty beds allowing for full patient verticalization (transition to a standing position using bed features); LE weight-bearing and front egress may assist these patients in earlier postoperative ambulation (prior to beginning stretching protocols)

Patient Adherence to Exercise Programs

Exercise interventions are most beneficial when they are performed as prescribed. Predictors with a positive influence on short-term adherence to physical activity include the following: supervised exercise, being physically active, having a high self-efficacy for physical activity, and overall good health. Based on this, it is likely that older adults with sedentary lifestyles and lower activity levels will need support in order to remain adherent to an exercise program.[74]

There are several related support strategies that clinicians can use to engage with their patients including *motivational interviewing* (MI), *action and coping planning* (ACP), and *brief action planning* (BAP). All have been shown to enhance patient adherence to different exercise programs.[74] MI was initially developed to help people discover and address ambivalence related to behavior change.[74] MI that consisted

TABLE 15-14 Postflap Considerations for Stretching and Activity

POD 14 65 degrees hip ✓	**POD 15** 70 degrees hip ✓	**POD 16** 75 degrees hip ✓	**POD 17** 80 degrees hip ✓	**POD 18** 85 degrees hip ✓	**POD 19** 90 degrees hip ✓	**POD 20** 95 degrees hip ✓
POD 21 100 degrees hip ✓	**POD 22** 105 degrees hip ✓	**POD 23** 110 degrees hip ✓	**POD 24** Begin sitting 30 min–Q15 min WS	**POD 25** Sitting 1 hour - Q15 min WS	**POD 26** Sitting 90 min - Q15 min WS	**POD 27** Sitting 2 hour - Q20 min WS
POD 28 Sitting 2½ hour Q20 min WS	**POD 29** Sitting 3 hour - Q20 min WS	**POD 30** Sitting 3½ hour - Q30 min WS	**POD 31** Sitting 4 hour - Q30 min WS			

✓, flexion; POD, postoperative day; Q, every; WS, weight shifts.

of a collaborative conversation using open-ended questions, affirmations, reflective listening, and summaries targeted at developing the patient's own motivation to change was added to balance-related home exercise programs. Patients who received instruction on activity habits and exercise combined with MI showed a significant adherence to the exercise program at 1-year follow-up.[74] Having a specific goal was also an important factor for patients in performing their prescribed exercises. Motivation for performing exercises showed a statistically significant difference at 3 months in the group that received MI, but did begin to decrease at the 9-month follow-up, indicating that some form of support is likely needed for longer than 3 months in order to sustain adherence.[74]

ACP encourages patients to specify when, where, and how an intended behavior (eg, exercise) will be executed in advance. Situational cues are also created that are meant to elicit responses automatically and with little conscious effort (eg, tennis shoes and exercise equipment set up the night before). Individuals are encouraged to proactively anticipate barriers to their plan and identify possible solutions in advance. This strategy has been used in relation to exercise with clinicians encouraging patients to complete ACP for their treatment plan at the end of a session and then following up at the start of the next session. Patients who participated in ACP reported greater improvement in symptoms than those who did not.[75]

The final support strategy is BAP which is grounded in MI theory (**FIGURE 15-7**). The overall goal of BAP is to assist patients in creating an action plan for a behavior that they feel confident they can achieve. BAP consists of three questions and five skills. All of the questions and three of the skills (ie, SMART plan, eliciting a commitment statement, and follow-up) are used during every BAP interaction. The skills of behavioral menu and problem solving for low confidence are used as needed.[76]

Regardless of the support strategy used, the most important thing for a clinician to remember in trying to increase patient adherence is the *patient*. An individualized exercise prescription that considers the patient's current level of function and activity, their goals and priorities, and their daily habits and routine will offer the patient the best chance for success. A variety of training plans exist including those that incorporate functional movement patterns (**TABLES 15-15** and **15-16**). Depending on the overall goals of treatment, different outcome measures can be used to track progress (**TABLE 15-17**).

The successful approach is to start small with two to three basic exercises that will make a significant impact in a short period of time, as well as build patient confidence and trust. Once that therapeutic rapport is established, progression of the patient's exercise plan is easier and future goals are more achievable.

CASE STUDY

CONCLUSION

Relative to the case in this chapter, questions that may be important for a clinician to ask regarding patient follow-up include:

1. Is exercise an appropriate addition for the patient?
2. Is exercise contraindicated?
3. If exercise is not contraindicated, would it be helpful to the overall health of the individual and would it facilitate wound healing?
4. What are possible special considerations for the patient?
   a. Are there parameters associated with their disease process that need to be included in the plan (eg, safe glycemic levels for exercise in people with diabetes)?
   b. Is the patient on medication that requires additional monitoring? (**TABLE 15-4**)
   c. Does the patient require exercise choices that allow for off-loading of the injured tissue?
   d. What protective strategies are necessary for safe exercise?
   e. What steps should be taken to prepare the patient for future mobility and positioning?
5. How might exercise added to the treatment plan improve the rate of healing?
6. Is this a patient who should be referred to an exercise specialist (eg, a physical therapist) for a specific exercise prescription?

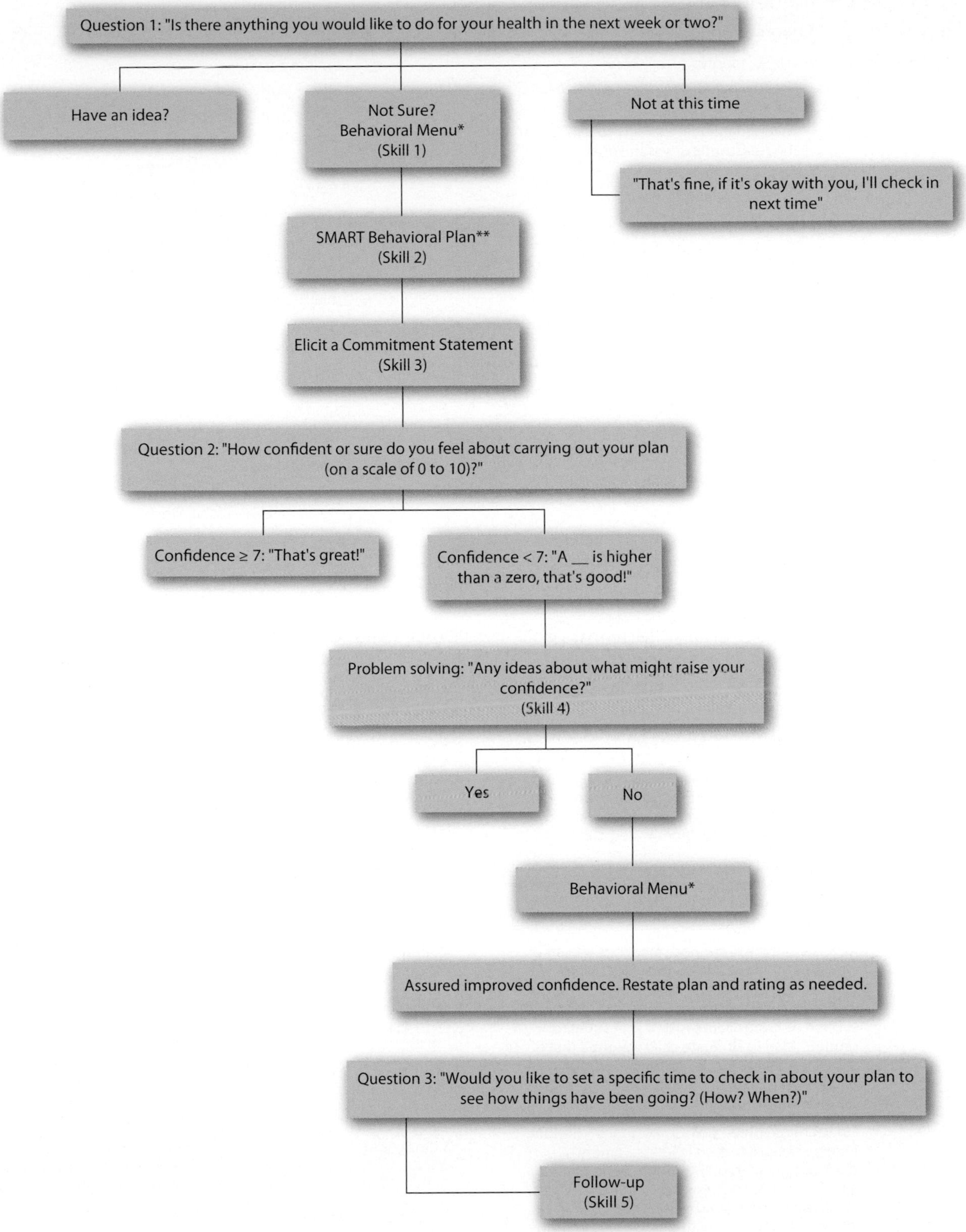

FIGURE 15-7 Brief action planning flowchart. [75] *Ask permission to share ideas with the patient; share two to three ideas; ask if any of these ideas or one of their own ideas might work. **What? When? Where? How often/long/much? Start date?

TABLE 15-15 Sample Training Plans[a]

Training Type	Characteristics	Example
Steady-state aerobic	▪ 20–30 minutes ▪ Cycle of aerobic activities and resistance repeated for a set period of time ▪ Assessment of RPE/ability to talk/HR throughout—moderate intensity is the goal	▪ 30-minute clock • Bike × 2 minutes • Single arm band press ([illegible]/arm) • Farmer's carry × 50 feet • Bent over band row (12/arm) • Row × 2 min
Interval training	▪ Equal time periods	▪ 30s/30s • 30 seconds bike at 80%/higher effort/RPE • 30 seconds bike at 50%/lower effort/ RPE
	▪ Every minute on the minute • 1-minute blocks of exercise are repeated cyclically. Goal is to do as many repetitions as possible for ~45 seconds and have 15 seconds rest prior to starting next minute of exercise	▪ 9-minute session • 1st minute—single arm band press (12/arm) • 2nd minute—banded lateral walks (10 each direction) • 3rd minute—Farmer's carry (45 s)
	▪ Incorporating active recovery • Goal is 2:1 work-"rest" ratio	▪ 5 sets, start every 3 minutes • Seated band row × 20 • Banded hinge × 12 • Suitcase carry × 30 feet • "rest" = easy walk/bike in remaining time before next set starts

[a]Exercises should be modified based on wound type and patient-specific needs.

TABLE 15-16 Functional Loading and Movement Training with Progressions

Push	Quadruped (alternate arm lefts, bird dogs) → modified plantigrade → resisted "punching" → landmine press → overhead press → sled pushes
Pull	Seated row (single arm vs. double arm) → standing row (single arm vs. double arm) → pull from elevated position/slightly lower position/ ground → rowing machine → sled pull
Squat	Sit back/counter/chair squat (UE support to start) → air squat (no UE support, vary height of surface or remove completely) → goblet/front squat
Rising from floor/ Split squat	Reverse lunge (UE support, foam block to step over and then rest knee on) → split stance supported standing (vary depth and UE support) → controlled/assisted split squat to elevated surface → controlled/assisted split squat to ground (load to simulate child weight if that is a goal) → assisted half-kneeling to standing → half-kneeling to standing (vary starting height, remove height, progress to resistance)
Hinge	Dowel hinge (three points of contact—occiput, t-spine, sacrum to help learn movement) → hip hinge banded pull-through (band behind and comes between knees) → stiff legged RDL → single leg RDL (load on side of LE that is extending, can start with single UE support for balance)
Carry	Farmer's carry (bilateral, upright posture, minimal sway) → suitcase carry (unilateral, upright posture, minimal sway) → goblet/front carry (to change center of gravity) → front rack carry → overhead carry (variations = 90/90, full overhead, vary gait from slow to marching to heel-toe)

Note: Use holds in positions to increase time under tension.

TABLE 15-17 Outcome Measures to Assess Physical Fitness

Functional Outcome Measure	Fitness Assessment	Resource
6-Minute Walk Test	Cardiorespiratory Fitness	https://www.sralab.org/rehabilitation-measures/6-minute-walk-test
Duke Activity Status Index (DASI)	Cardiorespiratory Fitness (rough estimate of patient's peak oxygen uptake)	https://www.mdcalc.com/duke-activity-status-index-dasi#next-steps
30-second chair stand	Strength	https://www.sralab.org/rehabilitation-measures/30-second-sit-stand-test
Arm curl	Strength	Rickli RE, Jones CJ. Test validity, reliability, and performance standards: identifying relevant fitness measures for older adults. In Rickli RE, Jones CJ. *Senior Fitness Test Manual*. Champaign, IL: Human Kinetics, 2001
5 times sit to stand	Power	https://www.sralab.org/rehabilitation-measures/five-times-sit-stand-test
Range of Motion	Flexibility	ACSM text 2022[6]
Timed Up and Go (TUG)	Balance	https://www.sralab.org/rehabilitation-measures/timed-and-go
Gait Speed	Balance	https://www.sralab.org/rehabilitation-measures/gait-speed

STUDY QUESTIONS

1. When a patient is taking a Beta blocker for blood pressure management, what is the best way to monitor intensity of exercise?
   a. Blood pressure readings during exercise
   b. Percent of heart rate max
   c. Percent of heart rate reserve
   d. Rating of perceived exertion
2. Which of the following is NOT included in the exercise guidelines for a patient with diabetes?
   a. 150 minutes of moderate to vigorous aerobic activity at least 3 days/week with no more than 2 consecutive days without activity
   b. Decrease sedentary time by interrupting sitting every 30 minutes
   c. Participate in balance and flexibility training two to three times per week
   d. Perform resistance training 2–3 consecutive days per week
3. For the patient with diabetes, what is the most appropriate glycemic level at which to begin exercise in order to minimize the risk of a hypoglycemic episode?
   a. 50–80 mg/dL
   b. >80–150 mg/dL
   c. 150–250 mg/dL
   d. >250–350 mg/dL
4. When prescribing exercise for a patient with VLU, which of the following is an important consideration?
   a. Avoid progressive resistance exercise
   b. Avoid walking or other exercise because of pain
   c. Inclusion of ankle ROM to address likely ROM limits from edema
   d. Limit exercise to a single type to maximize benefit
5. Exercise that improves pumping action at the calf may help improve venous return to the heart, thus mitigating calf muscle dysfunction that contributes to chronic venous insufficiency.
   a. True
   b. False
6. Which one of these conditions with lower extremity symptoms needs to be ruled out before making a diagnosis of PAD?
   a. Spinal stenosis
   b. Rheumatoid arthritis
   c. Restless leg syndrome
   d. Fibromyalgia
7. What additional modes of exercise (beyond walking) have been proven effective in treating intermittent claudication?
   a. Jumping rope
   b. Downhill skiing
   c. Upper extremity ergometry
   d. Lower extremity elevation
8. Patients who were least physically fit initially demonstrated the most improvement following strength training intervention for intermittent claudication.
   a. True
   b. False
9. Patients with which Stage of pressure injury severity are most likely to benefit from exercise prescription?
   a. Stage 1
   b. Stage 2
   c. Stage 3
   d. Stage 4
10. Patients with which type of surgical wound would benefit most from postural exercises?
    a. Trans-metatarsal amputation
    b. Median sternotomy
    c. Lower extremity bypass
    d. Fibular free flap
11. Which of the following exercises would best address the deficits of the patient with a pressure injury who was discussed in this chapter's case study?
    a. Hip/glut/proximal muscle strengthening in functional patterns
    b. High intensity interval training
    c. Plyometric exercises focusing on increasing single-limb stance
    d. Open chain upper extremity exercises

Answers: 1-d; 2-d; 3-c; 4-c; 5-a; 6-a; 7-c; 8-a;9-d;10-b;11-a.

REFERENCES

1. American Physical Therapy Association. APTA Guide to Physical Therapist Practice. Published online 2014. https://guide.apta.org/. Accessed November 16, 2022.
2. Latimer S, Chaboyer W, Thalib L, McInnes E, Bucknall T, Gillespie BM. Pressure injury prevalence and predictors among older adults in the first 36 hours of hospitalisation. *J Clin Nurs*. 2019;28(21-22):4119-4127.
3. Zellers JA, Mueller MJ, Commean PK, Chen L, Jeong HJ, Hastings MK. Multi-system factors associated with metatarsophalangeal joint deformity in individuals with Type 2 diabetes. *J Clin Med*. 2020;9(4):1012.
4. Powell KE, King AC, Buchner DM, et al. The scientific foundation for the physical activity guidelines for americans, 2nd edition. *J Phys Act Health*. 2019;16(1):1-11.
5. Piercy KL, Troiano RP, Ballard RM, et al. The physical activity guidelines for Americans. *JAMA*. 2018;320(19):2020-2028.
6. Liguori G. *ACSM's guidelines for exercise testing and prescription*. 11th ed. Wolters Kluwer; 2022.
7. Pack QR, Shea M, Brawner CA, et al. Exercise prescription methods and attitudes in cardiac rehabilitation: a national survey. *J Cardiopulm Rehabil Prev*. 2022;42(5):359-365.
8. Dempsey PC, Biddle SJH, Buman MP, et al. New global guidelines on sedentary behaviour and health for adults: broadening the behavioural targets. *Int J Behav Nutr Phys Act*. 2020;17(1):151.

9. World Health Organization. *WHO Guidelines on Physical Activity and Sedentary Behaviour*. 2020.
10. American Diabetes Association Profession Practice Committee. 5. Facilitating behavior change and well-being to improve health outcomes. Standards of Medical Care in Diabetes—2022. *Diabetes Care*. 2022;45(Supplement 1):S60-S82.
11. American Diabetes Association. 8. Pharmacologic approaches to glycemic treatment. *Diabetes Care*. 2022;45(Supplement_1): S125-S143.
12. Colberg SR, Sigal RJ, Yardley JE, et al. Physical activity/exercise and diabetes: a position statement of the American Diabetes Association. *Diabetes Care*. 2016;39(11):2065-2079.
13. Farzam K, Jan A. Beta blockers. In: *StatPearls [Internet]*. StatPearls Publishing; 2022.
14. Koracevic G, Micic S, Stojanovic M, et al. Beta blockers can mask not only hypoglycemia but also hypotension. *Curr Pharm Des*. 2022;28(20):1660-1668.
15. McKeever RG, Hamilton RJ. Calcium channel blockers. Published online; 2018.
16. Herman L, Padala S, Ahmed I, Bashir K. Angiotensin converting enzyme inhibitors(ACEI). In: *StatPearls [Internet]*. StatPearls Publishing; 2022. Available at: https://www.ncbi.nlm.nih.gov/books/NBK431051/#_NBK431051_pubdet. Accessed November 30, 2022.
17. Hill R, Vaidya P. Angiotensin II receptor blockers (ARB). In: *StratPearls [Internet]*. StatPearls Publishing; 2022. Available at: https://www.ncbi.nlm.nih.gov/books/NBK537027/. Accessed November 30, 2022.
18. evolve.elsevier.com/McCuistion/pharmacology/. Anticoagulants, Antiplatelets, and Thrombolytics. Basicmedical Key. https://basicmedicalkey.com/anticoagulants-antiplatelets-and-thrombolytics/#:~:text=The%20anticoagulants%20prevent%20the%20formation,clots%20that%20have%20already%20formed. Accessed November 30, 2022.
19. Ghlichloo I, Gerriets V. Nonsteroidal anti-inflammatory drugs (NSAIDs). In: *StatPearls*. StatPearls Publishing; 2022. Available at: https://www.ncbi.nlm.nih.gov/books/NBK547742/
20. Brutzkus JC, Shahrokhi M, Varacallo M. Naproxen. In: *StatPearls [Internet]*. StatPearls Publishing; 2022.
21. Ngo VTH, Bajaj T. Ibuprofen. In: *StatPearls [Internet]*. StatPearls Publishing; 2021.
22. Sizar O, Khare S, Jamil R, Talati R. Statin medications. In: *StatPearls [Internet]*. 2022. Available at: https://www.ncbi.nlm.nih.gov/books/NBK430940/.
23. Fluoroquinolones. In: *LiverTox: Clinical and research information on drug-induced liver injury [Internet]*. National Institute of Diabetes and Digestive and Kidney Diseases; 2018. https://www.ncbi.nlm.nih.gov/books/NBK548010/?report=reader. Accessed November 30, 2022.
24. Singh G, Correa R. Fibrate medications. In: *StatPearls [Internet]*. StatPearls Publishing; 2022. Available at: https://www.ncbi.nlm.nih.gov/books/NBK547756/. Accessed November 30, 2022.
25. Izquierdo M, Merchant RA, Morley JE, et al. International Exercise Recommendations in Older Adults (ICFSR): expert consensus guidelines. *J Nutr Health Aging*. 2021;25(7):824-853.
26. Renner R, Erfurt-Berge C. Depression and quality of life in patients with chronic wounds: ways to measure their influence and their effect on daily life. *Chronic Wound Care Manag Res*. 2017;4:143-151.
27. Walburn J, Weinman J, Norton S, et al. Stress, illness perceptions, behaviors, and healing in venous leg ulcers: findings from a prospective observational study. *Psychosom Med*. 2017;79(5): 585-592.
28. Campia U, Gerhard-Herman M, Piazza G, Goldhaber SZ. Peripheral artery disease: past, present, and future. *Am J Med*. 2019;132(10):1133-1141.
29. Harwood AE, Totty JP, Pymer S, et al. Cardiovascular and musculoskeletal response to supervised exercise in patients with intermittent claudication. *J Vasc Surg*. 2019;69(6):1899-1908.
30. Lane R, Harwood A, Watson L, Leng G, Lane R. Exercise for intermittent claudication. *Cochrane Database Syst Rev*. 2017;12(12):CD000990.
31. Hageman D, Fokkenrood H, Gommans L, van den Houten M, Teijink J. Supervised exercise therapy versus home-based exercise therapy versus walking advice for intermittent claudication. *Cochrane Database Syst Rev*. 2018;4(4):CD005263.
32. Jansen S, Abaraogu U, Lauret G, Fakhry F, Fokkenrood H, Teijink J. Modes of exercise training for intermittent claudication. *Cochrane Database Syst Rev*. 2020;8(8):CD009638.
33. Raffetto JD, Ligi D, Maniscalco R, Khalil RA, Mannello F. Why venous leg ulcers have difficulty healing: overview on pathophysiology, clinical consequences, and treatment. *J Clin Med*. 2020;10(1):29.
34. Kumar P, Khan IA, Das A, Shah H. Chronic venous disease. Part 1: pathophysiology and clinical features. *Clin Exp Dermatol*. 2022;47(7):1228-1239.
35. White-Chu EF, Conner-Kerr T. Overview of guidelines for the prevention and treatment of venous leg ulcers: a US perspective. *J Multidiscip Healthc*. 2014;7:111-117.
36. Qiu Y, Osadnik CR, Team V, Weller CD. Effects of physical activity as an adjunct treatment on healing outcomes and recurrence of venous leg ulcers: a scoping review. *Wound Repair Regen*. 2022;30(2):172-185.
37. Jull A, Slark J, Parsons J. Prescribed exercise with compression vs compression alone in treating patients with venous leg ulcers: a systematic review and meta-analysis. *JAMA Dermatol*. 2018;154(11):1304-1311.
38. *European Pressure Ulcer Advisory Panel, National Pressure Injury Advisory Panel and Pan Pacific Pressure Injury Alliance. Prevention and Treatment of Pressure Ulcers/Injuries: Clinical Practice Guideline.* The International Guideline. EPUAP/NPIAP/PPPIA; 2019.
39. Thiruvoth F, Mohapatra D, Sivakumar D, Chittoria R, Nandhagopal V. Current concepts in the physiology of adult wound healing. *Plast Aesthetic Res*. 2015;2(5):250.
40. Mueller MJ. Musculoskeletal impairments are often unrecognized and underappreciated complications from diabetes. *Phys Ther*. 2016;96(12):1861-1864.
41. Kluding PM, Bareiss SK, Hastings M, Marcus RL, Sinacore DR, Mueller MJ. Physical training and activity in people with diabetic peripheral neuropathy: paradigm shift. *Phys Ther*. 2017;97(1): 31-43.
42. Yaribeygi H, Butler AE, Sahebkar A. Aerobic exercise can modulate the underlying mechanisms involved in the development of diabetic complications. *J Cell Physiol*. 2019;234(8):12508-12515.
43. Lemaster JW, Mueller MJ, Reiber GE, Mehr DR, Madsen RW, Conn VS. Effect of weight-bearing activity on foot ulcer incidence in people with diabetic peripheral neuropathy: feet first randomized controlled trial. *Phys Ther*. 2008;88(11):1385-1398.
44. Tabibiazar R, Edelman SV. Silent ischemia in people with diabetes: a condition that must be heard. *Clin Diabetes*. 2003;21(1):5-9.
45. Krishnan S, Tokar TN, Boylan MM, et al. Zumba dance improves health in overweight/obese or type 2 diabetic women. *Am J Health Behav*. 2015;39(1):109-120.

46. Mendes R, Sousa N, Themudo-Barata J, Reis V. Impact of a community-based exercise programme on physical fitness in middle-aged and older patients with type 2 diabetes. *Gac Sanit.* 2016;30(3):215-220.
47. Stoa EM, Meling S, Nyhus LK, et al. High-intensity aerobic interval training improves aerobic fitness and HbA1c among persons diagnosed with type 2 diabetes. *Eur J Appl Physiol.* 2017;117(3): 455-467.
48. Senechal M, Johannsen NM, Swift DL, et al. Association between changes in muscle quality with exercise training and changes in cardiorespiratory fitness measures in individuals with Type 2 diabetes mellitus: results from the HART-D study. *PloS One.* 2015;10(8):e0135057.
49. de Sousa MV, Fukui R, Krustrup P, et al. Positive effects of football on fitness, lipid profile, and insulin resistance in Brazilian patients with type 2 diabetes. *Scand J Med Sci Sports.* 2014;24(Suppl 1): 57-65.
50. Karstoft K, Winding K, Knudsen SH, et al. The effects of free-living interval-walking training on glycemic control, body composition, and physical fitness in type 2 diabetic patients: a randomized, controlled trial. *Diabetes Care.* 2013;36(2):228-236.
51. Johannsen NM, Swift DL, Lavie CJ, Earnest CP, Blair SN, Church TS. Categorical analysis of the impact of aerobic and resistance exercise training, alone and in combination, on cardiorespiratory fitness levels in patients with type 2 diabetes: results from the HART-D study. *Diabetes Care.* 2013;36(10):3305-3312.
52. Maluf KS, Morley REJ, Richter EJ, Klaesner JW, Mueller MJ. Foot pressures during level walking are strongly associated with pressures during other ambulatory activities in subjects with diabetic neuropathy. *Arch Phys Med Rehabil.* 2004;85(2):253-260.
53. Mueller MJ, Maluf KS. Tissue adaptation to physical stress: a proposed "Physical Stress Theory" to guide physical therapist practice, education, and research. *Phys Ther.* 2002;82(4):383-403.
54. The International Working Group on the Diabetic Foot. IWGDF Guidelines on the prevention and management of diabetic foot disease. Published online at iwgdfguidelines.org. 2019:194. Accessed December 2, 2022.
55. Xiang J, Wang S, He Y, Xu L, Zhang S, Tang Z. Reasonable glycemic control would help wound healing during the treatment of diabetic foot ulcers. *Diabetes Ther.* 2019;10(1):95-105.
56. Lindberg K, Moller BS, Kirketerp-Moller K, Kristensen MT. An exercise program for people with severe peripheral neuropathy and diabetic foot ulcers - a case series on feasibility and safety. *Disabil Rehabil.* 2020;42(2):183-189.
57. Rodrigues M, Kosaric N, Bonham CA, Gurtner GC. Wound healing: a cellular perspective. *Physiol Rev.* 2019;99(1):665-706.
58. Rinkel WD, Luiten J, van Dongen J, et al. In-hospital costs of diabetic foot disease treated by a multidisciplinary foot team. *Diabetes Res Clin Pract.* 2017;132:68-78.
59. Mueller MJ. Mobility advice to help prevent re-ulceration in diabetes. *Diabetes Metab Res Rev.* 2020;36:1-5.
60. McGuire J, Coye T. EXPERT OPINION: Advances and alternatives in diabetic ulcer offloading. *Lower Extremity Review.* 2018. Available at: https://lermagazine.com/article/expert-opinion-advances-and-alternatives-in-diabetic-ulcer-offloading. Accessed March 13, 2023.
61. McGuire J. Transitional off-loading: an evidence-based approach to pressure redistribution in the diabetic foot. *Adv Skin Wound Care.* 2010;23(4):175-190.
62. Wendland D, Kline P, Simmons, Sinacore D. The effect of exercise, physical activity, stepping characteristics, and loading on diabetic foot ulcer healing: a systematic review. *Wounds.* In press.
63. Armstrong DG, Holtz-Neiderer K, Wendel C, Mohler MJ, Kimbriel HR, Lavery LA. Skin temperature monitoring reduces the risk for diabetic foot ulceration in high-risk patients. *Am J Med.* 2007;120(12):1042-1046.
64. Lavery LA, Higgins KR, Lanctot DR, Constantinides GP, Zamorano RG, Athanasiou KA. Preventing diabetic foot ulcer recurrence in high-risk patients. *Diabetes Care.* 2007;30.
65. Bus SA, Lavery LA, Monteiro-Soares M, et al. Guidelines on the prevention of foot ulcers in persons with diabetes (IWGDF 2019 update). *Diabetes Metab Res Rev.* 2020;36(Suppl 1):e3269.
66. Perry R, Herbert G, Atkinson C, et al. Pre-admission interventions (prehabilitation) to improve outcome after major elective surgery: a systematic review and meta-analysis. *BMJ Open.* 2021;11(9):e050806.
67. Umegaki H. Sarcopenia and frailty in older patients with diabetes mellitus. *Geriatr Gerontol Int.* 2016;16(3):293-299.
68. Fried L, Tangen C, Walston J, et al. Frailty in older adults: Evidence for a phenotype. *J Gerontol Biol Sci Med Sci.* 2001;56(3):M146-M156.
69. Grada A, Phillips T. Nutrition and cutaneous wound healing. *Clin Dermatol.* 2022;40(2):103-113.
70. Donald G, Ghaffarian A, Isaac F, et al. Preoperative frailty assessment predicts loss of independence after vascular surgery. *J Vasc Surg.* 2018;68(5):1382-1389.
71. Drudi L, Ades M, Landry T, et al. Scoping review of frailty in vascular surgery. *J Vasc Surg.* 2019;69(6):1989-1998.
72. Doughty D. Preventing and managing surgical wound dehiscence. *Adv Skin Wound Care.* 2005;18(6):319-322.
73. Holloway C, Pathare N, Huta J, et al. The impact of a less restrictive poststernotomy activity protocol compared with standard sternal precautions in patients following cardiac surgery. *Phys Ther.* 2020; 100(7):1074-1083.
74. Arkkukangas A, Hultgren S. Implementation of motivational interviewing in a fall prevention exercise program: Experiences from a randomized controlled trial. *BMC Res Notes.* 2019;12(1):270.
75. Hu H, Xu A, Gao C, Wang Z, Wu X. The effect of physical exercise on rheumatoid arthritis: An overview of systematic reviews and meta-analysis. *J Adv Nurs.* 2021;77(2):506-522.
76. Gutnick D, Reims K, Davis C, Gainforth H, Jay M, Cole S. Brief action planning to facilitate behavior change and support patient self management. *J Clin Outcomes Manag.* 2014;21(1):17-29.

CHAPTER SIXTEEN

Electrical Stimulation

Karen A. Gibbs, PT, PhD, DPT, CWS and Daryl Lawson, PT MPT, DSc

CHAPTER OBJECTIVES

At the end of this chapter, the learner will be able to:

1. **Describe current of injury and electrotaxis and their relationship to the use of electrical stimulation for wound healing.**
2. **Identify specific patient situations for which electrical stimulation might be indicated in wound management.**
3. **Describe the cellular and tissue effects of electrical stimulation on wounds and integrate this information into parameter selection.**
4. **Compare and contrast two application techniques for electrical stimulation and explain the advantages and disadvantages of both methods.**
5. **Explain precautions and contraindications for electrical stimulation in wound management.**

INTRODUCTION

Electrical stimulation (ES) technology has long been used in diagnostic and treatment procedures across multiple patient care settings including general medicine, cardiology, surgery, and physical therapy.[1,2] ES has clinical applications for electrocautery, neuromuscular electrical stimulation and muscle reeducation, pain control, improved blood flow, iontophoresis, and medication delivery, and as an adjunct therapy for chronic wound healing.[3–9] The mechanisms by which ES facilitates wound healing have been well documented and include cellular stimulation and migration, growth factor release, improved local angiogenesis and wound contraction, decreased bioburden and improved autolysis, and edema reduction.[3,10] At the time of publication, ES as an adjunct therapy for wound healing is considered an "off-label" use of medical bioelectric current, and there are no ES devices with U.S. Food and Drug Administration (FDA) approval.[6,11] However, due to an abundance of evidence,[11–16] ES for chronic wound healing is supported by multiple health profession organizations including the National Pressure Injury Advisory Panel and European Pressure Ulcer Advisory Panel,[17] the Wound, Ostomy and Continence Nurses Society,[18] and the American Physical Therapy Association's Academy of Clinical Electrophysiology and Wound Management.[19] This chapter discusses the therapeutic application of electrical current for chronic wound healing. (**TABLE 16-1** provides a brief review of ES-related terminology.)[1,20]

Standard ES equipment consists of an electric or battery-powered base unit with adjustments for parameters (eg, voltage, polarity, and treatment time), electrodes that conform to the wound or periwound surface, and lead wires that connect electrodes to the base unit. ES devices are available in various sizes from larger countertop units to small, hand-held, pocket-sized, portable units (**FIGURES 16-1** and **16-2**). In wound

TABLE 16-1 ES Terminology

Alternating current (AC)	Continuous bidirectional flow of current
Amperage	Rate of current flow: amperes (A), milliamperes (mA), microamperes (μA)
Amplitude (intensity)	Magnitude of current
Anode	Positively charged electrode
Balanced waveform	Opposite charges balance so no net charge is generated
Biphasic current	Current with two phases and constantly changing polarity
Cathode	Negatively charged electrode
Charge or current density	Amount of charge per surface area
Current	Flow of charged particles through a conductor
Direct current (DC)	Continuous, unidirectional flow of current
Duty cycle	Ratio of "on"-time to total cycle time
Electrotaxis (galvanotaxis)	Attraction of cells to an electrical charge
Impedance	Frequency-dependent opposition to current flow
Monophasic current	Current with one phase, either positive or negative
Polarity	Charge of an electrode: positive or negative
Pulse duration	Time elapsed from the beginning to the end of a pulse
Pulse frequency	Number of pulses per second
Pulsed current (PC)	Interrupted or pulsed current flow (each pulse is separated by a period of no current flow)
Unbalanced waveform	Opposite charges do not balance, resulting in a net charge in tissues
Voltage	Force of electricity
Waveform	Graphic representation of the flow of current

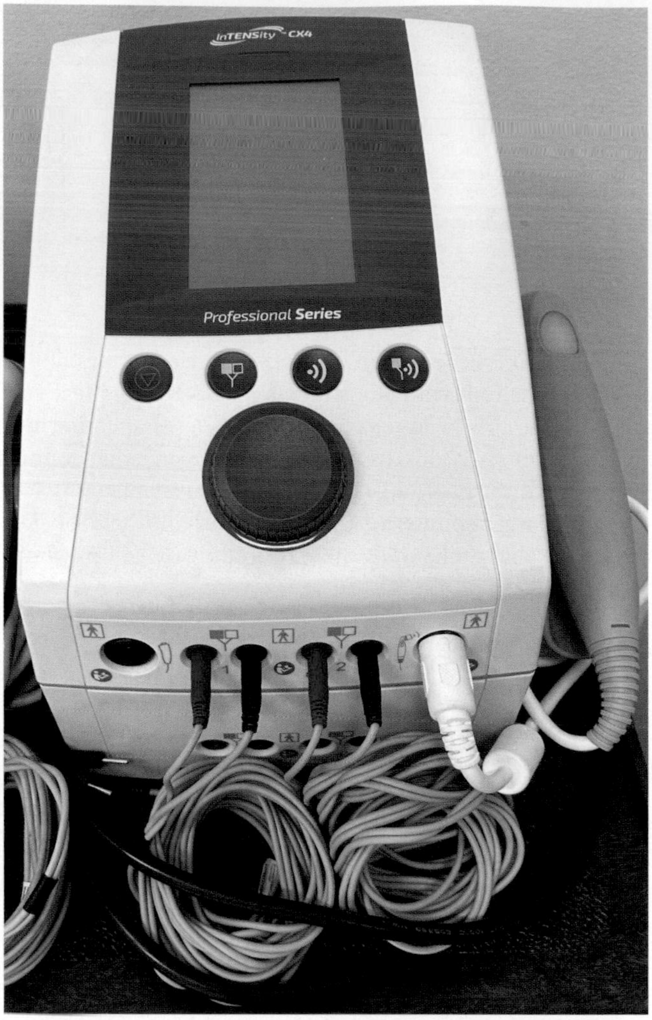

FIGURE 16-1 Example countertop electrical stimulation unit. This unit offers different types of biophysical energies including several types of ES for different diagnoses and intervention purposes. This type of unit, frequently used in clinics and hospitals, has ports for two sets of electrodes so that treatment can be applied to two different locations at the same time. Simultaneous treatment of wounds in proximity is not recommended as cells can be pulled from one wound location to the other, overall rendering simultaneous treatment ineffective.

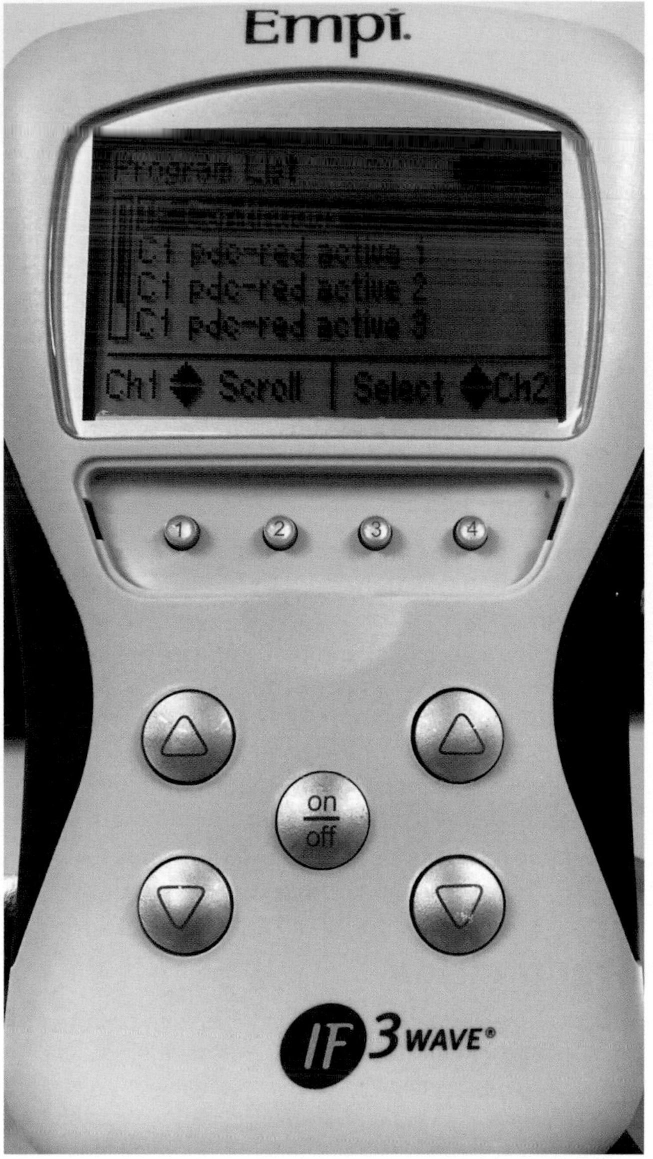

FIGURE 16-2 Example portable electrical stimulation unit. Smaller, handheld, portable units are less expensive than countertop units but may not offer all the same benefits as the larger devices. Portable units are useful for patients who can administer ES treatments at home and for hospitals and long-term care facilities where taking the unit from room to room is desired. This unit also has two channels for treating more than one site. All ES units are required to be checked by biomedical engineering at least once a year to ensure patient safety.

management, self-adhesive gel or carbon electrodes may be used depending on the application technique. Additionally, clinicians can create electrodes using saline-moistened gauze and aluminum foil paired with an alligator clip (**FIGURE 16-3A–C**), which provides wound-specific customization of electrodes. Lead wires, typically used in pairs, are available as single or bifurcated leads (**FIGURE 16-4**).

MECHANISM OF ACTION

Healthy, intact skin has a variable charge of approximately −23 mV, referred to as the transepithelial potential difference.[10,11,21] When a break in the skin occurs, the influx of positive charge (Na^+) from the wounded tissue and deeper layers of the epidermis interact with the negative charge (Cl^-) of adjacent intact skin, thereby creating a low-level bioelectric alert signal to the body that an injury has occurred (**FIGURE 16-6**).[3,22,23] This endogenous signal, referred to as the *current of injury*,[8] flows in a moist wound environment and continues to signal that repair is necessary until a new epidermis is established.[8,22,24,25] This natural, bioelectric signal

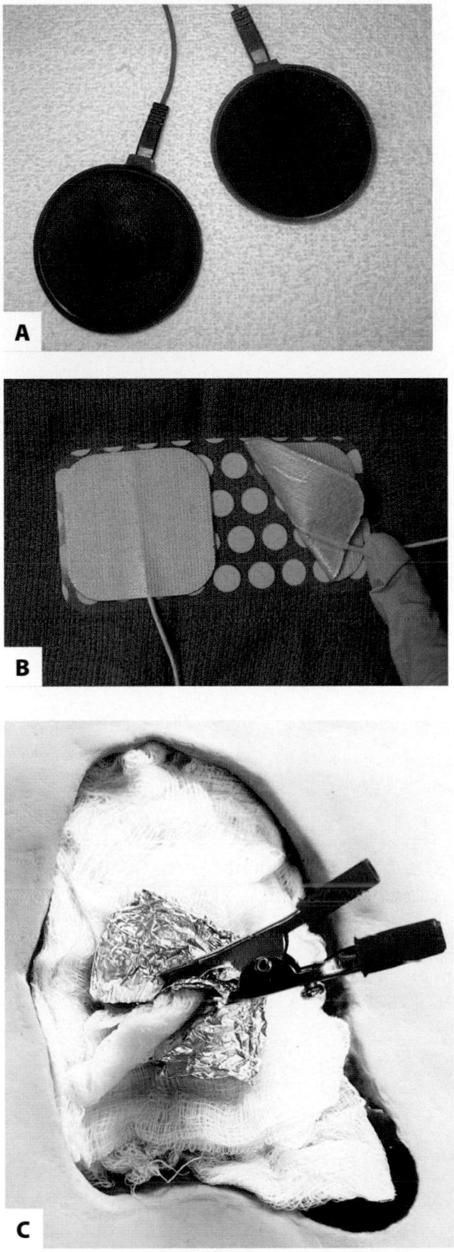

FIGURE 16-3 Types of electrodes used for electrical stimulation. Three types of electrodes that can be used for electrical stimulation include: **A.** Carbon electrodes that are combined with saline-moistened gauze and applied in either the direct or indirect method. If the active electrode is placed directly over the wound, the wound is first filled with a moist dressing or gel to ensure good conduction of the current into the wound surface. Electrodes are disinfected between every use. **B.** Gel electrodes are used only for the indirect or straddling technique and are used only on the same patient because they cannot be disinfected. **C.** Example of an improvised electrode with saline-moistened gauze, aluminum foil, and alligator clip. Aluminum foil is carefully placed in contact with moist gauze (but not in direct contact with intact skin or wound tissue) and held in place by the alligator clip. An electrode wire would be connected to the alligator clip and an appropriately sized dispersive pad would be used. This "homemade" gauze electrode can be adapted for a wound of any size and shape. The gauze and foil are discarded after each treatment, which is ideal when used for wounds with heavy bioburden or infection.

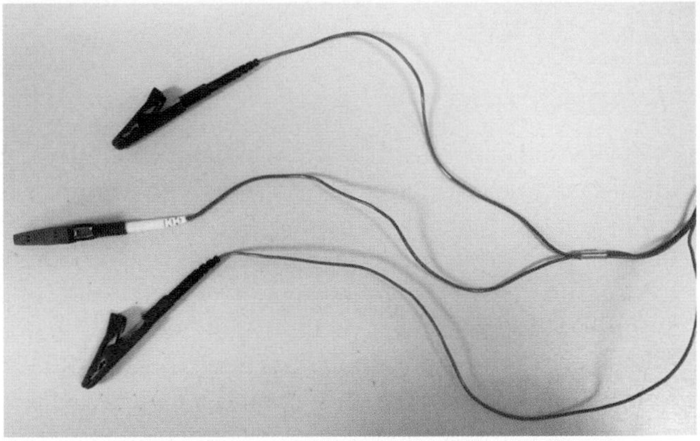

FIGURE 16-4 Lead wires used for electrical stimulation. Lead wires are either single or bifurcated, depending upon the desired method of application. The black alligator clips are attached to a bifurcating cable that is used for the straddling or indirect method; the red clip is attached to a single cable that would be used for the dispersive electrode. The direct method uses two single cables. Even though the clips are of different colors to correlate with polarity, the polarity is controlled by the negative/positive control on the stimulator.

for repair can be disrupted or halted in a low moisture or desiccated wound healing environment or with scab formation, resulting in reduced or stalled healing. Once a moist wound environment is re-established, the application of an exogenous electrical current can mimic the normal current of injury, resulting in the attraction of key cells involved in tissue healing, and essentially reinitiating the healing process.[8,22,25,26]

Additionally, through the action of electrotaxis (previously termed galvanotaxis), ES impacts wound healing by attracting cells (eg, macrophages, fibroblasts, and epithelial cells) necessary for repair into the wound bed (**FIGURE 16-7**, **TABLE 16-2**).[3,6,10,12,20,27,28] Improved cellular migration and up-regulation of cellular activity facilitate the current healing phase and encourage progression to the next phase of healing.[6,29]

EFFECTS AT THE CELLULAR AND TISSUE LEVELS

Although typically used for chronic wounds, ES has been shown to have beneficial cellular and tissue effects during all phases of tissue healing[3,30] (inflammation, proliferation, remodeling/maturation) regardless of wound etiology.[11,15,31] Primary cells active within each healing phase have different electrical charges and are therefore attracted to opposite current polarities. The individual phases of healing and primary cells in each phase drive decision-making for the application of the correct polarity to best facilitate specific actions within each phase. For more detailed descriptions of individual cell activity and roles in wound healing, see Chapter 2, Healing Response in Acute and Chronic Wounds.

CASE STUDY

INTRODUCTION

A 59-year-old patient with a history of type 2 diabetes, renal insufficiency, and hypertension presents with a nonhealing wound on the right plantar medial foot of more than 1-year duration. The wound began as a thick callus and progressed to necrotic tissue with underlying infection (**FIGURE 16-5**). Surgical debridement was performed about 1 month prior to the first visit, and the wound has been treated with wet-to-dry dressings at home since then. The patient works for the state department and is currently out on disability.

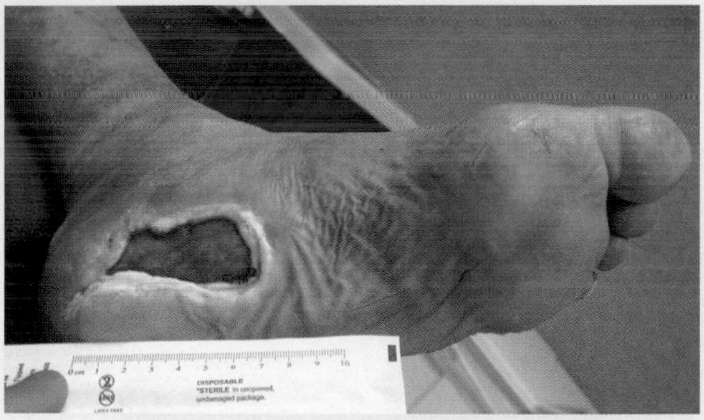

FIGURE 16-5 Case study. Wound on the left plantar foot of a patient who has a diabetic foot ulcer that has not responded to the standard of care for 30 days.

DISCUSSION QUESTIONS

1. What subjective information is needed to determine treatment for this patient?
2. What objective tests and measures are advised before initiating treatment?
3. What would be considered standard care for this type of wound?

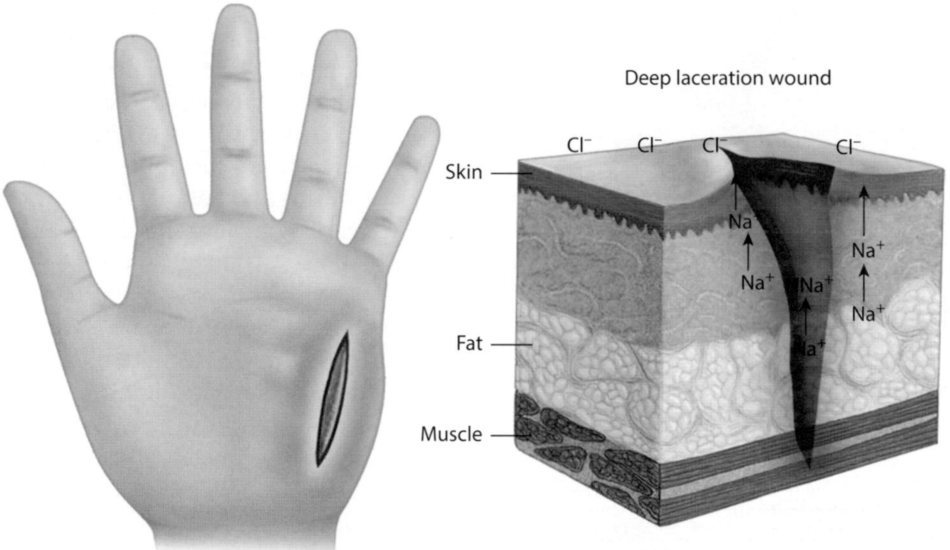

FIGURE 16-6 Current of injury. The current of injury, defined as a flow of negatively charged electrons from the deep tissue to the surface of the skin, occurs with any dermal injury. The flow of electrons serves as a signal to platelets and other cells that they are needed in the area to begin the healing response.

Inflammation

Primary cells active during the inflammatory phase of healing include neutrophils and macrophages. Since both cell types carry a negative ionic charge, exogenously applied electropositive (positive polarity) current encourages increased migration of neutrophils and macrophages into wounded tissue,[3,11,31] thereby facilitating, or in the case of chronic wounds, re-starting the inflammatory process. Increased numbers of macrophages also facilitate the debridement of nonviable tissue.[6,32] With an electropositive current, positively charged mast cells are repelled, which may result in decreased tissue fibrosis over the course of healing.[33–35] In the presence of wound infection, activated neutrophils become positively charged and the application of electronegative (negative polarity) current can encourage increased bacterial destruction.[3,36]

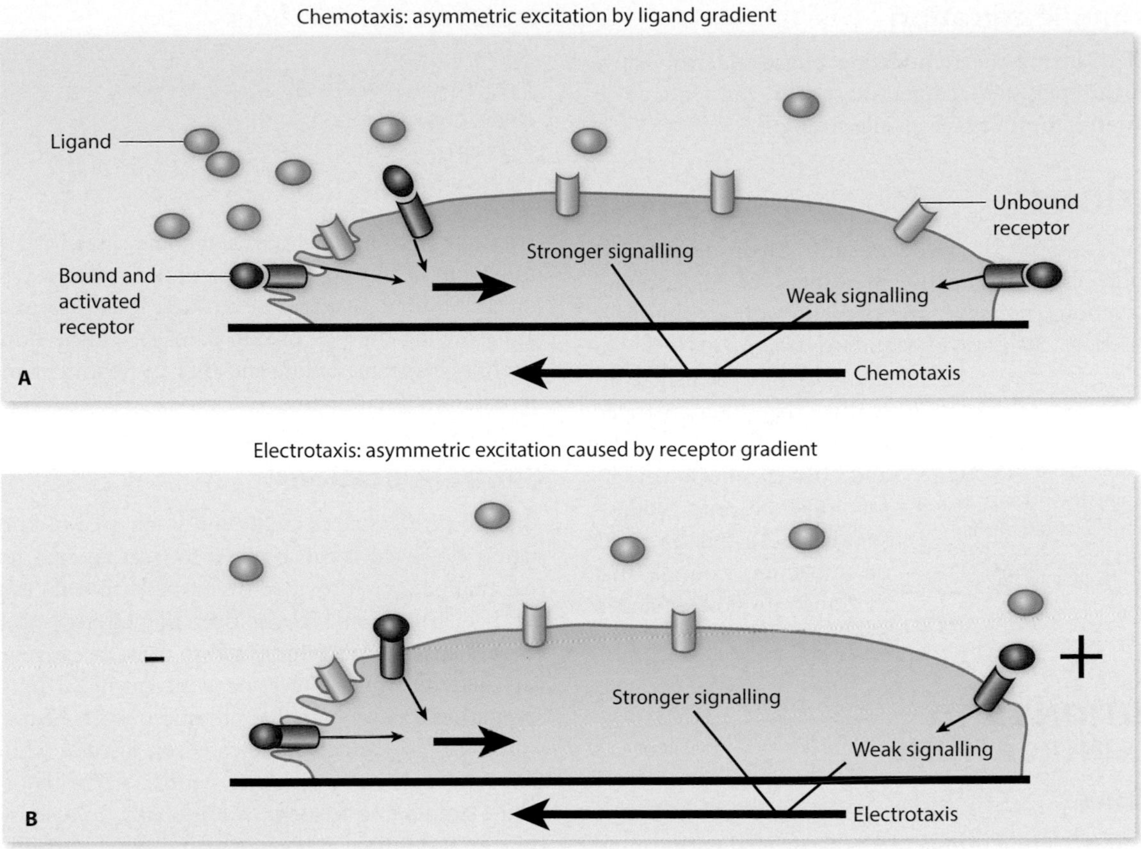

FIGURE 16-7 Chemotaxis and electrotaxis. Both chemotaxis **A.** (attraction of cells toward a chemical) and electrotaxis **B.** (attraction of cells toward an electrical field or charge) play a role in attracting cells necessary for wound healing to the injured tissue. During initial injury, chemicals and debris of destroyed bacteria and cells attract neutrophils needed to initiate the healing response. When the wound has stalled, electrotaxis can be used to attract the cells needed to progress a wound to the next healing phase.

TABLE 16-2 Cell Charge and Attracting Electrode

Cell Name	Healing Phase	Cell Charge	Attraction to Electrode
Platelets	Hemostasis and inflammatory	(Not reported)	
Macrophages	Inflammatory	(−)	Anode
Neutrophils (activated due to infection)	Inflammatory	(+)	Cathode
Neutrophils (inactive)	Inflammatory	(−)	Anode
Mast cells	Inflammatory	(−)	Anode
Fibroblasts	Proliferative	(+)	Cathode
Epidermal cells	Epithelialization/remodeling	(−)	Anode

Proliferation

Positively charged fibroblasts and negatively charged epithelial cells are the primary cells active during the proliferation phase. Electronegative charge increases the activity and number of fibroblasts migrating into the wound bed subsequently increasing protein synthesis, collagen deposition, and wound contraction.[3,10,12,36,37] ES, especially when combined with neutral warmth (eg, warm room temperatures), also encourages increased angiogenesis and local blood flow by facilitating increased capillary density and inhibiting local vasoconstriction, especially in people with diabetes.[3,11,33,38–40] When electropositive current is applied to an already granulated wound, epithelial cells can increase migratory distance and speed, resulting in faster re-epithelialization.[41] In addition, electrical current does not disrupt cellular adhesion between epithelial cells, and in fact, may actually augment the bonding or grouping of these cells, encouraging overall faster migration of large epithelial sheets across wound surfaces.[42,43]

Remodeling/Maturation

When applied during the remodeling phase, electropositive current, which repels like-charged mast cells, can reduce scar hypertrophy and improve scar tensile strength.[22,11,16]

INDICATIONS

In 2002, the Centers for Medicare and Medicaid Services (CMS) approved the adjunctive treatment of ES coverage for arterial, venous, pressure, and diabetic wounds that have not responded to 30 days of standard treatment.[27,36,47] For many years, published literature has demonstrated the beneficial cellular and tissue effects of ES for most chronic wounds (**TABLE 16-3**) and for acute or subacute wounds that demonstrate slow or stalled healing.[6–8,11–13,16,22,30,38,44,48]

CLINICAL CONSIDERATION

If a wound being treated with ES appears to stall in the healing process, changing the polarity of the treatment may be beneficial by attracting multiple cell types involved in overlapping healing phases.[39]

TABLE 16-3 ES Indications

Arterial wounds
Clean wounds with decreased or stalled healing
Diabetic foot ulcers
Pressure injuries
Venous ulcers

PRECAUTIONS AND CONTRAINDICATIONS

Precautions

In addition to attracting primary cells associated with wound healing, positive and negative currents also attract oppositely charged ions (Na^+, K^+, and H^+ to the negative pole and Cl^-, HCO_3^-; P^- to the positive pole).[3,20] Migrating ions under electrodes react with moisture in the skin causing alkaline (cathode) or acidic (anode) pH changes which can cause minor skin irritation or superficial burns in some cases.[20,26] However, the utilization of pulsed current parameter selections can reduce ion accumulation under electrodes, thus increasing comfort and reducing the risk of skin damage.[20,39] The skin should be carefully inspected before and after ES treatment and any signs of irritation documented.

Contraindications

The use of ES is contraindicated in an area of known malignancy; however, it can be used to treat an area remote from the malignancy provided metastasis to the targeted area has been ruled out. ES use over the anterior neck or upper chest is strictly contraindicated to prevent exogenous electrical currents from interfering with laryngeal muscles, parasympathetic nerve ganglia, phrenic nerves, heart, or carotid sinus.[1] ES is also contraindicated on anyone who has a cardiac pacemaker or implanted cardiac defibrillator regardless of the area being treated.[1] Additionally, ES use over the low back or abdominal area is contraindicated in patients who are pregnant.[1] ES is considered a precaution for use on children younger than 3 years since its effects on children in this age group have not been well documented. A full list of precautions and contraindications associated with ES is summarized in **TABLE 16-4**.[1,20,25,30,44]

CASE STUDY

CONTINUED

The patient reports the following subjective information:

- Wearing an athletic shoe and walking 2–3 miles a day to help manage diabetes.
- Blood glucose measurements taken every morning are usually 120–160.
- Medications include Glucophage, Norvasc, and Lasix.
- Currently working with a nephrologist to initiate peritoneal dialysis at home.

Objective information includes the following:

- Right plantar foot wound measures 5.8 cm × 3.1 cm × 0.4 cm with 3–5 mm of undermining at the medial proximal edge.
- Moderate serosanguineous drainage is interfering with the current lifestyle.
- Palpable pulses, 2+ (both DP and PT) bilaterally.
- "Yes" responses to 5.07 monofilament on bilateral dorsal feet, no responses on bilateral plantar feet.
- Diminished Achilles tendon reflexes bilaterally.
- Pitting edema on the Right lower extremity to the knee.
- Independent gait without an assistive device, wide base of support, minimal heel/toe sequence, and lateral trunk sway.
- Performs sit to stand without upper extremity assist, × 5 in 20 seconds.
- Unable to single-leg stance on either lower extremity.
- Lower extremity strength is 4-/5 bilaterally; Left plantarflexion ankle range of motion 5–30 degrees, 5–40 on the Right.

DISCUSSION QUESTIONS

1. Is ES an appropriate intervention for this patient?
2. What would be the optimal off-loading strategy for this patient?
3. What other physical therapy interventions (other than wound care) would be beneficial for overall function?

TABLE 16-4 ES Precautions and Contraindications

Precautions	Children <3 years of age Skin irritation or burns under electrodes Use in areas of impaired or absent sensation Skin irritation/burns from ion shifts
Contraindications	Malignancy in wound or periwound tissue Untreated osteomyelitis Over-implanted electrical devices or any patient with a pacemaker Over the heart In wounds with metallic ion residue (eg, povidone-iodine, silver, or zinc) In close proximity to a developing fetus Over areas of active bleeding Position such that current would flow through the anterior neck or upper chest Transcerebral application

PARAMETERS AND APPLICATION

Direct current, delivered as pulsed current (PC), is utilized for wound healing because it produces polarity changes in target tissues. Polarity is an important factor in utilizing ES for tissue healing, therefore alternating current, which generates a balanced, overall neutral charge, is not recommended for use in wound management (**FIGURE 16-8**).[3,28]

With PC, the flow of current is interrupted or pulsed at brief intervals with a finite "off" time between each pulse, making PC more comfortable and safer compared to direct current.[28] The choice of monophasic or biphasic PC is based on patient tolerance and skin status. The two most common types of pulsed current ES for wound management are (1) high-volt pulsed current (HVPC) and (2) low-volt pulsed current (LVPC); both are discussed below. Brief information regarding microcurrent and wireless electroceutical applications is also presented.

HVPC Monophasic HVPC provides a short pulse duration (5–20 μs) and high voltage (75–150 V), making ES delivery generally comfortable while decreasing the risk of skin damage from ion shifts typically associated with other monophasic modes of delivery.[8,28] The short duration, high-peaked waveform decreases skin resistance so current penetrates into deeper tissues without discomfort.[8] Monophasic HVPC is the best evidence-supported ES delivery for tissue healing.[3,8,26,49]

LVPC Low-volt devices offer either monophasic or biphasic waveforms with lower voltage and longer pulse durations compared to HVPC and may be initially better tolerated by patients who have severely painful wounds.[4] Monophasic delivery offers a single polarity selection; biphasic delivery offers a choice of polarity or delivery of an overall neutral or balanced charge. For biphasic LVPC delivery, transcutaneous electrical nerve stimulators (TENS units) that are commonly used in physical therapy practice for muscle and nerve stimulation can be used.[4,28] ES delivery using a TENS unit is typically comfortable and poses no risk of skin irritation due to ion shifts.[26] LVPC is used with electrodes at the periwound area with the goal of increasing blood flow.

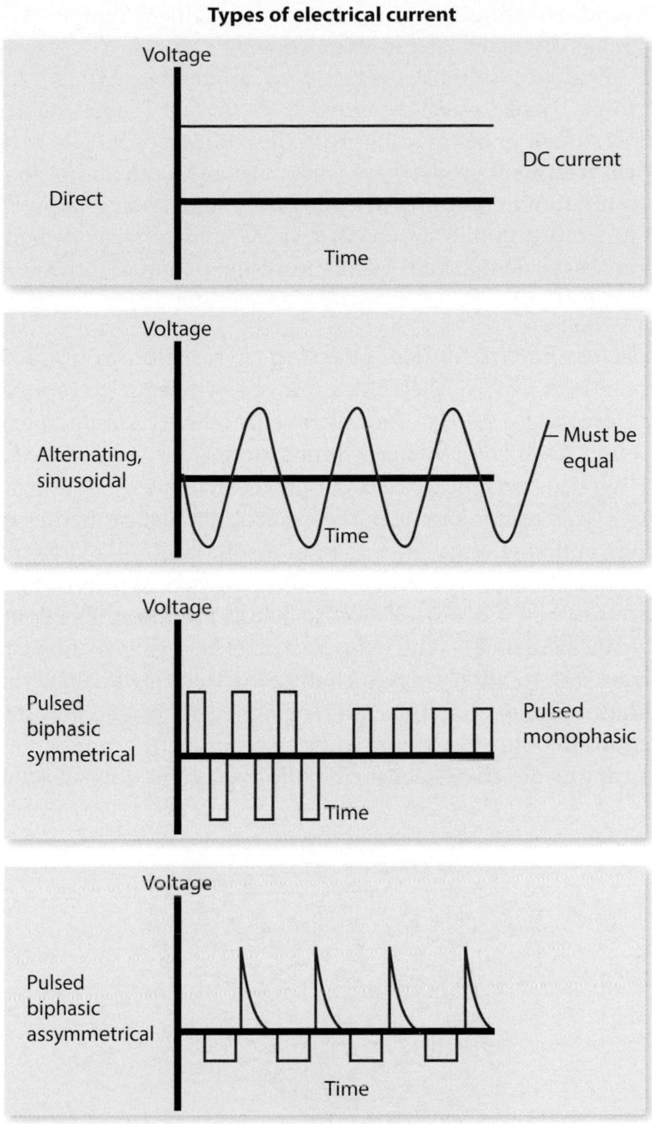

FIGURE 16-8 Direct and alternating currents. Types of electrical currents are as follows: direct, sinusoidal current, pulsed current, monophasic waveform, and biphasic waveform.

Microcurrent Microcurrent has gained recent interest for wound management and is conventionally defined as a current less than 1 mA, expressed in microamperes (μA).[50] Microcurrent, which mimics and enhances the skin's endogenous electrical field, offers amplitude ranges from 1.5 μA to 500 μA and causes little to no sensory perception of ES when applied to the skin.[51,52] Low-frequency, monophasic, pulsed microcurrent (MPMC) with an intensity of 200 μA, frequency of 2 Hz, and duty cycle of 50% has been shown to promote the migration, proliferation, and differentiation of human dermal fibroblasts.[53–55] It can be used as LVPC administered by a traditional ES unit or through a specialized fabric dressing embedded with silver and zinc microcells (Procellera Antimicrobial

Wound Dressing, Vomaris Innovations, Inc., Tempe, AZ) which is discussed later in this chapter.[56]

Evidence supports the use of adjunctive MPCM for chronic, hard-to-heal wounds.[53,55–59] In fact, some studies show similar or better results with the addition of MPCM even when treatment groups have worse overall health and/or longer duration nonhealing wounds than comparison groups.[57,60] While more studies are needed, these clinical trials demonstrate that microcurrent offers promising potential for wound management.

Wireless Electroceutical Dressing A variation from traditional forms of ES, the FDA approved, wireless electroceutical dressing (WED), Procellera (Procellera Antimicrobial Wound Dressing, Vomaris Innovations), provides an easily applied, evidence-based option to facilitate wound healing.[61] This technology uses the electrochemical properties of silver and zinc discs embedded in a soft, fabric-like dressing (**FIGURE 16-9A,B**).[61,62] When the dressing comes into contact with wound fluid, a weak electric field is produced.[62,63] Recent evidence documents the weak electric field negatively impacts bacteria in multiple ways, including interfering with bacterial communication, binding, and metabolism, essentially preventing biofilm formation when used in acute wounds and disrupting already established biofilm when used in subacute and chronic wounds.[61–63] Procellera also down-regulates inflammation and increases the rate of re-epithelialization.[62,63] WED produces no known antimicrobial resistance and works synergistically with antibiotics, facilitating their bactericidal properties.[61,62] The electric field is subsensory with no patient discomfort. The fabric-like nature of the dressing makes it easy to apply, placing the active side of the dressing in direct contact with the moist wound bed (a moist wound bed must be maintained to generate and sustain the electric field). Dressings can be cut to size, placed under compression bandaging, or used as the contact layer under negative pressure wound therapy,[60] and are disposable after use.[62]

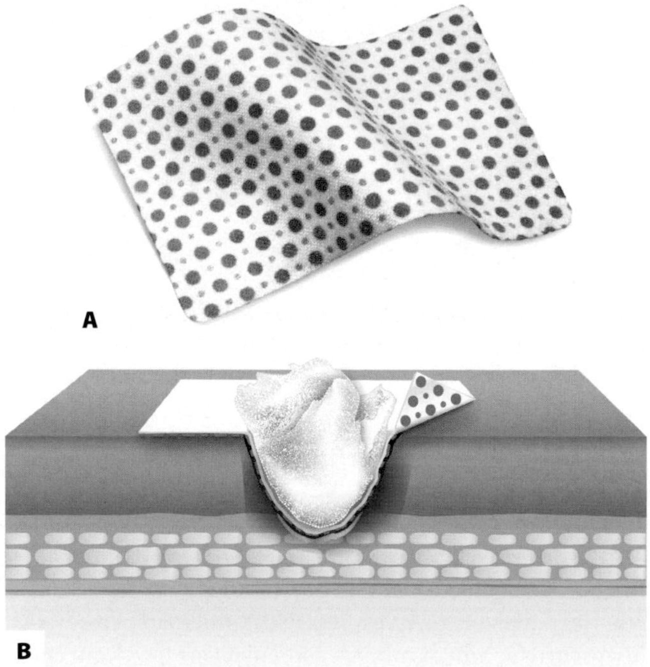

FIGURE 16-9 Low-volt pulsed frequency dressing. A. Procellera flexible, bioelectric dressing embedded with flat microcell batteries that produce a sustained low-level current (2–10 mV)[8] along the surface of the dressing after it is wet with wound fluid or normal saline solution. The soft Procellera dressing can be cut as needed to maintain good contact with the wound surface. **B.** Shows placement of the Procellera dressing in a wound with depth, using gauze or other filler to fill open space. (Courtesy of Vomaris Innovations, Inc., Tempe, AZ.)

Application

ES is applied to wound tissue by either *direct* or *indirect* (also called straddling or periwound) placement of electrodes.[3,8,11,30] In the *direct method,* the treatment electrode set to the desired polarity is placed directly in the wound bed (**FIGURE 16-10**). To ensure good contact between the electrode and all surfaces of the wound, saline-moistened gauze is commonly used as the electrode. Moist gauze conforms easily to irregular wound surfaces and can be wicked into tracts, tunnels, and areas of undermining so electrical current is distributed to all areas of the wound surface. The electrical charge is transferred from the lead wire to the gauze electrode via an alligator clip and a small piece of aluminum foil positioned so that the clip/foil attachment does not make contact with the wound or periwound tissue (**FIGURE 16-3C**). If the clip or foil touches the skin, the patient may experience a burning or painful sensation. The direct method is also referred to as *monopolar* because there is only one treatment or active electrode.[11]

For small wounds, the open area can be filled with sterile hydrogel, and the treatment electrode placed over the wound in direct contact with the hydrogel.[29] This method of application requires full contact between the electrode and the hydrogel. Once the wound is filled to the level of intact skin, the electrode is gently placed over the wound to prevent the

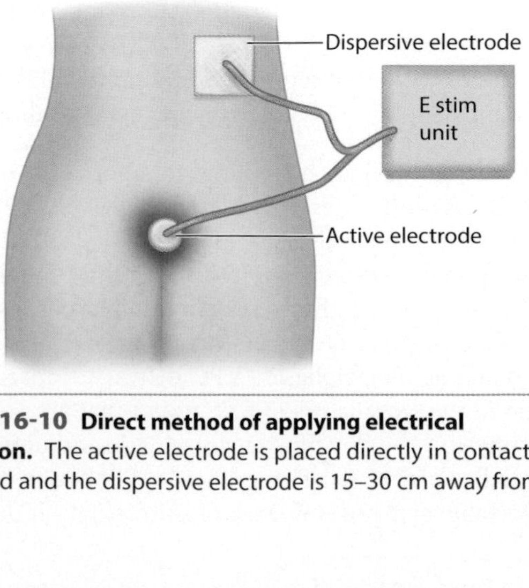

FIGURE 16-10 Direct method of applying electrical stimulation. The active electrode is placed directly in contact with the wound and the dispersive electrode is 15–30 cm away from the wound.

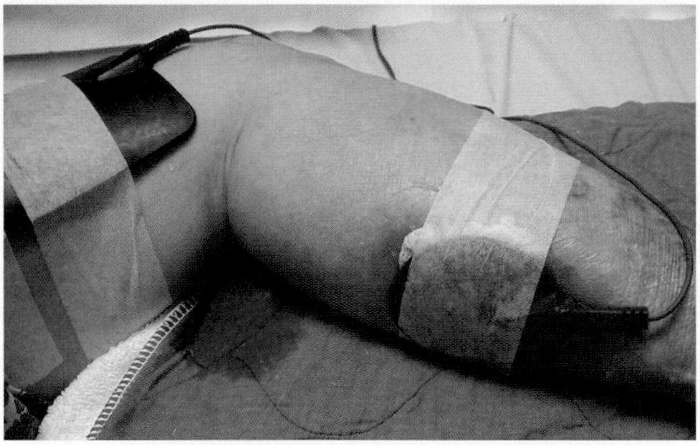

FIGURE 16-11 Placement of the electrodes to allow the flow of current to deep wound bed. For this wound, the carbon and gauze electrodes are used in the direct method for a deep wound on the calf. The dispersive electrode is placed on the lateral thigh, allowing the current to flow through muscle and subcutaneous tissue, and at a distance that will facilitate flow of the current to the deeper wound bed.

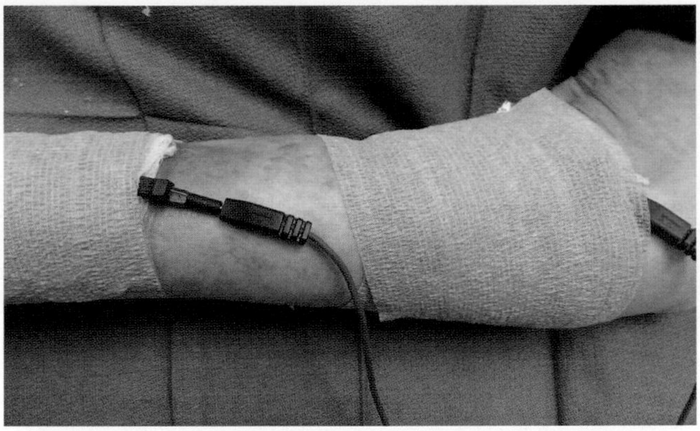

FIGURE 16-12 Placement of electrodes to facilitate the flow of current to superficial wound bed. The wound on the calf of a patient with spinal cord injury is shallow and the surrounding area has atrophied muscle and little subcutaneous tissue. Therefore, the dispersive electrode is placed closer to the wound so that current will flow to the superficial wounded tissue.

gel from being displaced onto the periwound skin. With this method, the treatment electrode must be of sufficient size to cover the wound opening and adhere to periwound skin.

To form a complete electrical circuit, ES applications require at least one treatment or active electrode and one dispersive electrode. For clear division of polar effects, the dispersive electrode is commonly placed 15–30 cm away from the wound site (**FIGURE 16-11**).[30] Placement of the dispersive pad can be changed between treatments to redirect current flow and target different wound areas. Positioning the dispersive pad over muscle is desirable because muscle has a high fluid content and therefore low impedance to electrical current. Tissues with low fluid content, such as bone or callus, are not good conductors and as such, skin overlying superficial bones and skin with callus are not desirable locations for dispersive electrodes. Since the depth of current penetration increases as the distance between treatment and dispersive electrodes increases, the depth of target tissues is taken into consideration in electrode placement (**FIGURE 16-12**). The presence of necrotic tissue in the wound must also be considered when placing electrodes because the high resistance of nonviable tissue can reduce or alter the flow of electrical current from target tissues.[64] Debridement of nonviable tissue prior to ES application helps optimize treatment outcomes.

Charge density is a consideration when selecting dispersive electrode size. The dispersive electrode needs to be approximately two times the size of the treatment electrode to ensure unidirectional current flow to the target tissue. This also distributes the return current across a larger surface area, improving comfort and reducing the risk of skin irritation under the dispersive electrode. Dispersive electrodes may be carbon or gel, or if larger sizes are needed, may be created using a combination of premade electrodes and a moist sponge cut to the desired size (**FIGURE 16-13**).

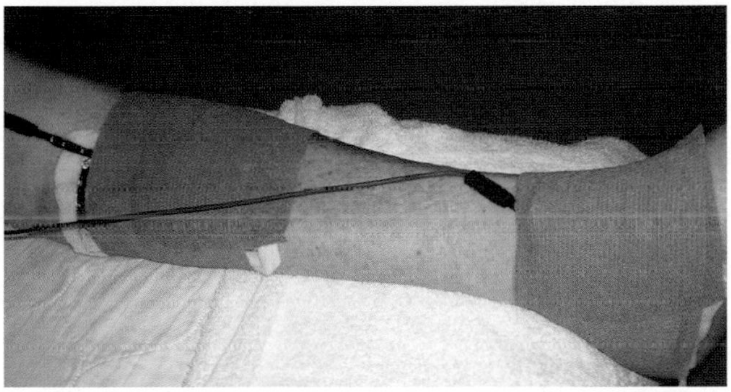

FIGURE 16-13 Improvised dispersive electrode. Dispersive electrodes can be a combination of carbon and gauze, aluminum foil and gauze, or large gel pads, and are at least twice the size of the active electrode. All electrodes need to have good contact with the skin and wound surface for both comfort and conductivity. They can be anchored with tape or self-adhesive bandages.

The *indirect, periwound,* or *straddling* technique uses a bifurcated lead wire and two same-polarity treatment electrodes that are placed on opposite sides of the wound (**FIGURE 16-14**). This simple technique can be beneficial when treating small or large wounds that do not accommodate one electrode or for home treatments. The dispersive electrode is placed the same as with the monopolar technique. The use of two treatment electrodes is also referred to as a *bipolar* application.[44] With this application, wound tissue is not covered with a treatment electrode; therefore, saline-moistened gauze is placed in the wound bed and the area is covered with an insulating dressing or dry towel so wound tissues are kept moist and protected from hypothermia during the treatment session. Since current flows between the treatment electrodes, they should be strategically placed based on wound needs and treatment goals. One concern with this application technique

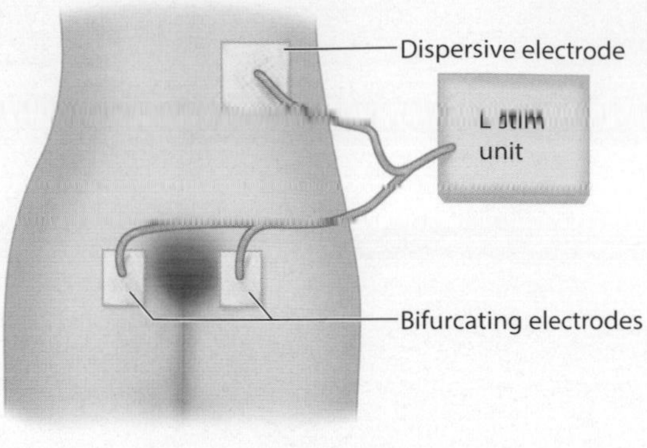

FIGURE 16-14 Straddling or indirect method of applying ES. The straddling or indirect method of applying ES uses two smaller electrodes on opposite sides of the wound and a larger dispersive electrode, placed 15–30 cm away, over soft tissue that will optimize current flow. Note that the dispersive electrode is placed over the paraspinal muscles and not directly over the vertebrae.

is that when treatment electrodes are placed on intact skin, the current must travel through nonhomogenous tissues (fat, muscle, blood vessels, etc.), and due to varying levels of resistance among these tissues, current flow between electrodes and into the wound can be reduced.[64]

Parameters

Determining optimal parameters for ES application based on research remains challenging due to the extensive variation in parameters used in published studies.[3,8,39] However, **TABLE 16-5** shows common parameters clinicians may use as a starting point and adjust based on patient comfort and wound response.[16,28] Once a decision on the mode of application has been made, direct parameter choices include voltage, polarity, pulse duration, pulse frequency, and overall frequency and duration of treatment.

Voltage For sensate patients, ES voltage, or intensity, is typically increased until a comfortable tingling is felt under the electrodes. For patients with impaired sensation in the target area, the voltage can be tested in another similar area with intact sensation or can be set just below a visible muscle twitch.[30] For patients with concomitant motor and sensory impairment in the treatment area, electrodes may be placed on an uninvolved area elsewhere in the body to establish estimated threshold levels. All patients should be monitored closely, especially during the first treatment. If skin irritation occurs under electrodes, the voltage should be reduced. If the patient's sensation of the current increases during treatment, the voltage needs to be decreased.

TABLE 16-5 ES Parameters

Type of ES	Recommended Parameter Ranges
HVPC	75–150 V 100 pps 20–100 μs pulse duration 45–60 min, 5–7 days per week
LVPC	30–35 milliamps (mA) 128 pps initially, can decrease to 64 pps after significant improvement 132 μs pulse duration 45–60 min, 5–7 days per week

Polarity Initial polarity is selected for a positive or negative charge based on treatment goal, phase of healing, and primary targeted cells.[8,65] However, research supports periodically (approximately every 3–7 days) switching polarity to combine positive and negative charge benefits, avoid healing plateaus, and maintain the progression of healing.[8,29,65] Overall, wound response guides adjustment of polarity, and clinicians must use clinical judgment as to when shifts in polarity need to occur.

Pulse Duration and Frequency As mentioned previously, shorter pulse durations are typically more comfortable. Typical pulse duration is set between 20 and 132 microseconds (μs) depending on the delivery method and specific ES units (**TABLE 16-5**). Pulse frequency ranges from 100 to 128 pulses per second (pps).[28]

Treatment Frequency and Duration ES is typically administered 5–7 days a week for 45–60 minutes a day; however, for outpatient settings, this frequency may not be practical. In this case, outpatients may be treated two to three times per week. After a treatment plan has been established, tolerance determined, and safe self-application techniques demonstrated, some patients may administer daily ES therapy at home using portable ES devices.[4,44]

INFECTION CONTROL GUIDELINES

Standard precautions apply anytime providers come into contact with body fluids, including wound drainage, and these same guidelines apply to the application of ES. Facility policies regarding infection control need to be adhered to when utilizing ES for wound management. With the direct application, gauze electrode material and foil are placed in regular waste, lead wires and the ES base unit are wiped with facility-approved disinfectant, and the alligator clip is thoroughly rinsed with disinfectant and air dried. Carbon electrodes, sometimes used as dispersive electrodes, are disinfected for repeat use per facility guidelines. Single-patient, self-adhesive electrodes utilized for indirect (periwound or straddle) applications and dispersive pads may be reused as long as the adhesive surface remains intact and provides even contact with periwound skin. Self-adhesive electrodes are not appropriate to use as the treatment electrode for the monopolar technique.

SUMMARY

Although there is extensive research supporting the use of ES for wound healing, variations in study design make determination of optimal treatment applications challenging.

CASE STUDY

CONCLUSION

After 30 days of standard care (including sharp debridement and advanced dressings to maintain a moist wound healing environment) and off-loading with a wound healing shoe (see Chapter 7, Diabetes and the Diabetic Foot), there was only a slight decrease in wound size and periwound callus. HVPC ES was initiated two times a week for 60 minutes at 100 pps and 120 V (patient unable to feel electrical charge) switching polarity at each treatment (**FIGURE 16-15A, B**). Other components of care included:

- Sharp debridement as indicated
- Absorbent cellulose dressings with foam reinforcement
- Modified compression to manage the edema using short stretch wraps
- Off-loading with the wound healing shoe (patient refused assistive device or total contact cast)
- Therapeutic exercise (designed to avoid shear or increased peak pressures) to increase ankle range of motion, lower extremity strength, and improve balance

Long-Term Goals:

- Full wound closure
- Patient was fitted with diabetic shoes with custom inserts to prevent a recurrence
- Patient ambulating with heel/toe sequence and no loss of balance on uneven surfaces
- Patient to return to part-time work as a consultant
- Patient compliant with daily foot care and inspection for recurrent skin breakdown

Outcomes:

- Wound was fully closed after 16 weeks of treatment
- Patient was fitted with diabetic shoes and inserts and demonstrated adherence to post-healing care to prevent recurrence
- Patient remained independent with gait and living but was unable to return to work due to the progression of renal failure and initiation of hemodialysis

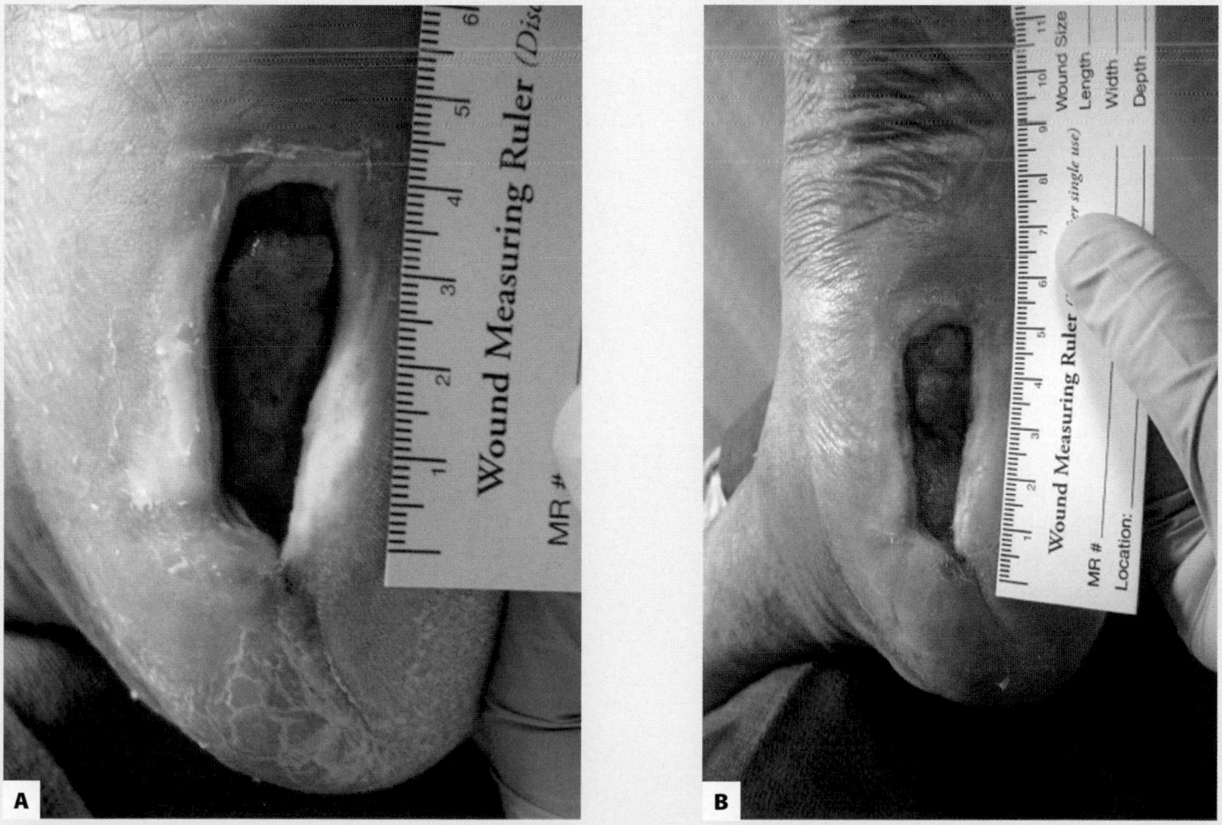

FIGURE 16-15 A. Patient's wound after 30 days of standard care. B. Noticeable responses to ES include decreased callus and adherence of the wound edges to the wound bed, thereby allowing epithelial migration to occur, and increased granulation tissue. Silver nitrate was used on the hypergranulation tissue to flatten the wound bed and facilitate full closure.

However, published applications and treatment recommendations provide a starting point for providers to initiate informed treatment. Because each patient, and indeed each wound, is different, understanding how electrical currents affect human cells and tissues can help guide clinical decisions in the safe application of ES for wound healing.

STUDY QUESTIONS

1. The mechanism of attracting cells to a specific area using electromagnetic fields is termed
   a. Chemotaxis.
   b. Electrotaxis.
   c. Current of injury.
   d. Electrocautery.
2. To facilitate the optimal migration of cells to the wounded area, it is advised to
   a. Have the electrodes of equal size and 15 cm apart.
   b. Have the active electrode distal to the wound and the dispersive proximal to the wound.
   c. Have the dispersive electrode twice the size of the active electrode and placed 10–15 cm apart from the active electrode.
   d. Have the active electrode over the wound and the dispersive electrode as far away as possible.
3. The intensity or voltage of the current is advised to be
   a. As high as the patient can tolerate.
   b. Equal to what the patient can tolerate on the opposite extremity.
   c. High enough to see visible fasciculations.
   d. High enough for the patient to feel a comfortable tingling sensation under the electrode.
4. ES as an adjunctive treatment for wounds is most frequently considered when a wound is at which stage?
   a. Acute
   b. Subacute
   c. Chronic
5. The primary goal of choosing LVPC for a wound is to
   a. Attract the negatively charged cells to the electrode.
   b. Attract the positively charged cells to the electrode.
   c. Increase blood flow in the wound area.
   d. Decrease slough at the wound area.
6. Monophasic HVPC provides generally comfortable treatment in part due to high voltage in the range of
   a. 25–50 volts.
   b. 50–75 volts.
   c. 75–150 volts.
   d. 150–250 volts.
7. An absolute contraindication for the use of ES to treat a wound is
   a. The patient has a pacemaker.
   b. The wound is suspected of having infection.
   c. The patient is insensate.
   d. The wound has been epithelialized for 1 week.

Answers: 1-b; 2-c; 3-d; 4-c; 5-c; 6-c; 7-a

REFERENCES

1. Cameron MH, Shapiro S, Ocelnik M. Introduction to electrotherapy. In: Cameron MH, ed. *Physical Agents in Rehabilitation: An Evidence-Based Approach to Practice*. 5th ed. St. Louis, MO: Saunders; 2018: 219-537.
2. Cambridge NA. Electrical apparatus used in medicine before 1900. *Proc R Soc Med*. 1977;70:635-641.
3. Rajendran SB, Challen K, Wright KL, Hardy JG. Electrical stimulation to enhance wound healing. *J Funct Biomater*. 2021;12(2):1-17.
4. Milne J, Swift A, Smith J, Martin R. Electrical stimulation for pain reduction in hard-to-heal wound healing. *J Wound Care*. 2021;30(7):568-580.
5. Arora M, Harvey LA, Glinsky JV, et al. Electrical stimulation for treating pressure ulcers. *Cochran Database Syst Rev*. 2020;1(1): CD012196.
6. Chen Z, Chen ZY, Liu WH, Li GS. Electrical stimulation as an effective adjunctive therapy for diabetic foot ulcer: A meta-analysis of randomized controlled trials. *Adv Skin Wound Care*. 2020;33:608-612.
7. Iskandar I, Dharmajaya R, Ariani Y. Increasing foot circulation with electrical stimulation in patients with diabetes mellitus. *Belitung Nurs J*. 2018;4(3):343-349.
8. Khouri C, Kotzki S, Roustit M, et al. Hierarchical evaluation of electrical stimulation protocols for chronic wound healing: An effect size meta-analysis. *Wound Repair Regen*. 2017;25(5):883-891.
9. Karaman M, Gun T, Temelkuran B, et al. Comparison of fiber delivered CO_2 laser and electrocautery in transoral robot assisted tongue base surgery. *Eur Arch Otorhinolaryngol*. 2017;274:2273-2279.
10. Ennis WJ, Lee C, Gellada K, Corbiere TF, Koh TJ. Advanced technologies to improve wound healing: Electrical stimulation, vibration therapy, and ultrasound-what is the evidence? *Adv Technol Wound Heal*. 2016;138(3S):94S-104S.
11. Lawson D, Tawfik J, Nolan T. Biophysical energies for wound healing: What is the evidence and when should we use them? presented at: American Physical Therapy Association's Combined Sections Meeting; February 2022; San Antonio, TX.
12. Atieh A, Zhang Z, Douville Y, Methot M, Rouabhia M. Effect of electrical stimulation on diabetic human skin fibroblast growth and the secretion of cytokines and growth factors involved in wound healing. *Biology*. 2021;10(7):641.
13. Cui S, Rouabhia M, Semlali A, Zhang Z. Effects of electrical stimulation on human skin keratinocyte growth and the secretion of cytokines and growth factors. *Biomed Mater*. 2021;16(6). Available at: doi: 10.1088/1748-605X/ac2bba. PMID: 34592730.
14. Uemura M, Sugimoto M, Yoshikawa Y, Hiramatsu T, Inoue T. Monophasic pulsed current Stimulation of duty cycle 10% promotes differentiation of human dermal fibroblasts into myofibroblasts. *Phys Ther Res*. 2021;24(2):145-152.
15. Polak A, Kucio C, Kloth L et al. A randomized, controlled clinical study to assess the effect of anodal and cathodal electrical stimulation on periwound skin blood flow and pressure ulcer size reduction in persons with neurological injuries. *Ostomy Wound Manage*. 2018;64(2):10-29.
16. Kloth L. Electrical stimulation technologies for wound healing. *Adv Wound Care*. 2013;3(2):81-90.
17. National Pressure Injury Advisory Panel and European Pressure Ulcer Advisory Panel. *Prevention and Treatment of Pressure Ulcers/ Injuries: Clinical Practice Guide*. The International Guideline 2019. Washington, DC: National Pressure Ulcer Advisory Panel; 2019.
18. Wound Ostomy and Continence Nurses Society. Wound Ostomy and Continence Nurses Society. *Venous, Arterial, and Neuropathic Lower-Extremity Wounds: Clinical Resource Guide. 2019*. Available at: https://cdn.ymaws.com/member.wocn.org/resource/resmgr/docs/Venous_Arterial__Neuropathic.pdf. Accessed November 6, 2022.

19. Academy of Clinical Electrophysiology and Wound Management. APTA's Academy of Clinical Electrophysiology and Wound Management Guide for Integumentary/Wound Management Content in Professional Physical Therapist Education. Available at: https://acewm.org/wp-content/uploads/2016/12/APTA-ACEWM-Wound-Recommendations-July-2014-Updates-2.pdf. Accessed November 6, 2022.
20. Frantz RA. Electrical Stimulation. In: Bryant RA, Nix DP, eds. *Acute & Chronic Wounds: Current Management Concepts*. 5th ed. St. Louis, MO: Elsevier; 2016:369-376.
21. Foulds IS, Barker AT. Human skin battery potentials and their possible role in wound healing. *Br J Dermatol.* 1983;109:515-522.
22. Kloth LC, McCulloch JM. Promotion of wound healing with electrical stimulation. *Adv Skin Wound Care.* 1996;9(5):42-45.
23. Jaffe LF, Vanable JW. Electric fields and wound healing. *Clin Dermatol.* 1984;2(3):34-44.
24. Hunckler J, de Mel A. A current affair: Electrotherapy in wound healing. *J Multidiscip Healthc.* 2017;10:179-194.
25. Woo K, Ayello EA, Sibbald RG. The edge effect: current therapeutic options to advance the wound edge. *Adv Skin Wound Care.* 2007;20(2):99-117.
26. Garcia-Perez, S, Garcia-Rios C, Perez-Marmol JM, et al. Effectiveness of transcutaneous electrical nerve stimulation energy in older adults: a pilot clinical trial. *Adv Skin Wound Care.* 2018;31(10):462-469.
27. Kloth LC. How to use electrical stimulation for wound healing. *Nursing.* 2002;32(12):17.
28. Kloth LC, Zhao M. Endogenous and exogenous electrical fields for wound healing. In: McCulloch JM, Kloth LC, eds. *Wound Healing: Evidence-Based Management.* 4th ed. Philadelphia, PA: FA Davis; 2012:150-513.
29. Recio AC, Felter CE, Schneider AC, McDonald JW. High-voltage electrical stimulation for the management of stage III and stage IV pressure ulcers among adults with spinal cord injury: Demonstration of its utility for recalcitrant wounds below the level of injury. *J Spinal Cord Med.* 2012,35(1):58-63.
30. Isseroff RR, Dahle SE. Electrical stimulation therapy and wound healing: where are we now? *Adv Skin Wound Care.* 2012;1(6):238-243.
31. Zhao M, Penninger J, Isseroff RR. Electrical activation of wound-healing pathways. *Adv Skin Wound Care.* 2010;23(1):567-573.
32. Thakral G, La Fontaine J, Kim P, et al. Treatment options for venous leg ulcers: Effectiveness of vascular surgery, bioengineered tissue, and electrical stimulation. *Adv Skin Wound Care.* 2015;28(4):164-172.
33. Jnger M, Arnold A, Zuder D, Stahl HW, Heising S. Local therapy and treatment costs of chronic, venous leg ulcers with electrical stimulation (Dermapulse®): A prospective, placebo controlled, double blind trial. *Wound Repair Regen.* 2008;16:480-487.
34. Gentzkow GD. Electrical stimulation to heal dermal wounds. *J Dermatol Surg Oncol.* 1993;19:753-758.
35. Reich LD, Cazzaniga AL, Mertz PM, Kerdel FA, Eaglstein WH. The effect of electrical stimulation on the number of mast cells in healing wounds. *J Am Acad Dermatol.* 1991;25:40-46.
36. Kloth LC. Electrical stimulation for wound healing: A review of evidence from in vitro studies, animal experiments and clinical trials. *Int J Low Extrem Wounds.* 2005;4(1):23-44.
37. Bourguignon GJ, Bourguignon LYW. Electrical stimulation of protein and DNA synthesis in human fibroblasts. *FASEB J.* 1987;1(5):398-402.
38. Karsli PB, Gurcay E, Karaahmet OZ, Cakci A. High-voltage electrical stimulation versus ultrasound in the treatment of pressure ulcers. *Adv Skin Wound Care.* 2017;30(12):565-569.
39. Lawson D, Petrofsky J. The effect of monophasic vs biphasic current on healing rate and blood flow in people with pressure and neuropathic ulcers. *J Acute Care Phys Ther.* 2013;4(1):26-33.
40. Petrofsky J, Schwas E, Lo T, et al. Effects of electrical stimulation on skin blood flow in controls and in and around stage III and IV wounds in hairy and non-hairy skin. *Med Sci Monit.* 2005;11(7):CR309-CR316.
41. Zhao M, Song B, Pu J, et al. Electrical signals control wound healing through phosphatidylinositol-3-OH kinase-γ and PTEN. *Nature.* 2006;442:457-460.
42. Li L, Hartley R, Reiss B, et al. E-cadherin plays an essential role in collective directional migration of large epithelial sheets. *Cell Mol Life Sci.* 2012;69(16):2779-2789.
43. Nishimura KY, Isseroff RR, Nuccitelli R. Human keratinocytes migrate to the negative pole in direct current electric fields comparable to those measured in mammalian wounds. *J Cell Sci.* 1996;109:199-207.
44. Haughton PE, Campbell KE, Fraser CH, et al. Electrical stimulation therapy increases rate of healing of pressure ulcers in community-dwelling people with spinal cord injury. *Arch Phys Med Rehabil.* 2010;91(5):669-678.
45. Weiss DS, Eaglstein WH, Falanga V. Exogenous electrical current can reduce the formation of hypertrophic scars. *J Dermatol Surg Oncol.* 1989;15(12):1272-1275.
46. Stromberg BV. Effects of electrical currents on wound contraction. *Ann Plast Surg.* 1988;21(2):121-123.
47. Burdge JJ, Hartman JF, Wright L. A retrospective study of high-voltage, pulsed current as an adjunctive therapy in limb salvage for chronic diabetic wounds of the lower extremity. *Ostomy Wound Manage.* 2009;55(8):30-38.
48. Hopf HW, Ueno C, Aslam R, et al. Guidelines for the treatment of arterial insufficiency ulcers. *Wound Repair Regen.* 2006;14:693-710.
49. Daeschlein G, Assadian O, Kloth L, et al. Antibacterial activity of positive and negative polarity low-voltage pulsed current (LVPC) on six typical gram-positive and gram-negative bacterial pathogens of chronic wounds. *Wound Repair Regen.* 2007;15(3):399-403.
50. Bellew JW, Nolan TP. *Michlovitz's Modalities for Therapeutic Intervention.* 7th ed. New York, NY: McGraw-Hill Education; 2022.
51. Ashrafi M, Alonso-Rasgado T, Baguneid M, Bayat A. The efficacy of electrical stimulation in lower extremity cutaneous wound healing: a systematic review. *Exp Dermatol.* 2017;26(2):171-178.
52. Kim H, Park S, Housler G, Marcel V, Cross S, Izadjoo M. An overview of the efficacy of a next generation electroceutical wound care device. *Mil Med.* 2016;181(suppl_5):184-190.
53. Yoshikawa Y, Hiramatsu T, Sugimoto M, Uemura M, Mori Y, Ichibori R. Efficacy of low-frequency monophasic pulsed microcurrent stimulation therapy in undermining pressure injury: a double-blind crossover-controlled study. *Prog Rehabil Med.* 2022;7:20220045.
54. Uemura M, Sugimoto M, Yoshikawa Y, Inoue R. Electrical shunting prevents the decline of galvanotaxis after monophasic pulsed microcurrent stimulation in human dermal fibroblasts. *Eplasty.* 2022;22:e27.
55. Lee BY, Wendell K, Al-Waili N, Butler G. Ultra-low microcurrent therapy: A novel approach for treatment of chronic resistant wounds. *Adv Ther.* 2007;24(6):1202-1209.
56. Ofstead CL, Buro BL, Hopkins KM, Eiland JE. The impact of continuous electrical microcurrent on acute and hard-to-heal wounds: a systematic review. *J Wound Care.* 2020;29(Sup 7):S6-S15.
57. Guest JF, Singh H, Rana K, Vowden P. Cost-effectiveness of an electroceutical device in treating non-healing venous leg ulcers: Results of an RCT. *J Wound Care.* 2018;27(4):230-243.
58. Ramadhinara A, Poulas K. Use of wireless microcurrent stimulation for the treatment of diabetes-related wounds: 2 case reports. *Adv Skin Wound Care.* 2013;26(1):1-4.

59. Young S, Hampton S, Tadej M. Study to evaluate the effect of low-intensity pulsed electrical currents on levels of oedema in chronic non-healing wounds. *J Wound Care*. 2011;20(8):368-373.
60. Ghatak PD, Schlanger R, Ganesh K, et al. A wireless electroceutical dressing lowers cost of negative pressure wound therapy. *Adv Wound Care*. 2015;4(5):302-311.
61. Khona DK, Roy S, Ghatak S, et al. Ketoconazole resistant *Candida albicans* is sensitive to wireless electroceutical wound care dressing. *Biochem*. 2021;142:1-19.
62. Barki KG, Das A, Dixith S, et al. Electric field based dressing disrupts mixed-species bacterial biofilm infection and restores functional wound healing. *Ann Surg*. 2019;269(4):756-766.
63. Sen CK, Mathew-Steiner SS, Das A, Sundaresan VB, Roy S. Electroceutical management of bacterial biofilms and surgical infection. *Antioxid Redox Signal*. 2020;33(10):713-724.
64. Petrofsky J, Schwab E. A re-evaluation of modeling of the current flow between electrodes: consideration of blood flow and wounds. *J Med Eng Technol*. 2007;31(1):62-74.
65. Balakatounis KC, Angoules AG. Low-intensity electrical stimulation in wound healing: review of the efficacy of externally applied currents resembling the current of injury. *J Plast Surg*. 2008;8:283-291.

CHAPTER SEVENTEEN

Negative Pressure Wound Therapy

Karen A. Gibbs, PT, PhD, DPT, CWS and Sonya Dick, PT, DPT, CWS

CHAPTER OBJECTIVES

At the end of this chapter, the learner will be able to:

1. **Explain the cellular and tissue effects of negative pressure wound therapy and link the effects to wound healing.**
2. **Identify the components of negative pressure wound therapy systems and their functions.**
3. **Describe the indications for negative pressure wound therapy in wound management.**
4. **Discuss precautions and contraindications for the use of negative pressure wound therapy and adaptation strategies.**
5. **Describe continuous and intermittent modes of negative pressure wound therapy and the advantages/disadvantages of both.**
6. **Explain the basic steps involved in the application of negative pressure wound therapy.**

INTRODUCTION

Negative pressure wound therapy (NPWT), also known as vacuum-assisted therapy,[1] was first documented as an adjunct treatment for open wounds in the early 1990s and by 2004 this active therapy was reported as a standard of care for a variety of acute and chronic wounds.[1–4] Through the application of a closed wound dressing with controlled, subatmospheric pressure to open wounds, the therapy provides the following benefits for wound healing:

- Promotion of moist wound healing and protection from the environment[5,6]
- Reduction of edema and interstitial fluid[7,8]
- Increased local perfusion[5,6]
- Approximation of wound edges with decreased wound volume[5,7]
- Stimulation of granulation tissue formation[9]
- Reduction in bacterial load[6,7]
- Reduction in the frequency of dressing changes[6,9]

Since its acceptance into evidence-based wound management, NPWT has been utilized to treat a wide variety of acute and chronic wounds including traumatic and surgical wounds healing by primary and secondary intention,[7,10,11] burns and skin grafts,[1,12–14] diabetic foot ulcers,[1,15] and pressure injuries.[1,16] Mass casualty events such as the devastating 2010 earthquake in Haiti[17] and mass casualty injuries during times of war[17–21] have also shown how the benefits of NPWT can positively influence limb salvage rates and decrease morbidity and mortality in mass casualty and high-energy injury situations.

A traditional NPWT system (**FIGURE 17-1**) consists of a subatmospheric pressure generating device, a wound filler that transfers negative pressure across the wound bed and allows for the flow of fluids away from the wound, a transparent occlusive sheet that covers the wound filler and creates a tight seal, and flexible tubing that delivers the negative pressure and serves as a conduit for removal of wound fluids and debris. Wound fluids are collected in a disposable container typically attached to the suction device (**TABLE 17-1**).[6] Advances in

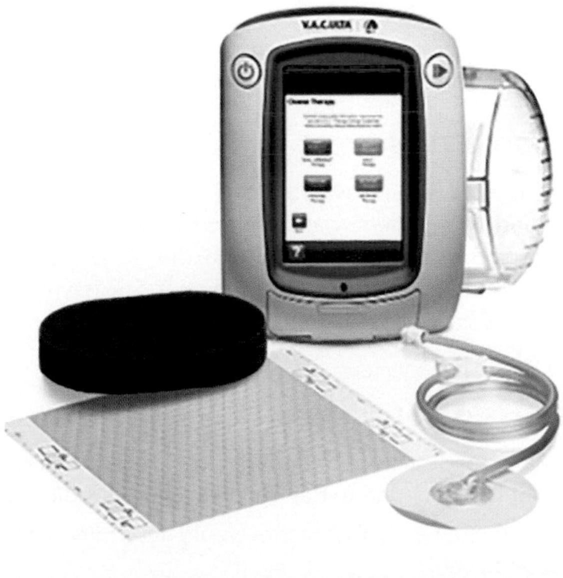

FIGURE 17-1 Negative pressure wound therapy. Wound fluid is suctioned from the wound, through the foam, into an attached tube, and into an airtight disposable canister. Although every system has its own unique characteristics, the basic functions of removing interstitial edema, stimulation of cellular activity, and reducing wound size are the same.

TABLE 17-1 Basic NPWT Components

Negative pressure device	Different sizes based on inpatient vs outpatient use Powered by electricity, battery, or mechanically Reusable *or* single-use and disposable Programmable for different parameters and negative pressure settings (mmHg) Alarms for full canister, leaks, interrupted suction, and/or low battery
Wound filler	Foam: black, white, green, blue reticulated open-cell with through holes or abdominal blue football shape with visceral protective spoke layer Gauze
Occlusive sheet cover	Semipermeable film or sheeting cut to size
Tubing	Delivers negative pressure and serves as a conduit for fluid removal Additional tubing utilized for fluid instillation
Collection canister	Various sizes depending upon the device and exudate amounts Single-use, disposable Changeable without necessitating a dressing change Disposable into red biohazard container or per facility guidelines

negative pressure technology now provide several variations of traditional units and are described later in this chapter.

Due to overwhelming evidence supporting NPWT for soft tissue healing,[1,3,5–7,11,13] an explosion in NPWT interest and development has occurred with multiple vendors offering devices in various sizes with some units specially designed for specific types of wounds (see **TABLE 17-2** for partial vendor list). Increased healing, portability, and ease of management can result in decreased length of hospital stay, faster return to function, healthcare economic benefits, and improved quality of life.[1,6,9,16]

MECHANISM OF ACTION

NPWT promotes wound healing through the removal of wound fluid, mechanical stimulation of cells improving the overall function, facilitation of wound contraction, maintenance of a moist wound environment, and protection from environmental contaminants. As fluid is removed from the wound, interstitial edema is reduced. Inflammatory mediators and bacteria are removed along with tissue fluids, thereby reducing wound inflammation and facilitating progression to the proliferative phase of healing. Mechanical stimulation at both the tissue (macrodeformation) and cellular (microdeformation) levels encourages increased cellular proliferation, granulation tissue formation, and wound contraction.[6,8–10,14,22] The occlusive sheeting maintains a moist wound environment, provides an optimal seal that sustains the vacuum-generated subatmospheric pressure, and protects the wound from the external environment. Despite differences in size and shape, all NPWT devices basically offer the same benefits, and selection of a device depends upon many factors including (1) wound type, size, and amount of drainage; (2) the patient's mobility level; (3) inpatient versus outpatient status; (4) the patient's medical coverage, and (5) availability of supplies. Because of the various NPWT devices, therapy can be individualized for optimal treatment and outcomes.

CASE STUDY

INTRODUCTION

A 59-year-old patient was referred for wound care of the left hand. The patient was admitted to the hospital with an infected human bite wound on the dorsal hand that required extensive surgical debridement. Surgery was performed 1 day prior to the initial consultation for wound care (**FIGURE 17-2**).

DISCUSSION QUESTIONS

1. What medical information from the patient's chart would be needed to determine if NPWT is indicated?
2. What wound characteristics would determine if NPWT is indicated?

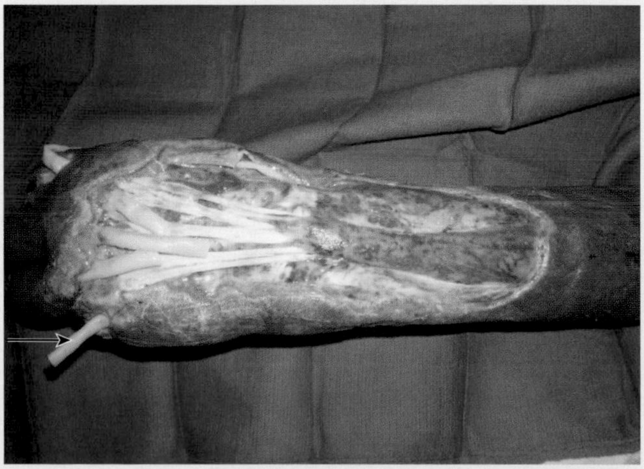

FIGURE 17-2 Wound for NPWT case study. Left-hand wound after surgical debridement of infected tissue. There are exposed tendons and muscles, and Penrose drains (at the arrow) have been placed to allow drainage from the deeper tissue.

TABLE 17-2 Partial NPWT Vendor List

American Medical Products	**extriCARE Compact (portable)** ▪ Uses peel-and-stick dressings in various sizes ▪ Operates on battery power **SVED Wound Treatment System** ▪ Uses black and white foam ▪ Provides instillation ▪ Operates on electrical and battery power
DeRoyal	**PRO-III and Prospera PRO-II (portable)** ▪ Uses black and white foam or gauze ▪ Operates on electrical and battery power
Genadyne Biotechnologies	**XLR8 (portable)** ▪ Offers various canisters and foam sizes ▪ Uses green foam and polyvinyl alcohol foam (PVA) ▪ Operates on battery power **XLRS plus (hospital and home care)** ▪ Operates on electrical and battery power **UNO (single-use system)**
Cardinal Health	**SVED (portable)** ▪ Uses black or white foam ▪ Provides instillation of topical fluids ▪ Operates on electrical and battery power
3M Kinetic Corporation, Inc. (KCI)	**V.A.C. Ulta Therapy** ▪ Used only for the instillation of topical fluids ▪ Operates on electrical and battery power **V.A.C. Via** ▪ Offers portable, disposable, 7-day therapy ▪ Operates on battery power **ActiV.A.C.** ▪ Operates on electrical power only **V.A.C. Freedom** ▪ Offers portability **V.A.C. ATS** **V.A.C. Simplicity** **InfoV.A.C.** ▪ Provides therapy for inpatient care only **Prevena therapy system** ▪ Offers portable, disposable, single-use therapy ▪ Used for surgical incisions ▪ Provides all-in-one, peel-and-stick dressings of various sizes ▪ Operates on battery power **SNAP therapy system** ▪ Offers portable, disposable therapy ▪ Operates on spring-power
Medela, Inc.	**Invia (portable, inpatient or outpatient)** ▪ Uses foam or gauze, various premade dressing kits ▪ Various canister sizes ▪ Multiple drain options ▪ Operates on electrical and battery power **Invia Motion (compact)** ▪ Operates on battery power
Mölnlycke Health Care	**Avance (portable, inpatient, or outpatient use)** ▪ Uses green foam, various canister sizes ▪ Operates on electrical and battery power **Avance Solo (portable)** ▪ Uses peel-and-stick dressings, can be combined with green foam ▪ Operates on battery power
Smith & Nephew, Inc.	**Renasys EZ Plus (inpatient use)** ▪ Uses gauze or foam, various canister sizes **PICO 1.6** ▪ Portable, single-use, all-in-one, canister free ▪ Uses "stick-on" dressings, in various sizes ▪ Treats 2 incisions simultaneously (PICO 7Y) ▪ Treats larger wounds (PICO 14) ▪ Operates on battery power
Talley Group Ltd	**Venturi Avanti (inpatient or outpatient use)** ▪ Uses gauze filler, a large canister **Venturi Compact** (portable) ▪ Uses foam or gauze **Venturi Mino** (very small) ▪ Uses peel-and-stick dressings

(Continued)

EFFECTS AT THE CELLULAR AND TISSUE LEVELS

NPWT has several documented effects at the cellular and tissue levels. Due to the close, interrelated nature of these effects, cellular and tissue changes associated with NPWT are discussed together and presented in the following main categories: occlusion, cellular deformation, fluid removal, vascular effects, contraction, and bioburden (**TABLE 17-3**).

Occlusion

The benefits of moist wound healing have been well established.[4,9,23–25] Since NPWT requires a tight seal in order to maintain a prescribed pressure setting, all devices require an occlusive adhesive sheet to be placed over the primary dressing. As long as the seal is preserved, a moist wound environment is created and vacuum-generated subatmospheric pressure is maintained. Most NPWT dressings are changed every 48–72 hours; thus, exposure of the wound to air (which can decrease wound bed moisture and temperature and subsequently slow the healing process) and the external environment is minimized.

Cellular Deformation

The mechanical force associated with NPWT causes the deformation of cells.[6,9,10,14,16] This pulling or stretching force, referred to as microstrain,[3] creates changes within the cells that result in increased release of growth factors and cytokines associated with cellular proliferation.[14] Increased cellular division and migration of macrophages, lymphocytes, and fibroblasts are

TABLE 17-3 Summary of NPWT Cellular and Tissue Effects

Occlusion and moisture balance	▪ Encourages moist wound healing (facilitates cell migration/proliferation, prevents tissue desiccation, normothermic, and minimizes wound associated pain[4,16,23–25] ▪ Protects tissues from outside contaminants decreasing the risk of infection[6,7,12]
Cellular deformation	▪ Increases growth factors and cytokines release[14] ▪ Facilitates cellular activity and macrophage, lymphocyte, and fibroblast migration[6,10,14,16] ▪ Increases angiogenesis and granulation tissue formation[9,14]
Promotes healing cascade	▪ Facilitates oxygen and nutrient diffusion[6,14] ▪ Decreases inflammation and sequesters excess MMPs[13] ▪ Removes harmful substances in chronic wound fluid[13,26] ▪ Facilitates lymphatic system engagement for reduction of interstitial edema via existing lymph vessels[27] ▪ Reduces open surface area[13]
Vascular effects	▪ Improves circulation through effects of cellular deformation and removal of fluid[6,13,14,28] • Improves local blood flow through decompression of blood vessels • Influences vasomotor tone through deformation of blood vessels • Increases dermal blood flow by opening vascular beds (use intermittent setting for wounds with compromised blood flow) • Increases angiogenesis through deformation and strain
Contraction	▪ Is improved through effects of removal of fluid ▪ Centripetal suction force approximates wound edges[6,7]
Bioburden	▪ Is decreased through effects of all of the following: • Occlusive dressing helps prevent outside contamination • Moist wound healing promotes healthy wound environment • Fewer dressing changes limit exposure to outside contamination • Removal of contaminated wound fluid decreases inflammatory cellular components • Improved blood flow facilitates delivery of systemic antibiotics

also facilitated.[10,14,16] Mechanical deformation caused by negative pressure results in increased angiogenesis and granulation tissue formation and is one of the most significant effects of NPWT.[9,14]

Fluid Removal

Timely and efficient removal of interstitial and exudative wound fluid is another important result of NPWT. Reduction of interstitial edema associated with acute injury and trauma facilitates oxygen and nutrient movement by decreasing the diffusion distance in the capillary beds.[6,14] Edema reduction also decreases inflammation when inflammatory mediators are removed from the wound fluid.[13,26] It has been well documented that chronic wound fluid has many pro-inflammatory mediators and is detrimental to wound healing,[13,29,30] thus making NPWT especially beneficial in the treatment of chronic wounds. Closed incision negative pressure therapy (ciNPT) is used to reduce surgical site complications and recently has been shown to effectively reduce post-operative hematoma and seroma formation.[31,32] Resolution of edema, as well as seromas or hematomas, is related to the function of the lymphatic system after surgery or tissue injury. Increased lymphatic clearance of fluids may explain the decrease in hematomas and seromas with ciNPT as compared to standard of care, even when fluid is not evacuated from subcutaneous or interstitial spaces into the attached canister.[27]

Vascular Effects

Local vascular function is improved with NPWT through the combined effects of cellular deformation and tissue fluid removal.[6,13,14,28] Mechanical stimulation of wound tissue promotes cellular migration, differentiation, and angiogenesis[6,26] while the resolution of tissue edema decreases interstitial pressure on capillaries, thereby decreasing diffusion distances for the exchange of oxygen, carbon dioxide and other cellular components, all of which can improve local circulation.[6,14,26] Some studies have shown NPWT can cause decreased blood flow at wound edges due to what appears to be compressive forces. As mildly hypoxic environments can trigger angiogenesis, these compressive forces may further stimulate new blood vessel formation.[22,33–35] In ischemic wounds, the use of lower negative pressure settings or the intermittent mode of NPWT is advised in order to reduce the risk of wound edge compression; in this case, wound status needs to be closely monitored (see the "Parameters" section for modes of NPWT delivery).

Contraction

The pulling force of NPWT assists in approximating wound edges, referred to as macrostrain,[3] and wound contraction.[5–7,13,14,28] This action combined with reductions in local tissue edema via fluid removal effectively reduces the wound surface area and volume.[6,13]

Bioburden

NPWT positively affects wound bioburden through all the mechanisms discussed above: promoting a warm, moist environment protected from outside contaminants; facilitating cellular migration and proliferation; evacuating bacteria along with wound fluids; increasing local vascular function; and by assisting in overall faster wound closure. Additionally some NPWT units provide for the instillation of topical solutions as another mechanism of combating pathologic bioburden (discussed later in this chapter).[3] Overall, NPWT is just one component in a treatment strategy for contaminated or infected wounds and should be appropriately combined with other standard therapies that may include sharp/surgical debridement, systemic antibiotics, and irrigation with pulsed lavage with suction (see Chapter 19, Pulsed Lavage with Suction).[36,37] NPWT is not indicated for all wounds (**FIGURE 17-3** and **TABLE 17-4**); safe and appropriate indications for NPWT are presented below.

INDICATIONS

TABLE 17-5 provides a list of wound etiologies for which NPWT is indicated (**FIGURES 17-4** to **17-11**). Cellular and tissue effects must be considered for each indication to obtain optimal patient outcomes.

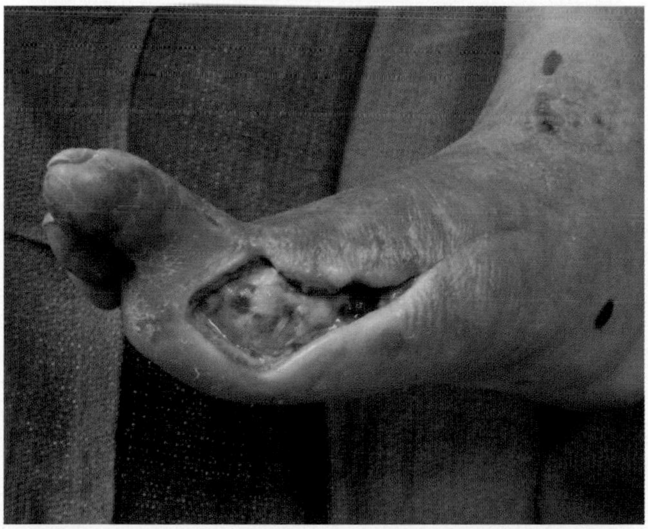

FIGURE 17-3 NPWT would not be placed on this wound until adequate tissue perfusion for wound healing is confirmed. There are no signs of neoangiogenesis in the wound bed and the residual toes are dusky. Moist wound dressings would be applied until vascular studies confirm that revascularization was successful.

TABLE 17-4 Prerequisites to NPWT in Infected Wounds

Patient is free of most systemic signs of gross infection.
Necrotic tissue is debrided and abscesses are drained.
Wound has adequate perfusion.

TABLE 17-5 Indications for NPWT

Acute surgical and traumatic	Meshed grafts and flaps[14,38]
	Wounds in need of additional physical stabilization[9]
	Fasciotomies performed for compartment syndrome[10]
	Full-thickness wounds with or without exposed structures or hardware prior to grafting, primary or secondary intention closure[3]
	Open abdominal wounds[3]
	At-risk surgical incisions[3,8]
	Deep partial- and full-thickness burns[28]
	Traumatic amputations and deep lacerations[3,11]
	Dermal substitutes, as a cover (Integra, Integra Sciences Corp, Plainsboro, NJ) and bioengineered skin substitutes (Apligraf, Organogenesis, Inc., Canton, MA)[39]
Chronic	Debrided neuropathic wounds and open amputation sites associated with diabetes[1,3,15,40]
	Stage III and IV pressure ulcers[9,16]
	Wounds associated with venous insufficiency[12,40,41]
	Wounds associated with arterial insufficiency with caution after adequate tissue perfusion has been achieved[42]
	Wounds treated as part of palliative care

Acute Wounds

Evidence supports the use of NPWT for most acute surgical wounds and for traumatic wounds that require increased granulation prior to surgical closure or grafting.[1,6,10,18,28,43] NPWT is especially beneficial for wounds with exposed bone, tendon, or hardware or those that require staged surgical procedures prior to final closure.[36] In many cases, the use of NPWT in acute wounds can efficiently reduce tissue edema resulting in faster delayed primary intention closure.[44] Due to the cellular and tissue effects of NPWT, placement over

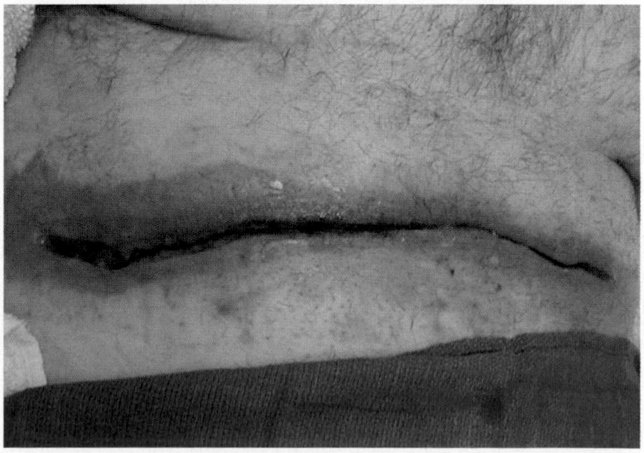

FIGURE 17-4 Abdominal incisional wound on a patient who has had a Whipple procedure for chronic pancreatitis. The erythema on the periwound skin is a result of copious drainage coming from the wound. NPWT is indicated to promote granulation, and wound closure, and to manage exudate in order to protect the periwound and surrounding skin.

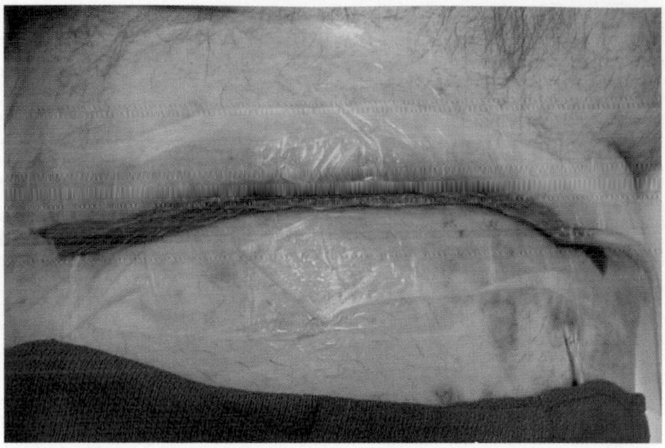

FIGURE 17-5 Abdominal wound with NPWT in place. NPWT is applied to the wound in **FIGURE 17-4** with a layer of Vaseline gauze under the adhesive drape to protect the inflamed skin and to help minimize pain when the drape is removed. Note the Chariker–Jeter or mesentery approach of applying the suction tube to the foam. This method is recommended for high-output wounds, small or narrow wounds where the round track pad may press on surrounding tissue, or gauze-filled wounds.

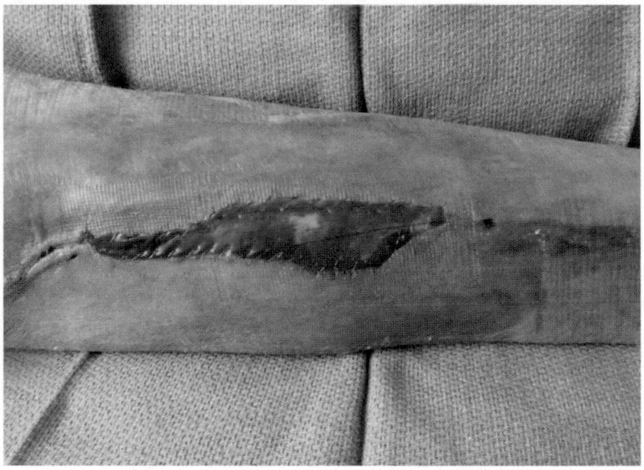

FIGURE 17-6 Wound with biologic dressing sutured in place. The NPWT will bolster the biologic dressing, will not disrupt new capillaries, will drain interstitial fluid, and will promote cellular activity.

a new split-thickness skin graft (STSG) has been shown to increase graft "take" through edema reduction and graft stabilization (see the "Precautions and Contraindications" and "Application" sections regarding how to apply NPWT over skin grafts).[13,14,28,38] Stabilization occurs once the therapy is turned on and the wound filler collapses on itself thereby transferring negative pressure to the graft. For skin grafts, the negative pressure force holds the skin graft and underlying granulation tissue tightly together, reducing the risk of shear, and it removes wound fluid which decreases the risk of edema and/or seroma formation.[14,28] These same mechanisms provide bone and soft tissue stabilization or splinting when NPWT is

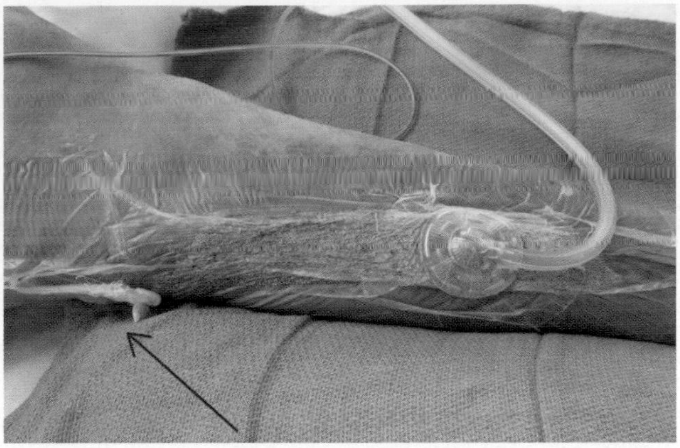

FIGURE 17-7 Wound with NPWT applied using silver-impregnated foam. Note how the drain at the proximal wound edge is incorporated into the dressing in order to ensure an adequate seal.

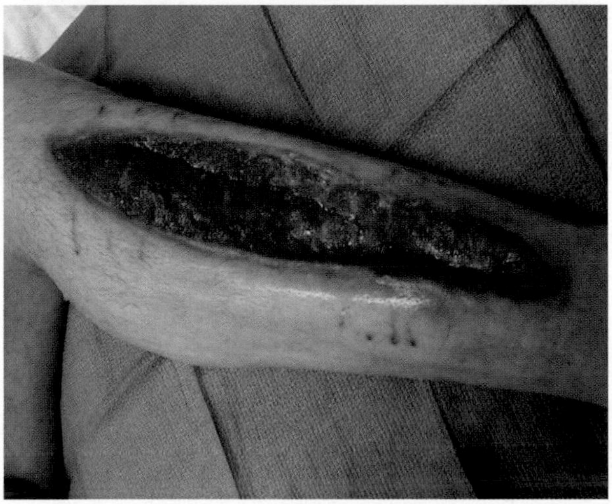

FIGURE 17-8 Lower extremity compartment syndrome after fasciotomy. Treatment with NPWT has provided *macrostrain* that is facilitating wound contraction and *microstrain* that is facilitating angiogenesis and enhanced granulation; both actions facilitate easier surgical closure or faster healing by secondary intention.

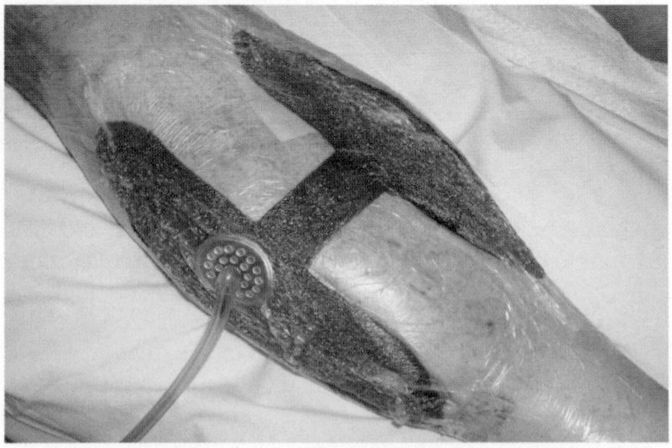

FIGURE 17-9 NPWT on medial and lateral lower extremity fasciotomies for compartment syndrome. The foam bridge (with a layer of drape beneath to protect the skin) allows both wounds to be connected to one pump.

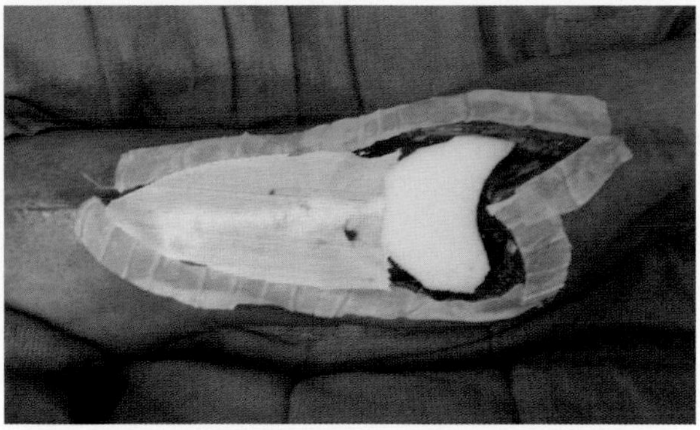

FIGURE 17-10 Traumatic wound on the lower extremity is prepared for NPWT application. White foam is placed over exposed bone, a nonadhesive, fine-meshed dressing is placed over muscle, and Xeroform strips are placed to protect the wound edges. These strategies minimize pain as well as damage to existing structures and new granulation tissue with dressing removal.

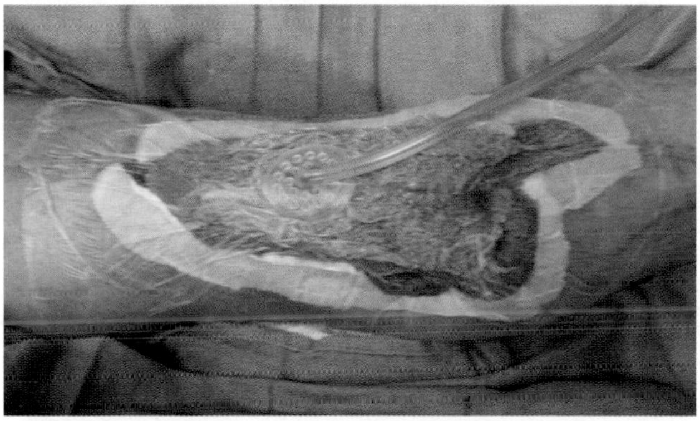

FIGURE 17-11 The wound in Figure 17-10 with the NPWT in place.

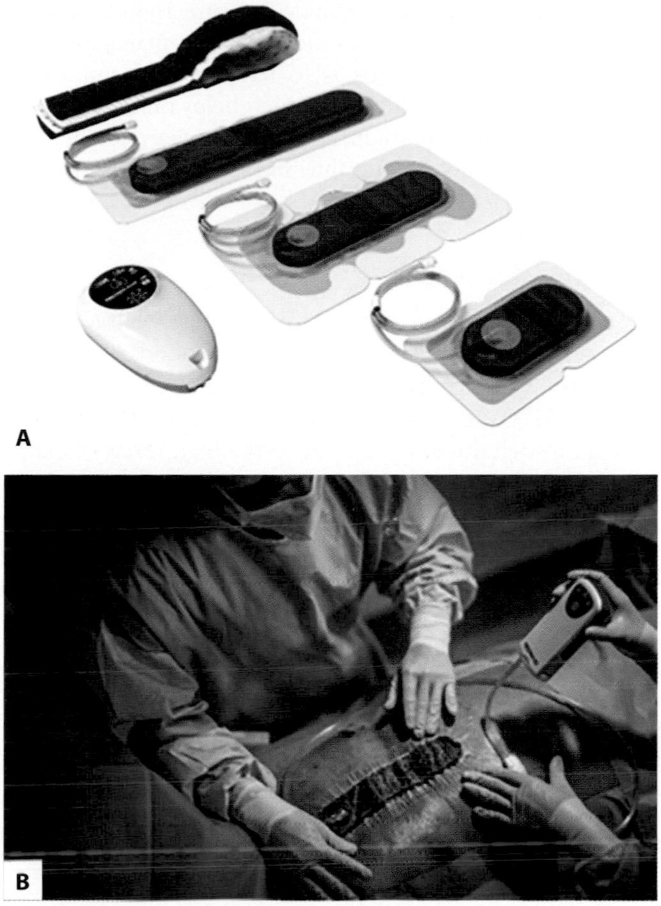

FIGURE 17-12 A. Negative pressure therapy for surgical incisions. The Prevena Incision Management System is a small ci-NPT unit that is placed over surgical incisions to help prevent dehiscence and surgical site infection. The disposable unit has a 45-mL canister and a peel-and-stick foam pad. It is applied over a clean surgical incision and left in place for the duration of the battery life. (Prevena Incision Management System; Courtesy of 3M/KCI Licensing, Inc., 2022.) **B.** The ci-NPT device and dressing applied to a sternal incision immediately after closure in the operating room which may be left in place for up to 7–14 days dependent on device and manufacturer instructions. (Courtesy of 3M/KCI Licensing, Inc., 2022.)

applied to surgical sites. These sites also benefit from extra external support, allowing increased patient mobility sooner in the recovery period.[14,45] In mass casualty or battlefield situations, NPWT has been used to stabilize and protect large open wounds until patients can be transported to advanced facilities for appropriate care.[17,20]

NPT (negative pressure therapy) is commonly placed over at-risk surgical incisions healing by primary intention, referred to as ciNPT.[3,8,46–48] Application over suture or staple lines improves wound integrity by maintaining wound edge approximation, decreasing lateral tension, removing wound fluids, improving lymphatic engagement, improving local blood flow, and protecting the site from environmental contaminants.[8,46,47,49] Single-use, disposable NPT devices especially constructed for ciNPT are available with various sizes of easy-to-apply, peel-and-stick dressings that are designed to stay in place for the first week after surgery, some up to 14 days post operatively.[1] Examples include Prevena (3M, Prevena Incision Management System, San Antonio, Texas) (**FIGURE 17-12A,B**) and PICO (PICO, Smith & Nephew, Inc., Andover, Massachusetts).

NPWT is sometimes indicated for acute partial-thickness burns or for full-thickness burns after debridement and skin graft placement (refer to NPWT for skin grafts previously presented).[1,28] Through the facilitation of a moist wound environment, edema removal, and improved circulation, NPWT can help prevent burn injury conversion to deeper tissue destruction.[28]

Abdominal wounds created when there is an acute or emergent need to perform abdominal surgery or perform repeated abdominal "wash outs" are difficult to manage; however, an application termed temporary abdominal closure (TAC) has been shown to improve outcomes compared to standard of care, including less time for patients in intensive care, decreased morbidity and mortality, and decreased overall cost.[50] The function of the TAC NPWT devices (3M AbThera Open Abdomen Negative Pressure Therapy and 3M ABTHERA 2.0, 3M, San Antonio, Texas) in managing complicated abdominal wounds is to remove fluid and reduce edema; provide medial tension, which helps minimize fascial retraction and loss of domain; and provide separation between abdominal wall and viscera, thus protecting abdominal contents (**FIGURE 17-13A, B**).[51,52]

Chronic Wounds

The cellular and tissue effects associated with NPWT make this intervention beneficial for chronic wounds.[1,3,6,13,36,45] Of particular benefit to chronic wounds is the removal of chronic wound fluid (CWF). The detrimental effects of CWF on tissue healing are well documented due to the high levels of matrix metalloproteinases (MMPs) and proinflammatory cytokines which result in the breakdown of extracellular matrix and cause sustained inflammation.[53,54] Sustained levels of pathologic bacteria or bioburden may also inhibit wound healing. With NPWT, MMPs, proinflammatory cytokines, and bioburden levels are reduced as they are efficiently removed along with wound fluid.

CLINICAL CONSIDERATION

Toe and forefoot amputation sites *after* vascular reconstruction need careful monitoring to ensure that perfusion is adequate for healing; otherwise, the pressure may occlude superficial capillaries and result in tissue necrosis.

Special Populations

Geriatrics. Dehydration is a special concern when using NPWT with older adults. Fluid intake and output need to be monitored, especially in geriatric patients with high-output wounds.[55] Other concerns in the elderly population that require close monitoring include confusion (when a patient may pull on or try to remove the NPWT dressing or device) and the use of anticoagulation medications.[56] Additionally, due to the normal aging process, elderly skin is less able to withstand shear,[57] so careful application of the adhesive NPWT occlusive sheeting is necessary to avoid skin tears. Consider the use of silicone-based occlusive sheeting (see the "Application" section) to avoid damage and pain for patients with fragile skin.

CLINICAL CONSIDERATION

The use of a skin protectant under the NPWT adhesive sheeting may decrease the risk of blistering or skin tears in elderly patients.

Pediatrics. Published literature regarding NPWT use in infants and children is limited compared to adult studies.[58,59] Santosa et al.[59] and others have documented the safe use of NPWT in the pediatric population for a variety of wounds including surgical (eg, traumatic, cardiothoracic, musculoskeletal, and closed incision lines), oncologic, pressure injuries, burns, and skin grafts.[44,58,60] In many cases, wound and

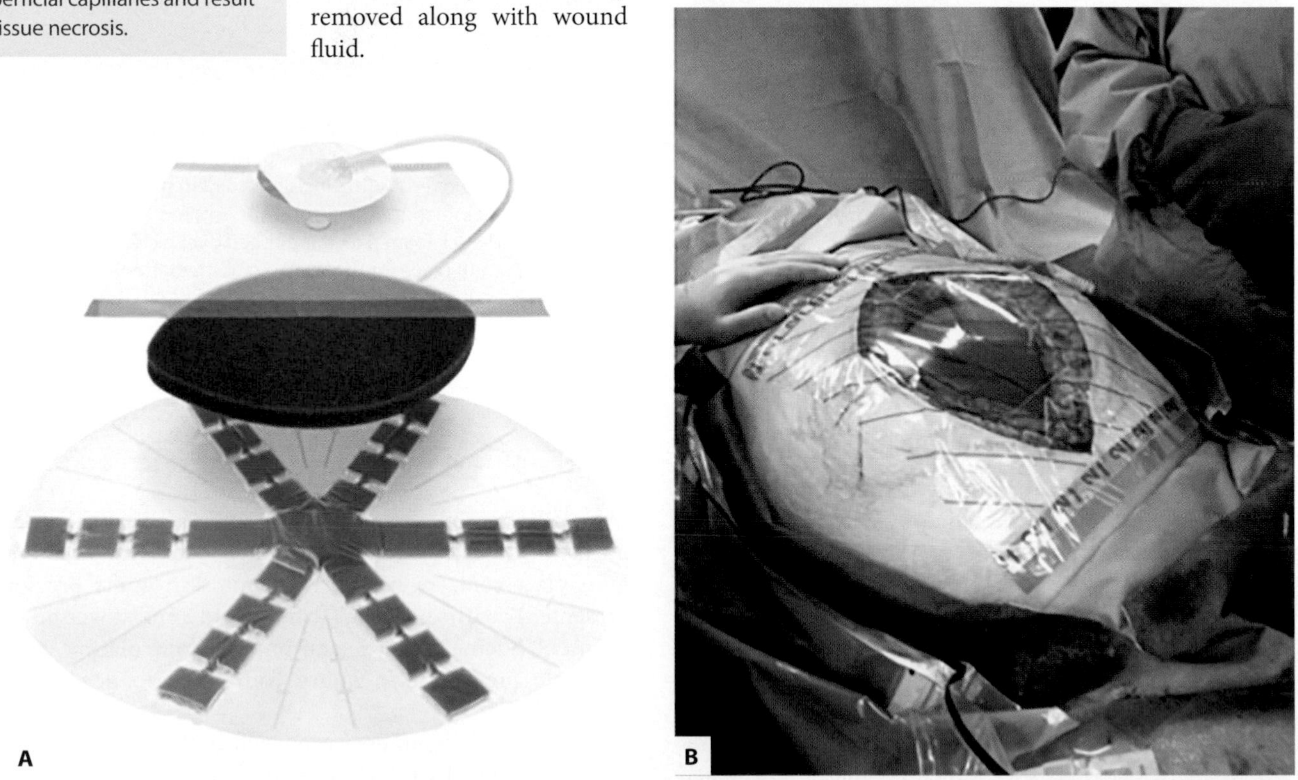

FIGURE 17-13 A. The ABTHERA Advance System is indicated for temporary bridging of abdominal wall openings where primary closure is not possible and/or repeated abdominal entries are necessary. The intended use of this system is for open abdominal wounds, with exposed viscera, including but not limited to abdominal compartment syndrome. Unique football shape with multiple slits allows passage of fluids from the paracolic gutters and the visceral protective layer prevents fistula formation when NPWT is applied directly over the abdominal contents. **B.** Temporary abdominal closure with the ABTHERA Advance dressing. (Courtesy of 3M-KCI Licensing, 2022.)

TABLE 17-6 NPWT Pressure Guidelines for Pediatric Patients[44,58–61]

	Negative Pressure Setting (mmHg)		
Wound Type/Condition	**Newborn/Infant (Birth–2 Years)**	**Child (>2–12 Years)**	**Adolescent (>12–21 Years)**
Sternal	−50 to −75 continuous	−50 to −75 continuous	−50 to −75 continuous
Omphalocele/gastroschisis	−50 to −75 continuous		
Enterocutaneous fistula	−50 to −75 continuous	−75 to −125 continuous	−75 continuous
Abdominal compartment syndrome	−50 to −75 continuous	−50 to −125 continuous	−75 to −125 continuous
Spinal	−50 to −75 continuous	−75 to −100 continuous	−75 to −125 continuous
Pilonidal disease	−50 to −75 continuous	−50 to −125 continuous	−75 to −125 continuous
Pressure ulcer	−50 to −75 continuous	−75 to −125 continuous	−75 to −125 continuous
Extremity wounds	−50 to −75 continuous	−75 to −100 continuous	−75 to −125 continuous
Fasciotomy wounds	−50 to −75 continuous	−75 to −100 continuous	−75 to −125 continuous
Burns	−50 to −75 continuous	−75 to −125 continuous	−75 to −125 continuous
Postgraft wounds	−50 to −75 continuous	−75 to −100 continuous	−75 to −125 Continuous

Reproduced with permission from Baharestani M, Amjad I, Bookout K, et al. V.A.C. Therapy in the management of paediatric wounds: clinical review and experience. *Int Wound J.* 2009;6 Suppl 1(Suppl 1):1-26.

graft stabilization provided by compressed NPWT dressings facilitates earlier mobilization and out-of-bed play for pediatric patients.[58] Evidence documenting NPWT use on the very young stresses the need for special consideration regarding patient size and weight as neonates, infants, and children are more susceptible to dehydration and are less tolerant of blood loss.[44,58,59,61] Therefore, the amount and type of evacuated fluid must be closely monitored. Storage of fluids in the NPWT device canister facilitates in/output monitoring and tailored rehydration interventions.[58] Immature immune systems, wound location, fragile skin, and impaired thermoregulation are additional factors that need to be considered.[44,58,60] Young patients may also experience fear or anxiety with NPWT and, on those too young to understand, the risk that they will try to remove or dislodge the dressing increases the chance of wound contamination or wound trauma.[59] Pain and psychological trauma may necessitate anesthesia or light sedation during NPWT dressing changes in some patients;[44,59] however, proper wound/periwound protection, use of silicone-based occlusive sheeting to prevent skin damage and minimize pain (see the "Application" section), and fewer dressing changes mean that NPWT may result in less pain and reduced use of pain medications compared to other types of dressings.[44,58,60] For pediatric patients, NPWT pressure settings range from −50 to −125 mmHg and are dependent on age, wound etiology, and location.[61] In 2009, Baharestani and expert colleagues[61] published detailed best practice guidelines for the use of NPWT in pediatric patients (**TABLES 17-6** to **17-8**). These guidelines are still supported by current literature.[44,58–60] Despite many published studies documenting the successful use of NPWT in pediatric patients, utilization of NPWT in this patient population is currently outside the U.S. Food and Drug Association's (FDA) indications. Medical directors from vendors of specific devices can provide more information on the use of a device in pediatric populations.

Palliative Care and Malignancy. NPWT can be effective in the palliative care of terminally ill patients with highly exudating and/or malignant wounds by reducing odor, controlling drainage, and decreasing the frequency of uncomfortable dressing changes (**FIGURE 17-14**).[62] The closed, secure NPWT system may also allow for easier patient mobilization by caregivers and/or more independent function. These benefits result in a better quality of life for the patient and make it more comfortable for family members to spend time with the patient. Generally, the use of NPWT in an area of malignancy is contraindicated[56] due to the resulting increase in local blood flow (see the "Precautions and Contraindications" section) but in the case of terminal illness, the benefits of NPWT in palliative care may outweigh the risk. As mentioned previously,

TABLE 17-7 NPWT Precautions for Pediatric Patients[44,58,59,61]

Precautions	
Spinal cord injury	Discontinue NPWT/ROCF to help minimize sensory stimulation
Bradycardia	Do not place dressing in proximity to the vagus nerve
Periwound tissue protection	Protect fragile/friable periwound skin with additional drape, thin hydrocolloid, petrolatum impregnated gauze, or other transparent film Repetitively applying and removing drapes may lead to stripping of periwound skin Do not allow foam to overlap onto intact skin
Temperature	Closely monitor and maintain temperature
Evacuated fluid	Closely monitor fluid intake and output to prevent dehydration

Reproduced with permission from Baharestani M, Amjad I, Bookout K, et al. V.A.C. Therapy in the management of paediatric wounds: clinical review and experience. *Int Wound J.* 2009;6 Suppl 1(Suppl 1):1-26.

TABLE 17-8 NPWT Guidelines for NPWT Foam Use for Pediatric Patients[58,59,61]

Wound Type/Condition	Black (Polyurethane) Foam	White (Polyvinylalcohol) Foam	Silver (Polyurethane) Foam
Sternal	X	X	X
Omphalocele/gastroschisis	X		
Enterocutaneous fistula	X	X	
Abdominal compartment syndrome	X		
Spinal	X	X	X
Pilonidal disease	X		X
Pressure ulcer	X		X
Extremity wounds	X		X
Fasciotomy wounds	X		X
Burns	X		X
Postgraft placement	X		X

Reproduced with permission from Baharestani M, Amjad I, Bookout K, et al. V.A.C. Therapy in the management of paediatric wounds: clinical review and experience. *Int Wound J.* 2009;6 Suppl 1(Suppl 1):1-26.

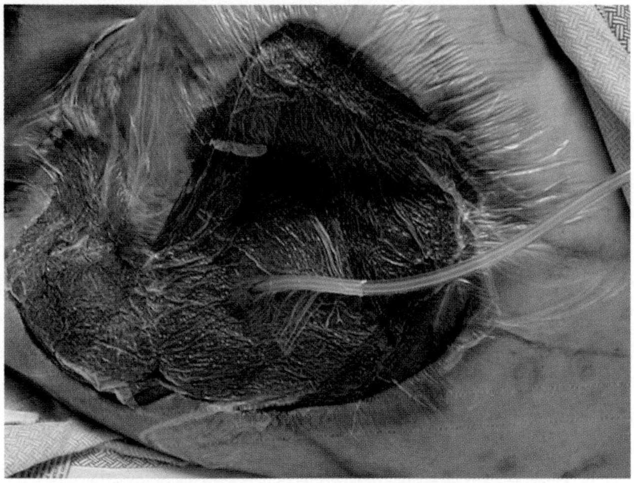

FIGURE 17-14 Palliative care. A patient receiving hospice care with an NPWT dressing on a large upper back wound where a malignant tumor was excised. The NPWT dressing is used to manage drainage with associated malodor, minimize pain, minimize dressing changes, and optimize the quality of life for both patient and family members during end-of-life care.

when NWPT is used outside of published indications, providers may wish to contact a vendor's medical or scientific affairs department for consultation.

PRECAUTIONS AND CONTRAINDICATIONS

Precautions and contraindications for NPWT are listed in **TABLE 17-9**. Wounds with low-level vascular compromise may benefit from NPWT and in this situation, research supports the use of intermittent mode therapy at lower pressure levels to reduce the risk of ischemia and ischemic pain.[22,33,35,42,64,69] In 2004, Banwell and Musgrave[4] reported that NPWT showed no benefit for wounds with significant ischemia. This was reported again in 2012 by McCallon[67] who stated that NPWT

TABLE 17-9 NPWT Precautions and Contraindications[51]

Precautions	Anticoagulants[13,63]
	Low platelet count
	Nonenteric and unexplored fistulas[44]
	Over named structures (bone, tendon, organs, vessels, etc.); requires placement of several layers of barrier dressing or use of white foam[44]
	Monitor for bleeding[13]
	Avoid circumferential occlusive sheeting application due to increased risk of ischemia[49]
	Monitor skin condition when dressing placed over bony prominences or prominent hardware due to compression[49]
	Debride sharp edges of exposed bone prior to application to protect soft tissues during compression[64]
	Irradiated vessels and tissues[13,63]
	Notify physician if drainage in collection canister is sanguineous, is filled with drainage in 1 hour, or if more than two canisters are filled within a 24-hour period
Contraindications	Untreated osteomyelitis[63,65]
	Gross infection with or without frank pus or sepsis[66]
	Malignancy in treatment area except in cases of palliative care[4,56,62]
	Lack of hemostasis[13,65]
	Blood dyscrasia such as with leukemia or hemophilia[66]
	Directly over exposed vessels, bypass grafts, organs, or other named structures[44,63,66]
	Ischemic wounds with significant proximal occlusion[1,59]
	Intermittent not used over grafting due to shear that increases risk for graft disruption[13,14,58]
	No suction devices/pumps in MRI, HBOT, or close to flammable anesthetics (see specific vendor specifications)[67]
	Any wound that shows a negative response to initial treatment
	NPWTi-d over skin grafts or dermal substitutes[68]

was ineffective on wounds with significant proximal arterial occlusion. NPWT has the potential to increase ischemia in wounds with vascular compromise leading to further tissue necrosis and ischemic pain, therefore initiation of treatment is deferred until blood flow is restored by revascularization surgery or endovascular procedures. If blood supply remains marginal, treatment is deferred until signs of granulation appear at the wound edges indicating there is sufficient oxygenation to support angiogenesis (**FIGURE 17-3**).

A study by Jung et al.[70] reinforced that caution is necessary with patients who have compromised vascularity, especially those with diabetes. $TcPO_2$ measurements were taken on the dorsal foot of patients with diabetes before, during, and after the application of −125 mmHg negative pressure with polyurethane foam. A significant decrease in surface $TcPO_2$ occurred during treatment (84%) and after discontinuation of therapy (40.3%). The rationale for this decrease was the presence of vasculopathy that affects both the macro- and microcirculation associated with diabetes. Their results suggest that minimal compression of the foam is recommended when applying NPWT to diabetic foot ulcers with compromised blood flow.

Precautionary measures are also critical when NPWT is placed over exposed named structures (eg, bone, tendon, muscle, organs), skin grafts, or surgical incision lines.[1,8,13,14,43,44,49,58,59] In most cases, NPWT may be placed over any body tissue provided an adequate protective covering is applied prior to the application of the wound filler. Several layers of nonadherent Vaseline/petrolatum- or paraffin-impregnated gauze,[44,49] ADAPTIC Non-Adhering Dressing (3M, St. Paul, Minnesota), nonadherent silicone or polyester film (Mepitel, Mölnlycke Health Care US, LLC, Peachtree Corners, Georgia),[44,69,71] or white dense foam are examples of protective dressings that may be used to protect vital structures (**FIGURE 17-15**). Nonadherent contact layers are also used between wound

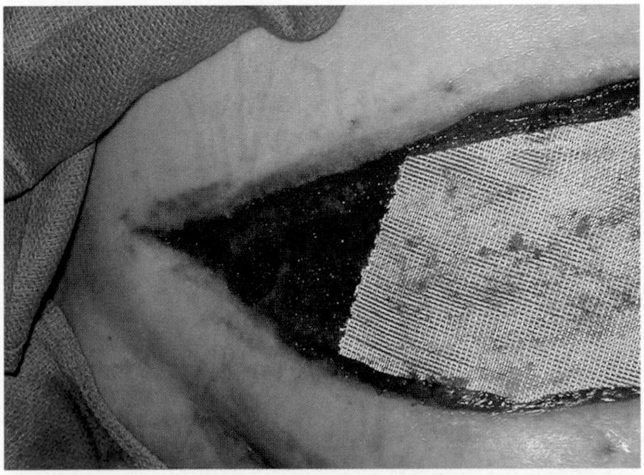

FIGURE 17-15 Protection of granulation tissue. Nonadherent mesh is placed over exposed muscle in a post-fasciotomy wound. On the left, a small piece of black foam is placed into a 1.5-cm sinus tract. Documentation includes all materials placed in the wound (interface materials, types of foam, and number of pieces) to ensure that all materials are removed at the next dressing change.

TABLE 17-10 Signs of Wound Deterioration[73]

▪ Increased periwound erythema
▪ Signs of periwound skin hypoxia
▪ Repeated need for sharp or surgical debridement
▪ Increased drainage or bleeding
▪ Newly observed infection or necrosis
▪ Increased pain
▪ Increased wound size
▪ Newly observed undermining or sinuses

fillers and skin grafts to protect the fragile new skin from being pulled into the filler via suction forces and to minimize graft disruption when removing NPWT dressings.[6,14,28,72]

Pain associated with wound filler removal is reduced by placing nonadherent dressings over freshly debrided tissue such as muscle or fascia. Strips of Xeroform (Coviden Xeroform Occlusive Petrolatum Gauze, Cardinal Health, Dublin, Ohio) or Vaseline-impregnated gauze placed over sensitive or inflamed wound edges will decrease pain associated with dressing changes and facilitate epithelial migration once granulation is level with surrounding skin (**FIGURES 17-10** and **17-11**). For all patients, wound tissues are assessed for signs of deterioration at each dressing change (**TABLE 17-10**).[69,73] Additionally, Kim et al.[68] recommend NPWT be discontinued after seven days if a wound fails to improve.

PARAMETERS AND TECHNIQUES FOR APPLICATION

Parameters

NPWT parameters are determined by the specific goals and needs of each patient. Although some devices have preset levels of pressure and vendor-specific wound fillers, providers have the flexibility to make adaptations for individualized therapy. Parameter considerations for NPWT include mode of delivery, wound fillers and interfaces, type of drain and/or connection port between the dressing and tubing, amount of subatmospheric pressure, frequency of dressing change, and initiation/discontinuation of the intervention.

Mode of Delivery NPWT devices offer the following modes of delivery: continuous, intermittent, variable, and instillation (**TABLE 17-11**).

With each mode, a wound filler and occlusive sheet dressing are applied along with tubing which connects the dressing to the NPWT device. When negative pressure is applied, the force collapses or compresses the filler into the wound bed (**FIGURES 17-16** and **17-17**). *Continuous mode* is the most commonly used delivery mode[74] in which the dressing is held at a constant, preset pressure (usually −125 mmHg)[5,11,44,61,69] until the next dressing change, which typically occurs every 48–72 hours.[61] This dressing change frequency is standard except when continuous NPWT is used over skin grafts and post-surgical incision lines in which the dressing is left in place and undisturbed for 5–7 days, or with some devices/dressings, up to 14 days.[1,7,13] Continuous mode is also typically chosen for

TABLE 17-11 Modes of Delivery[9,14,36,37,44,45,58,68,74]

Mode	Benefits	Disadvantages
Continuous	▪ Single compression cycle at each dressing change, thus decreasing risk of pain with multiple compressing/decompression cycles associated with intermittent therapy ▪ Continuous compression of dressing provides stability of wound (especially in sternal and abdominal wounds) and may allow for increased mobility for some patients ▪ Allows for continuous fluid collection in wounds that have heavy to copious drainage ▪ Decreases the risk of shear during the critical first days after placement of a split thickness skin graft	▪ Slower granulation tissue formation compared with intermittent therapy
Intermittent	▪ Cyclic compression of wound edge allows NPWT use for treating some wounds associated with decreased circulation ▪ Increases amount of mechanical stimulation and may facilitate faster granulation tissue formation compared to continuous therapy	▪ Airtight sheeting can loosen from skin with on/off cycles due to expansion/decompression of dressing ▪ Pooling of wound fluids resulting in leaks and periwound maceration ▪ Pooling during "off" time on wounds with copious exudates ▪ Potential for pain with cyclic compression/decompression of dressing ▪ Potential stress or irritation during cycles, may disrupt sleep
Variable	▪ Benefits of intermittent mode but maintenance of low pressure can prevent leakage and periwound maceration ▪ Maintenance of low pressure provides smooth pressure transition compared to hard on/off fluctuations with intermittent; can decrease pain associated with compression/decompression cycles	
Instillation	▪ Allows automatic periodic topical irrigation of wound tissues ▪ Solubilization, loosening, and removal of slough, infectious materials, and thick exudate ▪ Can prescribe the number and duration of instillations and dwell times ▪ May lead to increased granulation tissue formation due to frequent irrigation and removal of detrimental wound debris and fluids	

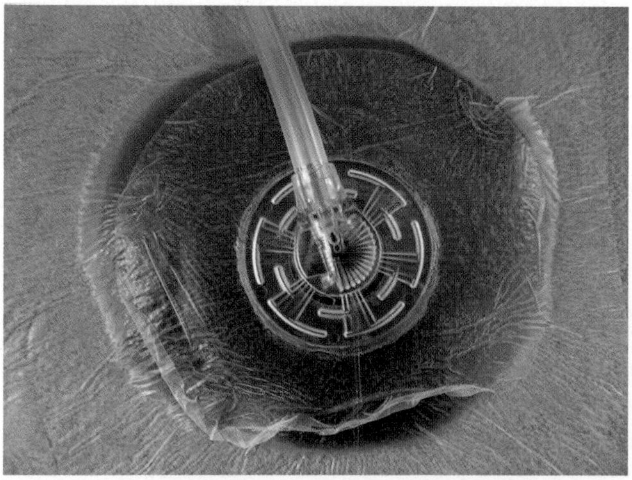

FIGURE 17-16 Puffy foam. Before application of the suction, the foam is puffy and after pressure application, it compresses. When applying the adhesive drape over the foam, care is taken to allow the foam to remain full and puffy. Pushing down on the foam with drape application will decrease the amount of wound contraction achieved with initial suction.

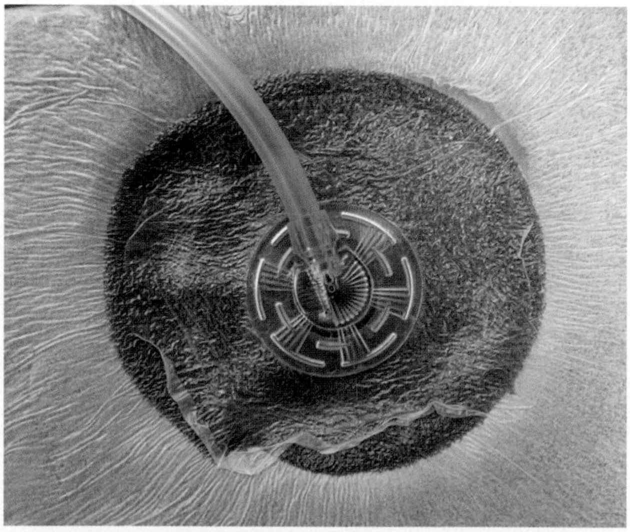

FIGURE 17-17 Compressed foam. After suction is applied, the foam is compressed firmly in place and noncompressible with external pressure.

CLINICAL CONSIDERATION

NPWT-induced wound edge hypoperfusion may have deleterious effects on wounds with compromised blood flow resulting in ischemic pain and tissue necrosis beneath the foam. These effects may be avoided by selecting the intermittent or variable modes of delivery and lower pressure levels so that both the time and force of tissue compression are reduced. This is of special concern in critically ill, hypotensive patients.

wounds with heavy drainage and/or high levels of tissue edema so wound fluids can be continuously removed. For wounds with large amounts of drainage or with difficulty maintaining a seal, changes may be required every 1–2 days.

With *intermittent mode*, negative pressure is delivered and released in cycles based on patient need (eg, 5 minutes "on" when the dressing is active followed by 2 minutes "off" during which time the dressing relaxes).[74,75] Research suggests that intermittent NPWT produces more changes in local blood flow and promotes faster granulation tissue formation compared to continuous mode.[74,76] However, patient discomfort and irritation from the constant active to relaxed cycles can be problematic, making continuous mode less painful and better tolerated by most patients.[74,76,77]

Variable mode is between continuous and intermittent in that it cycles from a maximum preset pressure of −125 mmHg to a low preset pressure typically set at −10 mmHg.[22] Since complete relaxation of the dressing is not achieved, a variable mode may help relieve some cyclic discomfort experienced with the intermittent mode.

Specially designed NPWT devices provide automatic instillation and removal of either irrigation or antiseptic topical solutions (eg, normal saline, hypochlorous acid, sodium hypochlorite, acetic acid, a combination of polyhexamethylene biguanide and betadine) through a second ingress tube.[9,37,68,78] Though other topical solutions are sometimes used, normal saline is the preferred irrigation fluid and is supported in published research as being as effective or better than other solutions in most situations.[68,78] However, for infected wounds when the patient is receiving appropriate debridement and antibiotics, the initial use of an antiseptic irrigation solution for the first 24–48 hours of treatment and then changing to normal saline has been shown to be effective.[68] Irrigation with antibiotic solutions is not recommended due to the risk of contact allergic reaction and the potential for antibiotic resistance.[68] With *instillation mode, referred to as NPWT instillation and dwell (NPWTi-d),* wound tissues are rinsed and soaked with irrigation fluid for prescribed periods of time (referred to as dwell time) before fluids are evacuated and negative pressure is resumed—all achieved without requiring dressing removal. Irrigation-dwell-evacuation cycles are programmed into the device to occur at regular intervals, temporarily interrupting negative pressure. NPWTi-d facilitates the solubilization and removal of slough, wound debris, bacteria, and thick exudate, thus allowing NPWT to be initiated when the wound has more than 30% nonviable tissue.[36,37,68,78] An international consensus guideline published in 2020 by Kim et al.[68] recommended NPWTi-d as an adjunctive treatment indicated for a variety of acute and chronic wounds, traumatic wounds, post-excision full-thickness burns, and wounds with exposed bone (**TABLE 17-12**). NPWTi-d is typically reserved for complex and/or infected wounds and/or wounds in patients with coexisting co-morbidities[78] that increase the risk of poor healing (see the "Precautions and Contraindications" section). Multiple studies have documented that when indicated, NPWTi-d results in fewer overall dressing changes, improved wound cleansing, fewer surgical debridements, shorter hospital stays, and earlier wound closure compared to standard NPWT.[3,9,36,37,45,68,78] One example of a NPWTi-d device is the 3M V.A.C. VERAFLO Therapy System with Smart Instill (3M, San Antonio, Texas)[79] which provides an automated system of periodic gravity-assisted instillation and suction removal of topical solutions (**FIGURE 17-18A, B**). A specially designed reticulated open-cell

CASE STUDY

CONTINUED

Pertinent medical information includes a 10-year history of type 2 diabetes controlled with oral medications; a human bite wound obtained during a physical altercation; wound cultures obtained during surgery were positive for oxacillin-sensitive *Staphylococcus aureus* and the patient is on IV antibiotics. Lab values include the following: hemoglobin—12 g/dL, hematocrit—35; platelets—200,000/mm², white blood cells—15,000/mm³; serum albumin—4 g/dL; fasting blood glucose—240 mg/dL; HbA1c—7.3; creatinine—0.7 mg/dL; and blood urea nitrogen—19 mg/dL. Vital signs are normal with no fever for the past 12 hours.

DISCUSSION QUESTIONS

1. Is this patient appropriate for NPWT?
2. Why or why not?

TABLE 17-12 Indications for NPWTi-d[36,37,45,68]

Traumatic wounds
Surgical and dehisced wounds
Diabetic wounds
Venous leg ulcers
Pressure injuries
Wounds with exposed bone
Wounds with underlying osteomyelitis (treated)
Infected/contaminated wounds with orthopedic fixation
Post-excision full-thickness burns
Wounds due to evacuation of a hematoma once hemostasis has been achieved
Wounds that are a bridge between staged or delayed amputation

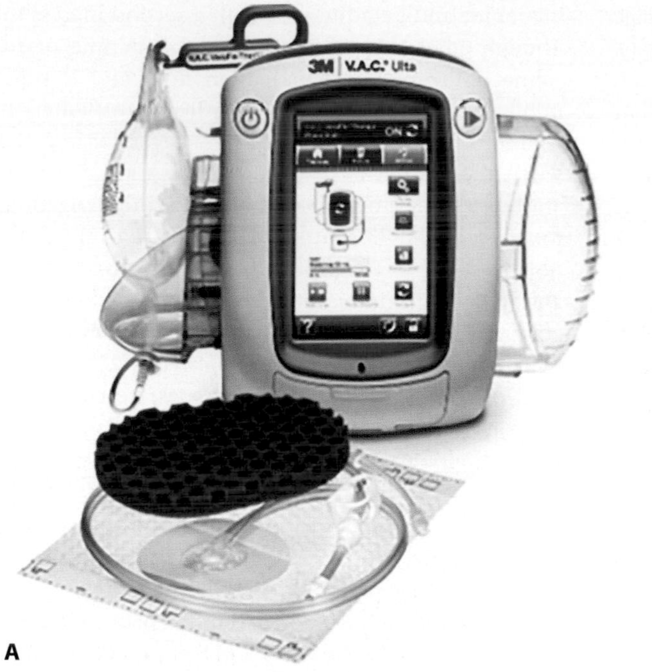

A

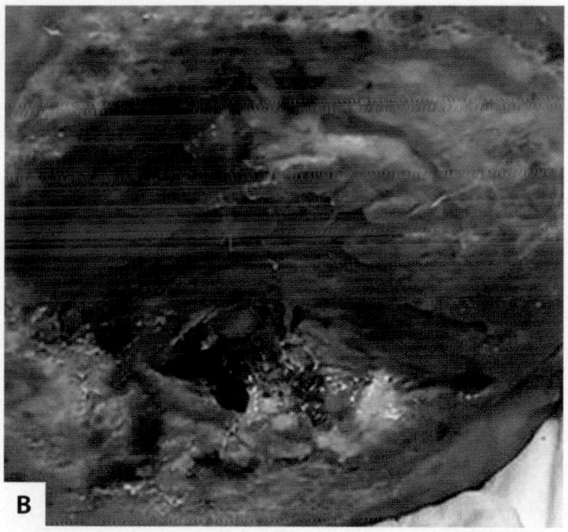

B

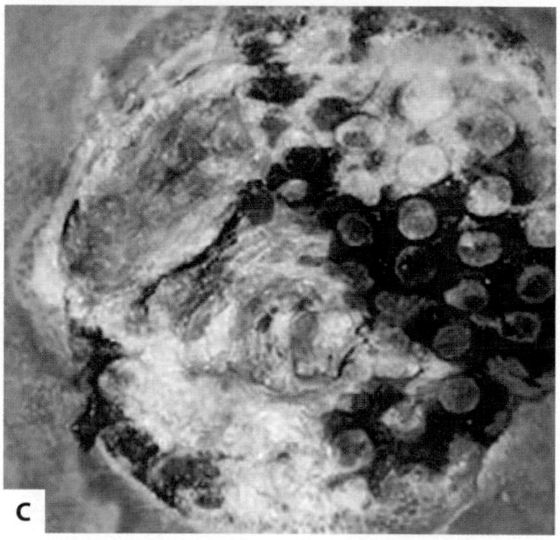

C

FIGURE 17-18 **A.** V.A.C. Instillation Therapy System and reticulated open-cell foam with through holes allows for the infusion of saline or topical antiseptics alternating with continuous suction for treatment of infected wounds or those with higher amounts of necrotic or nonviable tissue. (V.A.C. VERAFLO Cleanse Choice Complete dressing courtesy of 3M-KCI Licensing, Inc., 2018.) **B.** Sacral pressure injury prior to NPWT and **C**, wound treated with NPWT-id for three days. Initial placement on the left with a high amount of nonviable tissue and at dressing change day three with improved granulation tissue, enhanced vascularity, and through holes can be visualized on the tissue. (Courtesy of 3M-KCI Licensing, Inc., 2018.)

blue foam with a "through holes"[78] dressing (V.A.C. VERAFLO Cleanse Choice Complete Dressing, 3M, San Antonio, Texas)[79] enhances even distribution of instilled fluids across the wound bed and increases fluid clearance.[78]

Wound Filler Wound fillers are designed to evenly transfer negative pressure across the wound bed. Available devices utilize different types and colors of wound fillers depending on the kind of NPWT being delivered. Options for wound fillers include the following:

- Standard open-cell reticulated compressible foam (black, blue, or green) with or without silver
- Reticulated open-cell foam with through holes for NPWTi-d as previously described
- Noncompressible saline-soaked white foam
- Saline-moistened antimicrobial gauze Kerlix and Curity AMD gauze (Cardinal Health, Dublin, Ohio)[80]

Standard open-cell reticulated foams are shown in **FIGURE 17-19A, B**. NPWT devices utilized over intact incision lines or superficial wounds do not require a wound filler and instead use specially designed self-adherent peel-and-stick dressings. The Avance Solo NPWT system (Mölnlycke Health Care US, LLC, Peachtree Corners, Georgia) also includes film fixation strips to place along dressing edges for extra support in maintaining an undisturbed seal to protect against leakage (**FIGURE 17-20**). While research supports that gauze dressings can deliver some of the primary benefits of NPWT[41,69,72,81–83] and in some cases, may be used in conjunction with foam dressings, most units utilize some type of foam dressing. **TABLE 17-13** provides advantages and disadvantages of standard black and white foam and gauze wound fillers.

NPWT with black foam has been shown to promote granulation tissue formation faster than less active forms of wound dressings,[3,4,22,36,44] so much so that ingrowth of granulation tissue into the open-cell foam within 48 hours may occur. Black foam is hydrophobic (moisture repelling) which enhances exudate removal. A green polyurethane open-cell compressible foam (similar to black foam) is used with some devices, the lighter color allowing for easy visualization of any active bleeding (**FIGURE 17-19B**).[84,87] White foam, or polyvinylalcohol (PVA) foam, is softer and more dense compared to black foam and offers less aggressive therapy,

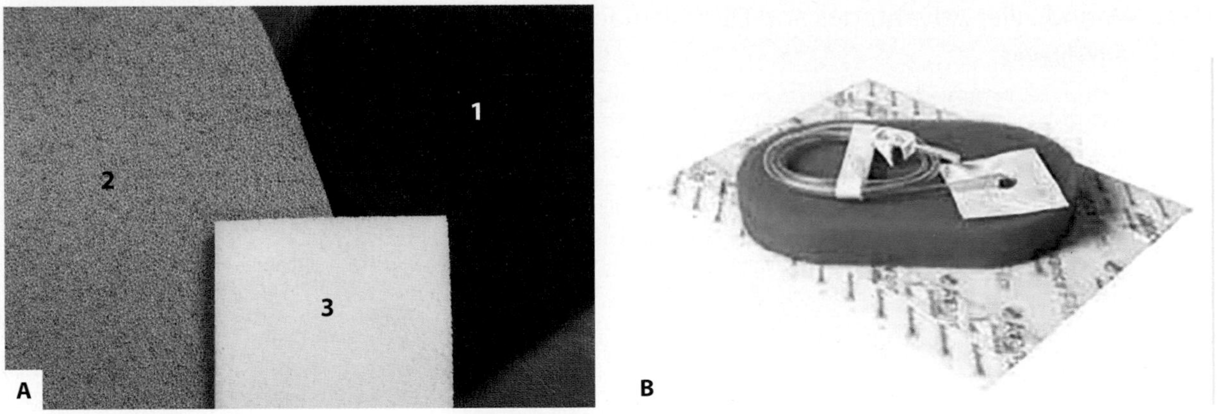

FIGURE 17-19 A. Standard foams. Commonly used for NPWT include (1) black reticulated open-cell polyurethane foam, (2) the same foam with impregnated silver ions, and (3) white polyvinylalcohol (PVA) foam. **B. Green foam.** Some systems use reticulated foam in green so that exudates and bleeding can be better visualized. The black foam is available in a variety of sizes, shapes, and thicknesses to accommodate different wound characteristics. (From Molnlycke Health Care US, LLC, Norcross, GA.)

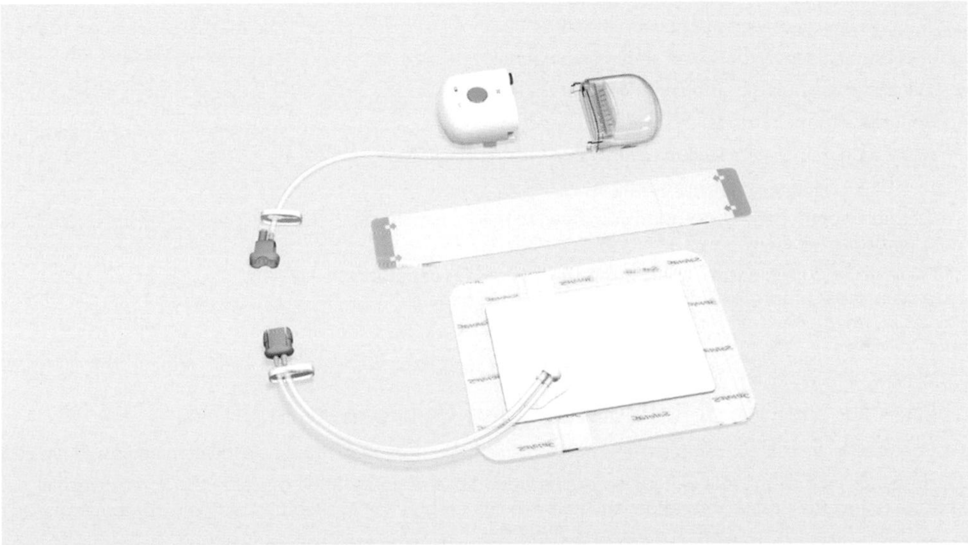

FIGURE 17-20 Avance Solo NPWT device. Single-use device indicated for closed incisions or chronic wounds, includes a canister and a dressing with handles for ease of fixation. (From Molnlycke Health Care US, LLC, Norcross, GA.)

less adherence, and less ingrowth of granulation tissue.[72,88] White foam is hydrophilic (moisture retentive), which makes it less likely to adhere to fragile wound tissues or structures such as bone, tendon, or ligaments. It also has a higher tensile strength compared to black foam, making it a safer and easier filler to remove from tight wound spaces such as tunnels, sinus tracts, and undermining (**FIGURE 17-19A**). The blue 3M reticulated open-cell foam-Cleanse Choice or ROCF-CC Complete foam (ROCF-CC Complete, 3M, San Antonio, Texas, **FIGURE 17-18A, B**), was developed for use with installation therapy. This two-sided, hydrophobic, specialty foam dressing has a flat side (that can be used to assist with leveling a wound bed) and a side with 1 cm through holes that allows for easier removal of thick exudate, infectious materials, and necrotic debris (**TABLE 17-14**).[68,90]

Two primary differences between open-cell reticulated foam and gauze wound fillers are (1) the type of granulation tissue formed and (2) the speed at which granulation tissue is synthesized. Black foam tends to produce thicker, less dense, less organized granulation tissue compared to gauze.[85,86] Granulation tissue is produced more quickly with foam fillers, thus facilitating faster skin graft application,[6] quicker resolution of wounds awaiting delayed primary closure, and faster overall closure of wounds healing by secondary intention.[3] There is some evidence indicating that while foam fillers promote faster overall wound closure, they may also result in increased scar tissue due to the thicker, unorganized granulation tissue produced.[84] With this consideration, the use of a gauze wound filler over facial wounds and in joints in preparation for grafting may be beneficial due to less scarring,

TABLE 17-13 Wound Filler Advantages and Disadvantages

	Advantages	Disadvantages
Black foam	▪ Open-cell reticulated foam shown to encourage granulation tissue formation faster than gauze due to increased tissue deformation[6,69] ▪ Superior compressibility assists in drawing wound edges together for quicker reductions in open wound size[5] ▪ Smaller foam dressings provide the highest levels of contraction[33,83–85] ▪ Due to faster wound closure, may be best for wounds when contraction/scarring is not a high concern[36] ▪ Can be used for deep or shallow wounds	▪ Granulation tissue can grow into open cells of foam, making removal painful and disruptive ▪ Requires more force for removal compared to gauze, resulting in pain and wound bed disruption[75,86] ▪ Disruption may be reduced by soaking foam with normal saline prior to removal ▪ Small pieces can break off in the wound due to decreased integrity of black foam and all pieces must be removed. Not recommended for tunnels, tracts, and undermining ▪ Cutting foam to fit exactly into open wound space can be time consuming
White foam	▪ Does not adhere in tunnels, tracts, or undermining because of the dense compact structure ▪ Can be used when less aggressive therapy is desired ▪ Less painful upon removal compared to black foam due to reduced likelihood that granulation tissue will grow into foam ▪ May have similar benefits as gauze due to less aggressive function[72] ▪ Protects viable structures (eg, bone, muscle, tendon)	▪ Slower granulation tissue formation compared to black foam ▪ Pressure under white foam will be less than at the sensor site ▪ Does not compress, therefore limits wound contraction
Antimicrobial gauze	▪ Contains polyhexamethylene biguanide (PHMB)[80] ▪ Produces thinner, denser, but more stable granulation[83–86] ▪ Typically easier to apply and mold into contours of a wound ▪ Appropriate for tunnels, tracts, and undermining ▪ Active bleeding more easily seen on white gauze versus black foam ▪ Can be used for deep or shallow wounds[72] ▪ Produces less wound edge hypofusion compared to black foam due to less compressive force[83] ▪ May be more comfortable with intermittent/variable modes of delivery due to decreased compressibility of dressing compared to foam[75]	▪ Potential for gauze fibers to shed into wound bed, especially if gauze has been cut to fit ▪ Produces less contraction and microstrain force on wound compared to black foam (could be beneficial depending on specific treatment goals)[33,83–85]

TABLE 17-14 Guidelines for the Use of Reticulated Open-Cell Foam with NPTWi-d,[36,78,79,89]

The ROCF-CC dressing is intended to be used in combination with negative pressure wound therapy instillation and dwell time (NPWTi-d).
Goals for using ROCF-CC dressings include the following: Cleanse the wound bed of slough and nonviable tissue, remove thick exudate, remove infectious materials, promote granulation tissue formation, and help provide progression to a defined endpoint for a clinical plan of care.
The ROCF-CC is appropriate for any wound that is indicated for NPWTi-d; however, it is not indicated as the sole treatment for infection.
Appropriate patients for the use of ROCF-CC include those who are not candidates for or refuse surgical debridement, those who have had surgical debridement but still have nonviable tissue in the wound bed, and those for whom surgical debridement is appropriate but not available.
Wounds for which ROCF-CC is appropriate are those with the majority (approximately 60%) of the wound bed nonviable, is large enough to accommodate at least 2 through holes.
Caution is advised for the following cases: patient has an increased risk of bleeding, signs of systemic infection or advancing infection at the wound site, exposed structures, and explored tunnels or undermining.
Wounds for which ROCF-CC is not recommended include those with 100% intact, dry eschar; unprotected vessels or organs; undrained abscess; smaller than 1.0 cm × 1.0 cm. in size; split-thickness skin grafts or dermal grafts; or acute ischemic wounds.[37,45,68]
Recommended settings are 10 minute dwell time and 2–2.5 hours of negative pressure at −125.[37,45,68]
ROCF-CC dressings may be used with or without the instillation option[79,90]

decreased fibrosis, and improved cosmesis.[84–86] Additionally, Mansoor et al.[19] reported greater ease in application using gauze filler as opposed to foams as gauze can quickly be molded inside irregularly shaped wounds.

Type of Drain: Tubing and Connection Port The type of tubing and the connection port between the NPWT device and the dressing is almost exclusively determined by the brand of NPWT device being used; their components are not generally interchangeable. With advances in NPWT technology, some connector ports and tubing are not just simple connectors between dressings and suction units but are multi-lumen communication devices designed to constantly monitor subatmospheric pressure and provide feedback to the unit for maintenance of desired pressure (eg, SensaT.R.A.C Pad, 3M, San Antonio, Texas; Invia NPWT System, Medela, LLC, Healthcare, McHenry, Illinois; Avance Solo, Molnlycke Health Care US, LLC, Peachtree Corners, Georgia).[87,91–93] Some drains or connectors help prevent and clear blockages and trigger alarms when clearance is unsuccessful[92] (**FIGURE 17-17**). Peel-and-stick, top mounted connecting ports typical of most foam-based dressing applications are easy to apply (**FIGURE 17-16**) and attached tubing simply snaps into tubing connected to the canister. NPWT applications with gauze as the wound filler typically use a flat, perforated drain similar to a Jackson Pratt hemovac drain in which the open-pore end of the drain is inserted into the gauze. Often referred to as the Chariker–Jeter or mesentery method, this technique is especially important when the gauze is utilized as the long, flexible drain can more efficiently draw fluid from different areas within the dressing.[19,69,82] Some researchers indicate this method of drain placement may be more appropriate for high-output wounds as fluids can be drawn from multiple areas at once (**FIGURE 17-5**).[19,69,82] With this method, it is important to fully surround the drain with the gauze filler to prevent direct suction contact between the drain and wound tissues.

Amount of Pressure Although pressure settings are highly dependent on patient comfort and desired outcomes, evidence supports that optimal granulation tissue formation is achieved with −125 mmHg[68] and that higher levels may decrease wound blood flow due to increased tissue compression. However, there are situations when exceeding −125 mmHg of pressure may be necessary, such as when multiple wound sites on the same patient are being treated with a single NPWT device or when there is excessive wound depth and/or undermining. Patients with abdominal wounds tend to experience discomfort with −125 mmHg which can be relieved by decreasing the pressure to −75 mmHg. If a patient is apprehensive about the NPWT, initiating treatment at a lower level of pressure may help alleviate those concerns. **TABLES 17-6** and **17-15** give evidence-supported NPWT pressure suggestions for pediatric and adult patients. Once an initial pressure has been selected, titration according to patient comfort, wound response, and treatment goals may be necessary. Reviewing device-specific manufacturer recommendations is also advised prior to application.

Frequency of Dressing Change NPWT dressings are typically changed every 48–72 hours. If there is a concern of granulation tissue ingrowth into the foam, a protective contact dressing as previously discussed can be used between the foam and granulation tissue. If the wound is infected, silver-impregnated foam, an antimicrobial dressing (eg, silver) placed under the foam, or NPWT with instillation may be advised. An initial 24-hour dressing change may be helpful in difficult or atypical wounds in order to monitor tissue response. Unless significant symptoms of tissue deterioration are present, NPWT used over skin grafts should not be changed for the first 3–5 days to ensure adequate graft stabilization.[13,14,28] Additionally, ciNPT dressings used for closed surgical incisions are typically left in place for 7 days and sometimes up to 14 days to allow for re-epithelialization and protection of the incision line before the dressing is removed.[3,17]

CLINICAL CONSIDERATION

When NPWT is applied to a fresh surgical wound at the time of surgery, the first dressing change is best performed 24 hours or less after surgery. The advantages of this protocol include less ingrowth of tissue into the foam, the ability to assess for possible bleeding, less adherence between the tissue and the foam and therefore less pain with the dressing change, and the opportunity to fill the wound with less foam due to the wound contraction that occurs with initial NPWT.

Initiation and Discontinuation In acute wounds, early placement of NPWT can decrease the risk of infection and maintain a moist wound-healing environment. NPWT is initiated immediately after the placement of a skin graft or primary surgical wound closure, which usually occurs in the operating room. **TABLE 17-16** lists recommendations for discontinuing NPWT.

TABLE 17-15 Pressure Recommendations for NPWT

Continuous mode	−75 to −125 mmHg over skin grafts for the first 3 to 5 days[14]
	−80 to −125 mmHg for most acute wounds and pressure injuries[37,45,68,69,86]
	80 mmHg for maximal effects on blood flow[22,34,35,42,69]
	−50 to −75 mmHg if pain is an issue
	−50 to −125 mmHg for chronic wounds[37,45,68]
	−40 to −50 mmHg for wounds with decreased circulation[83–85]
	−125 mmHg for abdominal wounds due to presence of pressure receptors in the abdomen[51]
Intermittent	−125 mmHg, 5 minutes on/2 minutes off[69]
	−40 to −75 mmHg for mild arterial wounds[83–85]
Variable	−10 to −125 mmHg depending on wound type and patient comfort[42]

TABLE 17-16 Recommendations for Discontinuation of NPWT

Goals of therapy have been met.
Wound depth less than or equal to 1 mm.
Good granular wound bed has been achieved and is even with skin surface.
No appreciable benefit is evident after 2 to 7 days of use.
Signs of wound deterioration occur.
Development of new infection after NPWT has been initiated.
Patient has discomfort/intolerance.
Other dressings more appropriate for current phase of healing.
Progression to little or no drainage has been achieved.
Sanguineous drainage (indicating hemostasis has not been achieved), fills canister in 1 hour or more than 2 canisters in 24 hours.

APPLICATION

While individual NPWT vendor application instructions should be reviewed and followed, there are some basic application steps common for acute and chronic wounds (TABLE 17-17). Some reusable or disposable devices specifically designed for uncomplicated, low exudating wounds eliminate some steps with peel-and-stick dressings. Periwound and surrounding skin covered by occlusive sheeting should be protected with a topical skin prep (eg, Mepiseal, Mölnlycke Health Care US, LLC, Peachtree Corners, Georgia; Skin-Prep, Smith & Nephew, Memphis, Tennessee), tincture of benzoin, hydrocolloid strips, Xeroform (FIGURE 17-10), petrolatum impregnated gauze, thin foam, or other protective dressing depending on skin condition with special consideration given to the patient's age (eg, pediatric, geriatric), other pathologies, and comorbidities (FIGURE 17-21).[44,49,58,67] This important step protects the skin from moisture and maceration and facilitates easier removal of the adhesive sheeting, decreasing skin stripping and pain at the next dressing change. As previously mentioned, white foam or several layers of nonadherent interface dressing (eg, ADAPTIC Non-Adhering Dressing, Mepitel) must be placed over named structures or fragile tissues (eg, blood vessels, nerves, muscle, organs) for protection (FIGURES 17-10 and 17-15).[44] If the wound has tunnels, sinus tracts, or undermining, these areas are wicked with either white foam or gauze wound filler.[65] Black foam or other ROCF are not advised for filling sinus tracts due to friction and granulation ingrowth can cause the foam to tear upon removal, leaving shreds of foam in the deep wound that may become infected, cause granuloma formation, or require surgical removal (denser white foam should be used instead). Wound filler is then placed inside the wound margins ensuring good contact with all wound surfaces as well as the ends of any filler placed in tunnels, sinus tracts, and undermining. Wound fillers are not tightly packed into wounds as this will occlude surface capillaries and limit the amount of wound contraction that occurs when suction is applied. The foam should extend above skin level to allow for good wound and sidewall coverage once negative pressure is applied and the filler compresses.

TABLE 17-17 Basic NPWT Application Steps

Prepare wound bed.
Prepare periwound skin with a topical moisture barrier or with strips of nonadherent gauze at the edges.
Apply a nonadherent protective layering over named or fragile structures (eg, bone, tendon, vessels, nerves, fragile granulation).
Apply wound filler (and perforated drain if using gauze).
Apply occlusive sheeting 3–5 cm past wound edge.
Apply top-mounted drain and tubing.
Connect tubing to NPWT suction device/canister.
Set parameters to desired settings.
Prepare patient for the noise and feeling that may be experienced with onset of pressure.
Turn on device and ensure airtight seal.
Educate patient and caregiver(s) on alarms and appropriate actions to take for each alarm.
Document the type and number of pieces of foam with each application to ensure all foam is removed at the next dressing change.

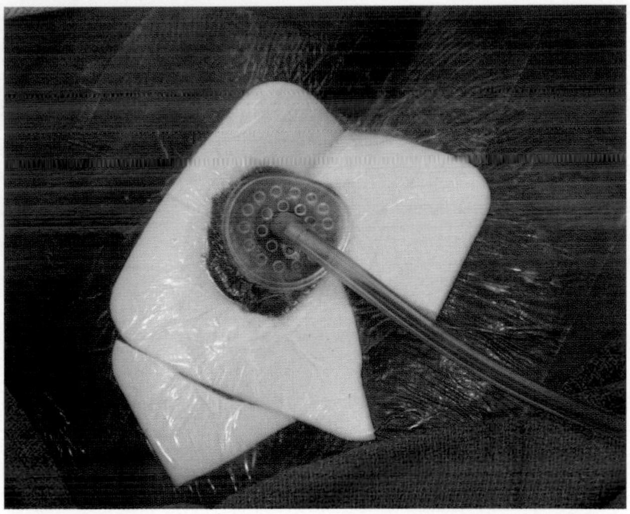

FIGURE 17-21 Use of thin foam under adhesive sheeting to protect periwound skin. If the wound has heavy exudate, the foam may absorb the fluid and hold it against the skin, causing maceration. In this case, the use of a topical moisture barrier may work better than a dressing. Trial and error, in addition to careful clinical decision-making, becomes part of the art of successful NPWT intervention.

Wound fillers should not overlap onto intact skin as they will cause maceration and skin deterioration.[44,58] Gauze molds easily into wound contours and foam fillers can be cut and shaped for appropriate filling. Foam dressings need to be cut away from the wound, and freshly cut edges gently rubbed to remove any loose particles, both to keep residue from falling into the wound bed. As long as pieces of foam or gauze are in contact with each other, negative pressure will be communicated between the pieces and into the wound base (FIGURE 17-22).[70] The number and type of foam and/or gauze pieces placed in the wound are documented at each application to ensure full removal at each subsequent dressing change.

When using gauze wound filler, the perforated drain is laid in the wound bed encircled by the gauze filler,[19] and the occlusive sheeting is placed over the wound accommodating for the drain. Top-mounted drains that require separate attachments are placed over a hole cut into the sheeting so the suction force can be transmitted to the wound filler.[49] The hole needs to be of sufficient size to accommodate the opening of the drain/connector port and to prevent occlusion when suction is applied. Drain tubing is then connected to the NPWT device and/or collection canister. In some disposable units used over surgical incisions and low exudating wounds, the wound peel-and-stick dressing may also serve as the collection canister and tubing is often pre-attached to the dressing.

Application of NPWT over a skin graft entails covering the graft with a nonadherent protective layer(s) (see previous examples of appropriate layers), placement of wound filler over the protective layer(s), appropriate skin preparation, coverage with occlusive sheeting, and drain placement. NPWT can

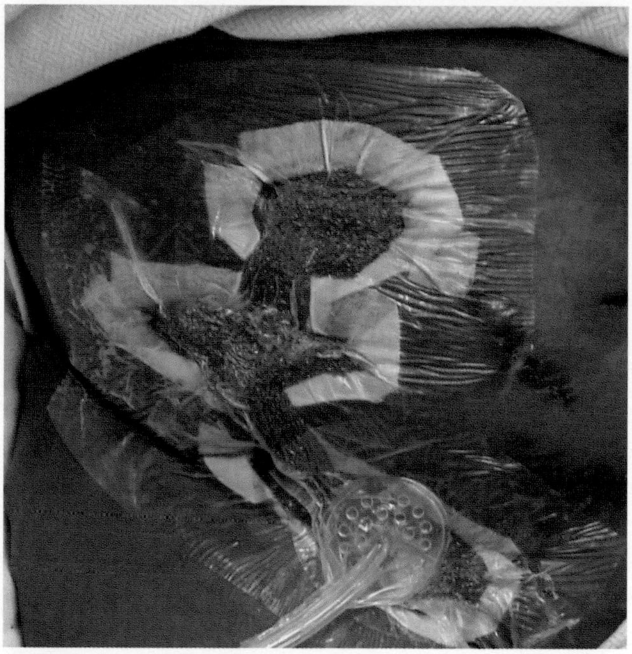

FIGURE 17-22 Use of multiple pieces of foam. Multiple wounds are connected with foam bridges, using numerous pieces of foam that connect to ensure that suction is applied to the entire wound base. A layer of adhesive sheeting or transparent film is placed between the skin and foam bridges to prevent skin maceration as fluid travels through the foam bridges.

also be used around external fixators with the greatest challenge being seal maintenance with occlusive sheeting wrapped around the fixator's posts.[36]

Some NPWT devices have sufficient suction to manage multiple wounds on the same patient; this is accomplished by using "Y" connecters to attach tubing from each wound to the NPWT device/collection canister (**FIGURE 17-23**). The technique of "bridging" is utilized for linking more than one wound together with a single device (**FIGURE 17-9**) and is accomplished by (1) placing occlusive sheeting over intact skin in areas between the wounds, (2) placing filler over the sheeting to bridge the gap between wounds, (3) ensuring bridge filler is in contact with filler in all wounds, and (4) placing occlusive sheeting over all the fillers to maintain a seal. As long as wound fillers are in contact with each other via the bridge, negative pressure will be transmitted throughout the dressing to all wounds. The bridging technique is also valuable when wound location, such as over a bony prominence or on a weight-bearing surface, necessitates offsetting top-mounted drain tube connections (**FIGURE 17-24**). Pre-made bridge or offset dressings offered by some vendors make this process convenient and efficient.

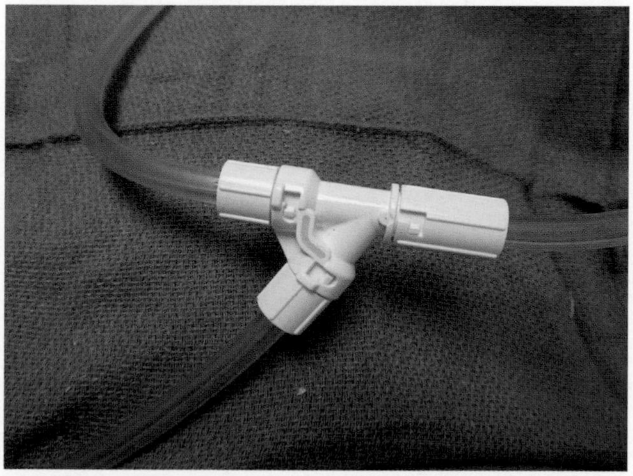

FIGURE 17-23 Y Connector to allow a single NPWT device to be used for more than one wound. A Y-connector allows collection tubes from two wounds to be connected to the single piece of tubing that goes to the collection canister.

CLINICAL CONSIDERATION

Note dermatitis of the periwound skin in **FIGURE 17-24**. Dermatitis can occur when wounds are draining, the patient has a reaction to the adhesive sheeting, or when NPWT is required for extended periods of time. Minimizing the amount of sheeting used, frequently changing the sheeting position when possible to allow the skin to "rest", ensuring a good seal, and using moisture barriers and/or protective layers are some strategies to help prevent, improve, or resolve dermatitis. In severe cases, topical powders, antifungal/yeast ointments, or anti-inflammatory ointments may be indicated. Dermatitis may be minimized or even prevented by using silicone-based occlusive sheeting (discussed below) instead of traditional, adhesive-based sheeting. If these strategies are not effective, the patient may need an NPWT "holiday."

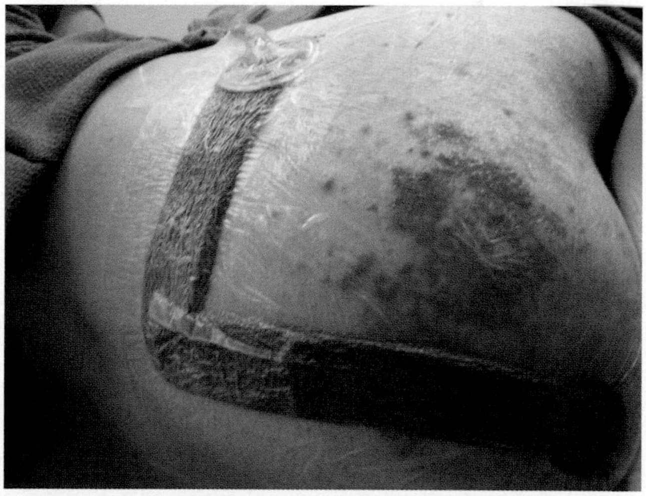

FIGURE 17-24 NPWT applied to a wound on the ischial tuberosity; a bridge of foam is carried to the lateral hip to prevent pressure from the connector and tubing being placed on the weight-bearing surface. Note the dermatitis of the periwound skin, a common complication, for example when wounds are draining, the patient has a reaction to the adhesive, or NPWT is required for extended periods of time. Minimizing the amount of drape that is used, ensuring a good seal, and using moisture barriers are some strategies to prevent dermatitis. In severe cases, topical powders, antifungal/yeast ointments, or anti-inflammatory ointments may be indicated.

When NPWT is used as an adjunct therapy for infected wounds, the addition of silver may be desirable for its antimicrobial properties.[72] Some nonadherent silver-impregnated dressings (eg, Acticoat Flex, Smith & Nephew, Memphis, Tennessee; Silverlon, Cura Surgical, Argentum Medical Co, Geneva, Illinois) can be placed under wound fillers in direct contact with the wound bed or suture line.[49,69] When nonadherent contact layers are inserted between wound fillers and the wound bed, slower rates of granulation tissue formation may occur due to reduced suction and tissue deformation.[69] The risk of fluid accumulation under contact layers in high-output wounds can be reduced by cutting slits in the interface; some fenestrated contact layers are available in various sizes and may be cut to fit (eg, Mepitel One, Mölnlycke Health Care US, LLC, Peachtree Corners, Georgia). NPWTi-d with topical antiseptic or normal saline solutions may be a better option for infected wounds without the addition of extra antimicrobial layers.[3,9,15,68,78]

Removal of the occlusive sheeting at dressing change can be painful and may result in skin stripping if intact skin is not adequately prepared with a protective skin barrier at the time of application. If periwound protective dressings are used, care should be taken to limit their contact with the foam as drainage may be pulled through the foam and into the dressings resulting in skin maceration. As mentioned earlier, skin protectants may be useful under protective dressings. The same technique used for the removal of semipermeable film is used when removing the occlusive sheeting: pull occlusive sheeting parallel to the skin and use adhesive remover pads to help decrease discomfort and skin irritation. Recent advances in occlusive sheeting have led to silicone-based products that allow for easy repositioning and prevent skin stripping and pain with removal (Avance Film with Safetac technology, Mölnlycke Health Care US, LLC, Peachtree Corners, Georgia; 3M Dermatac Drape, 3M, San Antonio, Texas)[94] (**FIGURE 17-25**). These easy-on-the-skin occlusive sheets provide excellent seal and leak prevention, even when used with NPWTi-d devices. The silicone-based sheets also decrease waste as they can be easily separated if they stick together during application. **TABLE 17-18** includes general tips regarding NPWT application and **TABLE 17-19** lists strategies for reducing pain with dressing removal.

Patient education regarding the use, application, and maintenance of NPWT is important, especially if there are alarms built into the system. **TABLE 17-20** lists recommended topics to cover with patients to maximize the benefits of NPWT and minimize its impact on patient quality of life. Some vendors offer online and video-based patient education as well as smartphone applications which allow patients and/or caregivers to communicate with trained healthcare professionals for trouble shooting and answering general questions.

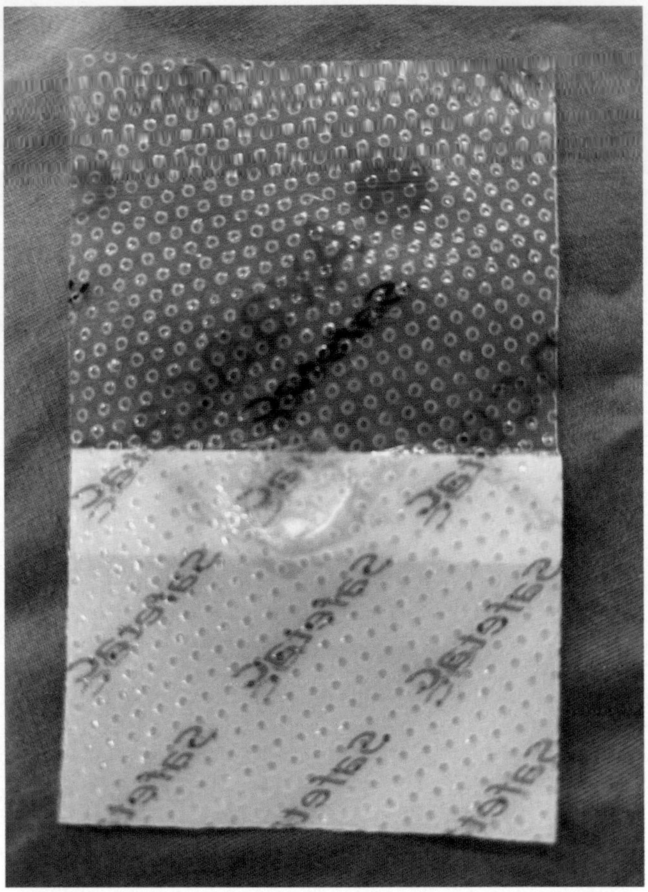

FIGURE 17-25 Avance Film with Safetac technology. (From Mölnlycke Health Care US, LLC, Norcross, Georgia.)

TABLE 17-18 General Tips for NPWT Application

- Monitor for bleeding, especially in first 24 hours.[49] Physician should be notified if drainage in collection canister is sanguineous, is filled with drainage in 1 hour, or if more than two canisters are filled within a 24-hour period.
- Leaks can be occluded by patching with an additional piece of occlusive sheeting.[49]
- Tubing should be placed such that the risk of pressure to intact skin is minimized and will allow for sitting and supine positions without the tube resting underneath the patient.
- Direction of drain placement should be considered, for example, if on lower leg, have tubing run out the waist or out the bottom of the pants leg.
- If foam wound filler must be cut, do so away from the wound to prevent foam residue from getting into the wound bed.
- Strips of Vaseline gauze or Xeroform at the edges make removal less painful, allow epithelial migration at the edges, and prevent skin maceration from any foam that overlaps the skin.
- Most skin protectants also remove oil from the skin surface, thereby improving adherence of occlusive sheeting and decreasing risk of leaks.[67]
- If odor develops with extended use, thorough irrigation should be completed at each dressing change and the wound assessed for infection or bleeding.

TABLE 17-19 Strategies for Reducing Pain at Dressing Change

- Infuse wound filler with normal saline and soak 3–5 minutes prior to change, can infuse directly or via tubing once disconnected from the canister.
- Place nonadherent protective layer(s) between wound tissue and foam fillers to prevent granulation tissue ingrowth.
- Use silicone-based occlusive sheeting to minimize skin stripping and pain with removal. If using non-silicone-based sheeting, remove by pulling parallel to the skin and release the seal with adhesive remover pads.
- Use skin protectant prior to occlusive sheeting application.
- Advise patients of the potential for pain or discomfort with initial pressure application and dressing compression.
- PVA white foam may be less painful upon removal compared to larger pore black foam.
- During dressing changes, prevent dehydration of granulation tissue by covering tissue with saline-soaked gauze.
- For larger wounds, have sufficient manpower to minimize treatment time.
- Provide pain medications at the appropriate time prior to dressing change (refer to Clinical Consideration, Chapter 14, page 426).

TABLE 17-20 Patient Education List

- Basic operation of NPWT unit
- Overview of how NPWT works and benefit to the wound
- When alarms may sound and what to do
- How to seal small leaks with occlusive sheeting
- Importance of keeping NPWT device "on" 24 hours a day
- Importance of keeping the tubing open and without kinks that may block suction
- 24-hour vendor troubleshooting assistance line
- Keeping the battery charged
- Action to take in the case of bleeding, increased pain, or other unexpected event
- Contact wound care provider to remove dressing as soon as possible if the suction is off for more than 2 hours

Adapted from Mouës CM, van den Bemd GJCM, Heule F, Hovius SER. Comparing conventional gauze therapy to vacuum-assisted closure wound therapy: a prospective randomized trial. *J Plast Reconstr Aesthet Surg*. 2007;60:672-681.

CASE STUDY

CONTINUED

Wound assessment shows the following:

1. Size: 28 cm × 10 cm × 0.4 cm deep.
2. Tissue consists grossly of 40% exposed muscle, 30% tendon with paratenon intact, 30% fascia, and subcutaneous tissue with 5 Penrose drains.
3. Drainage: moderate serosanguineous with no active bleeding; no evidence of pseudomonas.
4. Edges are clean with evidence of granulation and some epithelial migration at distal edges.
5. Periwound sensation intact.
6. Radial and ulnar pulses 3+.

DISCUSSION QUESTION

If NPWT were determined to be appropriate for this patient, what parameters, application materials, and guidelines should be used?

CASE STUDY

CONCLUSION

Plan of care:

- NPWT was used to facilitate tissue proliferation. Because of the exposed muscle and tendon, a nonadherent mesh dressing was placed over the majority of the wound bed; Xeroform strips were placed on the edges; black foam was used (because the patient had good circulation for delivery of systemic antibiotics, silver dressings were not necessary); suction was set at -125 mmHg, continuous mode. Dressing change frequency set for 3 times per week (**FIGURE 17-26A, B**).
- The patient was instructed in active finger exercises to help reduce finger edema and maintain tendon mobility. They were also instructed to keep the upper extremity and hand elevated on a pillow when supine.
- Even though the patient had a normal serum albumin level, protein supplements were recommended due to increased protein demands for wound healing.
- A sliding scale for insulin was initiated to ensure blood glucose levels were appropriate to optimize tissue proliferation.

Continued next page—

CASE STUDY *(Continued)*

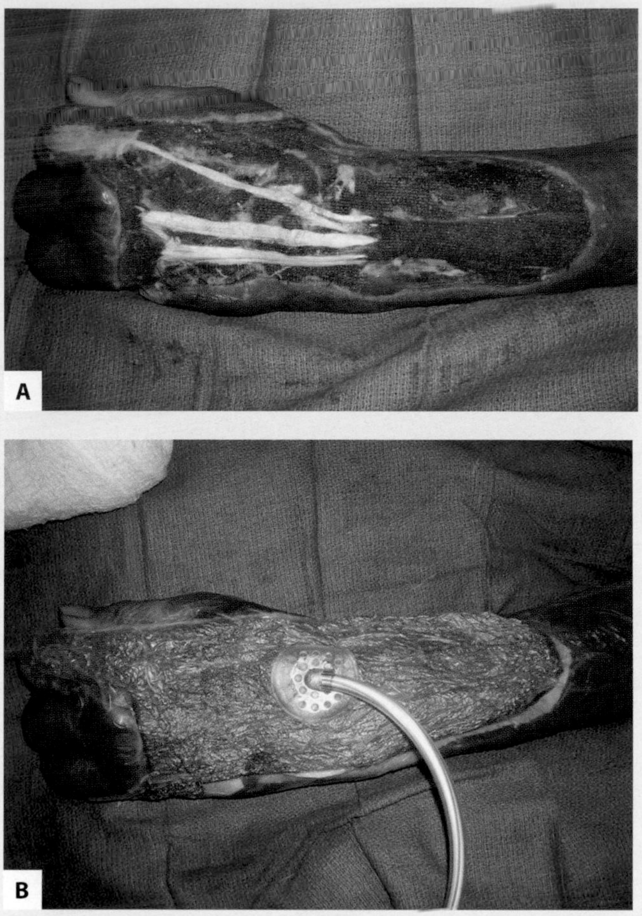

FIGURE 17-26 A. After 1 week of treatment. The patient responded well to the plan of care, and after 1 week was deemed appropriate for a split-thickness skin graft. **B.** Case study wound with NPWT in place.

Short-term goals:

- Increase granulation tissue to more than 90% of the wound bed
- Preserve integrity and function of the extensor tendons with no observable deterioration of tendons
- Prevent flexor contractions of the fingers with a patient having 75% of active range of motion in all fingers
- Decrease the bacterial load to minimize biofilm and effect on wound healing with no signs or symptoms of infection

Long-term goals:

- Full wound closure with a split-thickness skin graft
- Full range of motion of the fingers
- No adhesions to limit wrist function
- The patient to perform all activities of daily living independently
- The patient to return to work as a mechanic

Progress:
The patient responded well to NPWT and comorbidity management. After 1 week a split-thickness skin graft was applied with more than 95% take. The patient was discharged home with out-patient occupational therapy from a certified hand therapist.

SUMMARY

The evolution of NPWT continues as research and clinical knowledge advances and new devices with specialized features are developed. This chapter provides an overview of NPWT to assist providers in evaluating devices and in making informed decisions about when this intervention will benefit patients with wounds and prevent surgical site complications in high-risk patients. When used as one component in a complete wound management plan, NPWT has the potential to improve wound healing in a wide variety of patients.

STUDY QUESTIONS

1. The principle of ______________________ is defined as the stimulation of cells within the wound bed with mechanical force, thus stimulating them to reproduce.
   a. Macrostrain
   b. Microstrain
   c. Granulation
   d. Contraction
2. A patient referred for NPWT has a wound with a 7cm sinus tract at the lateral. Which of the following dressings is the *best* choice for filling the sinus?
   a. Black reticulated foam
   b. Iodoform gauze strip
   c. White, nonadherent foam
   d. No dressing needs to be put in the sinus
3. A clinician places an NPWT dressing on a patient with a large abdominal wound after hernia repair. The recommended pressure setting would be
   a. −125 mmHg—the pressure that is recommended as producing the fasted wound closure.
   b. −150 mmHg—recommended because of the wound size and the presence of hernia mesh in the wound bed.
   c. Between −125 and −175 mmHg—recommended to adequately remove exudate.
   d. Between −75 and −125 mmHg—based on patient comfort and adequate removal of exudate.

4. Which of the following is an indication to delay or discontinue the use of NPWT?
   a. The wound shows evidence of bleeding that does not stop with pressure.
   b. The patient complains of the inconvenience of carrying the pump.
   c. The wound size has decreased by 50%.
   d. The wound is more than 70% granulated.
5. A patient notifies the healthcare provider that the NPWT pump stopped working during the night, and they have not been able to reestablish good suction. The best advice for this patient is to
   a. Add extra occlusive sheeting to the edges and come in for the regularly scheduled appointment the next day.
   b. Remove the dressing, apply dry gauze, and come in the next day.
   c. Seal the wound with extra occlusive sheeting to prevent fluid leakage and come in as soon as possible so that the dressing can be removed, the wound cleansed and assessed, and a new NPWT dressing applied.
   d. Call the NPWT vendor as the problem is probably an equipment failure.
6. NPWT is to be applied with precautions on a patient who is on anticoagulants. Which of the following strategies is *best* for a patient who is at risk for bleeding?
   a. Lower the suction pressure to −50 mmHg.
   b. Apply a nonadherent interface dressing between the wound bed and foam to prevent ingrowth and granulation tissue disruption with dressing removal.
   c. Change the dressing every day.
   d. Reduce or discontinue the medication until the wound is closed.
7. NPWT placed over split-thickness skin grafts or dermal substitutes is usually changed the first time after
   a. 24 hours.
   b. 48 hours.
   c. 72 hours.
   d. 5 days.
8. The suction pressure recommended for newborns who are placed on NPWT is
   a. −50 mmHg.
   b. −100 mmHg.
   c. −125 mmHg.
   d. NPWT is contraindicated for patients less than 2 years of age.

Answers: 1-b; 2-c; 3-d; 4-a; 5-c; 6-b; 7-d; 8-a

REFERENCES

1. Fout B, Plotzke M. Comparing traditional and disposable negative-pressure wound therapy use by medicare home health patients. *Adv Skin Wound Care*. 2022;35(1):37-42.
2. Paglinawan R, Schwab P, Bechert K. Negative pressure wound therapy systems innovates standard of care via intelligent pressure control and dynamic exudate removal. *Wounds*. 2020;32 (10 Suppl.):S1-S8.
3. Singh D, Chopra K, Sabina J, Brown E. Practical things you should know about wound healing and vacuum-assisted closure management. *Plats Reconstr Surg*. 2020:145(4):839e-854e.
4. Banwell PE, Musgrave M. Topical negative pressure therapy: mechanisms and indications. *Int Wound J*. 2004;1(2):95-106.
5. Morgan-Jones R, Gefen A, Sandy-Hodgetts K. Surgical incision care-negative pressure wound therapy and advanced dressings. *Wounds Int*. 2022;13(2):34-39.
6. Shehata MSA, Bahbah E, El-Ayman Y, et al. Effectiveness of negative pressure wound therapy in patients with challenging wounds: a systematic review and meta-analysis. *Wounds*. 2022;34(12): e126-e134.
7. Kacmaz HY, Baser M, Sozuer EM. Effect of prophylactic negative-pressure wound therapy for high-risk wounds in colorectal cancer surgery: a randomized controlled trial. *Adv Skin Wound Care*. 2022;35:597-603.
8. Arellano ML, Serrano CB, Guedea M, et al. Surgical wound complications after colorectal surgery with single-use negative-pressure wound therapy versus surgical dressing over closed incisions: a randomized controlled trial. *Adv Skin Wound Care*. 2021;34:657-661.
9. Collinsworth AW, Griffin LP. The effect of timing of instillation therapy on outcomes and costs for patients receiving negative pressure wound therapy. *Wounds*. 2022(34(11):269-275.
10. Eceviz E, Cevik HB. Shoelace technique plus negative-pressure wound therapy closure in fasciotomy wounds. *Adv Skin Wound Care*. 2020;33(9):497-500.
11. Lavery LA, Davis KE, La Fontaine J, et al. Does negative pressure wound therapy with irrigation improve clinical outcomes? A randomized clinical trial in patients with diabetic foot infections. *Amer J Surg*. 2020;220(4):1076-1082.
12. James CV, Murray Q, Park SY, et al. Venous leg ulcers: potential algorithms of care. *Wounds*. 2022;34(12):288-296.
13. Lin DZ, Kao YC, Chen C, Wang HJ, Chiu WK. Negative pressure wound therapy for burn patients: a meta-analysis and systematic review. *Int Wound J*. 2021;18(1):112-123.
14. Rapp SJ, Dershem V, Zhang X, Schutte SC, Chariker ME. Varying negative pressure wound therapy acute effects on human split-thickness autografts. *J Burn Care Res*. 2020;41(1):104-112.
15. Davis KE, La Fontaine J, Farrar D, et al. Randomized clinical study to compare negative pressure wound therapy with simultaneous saline irrigation and traditional negative pressure wound therapy for complex foot infections. *Wound Repair Regen*. 2020;28(1):97-104.
16. Song YP, Wang L, Yuan BF, et al. Negative-pressure wound therapy for III/IV pressure injuries: a meta-analysis. *Wound Repair Regen*. 2020;29(1):20-33.
17. Gabriel A, Gialich S, Kirk J, et al. The Haiti earthquake: the provision of wound care for mass casualties utilizing negative-pressure wound therapy. *Adv Skin Wound Care*. 2011;24(10): 456-462.
18. Maury S, Bhandari PS. Negative pressure wound therapy in the management of combat wounds: a critical review. *Adv Wound Care*. 2016;5(9):379-389.
19. Mansoor J, Ellahi I, Junald Z, Habib A. Clinical evaluation of improvised gauze-based negative pressure wound therapy in military wounds. *Int Wound J*. 2015;12(5):559-563.
20. Hinck D, Franke A, Gatzka F. Use of vacuum-assisted closure negative pressure wound therapy in combat-related injuries—literature review. *Mil Med*. 2010;175(3):173-181.
21. Geiger S, McCormick F, Chou R, Wandel AG. War wounds: lessons learned from operation Iraqi Freedom. *Plast Reconstr Surg*. 2008;122(1):146-153.

22. Borgquist O, Ingemansson R, Malmsjö M. Wound edge microvascular blood flow during negative-pressure wound therapy: examining the effects of pressures from −10 to −175 mmHg. *Plast Reconstr Surg*. 2010;125(2):502-509.
23. Nuutila K, Eriksson E. Moist wound healing with commonly available dressings. *Adv Wound Care*. 2021;10(12):685-698.
24. Sathe PS, Prabhu DV, Ravikumar P, et al. Alternative wound management: translating science into practice. *Adv Skin Wound Care*. 2021;34(10):517-524.
25. Sibbald RG, Elliott JA, Persaud-Jaimangal R, et al. Wound bed preparation 2021. *Adv Skin Wound Care*. 2021;34(4):183-195.
26. Gao J, Wang Y, Song J, Li Z, Ren J, Wang P. Negative pressure wound therapy for surgical site infections: a systematic review and meta-analysis. *J Adv Nurs*. 2021;77:3980-3990.
27. Kilpadi DV, Cunningham MR. Evaluation of closed incision management with negative pressure wound therapy (CIM): Hematoma/seroma and involvement of the lymphatic system. *Wound Repair Regen*. 2011;19:588-596.
28. Cheng Y, Zhou Z, Hu Huan, et al. An application of negative-pressure wound dressing for partial- or full-thickness burn wounds. *Int J Low Extrem Wounds*. 2021;20(3):257-262.
29. Woo K, Ayello EA, Sibbald RG. The edge effect: current therapeutic options to advance the wound edge. *Adv Skin Wound Care*. 2007; 20(2):99-117.
30. Falange V. Growth factors and chronic wounds: the need to understand the microenvironment. *J Dermatol*. 1992;19:667-672.
31. Gombert A, Dillavou E, D'Agostino RD, Griffin L, Robertson J, Eells M. A systematic review and meta-analysis of randomised controlled trials for the reduction of surgical site infection in closed incision management versus standard of care dressings over closed vascular groin incisions. *Vascular*. 2020;28(3):274-284.
32. Pachowsky M, Gusinde J, Klein A, et al. Negative pressure wound therapy to prevent seromas and treat surgical incisions after total hip arthroplasty. *Int Orthop*. 2012;36(4):719-722.
33. Anesäter E, Borgquist O, Hedstrom E, Waga J, Ingemansson R, Malmsjö M. The influence of different sizes and types of wound fillers on wound contraction and tissue pressure during negative pressure wound therapy. *Int Wound J*. 2011;8(4):336-342.
34. Borgquist O, Gustafsson L, Ingemansson R, Malmsjö M. Micro- and macromechanical effects on the wound bed of negative pressure wound therapy using gauze and foam. *Ann Plast Surg*. 2010;64(6):789-793.
35. Borgquist O, Ingemansson R, Malmsjö M. The effect of intermittent and variable negative pressure wound therapy on wound edge microvascular blood flow. *Ostomy Wound Manage*. 2010;56(3): 60-67.
36. Kim P. Negative pressure wound therapy with instillation: an adjunctive therapy for infection management in orthopaedic trauma. *J Orthop Trauma*. 2022;36(9 Suppl.):S12-S16.
37. Kim PJ, Lavery LA, Galiano RD, et al. The impact of negative-pressure wound therapy with instillation on wounds requiring operative debridement: pilot randomised, controlled trial. *Int Wound J*. 2020;17(5):1194-1208.
38. Leong S, Lo ZJ. Use of disposable negative pressure wound therapy on split-thickness skin graft recipient sites for peripheral arterial disease foot wounds: a case report. *Int Wound J*. 2020;17:716-721.
39. Saab IR, Sarhane KA, Ezzeddine HM, Abu-Sittah GS, Ibrahim AE. Treatment of a paediatric patient with a distal lower extremity traumatic wound using a dermal regeneration template and NPWT. *J Wound Care*. 2014;23(10):S5-S8.
40. Sumpio B, Tahkor P, Mahler D, Blume P. Negative pressure wound therapy as postoperative dressing in below knee amputation stump closure of patients with chronic venous insufficiency. *Wounds*. 2011;23(10):301-308.
41. Tuncel U, Turan A, Bayraktar MA, Aydin U, Erkorkmaz U. Clinical experience with the use of gauze-based negative pressure wound therapy. *Wounds*. 2012;24(8):227-223.
42. Borgquist O, Anesäter E, Hedström E, Lee CK, Ingemansson R, Malmsjö M. Measurements of wound edge microvascular blood flow during negative pressure wound therapy using thermodiffusion and transcutaneous and invasive laser Doppler velocimetry. *Wound Repair Regen*. 2011;19:727-733.
43. Gabriel A, Camardo M, O'Rorke E, et al. Effects of negative-pressure wound therapy with instillation versus standard of care in multiple wound types: systematic literature review and meta-analysis. *Plast Reconstr Surg*. 2021;147(11):68S-76S.
44. de Jesus LE, Martins AB, Oliveira PB, et al. Negative pressure wound therapy in pediatric surgery: how and when to use *J Pediatr Surg*. 2018;53(4):585-591.
45. Kim PJ, Silverman R, Attinger CE, et al. Comparison of negative pressure wound therapy with and without instillation of saline in the management of infected wounds. *Cureus*. 2020;12(7);e9047.
46. Norman G, Goh EL, Dumville JC, et al. Negative pressure wound therapy for surgical wounds healing by primary closure. *Cochrane Database Syst Rev*. 2020;5:1-261
47. Gabriel A, Gupta S, Orgill DP. Challenges and management of surgical site occurrences. *Plast Reconstr Surg*. 2019;143(1S):7S-10S.
48. Willy C, Agarwal A, Andersen C, et al. Closed incision negative pressure therapy: International multidisciplinary consensus recommendations. *Int Wound J*. 2016;14(2):385-398.
49. DeCarbo WT, Hyer CF. Negative-pressure wound therapy applied to high-risk surgical incisions. *J Foot Ankle Surg*. 2010;49(3): 299-300.
50. Cheatham ML, Demetriades D, Fabian TC, et al. Prospective study examining clinical outcomes associated with a negative pressure wound therapy system and Barker's vacuum packing technique. *World J Surg*. 2013;37(9):2018-2030.
51. Atema JJ, Gans SL, Boermeester MA. Systematic review and meta-analysis of the open abdomen and temporary abdominal closure techniques in non-trauma patients. *World J Surg*. 2015;39(4): 912-925.
52. Kirkpatrick AW, Roberts DJ, Faris PD, et al. Active negative pressure peritoneal therapy after abbreviated laparotomy. The intraperitoneal vacuum randomized controlled trial. *Ann Surg*. 2015;262(1):38-46.
53. Widgerow AD. Chronic wound fluid-thinking outside the box. *Wound Repair Regen*. 2011;19(3):287-291.
54. Koenen P, Spanholtz T, Maegele M, et al. Acute and chronic wound fluids inversely influence adipose-derived stem cell function: molecular insights into impaired wound healing. *Int Wound J*. 2015;12(1):10-16.
55. Liu HR, Yang P, Han S, Zhang Y, Zhu HY. The application of enhanced recovery after surgery and negative-pressure wound therapy in the perioperative period of elderly patients with colorectal cancer. *BMC Surg*. 2021;21(1):336-342.
56. Cameron MH. Hydrotherapy. In: Cameron MH, ed. *Physical agents in rehabilitation: an evidence-based approach to practice*. 5th ed. St. Louis, MO: Elsevier; 2019:341-373.
57. Wysocki AB. Anatomy and physiology of skin and soft tissue. In: Bryant RA, Nix DP, eds. *Acute and Chronic Wounds: Current Management Concepts*. 5th ed. St. Louis, MO: Elsevier; 2016:40-62.

58. Pedrazzi NE, Naiken S, Scala GL. Negative pressure wound therapy in pediatric burn patients: a systematic review. *Adv Wound Care.* 2021;10(5):270-280.
59. Santosa KB, Keller M, Olsen MA, et al. Negative-pressure wound therapy in infants and children: a population-based study. *J Surg Res.* 2019;235:560-568.
60. Wong S, Eid A, Southerland W, Ver Halen JP. Use of negative pressure wound therapy in pediatric oncology patients: a single-center review of 66 patients. *Plast Aesthet Res.* 2016;3:248-253.
61. Baharestani MM, Amjad I, Bookout K, et al. V.A.C.® therapy in the management of paediatric wounds: clinical review and experience. *Int Wound J.* 2009;6:1-26.
62. Bryant RA. Managing wounds in palliative care. In: Bryant RA, Nix DP, eds. *Acute and Chronic Wounds: Current Management Concepts.* 5th ed. St. Louis, MO: Elsevier; 2016:531-540.
63. Pro-III Negative Pressure Wound System. Available at: https://www.deroyal.com/products/wound-care/npwt/npwt-item/wc-npwt-units-III. Accessed August 3, 2023.
64. Gabriel A, Shores J, Bernstein B, et al. A clinical review of infected wound treatment with vacuum assisted closure® (V.A.C.®) therapy: experience and case series. *Int Wound J.* 2009;6(2):1-25.
65. Kloth LC. Treatment options: 5 questions and answers about negative pressure wound therapy. *Adv Skin Wound.* 2002;15(5):226-229.
66. Gabriel A, Gupta S. Management of the wound environment with negative pressure wound therapy. In: Sussman C, Bates-Jensen B, eds. *Wound Care: A Collaborative Practice Manual for Physical Therapists and Nurses.* 4th ed. Baltimore, MD: Wolters Kluwer/Lippincott Williams & Wilkins; 2012.
67. McCallon SK. Negative-pressure wound therapy. In: McCulloch JM, Kloth LC, eds. *Wound Healing: Evidence-Based Management.* 4th ed. Philadelphia, PA: FA Davis Company; 2012.
68. Kim PJ, Attinger CE, Constantine T, et al. Negative pressure wound therapy with instillation: international consensus guidelines update. *Int Wound J.* 2020;17(1):174-186.
69. Glass GE, Nanchahal J. The methodology of negative pressure wound therapy: separating fact from fiction. *J Plast Reconstr Aesthet Surg.* 2012;65(8):989-1001.
70. Jung J, Yoo K, Han S, et al. Influence of negative-pressure wound therapy on tissue oxygenation in diabetic feet. *Adv Skin Wound Care.* 2016;29(8):364-370.
71. Krasner DL. Managing wound pain in patients with vacuum-assisted closure devices. *Ostomy Wound Manage.* 2002;48(5):38-43.
72. Birke-Sorensen H, Malmsjö M, Rome P, et al. Evidence-based recommendations for negative pressure wound therapy: treatment variables (pressure levels, wound filler and contact layer)—steps towards an international consensus. *J Plast Reconstr Aesthet Surg.* 2010;64:S1-S16.
73. Shirakawa M, Isseroff RR. Topical negative pressure devices: use for enhancement of healing chronic wounds. *Arch Dermatol.* 2005;141:1449-1453.
74. Sogorski A, Lehnhardt M, Goetrz O, et al. Improvement of local microcirculation through intermittent negative pressure wound therapy (NPWT). *J Tissue Viability.* 2018;27(4):267-273.
75. Malmsjö M, Gustafsson L, Lindstedt S, Gesslein B, Ingemansson R. The effects of variable, intermittent, and continuous negative pressure wound therapy, using foam, or gauze, on wound contraction, granulation tissue formation, and ingrowth into the wound filler. *ePlasty.* 2012;11:42-54.
76. Sundby OH, Hoiseth LO, Irgens I, et al. Intermittent negative pressure applied to the lower limb increases fort microcirculatory and microcirculatory blood flow pulsatility in people with spinal cord injury. *Spinal Cord.* 2018;56(4):382-391.
77. Aheam C. Intermittent NPWT and lower negative pressures—exploring the disparity between science and current practice: a review. *Ostomy Wound Manage.* 2009;55(6):22-28.
78. Faust E, Opoku-Agyeman JL, Behnam AB. Use of negative-pressure wound therapy with instillation and dwell time: an overview. *Plast Reconstr Surg.* 2020;147(1S-1):16S-26S.
79. Start Smart with 3M™ VerafloTM Therapy. 2022. Available at: https://www.3m.com/3M/en_US/medical-us/healthcare-professionals/wound-care/veraflo-therapy/. Accessed December 22, 2022.
80. Cardinal Health™ Curity™ AMD Antimicrobial Woven Sponges. 2022. Available at: https://www.cardinalhealth.com/en/product-solutions/medical/skin-and-wound-management/traditional-wound-care/woven-dressings/curity-amd-sponges.html. Accessed December 23, 2022.
81. Malmsjö M, Ingemansson R, Martin R, Huddleston E. Negative pressure wound therapy using gauze or open-cell polyurethane foam: similar early effects on pressure transduction and tissue contraction in an experimental porcine wound model. *Wound Repair Regen.* 2009;40(1):200-205.
82. Malmsjö M, Lindstedt S, Ingemansson R. Influence on pressure transduction when using different drainage techniques and wound fillers (foam and gauze) for negative pressure wound therapy. *Int Wound J.* 2010;7(5):406-412.
83. Malmsjö M, Ingemansson R. Effects of green foam, black foam, and gauze on contraction, blood flow and pressure delivery to the wound bed in negative pressure wound therapy. *J Plast Reconstruct Aesthet Surg.* 2011;64:289-296.
84. Malmsjö M, Ingemansoon R. Green foam, black foam, or gauze for NWPT: effects on granulation tissue formation. *J Wound Care.* 2011;20(6):294-299.
85. Malmsjö M, Gustafsson L, Lindstedt S, Ingemansson R. Negative pressure wound therapy-associated tissue trauma and pain: a controlled in vivo study comparing foam and gauze dressing removal by immunohistochemistry for substance P and calcitonin gene-related peptide in the wound edge. *Ostomy Wound Manage.* 2011;57(12):30-35.
86. Borgquist O, Gustafson L, Ingemansson R, Malmsjö M. Tissue ingrowth into foam but not into gauze during negative pressure wound therapy. *Wounds.* 2009;21(11):302-309.
87. Avance Solo. Molnlycke. Available at: https://www.avancesolo.com/our-npwt-system/. Accessed December 24, 2022.
88. Vowden P. Ten top tips…Using negative pressure wound therapy effectively. *Wounds Int.* 2014;5(2):13-15.
89. Kim PJ, Applewhite A, Dardano AN, Fernandez L, Hall K, McElroy E. Use of a novel foam dressing with negative pressure wound therapy and instillation: recommendations and clinical experience. *Wounds.* 2018;30(3):S1-S17.
90. 3M™ Veraflo™ Cleanse Choice Complete™ Dressing. 2022. Available at: https://www.3m.com/3M/en_US/p/d/b5005351004/. Accessed December 23, 2022.
91. Paglinawan R, Schwab P, Bechert K. Use of a double-lumen NPWT system with innovative technology outperforms a single-lumen NPWT system in accurate delivery of negative pressure and superior fluid removal. *Wounds.* 2022;34(2 Suppl):S1-S8.
92. SensaT.R.A.C.™ Pad. 3M Science Applied to Life™. 2022. Available at: https://www.3m.com/3M/en_US/p/d/b5005265161/. Accessed December 24, 2022.

93. Innovating the Standard of Care. Medela. 2021. Available at: https://www.medelahealthcare.com/en-US/solutions/negative-pressure-wound-therapy?creative=454653616304&keyword=pressure%20wound%20therapy&matchtype=p&network=g&device=c&utm_source=google&utm_medium=cpc&utm_campaign=npwt&utm_term=pressure%20wound%20therapy&gclid=Cj0KCQiA15qdBhD [illegible] a2yyaSiIYn-3eVbdukkCI7oznKiebMLu2lKfr8aAt3lEALw_wcB. Accessed December 24, 2022.

94. An Innovative Class of Negative Pressure Wound Therapy Drapes. 2022. Available at: https://engage.3m.com/dermatac-drape-sample?utm_term=hcbg-msd-icuroh-en_us-lead-cwc-cpc-google-na-sample-hderm-aug22-00000&gclid=CjwKCAiAhqCdBhB0EiwA1i0M_U [illegible] 06Wx-LHWGihoCo9UQAvD_BwE. Accessed December 25, 2022.

CHAPTER EIGHTEEN

Low-Frequency Ultrasound

Karen A. Gibbs, PT, PhD, DPT, CWS and Rose L. Hamm, PT, DPT, FACCWS

CHAPTER OBJECTIVES

At the end of this chapter, the learner will be able to:

1. **Define the following terms associated with the use of low-frequency ultrasound (LFUS): cavitation, frequency, intensity, and duty cycle.**
2. **Explain how the application of LFUS affects human tissue during different phases of healing.**
3. **Select specific patient indications appropriate for the use of noncontact and contact LFUS in wound management.**
4. **Explain precautions and contraindications associated with the use of LFUS.**
5. **Develop a care plan involving the use of LFUS in the treatment of a chronic wound.**
6. **Explain the benefits of extracorporeal shockwave therapy (ESWT) in wound management.**
7. **Identify indications and contraindications for the use of ESWT.**

INTRODUCTION

Healthcare providers have long utilized ultrasound (US) technology for both diagnostic and therapeutic purposes (**FIGURES 18-1**, **18-2**, and **TABLE 18-1**).[1–4] As a noninvasive diagnostic tool, ultrasonography is used to painlessly visualize medical images of fractures, patterns of blood flow, fetal sex and development, abscesses, soft tissue injuries, hematomas, and other internal anatomical and physiological events (**FIGURE 18-3**).[1,3–9] Once considered a hospital- or clinic-based modality, battery-powered, portable ultrasound units are now routinely used in point-of-care first aid, emergency care, and combat environments.[4,6,10] US technology is also utilized in invasive diagnostic procedures such as US-guided fine needle aspiration.[11]

As a treatment modality, US technology is used in lithotripsy, liposuction, tumor ablation, and many general surgical procedures.[12–15] Advances using ultrasound-mediated targeted delivery methods have shown improved tissue-specific delivery and uptake of cancer treatment medications.[16] Physical therapists use US for phonophoresis, thermotherapy, pain reduction, tissue evaluation and repair, noninvasive vascular testing, and wound management.[9,17–19] US provides the following benefits regarding wound healing: increased local vasodilation and increased angiogenesis, wound cleansing and reduction of bioburden, enhancement of all phases of wound healing, and debridement.[9,18,20–24]

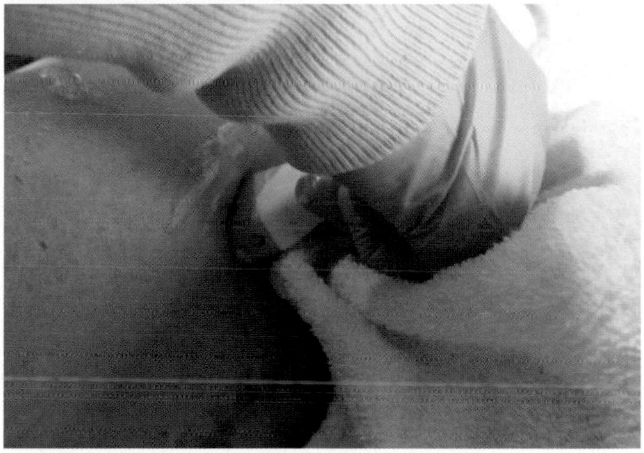

FIGURE 18-1 Diagnostic ultrasound being used on a medial thigh to detect vascular occlusion.

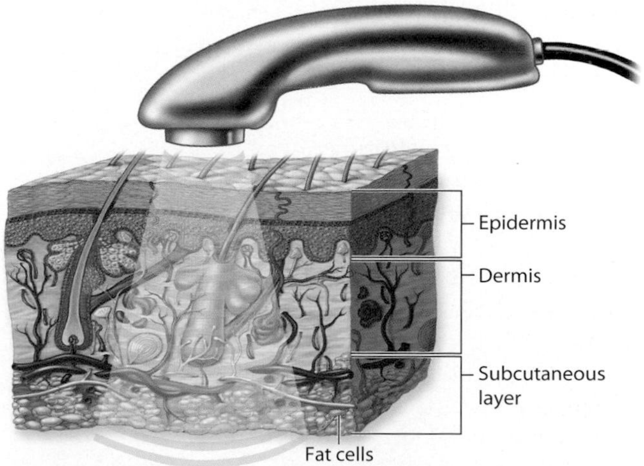

FIGURE 18-2 Transmission of sound waves. In traditional ultrasound, electric energy causes the piezoelectric crystal to vibrate and create sound waves that are transmitted to dermal/subdermal tissues via contact between the US head and overlying skin. For wound management, electrically generated sound waves penetrate tissues similarly to LFUS but are transmitted without making contact with wound tissues.

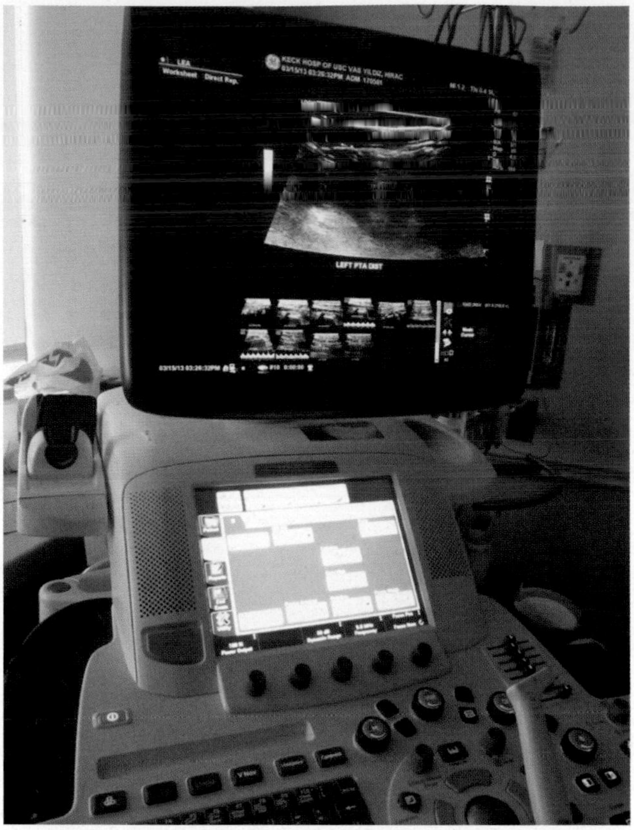

FIGURE 18-3 Diagnostic ultrasound equipment used for peripheral vascular studies. Diagnostic ultrasound is used both to detect occlusion of an artery affected by peripheral arterial disease and to confirm or rule out a deep vein thrombosis. The image created by the ultrasound waves can be visualized on the screen.

TABLE 18-1 US Technology Use

Diagnostic
High frequency (2–18.0 MHz)
Doppler/duplex scanning (tissue visualization)
Therapeutic
High frequency (1.0 or 3.0 MHz)
Thermotherapy, tissue repair, pain reduction, phonophoresis
Ablation (0.5–7.0 MHz)
Low frequency
Noncontact (40 kHz)
Tissue stimulation, wound cleansing, pain reduction
Contact
Wound debridement (20–50 kHz)
Lithotripsy (25–150 kHz)
Liposuction (20–30 kHz)
Surgical incisions (55.5 kHz)

MECHANISM OF ACTION

This chapter focuses on the use of noncontact and contact low-frequency ultrasound (LFUS) for wound healing. **TABLE 18-2** provides terminology and definitions used in the discussion of LFUS physics and application.[2,8,12,17,18,21,22] LFUS devices consist

TABLE 18-2 Ultrasound Terminology

Absorption	The tissue-dependent conversion of US energy into heat
Attenuation	Reduction in US intensity as sound waves move through different tissues and are reflected and scattered at different tissue interfaces
Banding	Separation of cells and plasma in circulating blood
Cavitation	Production, growth, and vibration of gaseous bubbles within tissue fluids formed due to local pressure changes with US application
-Stable cavitation	Gaseous bubbles are stable; they oscillate but do not rupture or burst
-Unstable cavitation	Gaseous bubbles are unstable; they oscillate but grow and implode releasing pressure sufficient to damage local cells
Continuous (thermal) US	Energy is continuously delivered with the goal of tissue heating
Duty cycle	The percentage of time that US energy is delivered during the total time of the treatment
Frequency	Number of US waves per second
Intensity	Amount of energy (W) per area of the sound head (cm^2) delivered during a treatment time, expressed as W/cm^2
Microstreaming	Movement or eddying of fluids caused by vibration of gaseous bubbles during cavitation
Piezoelectric crystal	The generation of sound waves when an electrical current is applied to a specific type of crystal, causing it to vibrate
Pulsed (nonthermal) US	Energy is delivered in pulses with the goal of cellular changes rather than tissue heating
Standing waves	Reflection of a sound wave back onto itself causing excess tissue heating and damage occurs if the sound head is not kept moving on tissue

of an electrically powered base unit with limited parameter adjustment, a method of saline delivery, and an attached soundwave-producing handpiece (**FIGURE 18-4**).[11]

US energy is used in wound healing due to its ability to affect changes in cellular activity. When therapeutic levels of US come into contact with tissues, two primary mechanical processes are produced: cavitation and microstreaming.[18,21,25] Acoustic *cavitation* refers to the generation of vibrating, microscopic bubbles in interstitial spaces. As they move through tissue fluids, bubble oscillations create compressive forces on surrounding cells which stimulate changes in cell membrane activity.[9,26] Cavitation is said to be *stable* when oscillating bubbles change in size but do not burst.[18] *Unstable cavitation* occurs when oscillating bubbles grow in size and implode causing free radical (OH^-, H^+) formation.[18] Unstable cavitation increases tissue temperature and pressure, which can cause local tissue damage (**FIGURES 18-5** and **18-6**).[18] Oscillating bubbles create eddies that produce unidirectional movement of tissue fluids potentiating mechanical stimulation to surrounding cells.[9,25] This type of fluid movement is

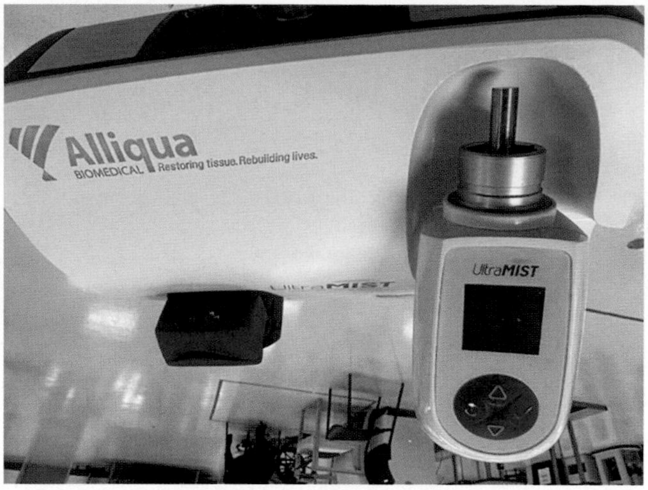

FIGURE 18-4 LFUS device. LFUS base unit showing the handpiece with the treatment wand exposed. A disposable applicator tip would be placed over the treatment wand (leaving only the very tip of the wand exposed) prior to patient use.

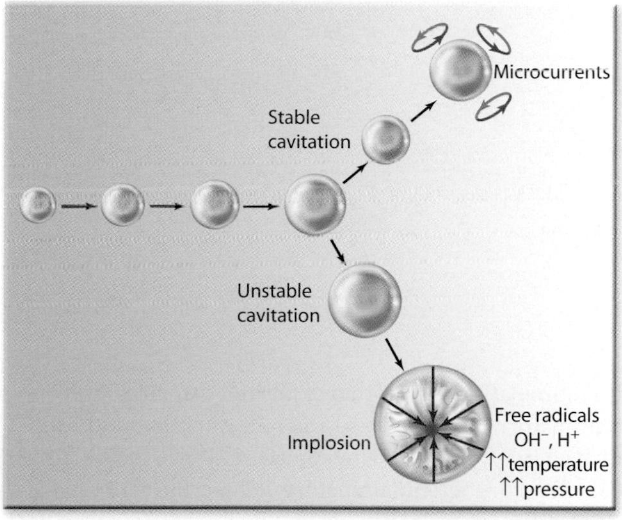

FIGURE 18-5 Illustration of microstreaming, stable cavitation, and unstable cavitation.

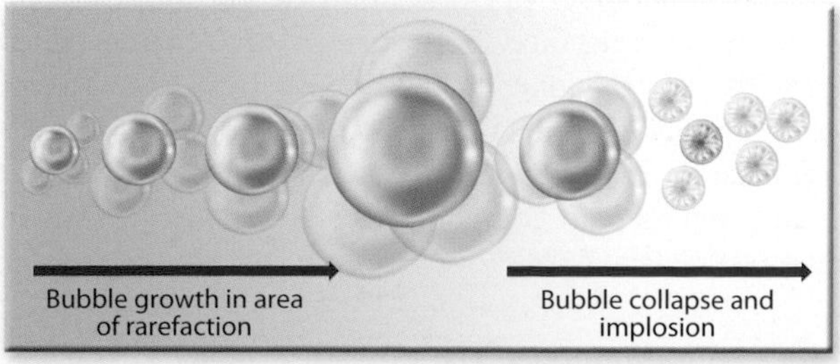

FIGURE 18-6 Unstable cavitation. Unstable cavitation occurs when transient gaseous bubbles implode causing tissue damage and free radical formation. This process may assist in the breakdown of necrotic tissue.

referred to as *microstreaming*. US-generated stable cavitation and microstreaming produce changes in cellular diffusion and growth factor production.[9,25]

EFFECTS AT THE CELLULAR AND TISSUE LEVELS

Noncontact LFUS has the potential to positively affect tissue during the inflammatory, proliferative, and remodeling/maturation phases of wound healing.[18,27] Low-frequency, pulsed energy produces nonthermal US, allowing for safe use during the acute inflammatory phase after hemostasis has been achieved.[18,28] The properties of cavitation and microstreaming change membrane permeability and facilitate the release of growth factors, enzymes, and chemotactic agents.[9,29,30] Activation of the inflammatory cells involved in autolysis facilitates the debridement of nonviable tissues.[31] Improved inflammatory response can result in earlier migration of proliferative cells and earlier onset of angiogenesis.[9,20,21] Noncontact LFUS has also been shown to decrease proinflammatory cytokines, hastening proliferation and decreasing pain.[32] In the proliferative phase, LFUS can accelerate granulation tissue formation and dermal repair by increased migration and activity of fibroblasts and endothelial cells.[27,30,33,34]

Positive effects of US seen during remodeling/maturation occur primarily when US is used during the acute inflammatory phase. Published data document stronger, more organized, and more elastic scar tissue with early application and suggest increased collagen production as the likely mechanism of action.[2,35,36] Since bacteria are present during all phases of wound healing, the role of LFUS in reducing bioburden applies throughout the entire healing process.[21,27,37] **TABLES 18-3** and **18-4** review the primary biophysical effects of US during each phase of healing and provide a general list of LFUS characteristics.[2,18,21,27,30,32–37]

Noncontact Low-Frequency US

Noncontact LFUS is the primary method of US delivery for wound management. At the time of publication, the UltraMIST System (**FIGURE 18-4**) is the only noncontact LFUS device specifically designed for promoting wound healing (Sanuwave Wound Care Technologies, Suwanee, GA). The UltraMIST System utilizes a thin mist of sterile saline as a coupling medium to transfer US energy to body tissues through the air without the need for physical contact (**FIGURE 18-7**).[28,30,37,38] UltraMIST therapy delivers continuous LFUS energy without tissue heating due to the low-intensity therapeutic treatment range, heat-dissipating saline mist, and noncontact method of delivery.[27]

Compared to therapeutic high-frequency US (1–3 MHz), LFUS (20–50 kHz) produces higher levels of cavitation and delivers greater amounts of US energy to tissues during comparable treatment times.[2] Using low-frequency (40 kHz) and low therapeutic intensities (0.1–0.6 W/cm^2), UltraMIST therapy has been shown to promote wound healing through

TABLE 18-3 Cellular and Tissue Biophysical Effects of Ultrasound by Phase of Healing

	Biophysical Effect	
Phase of Healing	**Cellular Level**	**Tissue Level**
Inflammation	Fluid movement in interstitial spaces Stimulation of growth factor release from platelets and macrophages Increase in mast cell degranulation and neutrophil recruitment Increase in chemotactic signals for fibroblast and endothelial cell migration Transition macrophages from proinflammatory to anti-inflammatory phenotypes	Edema reduction Decrease in exudate Facilitation of nonviable tissue breakdown by activated inflammatory cells
Proliferation	Stimulation of fibroblasts and endothelial cells Release of growth factors Increased production of nitric oxide Increased vasodilation	Increased angiogenesis, collagen formation (granulation tissue formation) Increased epithelialization Accelerated wound contraction
Remodeling/maturation	Effects due to initiation of US during the inflammatory phase	Improved scar organization, elasticity, and strength

TABLE 18-4 LFUS Characteristics

Characteristic	**LFUS**
Frequency range	20–50 kHz
Sound wave size	Long—low attenuation and absorption rates[6,18,22]
Tissue penetration	Noncontact 40 kHz ~3.0 mm[16] Contact debridement devices depend on application technique
Modes	Continuous and pulsed modes depending on the device Heat dissipated by noncontact and by saline irrigation
Application	Noncontact (facilitate wound healing) and contact (debridement) devices depending on the treatment goal
Therapeutic uses	Noncontact devices—tissue repair, wound cleansing, pain reduction Contact devices—debridement

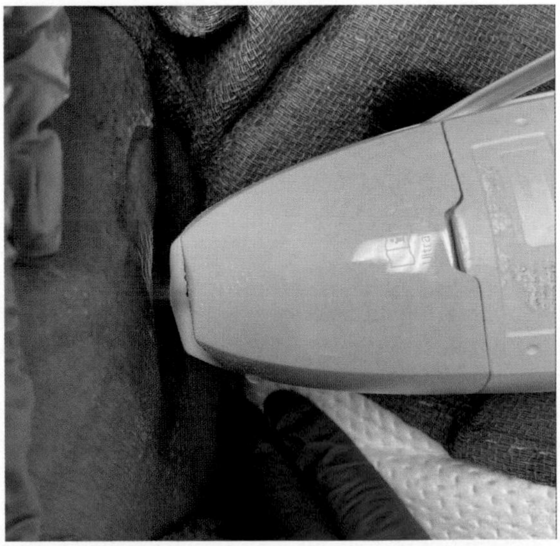

FIGURE 18-7 Saline is pulled from the IV bag, through the tubing, into the handpiece, and is delivered as a fine mist that serves as the conducting medium for noncontact LFUS. This picture shows the disposable applicator tip of the LFUS device in close proximity to but not in contact with wound tissue.

tissue stimulation, promotion of fibrinolysis, inhibition of pro-inflammatory cytokines, and the removal of wound exudates and bacteria.[23,24,27,31,34,37] Noncontact US also has a bactericidal effect through inflammatory cell recruitment during the inflammatory phase of healing and by direct damage to bacterial cell walls during all healing phases (**FIGURE 18-8**).[22,24,27,39] It has been proposed that LFUS may also alter the genetic code of certain bacteria, thus increasing antibiotic susceptibility and decreasing virulence. The simultaneous use of saline and noncontact LFUS is nontoxic and does not promote bacterial resistance. Both historic and current studies support the use of noncontact LFUS therapy as an adjunct to conventional wound management because of its ability to significantly reduce wound surface area, decrease bioburden, and reduce pain compared to standard treatment only (**TABLE 18-5**).[21,23,24,27,31,34,37,40]

Contact Low-Frequency US In wound management, contact LFUS devices are primarily used for selective debridement of nonviable tissue, reduction of bacteria, and removal of biofilm.[9,32,41] Various probes and/or modes are available for hard and soft tissue debridement. These devices produce highly

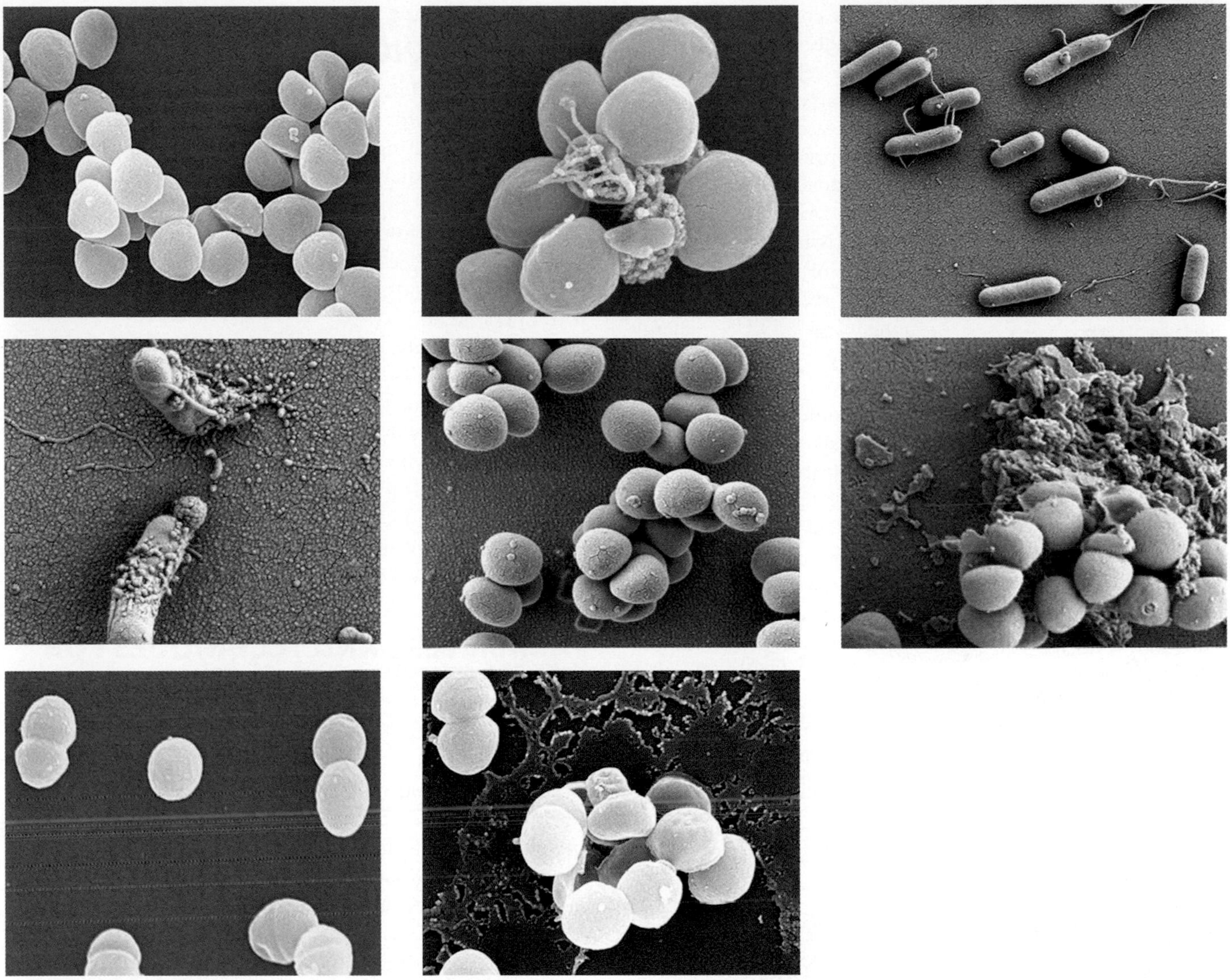

FIGURE 18-8 Treatment of bacteria with LFUS. Photographs showing the effect of noncontact LFUS on the cell membrane of bacteria that commonly cause wound infections. (From Kavros SJ, Schenck EC. Use of noncontact low-frequency ultrasound in the treatment of chronic foot and leg ulcerations: a 51-patient analysis. *J Am Pod Med Assn.* 2007;97(2):95–101. Used with permission.)

TABLE 18-5 Benefits of LFU

Cellular changes via cavitation and microstreaming
Overall increased US energy delivery compared to HFUS during the same treatment duration
Fluid mobilization in interstitial tissue
Decreased wound pain
Increased cellular permeability
Noncontact application for wound cleansing and tissue stimulation
Bacterial killing and removal
Effective, immediate, relatively painless debridement with contact applications

focused ultrasonic energy using irrigation fluid as a transfer medium that fragments or liquefies nonviable tissue by the production of unstable cavitation.[27,42] Portable devices such as the Qoustic Wound Therapy System (Arobella Medical, LLC, Minnetonka, MN), Sonoca Ultrasonic Debridement Device (Soring Medical Technology, Doral, FL), and the SonicOne (Bioventus, Inc., Farmingdale, NY) provide efficient, relatively painless, selective debridement without local anesthesia in both inpatient and outpatient settings.[43]

Contact LFUS devices may utilize continuous or pulsed mode depending on the specific manufacturer. Each device has some mechanism of simultaneous normal saline delivery so that debrided tissue can be quickly irrigated from the treatment site and any frictional heat generated by contact with vibrating treatment probes can be dissipated.[43–47] Although saline is typically used as the irrigation fluid, antimicrobial solutions such as hypochlorous acid can result in improved bacteria suppression.[48,49] The appropriate probe and/or mode of these devices is selected based on the type of tissue to be debrided, wound size, and wound location. During treatment, the probe is placed

CLINICAL CONSIDERATION

If LFUS is not available, traditional high-frequency ultrasound may be used to treat wounds by using *nonthermal parameters*: 3 MHz, 20% duty cycle, and 0.5 w/cm² for 1 minute over each cm² area of the wound bed. To prepare wound tissues to receive traditional contact, high-frequency US, apply a thin layer of hydrogel over the wound bed and cover it with a transparent film (**FIGURE 18-9**). US gel is then placed over the transparent film to allow for good transmission of US through the dressing and easy movement of the US head over the film. This technique provides a sterile transfer medium within the wound while also protecting the wound tissue and ultrasound head from cross-contamination. After treatment, the transparent film is removed and the wound is irrigated to remove the hydrogel transfer medium. The ultrasound head is disinfected per facility protocol.

in direct contact with nonviable tissue so the US energy can be selectively directed toward targeted tissues. While devices are marketed and utilized primarily as debridement modalities, when probes are held 1–10 mm away from wound tissues, they may also be used in low-intensity settings to secondarily transmit noncontact LFUS energy for tissue stimulation and irrigation.

In some cases, contact and noncontact methods of LFUS can be paired by using contact LFUS for efficient and safe removal of nonviable tissue and/or biofilm from the wound bed, followed by noncontact LFUS for overall wound stimulation, angiogenesis, and pain reduction.[27] Application and utilization of contact LFUS devices are presented in detail in Chapter 13, Wound Debridement, and their use is dictated by the providers' licensed scope of practice.

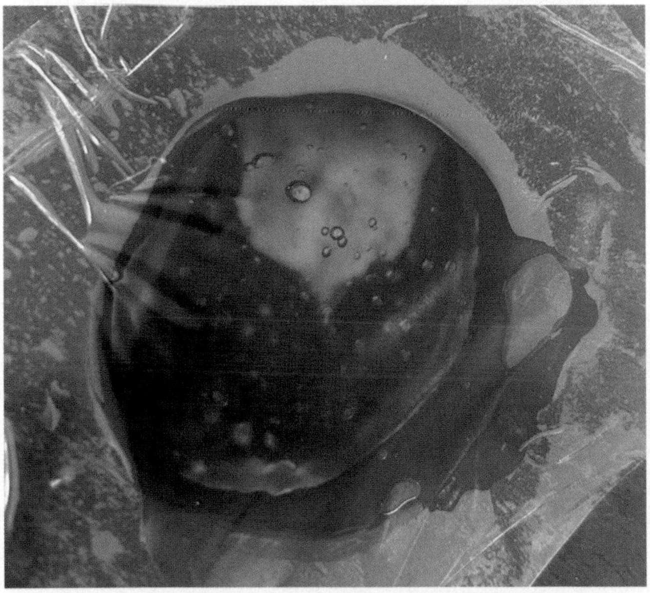

FIGURE 18-9 Set up technique for traditional contact US delivery. The wound bed is first filled with sterile hydrogel and covered with a transparent film dressing. Nonsterile US gel is then placed over the film dressing to provide good contact between the US head and facilitate the safe transfer of US energy through the film and into wound tissues.

INDICATIONS, PRECAUTIONS, AND CONTRAINDICATIONS

LFUS can be used in the treatment of most acute, subacute, and chronic wounds (**TABLE 18-6**).[32,37,38,43,50] Wounds associated with or resulting from vascular insufficiency, pressure, trauma, surgery, diabetes, burns, or skin grafts may benefit from the use of LFUS for tissue stimulation, reduction in bioburden and biofilm removal, tissue debridement, and pain reduction.[26,27,31,32,34,38–41,43,51,52] **FIGURE 18-10A–E** shows examples of wounds that are appropriate for the treatment with LFUS.

Before including LFUS as an adjunct treatment in a wound management plan of care, the clinician must first determine if US use is safe for the patient. **TABLE 18-7** lists general and wound management-specific precautions and contraindications associated with the use of LFUS.[2,18,29,30] However, some of the items on this list do not completely preclude the use of US. For example, LFUS is contraindicated for use near silicone breast implants but not contraindicated as long as the target tissue is located away from the chest.

PARAMETERS AND TECHNIQUES FOR APPLICATION

Parameters

Noncontact LFUS parameters are determined by wound surface area (cm²) and treatment time. The clinician using the UltraMIST system inputs the number of wounds to be treated and measurements for each wound. The amount of saline required for the surface area and the total treatment time are calculated by the device (**FIGURE 18-11**).[53] **TABLE 18-8** provides examples of predetermined UltraMIST treatment times.[25,30,54] Short treatment times for LFUS, compared to traditional high-frequency, therapeutic US devices, are due to higher amounts of US energy being transmitted via low-frequency sound waves. Frequency, duty cycle, and watts are preset in the UltraMIST System and are not changeable.[54]

Techniques for Application

The relatively small, noncontact, UltraMIST System has an electrical base unit and attached handpiece with an exposed

TABLE 18-6 Indications for LFUS

Specific Wound Etiology	General Indications
Traumatic	Debridement (contact LFUS)
Burns and friction injuries (skin tears)	Pain reduction
Pressure	Infection
Venous insufficiency	
Diabetic foot ulcers	
Inflammatory wounds (vasculitis)—pulsed only	
Split-thickness donor sites	
Neonatal extravasation injuries	

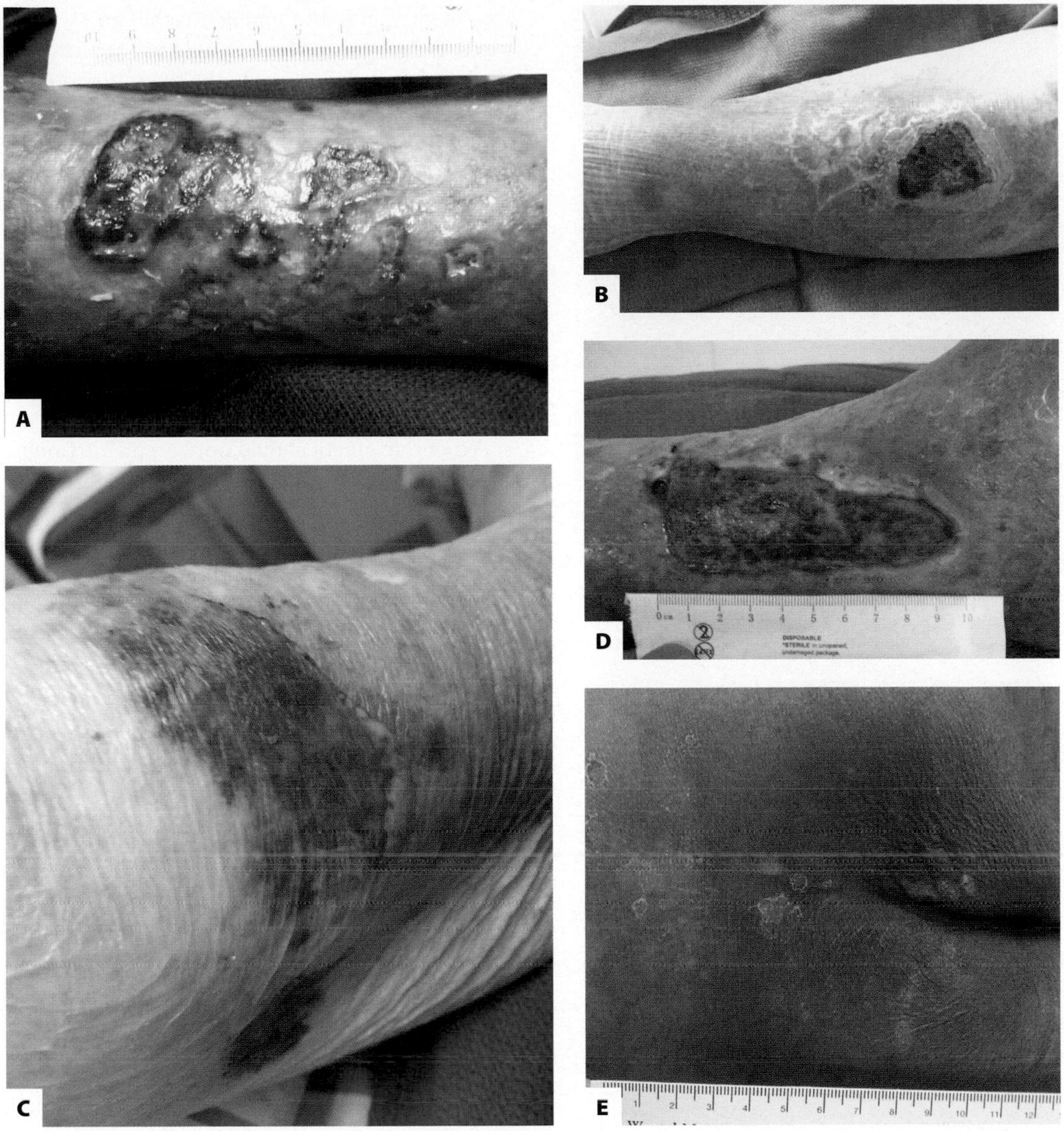

FIGURE 18-10 Ultrasound is indicated for the following wound diagnoses. A. Vasculitis. **B.** Trauma with edema. **C.** Skin tear with surrounding ecchymosis. **D.** Chronic venous insufficiency. **E.** Deep tissue injury.

TABLE 18-7 LFUS Precautions and Contraindications

General	Wound Management
Over growing epiphyseal plates	Acute inflammation (no thermal US)
Over breast implants	Pain associated with use over fracture site
Malignant tumor in treatment area (use only in conjunction with cancer treatment)	Untreated osteomyelitis
Gravid uterus (lower back/close proximity to developing fetus)	Profuse bleeding
Laminectomy (close proximity to exposed central nervous tissue)	Deep vein thrombosis
Joint cement	Thrombophlebitis
Plastics utilized for prosthetics (heat rapidly when exposed to US)	
Pacemaker (close proximity may cause interference) or near other types of electronic implants/prosthesis	
Near other types of electronic implants/prosthesis	
Eyes (cavitation may damage structures)	
Carotid sinus/cervical ganglia (may cause baroreceptor stimulation)	
Over the heart	

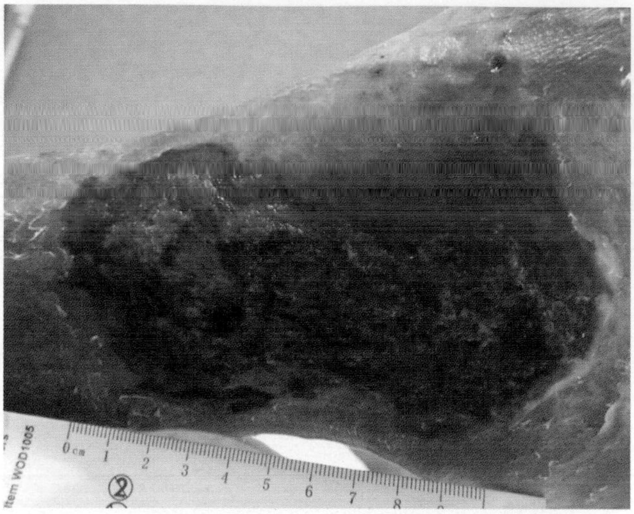

FIGURE 18-11 Calculation of ultrasound treatment time. The wound measures 11.5 cm × 5.0 cm with a total surface area of 57.5 cm². Noncontact LFUS application time would be determined by the equipment as 8 minutes.

TABLE 18-8 LFUS Treatment Parameters

Continuous mode, 100% duty cycle
Frequency: 20–40 kHz
Intensity: 0.1–0.5 W/cm²
Treatment duration, based on wound size ▪ <10 cm² = 3 minutes ▪ 10–19 cm² = 4 minutes ▪ 20–29 cm² = 5 minutes ▪ 30–39 cm² = 6 minutes ▪ 40–49 cm² = 7 minutes ▪ 50–59 cm² = 8 minutes ▪ 60–69 cm² = 9 minutes

treatment wand. The tubing attaches an IV bag to the handpiece. Before use, a sterile, single-use applicator is attached to the handpiece, leaving only the tip of the wand exposed.[55] An IV bag of sterile normal saline is attached to the device to serve as the transfer medium.[30] Clinical application of US requires *constant* movement of the US handpiece during sonation. Similar to traditional US, without constant movement, standing waves form due to sound wave reflection and have the potential to damage tissue (**FIGURE 18-12**).[17] The LFUS handpiece is held perpendicular to and 0.5 cm to 1.5 cm from the wound surface (**FIGURE 18-7**) and is moved slowly in both horizontal and vertical directions (creating a sort of checkerboard pattern).[17,53] As long as the handpiece is kept moving evenly within the predetermined treatment surface area, the exact speed of movement should not be a distraction from the overall application technique. Exceeding the predetermined treatment area will result in undersonation of the wound itself and less than optimal response. While the handpiece is held close to target tissues, there should never be direct contact between the treatment wand's metal tip (that extends slightly from the applicator) and wound tissue because the metal surface heats up during use, and contact can result in a burn.[20] **TABLE 18-9** shows application techniques for noncontact LFUS.[17,20,30,53,55] Application techniques for contact LFUS are presented in Chapter 13.

INFECTION CONTROL GUIDELINES

Clinicians using LFUS should follow facility guidelines regarding wearing personal protective equipment and infection control procedures (eg, ventilation) due to possible aerosolization of coupling mediums and potential vaporization of debrided tissue. Standard precautions apply anytime providers come into contact with body fluids, including drainage from open wounds. The noncontact LFUS device

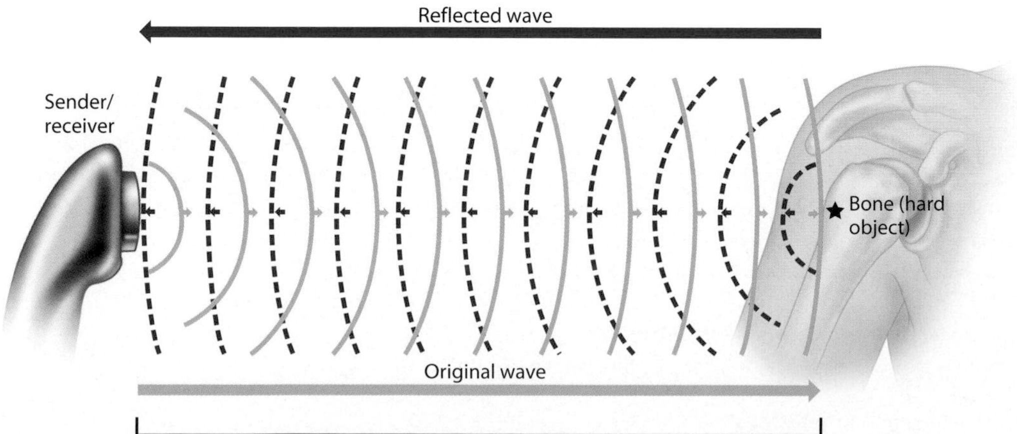

FIGURE 18-12 Illustration of reflected or standing sound waves.

CASE STUDY

INTRODUCTION

A 29-year-old patient is referred with nonhealing wounds on both lower extremities of more than 12 months' duration with a recent definitive diagnosis of polyarteritis nodosa. Polyarteritis nodosa is a vasculitic disease characterized by inflammation of the small arteries and arterioles that results in occluded vessels and subsequent skin necrosis. The wounds started as small, necrotic spots with surrounding tenderness and swelling and have now progressed to extensive wounds (**FIGURE 18-13 A-D**).

DISCUSSION QUESTION

1. What subjective and objective information is needed about this patient to develop a plan of care?

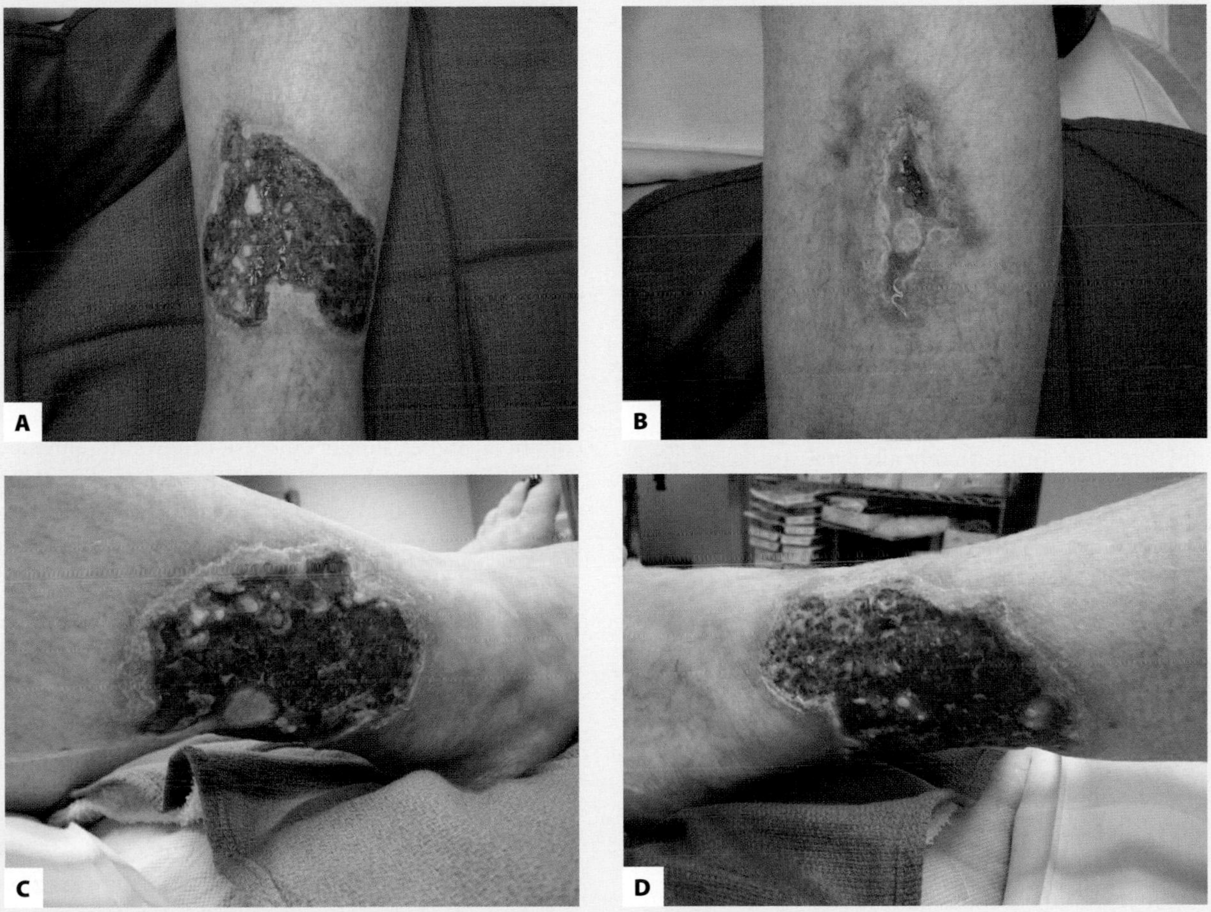

FIGURE 18-13 A–D. Photographs of the patient with lower extremity wounds due to polyarteritis nodosa at the time of initial evaluation.

TABLE 18-9 Noncontact LFUS Application Techniques

Points to Remember:
Keep US head moving at all times, and move evenly over the treatment area in overlapping vertical and horizontal lines.
Calculate wound surface area (cm^2) to determine treatment time.
Place an absorbent pad under the area being treated to absorb saline runoff during treatment.
Direct Application:
Expose the wound and appropriately drape the area.
Attach IV saline bag.
Direct the saline flow away from the wound initially until an even saline mist forms.
Hold the handpiece perpendicular to the wound with the disposable applicator 5–15 mm from the tissue.
Move the handpiece evenly and uniformly over the target tissue.
Avoid touching the applicator to the wound bed.

CASE STUDY

CONTINUED

The systems review (eg, cardiopulmonary, neurological, and musculoskeletal) for the patient was negative except for the integumentary evaluation, which revealed the following wounds:

Right lower extremity: 15 cm × 10 cm and 9.5 cm × 4.8 cm.

Left lower extremity: 10 cm × 8 cm and 5 cm × 1.7 cm.

Tissue: 70–80% granulation, 15–20% slough, and 5% fibrous. Edges are rolled and callused. Copious serous drainage is present from all wounds with 2+ pitting edema from the foot to the proximal calf. There are no signs of infection; however, pain levels were 8–10/10 with tactile stimulation.

Skin: Dry, no new nodules or lesions bilaterally.

Vascular assessment: 3+ dorsalis pedis and posterior tibialis bilaterally.

Sensation: Light touch, proprioception, and temperature are intact bilaterally.

Medications: Cytoxan, rituximab, methotrexate, Prednisone (40 mg/day), and Vicodin (as many as 8/day).

Nutrition: Good.

Social history: Lives with friends in a two-story house, works as a music executive.

Patient goals: Return to work 4 weeks after initiation of therapy, decrease pain medication, and participate in social functions.

DISCUSSION QUESTIONS

1. What aspects of this case make LFUS an appropriate possible intervention?
2. Are there any contraindications or precautions for using LFUS on this patient? Defend your answer.

utilizes a sterile, single-use, disposable applicator; however, the reusable handpiece and base unit are disinfected before and after use. Immediately after use, the used handpiece can be wrapped in a clean towel to reduce the risk of contact contamination of other surfaces until it can be disinfected.

LFUS SUMMARY

Multiple studies support the use of LFUS to enhance wound healing and tissue debridement. This evidence, combined with advances in application techniques and few strict contraindications, makes LFUS a valuable adjunct to facilitate the healing of both acute and chronic wounds.

CASE STUDY

CONCLUSION

Plan of care:

- Noncontact LFUS, initially 15 minutes bilaterally, decreases according to size as wounds progress.
- Selective debridement as pain allows.
- Nonadherent dressings (X-Cell, Medline Industries, Inc., Mundelein IL) to facilitate autolysis, maintain moisture balance, and reduce pain at dressing change.
- Multilayer compression bandages decrease edema and thereby decrease the drainage.
- Bilateral ankle active range of motion exercises to facilitate venous pump activity and decrease adhesions as healing occurs.

Frequency: 3 days a week, decreasing to 2 days a week as drainage and pain levels decrease.
Short-term goals:

- Decrease pain to less than 5/10 and pain medication to 1–2 per day.
- No pedal or lower extremity edema.
- Bilateral wounds in the proliferative phase of healing.
- At least 90% granulation tissue in all wounds.
- Visible epithelial migration at 75% of wound edges.
- Drainage controlled to allow participation in community activities.

Long-term goals:

- Full closure by secondary intention.
- No pain during normal daily activities.
- Able to wear compression stockings to prevent recurrent edema.
- Able to return to work.

Progress:
Week 1: Pain levels with treatment 1–2/10; discontinued pain medication at night; increased number of epithelial islands throughout bilateral wounds (**FIGURE 18-14 A-D**).

CASE STUDY (*Continued*)

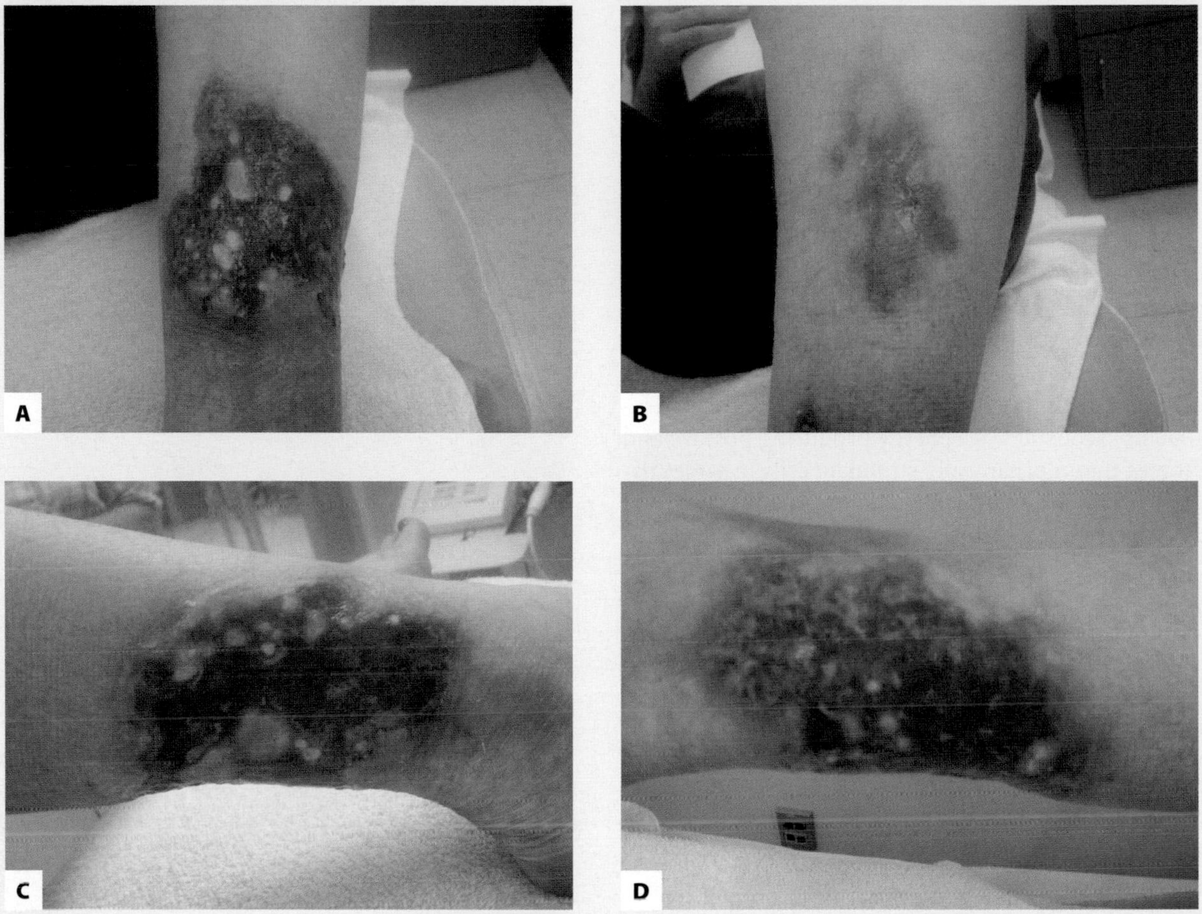

FIGURE 18-14 A–D. Photographs after 1 week of treatment with non contact LFUS and compression therapy.

Week 3: No pain during the day; sizes decreased to the following:

- Left lower extremity wounds: 6 cm × 4 cm (second wound closed and remodeling).
- Right lower extremity wounds: 8 cm × 3 cm and 9 cm × 7 cm.

Week 4: Returned to work, continued treatment two times/week.

Week 12: Wounds more than 50% re-epithelialized.

Week 24: All wounds re-epithelialized and remodeling except for a 1.2 cm × 0.3 cm opening on the left inferior wound, scant drainage present.

Week 26: All wounds closed and remodeling, transitioned to Class I compression stockings to prevent edema recurrence, initiated scar therapy with silicone sheeting (**FIGURE 18-15**).

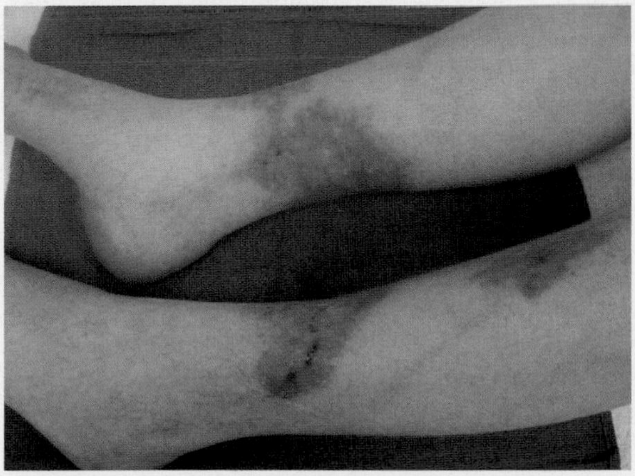

FIGURE 18-15 Photograph of the patient after full closure of all wounds, in the remodeling phase of healing.

EXTRACORPOREAL SHOCKWAVE THERAPY

Extracorporeal shockwave therapy (ESWT) has been used for many years in the treatment of various medical conditions including kidney stones (lithotripsy), bone healing, calcific tendinopathy, and plantar fasciitis.[55–57] Research on the use of ESWT as an adjunct therapy for wound healing began in 1986; however, it has experienced a somewhat slow, gradual implementation in the United States.[55,58,59] The ESWT dermaPACE System (Sanuwave, Inc., Eden Prairie, MN) was approved by the U.S. Food and Drug Administration in 2018 for the treatment of diabetic foot ulcers.[59,60] The following paragraphs provide a brief description of ESWT use for wound management.

ESWT devices utilize rapid rise, high peak, short duration (<1000 ns) acoustic wave energy producing positive and negative forces that mechanically stimulate cells in target tissues.[57,58,61,62] Depending upon application techniques, focused ESWT can penetrate as deep as 12 cm.[62]

Although the exact physiological mechanisms of shockwave therapy in wound healing are not yet fully understood, *mechanotransduction* is thought to be responsible for the biological changes that occur. Mechanotransduction is defined as the "transfer of mechanical stimuli into chemical signals."[63] With ESWT, cellular mechanosensory stimulation is an effect of cavitation[64] (similar to US) and results in the activation of gene expression of growth factors and cytokines, cellular proliferation, and cell differentiation.[65] The focus on ESWT clinical results thus far has been on the treatment of chronic wounds[56] for which ESWT has been shown to initiate an inflammatory response, stimulate fibroblasts, and upregulate the release of multiple growth factors.[56,60] Through these mechanisms, ESWT promotes quicker progression through inflammation, increases angiogenesis and epithelialization, decreases infection risk and pain, and can restart the healing cascade in chronic wounds.[56,59,60,66–68] Multiple studies document the potential benefit of including ESWT as an adjunct intervention in the treatment of hard-to-heal chronic wounds (eg, vascular insufficiency, diabetic foot ulcers, and pressure ulcers) and for the treatment of hypertrophic scaring.[56,57,59–61,69] At least some studies show possible application in acute/traumatic wounds and future studies may show benefit in burn wounds.[58,62,69] Some forms of ESWT may also disrupt the biofilm.[70,71]

A study in 2019 by Yang et al.[72] was aimed at demonstrating improved microcirculation in the feet of patients with diabetes and supported the results of earlier studies that demonstrated possible indications for ESWT to improve angiogenesis in skin flaps.[72] Similar to LFUS, ESWT is noninvasive, typically well tolerated, easy to use, and is relatively safe when applied appropriately.[56,59,66]

At the time of publication, the Sanuwave dermaPACE System is the primary ESWT device utilized for wound management. The device consists of a base unit and handpiece (**FIGURE 18-16A, B**). During application, the handpiece is covered with a single-use, sterile sleeve to prevent cross-contamination and uses proprietary sterile gel as the coupling medium.[60] The handpiece is held in contact with and perpendicular to wound tissue. The number of shocks is determined by wound surface area and patient comfort with treatments typically lasting 2–5 minutes one to three times a week. Indications and contraindications for dermaPACE System use for wound management are listed in **TABLE 18-10**.[62,73–75] Local erythema, petechiae, minimal pain, or small hematomas as well as nausea, dizziness, or migraine are possible short-term side effects of ESWT. Rare severe complications include local infection, muscle damage, thrombosis, or bleeding.[59,62,73]

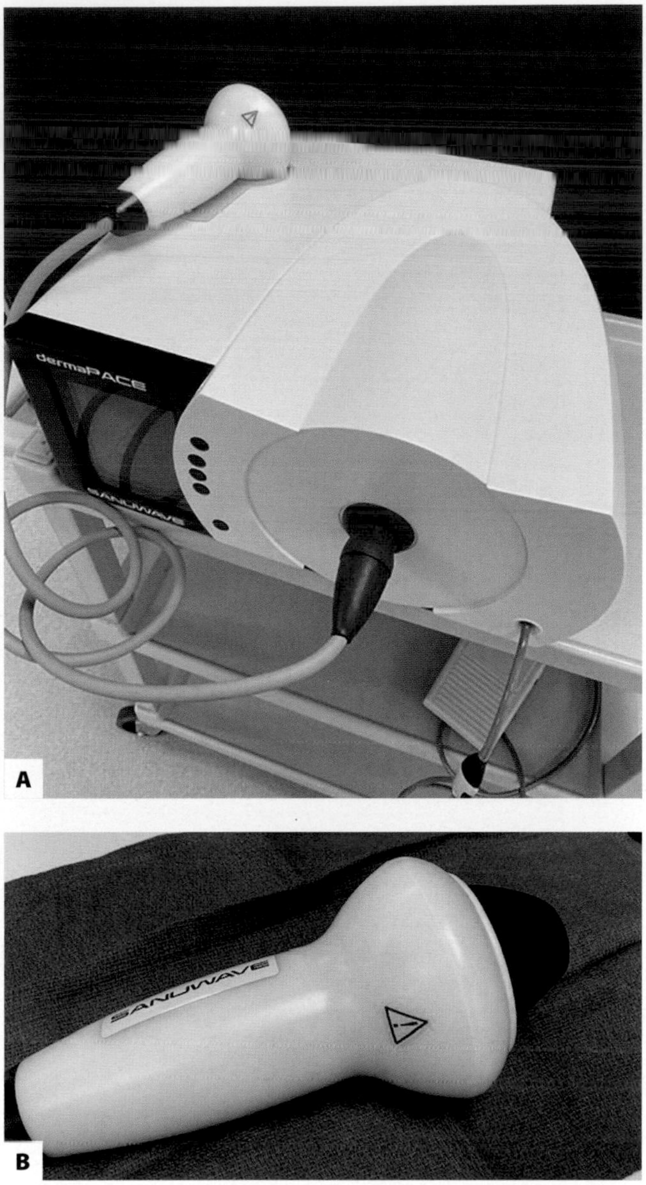

FIGURE 18-16 Sanuwave dermaPACE System. A. dermaPACE unit. B. dermaPACE handpiece. Sanuwave Wound Care Technologies, Suwanee, GA. (Pictures courtesy of Stephanie Woelfel, PT, DPT, CWS, Board Certified Wound Management Clinical Specialist.)

TABLE 18-10 Indications and Contraindications for ESWT

Indications	Contraindications (Not all-inclusive, check with the specific vendor prior to use)
▪ Chronic advanced-stage diabetic foot ulcers not responding to the standard of care for 30 days ▪ Full-thickness diabetic foot ulcers ▪ Wagner ulcer grade 1 or 2, stage A ▪ Wounds with <50% surface area reduction with the standard of care ▪ Wound area no larger than 16 cm^2 ▪ Adults 22 years and older	▪ Malignant changes in the treatment area ▪ Do not treat near the head, spine, lungs, bowels, gonads, fetus in a pregnant woman, or near electronic implants ▪ Presence of severe coagulopathy ▪ Not to be used on pediatric patients ▪ Do not use near oxygen-enriched environments, near flammable anesthetic gas mixtures, or other potentially explosive/flammable environments ▪ Possible increased risk of developing osteomyelitis when >7 treatments are given

STUDY QUESTIONS

1. The LFUS frequency range used to facilitate tissue repair and wound healing is
   a. Less than 20 kHz.
   b. 20–40 kHz.
   c. 3–7 MHz.
   d. 8–18 MHz.
2. The formation of gaseous bubbles that implode and release pressure that may cause tissue damage and facilitate the breakdown of necrotic tissue is termed
   a. Microstreaming.
   b. Stable cavitation.
   c. Unstable cavitation.
   d. Banding.
3. Which of the following conditions is an absolute contraindication for the use of noncontact LFUS?
   a. Vasculitis.
   b. Any painful wound.
   c. Arterial insufficiency.
   d. Malignant tissue.
4. Ultrasound is indicated in any of the wound healing phases except
   a. Hemostasis.
   b. Inflammation.
   c. Proliferation.
   d. Remodeling.
5. The mechanism by which ESWT produces cellular activity is
   a. Down-regulation.
   b. Extracellular signaling.
   c. Mechanotransduction.
   d. Microstreaming.

Answers: 1-b; 2-c; 3-d; 4-a; 5-c.

REFERENCES

1. Baril DT, Marone LK. Duplex evaluation following femoropopliteal angioplasty and stenting: criteria and utility of surveillance. *Vasc Endovasc Surg*. 2012;46(5):353-357.
2. Kloth LC, Niezgoda JA. Ultrasound for wound debridement and healing. In: McCulloch JM, Kloth LC, eds. *Wound Healing: Evidence-Based Management*. 4th ed. Philadelphia, PA: FA Davis Company; 2012.
3. Obata-Yasuoka M, Hamada H, Ohara R, Nakao A, Miyazono Y, Yoshikawa H. Alveolar capillary dysplasia associated with duodenal atresia: ultrasonographic findings of enlarged, highly echogenic lungs and gastric dilatation in a third-trimester fetus. *J Obstet Gynaecol Res*. 2011;37(7):937-939.
4. McNeil CR, McManus J, Mehta S. The accuracy of portable ultrasonography to diagnose fractures in an austere environment. *Prehosp Emerg Care*. 2009;13(4):50-52.
5. Deter RL, Lee W, Dicker P, et al. Third-trimester growth diversity in small fetuses classified as appropriate-for-gestational age or small-for gestational age at birth. *Ultrasound Obstet Gynecol*. 2021;58: 882-891.
6. Malik AN, Rowland J, Haber BD, et al. The use of handheld ultrasound devices in emergency medicine. *Curr Emerg Hosp Med Rep*. 2021;9:73-81.
7. Allen GM, Wilson DJ, Bullock SA, Watson M. Extremity CT and ultrasound in the assessment of ankle injuries: occult fractures and ligament injuries. *Br J Radiol*. 2020;93(1105):20180989.
8. Voss HJ, Voorneveld JD, Jebbink EG, et al. Contrast-enhanced high-frame-rate ultrasounds imaging of flow patterns in cardiac chambers and deep vessels. *Ultrasound Med Biol*. 2020;46(11): 2875-2890.
9. Kavros SJ, Coronado R. Diagnostic and therapeutic ultrasound on venous and arterial ulcers: a focused review. *Adv Skin Wound Care*. 2018;31(2):55-65.
10. Goldsmith AJ, Shokoohi H, Loesche M, et al. Point-of-care ultrasound in morbidity and mortality cases in emergency medicine: who benefits the most? *West J Emerg Med*. 2020; 21(6):172-178.
11. Horvath L, Kraft M. Evaluation of ultrasound and fine-needle aspiration in the assessment of head and neck lesions. *Eur Arch Otorhinolaryngol*. 2019;276(10):2903-2911.

12. Afif AM, Laroco OD, Lau SMD, et al. Usefulness of ultrasound fusion technology for hepatocellular carcinoma localization, pre- and post-thermal ablation. *Ultrasound*. 2022;30(3):194-200.
13. Zhang J, Li H, Lin L, Lu J, Wang H. Ultrasound guided microwave ablation for multiple benign breast lesions: a prospective study. *J Obstet Gynaecol Res*. 2021;47(9):3362-3369.
14. Elbaset MA, Elkarta A, Eraky A, Badawy M, Sheir KZ, Shokeir AA. [illegible] prediction of factors affecting stone-clearance post-shockwave lithotripsy for ureteral stones: a prospective study. *Int J Nephrol Urol*. 2020;52(9):1643-1649.
15. Duscher D, Maan ZN, Luan A, et al. Ultrasound-assisted liposuction provides a source for functional adipose-derived stromal cells. *Cytotherapy*. 2017;19(12):1491-1500.
16. Tian Y, Liu Z, Tan H, et al. New aspects of ultrasound-mediated targeted delivery and therapy for cancer. *Int J Nanomedicine*. 2020;15:401-418.
17. Buchanan V, Rawat M. Schwannoma of the posterior tibial nerve. *J Orthop Sports Phys Ther*. 2020;50(2):111.
18. Cameron MH. *Physical Agents in Rehabilitation: An Evidence-Based Approach to Practice*. 5th ed. St Louis, MO: Elsevier; 2018.
19. Hayes KW, Hall KD. *Manual for Physical Agents*. 6th ed. Upper Saddle River, NJ: Pearson Education, Inc; 2012.
20. UltraMIST®. Available at: https://www.woundsource.com/product/ultramist. Accessed November 13, 2022.
21. Wiegand C, Bittenger K, Galiano RD, Driver VR, Gibbons GW. Does noncontact low-frequency ultrasound therapy contribute to wound healing at the molecular level? *Wound Repair Regen*. 2017;25(5):871-882.
22. Conner-Kerr T, Alston G, Stoval A, et al. The effects of low-frequency ultrasound (35 kHz) on methicillin-resistant *Staphylococcus aureus* (MRSA) in vitro. *Ostomy Wound Manage*. 2010;56(5):32-43.
23. Li X, Liu S, Lai X, et al. A pilot study of ultrasonically assisted treatment of residual burn wounds. *Wounds*. 2009;21(10):267-272.
24. Serena T, Lee SK, Lam K, Attar P, Meneses P, Ennis W. The impact of noncontact, nonthermal, low-frequency ultrasound on bacterial counts in experimental and chronic wounds. *Ostomy Wound Manage*. 2009;55(1):22-30.
25. Ennis WJ, Valdes W, Gainer M, Meneses P. Evaluation of clinical effectiveness of MIST ultrasound therapy for the healing of chronic wounds. *Adv Skin Wound Care*. 2006;19(8):437-446.
26. Chenyu H, Du Y, Ogawa R. Chapter 15: mechanobiology and mechanotherapy for cutaneous wound-healing. In: Rawlinson SCF, ed. *Mechanobiology: Exploitation for Medical Benefit*. Hoboken, NJ: John Wiley & Sons; 2017:239-255.
27. Viana L, Pompeo M. Healing rate of chronic and subacute lower extremity ulcers treated with contact ultrasound followed by noncontact ultrasound therapy: the VIP ultrasound protocol. *Wounds*. 2017;29(8):231-253.
28. Voigt J, Wendelken M, Driver V, Alvarez OM. Low-frequency ultrasound (20-40 kHz) as an adjunctive therapy for chronic wound healing: a systematic review of the literature and meta-analysis of eight randomized controlled trials. *Int J Low Extrem Wounds*. 2011;10(4):190-199.
29. Ennis WJ, Lee C, Meneses P. A biochemical approach to wound healing through the use of modalities. *Clin Dermatol*. 2007;25(1):63-72.
30. Cordrey R. Chapter 24: Ultraviolet light and ultrasound. In Bryant RA, Nix DP eds. *Acute & Chronic Wounds: Current Management Concepts*. St. Louis, MO: Elsevier; 2016:377-385.
31. Driver VR, Yao M, Miller CJ. Noncontact low-frequency ultrasound therapy in the treatment of chronic wounds: a meta-analysis. *Wound Respir Regen*. 2011;19(4):475-480.
32. Kataoka Y, Kunimitsu M, Nakagami G, Koudounas S, Weller CD, Sanada H. Effectiveness of ultrasonic debridement on reduction of bacteria and biofilm in patients with chronic wounds: a scoping review. *Int Wound J*. 2021;18:176-186.
33. Altomare M, Nascimento A, Romana-Souza B, Amadeu TP, Monte-Alto-Costa A. Ultrasound accelerates healing of normal wounds but not of ischemic ones. *Wound Repair Regen*. 2009;17(6):825-831.
34. Bell AL, Cavorsi J. Noncontact ultrasound therapy for adjunctive treatment of nonhealing wounds: retrospective analysis. *Phys Ther*. 2008;88(12):1517-1524.
35. Jeremias SL, Camanho GL, Bassit ACF, Forgas A, Ingham SJM, Abdalla RJ. Low-intensity pulsed ultrasound accelerates healing in rat calcaneus tendon injuries. *J Orthop Sports Phys Ther*. 2011;41(7):526-531.
36. Fu SC, Shum WT, Hung LK, Wong MWN, Qin L, Chang KM. Low-intensity pulsed ultrasound on tendon healing: as study of the effect of treatment duration and treatment initiation. *Am J Sports Med*. 2008;36(9):1742-1749.
37. Kotronis G, Vas PRJ. Ultrasound devices to treat chronic wounds: the current level of evidence. *Int J Low Extrem Wounds*. 2020;19(4):341-349.
38. Wagner-Cox P, Duhame HM, Jamison DR, Jackson RR, Fehr ST. Use of noncontact low-frequency ultrasound in deep tissue pressure injury. *J Wound Ostomy Continence Nurs*. 2017;44(4):336-342.
39. Swoboda L. Biofilm-based wound management: implications for clinical practice. *Wound Manag Prev*. 2022;68(8):6-7.
40. Gibbons GW, Orgill DP, Serena TE, et al. A prospective, randomized, controlled trial comparing the effects of noncontact, low-frequency ultrasound to standard care in venous leg ulcers. *Ostomy Wound Manage*. 2015;61(1):16-29.
41. Vallejo A, Wallis M, McMillian D, Horton E. Use of low-frequency contact ultrasound debridement with and without polyhexamethylene biguanide in hard-to-heal leg ulcers: an RCT protocol. *J Wound Care*. 2021;30(5):372-379.
42. Granick MS, Paribathan C, Shanmugam M, Ramasubbu N. Direct-contact low-frequency ultrasound clearance of biofilm from metallic implant materials. *Eplasty*. 2017;29(17):128–134.
43. Murphy CA, Houghton P, Brandys T, Rose G, Bryant D. The effect of 22.5 kHz low-frequency contact ultrasound debridement (LFCUD) on lower extremity wound healing for a vascular surgery population: a randomized controlled trial. *Int Wound J*. 2017;15:460-472.
44. Qoustic Wound Therapy System™. 2022. Arobella Medical, LLC. Available at: http://arobella.com/products/. Accessed November 13, 2022.
45. SONOCA-185. Soring USA Web site. Available at: https://www.soering.de/en/products/soering-ultrasonic-generators/sonoca-185/. Accessed November 13, 2022.
46. Sonicone®O.R. Ultrasonic Debridement with Aspiration. Bioventus®, LLC. Available at: https://misonix.com/products/sonicone-or/. 2022. Accessed November 13, 2022.
47. Ultrasonic-assisted wound debridement (UAW). Available at: https://www.soering.de/en/applications/wound-debridement/. Accessed November 13, 2022.
48. Mallow PJ, Hiebert JM, Robson MC. Cost effectiveness of hypochlorous acid preserved wound cleanser versus saline irrigation in conjunction with ultrasonic debridement for complex wounds. *J Health Econ Outcomes Res*. 2021;8(2):76-81.
49. Hiebert JM, Robson MC. The immediate and delayed post-debridement effects on tissue bacterial wound counts of hypochlorous acid versus saline irrigation in chronic wounds. *Eplasty*. 2016;16:e32.

50. Chang YJR, Perry J, Cross K. Low-frequency ultrasound debridement in chronic wound healing: a systematic review of current literature. *Plast Surg*. 2017;25(1):21-26.
51. Ennis WJ, Formann P, Mozen N, et al. Ultrasound therapy for recalcitrant diabetic foot ulcers: results of a randomized, double-blind, controlled, multicenter study. *Ostomy Wound Manage*. 2005;51(8):24-39.
52. Prather JL, Tummel EK, Patel AB, Smith DJ, Gould LJ. Prospective randomized controlled trial comparing the effects of noncontact low-frequency ultrasound with standard care in healing split-thickness donor sites. *J Am Coll Surg*. 2015;221(2):309-318.
53. Reference Guide, UltraMIST Ultrasound Healing Therapy. Sanuwave Wound Care Technologies. 2021. Available at: UM_QuickRefGuide.pdf. Accessed October 20, 2022.
54. Honaker JS, Forston MR, Davis EA, Weisner MM, Morgan JA, Sacca E. The effect of adjunctive noncontact low frequency ultrasound on deep tissue pressure injury. *Wound Repair Regen*. 2016;24:1081-1088.
55. Mittermayr R, Antonic V, Hartinger J, et al. Extracorporeal shock wave therapy (ESWT) for wound healing: technology, mechanisms, and clinical efficacy. *Wound Repair Regen*. 2012;20:456-465.
56. Chuangsuwanich A, Kongkunnavat N, Kamanamool M, Maipeng G, Kamanamool N, Tonaree W. Extracorporeal shock wave therapy for hypertrophic scars. *Arch Plast Surg*. 2022;49:554-560.
57. Omar MTA, Gwada RFM, Shaheen AAM. Extracorporeal shockwave therapy for the treatment of chronic wound of lower extremity: current perspectives and systematic review. *Int Wound J*. 2017;14(6):898-908.
58. Zissler A, Stoiber W, Pittner S, Sanger, AM. Extracorporeal shockwave therapy in acute injury care: a systematic review. *Rehabil Process Outcome*. 2018;7:1-13.
59. Huang Q, Peijing Y, Xiong H, et al. Extracorporeal shock wave therapy for treating foot ulcers in adults with type 1 and type 2 diabetes: a systematic review and meta-analysis of randomized controlled trials. *Can J Diabetes*. 2020;44:196-204.
60. Snyder R, Galiano R, Mayer P, Rogers LC, Alvarez O. Diabetic foot ulcer treatment with focused shockwave therapy: two multicentre, prospective, controlled, double-blinded, randomized phase III clinical trials. *J Wound Care*. 2018;27(2):822-836.
61. Miller C, Kapp S, Green J, McGuiness W, Woodward M. Treating venous leg ulcers with extracorporeal shockwave technology (ESWT). *Wounds Int*. 2017;8(3):22-28.
62. Aguilera-Saez J, Munoz P, Serracanta J, Monte A, Barret JP. Extracorporeal shock wave therapy role in the treatment of burn patients. A systematic literature review. *Burns*. 2020;46(7):1525-1532.
63. Cayton T, Harwood AE, Smith GE, et al. Extracorporeal shockwave therapy for the treatment of lower limb intermittent claudication: study protocol for a randomised controlled trial (the SHOCKWAVE 1 trial). *Trials*. 2017;18:104.
64. Mariotto S. Extracorporeal shock wave therapy in inflammatory diseases: molecular mechanism that triggers anti-inflammatory action. *Curr Med Chem*. 2009;16(19):2366-2372.
65. Frairia R, Berta L. Biological effects of extracorporeal waves on fibroblasts: a review. *Muscles Ligaments Tendons J*. 2011;1(4):138-147.
66. Zhang L, Weng C, Zhao Z, Fu X. Extracorporeal shock wave therapy for chronic wounds: a systematic review and meta-analysis of randomized controlled trials. *Wound Repair Regen*. 2017;25:697-706.
67. Chen RF, Chang CH, Wang CT, et al. Modulation of vascular endothelial growth factor and mitogen-activated protein kinase-related pathway involved in extracorporeal shockwave therapy accelerate diabetic wound healing. *Wound Repair Regen*. 2019;27:69-79.
68. Fu S, Panayi A, Fan J, et al. Mechanotransduction in wound healing: from the cellular and molecular level to the clinic. *Adv Skin Wound*. 2021;34:67-74.
69. Aguilera-Saez J, dos Santos BP, Serracanta J, et al. The effect of extracorporeal shock wave therapy in the treatment of burn scars: a prospective, randomized, controlled trial. *Burns*. 2022;48(3):577-584.
70. Milstrey A, Rosslenbroich S, Everding J, et al. Antibiofilm efficacy of focused high-energy extracorporeal shockwaves and antibiotics in vitro. *Bone Joint Res*. 2021;10(1):77-84.
71. Yao W, Kuan EC, Grundfest WS, St John MA. Safety of lasser-generated shockwave treatment for bacterial biofilms in a cutaneous rodent model. *Lasers Med Sci*. 2021;36:1403-1410.
72. Yang JP, Lee YN, Son JW, Han SK. The impact of extracorporeal shock wave therapy on microcirculation in diabetic feet: a pilot study. *Adv Skin Wound*. 2019;32(12):563-567.
73. De Novo Classification Requests for dermaPACE System. Available at: https://www.accessdata.fda.gov/cdrh_docs/reviews/DEN160037.pdf. Accessed November 13, 2022.
74. Supercharge Your Patient Care and Reduce Costs: Heal Wounds With Energy First Using dermaPACE®. 2021. Available at: https://sanuwave.com/wp-content/uploads/2021/04/dermaPACE-Sales-Sheet-for-Wound-Care-Centers.pdf. Accessed November 13, 2022.
75. Galiano R, Snyder R, Mayer P, Rogers LC, Alvarez O. Focused shockwave therapy in diabetic foot ulcers: secondary endpoints of two multicentre randomized controlled trials. *J Wound Care*. 2019;28(6):383-395.

Pulsed Lavage with Suction

Karen A. Gibbs, PT, PhD, DPT, CWS and Rose L. Hamm, PT, DPT, FACCWS

CHAPTER OBJECTIVES

At the end of this chapter, the learner will be able to:

1. **Describe the mechanical effects of pulsed lavage with suction at the cellular and tissue levels.**
2. **Select patient situations when the use of pulsed lavage with suction might be indicated.**
3. **Relate advantages and disadvantages of using pulsed lavage with suction for wound healing.**
4. **Apply precautions during the use of pulsed lavage with suction for wound treatment.**
5. **Recall and explain infection control precautions used during pulsed lavage with suction treatment.**

INTRODUCTION

Pulsed lavage is a portable, battery-powered, handheld device that delivers pulsed, sterile irrigation fluid onto the wound surface. The handpiece is connected to either wall or portable suction which allows for simultaneous suction and removal of contaminated irrigation fluid and wound debris (**FIGURE 19-1**). The combination of pulsed lavage with concurrent suction, or pulsed lavage with suction (PLWS), can be used for wound cleansing, removal of topical agents, irrigation and tissue hydration, mechanical debridement, reduction of surface bacteria, and stimulation of cells associated with tissue healing and wound closure.[1–3]

PLWS has been used in healthcare for decades beginning in the 1960s when US Army physicians first modified WaterPik units for irrigating contaminated combat wounds.[4–7] Today, wall or portable suction facilitates the use of PLWS for surgical irrigation as well as wound management in inpatient, outpatient, and home health settings.[1,8] Battery-powered hand-pieces are easy to grip and maneuver and some systems offer an assortment of tips for different wound sizes and locations (**FIGURE 19-2**). The basic equipment requirements are essentially the same for any system and are listed in **TABLE 19-1**.

MECHANISM OF ACTION

PLWS delivers pulsed, positive-pressure irrigation at controlled pounds per square inch (psi) along with simultaneous negative pressure removal of contaminated irrigation fluid by suction, combining the benefits of both positive and negative pressures in one modality. The combination of these pressure forces facilitates wound cleansing, debridement of slough and loosening of nonviable tissue, reduction of surface bacteria, increased local perfusion, and stimulation of granulation tissue.[1–3,9]

Positive Pressure

Positive pressure hydrotherapy for the management of open wounds assists in general wound cleansing and tissue hydration; targeted, mechanical, nonselective debridement; and tissue stimulation (**TABLE 19-2**). Whirlpool (WP) therapy, once considered the primary method of hydrotherapy,[2,3,9,10] utilizes a turbine to generate positive pressure irrigation (**FIGURE 19-3**). However, unlike PLWS, the psi generated by the WP turbine cannot be predetermined and changes drastically depending on how close or far away from the turbine the body segment is positioned.[10,11] Research supports that positive pressure hydrotherapy delivered at less than 4 psi can be ineffective for wound cleansing and debridement; too high and wound tissues are damaged and surface bacteria may be pushed deeper into the wound bed.[2,3,11–14] For safe and effective delivery, the Agency for Health Care Policy and Research, the National Pressure Injury Advisory Panel, and the European Pressure Ulcer Advisory Panel recommend irrigation pressures between 4 and 15 psi for wound management.[2,15] PLWS units are designed so that providers select known psi settings within the safe 4–15 psi range (**FIGURE 19-4**).

Another benefit of PLWS over WP is the small, soft, pliable, cone-shaped applicator tip which allows delivery of sterile, positive-pressure hydrotherapy to specifically targeted tissues which reduce the risk of further wound contamination.[16]

Negative Pressure

Benefits associated with the negative pressure component of PLWS are tissue stimulation, locally increased perfusion, reduction of surface bacteria (**FIGURE 19-5**), and removal of irrigation fluid (**TABLE 19-3**).[9] The suction force generated from the negative pressure stimulates granulation tissue proliferation and epithelialization through the process of cellular deformation and strain.[17,18] Negative pressure also increases

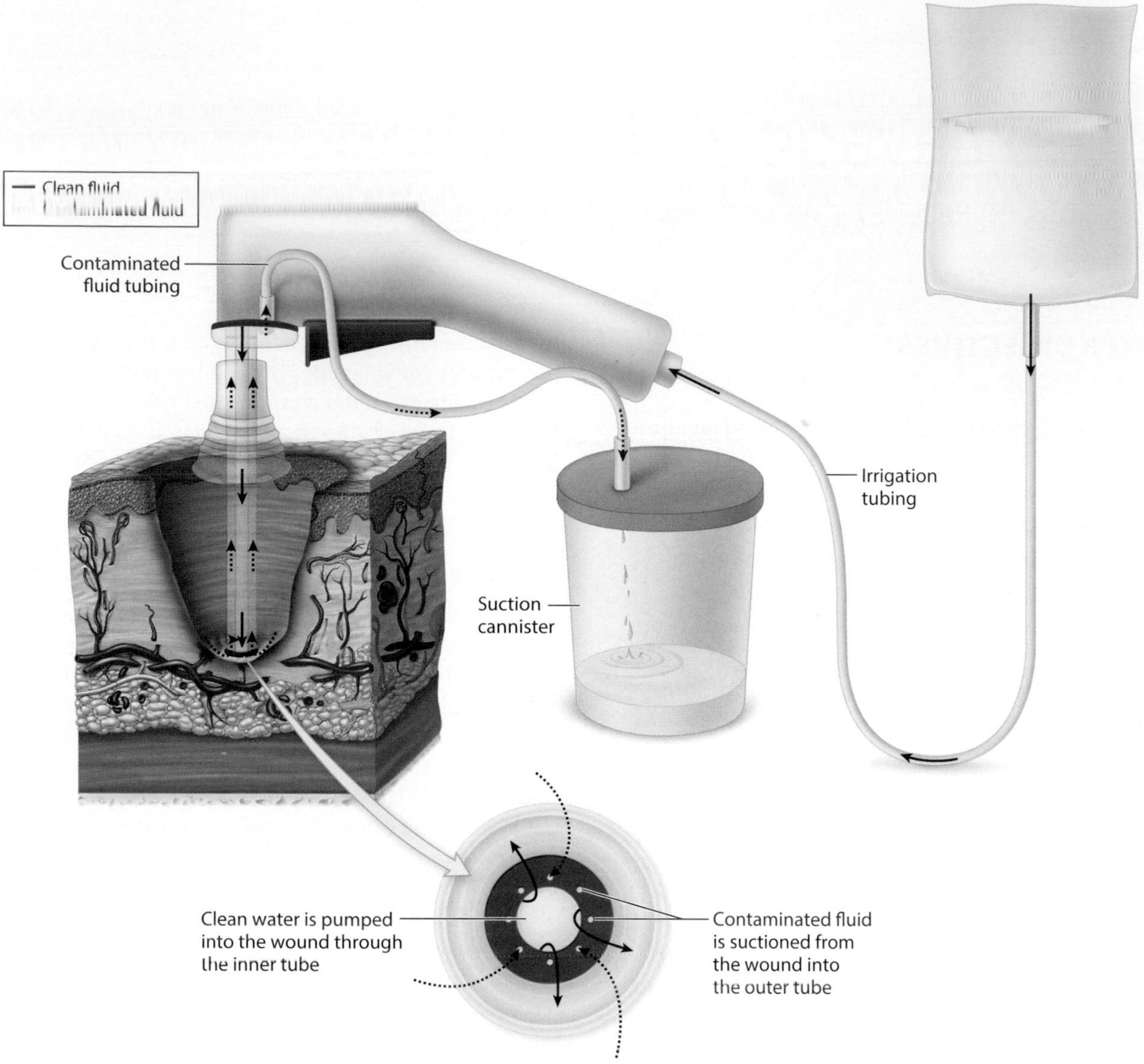

FIGURE 19-1 Components of pulsed lavage with suction. Irrigation fluid flows from the irrigation bag, through the tubing, into the handpiece, and through a central opening in the tip. As it is pulsed onto the wound bed, the contaminated fluid is suctioned through a concentric outer opening, into the return tubing, and into the fluid collection canister. Equipment setup includes connection of tubing to the irrigation bag and collection canister but also to a suction force, either wall or portable suction (suction force not pictured here).

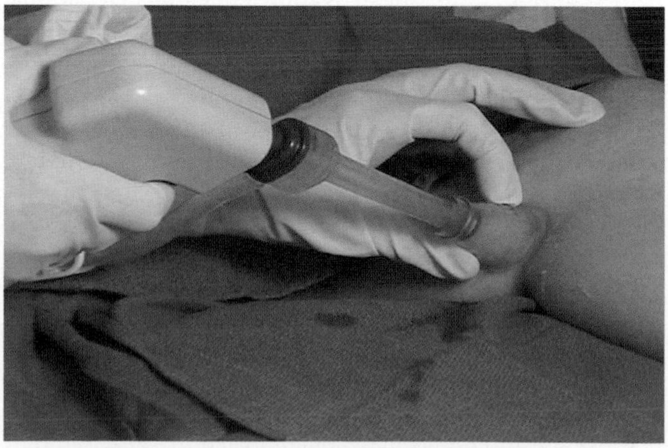

FIGURE 19-2 Photo of handpiece. The pulsed lavage handpiece *pulses* irrigation solution onto the wound with a known, controlled psi and *suctions* the contaminated fluid into collection canister. The therapist's fingers are used to maintain good contact between the tip and wound tissue. This helps prevent spillage and aerosolization of the fluid, directs the flow of the solution into the desired area, and provides maximum benefit of negative pressure stimulation. PLWS provides a sterile, closed system for irrigating open wounds in a variety of settings.

TABLE 19-1 PLWS Equipment Requirements

Irrigation fluid collection canister
IV bag of warm (37–38°C) irrigation solution Plastic tubing from suction to canister
PLWS single-use handpiece with tubing
Single-use tip with plastic tubing
Tubing connecting suction force to canister
Wall or portable suction

TABLE 19-2 Benefits of PLWS Positive Pressure

Hydration and loosening of adherent, nonviable tissue
Known safe psi for wound irrigation
Targeted, mechanical debridement of loose nonviable tissue and slough
Reduction of surface bacteria
Stimulation of healthy wound tissue
Wound cleansing and exudate removal

tissue perfusion by causing arterioles to dilate, thus increasing local blood flow.[17] Increased perfusion supports granulation tissue formation and enhances the body's ability to phagocytose bacteria in the wound.

PLWS also assists in reducing bioburden through the physical removal of loosened nonviable tissue and bacteria from the wound environment. Removal of nonviable tissue also decreases nutrients available for remaining bacteria.[2,19] Additionally, pressurized irrigation removes microorganisms from the wound surface and exudate as the irrigation fluid is evacuated. While normal saline is frequently used for irrigation, bioburden may also be decreased by adding topical antiseptics or antimicrobial solutions to irrigation fluids.[1–3] This can be especially beneficial when treating patients who are severely immunocompromised and/or have heavily contaminated, traumatic injuries with or without exposed bone.[1,2] There is no promotion of bacterial resistance (an increasing concern as drug resistance increases) when normal saline is used alone as the irrigation fluid.[1,20] When using other irrigation solutions (eg, bacitracin, sodium hypochlorite, etc.), the potential for allergic reactions to those medications or additives must be considered whereas normal saline has little to no allergic potential.[1] The selection of irrigation solution is based on systemic as well as local wound presentation.[2]

CLINICAL CONSIDERATION

Using normal saline is usually sufficient for wound cleansing and debridement; careful consideration is advised before adding agents to normal saline irrigation fluid. While antibiotic and toxic solutions temporarily decrease wound bioburden, they may damage tissues and kill healthy wound cells, allowing bacteria levels to rebound and causing delays in wound healing.[2,21]

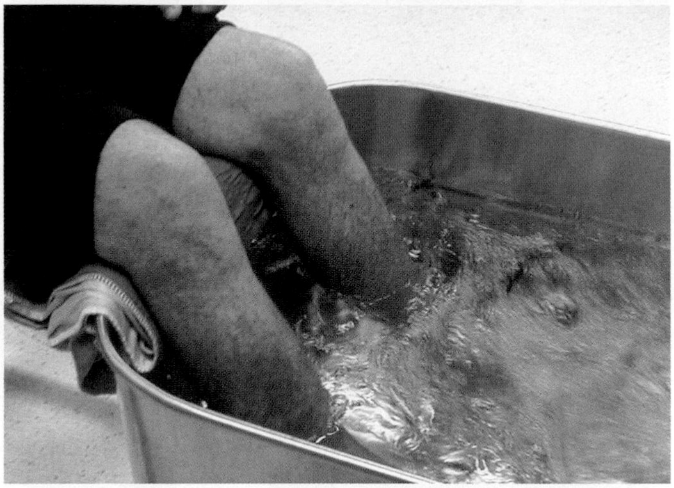

FIGURE 19-3 Whirlpool. The whirlpool turbine provides positive pressure to the treatment and surrounding area; however, the psi is undetermined. Detrimental effects of treating extremities in a dependent position, inability to isolate wounds during treatment and risk of cross contamination, and inability to treat patients who cannot be transported to or tolerate immersion hydrotherapy are just a few reasons whirlpool is no longer considered standard of care for the majority of wounds that require more than basic cleansing and irrigation.

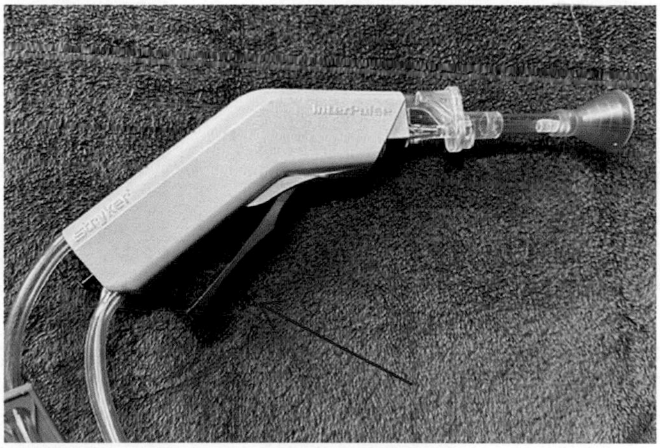

FIGURE 19-4 PLWS handpiece. PSI is controlled by the amount of pressure used to squeeze the trigger. The tip on this unit its a flexible cone that produces negative pressure when good contact is maintained with the wound or periwound tissue. One tube delivers the fluid to the wound; the other transports fluid from the wound bed to the collection container.

TABLE 19-3 Benefits of PLWS Negative Pressure

Convenient removal of irrigation fluid
Increased local perfusion
Reduction of surface bacteria
Stimulation of granulation tissue and epithelialization

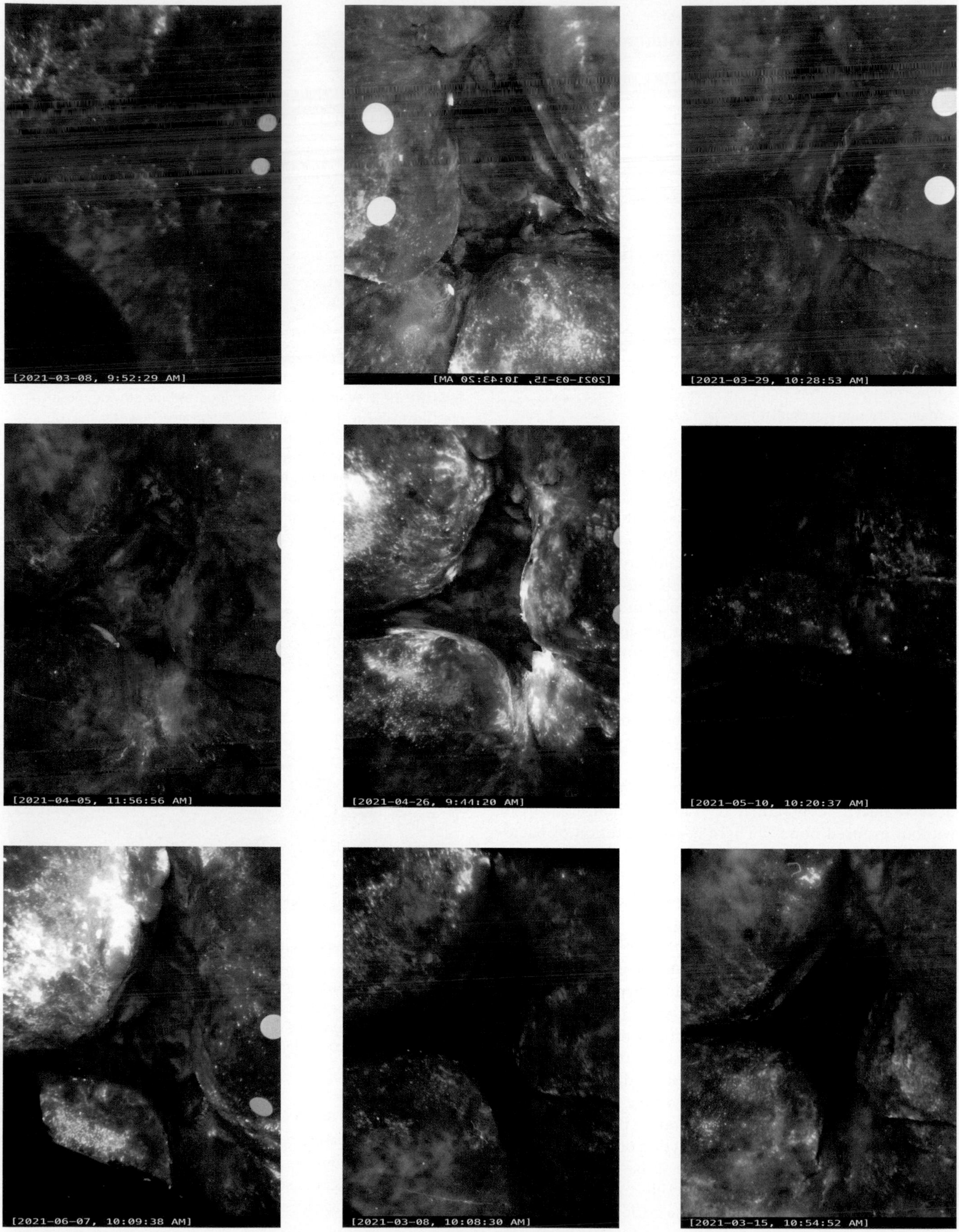

FIGURE 19-5 Bacteria load imaging on a wound using fluorescence imaging before and after treatment with pulsed lavage with suction. (Photographs complements of Dr. James Stiehl, used with permission.)

CASE STUDY

INTRODUCTION

A 34-year-old patient with a history of type 2 diabetes had gastric bypass surgery for morbid obesity followed by hernia repair with mesh reinforcement. The hernia repair incision, located in the right lower abdomen, became necrotic, dehisced, and ultimately required surgical incision and drainage (I&D) to remove infected tissue. The patient is referred for wound care evaluation and treatment in preparation for surgical closure. There is moderate serosanguinous drainage. The wound measures 18.5 cm × 12.7 cm × 3.8 cm and tunnels to a second (medial) opening measuring 3.6 cm × 1.7 cm (**FIGURE 19-6**).

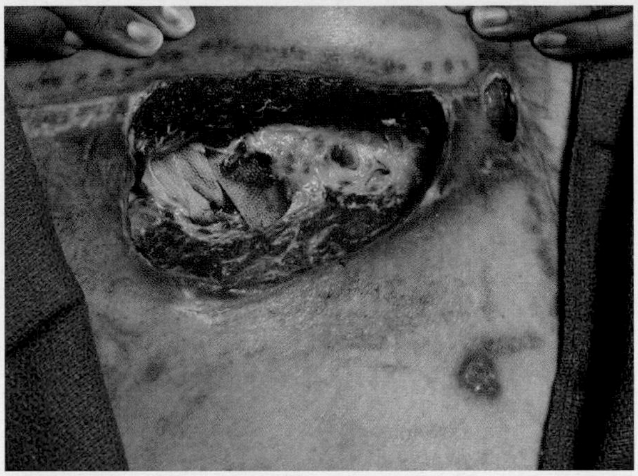

FIGURE 19-6 Patient picture. Right lower abdominal wound, secondary to dehisced hernia repair and subsequent I&D, at the time of wound evaluation.

DISCUSSION QUESTIONS

1. What subjective and objective information is needed to develop a plan of care?
2. What tissues (along with percentage of each) are visible in the wound beds?

EFFECTS AT THE TISSUE AND CELLULAR LEVELS

When a pulse of water strikes a tissue, the force of the pulse causes a brief compression of that tissue.[7,22] Between pulses, target tissues decompress or recoil. PLWS produces multiple, rapid iterations of tissue compression-decompression cycles that mechanically dislodge bacteria, nonviable tissue, and debris from the wound bed.[19] Adherent nonviable tissue remaining after a PLWS treatment is hydrated and loosened, thus facilitating natural phagocytosis and easier tissue-specific sharp debridement.[2,3] Compression–decompression mechanical manipulation also assists in exudate removal. Exudate removal is especially important as chronic wound fluid has long been known to damage healthy wound tissues and contribute to delayed healing (**FIGURE 19-7**).[23–29]

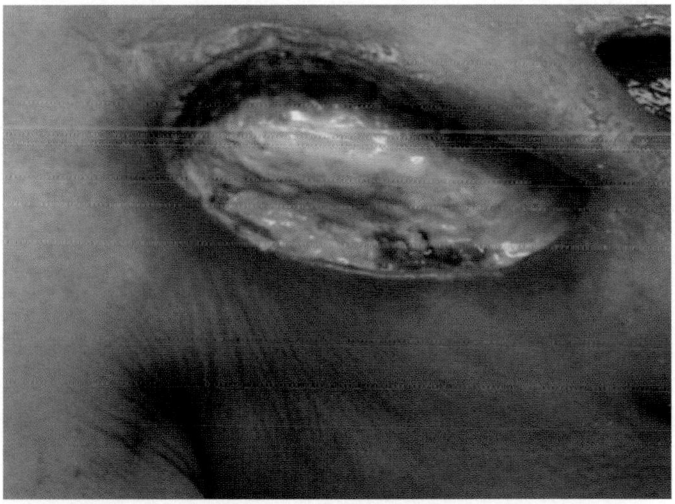

FIGURE 19-7 Wound with adhered fibrous tissue that can be loosened with PLWS, making selective debridement more effective. PLWS also removes wound exudate containing chronic wound fluid components such as matrix metalloproteases (MMPs) that are detrimental to healing.

The negative pressure component of PLWS also produces significant effects at the tissue and cellular levels via mechanical stress or stretch on structural components of extracellular matrix and local cells.[17,26,27,30] Cellular mechanical deformation promotes granulation tissue formation by stimulating increased protein synthesis by fibroblasts and by increasing cellular proliferation.[18,31]

The potential for wound hypothermia when using PLWS with cool irrigation fluid is a concern. Wounds heal faster when the wound temperature is close to normal body temperature (37–38°C) and it can take hours for wound tissue to recover from cool temperature irrigation. Warm irrigation fluids positively affect tissues by facilitating local increased vasodilation.[19,20] Necessary components for tissue healing are delivered through the blood and stimulating increased local blood flow delivers more leukocytes (white blood cells), antibodies, oxygen, and nutrients to the wound site.[19,20] Increased local vasodilation also improves the delivery of systemic antibiotics to the area and increases the removal of toxic waste products.

INDICATIONS

PLWS is indicated for atraumatic wound cleansing, tissue hydration, mechanical debridement, tissue stimulation, and bacterial reduction (**TABLE 19-4**). Etiologies appropriate for PLWS include wounds associated with neuropathy, pressure, venous insufficiency, post-surgical incisional dehiscence, or

TABLE 19-4 Indications for PLWS

Open amputation sites (for removal of coagulation and necrotic debris)
Presence of infection or necrotic tissue
Presence of thick or mucinous exudate
Presence of undermining, tunnels, or sinus tracts
Stage III and IV pressure injuries
Traumatic wounds with foreign debris
Wounds with decreased/stalled granulation due to high levels of bioburden

TABLE 19-5 PLWS Precautions

Anticoagulants or active bleeding (eg, low platelet count)
Facial wounds
Hypothermia with cool fluid irrigation
Near fistula or cavity linings
Near LVAD drive lines
Near recent bypass grafts or recent surgical closures
Near visible blood vessels
Overexposed bone or tendon
Poorly visualized wound spaces that may connect to body cavities (sinus tracts, tunnels)

amputation healing by secondary intention.[32] PLWS is also indicated for the removal of bacteria and debris in wounds associated with traumatic injury and bone exposure.[1,8] Utilization of flexible tips allows appropriate and safe use of PLWS for the irrigation and cleansing of tunnels, sinus tracts, and undermining unless there is concern that a wound extension leads into a body cavity (eg, thoracic or abdominal) (**FIGURE 19-8**).

PRECAUTIONS & CONTRAINDICATIONS

PLWS is contraindicated for use in overexposed blood vessels, nerves, tendons, or bone; over graft sites; or in the presence of active, profuse bleeding (**TABLE 19-5**).[2,9] Due to the presence of superficial vessels and nerves, caution is advised when treating facial wounds.[9]

Since PLWS is a method of nonselective, mechanical debridement, caution is also recommended when treating patients on anticoagulant therapy and treatment should be discontinued if active bleeding occurs.[9] PLWS encourages increased local blood flow and may cause increased blood loss from a wound with questionable or fragile hemostasis. The negative pressure can also increase blood loss in a wound that is bleeding. In situations of questionable hemostasis or easily damaged, exposed structures, selection of a lower psi (4–8 psi) is recommended. Further adaptation for painful wounds or friable tissue may include the use of a Yankauer suction tip for removal of irrigation fluids. Without contact negative pressure, Yankauer suction effectively removes irrigation fluids and decreases bleeding risk. However, the absence of contact negative pressure may result in less reduction of wound surface bacteria (**FIGURE 19-9**).

Caution is advised when the wound bed cannot be clearly visualized, as in the presence of tunneling, undermining, or sinus tracts. Knowledge of tract depth and possible tunnel connection with body cavities prior to administering PLWS is necessary in order to provide safe and effective treatment. Monitoring the amount of water that is pulsed in and suctioned out is recommended when treating wounds with sinus tracts to ensure removal of all irrigation fluids.

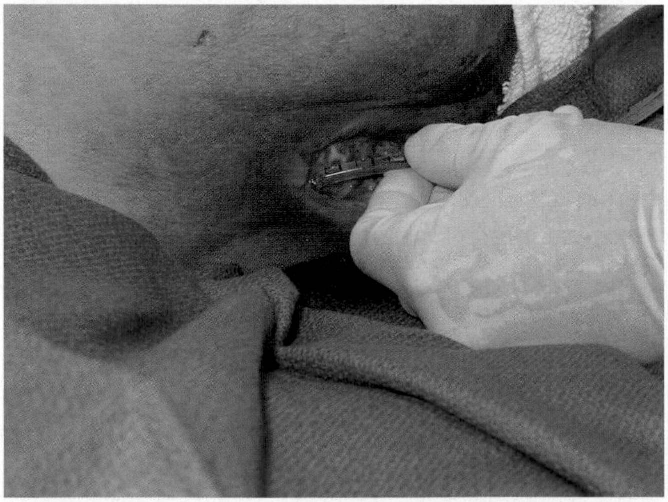

FIGURE 19-8 Pulsed lavage with suction using a flexible tip to irrigate deep undermining of a sacral pressure injury. Note the measuring guide on the tip, allowing for depth evaluation. The clinician's gently guides the flexible tip to ensure all areas are treated.

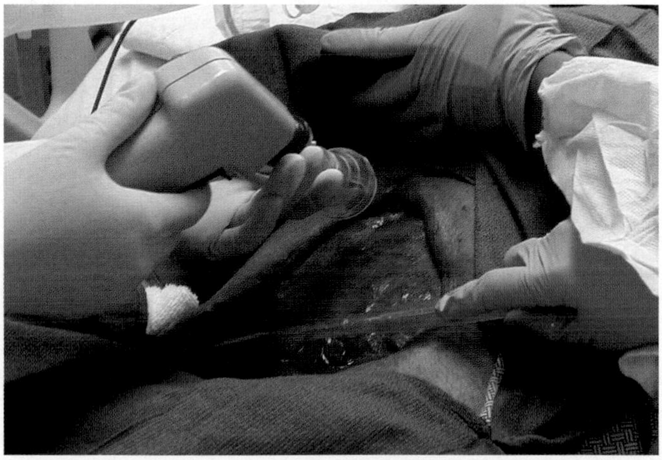

FIGURE 19-9 Yankaur suction. Large cavity wounds that enable irrigation fluid to pool or in wounds painful to tactile stimulation, a Yankauer tip can be used to evacuate fluid instead of suctioning through the PLWS tip. This method is less painful (albeit without the benefits of negative pressure tissue stimulation) and quickly evacuates larger amounts of irrigation fluid compared to the PLWS handpiece. In this application, the PLWS splash shield is held close to but not in contact with the wound bed to deliver positive pressure irrigation and minimize aerosolization.

As previously presented, the use of cool irrigation fluids (below normal body temperature) can result in tissue hypothermia and local vasoconstriction. IV bags designated for PLWS treatment can be heated to reach ideal temperatures (37–38°C) according to facility guidelines and may include placing IV bags in hot water or blanket warmers. Irrigation fluids at room temperature are not recommended for PLWS considering most clinical settings maintain ambient temperatures much cooler than normal body temperature.

PARAMETERS AND TECHNIQUES FOR APPLICATION

Parameters

Clinical judgment in selection and adjustment of treatment parameters is important due to the dynamic nature of wound healing with decisions based on patient tolerance and wound status. If the desired results are not realized, parameters should be adjusted to facilitate optimal patient response. Parameters for PLWS include type of irrigation tip, psi, suction force, irrigation fluid, and frequency and duration of treatment (**TABLE 19-6**).

Irrigation Force

Safe positive pressure irrigation for wound management is between 4 and 15 psi. Pressures greater than 15 psi may cause wound trauma and drive bacteria further into the wound bed.[2] Lower psi selections (4–8 psi) can be used for initial treatments to gauge patient tolerance and tissue response.[3,18] This also allows the patient to become familiar with the sensation and sound of active PLWS, and can help alleviate apprehension or anxiety associated with an unfamiliar method of treatment. In many cases, adequate wound cleansing and debridement can be achieved using 8–12 psi.[2,3,9] In the presence of anticoagulation therapy, fragile hemostasis, exposed named structures, or intense pain, lower psi settings should be used. Similarly, lower psi ranges (2–6 psi) are recommended for irrigation of tracts and tunnels. Higher forces (12–15 psi) are recommended for removal of infected tissue, thick mucinous exudate, or adherent necrotic tissue.[22,33] Generally, the lowest pressure that produces the desired response is recommended.

TABLE 19-6 Parameters for PLWS

Safe application range: 4–15 • 4–6 for sensitive areas • 8–9 to decrease bacterial load • 9–15 for noninfected wounds to remove debris
Continuous suction range: 60–100 mmHg • 60–80 for wounds that are painful or bleed easily • 80–100 for removal of exudate and necrotic debris
Irrigation temperature range: 37–38°C
Frequency range: • Daily for inpatients with infected, heavily draining wounds • 2–3 times a week for outpatients with moderate-to-heavy drainage and signs of high bioburden/local infection • 1–2 times per week for tissue stimulation for outpatients with minimal drainage and no infection

Suction Force

The recommended suction force is between 60 and 100 mmHg; low range pressures for patients with fragile hemostasis or pain and upper range pressures for increased debris removal and cellular stimulation.[34] As previously presented, Yankauer suction may also be used in specific situations.

Irrigation Fluid

The ideal wound irrigation fluid should be sterile, isotonic, non-hemolytic, nontoxic, transparent, and inexpensive (normal saline meets these requirements).[2] Antibacterial or antiseptic solutions can be used in cases of suspected high bioburden or infection. Skin loss in superficial wounds and insulating subcutaneous fat loss in deeper wounds causes loss of body heat; therefore, regardless of the irrigant used, solutions should be warmed to 37–38°C to help prevent further wound tissue hypothermia.[3,30] Reduced vasoconstriction, decreased pain, and overall patient relaxation are additional benefits of warm irrigation applications.[2,30] The amount of irrigation fluid used depends on wound size, characteristics, and level of bioburden. Sufficient volume to hydrate wound tissues and remove all visible, loose debris is recommended for contaminated wounds.

Frequency and Duration

For wounds with infection, odor, or greater than 50% necrotic tissue, daily PLWS applications may be beneficial in the inpatient setting.[3,9] For general cleansing and tissue stimulation, PLWS is applied based on wound characteristics and healing progress. PLWS should typically be discontinued after 1 week without improvement in wound status or when wound improvement allows for other less costly and time-consuming forms of intervention.[3] Overall, clinicians should apply sound clinical judgment in prescribing frequency and duration parameters based on patient preference, tissue response, clinical setting, and cost (**TABLE 19-6**).

APPLICATION

Personal Protective Equipment and Environmental Guidelines

To protect health professionals and patients from risks associated with aerosolization during PLWS use, standard personal protective equipment (PPE) is required (**FIGURE 19-10**).[3,9] Because PLWS delivers pressurized irrigation fluids, risk of fluid aerosolization and the potential for transporting bacteria is a concern.[3,5,35] PLWS aerosolization can transport bacteria as far as 8 feet away from the treatment area.[5] In 2004, Maragakis et al.[5] published data documenting a multidrug-resistant bacterial outbreak linked to PLWS aerosolization. Since that time, strict guidelines regarding PLWS use have been developed by the Center for Disease Control (TABLE 19-7).[2,3,9,36] Additionally, aerosolization risk and projectile contamination must be considered when PLWS is used during surgical procedures.[20,37,38]

Treatment Preparation and Application

If required, pain medications or topical analgesics are administered beforehand as appropriate. In preparation for PLWS treatment, the patient is positioned comfortably and draped appropriately (TABLE 19-7) with the targeted area exposed for easy access. A waterproof or water-resistant drape is placed under the treatment area along with extra toweling to absorb any irrigation fluid not evacuated by suction. If treating multiple areas during the same session, the patient is positioned (if possible) so that any irrigation runoff from one wound does not drain into other open wounds (FIGURE 19-11). Additionally, the cleanest wound is treated first; the most contaminated treated last to limit cross-contamination risk.

A warmed IV bag is suspended from an IV pole or hook with PLWS tubing inserted into the bag so fluid can be pulled from the bag into the hand-piece (FIGURE 19-12). Depending on wound characteristics, number of wounds, and treatment goals, more than one bag of irrigation fluid may be necessary. If so, extra irrigation bags wrapped in dry toweling to maintain warmth and extra suction canisters should be staged to facilitate transition of supplies with little interruption in treatment.

Wall or portable suction (FIGURE 19-13) is connected to the collection canister *and* to tubing from the PLWS hand-piece so that contaminated irrigation fluid is transported to the container (FIGURE 19-14). Any other openings in the collection canister lid are closed to prevent loss of suction.

CLINICAL CONSIDERATION

Maintaining good contact between the cone tip and wound tissue during treatment can help reduce aerosolization risk. This is facilitated by the healthcare provider using their non-dominate hand to gently mold the pliable cone tip to tissue contours (FIGURE 19-2). However, care must be taken not to occlude the small air hole on the side of the cone tip during application as this will increase suction force causing discomfort and/or tissue damage.[38] Continuous contact of the cone with targeted tissues improves containment of irrigation fluid during delivery, facilitates improved tissue stimulation, and enables good return (or collection) of used irrigation fluid. Additionally, continuing suction 1–2 seconds after discontinuing the delivery of irrigation fluid (releasing the hand-piece lever) facilitates good collection of any fluid remaining in the wound bed at the end of PLWS treatment.

CLINICAL CONSIDERATION

Placing absorbent pads and extra towels around the treatment area prevents runoff fluid from soiling linens, protects the patient and makes treatment more comfortable, and saves time with post-treatment cleanup.

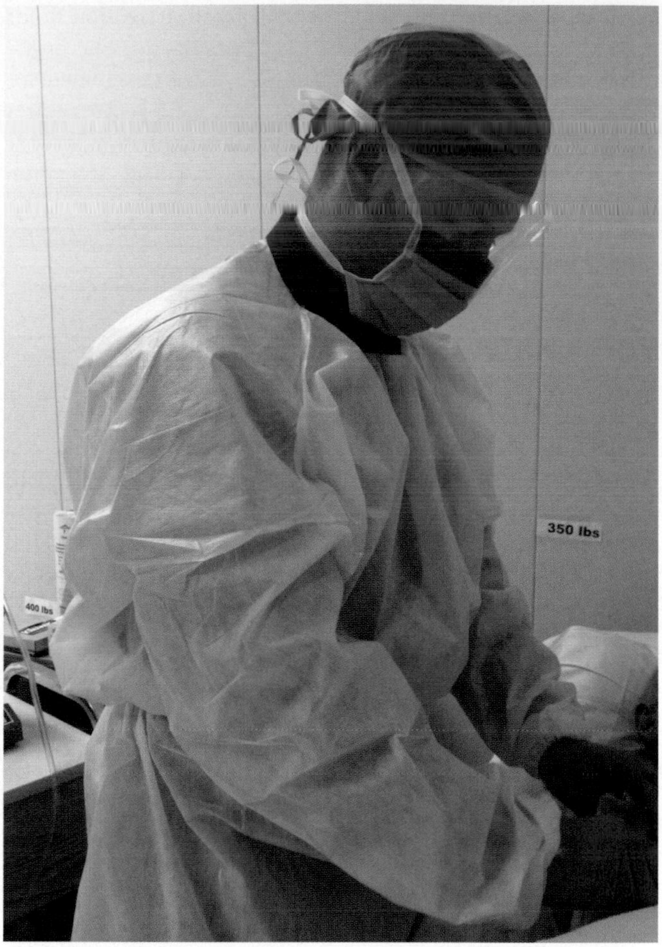

FIGURE 19-10 Photo of healthcare provider in PPE. Protective personal equipment for the healthcare provider using PLWS includes water resistant/waterproof gown, gloves, face mask with splash shield or mask with goggles, hair cover, and shoe covers.

TABLE 19-7 PLWS Infection Control Guidelines

Before Treatment	
	Allow only essential personnel in treatment room, no family
	Cover all patient lines, ports, or other wounds
	Cover all horizontal surfaces with sheets or towels
	Cover patient's personal items
	Have no open shelves in treatment area
	Have only essential equipment in treatment area
	Perform treatment in a single-patient room with nonfabric walls and doors that can be closed
	Place a mask on the patient and cover clothing/bed linens with a sheet
	Provider and any other personnel in the room wear appropriate PPE including hair cover, mask, face shield or goggles, water resistant/ waterproof gown, shoe covers, and gloves
After Treatment	
	Do not reuse single-use items
	Discard handpiece, tubing, and canister with contaminated fluid in a red biohazard container
	Disinfect all surfaces touched in the treatment area

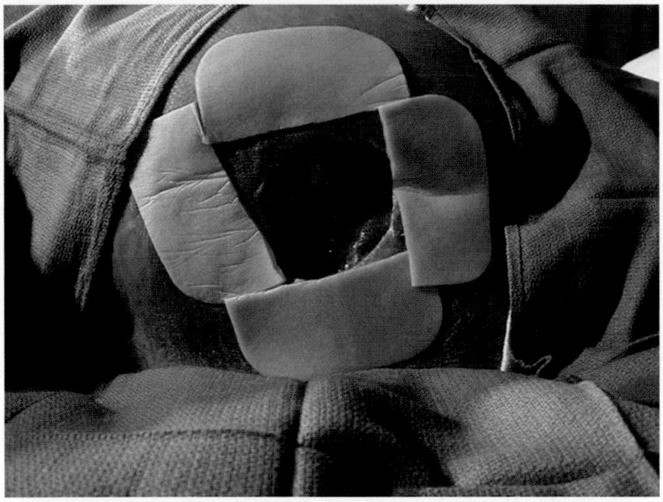

FIGURE 19-11 Patient with sacral ulcer is positioned in side-lying with pillow support for comfort and to protect vulnerable areas such as medial knees and malleoli. A sterile field is set up adjacent to the treatment site for placement of instruments during treatment. Extra towels and absorbent padding are positioned to collect fluids that spill during treatment. The hydrocolloid dressing placed around the wound prevents the use of tape or adhesives on the periwound skin when applying the new dressing.

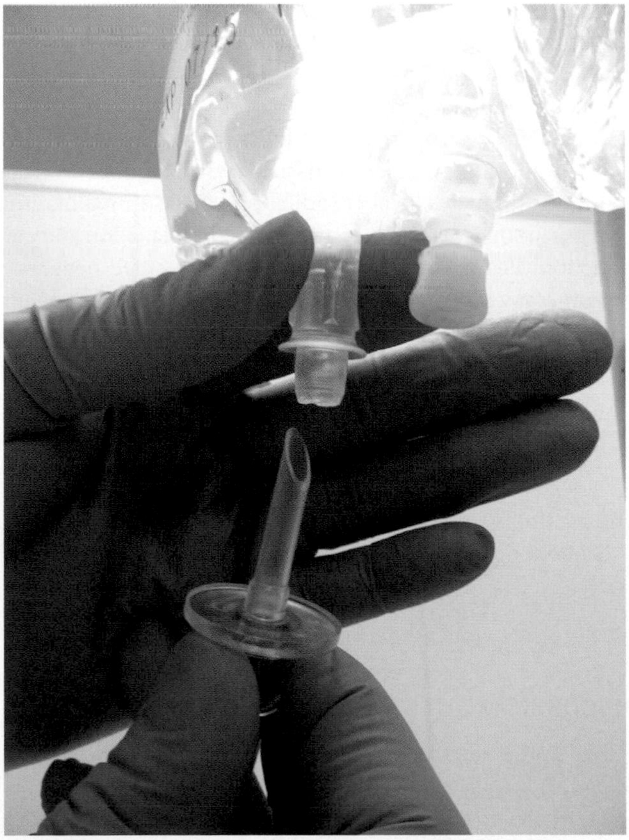

FIGURE 19-12 Piercing the irrigation bag with the tubing tip that goes to the handpiece.

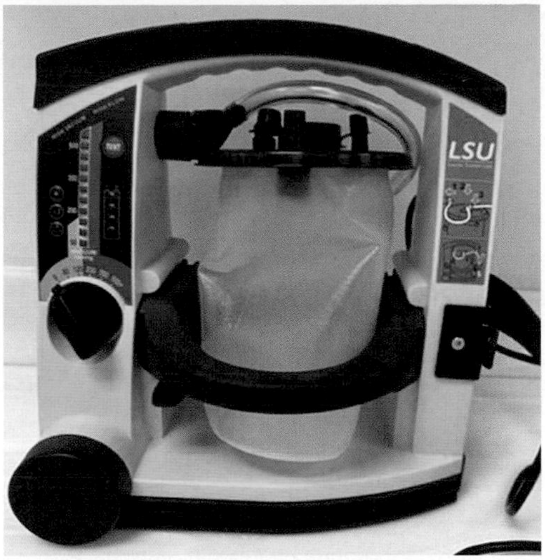

FIGURE 19-13 Example portable suction.

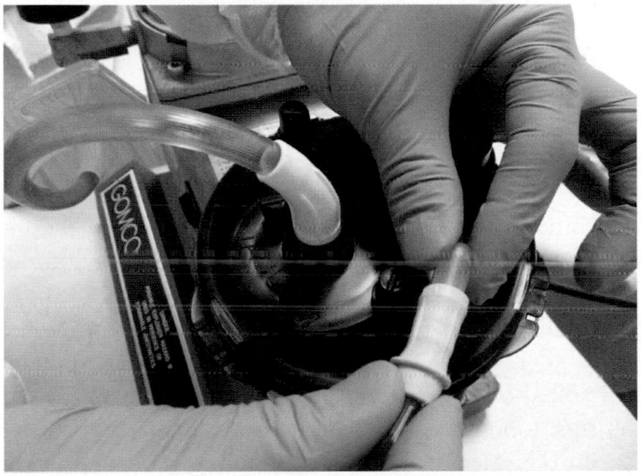

FIGURE 19-14 Top of the suction canister where the tube on the left leads to the suction pump and the tube on the right delivers the contaminated water from the treatment area into the canister.

A sterile field is prepared for the protection of and access to additional PLWS supplies (eg, different tips), sterile instruments for sharp debridement, dressings, and bandaging supplies. Silver nitrate sticks, surgical thrombin, or pressure with sterile gauze are recommended if bleeding occurs during treatment. As with any intervention, if bleeding cannot be stopped with local pressure (usually for at least 15 minutes without removal of pressure) or if arterial bleeding is suspected (detected by pulsating arterial flow), a physician should be contacted immediately.

CLINICAL CONSIDERATION

Each manufacturer has distinct device features and tips with advantages for specific patient and wound characteristics. The healthcare provider is advised to be familiar with equipment options and follow manufacturer's instructions.

TABLE 19-8 PLWS and WP Comparison

PLWS and WP Comparison	
PLWS	**WP**
Sterile, disposable, single use intervention	Nonsterile, multi-patient use intervention
Can be used with patient in various positions with few precautions	Requires immersion in a dependent position and contraindicated for venous insufficiency wounds
Known, adjustable psi	Unknown psi
Sterile normal saline, antibiotic, antiseptic, or antimicrobial irrigation fluids	Additives frequently added to tap water decrease risk of cross-contamination but may injure healthy cells
Site-specific	Risk of periwound/surrounding tissue maceration with general immersion
Portable	Patient must be transferred to WP area
Sterile IV irrigation fluids (typically 1–2 bags)	Can require multiple gallons of tap water
Quick cleanup	More time-intensive cleanup
Sterile, flexible tips for thorough irrigation of sinus tracts/tunnels/undermining	Sinus tracts/tunnels/undermining or skin fold wounds may not be thoroughly cleaned with turbine agitation
Risk of aerosolization but minimized with appropriate application techniques	Risk of aerosolization but minimized with appropriate application techniques
Requires use of appropriate PPE for provider and patient	Requires use of appropriate PPE for provider and patient

Openings on the flexible tips used for tunnels and sinus tracts are located at the end of the tip so moving the tips in and out of tunnels/tracts frequently during treatment ensures wound sidewalls are included in treatment. Using the index finger and thumb to help guide the tip during this procedure provides better control and ease of movement (**FIGURE 19-8**). Appropriate wound dressings should be applied as soon as possible after completing the PLWS treatment and removing all soiled or wet towels to minimize heat loss. The handpiece, tips, tubing, and closed suction canister are single-use items and must be placed in a biohazard container after use.[3,39] Documentation includes PLWS parameters used for treatment, type and amount of irrigation fluid, and patient response to treatment.

SUMMARY

The combination of positive and negative pressure benefits makes PLWS an effective and efficient method of hydrotherapy and mechanical debridement. Site-specific application and sterile, single-use supplies reduce hydrotherapy contraindications and risk of cross-contamination. Positive and negative pressure manipulation removes surface bacteria, nonviable tissue, and debris from the wound bed at safe, known psi levels while promoting granulation tissue formation. Warm irrigation fluid stimulates local vasodilation, assists in maintaining local normothermia, and promotes patient relaxation and pain reduction. PLWS combines the long-documented benefits of hydrotherapy into an advanced wound management modality with many advantages over traditional WP (**TABLE 19-8**).

CASE STUDY

CONTINUED

The patient's systems review was negative for cardiac, neuromuscular, or musculoskeletal issues. The patient is independent in all ADLs and IADLs and ambulates at a community level without an assistive device. The wound measures 18.5 cm × 12.7 cm × 3.8 cm and tunnels to a medial opening that is 3.6 cm × 1.7 cm. Drainage is moderate and tends to have a slight green tinge but there is no odor after cleansing.

Lab values: Hemoglobin A1C 6.1, albumin 2.2, hemoglobin 10.4.

Medications: Vitamins per gastric bypass protocol, just completed the course of Vancomycin.

Social history: Single parent, lives with two daughters who are in the second and third grades.

Patient goals:

1. Surgical closure of wound as soon as possible
2. Return to work as teacher's aide

DISCUSSION QUESTIONS

1. Is PLWS an appropriate intervention for this patient?
2. If so, what equipment and parameters would work best?

CASE STUDY

CONCLUSION

Plan of care

Due to insurance coverage, the patient was only approved for four visits. The physical therapist and patient agreed on biweekly treatments consisting of PLWS (using the flexible cone tip and 2,000 mL of warmed normal saline) followed by selective debridement of loose devitalized tissue. Care was taken to fully irrigate the mesh that tended to collect slough underneath it. Because advanced negative pressure wound therapy was not approved by the insurance, dressings consisted of a calcium alginate liner, sterile gauze fluffed to fill the remaining open wound space, and a semi-occlusive foam with adhesive borders to cover. The patient was instructed in dressing changes at home as needed to accommodate drainage.

Due to low albumin and the need for additional protein, the patient was advised to supplement meals with protein shakes. Blood glucose levels were monitored and kept below 120 mg/dL.

Three days after the first treatment, the wound was granulating and drainage had decreased to minimum with no green tinge or odor (**FIGURE 19-15**).

Two weeks after treatment was initiated, the wound was more than 90% granulated with very little visible mesh (**FIGURE 19-16**) and the patient was scheduled for surgical closure.

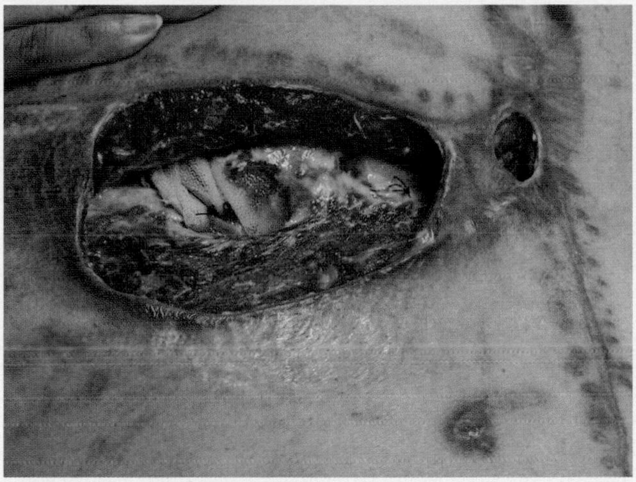

FIGURE 19-15 Case study 3 days after first treatment.

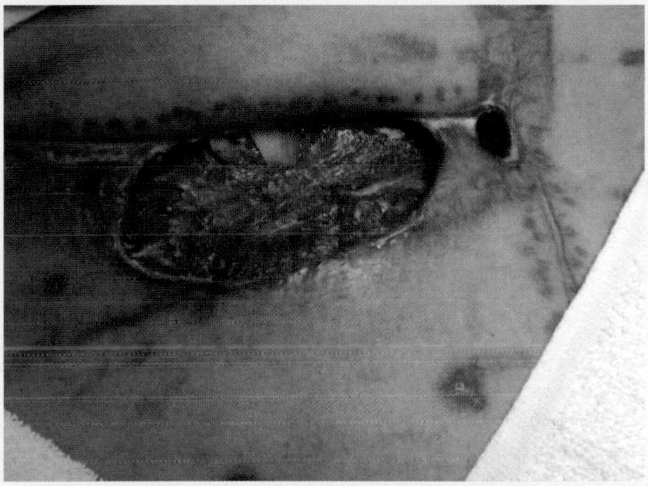

FIGURE 19-16 Case study after 4 treatments with PLWS (2 weeks after initiation of treatment).

STUDY QUESTIONS

1. A physical therapist is treating a patient with a Stage IV sacral pressure injury with a large amount of adherent fibrous tissue. The recommended psi to use in treating this patient with PLWS is
   a. 2.
   b. 6.
   c. 8.
   d. 15.
2. The solution most frequently used for PLWS is
   a. Ringer solution.
   b. Dakin's solution.
   c. Normal saline.
   d. Sterile water.
3. A physical therapist receives an order to provide wound care to a patient who has an open abdominal wound, cultured positive for pseudomonas, and wants to include PLWS as part of the care plan. The patient is in a semiprivate room with more than 6 feet between the beds and a curtain that can be pulled for privacy. The approach would be to
   a. Treat the patient with PLWS with all appropriate protective equipment and pliable cone tip to limit aerosolization.
   b. Request that the patient be moved to a private room before initiating treatment with PLWS.
   c. Transport the patient to the outpatient department for treatment to avoid treating in a room with curtains.
   d. Refuse to treat the patient until the other patient in the hospital room has been discharged.

4. What is the appropriate approach when treating a patient with multiple wounds?
   a. Use a different tip for each wound
   b. Treat only one wound in each treatment session
   c. Treat the infected wound first and then treat other wounds
   d. Treat the cleaner wounds first and the infected wound last
5. What is the range of suction recommended for most wounds treated with PLWS?
   a. 40–60 mmHg pressure
   b. 60–100 mmHg pressure
   c. 100–120 mmHg pressure
   d. 120–160 mmHg pressure
6. Which of the following patient conditions is a precaution for treating with PLWS?
   a. A tract more than 8 cm deep with a definite end-feel
   b. Transtibial amputation site
   c. Patient on isolation due to MRSA in the wound
   d. Patient with a mechanical heart valve on anticoagulants with an INR of 3.5

Answers: 1-d; 2-c; 3-b; 4-d; 5-b; 6-d

REFERENCES

1. Luck T, Zaki P, Michels R, Slotkin EM. The cost-effectiveness of normal-saline lavage for infection prophylaxis in total joint arthroplasty. *Arthroplast Today*. 2022;18:107-111.
2. Gabriel A. Wound irrigation. (2021). Available at: https://emedicine.medscape.com/article/1895071-overview. Accessed November 9, 2022.
3. Cameron MH. Hydrotherapy. In: Cameron MH, ed. *Physical Agents in Rehabilitation: An Evidence-Based Approach to Practice*. St. Louis, MO: Elsevier; 2018;341-373.
4. Granick MS, Tenenhaus M, Knox KR, Ulm JP. Comparison of wound irrigation and tangential hydrodissection in bacterial clearance of contaminated wounds: results of a randomized, controlled clinical study. *Ostomy Wound Manage*. 2007;53(4):64-72.
5. Maragakis LL, Cosgrove SE, Song X, et al. An outbreak of multidrug-resistant *Acinetobacter baumannii* associated with pulsatile lavage wound treatment. *JAMA*. 2004;292(24):3006-3011.
6. Keblish DJ, DeMaio M. Early pulsatile lavage for the decontamination of combat wounds: historical review and point proposal. *Mil Med*. 1998;163:844-846.
7. Bhaskar SN, Cutright DE, Hunsuck EE, Gross A. Pulsating water jet devices in debridement of combat wounds. *Mil Med*. 1971;136(3):264-266.
8. Bath MF, Suresh R, Davies J, Machesney MR. Does pulsed lavage reduce the risk of surgical site infection? A systematic review and meta-analysis. *J Hosp Infect*. 2021;118:32-39.
9. Ramundo JM. Wound debridement. In: Bryant RA, Nix DP, eds. *Acute & Chronic Wounds: Current Management Concepts*. St. Louis, MO: Elsevier; 2016:295-305.
10. Hunter S, Langemo D, Hanson D, Anderson J, Thompson P. The use of negative pressure wound therapy. *Adv Skin Wound Care*. 2007;20(2):90-95.
11. Hanz T, Butler JP, Luttrell T. The role of whirlpool in wound care. *J Am Coll Clin Wound Spec*. 2013;4(1):7-12.
12. Luedtke-Hoffman KA, Schafer DS. Pulsed lavage in wound cleansing. *Phys Ther*. 2000;80:292-300.
13. Lyder CH Pressure ulcer prevention and management. In: Fitzpatrick JJ, ed.. *Annual Review of Nursing Research: Geriatric Nursing Research*. New York, NY: Springer Publishing; 2002; 35-62
14. Rodeheaver GT, Pettry D, Thacker JG, Edgerton MT, Edlich RF. Wound cleansing by high pressure irrigation. *Surg Gyn Obstet*. [illegible]
15. National Pressure Injury Advisory Panel and European Pressure Ulcer Advisory Panel. *Prevention and Treatment of Pressure Ulcers/Injuries: Clinical Practice Guide*. The International Guideline 2019. Washington, DC: National Pressure Injury Advisory Panel; 2019.
16. American Physical Therapy Association. Choosing wisely: Five things physical therapists and patients should question. 2022. Available at: https://www.choosingwisely.org/societies/american-physical-therapy-association/. Accessed November 9, 2022.
17. Dong J, Qing C, Song F, et al. Potential molecular mechanisms of negative pressure in promoting wound healing. *Int Wound J*. 2020;17(5):1428-1438.
18. Bastawros DS. 5 Things you need to know about pulsed lavage. *Adv Skin Wound Care*. 2003;16(6):282.
19. Brown A. When is wound cleansing necessary and what solution should be used? *Nurs Times*. 2018;114(9):42-45.
20. Wynn M. The benefits and harms of cleansing for acute traumatic wounds: a narrative review. *Adv Skin Wound Care*. 2021;34:488-492.
21. Owens BD, White DW, Wenke JC. Comparison of irrigation solutions and devices in a contaminated musculoskeletal wound survival model. *J Bone Joint Surg Am*. 2009;91:92-98.
22. Bhandari M, Adili A, Schemitsch EH. The efficacy of low-pressure lavage with different irrigating solutions to remove adherent bacterial from bone. *J Bone Joint Surg Am*. 2001;83-A(3):412-419.
23. Boeringer T Gould L, Koria P. Protease-resistant growth factor formulations for the healing of chronic wounds. *Adv Wound Care*. 2020;9(11):612-622.
24. Stacey MC, Phillips SA, Farrokhyar F, Swaine JM. Evaluation of wound fluid biomarkers to determine healing in adults with venous leg ulcers: a prospective study. *Wound Repair Regen*. 2019;27(5):509-518.
25. Tati R, Nordin S, Abdillahi SM, Morgelin M. *J Wound Care*. 2018;27(4):199-209.
26. Shirakawa M, Isseroff RR. Topical negative pressure devices: use for enhancement of healing chronic wounds. *Arch Dermatol*. 2005;141:449-453.
27. Woo K, Ayello E, Sibbald RG. The edge effect: current therapeutic options to advance the wound edge. *Adv Skin Wound Care*. 2007;20(2):99-117.
28. Yager DR, Zhang LY, Liang HX, Diegelmann RF, Cohen IK. Wound fluids from human pressure ulcers contain elevated matrix metalloproteinase levels and activity compared to surgical wound fluids. *J Invest Dermatol*. 1996;107:743-748.
29. Falanga V. Growth factors and chronic wounds: The need to understand the microenvironment. *J Dermatol*. 1992;19:667-672.
30. Shetty R, Barreto E, Paul KM. Suction assisted pulse lavage: randomized controlled studies comparing its efficacy with conventional dressings in healing of chronic wounds. *Int Wound J*. 2012;10:1-11.
31. Gefen A. The influence zone: a critical performance measure for negative pressure wound therapy systems. *Br J Nurs*. 2022; 31(15):S8-S12.
32. Loehne HL. Pulsatile lavage with concurrent suction. In: Sussman C, Bates-Jensen B, eds. *Wound Care: A Collaborative Practice Manual for Physical Therapists and Nurses*. 4th ed. Baltimore, MD: Wolters Kluwer/Lippincott Williams & Wilkins; 2012.

33. Sibbald RG, Elliot JA, Persaud-Jaimangal R, et al. Wound bed preparation 2021. *Adv Skin Wound Care*. 2021;34(4):183-195.
34. Hamm R. Adjunct therapies – pulsed lavage with suction. 2019. Available at: https://www.accessmedicinenetwork.com/posts/56630-adjunct-therapies-pulsed-lavage-with-suction?channel_id=2015-weekly-wound-care-conundrum#:~:text=PLWS%20is%20the%20only%20cleansing,of%20exudate%20and%20necrotic%20debris. Accessed November 12, 2022.
35. Sonnergren HH, Strombeck L, Aldenborg F, Faergemann J. Aerosolized spread of bacteria and reduction of bacterial wound contamination with three different methods of surgical wound debridement: a pilot study. *J Hosp Infect*. 2013;85(2):112-117.
36. Fuller J. Help prevent deadly infections when using pulsed lavage. *LPN*. 2007;3:9.
37. Tobias AM, Chang B. Pulsed irrigation of extremity wounds: a simple technique for splashback reduction. *Ann Plast Surg*. 2002;48(4):443-444.
38. Simpuls™ SOLO. Available at: https://www.bd.com/en-us/products-and-solutions/products/product-page.0067500#overview. Accessed September 8, 2022.
39. Interpulse pulsed lavage system. 2022.Available at: https://www.stryker.com/us/en/orthopaedic-instruments/products/interpulse-pulsed-lavage-system.html. Accessed September 8, 2022.

CHAPTER TWENTY

Hyperbaric and Topical Oxygen Therapy

Lee C. Ruotsi, MD, CWS-P, ABWMS, UHM

CHAPTER OBJECTIVES

At the conclusion of this chapter, the learner will be able to:

1. **Relate the physiologic effect of hyperbaric oxygen therapy to wound healing.**
2. **Identify the diagnoses for which hyperbaric oxygen therapy is indicated.**
3. **Recognize the different types of chambers used for hyperbaric oxygen therapy.**
4. **Discuss the gas laws as they relate to the physics of pressurization.**
5. **State the contraindications for hyperbaric oxygen therapy.**
6. **Recognize the possible adverse effects of hyperbaric oxygen therapy.**
7. **Discuss Topical High Pressure Oxygen Therapy and its potential indications.**

INTRODUCTION

Hyperbaric oxygen therapy, in its simplest terms, means oxygen under pressure. Hyperbaric treatment pressures are compared to atmospheric or sea-level pressure. This chapter includes the history of air and oxygen under pressure, the physics and physiology of hyperbaric oxygen therapy (HBO_2), and the current uses of HBO_2 as it applies to wound healing. HBO_2, like any other treatment modality, has appropriate indications for its use that are supported by scientific evidence. Currently, the Undersea and Hyperbaric Medical Society has approved 14 indications for which there is adequate scientific basis for treatment with HBO_2 (**FIGURE 20-1**).

COMPRESSED AIR THERAPY

Hyperbaric therapy has been employed for hundreds of years for a multitude of purposes. The earliest reported uses of hyperbaric treatment date back to the 1600s. A British clergyman named Henshaw completed work that marked the beginning of the compressed-air era during which all hyperbaric treatments were performed only with compressed air, as oxygen was not discovered until 1775 by Priestley. In 1662, Henshaw built a sealed chamber that he called a "Domicilium."[1] Valved bellows controlled chamber pressures, which could be raised or lowered by the adjustment of the valve system. Henshaw believed that acute disease processes of all kinds would respond favorably to increased air pressure, while more chronic diseases would respond better to low pressure. If during treatment, a disease was felt to have become chronic, Henshaw readjusted the valves to create a slight vacuum. Given the small pressure changes possible with such an apparatus, any perceived effects on those patients treated were most certainly based on psychology and not physiology.

In 1879, French surgeon JA Fontaine constructed a mobile operating room on wheels that could be pressurized.[2] Surgical procedures were performed in this unit using nitrous oxide as the anesthetic agent. Due to the increased effective concentration of nitrous oxide and the increased partial pressure of oxygen at pressure, deeper and arguably safer surgical anesthesia was possible. According to the gas laws, compressed air at 2 atm (defined as pressure two times normal sea level air pressure) yields an effective oxygen percentage of 42% compared to 21% at 1 atm or sea-level pressures. In these surgical procedures, interesting physiologic and anatomic effects were observed. Patients did not have the usual cyanotic color while coming out of anesthesia and hernias were reduced more easily. Fontaine's experiments with hyperbaric surgery were the only semi-scientific efforts during the entire compressed-air era.

The end of the compressed-air era was marked by Orville J. Cunningham, a professor of anesthesia at the University of Kansas in Kansas City.[3] He noted, appropriately, that people with heart disease and other related disorders did poorly while living at altitude but improved upon return to sea level. With this concept in mind, Cunningham reasoned that exposing people to increased atmospheric pressures would be even more beneficial. During the flu epidemic of 1918, he placed a critically ill and hypoxic resident physician in a chamber that had been designed for animal studies. By compressing the chamber to 2 atm, he was able to keep the patient oxygenated through the hypoxic phase of his illness. Subsequently, Dr. Cunningham constructed a chamber 88 feet long and 10 feet in diameter and began to treat a multitude of diseases, most without any scientific evidence that HBO_2 would be an effective treatment.

In the 1920s, Henry Timken of the Timken Roller Bearing Company had a spontaneous recovery from a uremic illness while in Dr. Cunningham's chamber. In gratitude for his newly

UHMS approved indications

- Air or gas embolism
- Carbon monoxide poisoning
- Clostridial myositis and myonecrosis (gas gangrene)
- Crush injury, compartment syndrome and other acute traumatic ischemias
- Decompression sickness
- Arterial insufficiencies
- Severe anemia
- Intracranial abscess
- Necrotizing soft tissue infections
- Osteomyelitis (refractory)
- Delayed radiation injury (soft tissue and bony necrosis)
- Compromised grafts and flaps
- Acute thermal burn injury
- Idiopathic sudden sensorineural hearing loss

FIGURE 20-1 Indications for the use of hyperbaric oxygen therapy. The Undersea and Hyperbaric Medical Society has approved 14 indications for the use of hyperbaric oxygen therapy. These disorders have sound scientific evidence to support treatment with hyperbaric oxygen.

recovered health, Mr. Timken built for Dr. Cunningham the largest hyperbaric chamber ever constructed (**FIGURE 20-2**). It was a steel sphere, six stories high and 64 feet in diameter, featuring a dining room, individual patient rooms, and most interestingly, a smoking lounge on the top floor. It was capable of reaching 3 atm pressure.

Cunningham believed that there was an organism, unable to be cultured, that was responsible for a myriad of diseases including hypertension, uremia, diabetes, and cancer, and that treatment with increased atmospheric pressure helped control or inhibit this organism. Unfortunately, Dr. Cunningham was unable to provide any scientific evidence to support his treatments, and the Cleveland Medical Society, along with the American Medical Association (AMA), ultimately forced him to close in 1930.[4]

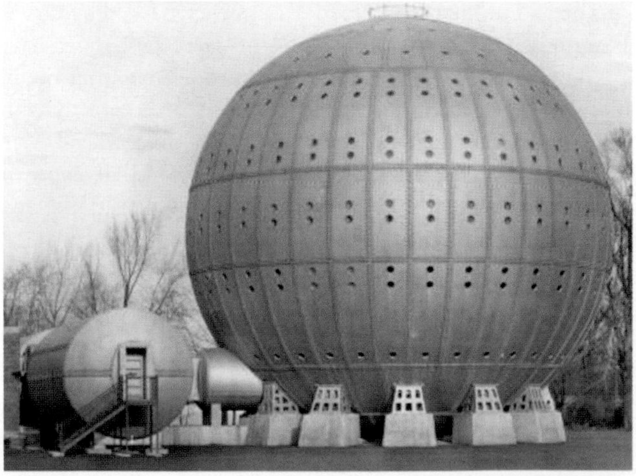

FIGURE 20-2 The largest chamber ever constructed. The largest chamber was six stories high, 64 feet in diameter, and had a smoking lounge on the top floor! The highest pressure was 3 atm; however, it was never able to meet scientific approval and was closed in 1930.

HYPERBARIC OXYGEN THERAPY

The use of hyperbaric oxygen therapy in clinical medicine began in 1955 with the work of I. Churchill-Davidson. He used increased oxygen environments to augment the effects of radiation therapy in cancer patients.[5] Also in 1955, Ite Boerema, Professor of Surgery at the University of Amsterdam in Holland, introduced the use of HBO_2 to improve outcomes in cardiac surgery patients. His initial work involved animal experiments using a chamber borrowed from the Royal Dutch Navy. These experiments yielded such promising results that Boerema had a large chamber built as an operating room at the University of Amsterdam, where he conducted surgery under pressure for a variety of cardiopulmonary conditions. The first publication of his work appeared in 1956.[6]

During this same period, W.H. Brummelkamp, also of the University of Amsterdam, found that hyperbaric oxygen inhibited the growth of certain anaerobic organisms, most importantly *Clostridium perfringens*, and his group published its first paper on the hyperbaric treatment of clostridial gas gangrene in 1961.[7] In 1962, George Smith and G.R. Sharp at the Western Infirmary in Glasgow, Scotland, studied the treatment of carbon monoxide poisoning.[8] Based on early favorable results from their work, a clinical chamber was constructed at Duke University, and another built later that same year at Mt. Sinai in New York City. Within a short period, similar chambers were constructed in large hospitals coast to coast.

Since the 1960s, HBO_2 therapy has seen tremendous growth. Based on the promising results seen for gas gangrene, cardiac surgery, and carbon monoxide poisoning, the search for new indications burgeoned. Patients suffering from a myriad of acute and chronic conditions were treated in chambers in the hope that hyperbaric oxygen would provide benefit in conditions for which conventional therapies had failed. Unfortunately, these efforts produced more anecdotal reports of positive outcomes than they did scientific data supporting those outcomes. Nevertheless, improvements in heart–lung machines and the use of hypothermia led to improved patient outcomes in cardiac surgery and essentially obviated the need for surgical hyperbaric units. As a result, by the early 1970s, many of the earlier chambers and programs had closed.

By the mid-1970s there was a need for structured and evidence-based guidelines for the use of HBO_2 therapy. Only one general textbook on hyperbaric, written by Eric Kindwall of St Luke's Hospital in Milwaukee in 1970, had been published. Dr. Kindwall remained a leader in the field of hyperbaric oxygen therapy and went on to author and edit three seminal volumes of the highly regarded text *Hyperbaric Medicine Practice*, which is in its fourth edition.[9]

The Undersea Medical Society (UMS) was founded in 1967 by a group of U.S. Navy Diving and Submarine Medical Officers and was conceived as an organization dedicated to diving and undersea medicine. In 1976, an 18-member ad hoc Committee on Hyperbaric Oxygenation was formed, with Eric Kindwall as chairman, to review the field of HBO_2 therapy.[10] In 1986, at the UMS annual meeting in Japan, the membership voted to change the name of the Undersea Medical Society to the Undersea and Hyperbaric Medical Society (UHMS), an organization that encompasses the fields of clinical use. The first "Report of the Committee on Hyperbaric Oxygenation" was published in 1977 and divided disorders treated with hyperbaric oxygen into four categories.[6] Category one contained disorders for which there was no question of the efficacy of HBO_2 and progressed in degrees of supporting evidence to category four, which comprised disorders for which there was no supporting evidence whatsoever. This report has been updated periodically. The most recent edition was published in 2014 and contains the 14 disorders presently approved for treatment with HBO_2 therapy (**FIGURE 20-1**).[11]

GENERAL PRINCIPLES OF HYPERBARIC OXYGENATION

Definition: Hyperbaric oxygen therapy is a treatment during which a patient who is inside a chamber breathes 100% oxygen intermittently, at a pressure higher than sea-level pressure.[11]

Any pressure above 1 atm absolute (sea-level pressure) can technically be considered hyperbaric; however, the pressure must be greater than 1.4 atm absolute (ATA) to be considered hyperbaric therapy. Most clinical treatment protocols call for ambient pressures between 2 and 3 ATA.

HBO_2 must be delivered systemically, with the patient in a chamber breathing elevated partial pressures of oxygen through an intact cardiopulmonary system. Topical high-pressure oxygen with containers enclosing individual limbs is not considered HBO_2 therapy; this treatment modality will be discussed later in this chapter.

EQUIPMENT

Using the above definitions and guidelines, HBO_2 therapy may be administered in either a monoplace chamber (able to treat one patient at a time) or a multiplace chamber (able to treat as many as 20 or more patients simultaneously). The physiology and partial pressures of oxygen are identical in either of the chamber types, but how the treatments are carried out varies significantly.

The monoplace chamber is a free-standing unit, typically with steel end caps and a thick, cylindrical acrylic hull (**FIGURE 20-3A, B**). There are variations on this design in terms of materials and configuration and some are designed to accommodate an inside attendant, although still a monoplace chamber with regard to patient treatment (**FIGURE 20-4**).

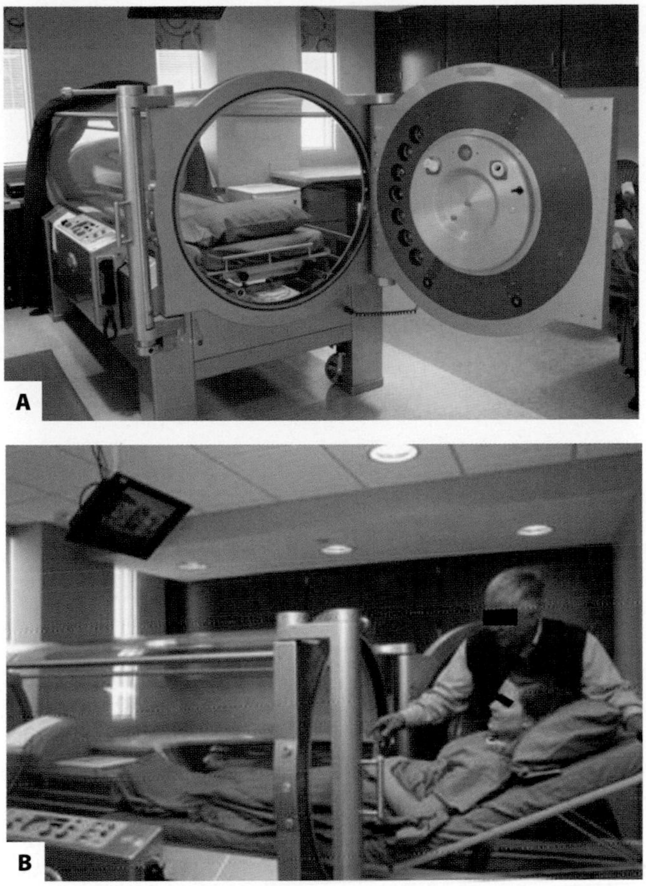

FIGURE 20-3 A, B. The monoplace hyperbaric oxygen chamber. The monoplace chamber is designed to treat one patient positioned supine on a stretcher.

Patients are treated in a supine or slightly inclined position on an adjustable bed, which slides into the chamber from a matted gurney on wheels. Depending on the age and sophistication of the chamber, pressures may be set and treatments run either manually or automatically by built-in computer systems. A monoplace chamber is compressed with 100%

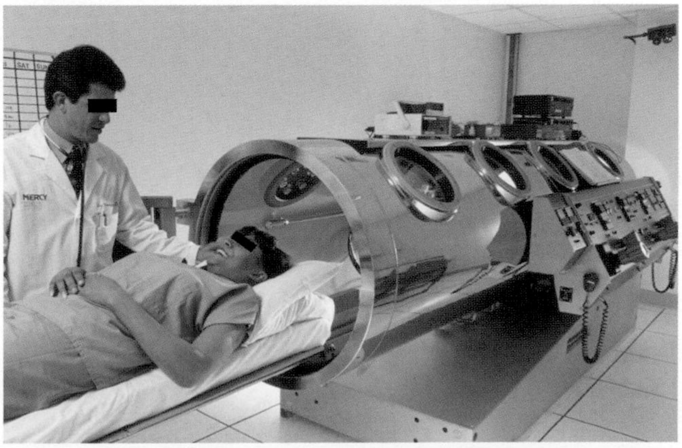

FIGURE 20-4 An enclosed monoplace chamber. A monoplace chamber that is enclosed may result in more claustrophobic reactions from patients. (Used with permission from Marc R. Kaiser, Boca Raton, FL.)

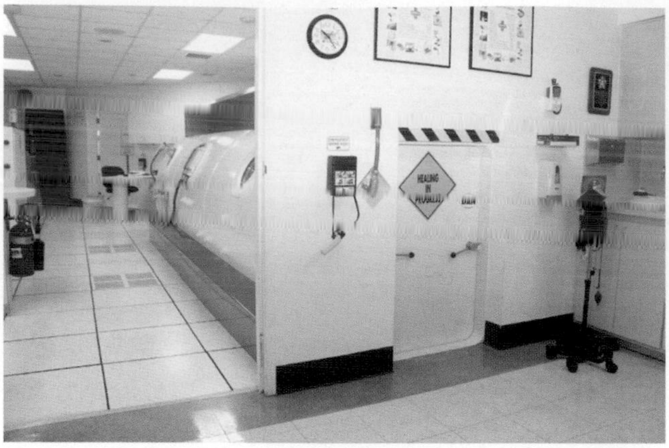

FIGURE 20-5 Multiplace chamber. Outside view of a multiplace chamber that can accommodate up to 30 patients who sit in medical grade air and breathe 100% oxygen through masks or hoods. These chambers require a certified attendant to be inside the chamber during treatment. (Used with permission from Marc R. Kaiser, Boca Raton, FL.)

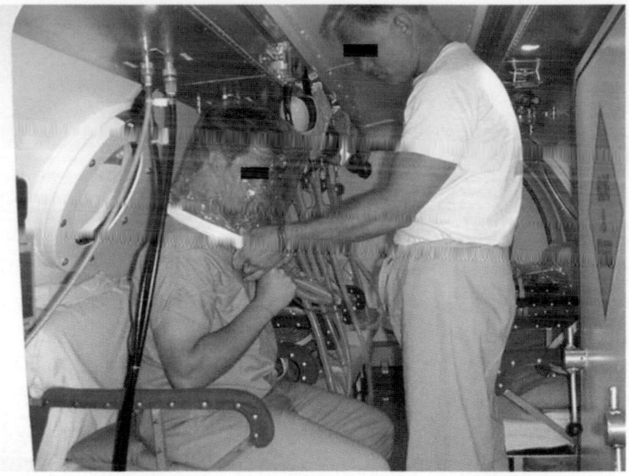

FIGURE 20-7 Patient in a multiplace chamber with an over-the-head hood providing the oxygen. (Used with permission from Marc R. Kaiser, Boca Raton, FL.)

oxygen, in contrast to the multiplace chamber, which is compressed with medical-grade air. It is possible to administer intravenous fluids, monitor blood pressures, and even mechanically ventilate an intubated patient within the monoplace chamber.[12,13]

Multiplace hyperbaric chambers can be cylindrical, spherical, or rectangular and vary greatly in their dimensions, from small two-person chambers to modern rectangular chambers that can seat 20–30 patients simultaneously (**FIGURE 20-5**). Patients are typically seated in special seats along the walls of the chamber. Due to the volume of gas required, these chambers are compressed with medical-grade air rather than with oxygen as in the monoplace chamber. 100% oxygen is then administered to the patients through built-in breathing (BIB) systems using either an air mask or an over-the-head hood (**FIGURES 20-6** and **FIGURES 20-7**). These consist of an oxygen-supply hose connected to either the mask or acrylic hood. A multiplace chamber is either single lock in configuration, with a single entrance to a single chamber room, or multilock, in which the chamber has two or three small chambers within it, each able to be pressurized independently. This enables the ingress and egress of patients, personnel, and supplies. An additional advantage of multiplace chambers is the presence of medical personnel within the chamber during each treatment, allowing hands-on or emergency care, if necessary, in addition to the ability to "lock-in" or "lock-out" extra personnel, equipment, and supplies.

Experimental chambers come in a wide variety of types and configurations, depending on their intended purpose. **FIGURES 20-8** and **20-9** illustrate a large double-lock chamber, and **FIGURE 20-10** illustrates a collapsible and portable chamber designed to be carried aboard a ship or dive boat.

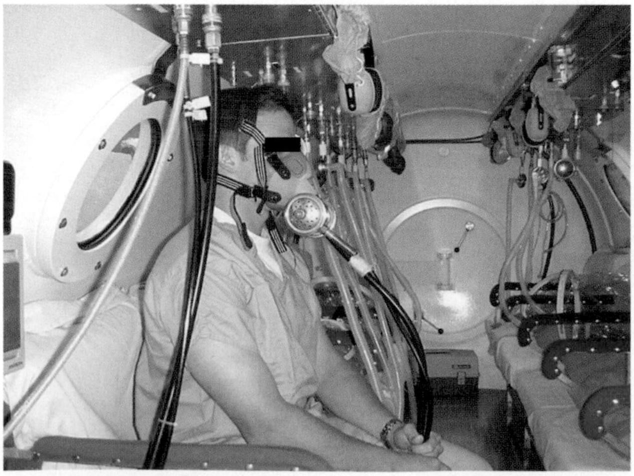

FIGURE 20-6 Patient in a multiplace chamber using a mask for breathing the oxygen. (Used with permission from Marc R. Kaiser, Boca Raton, FL.)

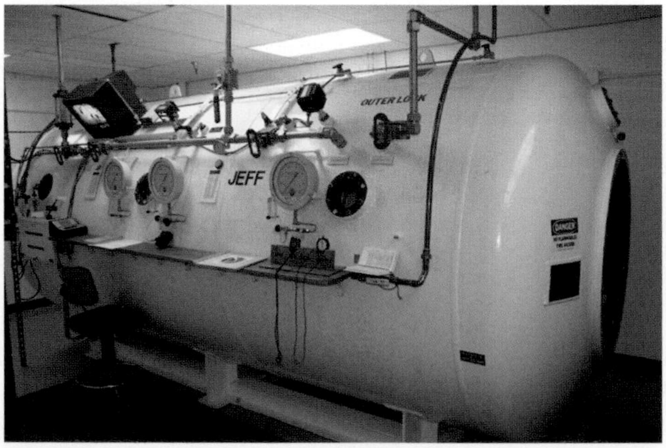

FIGURE 20-8 Outside view of a double-lock chamber.

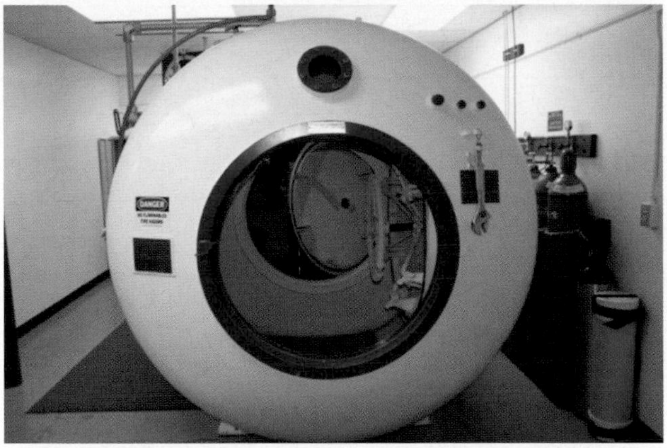

FIGURE 20-9 View of a double-lock chamber from the end.

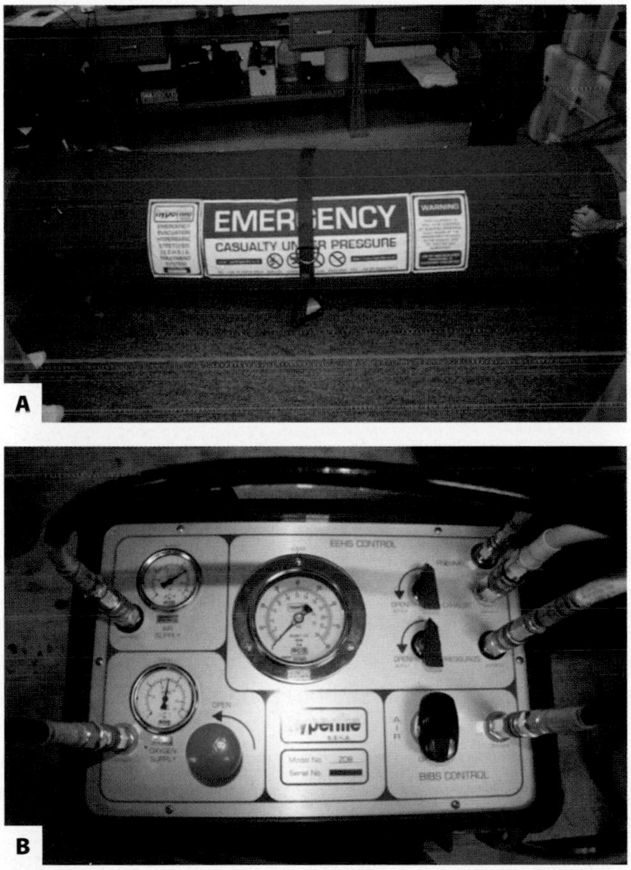

FIGURE 20-10 Portable, collapsible chambers that can be used on a ship or dive boat. (Used with permission of National Oceanic and Atmospheric Administration (NOAA).)

THE PHYSICS OF PRESSURIZATION

The Gas Laws

The principles of pressure and the behavior of gases under pressure are straightforward and governed by basic and well-accepted physical laws. While other gas laws come into play in HBO_2 therapy, understanding several of the most important principles is essential to understanding the effects of HBO_2 therapy.

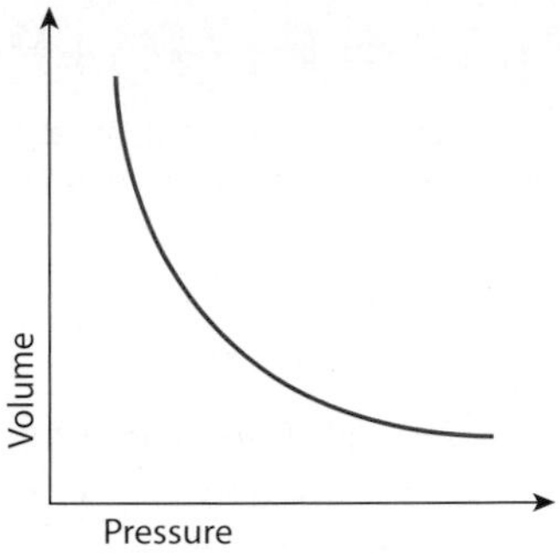

FIGURE 20-11 Boyle's law. As the pressure on a gas increases, the volume decreases.

Boyle's Law Boyle's law states that for a body of gas at a constant temperature, the volume of that body of gas is inversely proportional to the pressure. Essentially, as pressure increases, gas volume decreases (**FIGURE 20-11**). Boyle's law describes the behavior of gas bubbles and air within a sealed space.

Charles' Law Charles' law states that for a body of gas at constant pressure, the volume is directly proportional to the absolute temperature (**FIGURE 20-12**). In the clinical hyperbaric environment, it is the inverse of this that can become a concern; that is, compressing a gas makes it hotter. During the compression or pressurization phase of a hyperbaric treatment, the temperature inside the chamber can become uncomfortably warm if the airflow is not managed properly.

Dalton's Law Dalton's law states that in a mixture of gases, the sum of the partial pressures of the gases will equal the total pressure (**FIGURE 20-13**). Air is comprised of 21% oxygen and 79% nitrogen. It is well accepted that atmospheric pressure equals 760 mmHg. Using Dalton's law, oxygen at 21% has a partial pressure of 160 mmHg and nitrogen at 79% has a partial pressure of 600 mmHg, yielding a total system pressure of 760 mmHg. All gas mixtures obey this same principle.

Henry's Law Henry's law states that the partial pressure of a gas dissolved in a liquid is equal to the partial pressure of that gas exerted on the surface of the liquid at equilibrium (**FIGURE 20-14**). Gases can be dissolved in liquids. If constant

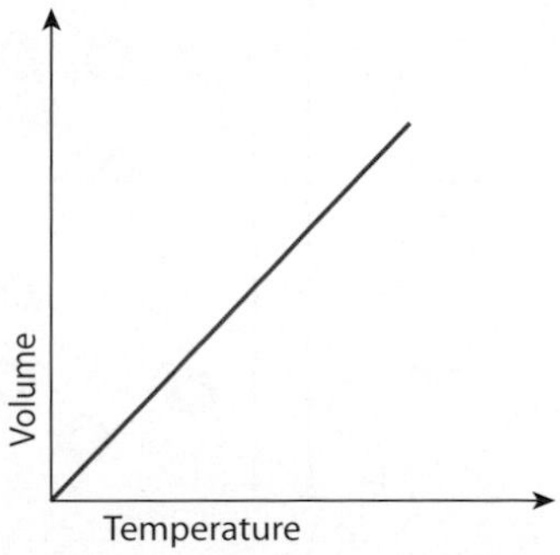

FIGURE 20-12 Charles' law. For a body of gas at constant pressure, the volume is directly proportional to the absolute temperature.

$$P_{Total} = P_1 + P_2 + P_3$$

The total pressure in a system of gases is equal to the sum of the partial pressures of the individual gases

FIGURE 20-13 Dalton's law.

pressure is applied to a liquid and gas solution, the gas will remain in solution. Higher pressures allow increased volumes of gas to be dissolved into the same volume of liquid. If the pressure on the system or solution is lowered, the gas will begin to come out of the solution and form bubbles. This law describes the oxygen-carrying ability of plasma at increased atmospheric pressures. The plasma portion of blood, under sea-level conditions, carries only 0.3 mL of oxygen per 100 mL of blood, in contrast with hemoglobin, which carries 20 mL of oxygen per 100 mL of blood.

Units of Pressure

In the United States, it is widely accepted that atmospheres absolute (ATA) is the unit of measure to describe ambient pressure in a hyperbaric environment. **FIGURE 20-15** illustrates the relationship between ATA and other commonly used units of measure: millimeters mercury (mmHg), pounds per square inch (psi), and feet of sea water (FSW). The maximum pressure typically utilized in clinical HBO_2 is 3 ATA.

The relationship between the ambient pressure in the hyperbaric chamber and the partial pressures of inspired oxygen and air when patients breathe these two gases is also an important concept (**FIGURE 20-16**). According to Dalton's law, the partial pressure of oxygen at sea level is illustrated by the simple equation (.21 × 760 mmHg) = 160 mmHg, where .21 is the percentage of oxygen in air at sea level and 760 mmHg is atmospheric pressure. As the pressure increases in the hyperbaric chamber, the effective concentration of inspired oxygen

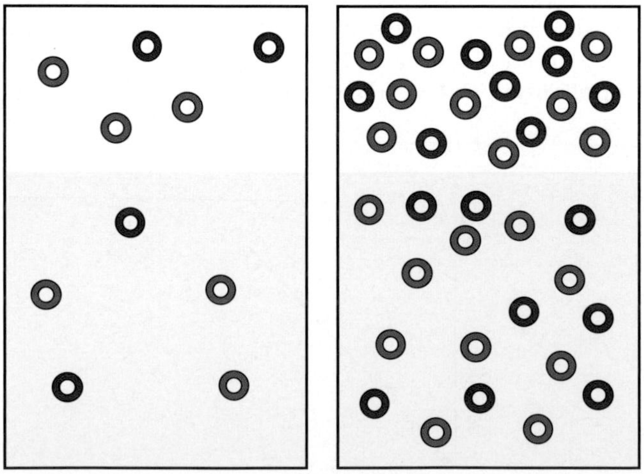

FIGURE 20-14 Henry's law. The partial pressure of a gas dissolved in a liquid is equal to the partial pressure of that gas exerted on the surface of the liquid at equilibrium.

1 ATA	760 mmHg	14.7 psi	0 FSW
2 ATA	1520 mmHg	29.4 psi	33 FSW
3 ATA	2280 mmHg	44.1 psi	66 FSW

FIGURE 20-15 Pressure equivalents. The relationship or relative values of ATA as compared to mmHg pressure, pounds per square inch (psi), and feet of sea water (FSW).

Air at sea-level	(.21 × 760) = 160 mmHg
Air at 2 ATA	(.21 × 1520) = 320 mmHg
Air at 3 ATA	(.21 × 2280) = 480 mmHg
100% O_2 at sea level	(1 × 760) = 760 mmHg
100% O_2 at 2 ATA	(1 × 1520) = 1520 mmHg
100% O_2 at 3 ATA	(1 × 2280) = 2280 mmHg

FIGURE 20-16 Effective inspired O_2 concentrations. Based on the equations of Dalton's law, the effective inspired O_2 concentration drastically increases when the individual is breathing in a hyperbaric oxygen chamber as compared to breathing at sea level.

increases as a function of pressure even though the partial pressure of oxygen in air remains constant at 21%. The numbers in the bottom part of the figure show the inspired gas pressure when the patient breathes 100% oxygen in the chamber. The magnitude of inspired oxygen concentrations possible within a hyperbaric environment is one reason that accepted guidelines in the use of HBO_2 therapy must be followed.

PHYSIOLOGIC EFFECTS OF HYPERBARIC OXYGENATION

Introduction

The physiologic effects, or mechanisms of action in hyperbaric oxygenation, are divided into two categories: the mechanical effects of reducing bubble size (occurring in decompression sickness or iatrogenic air emboli) and the effects of increased partial pressure of oxygen, which vary by the organ system and disorder being treated. At higher than atmospheric pressure, oxygen develops pharmacologic properties not present at atmospheric pressure, and thus, like any other drug, oxygen at pressure must be dosed appropriately to avoid complications.

Mechanical Effects on Gas Bubble Size

Gas bubbles within the intravascular or tissue compartments, as well as within any closed gas-containing body cavities, are affected by changes in pressure. The effects on bubble or body cavity size are governed by Boyle's law, which states that for a given body of gas at a constant temperature, the volume of gas is inversely proportional to the pressure. This law and its effect are used to treat any bubble-related disorders.

In the diving and undersea world, decompression sickness develops most frequently when a diver ascends from depth too rapidly, causing dissolved nitrogen to move from the

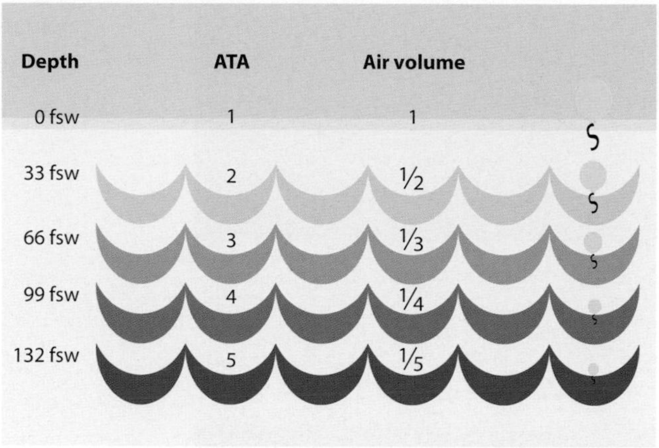

FIGURE 20-17 Factors affecting gas bubble size. Recompression of divers who ascend from depths too quickly and develop symptoms from the formation of gas bubbles. Note that at 2 ATA, the size of the bubbles is reduced by about half.

tissue compartment to the intravascular compartment where it forms bubbles. Depending on where the bubbles lodge, they can disrupt blood flow and cause "the bends." When this process occurs within the musculoskeletal system, it is referred to as type I decompression sickness (DCS I). If this phenomenon occurs within the brain or spinal cord, it is referred to as type II decompression sickness (DCS II), and devastating consequences, such as paralysis and death, may ensue. When an injured diver is recompressed at the surface in a recompression (hyperbaric) chamber, Boyle's law predicts that with recompression to 2 ATA, the size of the offending bubbles will be reduced to roughly one-half of their original size (**FIGURE 20-17**). Typically, with recompression and exposure to higher inspired levels of oxygen, the diver's symptoms are ameliorated and then, with slow decompression back to sea level, the nitrogen is allowed to remain harmlessly in solution. The bends is a complex disorder, but the principle of recreating the higher pressures found at depth for a diver in a chamber and then very gradually lowering that pressure to sea-level pressure will allow the diver to decompress slowly and the nitrogen to dissipate in a physiologically appropriate and harmless manner.

Another clinical application of hyperbaric therapy is in the urgent treatment of iatrogenic gas embolism. Occasionally, during cardiothoracic or vascular procedures, gas bubbles can inadvertently be introduced into either the venous or arterial system. Depending on the location of the event, the consequences can be mild to severe, as air bubbles within the arterial system can act as thrombotic emboli and lead to stroke-like events.

Mechanical Effects on Dissolved Oxygen in Plasma

While in a hyperbaric chamber, dissolved oxygen levels in plasma are dramatically increased more than tenfold. This is enough dissolved oxygen to meet the body's tissue-oxygen needs and to keep the hemoglobin fully saturated on the venous side of the circulation. This phenomenon was beautifully demonstrated by Dutch surgeon Ite Boerema in a 1960 study entitled, "Life Without Blood." In this study, Boerema exsanguinated pigs inside a hyperbaric surgical suite and replaced their blood with saline. The pigs remained alive and functioning in this environment essentially without any intravascular blood. After the experiment, the saline was replaced by the blood, and the pigs were returned to their usual normobaric existence.[14] This principle has occasionally been used as a lifesaving measure for human cases in which blood transfusions are not an option due to religious beliefs.

Effects Due to Elevated Partial Pressures of Oxygen

When under pressure, oxygen acts like a drug—it has pharmacologic properties and physiologic effects dependent on the exposure pressures and the duration of treatment, much like the serum concentrations of various medications that are dependent on drug dose and dosing interval. This principle is of paramount importance when administering HBO_2 in order to avoid adverse effects, which can range from very mild to catastrophic. The clinical administration of hyperbaric oxygen is limited to a maximal pressure of 3 ATA when breathing oxygen. Exceeding 3 ATA provides no additional benefit and only increases the potential toxic effects of oxygen under pressure.

Effect on Blood Flow to Tissues

Hyperbaric oxygen therapy is physiologically a vasoconstrictor. Bird and Telfer, as long ago as 1965, demonstrated a 20% reduction in flow to the extremities during hyperbaric oxygen breathing.[15] They concluded, however, that this was compensated for by the increased oxygen dissolved in the plasma and tissues, thus the tissues remained hyperoxic in spite of reduced blood flow. **FIGURE 20-18** illustrates the hyperoxygenation of plasma in the setting of an occluded artery secondary to thrombosis. Dooley and Mehm also demonstrated delivery despite vasoconstrictive reductions in peripheral blood flow as measured in the calf.[16] Using laser Doppler flowmetry, Hammarlund et al. demonstrated an oxygen-dose-dependent vasoconstriction in the skin of healthy volunteers while that same response was not seen in the skin surrounding a chronic venous leg ulcer even though the same subject demonstrated the expected vasoconstriction in the fingertip. After healing the venous leg ulcer, the expected dermal vasoconstriction in the area surrounding the wound was seen once again.[17]

Hypoxic Wounds

The ability of wounds to heal depends on an adequate supply of oxygen to the wound bed. The normal vascular supply to regional tissues and the wounds therein can be impaired in a macrovascular context, such as with peripheral arterial disease, or microvascular as with diabetes. Whatever the mechanism, wounds will not heal without oxygen. A critical step in wound healing is the production of collagen by fibroblasts. The process of forming new microcirculation (angiogenesis), collagen

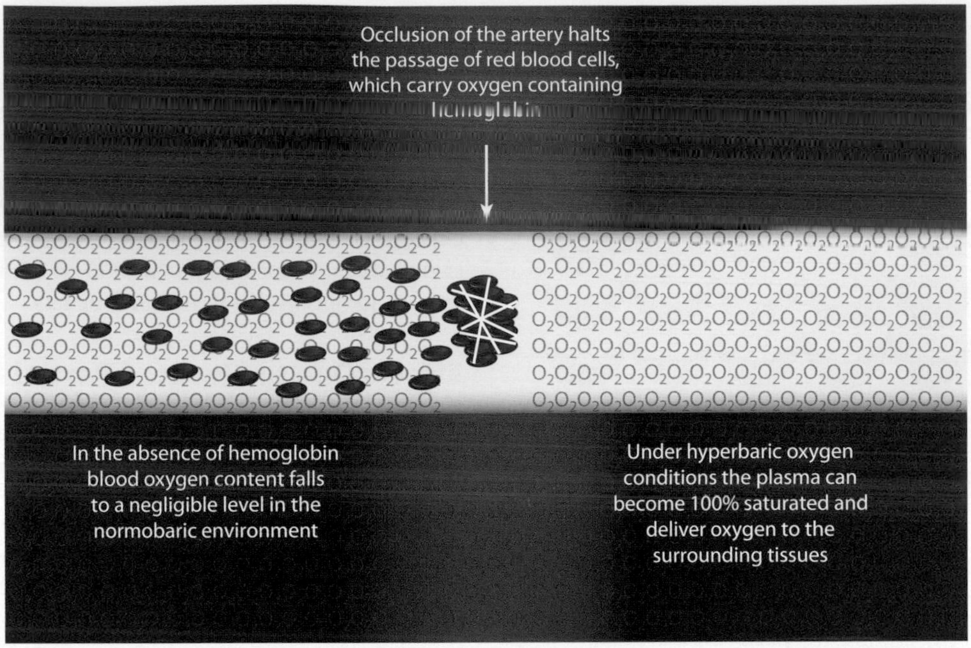

FIGURE 20-18 Oxygen delivery in the presence of an arterial occlusion. When the artery is occluded and red blood cells cannot carry oxygen to the distal tissue, hyperoxygenation of the plasma can provide compensatory oxygen to the tissue distal to the occlusion. This is the basic principle of healing diabetic foot ulcers with HBO_2.

deposition, and the ultimate closure and strength of wounds is dependent upon adequate oxygenation. Angiogenesis is accelerated in ischemic wounds by hyperoxygenation, and healing time is shortened.[18]

Inhibition of *Clostridium perfringens* in Gas Gangrene

Gas gangrene is a rapidly progressive and life-threatening bacterial disorder caused by the anaerobic, spore-forming, gram-positive rod, *C. perfringens*. Gas gangrene is usually initiated by the introduction of *C. perfringens* through a wound. The resultant spread through tissue planes is rapid, leaving necrotic, devitalized tissue in its wake. Hyperbaric oxygen inhibits the α-toxin produced by this bacterium and has a direct bactericidal effect due to polymorphonuclear leukocyte (PMN) activity.

Improvement in Viability of Skin Flaps

The survival of skin and tissue flaps has been studied extensively by numerous investigators. It appears that hyperbaric oxygen therapy increases the viability and ultimate survival of these flaps.[19,20] One of the primary mechanisms appears to be the increased production of superoxide dismutase (SOD) in the hyperbaric environment. SOD is an antioxidative defense mechanism and blocks the production of superoxide radicals from xanthine oxidase, which has been measured in increased quantities in preserved tissue flaps. Zamboni et al. demonstrated that hyperbaric oxygenation improved distal microvascular perfusion as measured by laser Doppler in ischemic skin flaps in the rat.[21]

HYPERBARIC OXYGEN THERAPY IN CLINICAL PRACTICE

According to the UHMS, there are presently 14 approved indications for the clinical application of HBO_2.[10] In nearly all applications, HBO_2 is an adjunctive to standard care and not intended to be stand-alone therapy. **FIGURE 20-19** illustrates categorically the applications of HBO_2. This section will focus

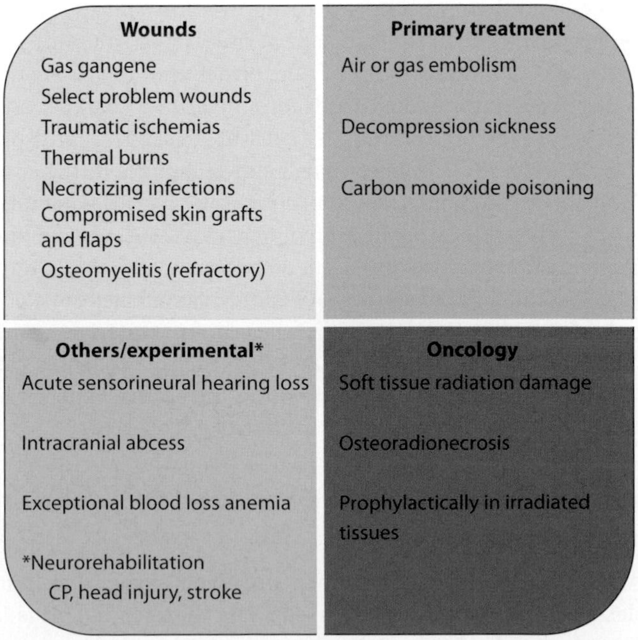

FIGURE 20-19 Categories of disorders that can be treated by HBO_2.

on the physiologic mechanisms and applications for hyperbaric oxygen therapy in wound healing.

General Principles

Research has shown that wounds need an adequate supply of oxygen in order to heal, and when tissue oxygen levels fall below the minimum levels necessary for healing, a number of detrimental effects occur. These include impairments in collagen production, fibroblast migration and proliferation, and reduced response to host infection. Ultimately, the result of these effects is a halt in angiogenesis and cessation of the wound healing cascade.[18]

Increase in Tissue Oxygen Levels with HBO_2 Therapy

Under normal sea-level conditions, the arterial partial pressure of oxygen in a person breathing air will be about 100 mmHg. Under these conditions, hemoglobin (hgb) is approximately 97% saturated with oxygen. Breathing increased concentrations of oxygen at sea level, therefore, has little effect on hemoglobin as it is already completely saturated. In a healthy person with a normal level of hemoglobin, the oxygen-carrying capacity is approximately 20 mL of oxygen for every 100 mL of blood, or 20 volumes percent (vol%). In contrast, the plasma portion of blood carries only about 0.3 mL of oxygen for every 100 cc of blood (0.3 vol%), so plasma, at sea-level conditions, makes no significant contribution to the oxygen-carrying capacity of blood. Therefore, under conditions of complete saturation of hemoglobin, the only way to increase the oxygen-carrying capacity of blood is to increase the amount of oxygen dissolved in plasma.

Looking again at Henry's law, the partial pressure of a gas dissolved in a liquid is equal to the partial pressure of that gas exerted on the surface of that liquid. Accordingly, as atmospheric pressure increases, so does the concentration of dissolved oxygen in the plasma. When breathing oxygen at 2 ATA, or twice the atmospheric pressure, the arterial partial pressure (pO_2) rises to approximately 1400 mmHg, representing over a tenfold increase in arterial oxygen content as compared to that seen at sea level, or 1 ATA. Along with the rise in arterial oxygen content comes a concomitant rise in tissue pO_2 levels, which rise to approximately 300 mmHg at 2 ATA. In the final analysis, at 2 ATA, the oxygen-carrying capacity of blood is increased from 20 vol% to about 24 vol%, an increase almost entirely due to an increase in dissolved plasma oxygen (**FIGURE 20-20**).

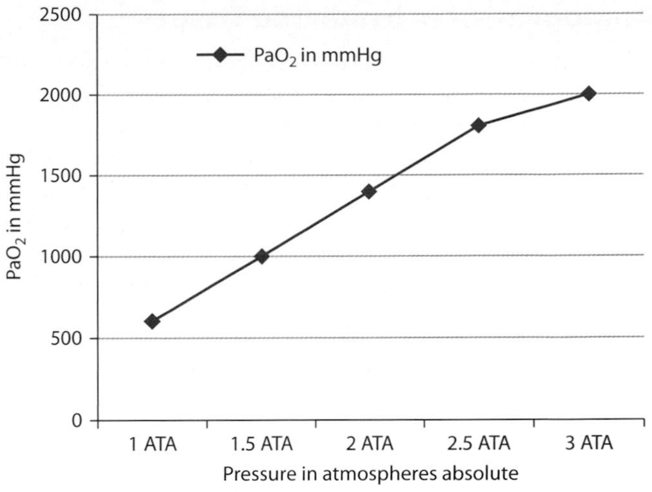

FIGURE 20-20 Arterial partial pressure increases are depicted as the ATA increases. At 2 ATA, the PaO_2 is approximately 1400 mmHg.

Physiological Impact of Oxygen in Wound Healing

The process of wound healing is an elegantly regulated cascade of cellular and biochemical events that work in concert to restore wounded tissue to a prewound condition through the encouragement of physical and physiologic processes. Once wounded, tissue and skin can never be restored to its precise normal anatomic and physiologic state, and tissue and tensile strength are not as high as in the prewound state, so the ultimate goal of the healing process is to restore tissue to an intact and functional status.

Collagen Deposition

Many studies have demonstrated that wound healing is dependent on adequate oxygenation of the vascularized tissue in the periwound area, the area immediately surrounding a wound. HBO_2 intermittently increases the tissue pO_2 as well as the diffusing distance of oxygen in this periwound area.[22] The increase in tissue pO_2 augments wound healing by accelerating fibroblast replication and the resultant collagen synthesis. This in turn leads to the process of granulation, neovascularization, and epithelialization.[23]

Immune Response

HBO_2 enhances the immune response of the host organism. Increased cellular oxygen levels increase leukocyte bactericidal activity, as well as gram-negative organisms, thereby potentially mitigating the extent of aggressive operative intervention in necrotizing bacterial infections.[24,25]

Mediation of Cytokine Activity

Hyperbaric oxygen therapy plays an important role in the production of platelet-derived growth factor (PDGF)-β receptor. This is an important finding, one supported by data reported by Bonomo et al.[26] and Buras et al.[27] These studies were done using dermal fibroblasts from individuals with type II diabetes and their nondiabetic siblings, and showed significantly increased fibroblast proliferation as well as expression of platelet-derived growth factor receptor (PDGFR). The fibroblast proliferation and PDGFR expression in the diabetic subjects were lower than in their nondiabetic siblings. These studies support yet another role of HBO_2 in angiogenesis.

Angiogenesis in Irradiated Tissues

HBO_2 enhances angiogenesis in ischemic, previously irradiated tissue as shown by Marx et al.[28] Delayed radiation soft tissue injuries are secondary to obliteration of end arteries and capillaries causing tissue hypoxia and fibrosis.[26] Marx and his colleagues also showed that dental extractions or other surgical procedures performed in previously irradiated mandibles have high rates of complication and failure unless these procedures are preceded by pre- and postoperative HBO_2.[29–32]

HYPERBARIC OXYGEN THERAPY IN SELECTED WOUND TYPES

Diabetic Wounds of the Lower Extremity

Diabetic foot wounds represent a problem of significant and increasing importance within our society and health care system. The incidence of new cases of diabetes tripled between 1990 and 2010[33] and the prevalence of diagnosed cases of diabetes in American adults and children is estimated to be 37.3 million as of 2022.[34] More than 60% of nontraumatic lower extremity amputations occur in people with diabetes, and in 2006 approximately 65,700 individuals with diabetes underwent such amputations. In addition, it has been reported that 10–15% of diabetics will have at least one foot ulcer at some point in their lives, so the stage is set for an epidemic of diabetic foot ulcers in our communities (**FIGURE 20-21**).[33]

Over the years, a number of clinical trials have been done in an effort to define the role of HBO_2 in the treatment of diabetic foot ulceration. A 2015 Cochrane Review[35] of randomized controlled clinical trials of HBO_2 treatment in chronic wounds concluded that "in people with foot ulcers due to diabetes, HBO treatment significantly improved the ulcers healed in the short term but not the long term." Short term was defined as "up to 6 weeks." The review also stated that HBO_2 may reduce the number of amputations in people with diabetes who have foot ulcers. However, this was not supported by a longitudinal cohort study of more than 6000 patients with diabetic foot ulcers and adequate arterial inflow by Margolis et al.[36] In 2002, Fife et al. conducted a retrospective, multicenter case series of 1144 patients and reported positive outcomes in 75.6% of subjects, all of whom had pretreatment hypoxic transcutaneous oximetry values.[37] In 1996, Faglia et al. studied 70 hospitalized patients with severe, ischemic, infected diabetic foot ulcers.[38] All patients underwent initial evaluation, radical surgical debridement, culture-directed antibiotic therapy, vascular evaluation, and revascularization if indicated. The subjects were then randomized with 35 in the hyperbaric arm and 33 in the control arm (no HBO_2). After a number of weeks, all were evaluated for major amputation by a surgeon unaware of their treatment status. There were fewer amputations, 3 out of 35, in the HBO_2 group than in the control group (11 out of 33); this difference was statistically significant ($p = 0.016$). Kalani et al. reported increased healing and decreased overall amputation rate with HBO_2 in a 12-week study.[39] Abidia et al. also reported improved healing with the use of HBO_2.[40] Unfortunately, statistical analyses were not performed on either of these two studies.

On April 1, 2003, the Centers for Medicare & Medicaid Services (CMS) made effective its decision to cover treatment of diabetic wounds of the lower extremities with hyperbaric oxygen in patients meeting the following criteria:

1. The patient has type 1 or 2 diabetes and has a lower-extremity wound due to diabetes.
2. The patient has a wound classified as Wagner grade III or higher.

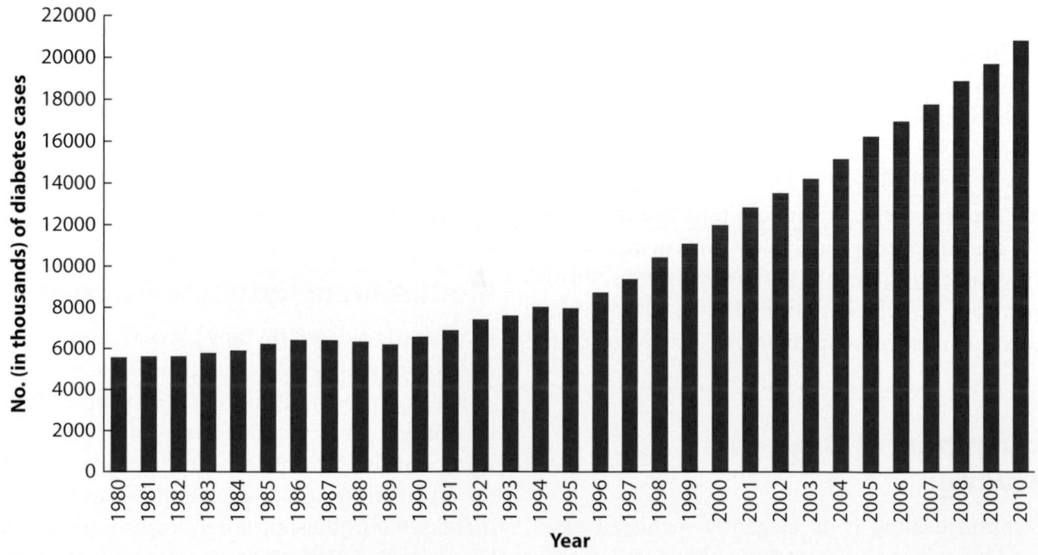

FIGURE 20-21 Annual number of U.S. adults aged 18–79 years with diagnosed diabetes, 1980–2000. The prevalence of diabetes has increased dramatically over the last three decades, making it a major problem for the healthcare system. HBO_2 has been shown to significantly decrease the number of amputations in patients with diabetes and improve healing rates.

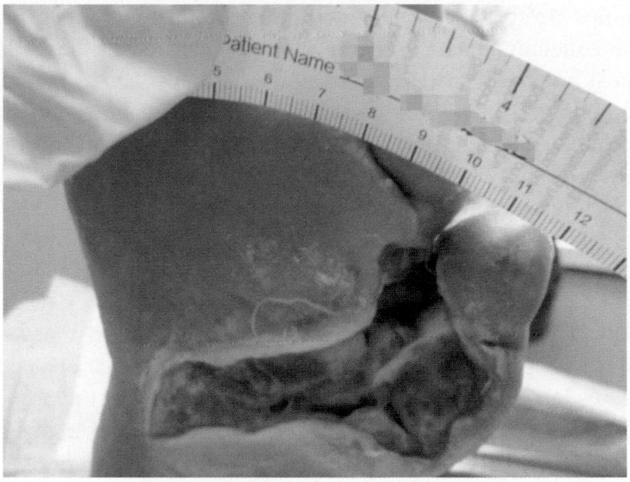

FIGURE 20-22 DFU prior to HBO_2 treatment. Presentation of a diabetic foot wound prior to initiation of standard care plus HBO_2 therapy.

3. The patient has failed an adequate course of standard wound therapy, defined as 30 days of standard treatment that includes the following components: assessment and correction of vascular abnormalities, optimization of nutritional status and glycemic control, debridement, moist wound dressing, offloading, and treatment of infection.

In order for HBO_2 to continue, reevaluation at 30-day intervals must show continued progress toward healing. **FIGURES 20-22** and **20-23** illustrate a diabetic foot ulcer at initial presentation and 8 weeks later following surgical debridement, appropriate wound care, offloading, and hyperbaric oxygen therapy.

Arterial Insufficiency due to Thrombosis

The primary objective in the treatment of a wound due to arterial insufficiency is restoration of adequate arterial flow. If revascularization for an ischemic wound has failed, or is not possible for any combination of reasons, HBO_2 may be beneficial because correction of tissue hypoxia with HBO_2 leads to fibroblast proliferation, collagen synthesis, angiogenesis, and the formation of granulation tissue.[22]

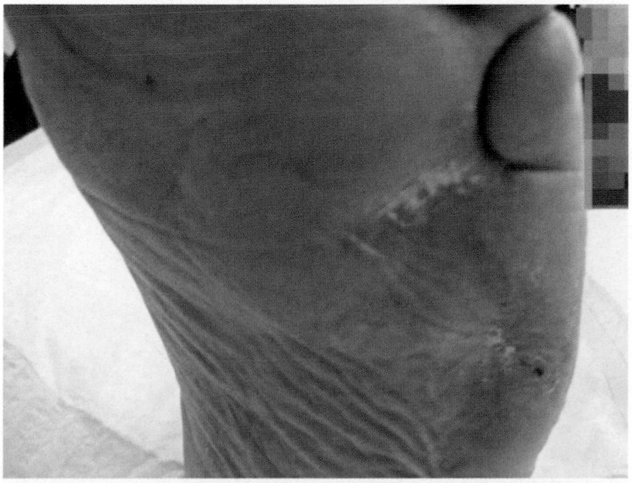

FIGURE 20-23 DFU after HBO_2 treatment. Presentation of the same wound after 8 weeks of standard care plus HBO_2 therapy. The wound is in the remodeling phase of healing.

When arterial insufficiency is the suspected etiology of a lower-extremity wound, transcutaneous oxygen measurement ($TcPO_2$) is performed to assess oxygen delivery to the periwound tissues. If the baseline $TcPO_2$ levels are abnormal, or if the medical history and/or clinical presentations suggest critical limb ischemia, the patient should be referred immediately for invasive arterial testing such as angiography or MRA. If revascularization is successful and tissue hypoxia is reversed, wound healing may then be expected to occur with standard wound care. If revascularization is unsuccessful or not possible due to medical concerns, HBO_2 may be beneficial in this critical limb-salvage situation. Before committing the patient to a full course of HBO_2 in this scenario, in-chamber $TcPO_2$ is performed and a minimum value of 200 mm at treatment depth must be observed in order for efficacy to be expected. It should be noted that the CMS has recently revised its guidelines, stating that the above-described arterial insufficiency must be due to thrombosis in order for HBO_2 to be a covered service. **FIGURE 20-24** illustrates an arterial insufficiency ulceration on the lateral lower leg with exposed tendon. (Refer to Chapter 4, Vascular Wounds, for more details on treating ischemic wounds.)

Delayed Radiation Injury—Soft Tissue and Bony Necrosis

Soft tissue radionecrosis and osteoradionecrosis typically develop months to years following exposure to external-beam radiation therapy, commonly used to treat cancer. In spite of numerous technological advances in the formulas and delivery of radiation therapy, the incidence of radiation injury remains problematic.

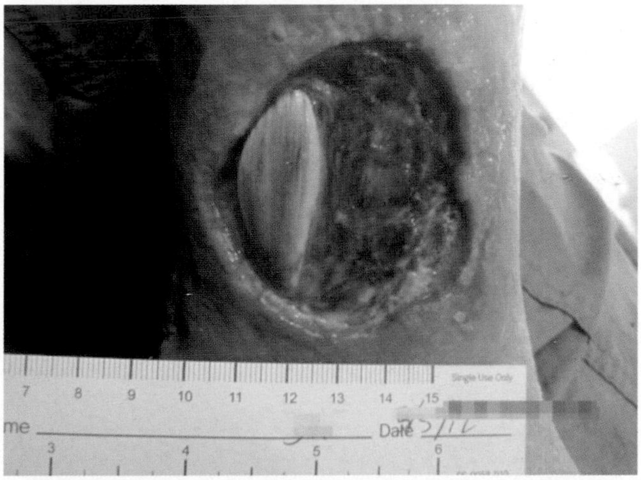

FIGURE 20-24 Arterial wound. An arterial wound with exposed tendon. The $TcPO_2$ at exposed depth is used as a criterion to determine if arterial wounds will benefit from HBO_2 therapy; a minimum value of 200 mmHg is the predictor of efficacy.

Both soft tissue and bony radionecrosis develop as a result of radiation therapy during which a beam of radiation is directed at the site of malignancy. It is impossible for the beam to strike only the cancerous target without affecting the surrounding tissue. With subsequent exposures, the radiation slowly obliterates the end arteries supplying the surrounding tissues leaving hypoxic, fibrotic tissue as a result. This tissue has been referred to as *triple H* tissue, which denotes hypoxic, hypovascular, and hypocellular (**FIGURE 20-25**).

With osteoradionecrosis, causative radiation is usually radiation therapy for cancers of the head and neck region. The zone of the radiation beam extends outward from the target beam and commonly affects the lower jaw (mandible). The affected bone becomes hypoxic, hypovascular, and hypocellular. The affected portion of the mandible may not become problematic for a number of years until a dental problem or oral surgery disrupts the bone, at which point healing of the bone will fail and the mandible may disintegrate. In more severe cases, the mandible may actually disintegrate spontaneously and the patient may present for dental care with exposed and fragmented bone.[41] Marx et al. studied this extensively and authored the treatment paradigms known as the Marx Protocols, which remain in use at this time.[28–30,32]

In the case of soft tissue radionecrosis, the mechanism of injury remains the same but the target tissues are typically different. External beam radiotherapy is commonly used on pelvic malignancies such as uterine and ovarian cancer in women and prostate cancer in men.[42] It is also commonly used in breast cancer treatment both before and after surgical intervention, depending on the type and size of the breast cancer. When a pelvic cancer is irradiated, the soft tissues typically affected are bowel and bladder, leading to conditions known as radiation proctitis and radiation cystitis. These are uncomfortable if not painful conditions characterized by episodic bleeding from the bladder or bowel. Clarke et al. published results of a randomized, controlled trial in 2008 establishing the efficacy of HBO_2 in the treatment of radiation proctitis.[43] Although this level of evidence does not yet exist for radiation cystitis, the mechanism is similar and the treatment is similarly accepted. Another relatively common location for soft tissue radionecrosis is the breast. Radiation therapy may be used preoperatively to reduce tumor size prior to surgery, or postoperatively with or without concomitant chemotherapy. Wound-related problems arise most frequently when surgery such as lumpectomy or mastectomy is performed in a previously irradiated field where, due to the impairment in tissue vascularity and cellularity, normal healing is not able to take place.

Radiation therapy can also lead to skin necrosis; 5–15% of the patients who undergo radiation therapy for cancer develop late radiation tissue injury. A systemic review by Borab et al. looked at eight articles on radiation induced skin necrosis treated with HBO_2 and concluded that it is a "safe intervention with promising outcomes; however, additional evidence is needed to endorse its application as a relevant therapy in the treatment of radiation-induced skin necrosis."[44] An observational cohort study of 2538 patients with radiation-induced injuries supported the use of HBO_2 as an adjunctive treatment to facilitate wound healing.[45] **FIGURES 20-26** and **20-27** illustrate such a wound that had failed to heal in the 15 months

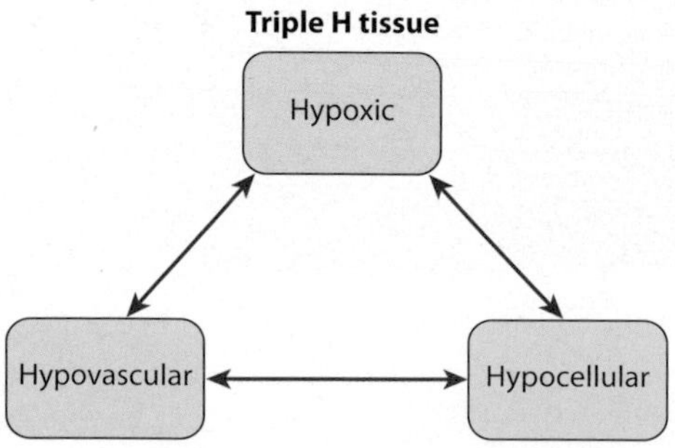

FIGURE 20-25 Radiation wound. Irradiated tissue has been described as Triple H because of the effects of the radiation. The loss of vascularity and oxygenation make the tissue vulnerable to both acute and chronic wounds that have been shown to respond to HBO_2 therapy.

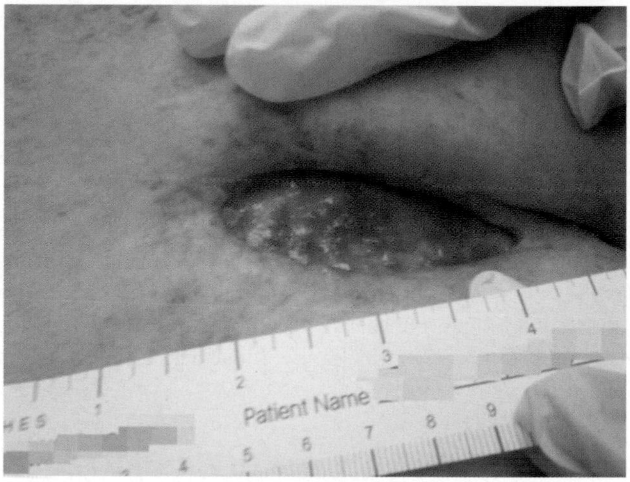

FIGURE 20-26 Radiation wound. Soft tissue necrosis with resulting nonhealing wound in radiated tissue. Note the pale granulation tissue that is indicative of the Triple H phenomenon.

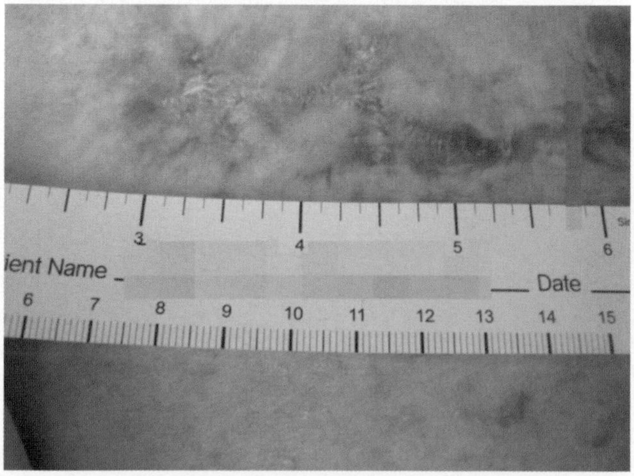

FIGURE 20-27 Radiation wound after HBO_2 treatment. The chronic radiation wound after 20 weeks of standard care and HBO_2 therapy.

following surgery in spite of good wound care. With a combination of appropriate topical wound care, negative-pressure wound therapy, and HBO_2 the wound progressed to complete closure in 20 weeks.

Clostridial Gas Gangrene

Gas gangrene is an uncommon condition caused by an anaerobic, gram-positive, spore-forming bacillus named *Clostridium perfringens*. This organism produces a toxin that creates a rapidly progressive, necrotizing infection of the muscles leading to grave illness, extensive tissue death, and production of gas, which can be palpated in the tissues and seen on X-ray. HBO_2 is used as an adjunct to surgery in the treatment of gas gangrene to attenuate toxicity and spread of infection. Exposure to HBO_2 halts the production of the α-toxin and is also bactericidal. HBO_2 has been shown to reduce morbidity and mortality and to lessen the degree of amputation due to tissue loss.

Chronic Refractory Osteomyelitis

Chronic osteomyelitis, refractory to conventional treatment, may benefit from HBO_2. Both chronicity and failure to respond to appropriate treatment must be documented. Oxygen levels in infected bone are usually significantly lower (20 mmHg) as compared to 30–40 mmHg in healthy tissues. Adjunct HBO_2, along with appropriate antibiotic and surgical management, can elevate bone oxygen levels to near-normal levels, stimulate osteogenesis, and catalyze the development of new capillary vasculature.

In a prospective trial of 32 patients designed to evaluate the efficacy of HBO_2 on postoperative sternal infections after median sternotomy, Barili et al. showed that relapse rates were lower, duration of antibiotic therapy was shorter, and hospital stays were less than in the non-HBO_2 treated group.[46] Although the two groups were not strictly randomized, they appeared well-matched from the perspective of their surgical and infection-related characteristics.

There are presently no randomized trials to support or refute the efficacy of HBO_2 in chronic refractory osteomyelitis; however, there is a robust collection of animal studies, human case series, and prospective clinical trials supporting the safety and efficacy of adjunct HBO_2 in its management.[47] The available evidence appears to support a reduction in the need for surgical procedures, antibiotic therapy, and overall health care expenditure (**FIGURE 20-28**).

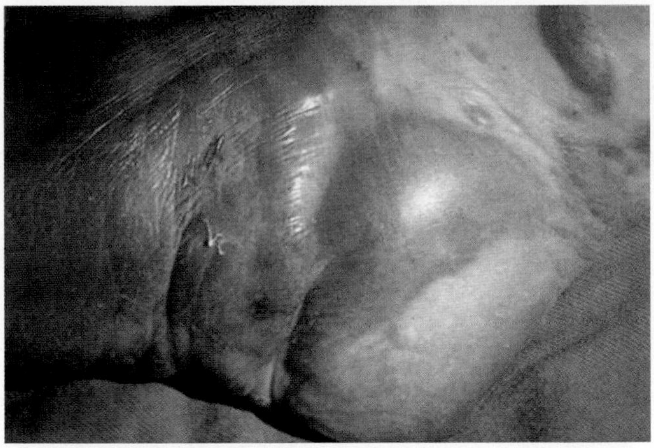

FIGURE 20-28 Chronic osteomyelitis. Blistering and other signs of chronic infection in the soft tissue are indicators of underlying osteomyelitis. In addition, any wound that can be probed to bone has a high probability of having osteomyelitis.

Compromised Skin Grafts and Flaps

HBO_2 has proven to be useful in the preservation and salvage of compromised or ischemic tissue flaps. There have, however, been no studies to support the use of HBO_2 for healthy, viable grafts and flaps. HBO_2 therapy has been studied extensively in grafts that are compromised by tissue hypoxia or involve previously irradiated tissue.

There are many causes for flap compromise, most resulting in an impairment of both blood flow and oxygenation to the flap. These causes range from arterial inflow compromise to edema caused by venous congestion. Ischemia-reperfusion injury can also lead to the compromise and ultimate failure of flaps. This is the condition in which a flap is exposed to a prolonged period of ischemia followed by reperfusion. Zamboni et al. examined and reported on the effect of HBO_2 during and immediately after ischemic periods in skin flaps in a rat model and found beneficial effects of HBO_2 when compared to the non-HBO_2 group.[48] These skin-flap studies were followed and supported by skeletal muscle studies, which in fact may be more important, as skeletal muscle is more sensitive to ischemia-reperfusion injury than is skin.[19]

Whatever the etiology of the ischemic insult, prompt recognition of the problem remains the most important factor in determining what measures can be taken. In some cases, surgical re-exploration will be able to identify and correct the cause, but in others, there may be no identifiable cause. In these cases, the prompt initiation of HBO_2 may assist in the salvage of a flap that otherwise may fail. The vasoconstrictive effects of HBO_2 leading to edema reduction and the saturation of tissues with oxygen are the primary protective hyperbaric mechanisms in the treatment of flaps. **FIGURE 20-29** illustrates amputation and ray resection of toes 2–5; **FIGURE 20-30** shows the surgical flap that has become totally nonviable.

Thermal Burn Injury

Hyperbaric oxygen therapy is indicated in the treatment of serious burns, defined as those covering more than 20% of total body surface area and/or involving the hands, face, feet, or perineum, and that are deep-partial or full-thickness injuries.[11] The burn wound is a complex and evolving injury characterized by a central area of coagulation due to capillary occlusion, with a surrounding area of stasis and a border of erythema. (Refer to Chapter 11, Burn Wound Management, for more details.) Local microcirculation appears to be maximally compromised in the 12–24 hours postburn and the

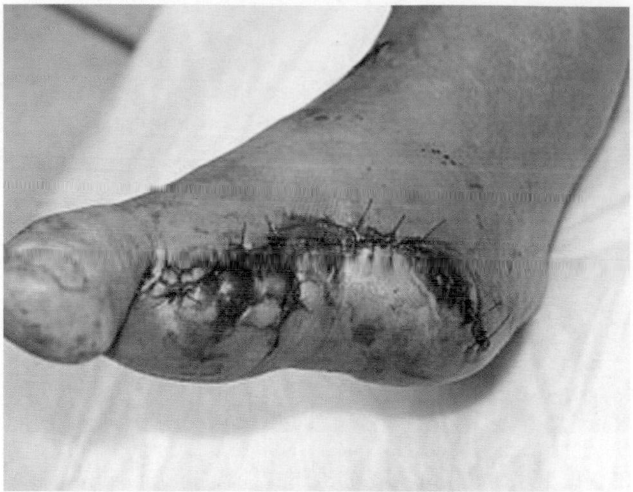

FIGURE 20-29 Amputation site immediately after surgery. Surgical incision after amputation and ray resection of toes 2–5. The blanching periwound skin and incisional necrosis are signs of hypoxia in the forefoot that may respond well to HBO_2 therapy.

central area of coagulation can increase by a factor of 10 over the first 48 hours. Burns are in this evolution process for up to 72 hours following the initial injury.[50]

Niezgoda et al. demonstrated reduced wound size, laser Doppler–measured hyperemia, and wound exudate in a UV-irradiated blister wound model.[51] This was the first prospective, randomized, controlled, double-blind trial comparing HBO_2 with sham controls in a human burn model. In a rat model study, deep second-degree burns were created, treated with silver sulfadiazine, and then assigned to either a normoxic placebo group or a 2.5 ATA HBO_2 group. The results were decreased burn edema, increased neoangiogenesis, increased number of regenerative skin follicles, and reduced time to healing.[52] In addition to the studies cited, there have been numerous others in both animal and human models supporting edema reduction, decreased need for grafting, faster healing, shorter hospital stays, and improved sepsis control.[53]

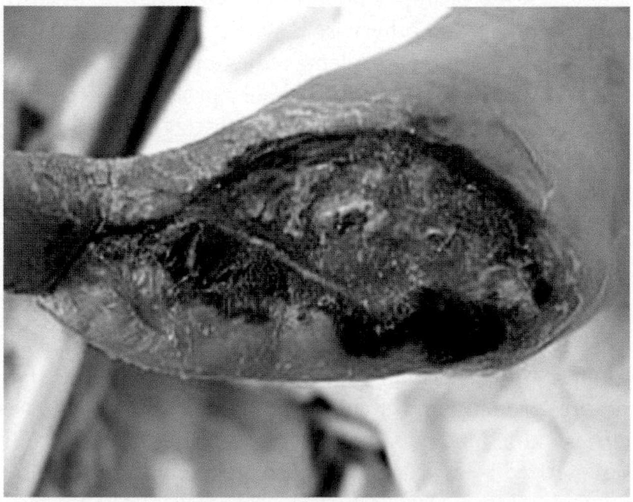

FIGURE 20-30 Necrotic amputation site. The same surgical incision will become a larger necrotic wound if the hypoxia cannot be reversed in time for the soft tissue to recover.

Although adjunct HBO_2 appears to markedly reduce the healing time in burn injuries, especially in deep second-degree injuries, more carefully controlled human studies are necessary in order to more completely define the role of HBO_2 in treating thermal burn injuries.

COVID-19

COVID-19 can cause pneumonitis with a massive inflammatory response that leads to hypoxemia, resulting in the need for ventilation therapy in the ICU. One RCT to study the "use of HBO_2 attenuates the inflammatory response" is being done in Great Britain[54]; however, numerous case studies have reported positive effects for treating patients with COVID-19 with HBO.[55–57] Treatment was reported for ICU patients to improve oxygenation, for hospitalized patients to prevent having to go to ICU, and for recovering patients with fatigue. Most of the studies reviewed by Oliaei et al. used less than 1.5-2 ATA for 90 minutes, decreasing to 60 minutes as the patients improved.[58] All of the authors cited state that more well-designed studies are needed to determine the efficacy and possible adverse effects of HBO_2 for COVID-19.

ADVERSE EFFECTS OF HYPERBARIC OXYGEN THERAPY

As a general rule, the adverse events and effects associated with HBO_2 are mild and relatively uncommon. As with any other treatment modality, both the clinician and the patient need to have an understanding of potential adverse effects associated with the treatment before initiation of therapy. As with the physiologic effects of HBO_2, some of the following adverse effects are associated purely with pressure and others with the combination of pressure and elevated partial pressures of oxygen. **FIGURE 20-31** illustrates some of the more common adverse effects of oxygen under pressure.

Middle-Ear Barotrauma

By far the most common adverse event associated with HBO_2 is middle-ear barotrauma and/or pain.[41] Under normal

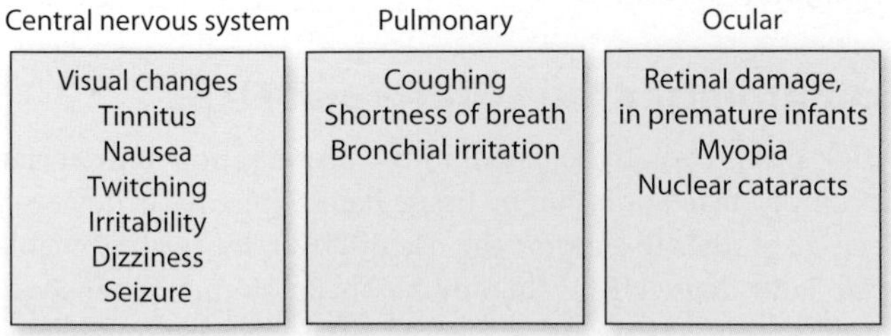

FIGURE 20-31 Adverse effects of O_2 under pressure. Trained personnel will observe the patient for any of these adverse effects and decompress the patient as soon as safely possible.

conditions, the middle-ear compartment communicates with or is ventilated to the external environment through the eustachian tube that connects the middle ear with the oral cavity (see **FIGURE 20-32**). The eustachian tube is normally closed in the resting condition and opens briefly and intermittently with yawning, swallowing, or various maneuvers such as the Valsalva maneuver. Normally air can exit the middle ear compartment passively; however, the entrance of air into the cavity is possible only with muscular contractions that open a portion of the eustachian tube. If for any reason the eustachian tube is unable to equilibrate pressure between the middle ear and the external environment during hyperbaric pressurization, pain develops, and if pressurization is allowed to continue, serious and permanent damage to the ear mechanism may result. Frequently, the use of decongestant nasal sprays is effective in allowing the eustachian tube to function well enough to equalize pressure. This process of equilibration is similar to the landing phase of an airplane flight. In most cases, careful coaching by the hyperbaric technologist is successful in helping the patient to perform appropriate maneuvers to equalize pressure. In cases where this is not successful, hyperbaric treatments should be curtailed until the patient is seen by an otolaryngologist and ventilation tubes inserted in the tympanic membranes to allow equilibration of pressure (**FIGURE 20-32**).

Sinus Squeeze

Sinus squeeze is another mechanical, pressure-related event and is the second most common adverse event associated with HBO_2. It occurs when upper respiratory infections or allergies create mucus and obstruction, thereby making the sinus cavities sealed cavities. Decongestants or steroid-containing nasal sprays are usually effective in clearing this problem so that HBO_2 treatments can continue. Under no circumstances should HBO_2 pressurization continue in the setting of pain.

Pulmonary Barotrauma

Pulmonary barotrauma is a less common but potentially life-threatening event associated with HBO_2. When this occurs, it is usually in the decompression phase of treatment and is due to an airway obstruction that does not allow passive re-expansion of the lungs, which have been compressed during the pressurization and treatment phase of therapy. A chest X-ray should be performed prior to HBO_2 in any patient with a known history or who is suspected of having a pulmonary disorder, and indeed, some practitioners advocate chest X-rays for all patients prior to pressurization regardless of age or medical/surgical history.[59]

Exacerbation of Congestive Heart Failure

Hyperbaric oxygenation causes vasoconstriction and, in so doing, can also cause exacerbations of congestive heart failure and pulmonary edema in patients with unstable cardiac disease. As systemic vascular resistance increases, the pressure against which the heart has to pump (afterload) also increases.[60] If an ailing heart is unable to pump against this increased pressure gradient, fluid can back up into the lungs and create acute pulmonary edema, which can be life-threatening. As always, HBO_2 is part of a team approach to patient care and a cardiologist should be involved whenever there is a history of cardiac disease.

Central Nervous System and Pulmonary Oxygen Toxicity

Exposure to 100% oxygen under pressure can in rare instances induce central nervous system (CNS) toxicity as well as pulmonary toxicity. Fortunately, the hyperbaric exposures in clinical hyperbaric medicine are not of sufficient duration or pressure to cause pulmonary toxicity. With prolonged exposures at higher pressures, the potential for pulmonary toxicity

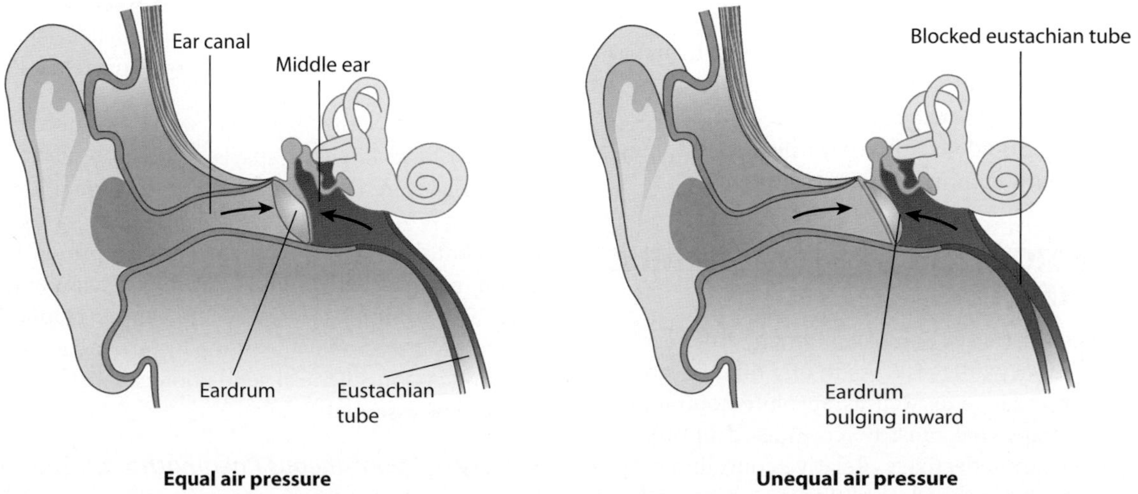

FIGURE 20-32 Middle-ear barotrauma. Diagram of middle-ear and eustachian tube illustrates barotrauma of the middle ear resulting in a bulging displaced eardrum that may cause pain and permanent damage to the ear. This is the most common adverse effect of HBO_2 therapy.

can be assessed using a formula and principle known as the unit pulmonary toxic dose (UPTD).

CNS toxicity can, however, occur in the clinical hyperbaric environment but it is rare. CNS toxicity most often manifests as a seizure, for example, in a diver who is at depth and under increased pressure. Recent studies including a total of 138,968 patients at three different facilities revealed a combined seizure incidence of about 0.03% for a standard oxygen breathing protocol at 2.4–2.5 ATA.[illegible] While seizures inside the hyperbaric chamber can be very disconcerting for patient and staff alike, they are self-limited and typically do not preclude continuation of the hyperbaric treatment regimen in the days to follow. In nearly all cases, the insertion of a 10-minute air-breathing period in the middle of the hyperbaric treatment eliminates the risk of further seizure activity.

Cataracts

The growth or maturation of preexisting cataracts can be stimulated by prolonged series of HBO_2 treatment. New cataracts have not been shown to develop in typical clinical hyperbaric regimens of 20–50 treatments but have been shown to develop in patients who were treated with 150–180 days of HBO_2. These cataracts, once formed, are not reversible and require surgical intervention for treatment.[64]

Myopia

Progressively worsening myopia (nearsightedness) has been shown to develop in some patients undergoing HBO_2 at standard treatment pressures in typical protocols of 20–40 daily treatments. The overall incidence appears to be between 20% and 40% with an increased incidence in diabetics and the elderly. Complete return of vision to baseline is normal, although there have been rare cases in which the myopia was not reversible.[64,65]

Claustrophobia

Patients who are predisposed to claustrophobia may experience some degree of discomfort while in the hyperbaric chamber. This confinement anxiety is more common in the monoplace chamber than in the multiplace, and patients so afflicted may require mild sedation with benzodiazepines in order to continue with their hyperbaric treatments.

CONTRAINDICATIONS TO HYPERBARIC OXYGEN THERAPY

Hyperbaric oxygen therapy is an exceptionally safe modality and overall carries very little risk. As in any other treatment, however, there are relative as well as absolute contraindications to HBO_2 therapy that must be considered in order for it to be used safely and effectively. Relative contraindications include those factors for which additional caution and risk assessment are needed but are not absolute contraindications. Absolute contraindications, as the name implies, are those conditions and medications with which HBO_2 is completely incompatible and for which there is a high risk of adverse outcome. Some contraindications are related to preexisting conditions, while others are related to prior or concurrent use of certain medications. For a complete and very detailed analysis of contraindications, the author suggests that the reader consult a hyperbaric medicine textbook.[66]

Absolute Contraindications

Untreated Pneumothorax Untreated pneumothorax is an absolute contraindication to HBO_2 therapy as there is risk of a simple pneumothorax becoming a tension pneumothorax when the patient is in the chamber.[22] A tension pneumothorax can worsen with decompression and lead to circulatory collapse and death. If HBO_2 is absolutely necessary for a patient with pneumothorax, chest-tube placement and a chest X-ray are considered mandatory prior to the initiation of therapy.

Relative Contraindications

Concomitant Treatment with Doxorubicin During investigation of HBO_2 for the treatment of tissue necrosis due to intravenous extravasation of doxorubicin, Upton et al. found 87% mortality in rats when this drug was combined with HBO_2.[67] The etiology of death in these cases appears to be cardiac. Subsequently, HBO_2 therapy has been used to aid in the healing of tissue necrosis secondary to doxorubicin extravasation. It is, however, recommended that 2–3 days be allowed to lapse between the discontinuation of the drug and the initiation of HBO_2.

Concomitant or Recent Treatment with Bleomycin Bleomycin sulfate is an antineoplastic drug commonly used in the treatment of testicular and certain squamous cell carcinomas. It has been thought, in the past, that exposure to HBO_2 at any point in time following the use of Bleomycin may lead to the development of a condition known as *bleomycin lung*. It is now felt that as long as the patient shows no signs of pulmonary fibrosis and the time interval between Bleomycin administration and HBO_2 exposure is longer than 3–4 months, there should be no Bleomycin-related problems related to HBO_2.[68,69]

Emphysema Some patients with advanced emphysema (COPD) have large air spaces known as blebs within their lungs. Blebs are due to destruction of normal lung tissue and are more prone to rupture during the decompression phase of treatment, leading to pneumothorax (ruptured lung). In addition, patients with emphysema may rely on chronic hypoxemia as a stimulus to breathe and can develop a dangerously low respiratory rate while in the hyperbaric environment. Intubation and mechanical ventilation can be employed if HBO_2 is felt to be essential.[70]

History of Spontaneous Pneumothorax Spontaneous rupture, or air leak, in a lung occurs without regard to activity level. Any patient with a history of spontaneous pneumothorax is at increased risk for recurrence, especially during the decompression phase of the treatment. While the management of pneumothorax in a staffed multiplace chamber is certainly feasible, the monoplace chamber presents a much greater challenge in that there is no inside attendant to perform needle thoracotomy should it become necessary. For this reason, HBO_2 for a patient with a history of spontaneous pneumothorax should be administered in a multiplace chamber if at all possible.

High Fever High fevers are a known risk factor for the development of oxygen toxicity seizures and every effort should be made to normalize body temperature prior to initiating HBO_2. In cases where HBO_2 must be initiated immediately, core cooling measures can be instituted.

Optic Neuritis There have been reports of blindness in patients who have a history of optic neuritis when they are exposed to HBO_2. Optic neuritis is a common component of the multiple sclerosis disease spectrum and ophthalmologic consultation should be sought prior to HBO_2 in any patient with a history of optic neuritis.[71]

Active Respiratory Infections and Sinusitis Respiratory infections and sinusitis typically create inflammation and increased mucus, making it more difficult for patients to equalize pressure in the middle ear. If the infection is significant, or if relief is not possible with nasal decongestants, suspension of HBO_2 until the problem clears is appropriate.

History of Ear Surgery In some ear surgeries, plastic or metallic components are placed into the middle ear mechanism to aid in sound conduction. If middle-ear pressure cannot be equalized during HBO_2, deformation of these components can occur with a resultant loss of hearing. Otolaryngology consultation is recommended for all such patients prior to initiation of HBO_2.

Seizure Disorders There is a concern that patients with preexisting seizure disorders may be more prone to seizures due to oxygen toxicity. It is not entirely clear when a patient's baseline antiepileptic regimen is adequate for seizure control in the setting of HBO_2. If possible, consultation with the patient's neurologist should be sought prior to initiating HBO_2.

Congestive Heart Failure In the majority of cases of stable congestive heart failure, HBO_2 is a very safe treatment. In some cases of unstable or labile congestive heart failure, however, even a slight increase in resistance to an already failing heart can cause the rapid development of an acute exacerbation of congestive heart failure. HBO_2 is a physiologic vasoconstrictor and, as such, can increase systemic vascular resistance and blood pressure, thereby increasing afterload or back pressure on the heart. Whenever a question arises regarding stability of congestive heart failure, it is prudent to consult with a cardiologist prior to initiating HBO_2.

Uncontrolled Hypertension Because HBO_2 is a physiologic vasoconstrictor, it can cause a rise in blood pressure. In most cases this increase is modest; however, in cases of uncontrolled or severe hypertension, an additional rise in pressure can lead to stroke or other related complications. Whenever possible in such cases, blood pressure should be brought under better control prior to proceeding with HBO_2.

Pregnancy The vasoconstrictive effects of HBO_2 can lead to the relative contraindication in pregnancy. Placental vasoconstriction can potentially lead to fetal hypoxia and the well-known associated complications. A commonly accepted exception to this guideline is in the case of carbon monoxide poisoning where the potential benefits of HBO_2 to mother and fetus are thought to outweigh the risks. An example is a young patient and her 16-month-old daughter who suffered carbon monoxide poisoning after spending a winter day driving in a van with faulty exhaust. They were treated by the author in a monoplace chamber. Of interest is that the patient was also pregnant at 16 weeks' gestational age at the time of these treatments so, in fact, there were three patients in the chamber rather than two. The mother did go on to deliver a healthy full-term infant.

SAFETY GUIDELINES

Safety is of the utmost importance in the use of hyperbaric oxygen therapy. While there has never been a hyperbaric chamber fire in a hospital-based hyperbaric department in the United States, the risk of fire and explosion remains ever-present due to the presence of 100% oxygen, which is intensely flammable and explosive. The two additional components needed are heat and an ignition source; therefore, hyperbaric chamber safety recommendations focus primarily on eliminating potentially static-producing materials from the chamber environment. Exhaustive lists of prohibited materials are available universally. The fundamental approach in most hyperbaric centers in the United States is to have a zero-tolerance policy for extraneous materials within the chamber. Daily checklists require patients to be recently bathed with no hair products, skin products, or jewelry, and to be clothed in 100% cotton scrubs. No outside clothing or shoes are allowed. Hearing aids, dentures, hairpieces, and any other nonanatomic items are removed and dressing products are to be carefully screened in order to avoid the introduction of petroleum products or any other synthetic materials that might potentially generate static electricity.[22]

The guidelines for multiplace chambers are in some instances less stringent than for monoplace chambers because the ambient gas environment in the multiplace chamber is air rather than 100% oxygen as in the monoplace chamber. Theoretically, using air rather than oxygen reduces the threat of fire or explosion. An additional safety strategy in the monoplace chamber is a grounding pad or bracelet worn by the patient and attached to the metal carriage of the chamber, which is in turn attached to an external ground.

This author's strong bias is that a daily culture of vigilance on the part of physicians, staff, and patients, coupled with a zero-tolerance policy, is the best defense against catastrophe and tragedy.

CASE STUDY 1

INTRODUCTION

A 45-year-old male with a 6-month history of diabetic foot ulcer present for approximately 6 months, was referred for HBO_2 consideration. He had been ambulating in standard shoes and wound care had consisted of topical applications of triple antibiotic ointment. Current vascular and radiographic studies have not been performed.

Past medical history:	Type 2 diabetes since age 27 Exogenous obesity Essential hypertension
Past surgical history:	Incision and drainage of right foot wound, 2000 Amputation of right third toe, 2003 Incision and drainage for right foot infection, 2008

At the time of initial visit to the clinic, the wound was full thickness, surrounded by copious hyperkeratosis, and probed to bone (**FIGURE 20-33A**). The third toe had been amputated 7 years prior.

DISCUSSION QUESTIONS

1. What subjective information is needed from this patient in order to make a diagnosis?
2. What tests and measures are indicated before initiating treatment?
3. What medical specialists would be helpful in caring for this patient?

The patient was admitted to the hospital on the day of initial evaluation and consultations were requested from Infectious Disease, Podiatry, and Vascular Surgery.

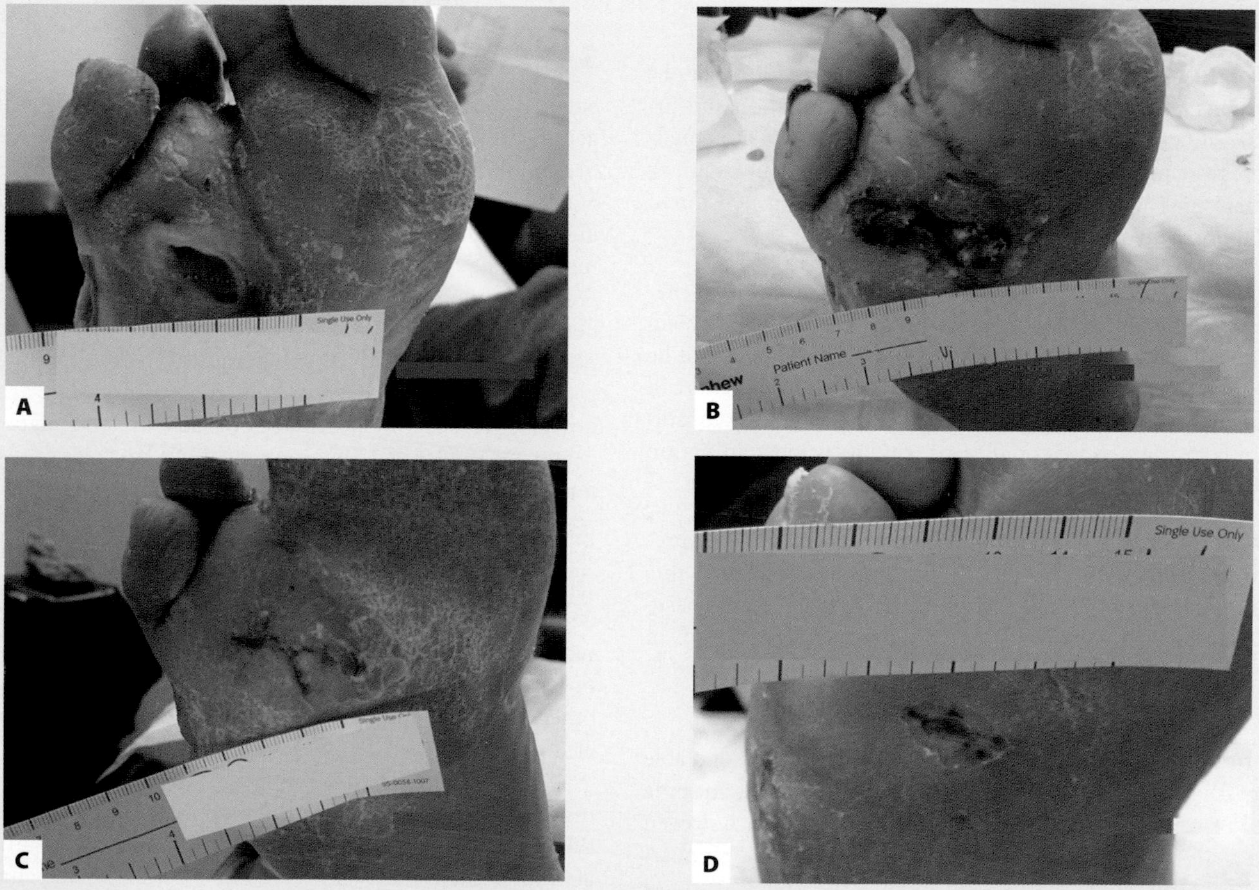

FIGURE 20-33 A–D. Case Study 1. A. Diabetic foot ulcer at the time of initial evaluation for HBO_2 therapy. **B.** Diabetic foot ulcer 10 days after debridement and standard care, including antibiotic therapy, antimicrobial dressings, and offloading. **C.** Diabetic foot ulcer 6 weeks after initial presentation and 4 weeks after initiation of HBO_2. **D.** Diabetic foot wound 3 months after the initial visit. The partial-thickness skin loss is from the debridement of hyperkeratosis that tends to form during and after the healing process for any diabetic foot ulcer. This callus formation requires that any patient with a history of diabetic foot ulcer, especially one that is difficult to heal, be followed periodically by a clinician experienced in caring for the diabetic foot.

CASE STUDY 1 *(Continued)*

Radiographs revealed osteomyelitis of the fourth and fifth metatarsal heads and, following vascular studies that confirmed no arterial insufficiency to interfere with wound healing, the patient was taken to surgery for debridement of bone and soft tissue. Intraoperative cultures of bone as well as soft tissue grew *Staphylococcus aureus* and the patient was placed on intravenous antibiotics which were continued for a period of approximately 6 weeks. The patient was discharged from the hospital 5 days after admission to continue with outpatient care. Initial offloading was accomplished with crutches. He was seen again in the wound center the following week. At that time, he was transitioned from crutches to a four-wheeled knee scooter and wound care was initiated with cadexomer iodine gel as a primary dressing and gauze as a cover dressing. **FIGURE 20-33B** shows the ulcer 10 days after debridement with a visible suture still in place.

Hyperbaric oxygen therapy was initiated and 30 daily treatments were carried out at 2 ATA for 2 hours per treatment. The patient maintained excellent compliance with offloading and wound care and the intravenous antibiotics were discontinued after a 6-week course of therapy. **FIGURE 20-33C** shows the ulcer approximately 6 weeks after initial presentation to the wound center and approximately 4 weeks after initiation of HBOT.

HBOT was discontinued at this time and the patient continued wound care with a silver hydrogel primary dressing and gauze cover; he also continued offloading with the knee scooter.

The patient was fitted with custom shoes and insoles and was seen for final follow-up 3 months after initial evaluation. The following week he returned to his job out of state and reported 3 months later that he remained completely healed. **FIGURE 20-33D** is the photo of the foot obtained on that final visit following debridement of a small callous.

CASE STUDY 2

INTRODUCTION

A 61-year-old female presented for evaluation of a scalp and cranial defect. The patient had undergone multiple craniotomies dating back to 1999 for treatment of recurrent cerebral meningioma. Prior to the original surgery in 1999 she underwent a 6-week course of external beam radiation therapy in an effort to shrink the tumor. In 2010, she underwent gamma knife surgery again followed by another open procedure later the same year. On initial presentation, the defect measured 2.6 cm × 2.4 cm × 1 cm deep. The base of the wound was exposed dura mater (**FIGURE 20-34A**).

Past medical history: Essentially unremarkable other than that associated with meningioma

Past surgical history:
- Open excision of meningioma, 1999
- External beam radiation therapy, 1999
- Gamma-knife excision of meningioma, 2010
- Open excision of meningioma, 2010
- Repair of scalp and cranial defect, 2010 and 2011
- Tonsillectomy, 1968
- Tubal ligation, 1991
- Rotator cuff repair, 1993
- Repair of ankle fracture, 2004

DISCUSSION QUESTIONS

1. Is this patient appropriate for HBO_2 and if so, why?
2. Are there any contraindications or precautions to HBO_2?
3. What tests would be indicated prior to initiation of therapy?
4. What parameters for treatment are recommended for this patient?

Treatment was initiated on day 1 with a synthetic collagen product applied directly to the wound bed every third day with a simple gauze covering. Hyperbaric oxygen therapy was initiated in late January and she received a total of 30 treatments of 90 minutes' duration at a pressure of 2.4 ATA through mid-March. **FIGURES 20-34B** to **20-34D** illustrate the wound progress during that time frame.

FIGURE 20-34E shows the wound after 1 year, fully epithelialized and remodeling.

Continued next page—

CASE STUDY 2 *(Continued)*

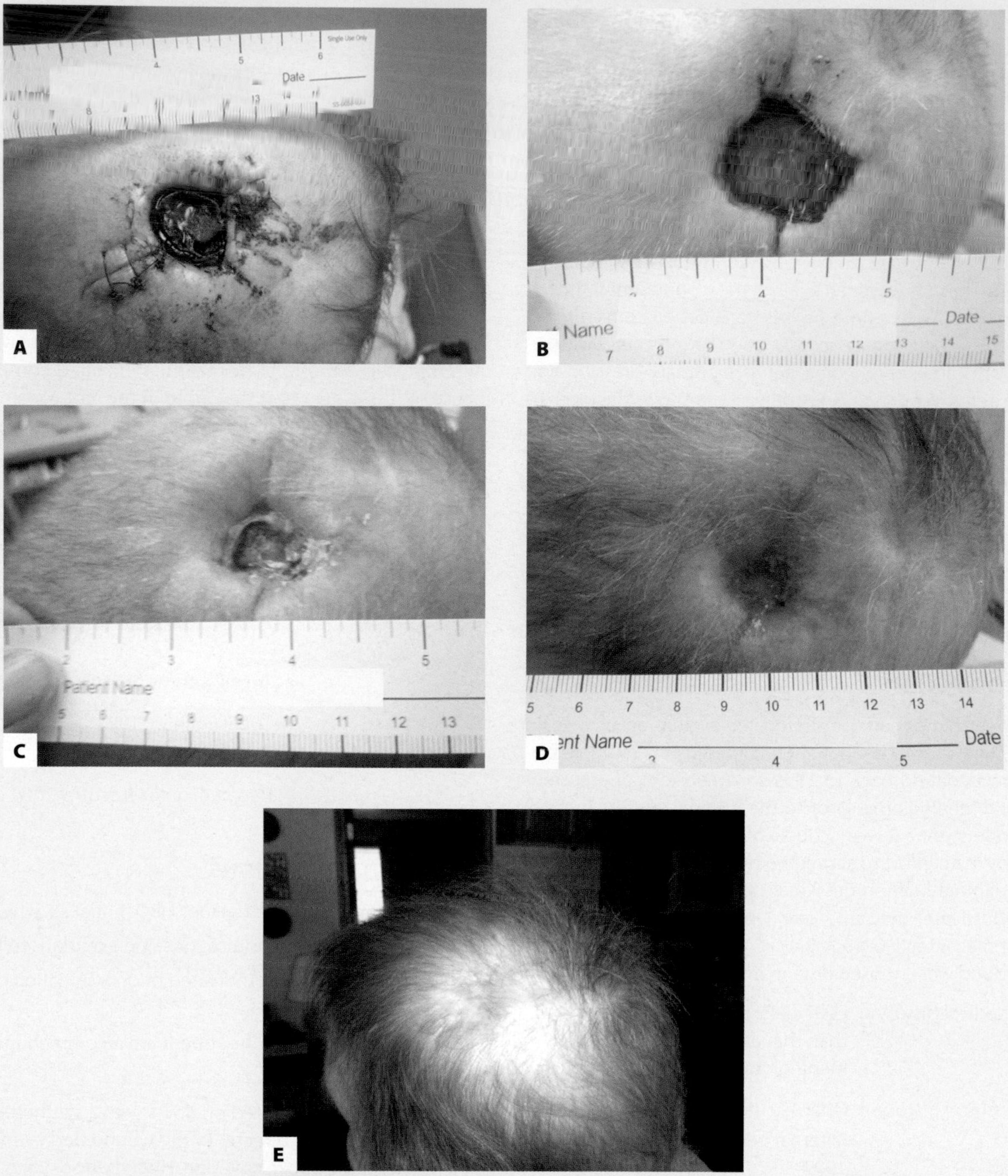

FIGURE 20-34 A–E. Case Study 2. A. Postradiation wound on the scalp of a patient who had multiple craniotomies, radiation therapy, and gamma-knife surgery. **B.** Signs of angiogenesis are visible in the deep wound bed. **C.** Wound contraction is evident by the decreased size. Note the healthy hair growth on the remaining scalp. **D.** Wound contraction is evident by the decreased size. Note the healthy hair growth on the remaining scalp. **E.** The radiation wound 1 year after initiation of therapy is fully epithelialized and in the remodeling phase of healing.

TOPICAL OXYGEN THERAPY

Introduction

Topical oxygen therapy (TOT) is a treatment modality that has gained much popularity, relevance, and scientific support over recent years. This therapy differs from hyperbaric oxygen therapy (HBO_2) in that 100% oxygen is delivered directly to the wound bed, with the affected limb enclosed in a boot or bag, rather than with the entire patient in a hyperbaric chamber. [72] The physiology of topical oxygen therapy differs significantly from hyperbaric oxygen therapy, so consequently the applications and indications vary as well. The advantage of TOT is that it does not have the risks associated with systemic hyperbaric oxygen therapy. As with any adjunctive therapy, standard wound care based on wound etiology is essential.

Physiology

The mechanism of topical oxygen therapy is based upon diffusion of oxygen into a moist wound bed, from an area of higher concentration to one of lower concentration. The partial pressure of oxygen (PO_2) in human tissue is approximately 50 mmHg at 3–4 mm below the surface for wounds exposed to air. Based on the discussion of Dalton's law air at normobaric pressure is 21% oxygen (160 mmHg). With the application of topical oxygen to the wound, the wound bed is exposed to 100% oxygen (760 mmHg) without an increase in pressure. A study has shown an increase in superficial wound tissue PO_2 from 10 mmHg in room air to 40%, within 4 minutes, when 100% oxygen at normobaric pressure is applied to the surface of a moist wound.[73]

There are three types of TOT delivery systems: (1) devices that provide continuous delivery of oxygen (CDO), (2) devices that provide low constant pressure in a contained chamber, and (3) devices that are cyclically pressurized and humidified in a contained chamber.[74] Research thus far has suggested that the CDO and cyclically pressurized devices in conjunction with standard care resulted in significant improvements in healing chronic DFUs. However, a systemic review by Sethi et al. concluded that most studies have a risk of bias and more stringent studies and RCTs are needed.[75]

Equipment

Wound treatment with topical oxygen therapy is typically delivered via a high-flow oxygen concentrator connected to a bag or other chamber which is sealed around the area of the wound (**FIGURE 20-35**). The treatment is most often intermittent, as with HBO_2; however, there are systems available that enable the continuous delivery of oxygen to the wound. With either system the oxygen must be delivered to a moist wound bed, otherwise the oxygen will desiccate the wound bed tissue and bring wound healing to a halt.

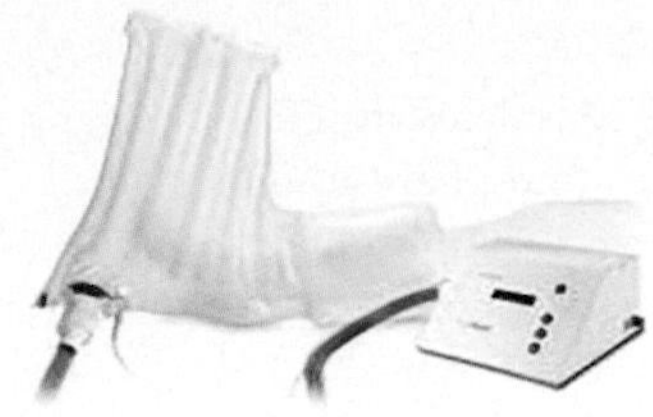

FIGURE 20-35 Equipment for topical oxygen therapy.

Indications

Wound types for which topical oxygen has been reported to be of benefit include the following:

- Diabetic foot ulcers
- Postsurgical wounds with dehiscence
- Pressure injuries
- Amputation sites
- Ischemic skin grafts
- Vascular ulcers: arterial and venous
- Augmented healing with cellular and tissue-based products (CTPs)
- Burns
- Frostbite

Contraindications

At this point, there are no known specific contraindications to topical oxygen therapy. Good clinical judgment, however, must prevail and other necessary and appropriate wound care measures must be in place.

SUMMARY

The science and practice of hyperbaric oxygen therapy is in its infancy. Hyperbaric oxygen has been in active clinical use only since 1955, and the preponderance of clinical research is much more recent than that. Over those years, a list of 14 indications that are approved for treatment by the UHMS has slowly and methodically been developed. The UHMS Committee, comprising hyperbaric medicine luminaries from around the world, regularly convenes to review the presently accepted indications for therapy and to carefully examine new potential indications for the use of HBO_2. These analyses serve to scrutinize the most recent scientific supporting evidence as well as a careful cost-effectiveness comparison relative to other accepted treatment modalities presently in use.

The increased study of, and evidence around topical oxygen therapy has added an additional oxygen-mediated modality to the wound care armamentarium and may allow increased access to oxygen therapy for those patients unable to access HBO_2 as well as for some wound etiologies for which there is presently no approved indication for HBO_2.

STUDY QUESTIONS

1. In order to be considered hyperbaric therapy, pressure must be
   a. Above one atmosphere absolute.
   b. Greater than 1.4 atmosphere absolute.
   c. Between [illegible] and [illegible] atmosphere absolute.
   d. Either inhaled or topical
2. Hyperbaric oxygen therapy is physiologically effective in increasing skin perfusion because it
   a. Causes vasodilation of the distal vessels.
   b. Increases the blood flow to the extremities by increasing the blood pressure.
   c. Increases the oxygen dissolved in the plasma and tissues.
   d. Dissolves the fibrinogen clots in occluded arteries.
3. Studies of HBOT on diabetic patients have shown that there is an increase in
   a. Platelet-derived growth factors and fibroblast production.
   b. Migration of macrophages to the injured tissue.
   c. Collateral circulation in the affected extremity.
   d. Histamine with resulting increased vasopermeability.
4. In order for Medicare to cover HBOT for a diabetic foot wound, it must be classified as a
   a. Wagner I.
   b. Wagner II.
   c. Wagner III.
   d. Wagner IV.
5. Which of the following is an absolute contraindication to HBOT?
   a. Emphysema
   b. Seizure disorder
   c. Congestive heart failure
   d. Untreated pneumothorax

Answers: 1-b; 2-c; 3-a; 4-c; 5-d.

REFERENCES

1. Henshaw IN, Simpson A. *Compressed Air as a Therapeutic Agent in the Treatment of Consumption, Asthma, Chronic Bronchitis and Other Diseases*. Edinburgh, Scotland: Sutherland and Knox; 1857.
2. Fontaine JA. Emploi chirurgical de l'air comprime. *Union Med*. 1879;28:445.
3. Cunningham OJ. Oxygen therapy by means of compressed air. *Analgesie*. 1927;6:64.
4. Williams HS. *Book of Marvels*. New York, NY: Funk & Wagnalls; 1931:12.
5. Churchill-Davidson I, Sanger C, Tomlinson RH. High pressure oxygen and radiotherapy. *Lancet*. 1955;1:1091-1095.
6. Boerema I, Kroll JA, Meijne NG, Lokin E, Kroonand B, Huiskes JW. High atmospheric pressure as an aid to cardiac surgery. *Arch Chir Neerl*. 1956;8:193-211.
7. Brummelkamp W, Hogendijk J, Boerema I. Treatment of anaerobic infections (*Clostridial myositis*) by drenching the tissues with oxygen under high atmospheric pressure. *Surgery*. 1961;49:299-302.
8. Smith G, Sharp GR. Treatment of coal gas poisoning with oxygen at two atmospheres pressure. *Lancet*. 1962;1:816-819.
9. Whelan HT, ed. *Hyperbaric Medicine Practice*. 4th ed. West Palm Beach, FL: Best Publishing; 2017.
10. Kindwall EP. *Report of the Committee on Hyperbaric Oxygenation*. Bethesda, MD: Undersea Medical Society; 1977.
11. Gesell LB. *Hyperbaric Oxygen Therapy Indications*. 12th ed. The Hyperbaric Oxygen Therapy Committee Report. Durham, NC: Undersea and Hyperbaric Medical Society; 2008.
12. Kot J. Staffing and training issues in critical care hyperbaric medicine. *Diving Hyperb Med*. 2015;45(1):47-50.
13. Lind F. A pro/con review comparing the use of mono- and multiplace hyperbaric chambers for critical care. *Diving Hyperb Med*. 2015;45(1):56-60.
14. Boerema I, Meyne NG, Brummerlkamp WH, et al. Life without blood. *Ned Tijdschr Geneeskd*. 1960;104(5):949-954.
15. Bird AD, Telfer ABM. Effect of hyperbaric oxygen on limb circulation. *Lancet*. 1965;13(1):355-356.
16. Dooley JW, Mehm WJ. Noninvasive assessment of the vasoconstrictive effects of hyperoxygenation. *J Hyperb Med*. 1990;4(4):177-187.
17. Hammarlund C, Castenfors J, Svedman P. Dermal vascular response to hyperoxia in healthy volunteers. In: Bakker DJ, Schmuts J, eds. *Proceedings of the Second Swill Symposium on Hyperbaric Medicine*. Basel, Switzerland: Foundation for Hyperbaric Medicine; 1988: 55–59.
18. Hunt TK. The physiology of wound healing. *Ann Emerg Med*. 1988;17:1265-1273.
19. Liang C, Liang W, Zhenxiang W, Qing G, Shirong L. Hyperbaric oxygen therapy for skin flap blood flow disorder: a care report. *J Med Coll PLA*. 2012;27(3):183-186.
20. Xiao D, Liu Y, Li J, et al. Hyperbaric oxygen preconditioning inhibits skin flap apoptosis in a rat ischemia reperfusion model. *J Surg Res*. 2015;199(2):732-739.
21. Zamboni WA, Roth AC, Russell RC, Smoot EC. The effect of hyperbaric oxygen on reperfusion of ischemic axial skin flaps: a laser Doppler analysis. *Ann Plast Surg*. 1992;28:339-341.
22. Lam G, Fontaine R, Ross FL, Chiu ES. Hyperbaric oxygen therapy: exploring the evidence. *Adv Skin Wound Care*. 2017;30(4):181-190.
23. Knighton D, Silver I, Hunt TK. Regulation of wound healing angiogenesis-effect of oxygen gradients and inspired oxygen concentration. *Surgery*. 1981;90:262-270.
24. Hohn DC. Oxygen and leukocyte microbial killing. In: Davis JC, Hunt TK, eds. *Hyperbaric Oxygen Therapy*. Bethesda, MD: Undersea Medical Society; 1977:101-110.
25. Knighton DR, Fiegel VD, Halverson T, Schneider S, Brown T, Wells CL. Oxygen as an antibiotic. The effect of inspired oxygen on infection. *Arch Surg*. 1990;125:97-100.
26. Bonomo SR, Davidson JD, Yu Y, Xia Y, Lin X, Mustoe TA. Hyperbaric oxygen as a signal transducer: upregulation of platelet derived growth factor-beta receptor in the presence of HBO_2 and PDGF. *Undersea Hyperb Med*. 1998;25:211-216.
27. Buras JA, Veves A, Orlow D, Reenstra W. The effects of hyperbaric oxygen on cellular proliferation and platelet-derived growth factor receptor expression in non-insulin dependent diabetic fibroblasts. *Acad Emer Med*. 2001;8:518-519.
28. Marx RE, Ehler WJ, Tayapongsak P, Pierce LW. Relationship of oxygen dose to angiogenesis induction in irradiated tissue. *Am J Surg*. 1990;160:519-524.
29. Marx RE, Ames JR. The use of hyperbaric oxygen in bony reconstruction of the irradiated and tissue-deficient patient. *J Oral Maxillofac Surg*. 1982;40:412-420.

30. Marx RE. A new concept in the treatment of osteoradionecrosis. *J Oral Maxillofac Surg*. 1983;41:351-357.
31. Marx RE, Johnson RP. Problem wounds in oral and maxillofacial surgery: the role of hyperbaric oxygen. In: Davis JC, Hunt TK, eds. *Problem Wounds: The Role of Oxygen*. New York, NY: Elsevier; 1988:65-123.
32. Marx RE, Johnson RP, Kline SN. Prevention of osteoradionecrosis: a randomized prospective clinical trial of hyperbaric oxygen versus penicillin. *J Am Dent Assoc*. 1985;111:49-54.
33. Reiber GE, Ledous WE. Epidemiology of diabetic foot ulcers and amputations: evidence for prevention. In: Williams R, Herman W, Kinmonth A-L, et al., eds. *The Evidence Base for Diabetes Care*. London: Wiley; 2002:641-665.
34. Centers for Disease Control and Prevention. National Diabetes Statistics Report website. https://www.cdc.gov/diabetes/data/statistics-report/index.html. Accessed February 2023.
35. Kranke P, Bennett MH, Martyn-St James M, Schnabel A, Debus SE, Weibel S. Hyperbaric oxygen therapy for treating chronic wounds. The Cochrane Library. June 24, 2015. Available at: https://www.cochrane.org/CD004123/WOUNDS_hyperbaric-oxygen-therapy-for-treating-chronic-wounds. Accessed September 10, 2018.
36. Margolis DJ, Gupta J, Hoffstad O. Lack of effectiveness of hyperbaric oxygen therapy for the treatment of diabetic foot ulcer and the prevention of amputation: a cohort study. *Diabetes Care*. 2013;36:1961-1966.
37. Fife CE, Buyukcakir C, Otto G, Sheffield P, Love T, Warriner RA. Factors influencing the outcome of lower-extremity diabetic ulcers with hyperbaric oxygen therapy. *Wound Repair Regen*. 2007;15: 322-331.
38. Faglia E, Favales F, Aldeghi A, et al. Adjunctive systemic hyperbaric oxygen therapy in treatment of severe prevalently ischemic diabetic foot ulcer: a randomized study. *Diabetes Care*. 1996;19:1338-1343.
39. Kalani M, Jörneskog G, Naderi N, Lind F, Brismar K. Hyperbaric oxygen (HBO) therapy in treatment of diabetic foot ulcers. Long-term follow-up. *J Diabetes Complications*. 2002;16(2):153-158.
40. Abidia A, Laden G, Kuhan G, et al. The role of hyperbaric oxygen therapy in ischemic diabetic lower extremity ulcers: a double-blind randomized-controlled trial. *Eur J Vasc Endovasc Surg*. 2003;25: 513-518.
41. Davis JC, Dunn JM, Heimbach RD. Hyperbaric medicine: patient selection, treatment procedures, and side effects. In: Davis JC, Hunt TK, eds. *Problem Wounds: The Role of Oxygen*. New York, NY: Elsevier; 1988:225-235.
42. Griffiths C, Howell RS, Boinpally H, et al. Using advanced wound care and hyperbaric oxygen to manage wound complications following treatment of vulvovaginal carcinoma. *Gynecol Oncol Rep*. 2018;24:90-93.
43. Clarke RE, Tenorio LM, Hussey JR, et al. Hyperbaric oxygen treatment of chronic refractory radiation proctitis: a randomized and controlled double-blind crossover trial with long-term follow-up. *Int J Radiat Oncol Biol Phys*. 2008;72(1):134-143.
44. Borab Z, Mirmanesh MD, Gantz M, Cusano A, Pu LLQ. Systematic review of hyperbaric oxygen therapy for the treatment of radiation-induced skin necrosis. *J Plast Reconstr Aesthet Surg*. 2017;70(4): 529-538.
45. Niezgoda JA, Serena T, Carter MJ. Outcomes of radiation injuries using hyperbaric oxygen therapy: an observational cohort study. *Adv Skin Wound Care*. 2016;29(1):12-19.
46. Barili F, Polvani G, Topkara VK, et al. Role of hyperbaric oxygen therapy in the treatment of organ/space sternal surgical site infections. *World J Surg*. 2007;31(8):1702-1706.
47. Skiek N, Porten BR, Isaacson E, et al. Hyperbaric oxygen treatment outcome for different indications from a single center. *Ann Vasc Surg*. 2015;29(2):206-214.
48. Zamboni WA, Roth AC, Russell RC, Nemiroff PM, Casas L, Smoot EC. The effect of acute hyperbaric oxygen therapy on axial pattern skin flap survival when administered before and after total ischemia. *J Reconstr Microsurg*. 1989;5:343-347.
49. Zamboni WA, Roth AC, Russell RC, Graham B, Suchy H, Kucan JO. Morphological analysis of the microcirculation during reperfusion of ischemic skeletal muscle and the effect of hyperbaric oxygen. *Plast Reconstr Surg*. 1993;91:1110-1123.
50. Atiyeh BS, Gunn SW, Hayek SN. State of the art in burn treatment. *World J Surg*. 2005;29(2):131-148.
51. Niezgoda JA, Cianci P, Folden BW, Ortega RL, Slade JB, Storrow AB. The effect of hyperbaric oxygen therapy on a burn wound model in human volunteers. *J Plast Reconstr Surg*. 1997;99(6):1620-1625.
52. Bilic I, Petri NM, Bota B. Effects of hyperbaric oxygen therapy on experimental burn wound healing in rats: a randomized controlled study. *Undersea Hyperb Med*. 2005;32(1):1-9.
53. Chiang H, Chen S, Huang K, Chou Y, Dai N, Peng C. Adjunctive hyperbaric oxygen therapy in severe burns. *Burns*. 2017;43(4): 852-857.
54. Kjellberg A, Douglas J, Pawlik MT, et al. Randomised, controlled, open label, multicentre clinical trial to explore safety and efficacy of hyperbaric oxygen for preventing ICU admission, morbidity and mortality in adult patients with COVID-19. *BMJ Open*. 2021;11(7):e046738.
55. Rubin P. Late effects of chemotherapy and radiation therapy: a new hypothesis. *Int J Radiat Oncol Biol Phys*. 1984;10:5-34.
56. Paganini M, Bosco G, Perozzo FAG, et al. The role of hyperbaric oxygen treatment for COVID-19: a review. *Adv Exp Med Biol*. 2021;1289:27-35.
57. Zant AE, Figueroa XA, Paulson CP, Wright JK. Hyperbaric oxygen therapy to treat lingering COVID-19 symptoms. *Undersea Hyperb Med*. 2022;49(3):333-339.
58. Oliaei S, SeyedAlinaghi S, Mehrtak M, et al. The effects of hyperbaric oxygen therapy (HBOT) on coronavirus disease-2019 (COVID-19): a systematic review. *Eur J Med Res*. 2021;26(1):96.
59. Brenna CT, Khan S, Djaiani G, Buckey JC Jr, Katznelson R. The role of routine pulmonary imaging before hyperbaric oxygen treatment. *Diving Hyperb Med*. 2022;52(3):197-207.
60. Whalen RE, Salzman HA, Holloway DH Jr, McIntosh HD, Sieker HO, Brown IW Jr. Cardiovascular and blood gas responses to hyperbaric oxygenation. *Am J Cardiol*. 1965;15:638-646.
61. Welslau W, Almeling M. Incidence of oxygen intoxication to the central nervous system in hyperbaric oxygen therapy. In: Marroni A, Oriani G, Wattel F, eds. *Proceedings of the International Joint Meeting on Hyperbaric and Underwater Medicine*. Milan: EUBS; 1996:211–216.
62. Plafki C, Peters P, Almeling M, Welslau W, Busch R. Complications and side-effects of hyperbaric oxygen therapy. *Aviat Space Environ Med*. 2000;71:119-124.
63. Hampson NB, Atik DA. Central nervous system oxygen toxicity during routine hyperbaric oxygen therapy. *Undersea Hyperbaric Med*. 2003;30:147-153.
64. Palmquist BM, Philipson B, Barr PO. Nuclear cataract and myopia during hyperbaric oxygen therapy. *Br J Opthalmol*. 1984;68:113-117.
65. Lyne AJ. Ocular effects of hyperbaric oxygen. *Trans Ophthalmol Soc U K*. 1978;98:66-68.
66. Whelan HP, Kindwall EP, eds. *Hyperbaric Medicine Practice*. 4th ed. Flagstaff, AZ: Best Publishing; 2017.

67. Upton PG, Yamaguchi KT, Myers S, Kidwell TP, Anderson RJ. Effects of antioxidants and hyperbaric oxygen in ameliorating experimental doxorubicin skin toxicity in the rat. *Cancer Treat Rep.* 1986;70(4):503-507.
68. Boude J, Cooper JS. Hyperbaric contraindicated chemotherapeutic agents. In: *StatPearls [Internet]*. Treasure Island (FL): StatPearls Publishing; 2023 Jan. 2022 Aug 8.
69. Torp KD, Carraway MS, Ott MC, et al. Safe administration of hyperbaric oxygen after bleomycin: a case series of 15 patients. *Undersea Hyperb Med.* 2012;39(5):873-879.
70. Dowell AR, Kylstra JA, Saltzman HA. Effects of a hyperbaric environment on gas exchange and ventilation in patients with chronic bronchitis and emphysema. *Am Rev Respir Dis.* 1967;96(3):389-399.
71. Register SD, Aaron ME, Gelly HB. Hyperbaric oxygen therapy and optic neuritis: case report and literature review. *Undersea Hyperb Med.* 2011;38(6):557-559.
72. Cates NK, Kim P. Topical oxygen therapy for wound healing: a critical evaluation. *Surg Technol Int.* 2022;19(5):33-36.
73. Fries RB, Wallace WA, Roy S, et al. Dermal excisional wound healing in pigs following treatment with topically applied pure oxygen. *Mutat Res.* 2005;579(1-2);172-181.
74. Frykberg RG. Topical oxygen therapy in the treatment of chronic diabetic foot ulcers. *Medicina(Kaunas).* 2021;57(9):917.
75. Sethi A, Khambhayta Y, Vas P. Topical oxygen therapy for healing diabetic foot ulcers: a systematic review and meta-analysis of randomized control trials. *Health Sciences Review.* 2022;3. Available at: https://doi.org/10.1016/j.hsr.2022.100028. Accessed March 11, 2023.

CHAPTER TWENTY-ONE

Ultraviolet C

Jaimee Haan, PT, MBA, CWS

CHAPTER OBJECTIVES

At the end of this chapter, the learner will be able to:

1. **Define terms describing the use of ultraviolet C including electromagnetic spectrum, ultraviolet radiation, minimal erythema dose (MED), and the cosine law.**
2. **Explain how the application of ultraviolet C to a chronic wound generates a bactericidal effect.**
3. **Develop safe and appropriate application parameters for ultraviolet C in wound healing.**
4. **Select specific patient indications appropriate for the use of ultraviolet C in wound management.**
5. **Identify precautions and contraindications for the use of ultraviolet C.**
6. **Select safe and appropriate treatment parameters for ultraviolet C application.**
7. **Develop and implement a care plan involving the use of ultraviolet C in the treatment of a chronic wound.**

INTRODUCTION

Although ultraviolet A (UVA) and ultraviolet B (UVB) have been used in health care for some time to treat dermatological conditions such as psoriasis and also have some evidence to support the use of ultraviolet radiation to promote wound healing, ultraviolet C is the ultraviolet light that is most commonly utilized today in the treatment of chronic wounds.[1,2] Specifically, ultraviolet C (UVC) is beneficial for the treatment of chronic wounds due to its bactericidal effects.[3] As the number of drug-resistant organisms continues to increase, wound clinicians are advised to consider treatment options that effectively destroy bacteria without damaging fibroblasts and other cells necessary for wound healing, as well as those that avoid the development of bacterial resistance.[4] UVC accomplishes both of these treatment goals and is a cost-effective, portable, and safe noncarcinogenic treatment modality.[5,6]

CASE STUDY

INTRODUCTION

A 63-year-old male is referred to the wound center for a failed split-thickness skin graft (STSG) on the left lower extremity. The original full-thickness wound resulted from a traumatic foot amputation that required multiple surgical procedures and eventually resulted in a below-knee amputation (**FIGURE 21-1**). The most recent debridement and STSG surgery was performed approximately 2 months prior to evaluation at an outpatient wound center. The patient initially received negative pressure wound therapy after his skin graft; however, at the time of his initial visit, he had been performing saline-moistened gauze dressing changes at home for 1 month.

DISCUSSION QUESTIONS

1. What subjective information is needed about this patient in order to develop a plan of care?
2. What tests and measures would be beneficial before implementing treatment?

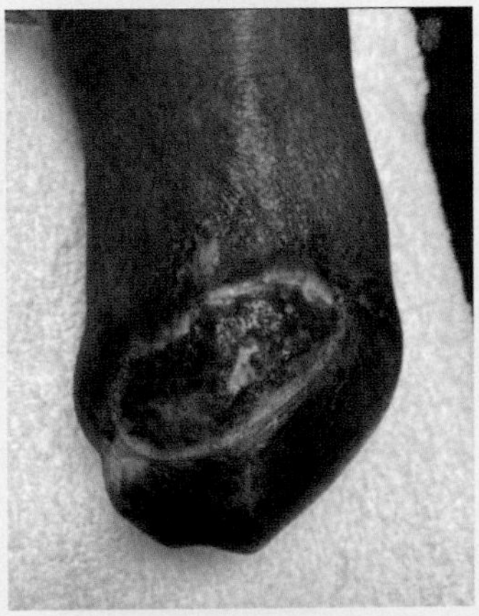

FIGURE 21-1 Patient's wound at the time of evaluation.

TABLE 21-1 Comparison of Ultraviolet A, B, and C[7]

Ultraviolet Light Characteristics	Ultraviolet A	Ultraviolet B	Ultraviolet C
Wavelength	320–400 nm	290–320 nm	100–290 nm
Effects	Hypodermal penetration Strong erythemal response High carcinogenic risk	Dermal penetration Moderate to strong erythemal response Moderate to high carcinogenic risk	Epidermal penetration No erythemal response Kills bacteria Kills viruses Low carcinogenic risk
Modes of delivery	Sun, penetrates through the atmosphere and through most sunscreens Whole-body cubicle	Sun, mostly absorbed by the atmosphere, but still a sufficient amount of UVB passes through to damage skin Whole-body cubicle Hand/foot cabinet	Sun, but completely filtered by the ozone layer Handheld wand

THEORY

Understanding the types of ultraviolet light is important in order to choose a wavelength that will deliver the desired outcome (**TABLE 21-1**, **FIGURE 21-2**). This chapter focuses on UVC, which has FDA approval for use on open wounds due to its bactericidal effects.[8] **TABLE 21-2** provides terminology and definitions used in the discussion of ultraviolet light. Handheld UVC devices consist of lamps that deliver ultraviolet light at a specific wavelength (254 nm), which falls within the optimal wavelength range for bacterial reduction.[12,13] These devices contain filters specific to UVC that reduce the risk of skin cancer and skin burns that are often associated with UVA and UVB.[14] Although studies have shown an increase in the risk of skin cancer associated with the use of ultraviolet B, there has been no link reported between skin cancer and UVC.[14,15]

A systematic review completed in 2021 supported the use of Ultraviolet Therapy as a safe adjunctive therapy to produce wound healing outcomes when using appropriate personal protective equipment.[16] When delivered at therapeutic levels, UVC can be used as an adjunct to antibiotic therapies and topical antimicrobial dressings in order to decrease the wound bioburden, especially in wounds with inadequate vascular supply which reduces the ability of systemic antibiotics to reach the infected tissues. When the UVC device is held 1 inch from the wound bed, the short-wave UVC is delivered at a precise nanometer (254 nm), resulting in a photochemical effect that leads to bacterial cell death.[3,6]

TABLE 21-2 Ultraviolet C Light Terminology

Bioburden	The number of bacteria living on a surface that has not been sterilized[9]
Cosine law	The cosine law states that the energy of illumination varies proportionately to the cosine of the degrees of deviation from the perpendicular[10]
Electromagnetic spectrum	A representation of various wave energies arranged in the order of their wavelength, frequency, or both[11]
Minimal erythema dose (MED)	Skin erythema (redness) that occurs 4–6 hours after exposure to ultraviolet light and disappears after 24 hours; exposure time for MED is determined for safe treatment times[10]
Ultraviolet radiation	Produced when the electrons in stable atoms are activated to move to higher orbits, thus creating an unstable state; the range of ultraviolet energy extending from 180 nanometers (nm) to 400 nm.[11] Electromagnetic waves with a frequency between 5.9×10^{15} and 7.5×10^{14} cycles per second or with a wavelength 180–400 nm[11]

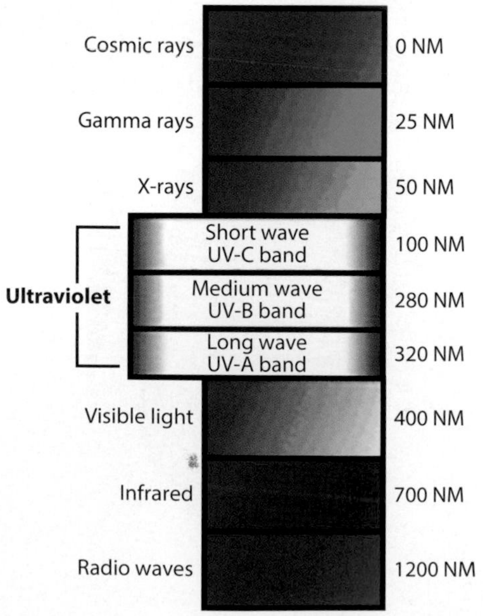

FIGURE 21-2 Ultraviolet light is electromagnetic radiation with a wavelength shorter than that of visible light, but longer than X-rays.

EFFECTS AT THE CELLULAR AND TISSUE LEVELS

Although a recent study demonstrated that UVC delivered at 222 nm can effectively eradicate *Candida* species and multiple bacteria species and has been proven to be a safe and effective treatment intervention in gluteal and sacral pressure ulcers, the 254 nm wavelength is the most commonly studied and used in wound management.[17] UVC delivered at 254 nm is strongly absorbed by organic molecules such as bacteria DNA, and a photochemical effect occurs in one

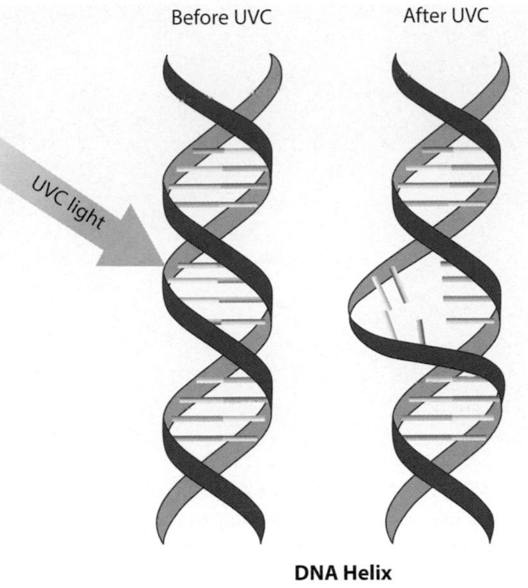

FIGURE 21-3 UVC alters the molecular structure of the DNA in bacteria and viruses, leading to cell death.

of the four proteins that make up the double-helix structure of cell DNA in bacteria. Where two thymine proteins are located next to each other on the double helix, the photochemical effect generated by the application of UVC causes the thymine proteins to fuse, thereby altering the DNA in the nucleus of the bacteria and rendering the cell useless. The bacteria cell is unable to metabolize or divide and eventually dies (**FIGURE 21-3**).[4] The inhibiting function of UVC radiation gives this technology the unique ability to kill bacteria without promoting resistance, unlike systemic and topical antibiotics.[18] While it can take days for antibiotics to eradicate microbes, UVC can accomplish similar results in less than an hour.[19] This same level of UVC light is much too low to have the same negative impact on mammalian keratinocytes and other healthy cells needed for wound healing.[5] The ability of UVC to selectively destroy bacteria cells without causing harm to healthy tissue enables the intervention to eradicate bacteria without negatively impacting wound healing.

INDICATIONS, PRECAUTIONS, CONTRAINDICATIONS, AND POSSIBLE ADVERSE EVENTS

Ultraviolet C is indicated in acute or chronic wounds where the presence of bacteria in the wound bed impedes wound healing. Wounds of many different etiologies may benefit from UVC in the presence of bacteria; however, the clinician must carefully consider the various contraindications and precautions for treatment. See **TABLE 21-3** for a list of contraindications, precautions, and possible adverse reactions. If a patient experiences an adverse reaction as a result of UVC treatment, the treatment is discontinued immediately.

TABLE 21-3 Ultraviolet C: Contraindications, Precautions, Possible Adverse Effects[7]

Contraindications	Precautions	Possible Adverse Effects
▪ Acute eczema, dermatitis, or psoriasis ▪ Cancerous growths ▪ Cardiac disease ▪ Diabetes ▪ Eyes, do not treat over ▪ Hepatic disease ▪ Herpes simplex ▪ Hyperthyroidism ▪ Pulmonary tuberculosis ▪ Renal disease ▪ Systemic lupus erythematosus	▪ Generalized fever ▪ Malignant wounds for palliative care ▪ Photosensitivity ▪ Photosensitizing medications ▪ Recent X-rays or other radiation therapies ▪ Skin cancer history	▪ Burning ▪ Itching ▪ Pain

PARAMETERS AND TECHNIQUES FOR APPLICATION

Parameters

Ultraviolet C parameters, when used to decrease wound bioburden, have been simplified over the past decade. Prior to 1999, safe treatment times for UV treatment were based on the minimal erythema dose (MED) specific to each patient.[20] However studies done by Sullivan et al.,[10] Sullivan and Conner-Kerr,[21] and Thai et al.[3] suggest a much shorter UVC treatment time is needed to achieve a bactericidal effect than those treatment times determined using the MED method.[2,13] In addition to time, the other treatment parameter is the distance of the UVC source from the wound bed, with a recommended distance of 1 inch or 2.54 cm from the wound surface.[13,20] See **TABLE 21-4** for UVC treatment parameters. Some UVC devices, such as the device seen in **FIGURE 21-4** (no longer available through the manufacturer, but are still in use), have a built-in guard that is placed against the periwound skin to ensure the UVC source is delivered 1 inch from and directly parallel to the wound bed, according to the cosine law.[7] Newer UVC models do not have a built-in guard bar; however, they provide a more compact and portable equipment option.

Techniques for Application

Clinical application of UVC requires that both the patient and the clinician wear eye protection, usually with UV protective

TABLE 21-4 UVC Treatment Parameters[13]

Time	30–60 seconds (180 seconds maximum)
Distance/Position	2.54 cm (1 inch) from and parallel to the wound bed
Frequency	Daily for 5 days; repeat treatment course if necessary

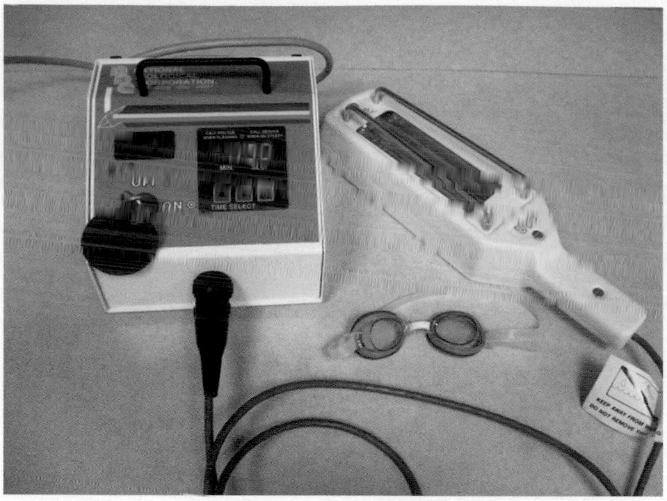

FIGURE 21-4 **Derma-Wand.**

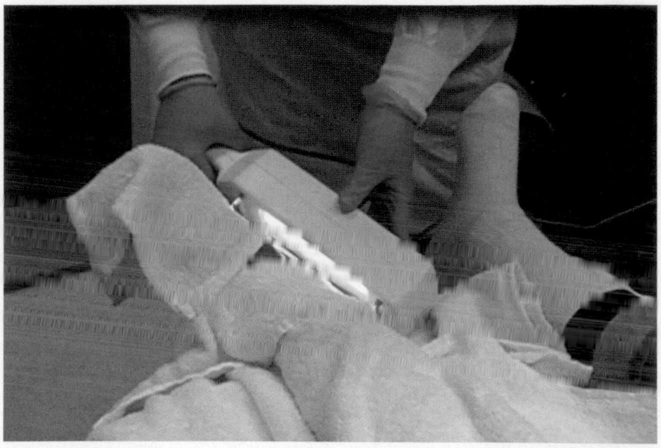

FIGURE 21-6 **The UVC light source is held directly parallel (so that the rays enter perpendicular to the wound surface) and 1 inch from the wound bed.**

goggles or with the patient's eyes draped with a cloth. The UVC equipment is cleansed prior to and after treatment per the manufacturer's guidelines. The patient is positioned comfortably to allow maximum exposure of the wound and to ensure that the UVC device can be placed directly parallel to and 1 inch from the wound bed. All dressings are removed from the wound prior to treatment as ultraviolet light does not penetrate any dressings, including transparent films.[2] After wound cleansing and debridement when indicated, a coat of nontoxic ointment that can block ultraviolet rays to the periwound skin is applied around the wound, avoiding the wound bed itself. Next, the patient's eyes are draped, the clinician's eyes are protected by goggles, and the skin surrounding the wound is protected with clean towels (FIGURE 21-5). Treatment then proceeds with the UVC device held 1 inch from the wound bed and the guard rails (if available) against the surrounding skin or drape to ensure the device is both the proper distance from and parallel to the wound bed (FIGURE 21-6). The UVC light is applied 30–180 seconds at each treatment, once a day for 5 days. This treatment course may be repeated after the initial 5 days of application if clinical signs of local infection are still present.[13] After each treatment is complete, the clinician's and patient's eye protection are removed. The drape and/or UV protective ointment from the periwound skin is removed and the appropriate dressing is applied to the wound. TABLE 21-5 lists key points to remember during UVC application.

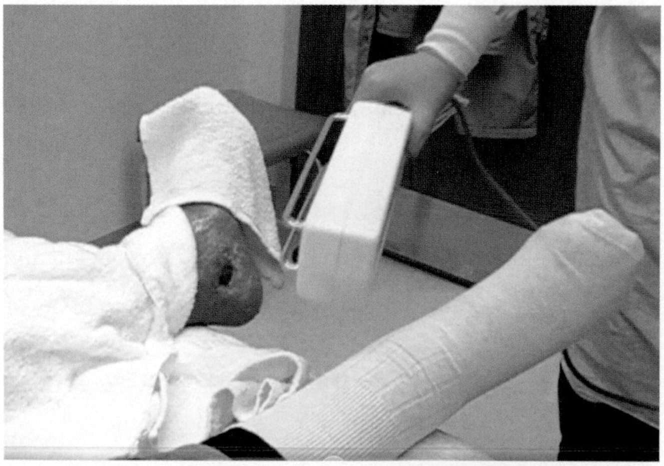

FIGURE 21-5 **Preparation for UVC treatment involves draping the wound and applying protective ointment to the periwound skin.**

TABLE 21-5 Application Techniques for UVC

Points to Remember:
▪ Eye protection is required for both the clinician and the patient.
▪ Skin surrounding the wound is completely protected using a UV-blocking ointment and/or drape.
▪ UVC source is held parallel and 1 inch from the wound bed.
▪ Only short treatment times of 30–60 seconds are needed to kill bacteria; do not treat more than 180 seconds.
▪ Treatment is terminated immediately if the patient experiences an adverse reaction.

SUMMARY

As more multidrug-resistant organisms are identified, alternative methods to manage the bacteria that commonly invade chronic wounds are needed to both reduce bacterial loads and facilitate wound healing. UVC is a treatment intervention that not only kills bacteria but does so without harming the healthy cells within the wound bed and without the carcinogenic risk of UVA and UVB. Recent studies show that UVC has a bactericidal effect on some of the most common and difficult-to-treat bacteria such as MRSA, VRE, and *Pseudomonas aeruginosa*.[2–4,6,22] This evidence, combined with advances in the UVC technology, makes UVC a necessary and feasible tool that wound clinicians can use to assist in the treatment of colonized or locally infected wounds.

CASE STUDY

CONTINUED

The patient had no pertinent past medical history except a penicillin allergy. Medications included an anticoagulant and narcotic for pain management. The patient reported good nutrition at the time of the evaluation but smokes daily. The review of the cardiopulmonary and neurologic systems was negative. The musculoskeletal examination revealed normal ROM and strength. The patient used crutches during ambulation due to the inability to use a prosthesis as a result of the wound. The patient was working as a concrete finisher prior to the accident. The integumentary examination revealed the following:

- Full-thickness wound on anterior residual limb after BKA: 7.2 cm × 3.8 cm × 0.2 cm
- Tissue: 10% yellow slough, 90% bright red granulation tissue with undefined wound edges
- Drainage: moderate green drainage from the wound with a sweet odor
- Edema: 1+ pitting edema left residual limb
- Wound tissue culture: positive 1+ *Pseudomonas*
- Pain: 5/10 on the pain scale at the wound site
- Skin: dry but no new nodules or lesions
- Vascular assessment: arterial screening using a PadNet was performed in the wound clinic which revealed no PAD of bilateral lower extremities; right ABI 1.23 TBI 0.59, normal waveforms bilaterally
- Sensation: intact to light touch, proprioception, and temperature

Patient goals:

1. Eliminate the need for all medications including antibiotics and pain medications.
2. Quit smoking to optimize wound healing and therefore allow independence with ADLs.
3. Ambulate at the community level with a prosthesis without the use of an assistive device and thus to participate in social functions more easily.

DISCUSSION QUESTIONS

1. Is ultraviolet C an appropriate intervention for this patient?
2. What other treatment interventions may be beneficial to facilitate healing and why?

CASE STUDY

CONCLUSION

Plan of care:

- UVC for 30 seconds, once a day for 5 days
- Acetic acid (0.25%) soaks 10 min/day for 5 days followed by rinsing with sterile water
- Selective debridement as pain allowed
- Nanocrystalline silver dressings moistened with sterile water and covered with an absorbent combination dressing to assist in the reduction of bacteria in the wound bed
- Long-stretch compression wrap applied in a figure-8 technique for edema management and residual limb shaping
- Initiate a smoking cessation program
- Frequency: 5 days for the first week, decreasing to 3 days a week the following week, and decreasing to 2 days a week as drainage and pain levels decreased

Short-term goals:

- Pain levels less than or equal to 3/10 so the patient can decrease pain medications
- No residual limb edema
- Wounds in the proliferative phase of healing
- Wound bed with 100% granulation tissue
- Wound edge adherence noted at more than 80% of the edges
- No green drainage and odor consistent with *Pseudomonas* infection

Long-term goals:

- Full closure by secondary intention
- No pain during normal daily activities resulting from the wound
- Patient able to wear stump shrinker to prevent recurrent edema
- Patient able to wear a prosthesis and ambulate without an assistive device at the limited community level

Progress:

Day 6 (**FIGURE 21-7**):

The patient reported a pain level of 3/10.

The patient was able to discontinue pain medication and is using gabapentin only to address phantom pain.

Wound surface area: 6.9 cm × 3.3 cm × 0.2 cm.

Continued next page—

CASE STUDY *(Continued)*

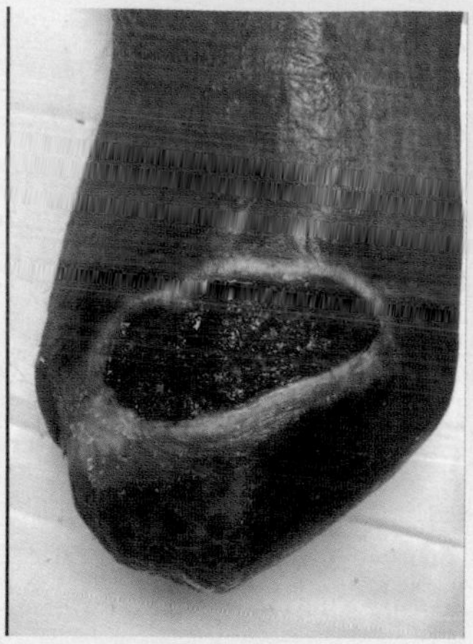

FIGURE 21-7 Patient's wound after treatment day 6.

Wound bed 100% granulated.

Minimal serosanguinous drainage with a slight green tinge.

No wound odor, which allowed the patient to participate in community activities.

Week 3 (FIGURE 21-8):

The patient reported 3/10 pain from phantom pain not specific to the wound.

Treatment frequency decreased to 2×/week.

Ultraviolet C discontinued due to a negative repeat tissue culture and the absence of green drainage.

Noncontact low-frequency ultrasound initiated and compression to the residual limb continued.

Wound edges approximately 70% adhered.

Left lower extremity wound size: 6.9 cm × 2.6 cm × 0.1 cm.

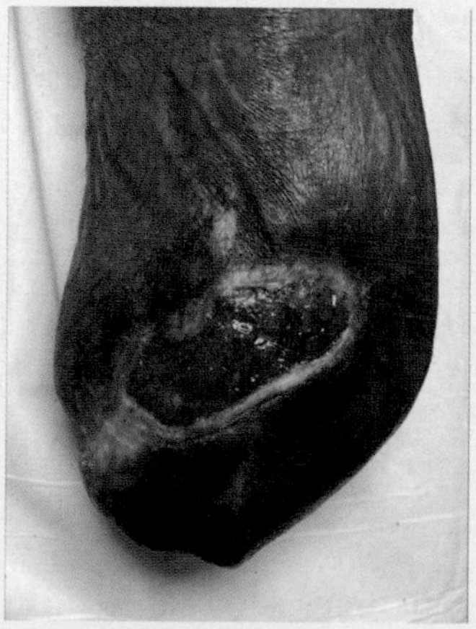

FIGURE 21-8 Patient's wound after treatment week 3.

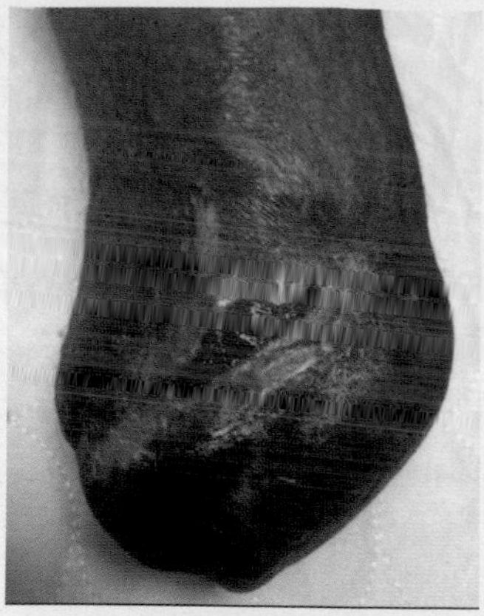

FIGURE 21-9 Patient's wound after treatment week 6.

Week 6 (FIGURE 21-9):

Patient reported 3/10 phantom pain and although he has cut back on smoking, he has not had success in quitting. Patient expressed an understanding of the consequences of this choice as it relates to wound healing.

Treatment frequency continued at 2×/week.

Noncontact low-frequency ultrasound, sharp selective debridement as tolerated, and compression were continued.

100% of wound edges adhered.

Left lower extremity wound now measuring: 4.2 cm × 1.7 cm × 0.1 cm.

Week 8 (FIGURE 21-10):

Patient continued to report 3/10 pain without need for pain medications.

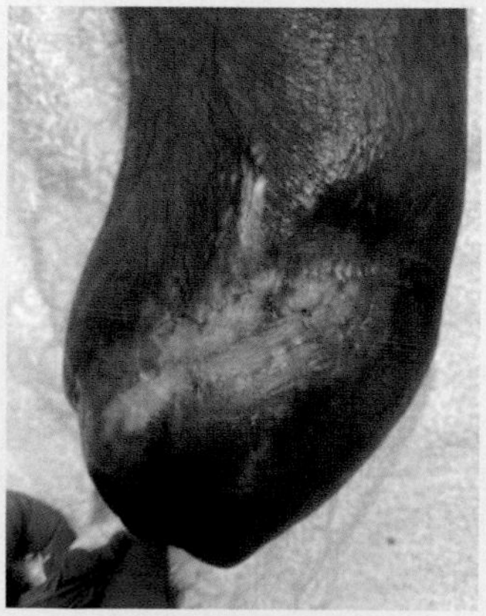

FIGURE 21-10 Patient's wound after treatment week 8.

CASE STUDY (*Continued*)

Patient treatment frequency decreased to 1×/week at week 8, at which time noncontact low-frequency ultrasound was discontinued.

Sharp selective debridement continued as tolerated to prevent biofilm and figure-8 compression continued for edema management and residual limb shaping.

Wound size decreased to 1 cm × 0.5 cm × 0.1 cm.

Conclusion of case study (**FIGURE 21-11**):

The patient's wound continued to epithelialize and was 100% closed by week 12. He was then fitted for a stump shrinker and returned to the amputee clinic to obtain a prosthesis and subsequently to ambulate independently without an assistive device. Treatment was discontinued, as all wound healing and functional goals were met despite continued smoking.

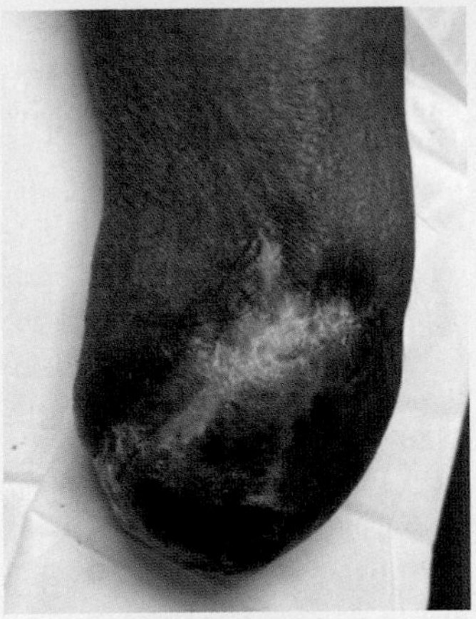

FIGURE 21-11 Patient's wound at week 12, wound closed.

STUDY QUESTIONS

1. The optimal wavelength used to kill bacteria in a wound bed using ultraviolet C is
   a. 124 nm.
   b. 254 nm.
   c. 354 nm.
   d. 424 nm.
2. The amount of time it takes to kill bacteria in a wound bed using UVC is
   a. 1–29 seconds.
   b. 30–180 seconds.
   c. 181–360 seconds
   d. Determined by the patient's MED.
3. The photochemical reaction caused by the application in UVC causes what proteins in the DNA of bacteria to bind, leading to cell death?
   a. Adenine
   b. Ferredoxin
   c. Guanine
   d. Thymine
4. How far should the UVC source be held from the wound bed?
   a. The distance the UVC light source is held from the wound bed is irrelevant.
   b. The UVC light source should be placed directly against the wound bed.
   c. 2.54 cm (1 inch) without any dressings in place.
   d. 2.54 cm (1 inch) with a transparent film covering the wound bed.
5. Which of the following conditions has been reported as a contraindication or precaution for the use of ultraviolet C in the treatment of wounds?
   a. Hyperthyroidism
   b. Renal disease
   c. Photosensitivity
   d. All of the above have been reported
6. According to the law of cosines, the ultraviolet source should be held
   a. At any angle to the wound bed.
   b. At a 90-degree angle to the wound bed.
   c. At a 30-degree angle to the wound bed.
   d. Directly parallel to the wound bed.

Answers: 1-b; 2-b; 3-d; 4-c; 5-d; 6-d

REFERENCES

1. Dogra S, De D. Narrowband ultraviolet B in the treatment of psoriasis: the journey so far! *Indian J Dermatol Venereol Leprol*. 2010;76(6):652-661.
2. Rao BK, Kumar P, Rao S, Gurung B. Bactericidal effect of ultraviolet C (UVC), direct and filtered through transparent plastic, on gram-positive cocci: an in vitro study. *Ostomy Wound Manage*. 2011;57(7):46-52.
3. Thai TP, Keast DH, Campbell KE, Woodbury MG, Houghton PE. Effect of ultraviolet light C on bacterial colonization in chronic wounds. *Ostomy Wound Manage*. 2006;51(10):1-5.
4. Dai T, Vrahas MS, Murray CK, Hamblin MR. Ultraviolet C irradiation: an alternative antimicrobial approach to localized infections? *Expert Rev Anti Infect Ther*. 2012;10(2):185-195.
5. Dai T, Murray CK, Vrahas MS, Baer DG, Tegos GP, Hamblin MR. Ultraviolet C light for *Acinetobacter baumannii* wound infections in mice: potential use for battlefield wound decontamination? *J Trauma Acute Care Surg*. 2012;73(3):661-667.
6. Conner-Kerr TA, Sullivan PK, Gaillard J, Franklin ME, Jones RM. The effects of ultraviolet radiation on antibiotic-resistant bacteria in vitro. *Ostomy Wound Manage*. 1998;44(10):50-56.
7. Bélanger A, Bélanger A. *Therapeutic Electrophysical Agents: Evidence Behind Practice*. 2nd ed. Philadelphia, PA: Wolters Kluwer Health/Lippincott Williams & Wilkins; 2010:xx, 504.

8. Irion G. Adjunct interventions. In: Irion G, ed. *Comprehensive Wound Management*. 2nd ed. Thorofare, NJ: Slack; 2009:253-268.
9. Babbush CA. *Mosby's Dental Dictionary*. 2nd ed. St Louis, MO: Mosby; 2008:x, 805.
10. Sullivan PK, Conner-Kerr TA, Smith ST. The effects of UVC irradiation on group A streptococcus in vitro. *Ostomy Wound Manage*. 1999;45(10):50-54, 56-58.
11. Hecox B. *Integrating Physical Agents in Rehabilitation*. 2nd ed. Upper Saddle River, NJ: Pearson/Prentice Hall; 2006:ix, 535.
12. Vermeulen N, Keeler WJ, Nandakumar K, Leung KT. The bactericidal effect of ultraviolet and visible light on *Escherichia coli*. *Biotechnol Bioeng*. 2008;99(3):550-556.
13. Conner-Kerr TA. Phototherapeutic applications for wound management. In: Sussman C, Bates-Jensen BM, eds. *Wound Care: A Collaborative Practice Manual for Health Professionals*. Philadelphia, PA: Wolters Kluwer/Lippincott Williams & Wilkins; 2011:669-678.
14. Houghton P. Therapeutic modalities in the treatment of chronic recalcitrant wounds. In: Krasner DL, Roseheaver GT, Sibbald RG, eds. *Chronic Wound Care: A Clinical Source Book for Healthcare Professionals*. Malvern, PA: HMP Communications; 2007:406-407.
15. Rigel DS. Cutaneous ultraviolet exposure and its relationship to the development of skin cancer. *J Am Acad Dermatol*. 2008;58 (5 suppl 2):S129-S132.
16. Inkaran J, Tenn A, Martyniuk A, Farrokhyar F, Cenic A. Does UV light as an adjunct to conventional treatment improve healing and reduce infection in wounds? A systematic review. *Adv Skin & Wound*. 2021;34:1-6.
17. Goh JC, Fisher D, Hing ECH, et al. Disinfection capabilities of a 222 nm wavelength ultraviolet lighting device: a pilot study. *J Wound Care*. 2021;30(2):96-104.
18. Dai T, Garcia B, Murray CK, Vrahas MS, Hamblin MR. UVC light prophylaxis for cutaneous wound infections in mice. *Antimicrob Agents Chemother*. 2012;56(7):3841-3848.
19. Goswami A, Basu S, Shukla V. Wound healing in the golden age: what we know and the possible way ahead. *Int J Low Extrem Wounds*. 2022;21(3):264-271.
20. Snyder-Mackler L, Seitz L. Therapeutic uses of light in rehabilitation. In: Michlovitz SL, ed. *Thermal Agents in Rehabilitation*. Philadelphia, PA: Davis; 1990:xxiii, 300.
21. Sullivan PK, Conner-Kerr TA. A comparative study of the effects of UVC irradiation on select prokaryotic and eukaryotic wound pathogens. *Ostomy Wound Manage*. 2000;46(10):28-34.
22. Thai TP, Houghton PE, Campbell KE, Woodbury MG. Ultraviolet light C in the treatment of chronic wounds with MRSA: a case study. *Ostomy Wound Manage*. 2002;48(11):52-60.

CHAPTER TWENTY-TWO

Photobiomodulation

Sharon Lucich, PT, CSPHA

CHAPTER OBJECTIVES

At the end of this chapter, the learner will be able to:

1. **Define photobiomodulation and describe the light spectrum of modalities using light energy to treat wounds.**
2. **Explain the cellular effects of light energy on wounded tissue.**
3. **Identify the most appropriate photobiomodulation device for wounds, based on their characteristics and expected outcomes.**
4. **Identify precautions and indications for the application of photobiomodulation therapy.**
5. **Demonstrate safe application parameters and procedures when using photobiomodulation devices for the treatment of chronic wounds.**

INTRODUCTION

The term ***Photobiomodulation (PBM)*** replaces older, limiting terminology, such as low-level laser therapy or low-level light therapy (LLLT), and broadens the use to the application of any low-power light (energy) source, such as light-emitting diodes (LEDs).[1] In 2014, the North American Association for Light Therapy and the World Association for Laser Therapy agreed by consensus to promote the term Photobiomodulation therapy, which they defined as *"a form of light treatment that utilizes nonionizing forms of light sources, including lasers, light-emitting diodes (LEDs) and broadband light, in the visible and infrared spectrum, involving a nonthermal process with endogenous chromophores eliciting photophysical (i.e., linear and nonlinear) and photochemical events at various biological scales." "This treatment results in beneficial therapeutic outcomes including, but not limited to, the alleviation of pain or inflammation, immunomodulation, and promotion of wound healing and tissue regeneration."*[2] An understanding of PBM provides a more focused approach to research and a new founded interest in therapeutic use, although it has been documented for some time that PBM stimulates the mitochondrial and cell membrane photoreceptors that increase cell viability and stimulate ATP synthesis.[3]

ELECTROMAGNETIC RADIATION AND THE LIGHT ENERGY SPECTRUM

Electromagnetic radiation, created by natural sources (ie, sun) and man-made sources (ie, manufactured devices), is known to emit wave-like patterns of both electric and magnetic fields, while traveling at the speed of light (**FIGURE 22-1**). The speed of light is a constant and is the product of the specific light wave frequency and wavelength. Electromagnetic waves can therefore be categorized equivalently, either according to their wavelength in meters (m) or frequency in Hertz (Hz).

Energy derived from electromagnetic radiation comes from the emission of *photons*, or packets of finite energy, that travel along the waves and transfer their energy onto matter. German physicist Max Plank quantified the amount of energy in a photon of light, which is referred to as *Planck's constant.* The energy of a particular photon wave can be calculated in Joules (J) by multiplying its frequency by Plank's constant. The energy associated with electromagnetic radiation is proportional to frequency and inversely proportional to wavelength; therefore, electromagnetic waves with longer wavelengths and lower frequencies have less energy and electromagnetic waves with shorter wavelengths and higher frequencies have more energy.[4,5]

Electromagnetic waves are categorized within the electromagnetic spectrum as nonionizing and ionizing, from lowest energy to highest energy. Nonionizing forms of radiation include radio waves, microwaves, infrared light, visible light, and ultraviolet light; ionizing forms, X-rays and gamma rays. Because of the broad range and effects at different levels of energy, photobiomodulation therapy is limited to nonionizing light in the infrared and visible light spectrum and is usually referenced by wavelength as opposed to frequency (**FIGURE 22-2**).

Treatment dose is commonly depicted by the *Energy density*, or *Energy fluence*, which is defined as the energy (J) delivered per unit surface area (cm^2), or J/cm^2.[6] *Power density*, or *Irradiance*, is the power (W) delivered per unit surface area, expressed as $watts/cm^2$.[6,7] 1 watt is equal to 1 joule per second.

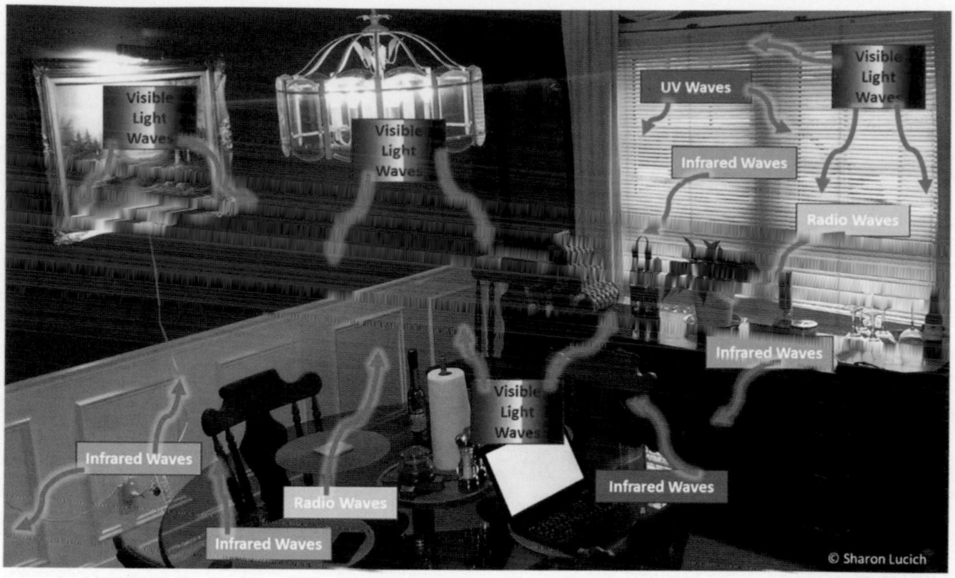

FIGURE 22-1 Various forms of electromagnetic radiation projected throughout a room. (Reproduced with permission from Sharon Lucich. © Sharon Lucich.)

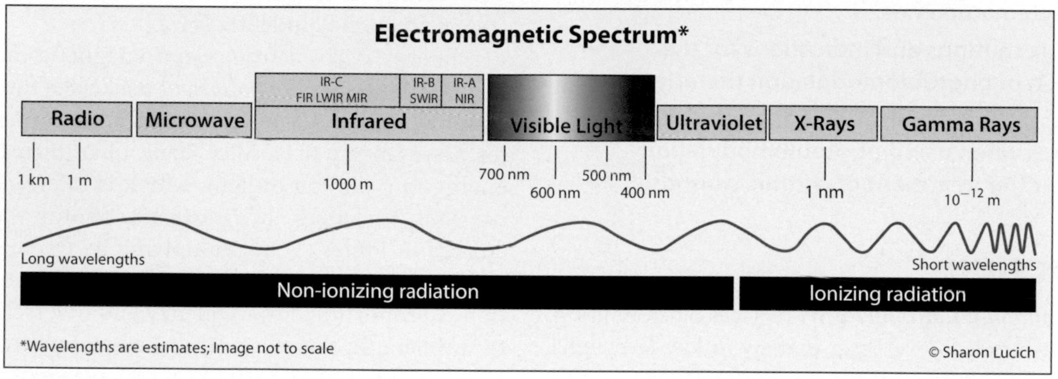

FIGURE 22-2 Electromagnetic spectrum.

Visible Light Spectrum

All electromagnetic radiation is light; however, the eyes can only perceive the colors that are within the visible light spectrum, as represented by a rainbow that occurs following a storm and consists of the colors Red, Orange, Yellow, Green, Blue, Indigo, and Violet (**FIGURE 22-3**). Each color has corresponding wavelengths (approximately 380–740 nm) and frequencies (approximately 405–790 THz). On a continuum, Red has higher wavelengths, lower frequencies, and lower energy levels; Violet has lower wavelengths, higher frequencies, and higher energy levels (**FIGURE 22-4**).

Infrared Spectrum

Infrared radiation (IR), also known as thermal radiation, is a form of electromagnetic radiation emitted particularly by heated objects and with temperatures measuring slightly warmer than visible light. This region of the spectrum is many times larger than the visible light spectrum and has a wavelength range longer than the red end of visible light, but shorter than microwaves. The infrared spectrum can be divided into IR-A (780 nm–1.4 μm) or Near- (NIR), IR-B (1.4–3 μm) or Short Wave (SWIR) and IR-C (3 μm–1 mm), which can further be divided into Medium Wave (MWIR), Long Wave (LWIR) and Far- (FIR). Infrared radiation has a wavelength from about 780 nm to 1,000,000 nm; however, near-infrared (NIR), which is the only level of infrared energy used in photobiomodulation, has the shortest of the infrared wavelengths and is between 780 and 2500 nm (**FIGURE 22-4**).[8–11]

PHOTOBIOMODULATION DEVICES

Lasers

Lasers are monochromatic (single color), coherent (of the same frequency and waveform), and collimated (going in the same direction) (**FIGURE 22-5**).[6] Unlike ordinary light, laser light has a specific wavelength, which when amplified and concentrated to a small area, can produce a focused, narrow beam of light with very high intensity.[12]

FIGURE 22-3 The colors of a rainbow depict the visible light spectrum.

Lasers used in PBM are often referred to as "low level" or "cold lasers" because of their low-energy densities as opposed to high-power lasers that use a photothermal effect to destroy tissue[13] (eg, ablation, cutting, thermally coagulating tissue, or when needing to produce heat within the tissue).[1] Only low-level lasers are used for wound healing; high-powered lasers are not appropriate for wound healing because of their thermal effects. The most common low-lever lasers use helium-neon, gallium arsenide, or gallium aluminum arsenide; a comparison of these three is listed in **TABLE 22-1**.

Laser classifications have been updated by the Center for Devices and Radiological Health (CDRH) and are classified according to their potential to cause biological damage (Class 1, 1M, 2, 2M, 3R, 3B, 4). The higher the classification number, the greater the potential risk presented by the laser or laser system.[12] Lasers used for PBM are usually Class 3B, previously referred to as type IIIb lasers, and have a power output between 5 and 500 mW. A few studies have used high-level lasers (type 4) with a power output of 500 mW or more.[3]

Light-Emitting Diodes (LEDs)

Light-emitting diodes (LEDs) are semiconductors that convert electrical energy into light energy. The color of the emitted light depends on the semiconductor material and composition. LEDs are generally classified by their color and/or wavelength, are efficient, small, and inexpensive.[14] LEDs are not laser diodes, and thus are not subject to the Federal laser product performance standard.[12]

Although LEDs produce light with wavelengths similar to those of lasers, they have broader output peaks (ie, they are less monochromatic) and lack the coherence that is a particular feature of laser light.[13] Therefore, they can treat a larger body surface area and do not have to be attended.

Broadband Light

Broadband or intense pulsed light (IPL) devices emit a white or polychromatic, incoherent, high-intensity light wave, producing light across a wide range of wavelengths. Most uses have been confined to treating dermatological conditions, including facial rosacea, acne, dyspigmentation, facial telangiectasia and dermal vascular lesions.[6,15–17]

PHOTOBIOMODULATION FOR WOUND TREATMENT

Background

Dr. Endre Mester (1903–1984) from Budapest, Hungary, who is considered to be the father of photobiomodulation, began his original work with lasers in 1965. After several years, he attempted to replicate other studies that used "high-power" lasers to destroy implanted malignant tumors, only to discover that the skin incisions created during the implantation healed faster and that the tumors did not respond as in other

	Red	Orange	Yellow	Green	Blue	Indigo	Violet
Wavelength	~625–740 nm	~590–625 nm	~565–590 nm	~520–565 nm	~445–520 nm	~425–445 nm	~380–425 nm
Frequency	~480–405 THz	~510–480 THz	~530–510 THz	~580–530 THz	~700–675 THz	~700–675 THz	~790–700 THz

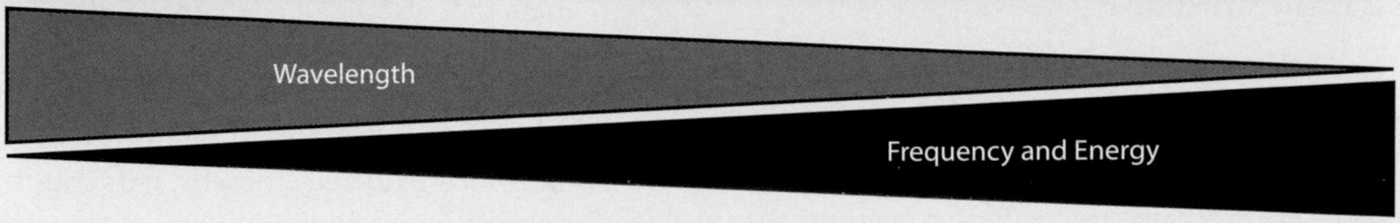

FIGURE 22-4 Approximate values for wavelength and frequency within the visible light spectrum.

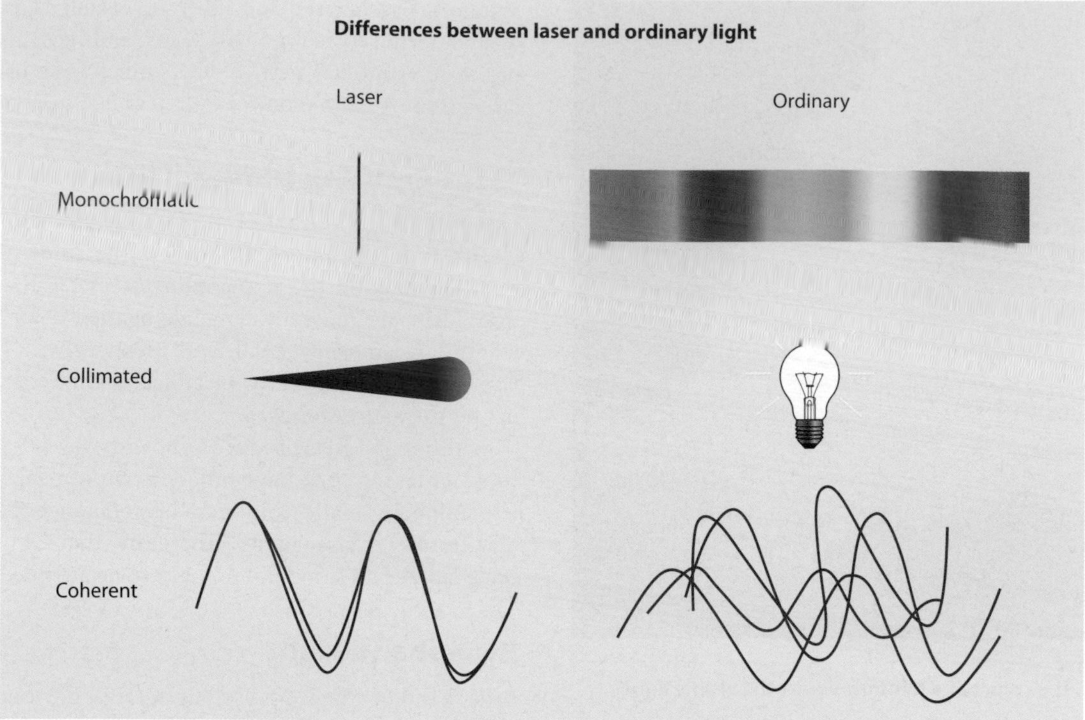

FIGURE 22-5 Comparison of laser and ordinary light. Laser is characterized by three distinct properties that make it different from conventional light.

TABLE 22-1 Comparison Between Common Low-Level Lasers

Laser Type	Medium	Wavelength	Electromagnetic Spectrum	Absorption Depth
Helium neon	Gas	632.8 nm	Red portion of visible light	2–5 mm
Gallium arsenide	Semiconductor	904 nm	Infrared	1–2 cm
Gallium aluminum arsenide	Semiconductor	830 nm	Infrared	3–5 cm

Source: From Conner-Kerr TA, Albaugh KW, Bell A. Phototherapeutic applications for wound management. In: Sussman C, Bates-Jensen BM, eds. *Wound Care: A Collaborative Practice Manual for Health Professionals*. Philadelphia, PA: Wolters Kluwer/Lippincott Williams & Wilkins; 2011:669–678.

reported research. It was discovered that his custom-designed ruby red laser was weak, and instead of being photoablative, the low-power light had no effect on the tumor; however, it stimulated the skin to heal faster. This encounter opened the field of monochromatic light treatment, or photobiomodulation, for dermal wound healing.[18] Chung et al. later reported that the application of light from low-power light sources was not only involved in promoting tissue repair but in decreasing inflammation and producing analgesia.[1] Because of the low-power, photobiomodulation causes no evident temperature rise in the treated tissue, and therefore, no significant change in the gross tissue structure.[19]

Mechanism of Action

Photons, which produce no heat, sound, or vibration,[13] are emitted from electromagnetic radiation within the visible light and NIR light spectrum, at wavelengths from approximately 600–1000 nm. The photons provide the energy in photobiomodulation therapy to stimulate a biological response, as the light triggers biochemical changes within cells. Cotler compared this process to what occurs during photosynthesis in plants, in which the photons are absorbed by cellular photoreceptors that trigger chemical changes.[20] Hashmi more specifically states that when light hits certain organic molecules, called ***chromophores***, the photon energy causes electrons to be excited and jump from low-energy orbits into higher-energy orbits.[13,21]

Several in vitro experiments demonstrated that the primary mechanism of action is at the level of the mitochondria, one of the organelles within the cell that are responsible for signals that stimulate cellular activity. Specifically, the principal chromophore affected within the mitochondria is Complex IV (cytochrome c oxidase or CCO), a heme protein needed for aerobic respiration. During photobiomodulation, CCO becomes oxidized, thereby reducing oxygen to water during respiration. Additionally, reactive oxygen species (ROS) production increases because ROS is a natural byproduct from part of the metabolized oxygen.[1,3,13,20,22]

In the wound healing process, the emitted light is absorbed by the cytochromes of the cells.[23] Cytochromes are mobile and help promote energy production of ATP which increases cellular metabolism.[23] In wound healing, this results in an increase in collagen synthesis due to an increase in fibroblast activity[24,25] and an increase in endothelial cell and keratinocyte production.[26] During the wound healing process, PBM also elicits a shifting of the cellular environment into a more oxidative state.[27] This shift has been seen to increase endorphin synthesis and decrease "C" fiber activity which is attributed to the sensation of pain.[28]

PBM treatment has resulted in other beneficial therapeutic outcomes including, but not limited to, alleviation of pain or inflammation, improvement in blood flow and tissue oxygenation, reduction of edema, and stimulation of stem cells.[2,29,30] Due to all these effects, PBM is an intervention that can be considered to promote the healing cascade in hard-to-heal or chronic wounds.[6]

PHOTOBIOMODULATION INDICATIONS AND CONTRAINDICATIONS

Determination of the indications and contraindications is dependent upon the goals of treatment. The biphasic dose-response states that there are optimal parameters (either energy density or power density) that are beneficial for particular diseases and exceeding these parameters in treatment can cause tissue damage, especially if the dosage is high.[31]

Whereas LLLT was routinely contraindicated over tumor tissue, evidence now supports the use of LED for the treatment of cancer therapy side effects, due to its large-area array, ability to deliver reasonable power densities (up to 100 mW/cm^2), and less concern of safety issues involved in its application (**TABLE 22-2**).[31,32] Other contraindications include the following:

- During the first trimester of pregnancy
- Over thyroid tissue
- Direct exposure to the eyes

TABLE 22-2 Cancer Therapy Side Effects That Can Be Treated with Photobiomodulation

▪ Oral mucositis
▪ Bisphosphonate-related osteonecrosis of the jaw (BRONJ)
▪ Lymphedema
▪ Radiation dermatitis
▪ Peripheral neuropathy
▪ Visceral pain
▪ Radiation fibrosis
▪ Tinnitus (ototoxicity)
▪ Muscle fatigue
▪ Wound healing
▪ Xerostoma (dry mouth)
▪ Trismus (muscle spasm in the temporomandibular joint)

Source: Adapted from Hamblin MR, Nelson ST, Strahan JR. Photobiomodulation and cancer: what is the truth? *Photomed Laser Surg.* 2018;36(5):241–245.

Indications for the use of PBM include skin rejuvenation, acne vulgaris, burns, chronic wounds, and diabetic foot wounds.[33–37] Although some studies have suggested PBM may be helpful for inflammatory skin disorders such as psoriasis and atopic dermatitis, ultraviolet therapy remains the gold standard for treating those disorders.[38]

The **patient and the clinician must wear protective glasses** during treatment to prevent possible damage to the retina. It has also been suggested that treatment be avoided over malignant lesions, artificial pacemakers, thyroid, or pregnant abdomen.[39]

Side Effects

No reports of adverse events can be directly attributed to laser or light therapy[1,13]; however, mild side-effects can occur, including cutaneous irritation, itching, and redness, which are not very harmful and do not result in a rise in temperature of the target tissue.[40]

PHOTOBIOMODULATION WOUND TREATMENT PARAMETERS

The effectiveness of PBM on the target tissue is dependent on the parameters used and includes the light source, wavelength, energy density, light pulse structure, and duration of the light application.[41]

It is now well documented that treatment with red or infrared lasers or LEDs in the wavelength range of 600–1100 nm, a power density (irradiance) of less than 0.2 W/cm^2, and an energy density (fluence) in the range of 0.1–5.0 J/cm^2 promotes wound healing.[1,40,42,43] Energy densities above 10–15 J/cm^2 are considered less effective or may result in cell death.[41,44] PBM generally requires at least two treatments a week for several weeks to achieve clinical significance, although treatment intervals are underexplored at this time.[1]

Specific parameters to promote the optimal wound healing environment are still being discussed in the literature,[6] and because of inconsistent reporting of key light parameters, there is uncertainty around optimal exposure profiles.[45] Hashmi et al. report that although several negative studies have been published, this should not necessarily imply that PBM in general does not work, but rather the parameters used in these studies may have been ineffective.[13]

Application Techniques for LLLT

Prior to application of the LLLT, the wound bed is cleansed and debrided if indicated, and the wound bed is covered with transparent film, extending the film at least ½ inch over the periwound skin. The laser beam can penetrate the film. Both the patient and the clinician don the goggles prior to initiating treatment (**FIGURE 22-6**). Using parameters recommended by the manufacturer of the device being used, the laser probe is placed in direct contact with the film, and treatment provided in one of the following techniques: (1) hold the probe still over the targeted tissue for the recommended time, repeat the procedure over different parts of the wound until the entire surface

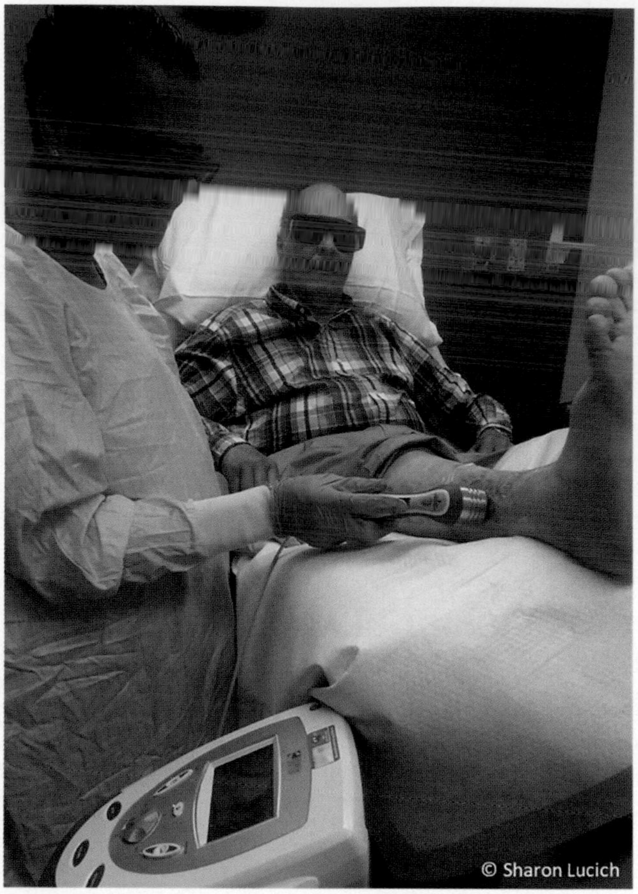

FIGURE 22-6 Protective equipment for both the clinician and the patient includes protective goggles, along with any personal protective equipment required when encountering body fluids. (Reproduced with permission from Sharon Lucich. © Sharon Lucich.)

has been treated or (2) slowly move the probe in a cross-hatching or tic-tac-toe pattern until every part of the wound bed has been exposed to the light for the recommended time. After treatment, remove the film and apply the appropriate dressing to the wound. As with any treatment device, following the manufacturer's recommendations for treatment application is necessary for optimal results and safety.

Future Advances/Opportunities

Although red and NIR are the most popular PBM wavelengths, recent data suggest that low doses of *blue light* demonstrate wound healing benefits. On the contrary, high doses (above 50 J/cm^2) appear to impair cell proliferation.[46] Additionally, blue light has been seen to take on more of an antimicrobial function.[47,48] This result may provide a promising modality for treating infected, nonhealing wounds, where the wound is initially exposed to blue light to reduce the bacterial load, followed by exposure to red light to promote wound closure.[45,49]

Shorter *red and blue wavelengths* demonstrate low penetration and high absorption, and longer NIR wavelengths provide low absorption and high penetration. It may be determined that red and blue wavelengths are targeted for treating superficial tissues, and NIR wavelengths are used to treat more deep-seated tissues.[6,46]

PBM is known for its stimulatory effects, promoting MMP activity and gene expression. Maintaining a dynamic balance between proteolytic activity and degradation could be a target for therapeutic advancement; however, its effect on various matrix proteins needs to be further understood.[50]

LIGHT ENERGY TECHNOLOGY FOR WOUND ASSESSMENT

Over the past decade, several light energy technologies have been developed to assist in wound assessment, providing the clinician with information that helps drive more efficacious treatment plans.

Fluorescence imaging uses LEDs to emit violet light (405 nm) to visualize bacterial fluorescence within and around wounds. The handheld device incorporates a built-in imaging sensor to obtain a digital image that reflects the bacterial load on a wound bed. Only signals from wavelengths associated with bacterial fluorescence (red and cyan) and from a narrow range of green tissue autofluorescence (for anatomical context) can pass through the optical filters to form the real-time image.[51,52] The interpretation of bacterial content and location indicates where debridement is most needed, when antimicrobial dressings or instillation with negative pressure may be indicated, and when bacterial loads have decreased to the point that interventions to promote proliferation and wound closure (eg, cellular/tissue products) can be applied.

Long-wave infrared thermography uses a handheld imaging device that measures the thermal energy emitted from the surface of the human body in the LWIR spectrum between 7 μm and 14 μm. The thermal image, along with a digital image, allows both physiologic and anatomic assessment of skin and subcutaneous tissue abnormalities and/or existing open wounds. The identification of a relative temperature differential near surrounding tissue may be directly correlated to the physiologic processes of circulation, micro perfusion, and metabolic activity, allowing a method for identifying soft tissue injury prior to visual identification.[53–55]

SUMMARY

Photobiomodulation (PBM) therapy refers to the use of nonionizing light in the NIR spectrum (780–2500 nm) to stimulate or inhibit biological processes in tissues by interacting with the chromophores within those tissues. The devices currently used for PBM therapy in wound management are low-level lasers and light-emitting diodes (LEDs). Because low-level laser light has to be monochromatic, coherent, and collimated, it targets a small area of tissue. LEDs produce light that is not monochromatic and coherent; therefore, it has a broader area of output and is not used in direct contact with the tissue. Research suggests that PBM therapy is beneficial for chronic wounds (including diabetic foot ulcers), burns, and some skin disorders such as acne vulgaris and radiation dermatitis.

STUDY QUESTIONS

1. The packets of finite energy that transfer the energy from light waves to tissue are termed
   a. Chromophores.
   b. Exosomes.
   c. Ions.
   d. Protons.
2. Which of the following infrared energy levels is used in photobiomodulation?
   a. 4–3 μm
   b. 3 μm–1 mm
   c. 780 nm–1,000,000 nm
   d. 780–2500 nm
3. The characteristic of lasers that describes the light waves being of the same frequency and waveform is termed
   a. Coherent.
   b. Collimated.
   c. Monochromatic.
4. Photobiomodulation appears to improve wound healing by which of the following mechanisms?
   a. Decreasing the oxidative state of the extracellular matrix
   b. Decreasing the pH of the wound environment
   c. Increasing the cellular activity that results in increased collagen synthesis
   d. Increasing the proinflammatory cytokines
5. Which of the following conditions is least recommended for the use of photobiomodulation?
   a. Acne vulgaris
   b. Atopic dermatitis
   c. Partial thickness burns
   d. Radiation dermatitis
6. The advantage of LED therapy over LLLT is
   a. LED has fewer complications and number of adverse events.
   b. LED is more effective for the treatment of small wounds.
   c. LED can be used to treat larger areas without direct supervision.
   d. LED is approved by FDA and reimbursable by Medicare.
7. When treating a wound with a LLLT device, the probe that delivers the light to the wound bed is held
   a. At a 45-degree angle to the wound bed.
   b. At least 1 cm from the wound surface.
   c. So that the light wave is visible to the clinician.
   d. In direct contact with the transparent film covering the wound.
8. Which of the light waves has shown promise for being antibacterial?
   a. Blue light
   b. Green light
   c. Red light
   d. Yellow light

Answers: 1-d; 2-d; 3-a; 4-c; 5-b; 6-c; 7-d; 8-a.

REFERENCES

1. Chung H, Dai T, Sharma SK, Huang YY, Carroll JD, Hamblin MR. The nuts and bolts of low-level laser (light) therapy. *Ann Biomed Eng.* 2012;40(2):516-533.
2. Anders JJ, Lanzafame RJ, Arany PR. Low-level light/laser therapy versus photobiomodulation therapy. *Photomed Laser Surg.* 2015; 33(4):183-184.
3. Dompe C, Moncrieff L, Matys J, et al. Photobiomodulation-underlying mechanism and clinical applications. *J Clin Med.* 2020;9(6):1724.
4. Funk RS, Stockham AL, Laack NNI. *Basics of Radiation Therapy.* Elsevier; 2016.
5. Fritzsche HP. *Electromagnetic Radiation.* Encyclopedia Britannica; 2022.
6. Mosca RC, Ong AA, Albasha O, Bass K, Arany P. Photobiomodulation therapy for wound care: a potent, noninvasive, photoceutical approach. *Adv Skin Wound Care.* 2019;32(4):157-167.
7. Yadav RK. Definitions in laser technology. *J Cutan Aesthet Surg.* 2009;2(1):45-46.
8. Infrared radiation. *Encyclopedia Britannica.* 2022.
9. CIE. Infrared Radiation. 2023; https://cie.co.at/eilvterm/17-21-004.
10. Viewsheen. *What is NIR/SWIR/MWIR/LWIR/FIR Spectral Range?* 2022; https://www.viewsheen.com/news/nir-swir-spectrum/.
11. ICNIRP. Infrared Radiation. 2023; https://www.icnirp.org/en/frequencies/infrared/index.html.
12. CDRH. Laser Products and Instruments. Center for Devices and Radiological Health 2021; https://www.fda.gov/radiation-emitting-products/home-business-and-entertainment-products/laser-products-and-instruments.
13. Hashmi JT, Huang YY, Osmani BZ, Sharma SK, Naeser MA, Hamblin MR. Role of low-level laser therapy in neurorehabilitation. *PM R.* 2010;2(12 Suppl 2):S292-S305.
14. Light-Emitting Diode. *Encyclopedia Britannica*, 2022.
15. Babilas P, Schreml S, Szeimies RM, Landthaler M. Intense pulsed light (IPL): a review. *Lasers Surg Med.* 2010;42(2):93-104.
16. Murtaza F, Toameh D, Al-Habib S, et al. Safety and efficacy of broadband intense pulsed light therapy for dry eye disease with meibomian gland dysfunction. *Clin Ophthalmol.* 2021;15:3983-3991.
17. Zhang-Nunes S, Guo S, Lee D, Chang J, Nguyen A. Safety and efficacy of an augmented intense pulse light protocol for dry eye syndrome and blepharitis. *Photobiomodul Photomed Laser Surg.* 2021;39(3):178-184.
18. Gaspar L. Professor Endre Mester: the father of photobiomodulation. *J Laser Dentistry.* 2009;17(3):146-148.
19. Caruso-Davis MK, Guillot TS, Podichetty VK, et al. Efficacy of low-level laser therapy for body contouring and spot fat reduction. *Obes Surg.* 2011;21(6):722-729.
20. Cotler HB, Chow RT, Hamblin MR, Carroll J. The use of low level laser therapy (LLLT) for musculoskeletal pain. *MOJ Orthop Rheumatol.* 2015;2(5):00068.
21. Britannica EoE. Cytochrome. *Encyclopedia Britannica*, 2018.
22. Held P. An introduction to reactive oxygen species, 2021. https://www.biotek.com/assets/tech_resources/ROS%20White%20Paper.pdf.
23. Hayes KW, Hall, K. *Manual for Physical Agents.* 6th ed. Pearson; 2011.
24. Cunha JLS, Carvalho FMA, Pereira Filho RN, Ribeiro MAG, de Albuquerque-Junior RLC. Effects of different protocols of low-level laser therapy on collagen deposition in wound healing. *Braz Dent J.* 2019;30(4):317-324.

25. Hopkins JT, McLoda TA, Seegmiller JG, David Baxter G. Low-level laser therapy facilitates superficial wound healing in humans: a triple-blind, sham-controlled study. *J Athl Train*. 2004;39(3): 223-229.
26. Vinck EM, Cagnie BJ, Cornelissen MJ, Declercq HA, Cambier DC. Increased fibroblast proliferation induced by light emitting diode and low power laser [illegible]. *Lasers Med Sci*. 2003;18(2):95-99.
27. Smith KC. The photobiological basis of low level laser [illegible] therapy. *Laser Ther*. 1991;3(1):19-24.
28. Laakso E, Cramond T, Richardson C, Galligan J. Plasma ACTH and beta-endorphin levels in response to low level laser therapy for myofascial trigger points. *Laser Therapy*. 1994;6:133-142.
29. Hamblin MR. Mechanisms and mitochondrial redox signaling in photobiomodulation. *Photochem Photobiol*. 2018;94(2):199-212.
30. Hamblin MR, Liebert A. Photobiomodulation therapy mechanisms beyond cytochrome c oxidase. *Photobiomodul Photomed Laser Surg*. 2022;40(2):75-77.
31. Hamblin MR, Nelson ST, Strahan JR. Photobiomodulation and cancer: what is the truth? *Photomed Laser Surg*. 2018;36(5):241-245.
32. Glass GE. Photobiomodulation: a review of the molecular evidence for low level light therapy. *J Plast Reconstr Aesthet Surg*. 2021;74(5):1050-1060.
33. Glass GE. Photobiomodulation: the clinical applications of low-level light therapy. *Aesthet Surg J*. 2021;41(6):723-738.
34. Keshri G, Kumar G, Sharma M, et al. Photobiomodulation effects of pulsated-NIR laser (810 nm) and LED (808±3 nm) with identical treatment regimen on burn wound healing: a quantitative label-free global proteomic approach. *J Photochem Photobiol*. 2021;6:100024.
35. Deana NF, Alves N, Zaror C, Del Sol M, Bagnato VS. Photobiomodulation therapy in burn wound healing: systematic review and meta-analysis of preclinical studies. *Photobiomodul Photomed Laser Surg*. 2021 Jul;39(7):439-452.
36. Leyane TS, Jere SW, Houreld NN. Cellular signalling and photobiomodulation in chronic wound repair. *Int J Mol Sci*. 2021;22(20):11223.
37. Jere SW, Houreld NN, Abrahamse H. Role of the PI3K/AKT (mTOR and GSK3β) signalling pathway and photobiomodulation in diabetic wound healing. *Cytokine Growth Factor Rev*. 2019;50:52-59.
38. Kemény L, Varga E, Novak Z. Advances in phototherapy for psoriasis and atopic dermatitis. *Expert Rev Clin Immunol*. 2019 Nov;15(11):1205-1214.
39. Dhobley A, Thombre AS, Sharma A, Deoghare A, Billaiya P, Dhopte A. Healing with low level laser therapy: a review. *Ann Romanian Soc Cell Biol*. 2021;25(4):3918-3921.
40. Zamani ARN, Saberianpour S, Geranmayeh MH, Bani F, Haghighi L, Rahbarghazi R. Modulatory effect of photobiomodulation on stem cell epigenetic memory: a highlight on differentiation capacity. *Lasers Med Sci*. 2020;35(2):299-306.
41. deAbreu PTR, de Arruda JAA, Mesquita RA, et al. Photobiomodulation effects on keratinocytes cultured in vitro: a critical review. *Lasers Med Sci*. 2019;34(9):1725-1734.
42. Kujawa J, Pasternak K, Zavodnik I, Irzmanski R, Wrobel D, Bryszewska M. The effect of near-infrared MLS laser radiation on cell membrane structure and radical generation. *Lasers Med Sci*. 2014;29(5):1663-1668.
43. Hamblin MR. Shining light on the head: photobiomodulation for brain disorders. *BBA Clin*. 2016;6:113-124.
44. Hawkins DH, Abrahamse H. The role of laser fluence in cell viability, proliferation, and membrane integrity of wounded human skin fibroblasts following helium-neon laser irradiation. *Lasers Surg Med*. 2006;38(1):74-83.
45. Sutterby E, Chheang C, Thurgood P, Khoshmanesh K, Baratchi S, Pirogova E. Investigating the effects of low intensity visible light on human keratinocytes using a customized LED exposure system. *Sci Rep*. 2022;12(1):18907.
46. Purbhoo-Makan M, Houreld NN, Enwemeka CS. The effects of blue light on human fibroblasts and diabetic wound healing. *Life*. Sep 14 2022;12(9):1431.
47. Masson-Meyers DS, Bumah VV, Enwemeka CS. Blue light does not impair wound healing in vitro. *J Photochem Photobiol B*. 2016; 160:53-60.
48. Bumah VV, Masson-Meyers DS, Enwemeka CS. Pulsed 450 nm blue light suppresses MRSA and propionibacterium acnes in planktonic cultures and bacterial biofilms. *J Photochem Photobiol B*. 2020;202:111702.
49. Chellini F, Zecchi-Orlandini S, Giannelli M, Sassoli C. In vitro evidences of different fibroblast morpho-functional responses to red, near-infrared and violet blue photobiomodualation: clues for addressing wound healing. *Appl Sci*. 2020;10(21):7878.
50. Ayuk SM, Abrahamse H, Houreld NN. The role of matrix metalloproteinases in diabetic wound healing in relation to photobiomodulation. *J Diabetes Res*. 2016;2016:2897656.
51. Andersen CA, McLeod K, Steffan R. Diagnosis and treatment of the invasive extension of bacteria (cellulitis) from chronic wounds utilising point-of-care fluorescence imaging. *Int Wound J*. 2022;19(5):996-1008.
52. Rennie MY, Lindvere-Teene L, Tapang K, Linden R. Point-of-care fluorescence imaging predicts the presence of pathogenic bacteria in wounds: a clinical study. *J Wound Care*. 2017;26(8):452-460.
53. Langemo D, Spahn JG. A Multimodality imaging and software system for combining an anatomical and physiological assessment of skin and underlying tissue conditions. *Adv Skin Wound Care*. 2016;29(4):155-163.
54. Langemo DK, Spahn JG. A reliability study using a long-wave infrared thermography device to identify relative tissue temperature variations of the body surface and underlying tissue. *Adv Skin Wound Care*. 2017;30(3):109-119.
55. Koerner S, Adams D, Harper SL, Black JM, Langemo DK. Use of thermal imaging to identify deep-tissue pressure injury on admission reduces clinical and financial burdens of hospital-acquired pressure injuries. *Adv Skin Wound Care*. 2019;32(7):312-320.

Index

Note: Page numbers followed by *f* indicate figures; and page numbers followed by *t* indicate tables.

B

C

D